COMPLETE GUIDE TO
PEDIATRIC SYMPTOMS, ILLNESS & MEDICATIONS

Cindy

Hope you never need
to use this, but
just in case...
Best wishes!
Love,
Lynn

COMPLETE GUIDE TO PEDIATRIC SYMPTOMS, ILLNESS & MEDICATIONS

H. Winter Griffith, M.D.

THE BODY PRESS/PERIGEE

Notice: The information in this book is true and complete to the best of our knowledge. The book is intended only as a supplementary guide to medical treatment and to drugs used for medical treatment. It is not intended as a replacement for sound medical advice from a doctor. Only a doctor can include the variables of a child's age, sex and past medical history needed for proper medical care and for wise drug prescription. This book does not contain every possible factor relating to medical symptoms, illnesses, or treatments, nor does it contain every possible side effect, adverse reaction or interaction with other drugs or substances. Important decisions about treating an ill child should be made by the parent and the doctor. All recommendations herein are made without guarantees on the part of the author or the publisher. The author and publisher disclaim all liability in connection with the use of this information.

The Body Press/Perigee Books
are published by
The Berkley Publishing Group
200 Madison Avenue
New York, NY 10016

Library of Congress Cataloging-in-Publication Data

Griffith, H. Winter (Henry Winter), date.
Complete guide to pediatric symptoms, illness & medications.

Includes index.
1. Pediatrics—Popular works. 2. Children—Heath and hygiene. I. Title.
RJ61.G83 1989 618.92 89-946
ISBN 0-89586-816-4

Printed in the United States of America

4 5 6 7 8 9

Contents

About the Author

H. Winter Griffith has authored many medical books, including the *Complete Guide to Symptoms, Illness & Surgery*, *Complete Guide to Prescription & Non-Prescription Drugs* and *Complete Guide to Sports Injuries*, all published by The Body Press. Others include *Instructions for Patients, Drug Information for Patients, Instructions for Dental Patients, Information and Instructions for Pediatric Patients, Vitamins, Minerals and Supplements*, and *Medical Tests—Doctor Ordered and Do-It-Yourself*. Dr. Griffith received his medical degree from Emory University in 1953. After 20 years in private practice, he established a basic medical-science program at Florida State University. He then became an associate professor of family and community medicine at the University of Arizona College of Medicine. Dr. Griffith now devotes all of his time and attention to his writing.

Technical Consultants

Ruth Becker-Schaller, R.N.
Nurse Practitioner

Daniel O. Levinson, M.D.
Associate Professor of Medicine, University of Arizona College of Medicine. Fellow of the American Board of Family Practice.

Steven Moore, M.D.
Private Medical Practice, Tucson, Arizona. Fellow of the American Board of Family Practice.

Preface

Illnesses and injuries, especially when they occur in your own children, can be frightening experiences. Next to worrying about the illness itself, I think a parent's biggest fear, on leaving a doctor's office or emergency room, is "Am I going to remember what the doctor told me?"

It's a legitimate fear. Studies show that in most cases, doctors aren't very good communicators. Sometimes a doctor's office is not the best place to learn anything. However, as a doctor myself, I didn't learn that overnight.

When I was a general practitioner in Dade County, Florida, in the 1950s and '60s, I reached a point where I was so dissatisfied with my practice I was ready to give it up. I was saying the same things over and over again to patients in the office and then getting phone calls from anxious parents about things I thought I had already explained. Sometimes, I couldn't remember exactly what I had told one patient or parent and what I had told another.

I began to examine what was wrong, and I found that I needed a better way to convey medical information to my patients. At that time—the early '60s—office copiers were first coming on the scene, and I immediately saw their potential as an educational tool.

I wrote and copied over 300 patient instruction sheets covering the highlights of the most common complaints seen in our office, with information about what to expect, when to call the doctor, and how to prevent complications and recurrences of the problem.

The instruction sheets were a hit! Patients really appreciated having something written to take home and refer to. Many a mother folded the instruction sheet and carefully slipped it into her purse, bringing it with her to her child's next appointment. My "nuisance" phone calls diminished by about 50 percent, while the phone calls I really needed to get, increased.

I remember one mother whose fifth child had measles (this was before the measles vaccination). She called, somewhat embarrassed, and said, "I've had four other kids and nursed them through the measles, and I know how to take care of them, but I read on this paper to watch for a worsening cough and dusky fingernail beds, and that's what my daughter has." It turned out the child had a serious case of measles bronchopneumonia. That simple instruction sheet may have saved the child's life.

Still, I only used the instruction sheets with my own patients. I had never thought of doing anything else with them until one day in the mid-'60s. A visiting cousin who had some experience with book publishing saw the instruction sheets and suggested that they could be published and made available to other physicians for use with their patients. In 1969, that collection of instruction sheets (somewhat edited and modified, of course) was published. It was sold only to medical personnel and was not available in general bookstores.

By the 1970s, patients and parents of patients not only wanted to know more about their health care, but felt they had a right to know more. The books I wrote during the '70s and '80s were for the general public and were written to enable people to exercise that right. This book is in the same tradition of making patients—in this case, parents—partners in the health care of their children. I hope it serves you well.

H. Winter Griffith, M.D.

Caring for Your Sick Children

Consider the following scenarios:

Your toddler comes out of the bathroom carrying an empty bottle of acetaminophen or aspirin. Besides calling your poison control center, what do you do? What signs and symptoms do you watch for? . . . Your adolescent daughter complains of heavy menstrual bleeding. What are the possible reasons? Should she see a doctor? Can it be treated at home? . . . Your physician has prescribed a new antibiotic for your son's latest ear infection, and you think it's making him nauseated. Is that one of the side effects of this drug? Are there alternative medications you can ask about?

This book is intended to help you find the answers.

PARTNERS: DOCTORS AND PARENTS

Early in my practice as a family doctor, patients and parents came to me with the attitude, "Please do something to make me (or my child) better." Either verbally or by body language, my response (and typical of most of my colleagues) was, in effect, "Do what I tell you, but don't ask too many questions." In those days, doctors thought a little knowledge was a dangerous thing for patients to deal with. We had been trained to be authoritarian in our dealings with patients and parents.

Fortunately, times have changed. Most physicians and other health care professionals now welcome—indeed, depend on—informed parents to help them diagnose and treat a sick or injured child, and to prevent illness when possible.

Many thoughtful and assertive parents have taught us they wish to be more involved. They don't wish to be passive and powerless in matters that affect their children's health. They don't want incomplete guidance. Instead, they want enough information so they can think for themselves and make certain decisions to help a sick child get well.

Several years ago, I set a personal goal to translate complicated, technical medical information into up-to-date, easily understood information that any interested layman could use. Toward that end, I wrote *Complete Guide to Prescription & Non-Prescription Drugs; Complete Guide to Symptoms, Illness and Surgery;* and *Complete Guide to Sports Injuries,* all published by The Body Press, a division of Price Stern Sloan, Inc.

This book is another major step toward that goal. It evolves from personal experience during more than 25 years as a family doctor treating not only children but their families as well, from my years of teaching medical students, and from my own experience as a parent of five children.

The following sections contain far more than mere "baby care" tips. You'll find information on topics ranging from colic and cold sores to serious childhood cancers, drug addiction, and AIDS. The topics are conveniently arranged for easy access and apply to children from premature birth through adolescence.

TRANSLATING THE WISDOM

Doctors have a lot of knowledge and training, and new information becomes available to them every day. Along the way, most doctors also acquire some wisdom and intuitive judgment. Ideally, they develop compassion for the children and parents they treat, and a sincere desire to communicate with them.

But unfortunately, a doctor sometimes does not translate medical advice into usable form to the most important member of the child's health care team—the parent.

Even when information *is* competently conveyed, the parent or child usually has no follow-up written checklist to remind and reinforce what needs to be learned or remembered.

This book is intended to provide the translation and the missing checklist. It is intended to supplement, though not replace, the information you receive from your physician or other health care professional. My hope is that it will make you a better, more informed consumer of health care for your children, and that it will help you communicate more effectively with your physician.

A SIMPLIFIED APPROACH

Condensing a broad field of child care knowledge into one volume has required much simplification. I have tried not to omit major facts and concepts, but, of necessity, many details have been left out. This book is not a substitute for your doctor's knowledge and experience.

There is no way to include *all* the factors and circumstances that affect each child's health. Your physician has the opportunity and obligation to take into account many factors not included here (such as your child's age, sex, and previous medical history) when he or she makes a precise diagnosis or recommends a particular treatment.

This book is not meant to be the definitive answer for every medical problem. When the treatment outlined in the book differs from what your doctor advises, feel free to explore the options with him or her. Doctors do not always agree on the best course of treatment for a particular illness, and new knowledge is added to the medical literature every day. Your doctor should welcome your questions. (If he or she doesn't, I would consider consulting someone else.)

ORGANIZED FOR EASY ACCESS

I have organized simple, concise information into three major sections: Symptoms; Illnesses and Disorders; and Medications. The book also contains appendices on a variety of important topics; glossaries where you can look up information about medical terms and drugs used for treatment; a reading list for further, more in-depth information about particular conditions; and a list of organizations and resources with many toll-free hotline numbers.

Armed with the introductory knowledge about symptoms, illnesses, and drugs discussed in this book, you are in a strong position in the following ways:

- You can better understand the nature of your child's condition.
- You can more easily recognize circumstances where a physician's help is necessary—and how urgently.
- You can learn useful facts about how to prevent disease and injury or how to prevent their recurrence.
- You can refresh your memory about facts regarding your child's medical problems.
- You can review a checklist of ways to care for your child away from professional medical supervision.
- You can discuss issues with your doctor when treatment outlined in the book differs from what your doctor advises.

I believe the best way to achieve and maintain optimal health is to participate fully in taking care of your own family. I hope this book provides you with a tool to help you reach that goal.

Guide to Illness & Disorder Charts

The information in this book about illnesses, disorders, and injuries is organized in condensed, easy-to-read charts. Each one is described in the format shown in the sample chart, **CHICKENPOX (Varicella)**, on page xii and xiii. The major parts of the chart format are numbered and explained in the next few pages.

Most of the charts in this section refer to an illness or an injury. In some cases, however, charts refer to disorders or problems that are not really illnesses. For example, the chart on **TEETHING** is not about a disease—or even a disorder. It deals with a normal process that all children experience. It would be a disorder only if it did *not* occur.

But teething can be a medical problem. It often affects an infant's sense of well-being, and it may require treatment. Because teething is so common, and because some treatments for it are appropriate and others are not, it is included with the illness charts.

1—CHART NAME

Charts are arranged alphabetically by the most common name for the illness, disorder, or medical problem. Other names appear in parentheses below or beside the main heading. **CHICKENPOX** has another name, **Varicella**, so it appears in parentheses. However, a disease such as **MUMPS** has only that name, so it appears alone. Sometimes names for various medical problems vary in different geographic regions. All names in this book, including alternate names, are cross-referenced in the index.

To find information about a medical problem, check the index. You may also look up its major symptoms in the symptoms section.

2—GENERAL INFORMATION

This section includes five topics: DESCRIPTION; SIGNS & SYMPTOMS; CAUSES; RISK FACTORS; and PREVENTING COMPLICATIONS OR RECURRENCE. Each is discussed separately.

3—DESCRIPTION

First, a definition of the problem or disease is provided. Sometimes the definition must include other categories, such as causes, body parts involved, and other information. The definition may also include information of general interest, such as how common a disease is, or whether it is contagious, cancerous, or inherited.

The next part of the DESCRIPTION highlights the body parts involved. This is usually a list of specific body parts or organs, such as bones, skin, or liver. Sometimes general body systems such as the central nervous system, genitourinary system, or gastrointestinal system will be listed. The list usually includes only those body parts affected at the beginning of the disease, because many diseases spread to other body parts as they progress.

The third part of DESCRIPTION delineates the sex or age most affected, unless there is no differentiation to note. This section may explain whether the medical problem occurs more often in males or females, or whether the condition affects both sexes. It may also list the age group usually affected. These are generalizations, and variations can occur with specific individuals. Sometimes labels such as "newborns" or "adolescents" are used to describe age ranges. These labels are arbitrary names for specific ages, but they are commonly used in medical texts. Following are the age classifications applicable to this book.

- Newborns (0 to 2 weeks)
- Infants (2 weeks to 1 year)
- Young children (1 to 5 years)
- Older children (5 to 12 years)
- Adolescents (12 to 20 years)

The last part of DESCRIPTION includes mention of some of the forms of appropriate health care for the problem under consideration. Self-care or home care is often listed as the form of appropriate health care. These are important for almost all disorders. Sometimes home care suffices if you have previous experience with a particular medical problem and a resource such as a book to review important points in treatment.

Usually, however, your child's medical problem should be diagnosed by a doctor before you attempt home care. Once your doctor diagnoses an illness and outlines a treatment program, self-care or home care is often important. Treatments outlined in this book are designed to guide you in taking care of your child.

To make self-care effective, your child must maintain a positive attitude and be determined to improve or heal. During illness, a sense of humor and a positive outlook are frequently just as helpful as medication or other treatment measures.

A doctor's care is often necessary, not only to diagnose and prescribe treatment for a medical problem, but to supervise self-care (or hospitalization, when necessary) and to provide additional medical treatment such as surgery.

In addition, even the simplest medical problems sometimes develop complications and require a doctor's care. In those cases, a doctor's treatment can be appropriate even though it applies to a small fraction of cases. Find a competent personal physician who communicates well with you and your child and with whom you can establish mutual respect.

Psychotherapy, counseling, or biofeedback training may be useful for a medical problem caused mainly by stress or emotional problems. Counseling and therapy are also helpful in providing personal and family support, especially with illnesses that are terminal or represent major lifestyle adjustments.

Rehabilitation is often helpful for illnesses or injuries that cause temporary or permanent disability. Rehabilitation may be provided by trained physical therapists or physiatrists (medical doctors who specialize in physical therapy). If rehabilitation is mentioned as appropriate health care, ask your doctor for information specific to your child's disability.

4—SIGNS AND SYMPTOMS

Signs are observed. *Symptoms* are felt or experienced. A sign may be observed by the patient or by someone else, or it may represent physical findings determined by laboratory tests, X-rays, and other diagnostic measures. Symptoms are feelings only the patient can describe. Signs and symptoms are listed together in this book; no attempt is made to separate the two. On most charts, a wide range of possible signs and symptoms is listed. *It is unlikely that any patient will have all, or even most, of the possible signs and symptoms.* The presence or absence of signs and symptoms may vary according to:

- Age and sex of the child.
- Extent of the illness.
- Stage of the illness.
- Medical and family history.
- Current state of health.

5—CAUSES

Many times the cause of a disorder is unknown. Causes for most medical problems include the following:

- Inherited (congenital) defects.
- Infections from bacteria, viruses, parasites, yeasts, or fungi. All of these are sometimes referred to as "germs," but most people associate "germs" with bacteria only.
- Physical injury.
- Toxins (poisons) from a wide range of sources, such as contaminated food, environmental pollution, and bites from poisonous snakes or insects.
- Allergies.
- Tumors. These may be benign or malignant. Benign tumors do not spread to adjacent or distant organs. Malignant (cancerous) tumors can.

1 # CHICKENPOX (Varicella)

2 ## GENERAL INFORMATION

3 **DESCRIPTION**

Chickenpox is a very contagious, mild disease caused by the herpes zoster virus. The skin and mucous membranes are involved.

Appropriate health care includes:

- Self-care after diagnosis.
- Physician's monitoring of general condition and medications, if complications arise.

4 **SIGNS & SYMPTOMS**

The following are usually mild in children, severe in adults:

- Fever.
- Abdominal pain or a general ill feeling that lasts 1 or 2 days.
- Skin eruptions that appear almost anywhere on the body, including the scalp and penis, and inside the mouth, nose, throat, or vagina. They may be scattered over large areas, and they occur least on the arms and legs. Blisters collapse within 24 hours and form scabs. New crops of blisters erupt every 3 to 4 days. (Adults have additional symptoms that resemble influenza.)

5 **CAUSES**

- Infection with the herpes zoster virus. Incubation after exposure is 7 to 21 days.
- A newborn is protected for several months from chickenpox if the mother had the disease prior to or during pregnancy. The immunity diminishes in 10 to 12 months.

6 **RISK FACTORS**

Use of immunosuppressive drugs.

7 **PREVENTING COMPLICATIONS OR RECURRENCE**

Cannot be prevented at present. An experimental vaccine is available for high-risk persons, such as those who take anti-cancer or immunosuppressive drugs.

8 ## WHAT TO EXPECT

9 **MEDICAL TESTS**

- Your own observation of symptoms.
- Medical history and physical exam by a doctor.

10 **POSSIBLE COMPLICATIONS**

- Secondary bacterial infection of chickenpox blisters.
- Encephalitis (rare).
- Shingles many years later in adulthood (possibly).
- Scarring (rare). This is more common if blisters become infected.

11 **PROBABLE OUTCOME**

- Spontaneous recovery. Children usually recover in 7 to 10 days. (Adults take longer and are more likely to develop complications.) After recovery, a person usually has lifelong immunity against a recurrence of chickenpox.
- After chickenpox runs its course, the virus remains dormant in the body (probably in the roots of nerves near the spinal cord). The same virus may later cause shingles.

208

CHICKENPOX
(Varicella)

TREATMENT 12

HOME CARE

- Use cool-water soaks or cool-water compresses to reduce your child's itching.
- Keep the patient as quiet and cool as possible. Heat and sweat trigger itching. 13
- Keep the child's nails short to discourage scratching, which can lead to secondary infection.

MEDICATION

- The following non-prescription medicines may decrease your child's itching:
  - — Steroid lotion, ointment, or cream. This reduces inflammation and relieves itching in 24 to 48 hours.
  - — Topical anesthetics and topical antihistamines, which provide quick, short-term relief. Preparations containing lidocaine and pramoxine are least likely to cause allergic skin reactions.
  - — Lotions that contain phenol, menthol, and camphor (such as calamine 14 lotion). These are soothing, but use with care. Large amounts may be absorbed through the skin into the bloodstream, and they can be toxic.
- If you must reduce fever, use acetaminophen instead of aspirin. Aspirin may contribute to the development of Reye's syndrome, a form of encephalitis, when given to children during a viral illness.
- See Medications section for information regarding medicines your doctor may prescribe.

ACTIVITY

Bed rest is not necessary. Allow quiet activity in a cool environment. Your child 15 may play outdoors in the shade during nice weather. Keep an ill child away from others until all blisters have crusted.

DIET & FLUIDS 16

No special diet.

OK FOR SCHOOL, PRESCHOOL, OR NURSERY?

The child can return when lesions have all scabbed over, temperature is normal, 17 and sense of well-being has returned.

CALL YOUR DOCTOR IF 18

- Your child has symptoms of chickenpox.
- Lethargy, headache, or sensitivity to bright light develop.
- Fever rises over 103F (39.4C).
- Chickenpox lesions contain pus or otherwise appear infected.

209

• Endocrine disorders. This means too many or too few hormones are produced from the pituitary gland, thyroid gland, parathyroid gland, pancreas, adrenal glands, ovaries, testicles, or thymus gland.
• Diseases caused by defects in the body's immune system. These include disorders of hypersensitivity, such as rheumatic fever, rheumatoid arthritis, systemic lupus erythematosus, and many others.

6—RISK FACTORS

Many disorders have known risk factors that can trigger the problem, make it more likely to occur, or increase its duration and intensity. The most common risk factors include:

• Age. For example, infections during the first few days or weeks of life are more likely to occur and more likely to be life-threatening than when the child grows older.
• Genetic factors, such as family or ethnic tendency toward a disease.
• Stress—either physical or emotional.
• Anxiety, depression, and other mental or emotional problems.
• Fatigue or overwork.
• Poor nutrition due to improper diet or disease.
• Obesity.
• Recent or chronic illness that can lower the child's resistance to other diseases.
• Recent surgery or injury.
• Use of drugs, such as alcohol, tobacco, caffeine, narcotics, psychedelics, hallucinogens, marijuana, sedatives, hypnotics, or cocaine.
• Use of medications, whether prescription or non-prescription. Even necessary drugs cause adverse reactions and side effects that can complicate the treatment and outcome of your child's medical problems.
• Exposure to allergens, environmental pollutants, or poisons.
• Geographic areas. For example, Valley fever is more likely to occur in central California and Arizona than in other areas.
• Crowded or unsanitary living conditions.
• Socioeconomic factors.

7—PREVENTING COMPLICATIONS OR RECURRENCE

Prevention can be of two types—prevention of the initial disease or prevention of a relapse or recurrence after recovery.

Prevention of any medical problem is the *best treatment.* Researchers continue to discover ways to prevent, delay, or diminish some illness, pain, disability, and untimely deaths. These ways are included whenever available.

Proper and complete treatment of the disorder may be necessary to prevent recurrence or complication. For example: Adequate antibiotic treatment of a streptococcal throat infection is necessary to assure the prevention of two possible complications, rheumatic fever and glomerulonephritis. Adequate treatment must be carried out for a sufficient amount of time to prevent recurrences of urinary tract infections.

The causes and risk factors for a disease often provide the best clues for prevention. Many diseases, however, cannot be prevented at present.

8—WHAT TO EXPECT

This section includes three topics: MEDICAL TESTS, POSSIBLE COMPLICATIONS, and PROBABLE OUTCOME. Each is discussed separately below.

9—MEDICAL TESTS

Your own observation of your child's symptoms is usually the first—and often, most important—diagnostic measure. It is the first step toward medical treatment. For that reason, it is listed under the heading on almost all illness charts. A medical history and physical exam by a doctor are also almost universal requirements before treatment for any disorder can begin. Even if a medical problem is usually treated at home, a history and exam will be necessary if complications develop that require medical treatment.

Additional diagnostic measures include laboratory studies and other medical tests. The most common include:

- Studies of body fluids, such as blood, serum, plasma, or spinal fluid.
- Microscopic and chemical examination of excreted material, such as urine or stools.
- CT or CAT (computerized axial tomography) scans or X-rays of the affected body part.
- Magnetic Resonance Imaging (MRI)—a very precise and expensive new diagnostic tool, particularly useful in locating abnormal growths in the brain.
- EKG (electrocardiogram), EEG (electroencephalogram), and EMG (electromyogram).
- Nuclear medicine studies to define both anatomical structure and physiological function.
- Therapeutic trial of medication. This is used sometimes for a critically ill patient without a specific diagnosis while awaiting laboratory results.

Your child may not undergo every diagnostic test listed on the chart, and conversely, the child may undergo tests not listed. Some tests are performed only if previous tests have not provided enough information. Others are performed only when complications develop. All medical diagnostic tests mentioned in this book are defined in the Glossary.

When your child is to have tests performed, learn as much as you can about these tests. Ask questions of your doctor or technician. Learn how much a test will cost, and whether or not it will cause your child embarrassment or pain. Ask what foods or medications will affect the results. Ask for a full report—in writing—and make sure you know what the test results mean and what you are supposed to do if they are abnormal.

10—POSSIBLE COMPLICATIONS

Complications are additional medical problems triggered by or as a result of the original illness. Complications sometimes occur, despite accurate diagnosis and competent treatment. Some are preventable, a few are inevitable—but most are rare.

11—PROBABLE OUTCOME

A very important concern in any illness is the question, "What is going to happen to my child? How will this disease or injury affect my child's life?" No one can completely predict the outcome of an illness or accident. The predictions in this section are guesses based on averages. Patients and doctors work toward optimal results, but medicine is an inexact science. Response to treatment depends on many variables, and there are many unanswered questions about health and disease.

Some illnesses are considered incurable at present. The term "incurable" is a general one that may apply to insignificant conditions that are mere annoyances to fatal diseases that bring certain death in a short time. For that reason, additional information about life expectancy is usually included for incurable illnesses. Again, individual variations are common, but the predictions are an attempt to answer some important questions. We hope they help you and your child adopt optimistic but realistic expectations.

In almost all cases—no matter how serious the illness—symptoms can be relieved or controlled to minimize your child's pain and discomfort.

12—TREATMENT

This section provides a checklist that reminds you of instructions your doctor may have given. The information should not replace your doctor's instructions, because treatments vary a great deal. If the instructions don't seem to fit your problem, ask your doctor or nurse for answers that apply uniquely to your child. The five major headings include: HOME CARE, MEDICATION, ACTIVITY, DIET & FLUIDS, and OK FOR SCHOOL, PRESCHOOL, OR NURSERY?

13—HOME CARE

The instructions under this heading apply to home treatment. They cover common matters such as soaks for skin problems, use of crutches, appropriate clothing, bandages, or bathing. They are not complete and may not apply to every child, but they provide a good review of general measures helpful for most patients.

14—MEDICATION

Information under this heading is generally of two types—medications your doctor may prescribe, and non-prescription drugs your child can safely take. Prescription medications are named by generic name or drug class. A brief description of a drug's purpose and effect is given. For more information about a specific medication, see the Drugs Glossary and the Medications section. They contain entries for generic drugs and drug classes mentioned in this book.

Additionally, you may refer to my book, *Complete Guide to Prescription and Non-Prescription Drugs,* published by The Body Press, a division of Price Stern Sloan, Inc. For general instructions about the safe use of medicine, see Appendix 18.

15—ACTIVITY

Parents are often confused about whether their children must stay in bed during an illness. They are concerned about when the child can return to school, and whether the child's activity will be restricted after recovery. These questions are answered under this heading. Exercise references are often included, and when not specified otherwise, references to regular physical exercise mean *aerobic* exercise (see Appendix 36).

16—DIET & FLUIDS

Diet information can vary from "no special diet" to references to the following diets included in the Appendix section:

- Regular, well-balanced diet that is high in fiber.
- Pregnancy and lactation (breast-feeding) diet.
- Milk-restricted diet.
- Allergy diet.
- Low-fat diet.
- Low-salt diet.
- Weight-loss diet.

For additional specialized diets, consult your doctor or a dietitian.

Maintaining an adequate fluid intake is one of the most important parts of treating many diseases of newborns and children, particularly those associated with serious vomiting or diarrhea, or during a post-operative period.

17—OK FOR SCHOOL, PRESCHOOL, OR NURSERY?

Young children are quite susceptible to minor respiratory infections. Keeping them isolated seldom protects other children, because exposure to others usually occurs before symptoms begin. There are no general rules about returning to school, preschool, or nursery. Some estimate as to the appropriate time to return regarding the medical problem in question is listed in this information block. These suggestions should be tempered with your own common sense and the advice you receive from your physician.

18—CALL YOUR DOCTOR IF

For most medical problems, a phone call or visit to your doctor is recommended to establish a diagnosis. After diagnosis, when the course of an illness differs from what is expected, your doctor wants to know. Many developing complications can be averted with prompt medical treatment. Specific symptoms are usually listed that indicate complications.

Of course, if any other symptoms begin that you believe are related to your child's illness or to any medications, call your doctor about them, too.

Symptoms Guide

Symptoms Guide

A *symptom* is a physical phenomenon that is interpreted by the person experiencing it as a departure from normal function, sensation, or feeling. Symptoms are subjective. *Signs*, on the other hand, are departures from normal appearance or function as observed by someone other than one who is experiencing symptoms. The difference between signs and symptoms is usually quite thin, so in this book they are presented in the following combined list.

This index of symptoms and signs can lead you to most of the disorders, illnesses, and injuries described in this book. This list (or any of the disorders the list may lead you to) is not intended to be used as a guide to *diagnosis*. Rather, it is a categorized table of contents that can lead to finding more information about the disorders with which these signs and symptoms are associated.

This list should not be used as a substitute for your family physician or pediatrician. If you are worried about a symptom that your child has, consult your physician. All the information listed here is merely to guide you to more information, to serve as a reminder for what you and your physician have decided together, and to provide checklists of things you may do to help your child's recovery or state of well-being.

To use this list effectively, first look up a child's symptoms or signs alphabetically (see the bold headings). You may need to look for similar or synonymous headings. For example, if you don't find an entry under "Stomach ache," look under "Abdomen." Also, use the main index in the back of the book to help you find illnesses or other topics.

The bold headings in this list are symptoms or signs. The alphabetized lists following each bold entry are possible illnesses or disorders that the symptom may indicate. You can find these in the Illnesses & Disorders section of this book.

A

Abdomen, audible or rumbling noises from
- Colic in Infants
- Intestinal Obstruction
- Intussusception
- Lactose Intolerance

Abdomen, bloated or swollen
- Alcoholism
- Appendicitis
- Celiac Disease
- Colitis, Ulcerative
- Congestive Heart Failure
- Constipation
- Cor Pulmonale
- Endocarditis
- Fluid & Electrolyte Disorder
- Gallstones
- Gastritis
- Histoplasmosis
- Hypochondriasis
- Indigestion
- Intestinal Obstruction
- Intussusception
- Lactose Intolerance
- Liver Cancer
- Nephrosis
- Ovarian Cyst
- Premenstrual Syndrome
- Scleroderma
- Vitamin E Deficiency

Abdomen, burning, gnawing pain in upper
- Ulcer, Peptic

Abdomen, burning pain in skin of
- Shingles (Herpes Zoster)

Abdomen, colicky pain in upper right region, with nausea and fever
Gallstones

Abdomen, enlarged
Acetaminophen Poisoning
Congestive Heart Failure
*Metastatic Cancer
Spleen Rupture
Wilm's Tumor

Abdomen, enlarged, hard, sometimes tender mass in
Ovarian Cancer

Abdomen, faint rash on (pale pink or brown)
Dermatitis, Contact
Pityriasis Rosea

Abdomen of infant who cries out and brings legs up
Intussusception

Abdomen, mass in
Fecal Impaction
Intussusception
Kidney, Polycystic
Liver Cancer
*Metastatic Cancer
Ovarian Cancer
Pyloric Stenosis, Congenital
Wilm's Tumor

Abdomen, muscle weakness in
Guillain-Barré Syndrome

Abdomen, pain on left side (improves after bowel movements)
Colitis, Ulcerative
*Diverticulitis
*Diverticulosis

Abdomen, pain in right lower quadrant
Appendicitis

Abdomen, rash on
Dermatitis, Contact
Diaper Rash
Pityriasis Rosea
Purpura, Allergic
Rheumatic Fever
Rocky Mountain Spotted Fever
Typhoid Fever

Abdomen, rumbling, audible sounds from
Colic in Infants
Intestinal Obstruction
Intussusception
Lactose Intolerance

Abdomen, see-saw movements of, with breathing difficulty
Bronchiolitis

Abdomen, tenderness over right side
Amebiasis
Appendicitis

Abdominal cramps
Amebiasis
Appendicitis
Cholecystitis or Cholangitis, Acute
Dysentery, Bacillary
Dysmenorrhea
Ectopic Pregnancy
Fecal Impaction
Gastritis
Giardiasis
Intestinal Obstruction
Intussusception
Lactose Intolerance
Peritonitis
Pseudomembranous Enterocolitis
Salmonella, Infectious
Shingles
Trichinosis
Typhoid Fever

* No chart in this book for this disorder.

Abdominal pain or discomfort
Addison's Disease
Anemia, Iron-Deficiency
Appendicitis
Bladder Infection
Bladder or Urethra Injury
Celiac Disease
Chickenpox
Decompression Disease
Diarrhea, Acute
DIC
Ectopic Pregnancy
Fecal Impaction
Gallstones
Gastritis
Hand, Foot & Mouth Disease
Heartburn
Hepatitis, Acute Viral
Herpangina
Hyperparathyroidism
Indigestion
Intestinal Obstruction
Intussusception
Kidney Failure, Chronic
Kidney Infection, Acute
Lead Poisoning
Leukemia, Acute
Liver Cancer
Malabsorption
Ovarian Cancer
Ovarian Cyst
Pelvic Inflammatory Disease
Peritonitis
Pica
Pneumonia, Bacterial
Pneumonia, Mycoplasma
Polyarteritis
Porphyria
Purpura, Allergic
Roundworms
Sickle-Cell Anemia
Spleen Rupture
Tapeworm
Ulcer, Peptic
Vitamin B Deficiencies
Wilm's Tumor

Abdominal tenderness
Amebiasis
Appendicitis
Celiac Disease
Cholecystitis or Cholangitis, Acute
*Colitis, Spastic
Colitis, Ulcerative
*Diverticulitis
*Diverticulosis
Ectopic Pregnancy
Fecal Impaction
Hepatitis
Intestinal Obstruction
Intussusception
Leukemia, Acute
Liver Cancer
*Migraine, Abdominal
Pelvic Inflammatory Disease
Peritonitis

Abdominal wall, large, firm, smooth tumor (can be felt)
Wilm's Tumor

Aches and pains
Blood-transfusion Reaction
Endocarditis

Achilles tendon, painful inflammation of
Tendinitis

Aching, general body
Agranulocytosis
Anxiety
Arthritis, Juvenile Rheumatoid
Cold, Common
*Fever from any cause
Influenza
Kidney Infection, Acute
Mononucleosis, Infectious
Pharyngitis

Acid taste in mouth
Heartburn
Indigestion

* No chart in this book for this disorder.

Acne outbreak
Acne Vulgaris
Premenstrual Syndrome

Adenoids, enlarged
APC Disease
Pharyngitis

Aggressive behavior
Addison's Disease
*Many mental and emotional disorders

Airways obstructed
Bronchiolitis ("Croup")
Diphtheria

Alcohol, pain in diseased area after drinking
Hodgkin's disease

Amnesia
Head Injury
Hypothermia
*Many mental and emotional disorders

Anal area, irritation of skin associated with frequent bowel movements
Diarrhea, Chronic, Non-Specific, of Childhood
*Diarrhea from any cause

Anaphylaxis (sudden itching, difficulty in breathing, or loss of consciousness)
Bee Stings
Drug Hypersensitivity

Anemia
Anemia, Iron Deficiency
Ankylosing Spondylitis
Arthritis, Juvenile Rheumatoid
Bronchiectasis
Celiac Disease
*Excessive bleeding from any cause
Hodgkin's Disease
Kidney Failure, Chronic
Kidney Infection, Chronic
Lead Poisoning
Leukemia, Acute
Lupus Erythematosus, Systemic
Lymphoma, Non-Hodgkin's
Ovarian Cancer
Radiation Sickness
Sickle-Cell Anemia
Ulcer, Peptic
Vitamin C Deficiency
Vitamin E Deficiency

Anemia, hemolytic
Drug Hypersensitivity

Anger
*Many mental and emotional disorders
Rape Crisis Syndrome

Ankles, inflammation and pain in
Ankle Sprain
*Any injury to ankle
Arthritis, Juvenile Rheumatoid
Rheumatic Fever
Thrombosis, Deep-Vein

Ankles, stiffness in
Arthritis, Juvenile Rheumatoid

Ankles, swelling of
Ankle Sprain
Arthritis, Juvenile Rheumatoid
Congestive Heart Failure
Cor Pulmonale
Erythema Nodosum
Glomerulonephritis
Idiopathic Hypertrophic Subaortic Stenosis
Kidney, Polycystic
Myocarditis
Nephrosis
Premenstrual Syndrome
Thrombosis, Deep-Vein
Vitamin E Deficiency

Ankles, tender, red, hard bumps on
Erythema Nodosum

Anus, itching around
Hemorrhoids
Pinworms
Pruritis Ani

* No chart in this book for this disorder.

Anus, itchy rash
- Dermatitis, Atopic
- Diaper Rash

Anxiety, unusual
- Alcoholism
- Drug Abuse & Addiction
- Drug Hypersensitivity
- Hypochondriasis
- *Many heart diseases
- *Many mental and emotional disorders
- Pericarditis, Acute
- Shock
- Sodium Imbalance

Appetite increased (but still have weight loss)
- Diabetes Mellitus, Insulin-Dependent
- Hyperthyroidism
- *Many mental and emotional disorders

Appetite, loss of
- Addison's Disease
- Anxiety
- *Any gastrointestinal disorder
- Arthritis, Juvenile Rheumatoid
- Anemia, Iron-Deficiency
- Calcium Imbalance
- Celiac Disease
- Cold, Common
- Colitis, Ulcerative
- Depression
- Gastritis
- Gastroenteritis
- Glomerulonephritis
- Hand, Foot & Mouth Disease
- Hepatitis, Acute Viral
- Histoplasmosis
- Kidney Failure, Acute
- Kidney Infection, Chronic
- Lead Poisoning
- Liver Cancer
- *Many mental and emotional disorders
- Measles
- Nephrosis
- Pinworms
- Pneumonia, Viral
- Psittacosis
- Pulmonary-Valve Stenosis
- Rheumatic Fever
- Roundworms
- Trichinosis
- Ulcer, Peptic
- Zinc Deficiency

Armpits, skin infection under
- Hidradenitis Suppurativa

Armpits, small raised bumps on skin
- Lyme Disease

Armpits, swollen lymph glands
- Hodgkin's Disease
- Lymphoma, Non-Hodgkin's
- Syphilis

Arms, inability to move
- Encephalitis, Viral or Aseptic
- Extradural Hemorrhage
- Paraplegia or Quadriplegia
- Subarachnoid Hemorrhage

Arms, itchy rash on
- Polymyositis & Dermatomyositis

Arms, loss of sensation in
- Paraplegia or Quadriplegia

Arms, muscle weakness in
- Guillain-Barré Syndrome

Arms, numbness in
- Calcium Imbalance
- Encephalitis, Viral or Aseptic
- *Hyperventilation Syndrome
- Subarachnoid Hemorrhage

Arms, pain in
- Shoulder, Frozen

Arms, pain, tingling or burning
- Frostbite

Arms, small white patches on skin
- Pityriasis Alba

* No chart in this book for this disorder.

Arms, tingling sensation in
Calcium Imbalance
Frostbite
Hyperaldosteronism
*Hyperventilation Syndrome

Arms, twitching of (lasting 2-3 minutes)
Convulsions, Febrile
Epilepsy

Arms, weakness in
*Any injury
Encephalitis, Viral or Aseptic
Subarachnoid Hemorrhage

B

Back pain
*Any injury to back
Arthritis, Juvenile Rheumatoid
Blood-Transfusion Reaction
Bladder Infection
Brain or Epidural Abscess
Brucellosis
Cholecystitis or Cholangitis, Acute
DIC
*Herniated Vertebral Disc
Hyperparathyroidism
Influenza
Kidney Infection, Chronic
Kidney or Ureter Injury
Kidney, Polycystic
Reiter's Syndrome
Sickle-Cell Anemia
Spinal-Cord Tumor

Back, skin rash on
Rheumatic Fever
Scarlet Fever

Back, stiff
Meningitis
Rocky Mountain Spotted Fever

Back, tenderness in
Kidney or Ureter Injury
Urinary Tract Infection

Back (upper), fat accumulation over, accompanied by red stretch marks
Cushing's Syndrome

Backache, low
Ankylosing Spondylitis
*Any bone or muscle injury in back region
Kidney Infection, Acute
*Ruptured Intervertebral Disc

Balance, poor
Alcoholism
Brain Tumor
Cerebral Palsy
*Drug Intoxication
Hypoglycemia
*Labyrinthitis
Otitis Media (affecting inner ear structures)
*Polymyalgia
Syphilis

Barking cough
Croup

Barrel chest
Bronchitis, Chronic
Emphysema

Beard, lesions causing itchy, scaling rash under
Ringworm

Bed-wetting at night
Bed-wetting (Enuresis)

Belching
Anxiety
Cholecystitis or Cholangitis, Acute
Gallstones
Gastritis
Heartburn
Hiatal Hernia
Hypochondriasis
Indigestion
*Many mental and emotional disorders
*Swallowing air

* No chart in this book for this disorder.

Binge eating
Bulimia

Birth weight, low (less than 5-1/2 lbs.)
Premature Infants

Bite marks, red
Creeping Eruption
Lice

Bizarre behavior
*Many mental and emotional disorders

Blackheads
Acne

Blackouts
Alcoholism
Fainting (Syncope)

Bladder, difficulty in emptying completely
Bladder Infection
Ovarian Cyst
Urethritis

Bladder, loss of control of
Bladder Infection
Convulsions, Febrile
Epilepsy
Hemiplegia
Hypoglycemia of Diabetes
Incontinence, Stress
Paraplegia or Quadriplegia

Bladder, pain in abdomen over
Bladder Infection

Bleeding, arms or legs & swelling at the joints
Hemophilia
Purpura, Henoch-Schönlein

Bleeding, excessive, from minor cuts
Hemophilia
Vitamin C Deficiency

Bleeding, from any or several body areas
Aspirin Poisoning
DIC

Bleeding, from gastrointestinal tract
Aspirin Poisoning
Colitis, Ulcerative
*Diverticulitis
Hodgkin's Disease
*Large-intestine Cancer
Ulcer, Peptic

Bleeding, from rectum
Anal Fissure
Hemorrhoids
*Injury to rectum from foreign bodies or anal intercourse
Intestinal Obstruction
Intussusception
Vagina or Vulva, Cancer of

Bleeding, spontaneous from any organ or skin
*Adverse reactions to drugs or medications
Anemia, Aplastic
Kidney Failure, Acute
Leukemia, Acute

Blindness
Brain Tumor
Diabetes Mellitus
Glaucoma
Tay-Sachs Disease

Blisters on skin, discharge of blood-stained pus
Folliculitis, Bacterial

Blisters, forming into scabs
Chickenpox

Blisters, in mouth and throat
Herpangina

Blisters, painful and red
Shingles

Blisters, painful, around genitals
Herpes, Genital

Blisters, painful, around mouth
Cold Sores (Herpes Simplex)

Blisters, pierced by hair, or near hair follicles
Folliculitis, Bacterial

* No chart in this book for this disorder.

Blisters, progressing to ulcers
Sores, Pressure

Blisters, small and filled with fluid
"Id" Reaction
Prickly Heat

Blisters, small, appearing on hands or feet
Athlete's Foot
Dyshidrosis

Blisters, small, containing pus
Folliculitis, Bacterial
Impetigo

Blisters, small, itchy (break easily when scratched)
Scabies

Blisters, small, that don't break easily
Dyshidrosis

Blisters, small, forming yellow crusts when broken
Impetigo

Blisters, small, progressing to thin, raised, red or white lines on skin
Larva Migrans, Cutaneous

Blisters, small, that come together and form larger blisters
Dyshidrosis

Blisters, small and oozing
Eczema

Blisters, small, yellow-white, and surrounded by red rings
Folliculitis, Bacterial

Blisters, surrounded by a red ring, and filled with fluid
Cold Sores

Blisters, when broken, leave scratch marks and thickened skin
Scabies

Blisters, with itchy lesions
Dermatitis Herpetiformis

Blood pressure, drop in
Blood Poisoning
Ectopic Pregnancy
Fainting
Heart-Rhythm Irregularity (Arrhythmia)
*Internal or external brisk bleeding
Pseudomembranous Enterocolitis

Blood pressure, high
Calcium Imbalance
Cushing's Syndrome
Glomerulonephritis
Heart-Valve Disease
Hyperaldosteronism
Kidney Failure, Acute
Kidney Failure, Chronic
Wilm's Tumor

Blood pressure, excessively low (under 80 systolic)
Addison's disease
Congestive Heart Failure
Dehydration
Diphtheria
Heart-Valve Disease
Kidney Failure, Acute
Peritonitis
Pituitary Tumor
Potassium Imbalance
Shock
Snakebite
Toxic Shock Syndrome

Blood streaks, on toilet paper, underwear or diaper
Anal Fissure

Blood sugar, low
Pituitary Tumor
*Too much sugar

Body image, distorted
Anorexia Nervosa
*Many mental and emotional disorders

* No chart in this book for this disorder.

Body movements, agitated or bizarre
Epilepsy
*Many mental and emotional disorders

Body movements, purposeless
Cerebral Palsy

Body odor, unpleasant
*Excessive garlic intake
Hyperhidrosis
*Uncleanliness

Body postures, unusual
Cerebral Palsy
*Many mental and emotional disorders

Body temperature, drops
Hypothermia

Body temperature, low
Hypothermia
Premature Infants

Body, wasting of
Anorexia Nervosa

Bone fractures, easy
*Genetic disorders
Hyperparathyroidism
Kidney Failure, Chronic

Bone pain
Celiac Disease
Kidney Failure, Chronic
Osteomyelitis
Vitamin D Deficiency

Bone softening
Hyperparathyroidism

Boredom
Depression
*Many mental and emotional disorders

Bowel movements, absence of normal
Fecal Impaction
Intestinal Obstruction

Bowel movements, infrequent and/or difficult to pass
Constipation

Bowel movements, loss of control of
*Cardiac Arrest
Convulsions, Febrile
Diarrhea, Acute
Encopresis
Epilepsy
Paraplegia or Quadriplegia
Spinal-Cord Tumor

Bowel movements, pain or bleeding with
Anal Fissure
Constipation

Bowel movements, straining during
Constipation

Breast nipples, darkening of
Addison's Disease

Breast pain, redness or hardness
Breast Abscess
Breast Cancer

Breast tenderness
Breast Abscess
Premenstrual Syndrome

Breasts, swollen
*Pregnancy
Premenstrual Syndrome

Breasts, swollen in males
Gynecomastia

Breastbone, burning sensation behind
*Angina Pectoris
Decompression Disease
Indigestion

Breastbone, burning, gnawing pain below
Ulcer, Peptic

* No chart in this book for this disorder.

Breastbone, feeling of pressure behind
- Bronchitis, Acute

Breath, bad
- Empyema
- *Food indiscretion
- Gingivitis
- Hepatitis, Acute Viral
- Kidney Failure, Chronic
- Kidney, Polycystic
- Lung Abscess
- Tooth Abscess
- Tooth Decay
- Trench Mouth

Breath, shortness of
- Alcoholism
- Anemia, Folic-Acid Deficiency
- Atelectasis
- Asthma
- Blood-Transfusion Reaction
- Bronchiectasis
- Bronchitis, Chronic
- Congestive Heart Failure
- Cor Pulmonale
- Decompression Disease
- Endocarditis
- Glomerulonephritis
- Heart-Rhythm Irregularity
- Heart-Valve Disease
- Hypertension
- Idiopathic Hypertrophic Subaortic Stenosis
- Kidney, Polycystic
- Lupus Erythematosus, Systemic
- Myocarditis
- Nosebleed
- Pneumonia, Bacterial
- Pneumothorax
- Polyarteritis
- Psittacosis
- Radiation Sickness
- Rheumatic Fever
- Shock
- Sickle-Cell Anemia
- Tapeworm
- Tuberculosis
- Valley Fever

Breathing, difficult
- Anaphylaxis
- Asthma
- Bronchiolitis
- Croup
- Diphtheria
- Drug Hypersensitivity
- Epiglottitis, Acute
- Guillain-Barré Syndrome
- Histoplasmosis
- Hypoparathyroidism
- Myocarditis
- Premature Infants
- Snakebite
- Tetanus
- Thyroid Tumor

Breathing, rapid
- Anxiety
- Aspirin Poisoning
- Asthma
- Bronchiolitis
- Empyema
- Esophageal Stricture or Corrosive Esophagitis
- Fainting
- Hyperventilation Syndrome
- Malaria
- Pericarditis, Acute
- Pleurisy
- Pneumonia, Bacterial
- Pneumonia, Viral
- Shock
- Subarachnoid Hemorrhage

Breathing, shallow
- Asthma
- Bronchiolitis
- Empyema
- Pleurisy

Breathing stops (during sleep)
- Sleep Apnea in Infants

* No chart in this book for this disorder.

Bright light, sensitivity to (photophobia)
Conjunctivitis
Corneal Ulcer
Drug Abuse & Addiction
Keratitis
Porphyria
Sty
Subarachnoid Hemorrhage

Bright light, vision worse
Cataract Bruises
*Any musculo-skeletal injury
*Drug effect (anticoagulants)
Hemophilia
Rape Crisis Syndrome
Sprains & Strains

Bruising, unexplained, easy or unexpected
Anemia, Aplastic
DIC
Drug Hypersensitivity
Kidney Failure, Acute
Leukemia, Acute
Thrombocytopenia
Vitamin K Deficiency

Bump, slightly swollen, warm and tender, below knee
Osgood-Schlatter Disease

Bumps, firm, smooth, domed, and skin-colored or white
Molluscum Contagiosum

Bumps, pin-sized
Granuloma, Pyogenic
Warts, Plantar

Bumps, pin-sized, but grow rapidly
Granuloma, Pyogenic

Bumps, purplish with a whitish surface
Lichen Planus

Bumps, small, firm, clustered at the openings of hair follicles
Keratosis Pilaris

Bumps, small, firm, and containing a coiled hair
Keratosis Pilaris

Bumps, small, raised, and itchy
Hives
Lichen Planus

Bumps, small, raised on skin
Granuloma Annulare
Granuloma, Pyogenic
Hives
Lichen Planus
Lyme Disease
Warts

Bumps, small, raised, that are domed or slightly flat shaped
Granuloma Annulare

Bumps, small, raised, firm, white, with a "sandpaper" feeling
Keratosis Pilaris

Bumps, small, raised, that bleed easily when injured
Granuloma, Pyogenic

Bumps, small, raised, that don't itch or hurt
Granuloma Annulare
Granuloma, Pyogenic
Keratosis Pilaris
Molluscum Contagiosum
Rheumatic Fever
Warts

Bumps, pink or violet, that appear in shape of a ring
Granuloma Annulare

Buttocks, one side more creases than other
Hip Dislocation, Congenital

Buttocks, pain in
Arthritis, Infectious

Buttocks, small raised bumps on skin
Lyme Disease

* No chart in this book for this disorder.

C

Calf, swollen and painful
Thrombosis, Deep-Vein

Cavities in teeth
Tooth Decay

Cervix, painless red sore on
Syphilis

Cheek pain, that may resemble a toothache
Sinus Infection

Cheeks, flat rash on, in shape of a butterfly
Lupus Erythematosus, Systemic

Cheeks, skin lesions, red and raised
Lupus Erythematosus, Discoid

Cheeks, small white patches on
Pityriasis Alba

Cheeks, ulcers on inner
Canker Sores

Chest blisters, painful and red
Shingles

Chest, burning, gnawing pain in lower
Ulcer, Peptic

Chest, enlarged
*Any chronic lung disease
Asthma
Emphysema

Chest, feeling that food sticks in the
*Esophageal stricture
Scleroderma

Chest, heavy, uncomfortable sensation in
*Heart disease
Heartburn

Chest, muscle weakness
Guillain-Barré Syndrome

Chest pain, in front, that worsens with movement
Pericarditis, Acute

Chest pain or discomfort
APC Disease
Arthritis, Juvenile Rheumatoid
Atelectasis
Blood-Transfusion Reaction
Cholecystitis or Cholangitis, Acute
Cor Pulmonale
Croup
Decompression Disease
Depression
Empyema
Esophageal Stricture or Corrosive Esophagitis
Gastritis
Heart-Valve Disease
Heartbeat, Rapid
Idiopathic Hypertrophic Subaortic Stenosis
Kidney, Polycystic
Lung Abscess
Lupus Erythematosus, Systemic
Pleurisy
Pneumonia, Mycoplasma
Pneumonia, Viral
Pneumothorax
Polyarteritis
Pulmonary-Valve Stenosis
Radiation Sickness
Rib Fracture (hurts with coughing, sneezing, or deep breathing)
Shingles
Sickle-Cell Anemia

Chest pain, that worsens with breathing or coughing
Pericarditis
Pleurisy
Pneumonia, Bacterial

Chest, rash that is faint pale pink or brown
Pityriasis Rosea

Chest, see-saw movements of
Bronchiolitis

* No chart in this book for this disorder.

Chewing, extreme pain upon
Tooth Abscess

Chewing movements, odd
Epilepsy
*Many mental and emotional disorders

Chewing, tenderness of the muscles used in
Temporo-Mandibular Joint Syndrome (TMJ)

Chills and fever, see Fever

Chills, shaking
Blood Poisoning
Kidney Infection, Acute
Malaria
Pneumonia
Virus Infection

"Chokes"
Decompression Disease

Clitoris, enlarged
Cushing's Syndrome
Ovarian Tumors

Cold, intolerance to
Anorexia Nervosa
*Many infections

Coma
*Adverse drug reaction
Alcoholism
Brain Tumor
Calcium Imbalance
Decompression Disease
Dehydration
DIC
*Drug or medication overdose
*Electrolyte imbalance
Encephalitis, Viral or Aseptic
Kidney Failure, Acute
Reye's Syndrome
Rocky Mountain Spotted Fever
Sodium Imbalance
Subarachnoid Hemorrhage

Complexion, ruddy red
Alcoholism
Cushing's Syndrome

Confusion
Alcoholism
Aspirin Poisoning
Asthma
Blood Poisoning
Brain or Epidural Abscess
Drowning, Near
Epilepsy (following an episode)
Fluid or Electrolyte Disorders
Head Injury
Hypertension
Hypoglycemia, Functional
Hypothermia
Kidney Failure, Chronic
Lead Poisoning
*Many mental and emotional disorders
Meningitis, Aseptic
Meningitis, Bacterial
Rabies
Reye's Syndrome
Rocky Mountain Spotted Fever
Shock
Sodium Imbalance
Subdural Hemorrhage & Hematoma
Toxic Shock Syndrome
Vitamin B Deficiencies

Consciousness, loss of
Anaphylaxis
Decompression Disease
Epilepsy
Head Injury
Heart Block
Hypoglycemia, Functional (due to excessive insulin)
Hypothermia

* No chart in this book for this disorder.

Constipation
- Amebiasis
- Anorexia Nervosa
- Appendicitis
- Botulism
- Brucellosis
- Depression
- Diabetes Insipidus
- Lead Poisoning
- Paraplegia or Quadriplegia
- *Poor dietary habits
- Premenstrual Syndrome
- Pyloric Stenosis, Congenital
- Tay-Sachs Disease

Convulsions
- Brain or Epidural Abscess
- Brain Tumor
- Cerebral Palsy
- DIC
- Epilepsy
- Head Injury
- Heart Block
- Hypoglycemia of Diabetes
- Kidney Failure, Acute
- Subarachnoid Hemorrhage
- Vitamin B Deficiencies

Cough
- APC Disease
- Asthma
- Atelectasis
- Bronchiolitis
- Bronchitis, Chronic
- Congestive Heart Failure
- Decompression Disease
- Hay Fever
- Heartbeat, Rapid
- Histoplasmosis
- Pericarditis, Acute
- Pleurisy
- Pneumonia, Mycoplasma
- Psittacosis
- Rabies
- Roundworms
- Scarlet Fever
- Sinus Infection
- Snakebite
- Tonsillitis
- Valley Fever
- Whooping Cough

Cough, chronic
- Cystic Fibrosis

Cough, dry
- Pneumothorax
- Radiation Sickness

Cough, harsh, hacking
- Measles
- Pneumothorax

Cough with sputum
- Lung Abscess
- Pneumonia, Bacterial
- Pneumonia, Mycoplasma
- Psittacosis
- Pulmonary-Valve Stenosis
- Tuberculosis
- Whooping Cough

Cough with very little or no sputum
- Bronchitis, Acute
- Cold, Common
- Influenza

Coughing blood
- Hypertension

Coughing bouts
- Whooping Cough

Coughing, frequent
- Bronchiectasis

Coughing spasms
- Bronchitis, Chronic

Cramps in legs
- *Calcium deficiency
- Hypochondriasis
- *Sodium deficiency

Craving for ice, paint or soil (especially red clay)
- Anemia, Iron-Deficiency

Crawling, delayed
- Vitamin D Deficiency

* No chart in this book for this disorder.

Crying bouts in infants
Colic in Infants
*Hunger
*Many mental and emotional disorders

Curvature of spine of upper body
Scoliosis

Cyst that becomes bright red and painful (if infected or injured)
Sebaceous Cyst

Cyst, dome-shaped, nodular appearance, with a smooth surface
Sebaceous Cyst

Cyst, sloped shoulders
Sebaceous Cyst

Cyst, smooth, containing a hair, at the base of spine
Pilonidal Cyst

Cyst, whitish or skin-colored
Sebaceous Cyst

D

Death, feeling of impending, with shortness of breath
Heartbeat, Rapid

Decisions, difficulty making
Depression
*Many mental and emotional disorders

Delirium
Asthma
Blood Poisoning
Brain or Epidural Abscess
Brain Tumor
Sunburn

Delirium tremens
Alcoholism

Depression
Addison's Disease
*Adverse reaction to drugs or medications
Anorexia Nervosa
Brucellosis
Bulimia
Hyperparathyroidism
*Many mental and emotional disorders
Porphyria
Rape Crisis Syndrome
Valley Fever

Depth perception, loss of
Strabismus (crossed eyes)

Development, retarded
Down Syndrome

Development, slow
Cerebral Palsy
Failure to Thrive
Lactose Intolerance
*Many mental and emotional disorders
Sickle-Cell Anemia

Diarrhea
Addison's Disease
AIDS
Amebiasis
Anemia, Folic-Acid Deficiency
Anxiety
Appendicitis
Botulism
Calcium Imbalance
Drug Hypersensitivity
Dysentery, Bacillary
Dysmenorrhea
Ear Infection, Middle
Gastritis
Gastroenteritis
Giardiasis
Hepatitis, Acute Viral
Histoplasmosis
Intestinal Obstruction (partial obstruction only)
Kidney Failure, Acute
Kidney, Polycystic

* No chart in this book for this disorder.

Diarrhea, continued
- Lactose Intolerance
- Malabsorption
- Premenstrual Syndrome
- Pruritis Ani
- Radiation Sickness
- Roundworms
- Salmonella Infections
- Shingles
- Sodium Imbalance
- Tapeworm
- Trichinosis
- Typhoid Fever
- Vitamin B Deficiencies
- Whooping Cough

Diarrhea, bloody
- *Colon Cancer
- *Diverticulitis
- Pseudomembranous Enterocolitis

Diarrhea, bloody with mucus
- Colitis, Ulcerative

Diarrhea, foamy
- Lactose Intolerance

Diarrhea, watery
- Dysentery, Bacillary
- Pseudomembranous Enterocolitis
- Salmonella Infections
- Toxic Shock Syndrome
- Typhoid Fever

Disorientation
- *Many mental and emotional disorders
- Pseudomembranous Enterocolitis
- Shock

Distortion, severe, of the body
- Muscular Dystrophy

Dizziness
- Addison's Disease
- Atelectasis
- Barotitis Media
- Brain Tumor
- Eardrum, Ruptured
- Ectopic Pregnancy
- Heart-Valve Disease
- Intestinal Obstruction
- *Labyrinthitis (inflamed inner ear)
- Peritonitis
- Pituitary Tumor
- Premenstrual Syndrome
- Pulmonary-Valve Stenosis
- Subarachnoid Hemorrhage
- Subdural Hemorrhage & Hematoma
- Sun Poisoning
- Whiplash

Dreams, vivid
- *Adverse reaction to drugs or medications
- Narcolepsy

Drooling
- Epiglottitis, Acute

Drowsiness
- *Adverse reaction to drugs or medications
- Encephalitis, Viral or Aseptic
- Extradural Hemorrhage
- Glomerulonephritis
- Head Injury
- Hypertension
- Kidney Failure, Acute
- Kidney Failure, Chronic
- *Many mental and emotional disorders
- Meningitis, Aseptic
- Meningitis, Bacterial
- Reye's Syndrome
- Roseola Infantum
- Subarachnoid Hemorrhage
- Subdural Hemorrhage & Hematoma

E

Ear, bleeding from
- Eardrum, Ruptured

Ear, discharge or leakage from
- Ear Infection, Middle-
- Ear Infection, Outer-
- Eardrum, Ruptured

* No chart in this book for this disorder.

Ear, feeling of fullness in
Ear Infection, Middle-

Ear pain
Ear Infection, Middle-
Ear Infection, Outer-
Earwax Blockage
Strep Throat
Tonsillitis

Ear pain, behind, with facial paralysis
Bell's Palsy

Ear pain, sudden
Eardrum, Ruptured

Ear, plugged feeling in
Barotitis Media
Earwax Blockage

Ear, pulling at the
Ear Infection, Middle-

Ear, ringing noises in
Barotitis Media
Eardrum, Ruptured
Earwax Blockage
Hearing Impairment or Loss
*Labyrinthitis (inflamed inner ear)
Otosclerosis

Earache
Ear Infection, Inner-
Earwax Blockage
Ear Infection, Middle-
Strep Throat
Tonsillitis
Tooth Abscess

Ears, swollen lymph glands behind
Measles, German

Eating, difficulty in self-feeding
Hemiplegia

Eating non-food substances (such as clay, hair, gravel, and paint)
Pica

Eating, pain immediately after
Ulcer, Peptic

Eating, pain in mouth and chest after
Esophageal Stricture or Corrosive Esophagitis

Eating patterns, abnormal (gorging or fasting)
Bulimia

Eggs in stools (microscopic-sized)
*Other intestinal parasites
Tapeworm

Eggs on hair shafts (''nits'')
Lice

Elbows, painful inflammation of tendon
Tendinitis

Elbows, inflammation of joints
*Following injury
Rheumatic Fever

Elbows, itching rash
Dermatitis, Atopic

Elbows, pain, swelling, and stiffness in
Arthritis, Juvenile Rheumatoid

Elbows, yellowish nodules of fat in skin beneath
Hyperlipidemia, Types I, II, III, IV, V

Emotional instability
Hypoglycemia of Diabetes
*Many mental and emotional disorders
Premenstrual Syndrome

Eyelids, crusted after sleeping
Conjunctivitis
Keratitis

Eyelids, drooping
Botulism
Pituitary Tumor
Ptosis

Eyelids, paleness in lining
Anemia, Iron-Deficiency

Eyelids, redness, swelling, pain, warmth or tenderness of
Sty

* No chart in this book for this disorder.

Eyelids, spasm
Corneal Ulcer

Eyelids, swollen
Conjunctivitis
Sty

Eyes, almond-shaped and slanting
Down Syndrome

Eyes, bleeding in whites of
Subconjunctival Hemorrhage

Eyes, blinking reflexes poor
Ptosis

Eyes, bloodshot
*Adverse reaction to marijuana
Conjunctivitis
Corneal Ulcer
Headache, Migraine
Toxocara

Eyes, bright spots appear
Headache, Migraine

Eyes, bruising in or around the
Eye Contusion or Laceration

Eyes, bulging
Exophthalmos
Eye Tumor

Eyes, crossed
Cerebral Palsy
Eye Tumor
Strabismus

Eyes, discharge from
Conjunctivitis
Toxocara

Eyes, feeling like something is in
*Chalazion
Cold Sores
Conjunctivitis
Eye, Foreign Body in
Toxocara

Eyes, irritation in the
Eye, Foreign Body in

Eyes, itchy
Hay Fever

Eyes, movements uncoordinated
Strabismus (crossed eyes)

Eyes, pain and redness in
APC Disease
Arthritis, Juvenile Rheumatoid
Cold Sores
Eye Contusion or Laceration
Eye, Foreign Body in
Glaucoma, Acute Infantile

Eyes, pain below the
Tear Duct, Infection or Blockage of

Eyes, pain in
APC Disease
Arthritis, Juvenile Rheumatoid
Cold Sores
Conjunctivitis
Contusion or Laceration
Corneal Ulcer
Exophthalmos
Eye Contusion or Laceration
Eye, Foreign Body in
Keratitis
Subarachnoid Hemorrhage

Eyes, puffy
Cushing's Syndrome
Glomerulonephritis
Nephrosis

Eyes, red
*Adverse reaction to marijuana
APC Disease
Arthritis, Juvenile Rheumatoid
Cold Sores
Eye Contusion or Laceration
Eye, Foreign Body in
Measles
Reiter's Syndrome

Eyes, redness and gritty feeling in
Conjunctivitis
Sty

* No chart in this book for this disorder.

Eyes, sensitive to light
Cold Sores
Conjunctivitis
Corneal Ulcer
Drug Abuse & Addiction
Glaucoma, Acute Infantile
Measles
Meningitis, Aseptic
Meningitis, Bacterial

Eyes, sunken
Dehydration

Eyes, swelling around
Eye Contusion or Laceration
Kidney, Polycystic

Eyes, tearing
Conjunctivitis
Corneal Ulcer
Hay Fever
Keratitis

Eyes, tumor (visible through the pupil)
Eye Tumor

Eyes, watery
Anaphylaxis
Cold, Common
Cold Sores
Corneal Ulcer
Hay Fever
Keratitis

Eyes, yellowish nodules of fat in skin beneath
Hyperlipidemia, Types I, II, III, IV, V

F

Face becomes tight and loses elasticity
Scleroderma

Face, bright, flat, red rash on
Scarlet Fever

Face, crackling feeling when touched
Facial Bones, Fracture of

Face, feeling of fullness in
Nasal Polyps

Face, flat, with expressionless features on one side
Bell's Palsy

Face, itchy rash
Dermatitis, Atopic
Drug Hypersensitivity
Polymyositis & Dermatomyositis

Face, puffiness in
Fluid & Electrolyte Disorders
Glomerulonephritis
Nephrosis
Premenstrual Syndrome
Trichinosis

Face, redness that becomes multi-colored
Facial Bones, Fractures of

Face, round
Cushing's Syndrome

Face, swelling of
Facial Bones, Fracture of
Lupus Erythematosus, Systemic
Vitamin E Deficiency

Face, swelling and tenderness
Facial Bones, Fracture of
Sinusitis
Tooth Abscess

Face, twitching of (that lasts 2-3 minutes)
Convulsions, Febrile

Facial grimacing (that disappears when sleeping)
St. Vitus' Dance

Facial hair, growth of, in females
Cushing's Syndrome

Facial pain
Facial Bones, Fracture of
Nasal Polyps
Shingles
Sinusitis

* No chart in this book for this disorder.

Fainting
Cor Pulmonale
Drug Hypersensitivity
Ectopic Pregnancy
Hyperventilation Syndrome
Idiopathic Hypertrophic Subaortic Stenosis
Intestinal Obstruction
*Many mental and emotional disorders
Premenstrual Syndrome

Faintness
Addison's Disease
Anemia, Aplastic
Anemia, Iron-Deficiency
Bladder or Urethra Injury
Congestive Heart Failure
Drug Hypersensitivity
Guillain-Barré Syndrome
Heart-Rhythm Irregularity
Heart-Valve Disease
Heartbeat, Rapid
Hyperventilation Syndrome
Hypoglycemia, Functional
Pulmonary-Valve Stenosis

Falling with difficulty getting up
Muscular Dystrophy
Polymyositis & Dermatomyositis

Fang marks
Snakebite

Fatigue
Addison's Disease
AIDS
Amebiasis
Anemia
Anemia, Folic-Acid Deficiency
Anemia, Iron-Deficiency
Ankylosing Spondylitis
Anxiety
Bronchiectasis
Brucellosis
Cat-Scratch Fever
Celiac Disease
Cold, Common
Congestive Heart Failure
Cor Pulmonale
Depression
Diabetes Mellitus, Insulin-Dependent
Empyema
Endocarditis
Fluid & Electrolyte Disorders
*Heart Disease
Heart-Valve Disease
Hepatitis, Acute Viral
Hyperaldosteronism
Influenza
Kidney Failure, Chronic
Kidney Infection, Acute
Kidney, Polycystic
Lead Poisoning
Leukemia, Acute
Lyme Disease
Malaria
*Many mental and emotional disorders
Measles
Measles, German
Myocarditis
Pityriasis Rosea
Pneumonia, Bacterial
Pneumonia, Viral
Pulmonary-Valve Stenosis
Rabies
Radiation Sickness
Rheumatic Fever
Roundworms
Scleroderma
Sickle-Cell Anemia
Small-Intestine Tumor
Sun Poisoning
Tapeworm
Thalassemia
Thrombocytopenia
Toxic Shock Syndrome
Tuberculosis
Vitamin B Deficiencies
Vitamin C Deficiency

Feces, see Stools

Feeling that something bad is going to happen
Anxiety

* No chart in this book for this disorder.

Feet, burning sensation in
Alcoholism
Kidney Failure, Chronic
Neuropathy, Peripheral

Feet, cold
Guillain-Barré Syndrome
Neuropathy, Peripheral
Polymyositis & Dermatomyositis
Shock

Feet, damp musty odor
Athlete's Foot

Feet, moist, soft, gray-white or red scales on
Athlete's Foot

Feet, muscle spasms in
*Adverse reactions to drugs or medications
Hyperventilation Syndrome
Hypoparathyroidism

Feet, muscle weakness in
Guillain-Barré Syndrome
*Neuritis, Peripheral

Feet, numbness in
Alcoholism
Calcium Imbalance
Hypertension
Hyperventilation Syndrome
Kidney Failure, Chronic
*Neuritis, Peripheral
Polyarteritis
Porphyria
Snakebite

Feet (of newborn) point down, turn inward and curl under
Clubfoot

Feet, skin lesions on soles and toenails
Reiter's Syndrome

Feet, small blisters on
Athlete's Foot

Feet, swollen
*Adverse reactions to drugs or medications
Alcoholism
Cor Pulmonale
Endocarditis
*Fluid Retention
Idiopathic Hypertrophic Subaortic Stenosis
Myocarditis
Premenstrual Syndrome
Pulmonary-Valve Stenosis

Feet, tingling sensation in
*Adverse reactions to drugs or medications
Alcoholism
Calcium Imbalance
Diabetes
Hyperaldosteronism
Hypertension
Hyperventilation Syndrome
Kidney Failure, Chronic
*Neuritis, Peripheral
Porphyria
Snakebite

Feet, warts appear on soles of
Warts, Plantar

Fever
Agranulocytosis
AIDS
Amebiasis
APC Disease
Appendicitis
Arthritis, Infectious
Arthritis, Juvenile Rheumatoid
Aspirin Poisoning
Atelectasis
Balanitis
Bladder Infection
Blood-Transfusion Reaction
Boils
Breast Abscess
Bronchitis, Acute
Brucellosis
Burns

* No chart in this book for this disorder.

Fever, continued

Cat-Scratch Fever
Cellulitis
Chickenpox
Cholecystitis or Cholangitis, Acute
Cold, Common
Colitis, Ulcerative
Diarrhea, Acute
Diphtheria
Drug Hypersensitivity
Dysentery, Bacillary
Ear Infection, Middle-
Ear Infection, Outer-
Empyema
Encephalitis, Viral or Aseptic
Endocarditis
Epiglottitis, Acute
Erythema Nodosum
Fecal Impaction
Fever of Undetermined Origin (FUO)
Gangrene
Gastritis
Gastroenteritis
Gingivitis
Hand, Foot & Mouth Disease
Hepatitis, Acute Viral
Herpangina
Herpes, Genital
Histoplasmosis
Hodgkin's Disease
Impetigo
Influenza
Intestinal Obstruction
Kidney Infection, Acute
Kidney or Ureter Injury
Laryngitis
Leukemia, Acute
Liver Cancer
Lung Abscess
Lyme Disease
Malaria
Measles, German
Meningitis, Aseptic
Meningitis, Bacterial
Mononucleosis, Infectious
Mumps
Myocarditis
Osteomyelitis
Ovarian Cyst
Pelvic Inflammatory Disease
Pericarditis, Acute
Peritonitis
Pharyngitis
Pilonidal Cyst
Pityriasis Rosea
Pleurisy
Pneumonia, Bacterial
Pneumonia, Mycoplasma
Pneumonia, Viral
Polymyositis & Dermatomyositis
Polyarteritis
Pseudomembranous Enterocolitis
Psittacosis
Purpura, Allergic
Rabies
Reiter's Syndrome
Rheumatic Fever
Rocky Mountain Spotted Fever
Roseola Infantum
Salmonella Infections
Scarlet Fever
Shingles
Sinus Infection
Snakebite
Sodium Imbalance
Strep Throat
Subarachnoid Hemorrhage
Sun Poisoning
Sunburn
Surgical-Wound Infection
Syphilis
Tetanus Thrombophlebitis, Superficial
Thrombosis, Deep-Vein
Tonsillitis
Tooth Abscess
Toxic Shock Syndrome
Toxocara
Trichinosis
Tuberculosis
Typhoid Fever
Valley Fever
Vitamin C Deficiency
Whooping Cough
Wilm's Tumor

* No chart in this book for this disorder.

Fever, prolonged (2-3 weeks)
Fever of Undetermined Origin (FUO)

Fingernails, blue
Pneumonia

Fingernails, pitted
Psoriasis

Fingers, burning sensation in
*Adverse reactions to drugs or medications
Diabetes
Frostbite
Hyperventilation Syndrome
*Neuritis, Peripheral

Fingers, hardening and thickening of skin
Scleroderma

Fingers, numbness around
Frostbite
Hypoglycemia of Diabetes
Raynaud's Disease

Fingers, pain
Arthritis, Juvenile Rheumatoid
Paronychia
Raynaud's Disease

Fingers, pain, tenderness, redness, swelling, and warmth
Paronychia

Fingers, pale then followed by bluish tint, then redness
Raynaud's Disease
Raynaud's Phenomenon

Fingers, stiffness, poor circulation, numbness, and ulceration
Scleroderma

Fingers turn pale when exposed to cold or stress
Raynaud's Disease
Raynaud's Phenomenon

Fingers, purple
Frostbite
Hypothermia

Fingertips, tingling
Frostbite
Hyperventilation Syndrome
Hypoparathyroidism

Fingertips, ulcers on
Raynaud's Disease
Raynaud's Phenomenon

Flank pain
Hyperparathyroidism
Kidney Infection, Acute
Kidney Infection, Chronic

Fluid retention
Cor Pulmonale
Kidney Infection, Chronic
Kidney, Polycystic
Liver Cancer
Nephrosis
Premenstrual Syndrome
Rheumatic Fever

Foot, pain when raising or flexing
Thrombosis, Deep-Vein

Forehead, reddish rash on
Drug Hypersensitivity
Measles

Fracture, bleeding or bruising
Bone Fracture (compound, with broken bone protruding through skin)

Freckles, darkening of
Addison's Disease

Freckles, flat, brownish spots
Skin Lesions, Benign

Frenzy
Drug Abuse & Addiction

Frowns, distorted
Bell's Palsy

Fullness, feeling of
Indigestion
Ulcer, Peptic

* No chart in this book for this disorder.

* No chart in this book for this disorder.

SYMPTOMS

Gums, painful
Trench Mouth

Gums, swollen
Gingivitis
Vitamin C Deficiency

Gums, swollen, red, and soft around teeth
Gingivitis

Gums, ulcers on
Canker Sores
Kidney Failure, Chronic
Trench Mouth

H

Hair follicles, infected
Folliculitis, Bacterial
Folliculitis, Fungal

Hair growth, excessive
Ovarian Cancer
Ovarian Cyst (functioning)

Hair growth, sparse
Zinc Deficiency

Hair loss
Addison's Disease
*Adverse reactions to drugs or medications
Alopecia Aereata
Lichen Planus
Lupus Erythematosus, Systemic
Radiation Sickness
Telogen Effluvium

Hair, matted
Lice

Hair shafts, eggs on
Lice

Hallucinations
*Adverse reactions to drugs or medications
Alcoholism
Drug Abuse & Addiction
*Many mental and emotional disorders
Narcolepsy
Schizophrenia
Vitamin C Deficiency

Hamstring, painful inflammation of tendon
*Athletic Injury
Tendinitis

Hands, broad, with large, unusual palm creases
Down Syndrome

Hands, cold
*Adverse reactions to drugs or medications
Anxiety
Guillain-Barré Syndrome
Polymyositis & Dermatomyositis
Shock

Hands, dry
Diabetes Insipidus

Hands, muscle spasms in
Hyperventilation Syndrome
Hypoparathyroidism

Hands, muscle weakness in
Guillain-Barré Syndrome

Hands, numbness in
*Adverse reactions to drugs or medications
Alcoholism
Calcium Imbalance
Hypertension
Hyperventilation Syndrome
*Many mental and emotional disorders
Polyarteritis
Porphyria
Snakebite

Hands, paleness in
Anemia, Iron-Deficiency

Hands, puffiness in
Fluid & Electrolyte Disorders
Premenstrual Syndrome

* No chart in this book for this disorder.

Hands, rash that's itchy
Dermatitis, Atopic

Hands, rash with blisters on
Hand, Foot & Mouth Disease

Hands, red
Lupus Erythematosus, Systemic
*Many mental and emotional disorders

Hands, skin lesions on palms and fingernails
Reiter's Syndrome

Hands, tingling
*Adverse reactions to drugs or medications
Alcoholism
Calcium Imbalance
Hyperaldosteronism
Hypertension
Hyperventilation Syndrome
*Many mental and emotional disorders
Polyarteritis
Porphyria
Snakebite

Hands, trembling
Hypoglycemia, Functional
*Overactive Thyroid

Hangover
Alcoholism

Head, delayed closing of "soft spots"
Brain Tumor
Subdural Hematoma
Vitamin D Deficiency

Head, feeling of pressure inside
Sinus Infection

Head, feeling that a vise is over the back of
Headache, Tension or Vascular

Head injury
Extradural Hemorrhage

Head pain
Headache, Migraine
Headache, Tension or Vascular

Head posture, odd, with severe breathing difficulty
Epiglottitis, Acute

Head, throbbing pain all over
*Adverse reactions to drugs or medications
Headache, Tension or Vascular
*Many mental and emotional disorders

Head, turns sideways and bends down
Torticollis

Headache
*Adverse reactions to drugs or medications
Anxiety
Blood-Transfusion Reaction
Brain or Epidural Abscess
Brain Tumor
Brucellosis
Cat-Scratch Fever
Depression
Encephalitis, Viral or Aseptic
Extradural Hemorrhage
Glomerulonephritis
Head Injury
Hepatitis, Acute Viral
Histoplasmosis
Hypertension
Hypoglycemia of Diabetes
Influenza
Kidney Infection, Acute
Kidney, Polycystic
Lead Poisoning
Leukemia, Acute
Lyme Disease
Malaria
*Many mental and emotional disorders
Measles, German
Meningitis, Aseptic
Meningitis, Bacterial

* No chart in this book for this disorder.

Headache, continued
- Mononucleosis, Infectious
- Mumps
- Nasal Polyps
- Pituitary Tumor
- Pityriasis Rosea
- Premenstrual Syndrome
- Radiation Sickness
- Rocky Mountain Spotted Fever
- Sinus Infection
- Snakebite
- Strep Throat
- Subarachnoid Hemorrhage
- Subdural Hemorrhage & Hematoma
- Syphilis
- Tooth-Grinding
- Toxic Shock Syndrome
- Typhoid Fever
- Valley Fever
- Whiplash

Hearing, decreased
- Earwax Blockage

Hearing loss
- Barotitis Media
- *Congenital Deafness
- Ear Infection, Middle-
- Ear Infection, Outer-
- Encephalitis, Viral or Aseptic
- Otitis, Serous
- Otosclerosis
- Reye's Syndrome

Hearing loss, partial
- Eardrum, Ruptured

Hearing that is better in a noisy environment
- Otosclerosis

Heart, enlarged
- *Congenital Heart Disease
- Congestive Heart Failure
- Lyme Disease

Heart failure, congestive
- *Adverse reactions to drugs or medications
- Alcoholism
- Pulmonary-Valve Stenosis
- Vitamin B Deficiencies

Heart inflammation
- AIDS
- Radiation Sickness
- *Virus infections, many

Heart murmur
- Down Syndrome
- *Congestive Heart Disease
- Endocarditis
- Heart-Valve Disease
- Idiopathic Hypertrophic Subaortic Stenosis

Heart, palpitations
- Heartbeat, Rapid

Heart, pounding
- *Adverse reactions to drugs or medications
- Anaphylaxis
- Blood Poisoning
- Heartbeat, Rapid
- Hypoglycemia of Diabetes
- *Many mental and emotional disorders

Heartbeat, aware of one's own
- Heart-Rhythm Irregularity

Heartbeat, irregular
- *Adverse reactions to drugs or medications
- Calcium Imbalance
- Congestive Heart Failure
- Endocarditis
- Fluid & Electrolyte Disorders
- Heart Block
- Heart-Rhythm Irregularity
- Heart-Valve Disease
- Idiopathic Hypertrophic Subaortic Stenosis
- Lupus Erythematosus, Systemic
- Lyme Disease

* No chart in this book for this disorder.

Heartbeat, irregular, continued
*Many mental and emotional disorders
Myocarditis
Potassium Imbalance
Rabies
Thalassemia

Heartbeat, rapid
Alcoholism
Anemia, Iron-Deficiency
Anxiety
Aspirin Poisoning
Congestive Heart Failure
Diphtheria
Ectopic Pregnancy
Endocarditis
Fainting
Guillain-Barré Syndrome
Heart-Rhythm Irregularities
Lupus Erythematosus, Systemic
Myocarditis
Nosebleed
Peritonitis
Potassium Imbalance
Pseudomembranous Enterocolitis
Radiation Sickness
Rheumatic Fever
Sickle-Cell Anemia
Subarachnoid Hemorrhage
Testicle Torsion

Heartbeat, skips
*Adverse reactions to drugs or medications
Heart-Rhythm Irregularity

Heartbeat, slow
*Adverse reactions to drugs or medications
Heart Block
Heart-Rhythm Irregularity

Heartburn
Hiatal Hernia
Indigestion
Scleroderma
Ulcer, Peptic

Hip, pain and stiffness in
Arthritis, Juvenile Rheumatoid
Legg-Perthes Disease

Hips, pain in joints
Decompression Disease
Reiter's Syndrome

Hives
*Adverse reactions to drugs or medications
Anaphylaxis
Blood-Transfusion Reaction
Drug Hypersensitivity
Lice
*Many mental and emotional disorders
Purpura, Allergic
Serum Sickness

Hoarseness
Anxiety
Cold, Common
Croup
Epiglottitis, Acute
Influenza
Laryngitis
Thyroid Tumor

Hunger
*Adverse reactions to drugs or medications
*Many mental and emotional disorders
Ulcer, Peptic

Hunger, excessive
*Adverse reactions to drugs or medications
Hypoglycemia, Functional
Hypoglycemia of Diabetes
*Many mental and emotional disorders

Hypertension
*Congenital Heart Disease
Kidney Infection, Chronic
Kidney, Polycystic

* No chart in this book for this disorder.

Hyperthyroidism, symptoms of (rapid heartbeat, weight loss)
Thyroid Tumor

Hyperventilation
Anxiety

I

Ill feeling, general
*Adverse reactions to drugs or medications
Blood Poisoning
Bronchiectasis
Breast Abscess
Cellulitis
Chickenpox
Encephalitis, Viral or Aseptic
Glomerulonephritis
Hepatitis, Acute Viral
Herpangina
Herpes, Genital
Hodgkin's Disease
Leukemia, Acute
Lymphoma, Non-Hodgkin's
*Many mental and emotional disorders
Nephrosis
Osteomyelitis
Pelvic Inflammatory Disease
Psittacosis
Rheumatic Fever
Shingles
Strep Throat
Tooth Abscess
Valley Fever

Imaginary illnesses
Hypochondriasis

Incision, fluid collecting around
Surgical-Wound Infection

Indigestion
Gallstones
Ulcer, Peptic
Vitamin B Deficiencies

Infections, frequent
Anemia, Iron-Deficiency
Cushing's Syndrome
Diabetes Mellitus, Insulin-Dependent
Failure to Thrive
Leukemia, Acute
Premature Infants
Premenstrual Syndrome
Sickle-Cell Anemia
Vitamin C Deficiency

Inhalations, noisy, high-pitched, squeaky
Epiglottitis, Acute

Insomnia
*Adverse reactions to drugs or medications
Alcoholism
Depression
Hypochondriasis
*Many mental and emotional disorders

Interest in life, loss of
Depression

Irritability
*Adverse reactions to drugs or medications
Anxiety
Depression
Ear Infection, Middle-
Gastroenteritis
Head Injury
Kidney Failure, Acute
*Many mental and emotional disorders
Meningitis, Aseptic
Meningitis, Bacterial
Premenstrual Syndrome
Rabies
Roseola Infantum
Roundworms

* No chart in this book for this disorder.

Itching
*Adverse reactions to drugs or medications
Anaphylaxis
*Any skin irritation
Blood-Transfusion Reaction
Conjunctivitis
Dermatitis, Atopic
Dermatitis, Contact
Drug Sensitivity
Hodgkin's Disease
Id Reaction
Insect Bites & Stings
Jock Itch
Kidney Failure, Acute
Lice
*Many mental and emotional disorders
Pityriasis Rosea

J

Jaundice
Acetaminophen Poisoning
Alcoholism
Amebiasis
Cholecystitis or Cholangitis, Acute
Gallstones
Gilbert's Syndrome
Hodgkin's Disease
Liver Cancer
Lymphoma, Non-Hodgkin's
*Metastatic Cancer
Mononucleosis, Infectious
Premature Infants
Sickle-Cell Anemia
Thalassemia

Jaw, bleeding under the skin, pain and swelling in
Jaw Dislocation

Jaw, inability to open completely
Temporo-Mandibular Joint Syndrome (TMJ)

Jaw pain, dull, aching on one side of
Temporo-Mandibular Joint Syndrome (TMJ)

Jawline, skin lesions, red and raised
Lupus Erythematosus, Discoid

Jerking uncontrollably
Epilepsy
*Fungus infection of the skin
Jock Itch

Joints, bleeding or bruising under
*Athletic Injury
Vitamin C Deficiency

Joints, deformity (after an injury)
Dislocation or Subluxation

Joint inflammation
Arthritis, Juvenile Rheumatoid
*Gout (rare in children)
Reye's Syndrome

Joint, movement limited, or no movement
Dislocation or Subluxation
Sprains & Strains

Joint pain
*Adverse reactions to drugs or medications
Arthritis, Infectious
Arthritis, Juvenile Rheumatoid
Decompression Disease
Dislocation or Subluxation
Drug Hypersensitivity
Hemophilia
Lupus Erythematosus, Systemic
Lyme Disease
*Many mental and emotional disorders
Measles, German
Osteomyelitis
Polymyositis & Dermatomyositis
Psoriasis
Reiter's Syndrome
Rheumatic Fever
Scleroderma
Sickle-Cell Anemia
Sprains & Strains

* No chart in this book for this disorder.

Joints, redness, tenderness (inflammation), pain
Arthritis, Infectious
Arthritis, Juvenile Rheumatoid
Lupus Erythematosus, Systemic
Osteomyelitis
Rheumatic Fever
Serum Sickness
Sprains & Strains

Joints, swelling
Arthritis, Infectious
Arthritis, Juvenile Rheumatoid
Hemophilia
Lupus Erythematosus, Systemic
Osteomyelitis
Rheumatic Fever
Scleroderma
Sprains & Strains

Joints, swelling (following an injury)
Dislocation or Subluxation
Sprains & Strains

K

Kidney infections, repeated
Diabetes Mellitus
Kidney, Polycystic

Kidney Stones
Hyperparathyroidism

Knee, slightly swollen, with warm and tender bump below
Osgood-Schlatter Disease

Knees, pain in joints (without redness or tenderness)
Decompression Sickness
Legg-Perthes Disease

Knees, rash that's itchy on skin
*Adverse reactions to drugs or medications
Dermatitis, Atopic

Knees, red, tender, and swollen, with small bumps
Erythema Nodosum

Knees, swelling and stiffness in
Arthritis, Juvenile Rheumatoid

Knees, yellowish nodules of fat in skin under
Hyperlipidemia, Types I, II, III, IV, V

Knock-knees
Vitamin D Deficiency

L

Larynx, spasms of the
Hypoparathyroidism

Laughing for no reason
Epilepsy
*Many mental and emotional disorders

Legs, bowed
Vitamin D Deficiency

Legs, burning sensation in
Frostbite
Kidney Failure, Chronic
Thrombophlebitis

Legs, clicking sound when pulled apart (newborn)
Hip Dislocation, Congenital

Legs, drawing up as if in pain
Colic in Infants

Legs, inability to move
Brain Tumor
Encephalitis, Viral or Aseptic
Extradural Hemorrhage
Spinal-Cord Tumor
Subarachnoid Hemorrhage

Legs, loss of movement
Paraplegia or Quadriplegia

Legs, loss of sensation
Paraplegia or Quadriplegia
*Neuritis, Peripheral
Vitamin B Deficiencies

Legs, muscle weakness in
*Following injury
Guillain-Barré Syndrome

* No chart in this book for this disorder.

Legs, nodules, painful and red
Erythema Nodosum

Legs, numbness in
Calcium Imbalance
Encephalitis, Viral or Aseptic
Kidney Failure, Chronic
*Neuritis
Subarachnoid Hemorrhage

Legs, one that appears shorter
Hip Dislocation, Congenital

Legs, pain in
*Following injury
Frostbite
Legg-Perthes Disease
Syphilis
Thrombophlebitis
Thrombosis, Deep-Vein

Legs, pain when raising
Thrombosis, Deep-Vein

Legs, rash on
*Adverse reactions to drugs or medications
Purpura, Allergic
Rocky Mountain Spotted Fever

Legs, swelling of
Congestive Heart Failure
Endocarditis
Fluid & Electrolyte Disorders
Lupus Erythematosus, Systemic
Rheumatic Fever
Vitamin C Deficiency

Legs, tingling in
Calcium Imbalance
Frostbite
Hyperaldosteronism
Kidney Failure, Chronic
*Neuritis
Vitamin B Deficiencies

Legs, twitching of (lasting 2-3 minutes)
Convulsions, Febrile

Leg ulcers
Sickle-Cell Anemia
Thalassemia

Lesions, itchy
Dermatitis Herpetiformis
Hives
Pityriasis Alba

Lesions, red or pink, with swelling
Hives

Lesions, red, raised, with clearly defined borders
Lupus Erythematosus, Discoid

Lesions, scar as they heal
Lupus Erythematosus, Discoid

Lesions, small white patches with vague borders
Pityriasis Alba

Lesions, with blisters
Dermatitis Herpetiformis
Herpes Virus Infections

Lesions, with round, flat-topped patches
Winter Itch

Lesions, with small raised bumps
Pityriasis Alba

Lethargy
*Adverse reactions to drugs or medications
Aspirin Poisoning
Calcium Imbalance
Leukemia, Acute
*Many infections, particularly those involving the central nervous system
*Many mental and emotional disorders
Meningitis, Aseptic
Meningitis, Bacterial
Reye's Syndrome

Lightheadedness
Fainting
Nosebleed

* No chart in this book for this disorder.

Limp
- Hip Dislocation, Congenital
- Legg-Perthes Disease
- Osteomyelitis

Lips, bluish
- *Congenital Heart Disease
- Croup
- Measles
- Pneumonia, Bacterial

Lips, cracked
- Vitamin B Deficiencies

Lips, ulcers on
- Canker Sores
- Herpes Virus Infections

Listlessness
- *Adverse reactions to drugs or medications
- Congestive Heart Failure
- Depression
- Kidney Failure, Chronic
- *Many mental and emotional disorders
- Vitamin Deficiency

Liver, enlarged
- Congestive Heart Failure
- Cor Pulmonale
- Cystic Fibrosis
- Hyperlipidemia, Types I, II, III, IV, V
- Idiopathic Hypertrophic Subaortic Stenosis
- Mononucleosis, Infectious

Liver, swollen
- Hepatitis, Acute Viral

Liver, tender
- Amebiasis
- Congestive Heart Failure
- Hepatitis, Acute Viral
- Idiopathic Hypertrophic Subaortic Stenosis

Lump, in groin, that returns to normal position when lying down
- Hernia

Lump, mild discomfort or pain at groin
- Hernia

Lumps, red, in skin (scattered)
- Insect Bites & Stings

Lung infections, repeated
- AIDS
- Bronchiectasis

Lymph glands under the jaw, swollen
- Tonsillitis

Lymph glands, swollen, generalized or in proximity to disorder
- AIDS
- Arthritis, Juvenile Rheumatoid
- Boils
- Cat-Scratch Fever (underarm glands)
- Cellulitis
- Herpetic Whitlow (underarm glands)
- Hodgkin's Disease
- Lupus Erythematosus, Systemic
- Lymphoma, Non-Hodgkin's
- Measles, German
- Mononucleosis, Infectious
- Serum Sickness

M

Malabsorption
- Vitamin E Deficiency

Mania
- *Adverse reactions to drugs or medications
- *Many mental and emotional disorders
- Porphyria

Marks, strawberry-colored on skin
- Skin Lesions, Benign

* No chart in this book for this disorder.

Memory loss
- *Adverse reactions to drugs or medications
- Alcoholism
- Brain Tumor
- Frostbite
- Hypoglycemia of Diabetes
- Lead Poisoning
- *Many mental and emotional disorders

Menstrual flow, heavy
- *Miscarriage
- Pelvic Inflammatory Disease

Menstrual period, absence of (3 months or more)
- Amenorrhea, Secondary
- *Pregnancy

Menstrual period, absent after puberty
- Amenorrhea, Primary
- *Pregnancy

Menstrual period, foul-smelling, frothy discharge
- Vaginitis, Trichomonal

Menstrual period, irregular
- Cushing's Syndrome
- Ovarian Cancer
- Ovarian Cyst

Menstrual period, missed
- Ectopic Pregnancy
- *Pregnancy

Menstrual periods, pain in pelvis
- Pelvic Inflammatory Disease

Menstrual periods, painful cramps during
- Dysmenorrhea

Menstrual periods, stoppage of
- Anorexia Nervosa
- *Athletic "over-training"
- Cushing's Syndrome
- Kidney Failure, Chronic
- Kidney, Polycystic

Mental abilities, impaired
- Asthma
- Blood Poisoning
- Lead Poisoning

Mental changes
- *Adverse reactions to drugs or medications
- Cushing's Syndrome
- Kidney Failure, Acute
- Lupus Erythematosus, Systemic
- *Many mental and emotional disorders
- Porphyria
- Subdural Hemorrhage & Hematoma
- Toxic Shock Syndrome
- Vitamin B Deficiencies
- Vitamin C Deficiency

Mental Deterioration
- Brain Tumor
- *Metastatic Cancer
- Syphilis

Mental development, delayed
- Failure to Thrive
- Lead Poisoning

Mental retardation
- Cerebral Palsy
- Down Syndrome
- Hypoparathyroidism

Moles, black, blue, brown, red or yellow
- Skin Lesions, Benign

Moles, changes in appearance of
- Malignant Melanoma

Mood changes
- Addison's Disease
- *Adverse reactions to drugs or medications
- Cushing's Syndrome
- *Many mental and emotional disorders
- Premenstrual Syndrome

Mood, pleasant (temporary)
- Drug Abuse & Addiction

* No chart in this book for this disorder.

Mouth, abnormal bleeding in
*Adverse reactions to drugs or medications
Thrombocytopenia

Mouth, acid taste in
Gastritis

Mouth, blisters in
Hand, Foot & Mouth Disease

Mouth, blisters around that are painful
Cold Sores

Mouth, burning
Vitamin B Deficiencies

Mouth, clicking or popping sounds when opening
Temporo-Mandibular Joint Syndrome

Mouth, dry
Anxiety
Botulism
Dehydration
Fluid & Electrolyte Disorders
Radiation Sickness
Thrush

Mouth, foul taste in
Tooth Abscess
Tooth Decay

Mouth, inability to close
Jaw Dislocation

Mouth, irregular whitish line inside
Lichen Planus

Mouth, itching in the roof of
Hay Fever

Mouth, numbness or tingling around
*Adverse reactions to drugs or medications
Anaphylaxis
Hyperventilation Syndrome
Hypoglycemia of Diabetes
Snakebite

Mouth, pain in after eating
Esophageal Stricture or Corrosive Esophagitis

* No chart in this book for this disorder.

Mouth patches that are white to creamy yellow, slightly round
Thrush

Mouth patches that when rubbed off, leave painful ulcers
Thrush

Mouth, rash with small, red scaly bumps on
Syphilis

Mouth, small
Down Syndrome

Mouth, sore
Vitamin B Deficiencies

Mouth sores
*Adverse reactions to drugs or medications
Canker Sores (Aphthous Ulcers)
Herpes Virus Infections
Leukemia, Acute
Syphilis
Thrush

Mouth, swelling or itching in back of
Anaphylaxis

Mouth, tiny white spots in
Measles

Mouth, ulcers in
Agranulocytosis
Anemia, Aplastic
Canker Sores
Celiac Disease
Hand, Foot & Mouth Disease
Leukemia, Acute
Lupus Erythematosus, Systemic
Reiter's Syndrome
Thrush

Mouth ulcers, small, painful, shallow
Canker Sores

Movements, uncontrollable, purposeless and non-repetitive
St. Vitus' Dance

Movements, wandering or jerky
St. Vitus' Dance

Muscle aches
- *Adverse reactions to drugs or medications
- Amebiasis
- Dysentery, Bacillary
- Hepatitis, Acute Viral
- Influenza
- Lyme Disease
- Measles, German
- Pneumonia, Viral
- Rocky Mountain Spotted Fever
- Scleroderma
- Typhoid Fever
- Valley Fever

Muscle, tight contraction of
- Muscle, Pulled or Torn

Muscles, contraction of, on the face
- Tooth-Grinding

Muscle cramps
- *Adverse reactions to drugs or medications
- Kidney Failure, Chronic
- Muscle Cramps
- Porphyria
- Sodium Imbalance
- Vitamin E Deficiency

Muscle deterioration (requiring confinement to a wheelchair by age 9-12)
- Muscular Dystrophy

Muscle pain
- Brucellosis
- Dysentery, Bacillary
- *Following injury
- Kidney Failure, Chronic
- Lyme Disease
- Muscle, Pulled or Torn
- Tetanus
- Trichinosis

Muscles, rigid
- Hypothermia

Muscle spasms
- *Adverse reactions to drugs or medications
- Calcium Imbalance
- Cerebral Palsy
- Electric Shock
- *Following injury
- Hyperaldosteronism
- Hyperventilation Syndrome
- Hypoparathyroidism
- Tetanus

Muscle spasms in neck
- *Following injury
- Torticollis

Muscle stiffness
- *Following injury
- Measles, German
- Muscle, Pulled or Torn

Muscles, swelling, redness or bruising at injured area
- Muscle, Pulled or Torn

Muscle, tenderness
- Muscle, Pulled or Torn

Muscle tension
- Anxiety
- Hypoparathyroidism

Muscle tone, lack of
- Cerebral Palsy
- Down Syndrome
- Tay-Sach's Disease

Muscle twitching
- *Adverse reactions to drugs or medications
- Calcium Imbalance
- Hypoglycemia of Diabetes
- *Peripheral Neuritis

Muscles, wasting of
- Spinal-Cord Tumor

Muscles, weaker than normal
- Muscular Dystrophy
- Spinal-Cord Tumor

* No chart in this book for this disorder.

Muscle weakness
Guillain-Barré Syndrome
Muscle Weakness
Polymyositis & Dermatomyositis
Vitamin D Deficiency
Vitamin E Deficiency

N

Nails, blisters that are barely visible around
Herpetic Whitlow

Nails, bluish
Bronchiolitis
Pneumonia, Bacterial
Pneumonia, Viral

Nails, chronic infections of
Raynaud's Disease
Raynaud's Phenomenon

Nails, deformed
Zinc Deficiency

Nails, painless splitting of
Nail Splitting

Nails, purple
Epiglottitis, Acute
Hypothermia
Pneumonia

Nails, redness and swelling
Paronychia

Nails, redness, swelling, and warmth around
Herpetic Whitlow
Paronychia

Nails, separation between the end of nail and nail bed
Nails, Ringworm Infection of

Nails, soft yellow material build-up
Nails, Ringworm Infection of

Nails, splitting
Hypoparathyroidism
Nail Splitting

Nails, sudden pain around
Herpetic Whitlow

Nails (fingers and toes), yellow and misshapen
Nails, Ringworm Infection of

Nasal congestion
Cold, Common
Hay Fever
Nasal Polyps
Sinus Infection

Nausea
Addison's Disease
*Adverse reactions to drugs or medications
Anemia, Folic-Acid Deficiency
Anxiety
Appendicitis
Bladder or Urethra Injury
Brain or Epidural Abscess
Brain Tumor
Cholecystitis or Cholangitis, Acute
Colitis, Ulcerative
Dysentery, Bacillary
Dysmenorrhea
Extradural Hemorrhage
Fainting
Gallstones
Gastritis
Glomerulonephritis
Head Injury
Headache, Migraine
Hepatitis, Acute Viral
Indigestion
Intestinal Obstruction
Kidney Failure, Acute
Kidney, Polycystic
Lactose Intolerance
Lyme Disease
Malaria
*Many mental and emotional disorders
Motion Sickness
Pituitary Tumor
Pseudomembranous Enterocolitis
Pulmonary-Valve Stenosis
Radiation Sickness
Rocky Mountain Spotted Fever
Shingles
Sunburn

* No chart in this book for this disorder.

Nausea, continued
Testicle Torsion
Trichinosis
Vitamin B Deficiencies
Whiplash

Neck glands, swollen
Diphtheria
Lymphoma, Non-Hodgkin's
Measles, German
Mononucleosis, Infectious
Pharyngitis
Pneumonia, Viral
Scarlet Fever
Strep Throat
Syphilis
Tooth Abscess

Neck glands, tenderness in
Tooth Abscess

Neck joints, pain, swelling, and stiffness in
Arthritis, Juvenile Rheumatoid

Neck muscle spasm
Torticollis

Neck muscles, tight
Headache, Tension or Vascular
Measles, German

Neck, pain on movement
Encephalitis, Viral or Aseptic
Lyme Disease
Measles, German
Meningitis, Aseptic
Meningitis, Bacterial
Subarachnoid Hemorrhage
Valley Fever
Whiplash

Neck, stiff
Encephalitis, Viral or Aseptic
Lyme Disease
Measles, German
Meningitis, Aseptic
Meningitis, Bacterial
Subarachnoid Hemorrhage
Valley Fever
Whiplash

Neck veins, distended
Congestive Heart Failure
Cor Pulmonale
Idiopathic Hypertrophic Subaortic Stenosis
Myocarditis

Nerve damage
Drug Hypersensitivity

Nervousness
*Adverse reactions to drugs or medications
Hypoglycemia, Functional
Hypoglycemia of Diabetes
*Many mental and emotional disorders
Premenstrual Syndrome

Nightmares
*Adverse reactions to drugs or medications
Alcoholism
Anxiety
*Many mental and emotional disorders

Nodules, change color from pink to red to blue to brown
Erythema Nodosum

Nodules, dome-shaped, non-tender, that feel "doughy"
Lipomas

Nodules, firm, tender, domed (located in underarm area)
Hidradenitis Suppurativa

Nodules, large and warm (on legs)
Erythema Nodosum

Nodules, large, that when pressed feel like an overfilled inner tube (located in underarm area)
Hidradenitis Suppurativa

Nodules, painful, tender, red
Boils
Erythema Nodosum

* No chart in this book for this disorder.

Nodules, pus on the surface
Boils

Nodules that soften in center and become painful
Boils
Hidradenitis Suppurativa

Noises, hearing strange
*Adverse reactions to drugs or medications
Epilepsy
*Many mental and emotional disorders

Nose, bleeding from
Nose Injury
Nosebleed
Vitamin K Deficiency

Nose, crooked
Nose Fracture
Nose Injury

Nose, inability to breathe through
Cold, Common
Nasal Polyps
Nose Fracture
Nose Injury

Nose, loss of sensation in
Facial Bones, Fractures of

Nose, gradual numbness, hardness, and paleness in
Frostbite

Nose, obstruction of air through
Nasal Polyps

Nose, pain and tingling or burning
Frostbite

Nose, runny
APC Disease
Cold, Common
Headache, Migraine
Influenza
Measles
Nasal Polyps
Pituitary Tumor
Whooping Cough

Nose, skin lesions on bridge of, red and raised
Lupus Erythematosus, Discoid

Nose, stuffy
Cold, Common
Hay Fever
Nasal Polyps

Nose, swollen, discolored, following injury
Nose Fracture

Nosebleed
Nose Fracture
Nose Injury
Nosebleed

Nosebleeds, spontaneous
*Adverse reactions to drugs or medications
Hemophilia
Leukemia, Acute
Thrombocytopenia

Numbness on one side of body
Subdural Hemorrhage & Hematoma

O

Obesity, fear of
Anorexia Nervosa
Bulimia

Odors, sensations of unpleasant
Epilepsy
Zinc Deficiency

Overeating
*Adverse reactions to drugs or medications
Bulimia
Depression
*Many mental and emotional disorders

P

Pain, see various organs and regions of the body

* No chart in this book for this disorder.

Pain, close to navel, then moving to right lower abdomen
Appendicitis

Pain, spreading
Ankylosing Spondylitis

Pain, when passing a hard or bulky stool
Anal Fissure
Constipation

Palate, ulcers on
Canker Sores

Paleness
Anemia, Aplastic
Anemia, Folic-Acid Deficiency
Anemia, Iron-Deficiency
Celiac Disease
Diphtheria
Drowning, Near
Ectopic Pregnancy
Fainting
Headache, Migraine
Histoplasmosis
Intussusception
Kidney Failure, Chronic
Leukemia, Acute
Nosebleed
Pinworms
Rheumatic Fever
Small-Intestine Tumor
Thalassemia
Thrombocytopenia
Vitamin B Deficiencies

Palms, red
Alcoholism
*Liver Disease
Lupus Erythematosus, Systemic

Paralysis
*Adverse reactions to drugs or medications
Botulism
Brain or Epidural Abscess
Brain Tumor
Decompression Disease
*Following injury
Guillain-Barré Syndrome
Hemiplegia
*Many mental and emotional disorders
Potassium Imbalance
Reye's Syndrome
Spinal-Cord Tumor

Parotid glands, inflammation, swelling, and pain
Mumps

Parotid glands, pain increases with chewing or swallowing
Mumps

Patches on skin, flat and white on both sides of body
Vitiligo

Patches on skin, with blisters that are small and white
Folliculitis, Fungal

Patches on skin, round, flat-topped
Winter Itch

Patches on skin, small, white with vague borders
Pityriasis Alba

Patches on skin, with clearly defined borders, blistered, with pus
Folliculitis, Fungal

Patches on skin, with small raised bumps
Pityriasis Alba

Pelvic bones, shortening of
Vitamin D Deficiency

Pelvic girdle, muscle weakness in
*Following injury
Polymyositis & Dermatomyositis

Pelvis, aching in
*Following injury
Pelvic Inflammatory Disease
Reiter's Syndrome

Pelvis, pain on one or both sides
*Following injury
Pelvic Inflammatory Disease

* No chart in this book for this disorder.

Penis, discharge from
Balanitis
Gonorrhea
*Non-Specific Urethritis

Penis, inability to retract the foreskin
Circumcision

Penis, inflammation of the foreskin
Balanitis
Circumcision

Penis, itching and irritation of
Herpes, Genital

Penis, pain, redness, and swelling of the head
Balanitis

Penis, painful blisters
Herpes, Genital

Penis, painless red sore on
Syphilis

Penis, rash with small, red, scaly bumps on
Syphilis

Penis, red, raw, occasionally bloody area around the opening at tip of
Diaper Rash (in infant males)

Penis, ulceration of
Balanitis

Penis, ulcers on the tip
Reiter's Syndrome

Penis, warts on
Warts, Venereal

Perineum, swelling, pain, tenderness of,
Perineal Contusion

Personality changes
*Adverse reactions to drugs or medications
Brain Tumor
Encephalitis, Viral or Aseptic
Hypoglycemia, Functional
*Many mental and emotional disorders
Reye's Syndrome

Perspiration, see Sweating

Photosensitivity (skin reaction to sunlight)
*Adverse reactions to drugs or medications
Drug Hypersensitivity

Physical development (height, weight) not normal
Failure to Thrive

Physical skills, slow to develop
Failure to Thrive

"Pigeon Breast"
Vitamin D Deficiency

Plaques on skin, large, flat, raised, skin-colored lesions
Hives

Plaques on skin, surrounded by small white blisters with pus inside
Candidiasis of Intertriginous Skin

Post-nasal drip
Hay Fever
Sinus Infection

"Pot Belly"
Vitamin D Deficiency

Psychosis
*Adverse reactions to drugs or medications
Cushing's Syndrome
Hypoparathyroidism
Lupus Erythematosus, Systemic
*Many mental and emotional disorders
Vitamin B Deficiencies

Pulse, loss of (below a fracture)
Bone Fracture

* No chart in this book for this disorder.

Pulse, rapid and/or weak
- *Adverse reactions to drugs or medications
- *Any heart disease
- Bladder or Urethra Injury
- Congestive Heart Failure
- *Following injury
- *Many mental and emotional disorders
- Shock (from any cause, such as bleeding)
- Toxic Shock Syndrome

Pupils, dilated
- Glaucoma, Acute Infantile

Pupils, opaque, milky, white
- Cataract

Pupils that may be different sizes
- Encephalitis, Viral or Aseptic
- Extradural Hemorrhage
- Head Injury
- Meningitis, Bacterial
- Subdural Hemorrhage & Hematoma

Pupils, whitish ring around
- Hyperlipidemia, Types I, II, III, IV, V

Pus, discharge of
- Folliculitis, Bacterial
- Pilonidal Cyst

Pus drainage, through a skin abscess
- Osteomyelitis

Pus that can be squeezed out from a fingernail
- Paronychia

Pus-filled lesions, large
- Boils

Pus-filled lesions, small
- Acne

R

Rash
- *Adverse reactions to drugs or medications
- *Almost any skin disorders
- Celiac Disease
- Drug Hypersensitivity
- Lupus Erythematosus, Systemic
- Measles
- Measles, German
- Prickly Heat
- Scarlet Fever
- Thrombocytopenia
- Toxic Shock Syndrome

Rash, faint, found in skin creases
- Pityriasis Rosea

Rash with blisters on hands, feet, and groin
- Hand, Foot & Mouth Disease

Rash with small blisters that may itch
- Impetigo

Rectal bleeding
- Anal Fissure
- *Injury to rectum
- Intestinal Obstruction
- Intussusception
- Vagina or Vulva, Cancer of

Rectal discomfort and discharge
- Constipation
- Gonorrhea
- *Proctitis

Rectal tears
- Anal Fissure
- Rape Crisis Syndrome

Rectum, cramps and pain around
- Colitis, Ulcerative
- Constipation

Rectum, involuntary contraction of muscles around
- Vaginismus

Rectum, itching around
- Anal Fissure
- Pinworms
- Pruritis Ani

Rectum, painless red sore on
- Syphilis

* No chart in this book for this disorder.

Rectum, sense of fullness in, but inability to pass stool
Fecal Impaction

Rectum, thin watery discharge from
Fecal Impaction

Rectum, ulcers in
Anemia, Aplastic

Rectum, warts on the entrance to
Warts, Venereal

Regurgitation (slight) of stomach contents into mouth
Heartburn
Hiatal Hernia

Respiratory infections, recurrent
AIDS
Bronchiectasis
Cystic Fibrosis
Failure to Thrive
Immunodeficiency Disease
Lung Abscess
Muscular Dystrophy

Restlessness
*Adverse reactions to drugs or medications
Asthma
Insomnia
*Many mental and emotional disorders
Pinworms
Rabies
Roundworms
Sodium Imbalance
Vitamin D Deficiency

Ribs, tender
*Following injury
Vitamin C Deficiency

S

Saliva, increased
Esophageal Stricture or Corrosive Esophagitis
Rabies
Teething

Salivation, changes in
Bell's Palsy

Scales on skin, white flaking over reddish patches
Dermatitis, Seborrheic

Scalp, enlarged lymph glands at back of
Lice
Measles, German

Scalp, inflamed
Lice
Psoriasis
Seborrheic Dermatitis

Scalp lesions causing hair loss and scaling
Ringworm

Scalp lesions with localized patches of hair loss
Lupus Erythematosus, Discoid

Scalp muscles, tight
Headache, Tension or Vascular

Scars, darkening of
Addison's Disease

Scars with thick, pale, irregular growths
Skin Lesions, Benign

Sciatic nerve (located in back of leg), pain along
*Adverse reactions to drugs or medications
Ankylosing Spondylitis

Scratching
Lice

Scratching, uncontrolled
Dermatitis, Atopic

Scrotal contents, tender and swollen
Epididymitis
*Following injury
Hernia
Testicle Torsion

* No chart in this book for this disorder.

Scrotum, appears underdeveloped on one or both sides
Testes, Undescended

Scrotum, itching around base of
Pruritis Ani

Seizures
*Adverse reactions to drugs or medications
Aspirin Poisoning
Brain Tumor
Calcium Imbalance
Encephalitis, Viral or Aseptic
*Following injury
Hypoglycemia, Functional
Hypoparathyroidism
Lead Poisoning
*Many mental and emotional disorders
Pituitary Tumor
Reye's Syndrome
Snakebite
Tay-Sachs Disease

Self-confidence, false feelings of
Drug Abuse & Addiction

Sensations, loss of normal
Decompression Disease
Hemiplegia

Sex drive, decreased
*Adverse reactions to drugs or medications
Alcoholism
Anorexia Nervosa
Kidney Failure, Chronic
*Many mental and emotional disorders
Premenstrual Syndrome

Sex drive, increased
Premenstrual Syndrome

Sexual function, impaired
*Adverse reactions to drugs or medications
*Following injury
*Many mental and emotional disorders
Paraplegia or Quadriplegia

Sexual impotence
*Adverse reactions to drugs or medications
Alcoholism
*Following injury
*Many mental and emotional disorders
Syphilis

Sexual intercourse, bleeding with
*First intercourse
Vagina or Vulva, Cancer of
*Vaginal injury

Sexual intercourse, pain or tenderness with
Gonorrhea
Ovarian Cancer
Vaginitis

Shin splints
Shin Splints

Shoulders that become uneven
Scoliosis

Shoulder, colicky pain between shoulder blades
Ectopic Pregnancy
Gallstones

Shoulder, deformed
Shoulder Dislocation

Shoulder girdle, muscle weakness in
Polymyositis & Dermatomyositis

Shoulder, inability to move
Shoulder Bursitis, Subachromial
Shoulder, Frozen

Shoulder pain
Arthritis, Juvenile Rheumatoid
Decompression Disease
Ectopic Pregnancy
*Following injury
Peritonitis
Shoulder Bursitis, Subachromial
Shoulder Dislocation
Shoulder, Frozen
Tendinitis

* No chart in this book for this disorder.

Shoulders, pain and stiffness in
Arthritis, Juvenile Rheumatoid
Shoulder Bursitis, Subachromial
Shoulder, Frozen

Shoulders, swelling in
Arthritis, Juvenile Rheumatoid

Sights and sounds, increased sensitivity to
Drug Abuse & Addiction

Sinus, pain and complete blockage of
Sinus Infection

Skin, black with dead underlying muscle and bone
Gangrene

Skin, bleeding spots under
Kidney Failure, Acute
Purpura, Allergic
Radiation Sickness
Snakebite
Thrombocytopenia

Skin, blistered
Burns
Frostbite
Porphyria
Sun Poisoning
Sunburn
Vitamin B Deficiencies

Skin, brownish, with white patches
Addison's Disease

Skin, bruising under
Vitamin C Deficiency

Skin, burning inflammation
Radiation Sickness

Skin, clammy
Hypoglycemia of Diabetes

Skin, cold
Atelectasis
Bladder or Urethra Injury
Diphtheria
Hypoglycemia of Diabetes
Shock

Skin, crackling feeling upon touching
Gangrene

Skin, cracks and fissures in
Dermatitis, Contact
Diaper Rash
Winter Itch

Skin darkening, all over body
Addison's Disease
*Tanning from exposure to sun
Zinc Deficiency

Skin darkening, permanent
Radiation Sickness

Skin eruptions, appearing first as blisters, then forming scabs
Chickenpox

Skin eruptions, redness and inflammation around
Acne ("zits" or pimples)

Skin, flat-topped patches that itch, burn, and sting
Winter Itch

Skin, flushed
Drug Hypersensitivity

Skin, hardening and thickening of
Scleroderma

Skin, itchy
*Adverse reactions to drugs or medications
Candidiasis of Intertriginous Skin
Cholecystitis or Cholangitis, Acute
Dermatitis, Seborrheic
Drug Hypersensitivity
Eczema
Kidney Failure, Chronic
Kidney, Polycystic
*Liver disorders
*Many mental and emotional disorders
Polymyositis & Dermatomyositis
Porphyria
Psoriasis
Purpura, Allergic
Trichinosis

* No chart in this book for this disorder.

Skin lesions, raised, black, brown, with irregular borders
Skin Cancer
Malignant Melanoma

Skin lesions, red, circular, flat, and scaling
Ringworm

Skin, loss of pigmentation in patches
Vitiligo

Skin, moist, painful, red, spotty, and itchy in diaper area
Diaper Rash

Skin, pale and moist all over
Atelectsis
Bladder or Urethra Injury
Shock

Skin patches, moist and crusted
Candidiasis of Intertriginous Skin

Skin patches, see also Plaques

Skin, peeling
Scarlet Fever
Sunburn

Skin rash, progressing to thin raised lines
Larva Migrans, Cutaneous

Skin rash, red or purple
Meningitis, Bacterial

Skin, red dots of bleeding under
Anemia, Aplastic

Skin, red lumps in (painful)
Erythema Nodosum
Insect Bites & Stings

Skin, red patches with poorly defined borders (in groin and under breasts)
Candidiasis of Intertriginous Skin

Skin, red, swollen, painful
Sunburn

Skin, red, weeping areas
Dermatitis, Contact

Skin, redness (slight)
Dermatitis, Contact
Sunburn (mild)

Skin, redness, most pronounced in small cracks and fissures
Winter Itch

Skin, redness, tenderness, pain, swelling
Burns
Sun Poisoning

Skin, redness, tenderness, swelling
Cellulitis

Skin, rough
Corn or Callus
Dermatitis, Atopic
Eczema
Psoriasis
Vitamin C Deficiency

Skin, scaling
Hypoparathyroidism
Psoriasis

Skin, scarring of
*Following injury (after healing)
Radiation Sickness

Skin, severely chapped, that becomes cracked and inflamed
Winter Itch

Skin, soft, flesh-colored buds, often on stalks
Skin Lesions, Benign

Skin, areas that are red, shiny, and frequently ulcerate
Sores, Pressure

Skin, peeling or tanning after sun or ultra-violet light exposure
Sunburn

Skin, thickened
Corn or Callus
Dermatitis, Atopic
Eczema

* No chart in this book for this disorder.

Skin ulcers
Gangrene
Sickle-Cell Anemia
Sores, Pressure

Skin, warm and flushed
Blood Poisoning
*Fever from any cause

Skin, white scales over reddish patches
Dermatitis, Seborrheic

Skin, wrinkled
Dehydration
Fluid & Electrolyte Disorders

Skin, yellowish nodules of fat beneath eyes, elbows, knees, and in tendons
Hyperlipidemia, Types I, II, III, IV, V

Sleep attacks
Narcolepsy

Sleep, breathing that stops during
Sleep Apnea in Infants

Sleep, brief, followed by wakefulness
*Adverse reactions to drugs or medications
Insomnia
*Many mental and emotional disorders

Sleep, deep (following a seizure)
Epilepsy

Sleep habits, poor
*Adverse reactions to drugs or medications
*Many mental and emotional disorders
Vitamin D Deficiency

Sleep, restless
*Adverse reactions to drugs or medications
*Many mental and emotional disorders
Pinworms
Sinus Infection

Sleepiness at inconvenient times
Insomnia
Narcolepsy

Sleeping, excessive
*Adverse reactions to drugs or medications
Depression
*Many mental and emotional disorders

Sleeplessness
Anxiety
Insomnia

Sleeplike states
Drug Abuse & Addiction

Slurred speech
Alcoholism
Bell's Palsy
Botulism
Brain Tumor

Smell, decreased sense of
Zinc Deficiency

Smell, impaired sense of
Brain Tumor
Nasal Polyps

Smile, distorted
Bell's Palsy

Sneezing
Anaphylaxis
Cold, Common
Hay Fever
Measles

Social isolation
Depression
Hypochondriasis
*Many mental and emotional disorders

Social skills, delayed in infant or child
Failure to Thrive

Sodium, high blood levels of
Hyperaldosteronism

Sore throat, see Throat, sore

* No chart in this book for this disorder.

Sounds, difficulty in listening selectively to
Hearing Impairment or Loss

Sounds, lack of response to
Hearing Impairment or Loss

Sounds, vivid (at beginning of a sleep attack)
Narcolepsy

Spasmodic contractions of the diaphragm
Hiccup

Speaking difficulty
Brain or Epidural Abscess
Brain Tumor
Encephalitis, Viral or Aseptic
Failure to Thrive
Frostbite
Hemiplegia
Polymyositis & Dermatomyositis
Reye's Syndrome
Stuttering (see Appendix)
Trench Mouth

Spine that becomes S-shaped
Scoliosis

Spine with pain, redness, tenderness, and swelling at base, close to rectum
Pilonidal Cyst

Spinning sensation
*Labyrinthitis
Motion Sickness

Spleen, enlarged
AIDS
Cystic Fibrosis
Hyperlipidemia, Types I, II, III, IV, V
Leukemia, Acute
Lyme Disease
Mononucleosis, Infectious
Thalassemia

Sputum, bad-smelling, green or yellow
Bronchiectasis
Lung Abscess

Sputum containing blood or blood streaks
Pneumonia, Bacterial or Viral
Pulmonary-Valve Stenosis
Tuberculosis

Sputum, hard to cough up
Bronchitis, Chronic
Cystic Fibrosis

Sputum, yellow, thick or gray
Tuberculosis

Staring blankly (unaware of what is happening)
Epilepsy

Staring expression
Hypoglycemia of Diabetes

Stiffness in muscles
Ankylosing Spondylitis
Cerebral Palsy
*Following injury
Measles, German
Muscle, Pulled or Torn

Stools, bad-smelling
Amebiasis
Celiac Disease
Cystic Fibrosis
*Dietary indiscretion
Giardiasis
Malabsorption

Stools, black, tarry or bright red (indicating bleeding somewhere in the gastrointestinal tract)
DIC
*Diverticulitis
Dysentery, Bacillary
Gastric Erosion
Hemorrhoids
Salmonella Infections
Small-Intestine Tumor
Thrombocytopenia
Typhoid Fever
Ulcer, Peptic

* No chart in this book for this disorder.

Stools, bulky
Celiac Disease
Giardiasis

Stools, copious
Malabsorption

Stools, frequent or loose
Celiac Disease
Diarrhea, Acute
Diarrhea, Chronic, Non-Specific, of Childhood
Giardiasis
Typhoid Fever

Stools, hard
Constipation

Stools, large, fatty, and smelling bad
Cystic Fibrosis

Stools, light, "clay-colored" or whitish
Hepatitis, Acute Viral

Stools, mucus and blood in
Amebiasis
Colitis, Ulcerative
Dysentery, Bacillary

Stools, pale or "clay-colored"
Celiac Disease
Cholecystitis or Cholangitis, Acute
Hepatitis

Stools, pus in
Colitis, Ulcerative
Dysentery, Bacillary

Stools, thick and sticky
Cystic Fibrosis

Stools, worms or worm eggs in (sometimes only visible through a microscope)
Pinworms
Tapeworm

Stupor
*Adverse reactions to drugs or medications
Alcoholism
Drug Abuse & Addiction
Kidney Failure, Acute
*Many mental and emotional disorders
Sodium Imbalance

Sucking, weak
Premature Infants

Sun, increased sensitivity to
*Adverse reactions to drugs or medications
Lupus Erythematosus, Systemic

Surroundings, unaware of
Epilepsy
Hypoglycemia of Diabetes

Swallowing difficulty
Anxiety
Botulism
Hiatal Hernia
Laryngitis
Pharyngitis
Polymyositis & Dermatomyositis
Radiation Sickness
Scleroderma
Tetanus
Thyroid Tumor
Trench Mouth
Tonsillitis

Swallowing, impossible
Rabies

Swallowing, painful
*Any throat infection
Herpangina
Mononucleosis, Infectious
Strep Throat

Swallowing reflexes, weak
Premature Infants

Swallowing, sudden or gradual decrease in ability
Esophageal Stricture or Corrosive Esophagitis

* No chart in this book for this disorder.

Sweat, salty
Cystic Fibrosis

Sweating
Alcoholism
Anxiety
Bladder or Urethra Injury
Brucellosis
Cellulitis
Colitis, Ulcerative
Diphtheria
Dysmenorrhea
Endocarditis
Fainting
Guillain-Barré Syndrome
Hyperhidrosis
Hypoglycemia, Functional
Hypoglycemia of Diabetes
Lung Abscess
Malaria
Meningitis, Bacterial
Snakebite
Sodium Imbalance
Testicle Torsion
Trichinosis
Tuberculosis
Valley Fever
*Vigorous exercise
Vitamin D Deficiency

T

Taste, changes in
Bell's Palsy

Taste, decreased sense of
Zinc Deficiency

Taste, loss of
Radiation Sickness

Taste, sensation of unpleasant
Zinc Deficiency

Tear duct, drainage of mucus and pus, instead of tears
Tear Duct, Infection or Blockage of

Tear duct, redness and swelling of
Tear Duct, Infection or Blockage of

Tear formation, changes in
Bell's Palsy

Tears
Conjunctivitis
Corneal Ulcer
Keratitis
Rabies
Sty
Tear Duct, Infection or Blockage of

Teeth, damaged
Tooth-Grinding

Teeth, loss of
Vitamin C Deficiency

Teeth, protruding front
Thumb-Sucking

Teeth, sensitive to heat or cold
Tooth Decay

Temples, constant pain over
Headache, Tension or Vascular

Temples, dull, boring pain in
Headache, Migraine

Tendons, movement restricted, tenderness and swelling
Tendinitis

Tendon, weakness in
Tendinitis

Tendons, yellowish nodules of fat beneath
Hyperlipidemia, Types I, II, III, IV, V

Tense feeling
Epilepsy

Testicle that can't be felt in scrotum
Testes, Undescended

Testicle, enlarged, hardened, with tenderness
Epididymitis

Testicle, firm swelling in one
Testicle, Cancer of

* No chart in this book for this disorder.

Testicle, painful, swollen
Mumps

Testicle, sudden pain in one
Testicle Torsion

Thigh bone that rides up behind the hip socket
Hip Dislocation, Congenital

Thighs, pain in
Arthritis, Infectious
*Following injury
Legg-Perthes Disease

Thighs, swelling and pain in
Thrombosis, Deep-Vein

Thighs, small raised bumps on skin of
Lyme Disease

Thighs, stiffness in
Legg-Perthes Disease

Thirst, excessive
Calcium Imbalance
Diabetes Insipidus
Electrolyte Imbalance
Hyperaldosteronism
Pituitary Tumor
Toxic Shock Syndrome

Throat that feels like a "lump" in it
Pharyngitis

Throat muscles, spasms of
Hypoparathyroidism

Throat pain
Croup
Herpangina
Strep Throat
Tonsillitis

Throat, red
Croup
Herpangina
Pharyngitis
Scarlet Fever
Strep Throat
Tonsillitis

Throat, red or covered with a grayish membrane
Diphtheria
Pharyngitis

Throat, sore
*Adverse reactions to drugs or medications
Agranulocytosis
APC Disease
Cold, Common
Croup
Diphtheria
Epiglottitis, Acute
Gonorrhea
Hand, Foot & Mouth Disease
Herpangina
Influenza
Laryngitis
Lyme Disease
Meningitis, Bacterial
Mononucleosis, Infectious
Mumps
Pharyngitis
Pneumonia, Viral
Purpura, Allergic
Rabies
Scarlet Fever
Strep Throat
Tonsillitis
Toxic Shock Syndrome
Valley Fever

Throat, swelling or itching in
Anaphylaxis
Hay Fever

Throat, tiny white spots in
Measles

Throat, ulcers in
Agranulocytosis
Anemia, Aplastic
Canker Sores
Herpangina

* No chart in this book for this disorder.

Tiredness
- Addison's Disease
- AIDS
- Amebiasis
- Anemia
- Anemia, Folic-Acid Deficiency
- Anemia, Iron-Deficiency
- Ankylosing Spondylitis
- Anxiety
- Bronchiectasis
- Brucellosis
- Cat-Scratch Fever
- Celiac Disease
- Cold, Common
- Congestive Heart Failure
- Cor Pulmonale
- Depression
- Diabetes Mellitus, Insulin-Dependent
- Empyema
- Endocarditis
- Fluid & Electrolyte Disorders
- *Heart Disease
- Heart-Valve Disease
- Hepatitis, Acute Viral
- Hyperaldosteronism
- Influenza
- Kidney Failure, Chronic
- Kidney Infection, Acute
- Kidney, Polycystic
- Leukemia, Acute
- Lyme Disease
- Malaria
- *Many mental and emotional disorders
- Measles
- Measles, German
- Myocarditis
- Pityriasis Rosea
- Pneumonia, Bacterial
- Pneumonia, Viral
- Pulmonary-Valve Stenosis
- Rabies
- Radiation Sickness
- Rheumatic Fever
- Roundworms
- Scleroderma
- Sickle-Cell Anemia
- Small-Intestine Tumor
- Sun Poisoning
- Tapeworm
- Thalassemia
- Thrombocytopenia
- Toxic Shock Syndrome
- Tuberculosis
- Vitamin B Deficiencies
- Vitamin C Deficiency

Tissues, wasting away
- Polyarteritis

Toenail, inflamed, then infected and painful
- Toenail, Ingrown

Toes, dead skin between
- Athlete's Foot

Toes, gradual numbness, hardness, and paleness in
- Frostbite

Toes, moist, soft, gray-white or red scales between
- Athlete's Foot

Toes, pain
- Arthritis, Infectious
- Arthritis, Juvenile Rheumatoid
- Frostbite
- *Gout
- Toenail, Ingrown

Toes, painful raised bump on the side or over the joint
- Corn or Callus

Toes, purple
- Frostbite
- Hypothermia

Toes, sharp toenail that pierces the surrounding fold of tissue
- Toenail, Ingrown

Toes, stiffness in
- Arthritis, Juvenile Rheumatoid

Toes, swelling
- Arthritis, Juvenile Rheumatoid
- Toenail, Ingrown

* No chart in this book for this disorder.

Toes, tenderness, redness, and heat
Toenail, Ingrown

Toes, tingling or burning in
Frostbite
*Peripheral Neuritis

Tongue, burning
Vitamin B Deficiencies

Tongue, hairy-looking
Tongue Inflammation

Tongue, inflammation of
Anemia, Iron-Deficiency
Tongue Inflammation

Tongue, protruding
Down Syndrome

Tongue, red
Anemia, Folic-Acid Deficiency
Scarlet Fever
Tongue Inflammation

Tongue, sore
Anemia, Folic-Acid Deficiency
Vitamin B Deficiencies

Tongue, swollen and bright red
Tongue Inflammation (Glossitis)

Tongue, ulcers on
Canker Sores
Reiter's Syndrome
Tongue Inflammation

Tonsils, bright red, sometimes with specks of pus
Strep Throat
Tonsillitis

Tonsils, enlarged
APC Disease
Mononucleosis, Infectious
Strep Throat
Tonsillitis

Tooth development, poor
*Adverse reactions to drugs or medications
Hypoparathyroidism
*Vitamin deficiency

Tooth pain
Tooth Abscess
Tooth Decay

Trembling
*Adverse reactions to drugs or medications
Anxiety
*Many mental and emotional disorders

Tremors
Alcoholism
*Any disorder involving the central nervous system
Brain Tumor

Trunk with fat accumulation and red "stretch marks"
Cushing's Syndrome

Tumors, benign, small
Warts, Flat

Tumor, in the eye
Eye Tumor

Tumor, large, firm, smooth, that can be felt in either flank of the abdominal wall
Wilm's Tumor

U

Ulcers in dead tissue, bad-smelling discharge from
Gangrene

Ulcers in mouth
Agranulocytosis
Anemia
Canker Sores
Celiac Disease
Herpes
Reiter's Syndrome

Ulcers in rectum
Anemia, Aplastic

Ulcers in throat
Agranulocytosis
Anemia, Aplastic
Canker Sores

* No chart in this book for this disorder.

Ulcers on cheek
Canker Sores

Ulcers on gums
Canker Sores

Ulcers on legs
Sickle-Cell Anemia
Pressure Sores
Thalassemia

Ulcers on lips
Canker Sores

Ulcers on palate
Canker Sores

Ulcers on tip of penis
Reiter's Syndrome

Ulcers on tongue
Canker Sores
Reiter's Syndrome
Tongue Inflammation

Ulcers in mouth, preceded by tingling or burning
Canker Sores

Unconsciousness
*Adverse reactions to drugs or medications
Aspirin Poisoning
Convulsions, Febrile
Drowning, Near
Encephalitis, Viral or Aseptic
Extradural Hemorrhage
*Following injury
Hypoglycemia of Diabetes
*Many mental and emotional disorders
Meningitis, Bacterial
Subarachnoid Hemorrhage

Underarms, swollen lymph glands in
Cat-Scratch Fever
Mononucleosis, Infectious

Undernourished appearance
Anorexia Nervosa
Bulimia
Celiac Disease

Urethra, bloody discharge from
Bladder or Urethra Injury
Cystitis
Urethritis

Urethra, cloudy, yellow-green mucus discharge from
Cystitis
Gonorrhea
Urethritis

Urinary-tract infections, unusual susceptibility to
Diabetes Mellitus, Insulin-Dependent

Urine, bad-smelling
Bladder Infection
Kidney Infection, Acute
Kidney Infection, Chronic

Urine, blood in
Bladder Infection
Blood-Transfusion Reaction
Glomerulonephritis
Hemophilia
Kidney Infection, Acute
Kidney Infection, Chronic
Kidney or Ureter Injury
Kidney, Polycystic
Polyarteritis
Purpura, Allergic
Thalassemia
Thrombocytopenia
Tuberculosis
Wilm's Tumor

Urine, cloudy (indicating small amount of blood)
*Any disorder of kidney, ureter, bladder or urethra

Urine, dark
Hepatitis, Acute Viral
Porphyria
Thalassemia

Urine, passage of little or none
Fluid & Electrolyte Disorders
Kidney Failure, Acute

* No chart in this book for this disorder.

Urine, passage of large amounts, diluted and colorless
*Adverse reactions to drugs or medications
Diabetes Insipidus

Urine, protein in the
Glomerulonephritis
Kidney Infection, Acute
Kidney Infection, Chronic
Lupus Erythematosus, Systemic
Nephrosis
Purpura, Allergic

Urine, unintentional loss of (with lifting, sneezing, etc.)
Incontinence, Stress

Urination, burning and stinging
Balanitis
Bladder Infection
Gonorrhea
Kidney Infection, Acute
Ovarian Cyst
Urethritis
Vaginitis, Monilial

Urination, decreased
Dehydration
Fluid & Electrolyte Disorders
Glomerulonephritis
Nephrosis
Premenstrual Syndrome
Shock

Urination, difficult
Decompression Disease
Gonorrhea
Herpes, Genital
Spinal-Cord Tumor

Urination, frequent
Anxiety
Bladder Infection
Diabetes Mellitus, Insulin-Dependent
Heartbeat, Rapid
Hyperaldosteronism
Kidney Infection, Acute
Kidney, Polycystic
Pelvic Inflammatory Disease
Reiter's Syndrome

Urination, inability
Bladder or Urethra Injury
Dehydration

Urination, increased urge
Bladder Infection
Reiter's Syndrome
Spinal-Cord Tumor
Urethritis

Urination, lack of control of
Bladder Infection
Convulsions, Febrile
Fecal Impaction
Hemiplegia
Hypoglycemia of Diabetes
Incontinence, Stress
Paraplegia or Quadriplegia
Spinal-Cord Tumor
Vitamin B Deficiencies

Urination, painful
Bladder or Urethra Injury
Gonorrhea
Herpes, Genital
Pelvic Inflammatory Disease
Urethritis
Vaginitis, Trichomonal
Vulvovaginitis Before Puberty

V

Vagina changing color from pale pink to red
Vagina, Foreign Body in
Vaginitis, Gardnerella or Non-Specific
Vaginitis, Monilial

Vagina, involuntary contraction of muscles around
Vaginismus

Vagina, irregular whitish line inside
Lichen Planus

Vagina, painless red sore on
Syphilis

Vagina, rash with small, red, scaly bumps on
Syphilis

* No chart in this book for this disorder.

Vagina, redness, pain, and itching
Vulvovaginitis Before Puberty

Vagina, skin atrophy
Pruritis Ani

Vagina, spasms of the muscles around
Vaginismus

Vagina, warts on the entrance to
Warts, Venereal

Vaginal bleeding (other than normal menstruation)
Cervical Erosion
DES Exposure
DIC
Ectopic Pregnancy
Thrombocytopenia
Uterine Bleeding, Abnormal
Vagina or Vulva, Cancer of
Vaginitis in Female Athletes
Vulvovaginitis Before Puberty

Vaginal bleeding, painful, prolonged
Uterine Bleeding, Abnormal

Vaginal discharge
Cervical Erosion
Chlamydia
DES Exposure
Gonorrhea
Pruritis Ani
Vagina, Foreign Body in
Vaginitis in Female Athletes
Vaginitis, Monilial
Vaginitis, Trichomonal
Vulvovaginitis Before Puberty

Vaginal discharge, bad-smelling
Chlamydia
Gonorrhea
Pelvic Inflammatory Disease
Vagina, Foreign Body in
Vaginitis, Gardnerella or Non-Specific
Vaginitis, Monilial
Vaginitis, Trichomonal

Vaginal discharge, brownish
Chlamydia
Gonorrhea
Ovarian Cyst
Vaginitis, Monilial
Vaginitis, Trichomonal

Vaginal discharge, frothy
Chlamydia
Gonorrhea
Vaginitis, Monilial
Vaginitis, Trichomonal

Vaginal discharge, itching and discomfort
Chlamydia
Gonorrhea
Pinworms
Vaginitis, Gardnerella or Non-Specific
Vaginitis, Monilial
Vaginitis, Trichomonal

Vaginal discharge, white, "curdy," resembling cottage cheese
Chlamydia
Gonorrhea
Vaginitis, Monilial
Vaginitis, Trichomonal

Vaginal lips, firm, ulcerated, painless lesion of
Syphilis
Vagina or Vulva, Cancer of

Vaginal lips, irritation of
Dermatitis, Seborrheic
Diabetes Mellitus
Herpes, Genital

Vaginal lips, itching around
Diabetes Mellitus
Herpes, Genital
Pruritis Ani
Vaginitis, Monilial
Vaginitis, Trichomonal

Vaginal lips, painful blisters
Herpes, Genital

Vaginal lips, painless sores on
Syphilis
Vagina or Vulva, Cancer of

* No chart in this book for this disorder.

SYMPTOMS

Vaginal lips, redness of
Vaginitis, Monilial
Vaginitis, Trichomonal

Vaginal lips, swollen, tender
*Following injury
Vaginitis, Monilial

Vaginal lips, thin adhesive membrane forming between
Diaper Rash (female infants)

Vaginal spotting, unexplained
Ectopic Pregnancy
*Following injury

Vaginal tears
Rape Crisis Syndrome

Vein, blood clot that forms inside
Thrombosis, Deep-Vein

Vein, superficial, hard (feels like a cord)
Thrombophlebitis, Superficial

Vein, superficial, red, tender, and painful
Thrombophlebitis, Superficial

Vein, swollen and painful
Thrombosis, Deep-Vein

Vision, blurred
Botulism
Brain Tumor
Cataract
Corneal Ulcer
Facial Bones, Fracture of
Fainting
Glaucoma, Acute Infantile
Head Injury
Hemiplegia
Pituitary Tumor
Retinal Detachment
Snakebite

Vision, disturbances in
Diabetes Mellitus
Epilepsy
Eye Contusion or Laceration
Glomerulonephritis
Headache, Migraine
Hyperaldosteronism
Subdural Hemorrhage & Hematoma

Vision, double
Botulism
Brain Tumor
Cataract
Encephalitis, Viral or Aseptic
Exophthalmos
Facial Bones, Fracture of
Hemiplegia
Hypoglycemia of Diabetes
Pituitary Tumor
Reye's Syndrome
Strabismus (Crossed Eyes)

Vision, floating spots in the field of
Retinal Detachment

Vision, gradual loss of
Diabetes
Eye Tumor
Retinal Detachment
*Retinitis Pigmentosa

Vision, in one eye only
Strabismus (Crossed Eyes)

Vision, light flashes in the field of
Retinal Detachment

Visual images, wavy
Retinal Detachment

Voice, loss of
Laryngitis

Vomiting
Addison's Disease
*Adverse reactions to drugs or medications
Anemia, Folic-Acid Deficiency
Appendicitis
Aspirin Poisoning
Botulism
Brain or Epidural Abscess
Brain Tumor
Calcium Imbalance
Cholecystitis or Cholangitis, Acute
Drug Hypersensitivity
Dysentery, Bacillary
Dysmenorrhea

* No chart in this book for this disorder.

Vomiting, continued
- Encephalitis, Viral or Aseptic
- Esophageal Stricture or Corrosive Esophagitis
- Extradural Hemorrhage
- Gallstones
- Gastritis
- Gastroenteritis
- Glomerulonephritis
- Head Injury
- Headache, Migraine
- Heartburn
- Hepatitis, Acute Viral
- Hernia
- Herpangina
- Intestinal Obstruction
- Intussusception
- Kidney Failure, Acute
- Kidney, Polycystic
- Lactose Intolerance
- Lead Poisoning
- Lyme Disease
- *Many mental and emotional disorders
- Meningitis, Aseptic
- Meningitis, Bacterial
- Motion Sickness
- Ovarian Cyst
- Pituitary Tumor
- Porphyria
- Pseudomembranous Enterocolitis
- Purpura, Allergic
- Radiation Sickness
- Rocky Mountain Spotted Fever
- Salmonella Infections
- Scarlet Fever
- Sodium Imbalance
- Subarachnoid Hemorrhage
- Subdural Hemorrhage & Hematoma
- Sunburn
- Testicle Torsion
- Tonsillitis
- Toxic Shock Syndrome
- Trichinosis
- Typhoid Fever
- Ulcer, Peptic
- Vitamin B Deficiencies
- Whiplash
- Whooping Cough
- Wilm's Tumor

Vomiting, bloody
- *Adverse reactions to drugs or medications
- DIC
- Esophageal Stricture or Corrosive Esophagitis
- Gastric Erosion
- Ulcer, Peptic

Vomiting, recurrent
- *Adverse reactions to drugs or medications
- Failure to Thrive
- Pyloric Stenosis, Congenital
- Ulcer, Peptic

Vomiting, self-induced
- Bulimia

Vomiting, with mucus
- Esophageal Stricture or Corrosive Esophagitis

Vulva, see Vaginal Lips

W

Wakefulness
- Insomnia

Walking, delayed
- Failure to Thrive
- Vitamin D Deficiency

Walking, limping or favoring one side
- Hip Dislocation, Congenital

Walking with soreness or pain
- Thrombosis, Deep-Vein
- Warts, Plantar

Warts
- Warts
- Warts, Flat
- Warts, Plantar
- Warts, Venereal

Warts, flat-topped, barely raised on skin
- Warts, Flat

* No chart in this book for this disorder.

Warts, thin, flexible, solid, taller than wide
Warts, Venereal

Weakness
Anemia, Aplastic
Anemia, Folic-Acid Deficiency
Anemia, Iron-Deficiency
Atelectasis
Congestive Heart Failure
Cor Pulmonale
Decompression Disease
Endocarditis
Fainting
Fluid & Electrolyte Disorders
Gastritis
Guillain-Barré Syndrome
Heart-Rhythm Irregularity
Heart-Valve Disease
Hyperaldosteronism
Hyperventilation Syndrome
Hypoglycemia, Functional
Hypoglycemia of Diabetes
Intestinal Obstruction
Kidney Infection, Chronic
Kidney, Polycystic
Lead Poisoning
Malabsorption
Motion Sickness
Muscular Dystrophy
Nephrosis
Pericarditis, Acute
Peritonitis
Porphyria
Potassium Imbalance
Rocky Mountain Spotted Fever
Scleroderma
Sodium Imbalance
Tapeworm
Thrombocytopenia
Toxic Shock Syndrome
Vitamin B Deficiencies
Vitamin C Deficiency

Weakness and inability to bear weight
Bone Fracture

Weakness on one side of body
Brain or Epidural Abscess
Brain Tumor
Hemiplegia
Subdural Hemorrhage & Hematoma

Weight 20% more than normal
Obesity

Weight gain, slowed
Celiac Disease
Cystic Fibrosis
Failure to Thrive
Lactose Intolerance
Roundworms

Weight gain, unexplained
Pituitary Tumor

Weight loss (not by dieting)
Addison's Disease
AIDS
Ankylosing Spondylitis
Anorexia Nervosa
Anxiety
Arthritis, Juvenile Rheumatoid
Brucellosis
Celiac Disease (in infants)
Colitis, Ulcerative
Diabetes Mellitus, Insulin-Dependent
Empyema
Histoplasmosis
Hodgkin's Disease
Liver Cancer
Lung Abscess
Lymphoma, Non-Hodgkin's
Malabsorption
Ovarian Cancer
Polymyositis & Dermatomyositis
Pyloric Stenosis, Congenital
Polyarteritis
Roundworms
Scleroderma
Small-Intestine Tumor
Tapeworm
Tuberculosis
Ulcer, Peptic
Valley Fever
Wilm's Tumor

* No chart in this book for this disorder.

Wheezing
- *Adverse reactions to drugs or medications
- Anaphylaxis
- Asthma
- Bronchitis, Acute
- Bronchiolitis
- Congestive Heart Failure
- Croup
- Drug Hypersensitivity
- Hay Fever
- Roundworms

Whiteheads
- Acne ("zits" or pimples)

Whooping sound when coughing
- Whooping Cough

Withdrawal symptoms
- *Adverse reactions to drugs or medications
- Alcoholism
- Drug Abuse & Addiction

Words, difficulty speaking, understanding or recognizing
- Hemiplegia

Wound, pain and redness around (following surgery)
- Surgical-Wound Infection

Y

Yeast infections of skin, repeated
- Diabetes Mellitus, Insulin-Dependent
- Immunodeficiency Disease
- Pruritis Ani
- Radiation Sickness

* No chart in this book for this disorder.

Illnesses & Disorders

ABDOMINAL MASSES

GENERAL INFORMATION

DESCRIPTION

Abdominal masses are lumps or swollen areas anywhere in the abdomen (below the ribs, above the legs). They may be associated with the kidneys, intestinal tract, adrenal glands, genitals, or spleen. Abdominal masses may appear at any age. They usually do not look discolored, but they may cause pain when touched.

Appropriate health care includes:

Doctor's diagnosis and treatment, including hospitalization for extensive studies and possibly surgery.

SIGNS & SYMPTOMS

- A slight swelling or a substantial bulge above the surface of the child's abdomen, but the mass may be so deep that it is not visible.
- Pain upon pressing the mass (usually).

CAUSES

- Abnormal growths on the kidneys, genitals, stomach, intestines, liver, adrenals, and bile ducts.
- Results of injury.
- Some growths are congenital (present at birth).
- More than half the growths present in newborn babies are caused by hydronephrosis (a condition existing when urine is blocked from release from a kidney).

RISK FACTORS

- Prematurity.
- History of similar masses in other children in the family.

PREVENTING COMPLICATIONS OR RECURRENCE

No specific preventive measures.

WHAT TO EXPECT

MEDICAL TESTS

- Your own observation of symptoms.
- Medical history and physical exam by a doctor.
- Blood and urine studies.
- Intravenous pyelograms (see Glossary).
- Voiding cystourethrography (see Glossary).
- X-ray exams of the gastrointestinal tract.
- Ultrasound studies (see Glossary).
- Computerized tomography (CAT or CT scan—see Glossary).
- Nuclear medicine studies (see Glossary).

POSSIBLE COMPLICATIONS

- Some congenital masses may be malignant.
- Failure to treat quickly and effectively may cause permanent damage.

PROBABLE OUTCOME

Varies according to the location and nature of the mass in your child's abdomen. Curable if underlying causes can be eliminated or modified.

TREATMENT

HOME CARE

Varies according to the nature of the mass. Follow your doctor's instructions.

MEDICATION

- Your doctor will prescribe medications according to the nature of the mass.
- See Medications section for information regarding medicines your doctor may prescribe.

ACTIVITY

Your child should resume activities as your doctor advises.

DIET & FLUIDS

Depending on the nature of the mass, your doctor will determine the proper diet and fluid intake.

OK FOR SCHOOL, PRESCHOOL, OR NURSERY?

Only after problems of diagnosis and treatment are solved.

CALL YOUR DOCTOR IF

You discover any mass in your child's abdomen.

ABDOMINAL PAIN, CHRONIC

GENERAL INFORMATION

DESCRIPTION

Chronic abdominal pain means recurrent, vague abdominal pain in a child over a period of days, weeks, or even months. This pain is frequently associated with headache, paleness, and tiredness. It is a frequent problem, sometimes estimated to periodically affect as many as one in ten children. Sometimes a specific treatable cause can be found. More often, it is hard to establish a specific medical or surgical diagnosis of the problem. Parents and friends frequently suspect that the child is faking the symptom. However, it is more likely that a child uses the symptom of abdominal pain to express troubled feelings. Parents should consider that the pain is very real and not "put on." Chronic abdominal pain is more likely to occur in intelligent, competitive, overachieving children of both sexes. It is not contagious or cancerous. Appropriate health care includes a doctor's care until the problem is resolved.

SIGNS & SYMPTOMS

Vague pain usually perceived to be located around the navel. Pain is a sensation that indicates an abnormality which might otherwise be overlooked. Because pain can be felt only by the patient, you and your child's physician learn of its features only through the child's description or your observation of the child's reactions.

CAUSES

Unknown. Possibly anxiety or tension.

RISK FACTORS

Outside pressure on the child from any source.

PREVENTING COMPLICATIONS OR RECURRENCE

Avoid excessive pressure on the child when possible.

WHAT TO EXPECT

MEDICAL TESTS

- Your own observation of symptoms.
- Medical history and physical exam by a doctor.
- Diagnostic measures including urinalysis, blood counts, and stool exams.

POSSIBLE COMPLICATIONS

None expected.

PROBABLE OUTCOME

Complete recovery.

ABDOMINAL PAIN, CHRONIC

TREATMENT

HOME CARE

- Don't discuss the illness with friends or neighbors in the presence of your child. You may thoughtlessly transfer your fears to your child.
- Keep a weight chart. A steady weight gain is evidence of a healthy child.

MEDICATION

- Medicines must be fitted to your child's own particular needs. Do not give any medicine (not even medicine you buy without prescription) without telling your doctor. If your doctor does prescribe drugs, carefully follow the instructions on the label.
- Usually your doctor will not prescribe any medication unless a specific cause can be discovered.
- See Medications section for information regarding medicines your doctor may prescribe.

ACTIVITY

Try to encourage your child to participate in normal activities, but avoid tension and too much excitement or stimulation. Children with recurrent abdominal pain are frequently intelligent, competitive, and apt to be overachievers.

DIET & FLUIDS

No change is necessary unless the situation changes dramatically. If mild, continuous pain becomes progressively worse, or if your child becomes incapacitated, then give nothing to eat or drink (particularly avoid laxatives) until your doctor re-examines the child and finds the cause.

OK FOR SCHOOL, PRESCHOOL, OR NURSERY?

Yes, if the child's condition and feeling of well-being will allow.

CALL YOUR DOCTOR IF

Your child experiences any of the following:

- Painful or frequent urination.
- Fever over 101 degrees.
- Blood in bowel movements.
- Black, tarry-appearing bowel movements.
- Weight loss.
- Paleness.
- Pain that interferes with sleep and normal activity or becomes incapacitating.

ACETAMINOPHEN POISONING

GENERAL INFORMATION

DESCRIPTION

Acetaminophen poisoning is an acute emergency in childhood. It is caused by swallowing a large amount of acetaminophen. Poisoning may cause great harm to young children if treatment is inadequate. Tylenol is the best-known brand name; other brand names include A'Cenol, Acephen, Aceta, Ace-Tabs, Acetaminophen Uniserts, Actamin, Anacin-3, Anuphen, Apacet, APAP, Apo-Acetaminophen, Aspirin-Free Pain Relief, Atasol, Banesin, Bromo-Seltzer Buffered Acetaminophen, C2A, Cafadol, Campain, Conacetol, Dapa, Datril, Dolanex, Dorcol Children's Fever and Pain Reducer, Exdol, Genapap, Genebs, Genetabs, Halenol, Liquiprin, Meda Cap, Meda Tab, Myapap, Neopap, Oraphen-PD, Panadol, Panasorb, Panex, Paracetamol, Paraphen, Pedric, Phenaphen, Robigesic, Rounox, St. Joseph Aspirin-Free, Summit, Suppap, Tapanol, Tempra, Tenol, Ty Caplets, Ty Pap, Ty Tab, Valadol, and Valorin.

Appropriate health care includes hospitalization (sometimes) to have the child's stomach pumped out and to give other supportive treatment.

SIGNS & SYMPTOMS

- Paleness.
- Nausea.
- Perspiration.
- Vomiting.
- Tenderness of the liver.
- Mental confusion.
- Jaundice (yellow skin and eyes).
- Abdominal swelling.

CAUSES

Swallowing excessive amounts of acetaminophen either in tablet form or liquid form or as a component of other medicines. The minimum toxic dose is approximately 150 milligrams of acetaminophen per 2.2 pounds of weight of a child. The average children's tablet contains 70 mg of acetaminophen and a regular-strength adult-size tablet contains 325 mg. Example: A 50-pound child will be poisoned after swallowing 50 children's tablets or 10 adult tablets.

RISK FACTORS

A curious child who likes to explore.

PREVENTING COMPLICATIONS OR RECURRENCE

- Keep medications out of sight and reach of all children.
- Use medicines with child-proof bottles only.
- Limit the number of tablets in any container of medicine.

? WHAT TO EXPECT

MEDICAL TESTS

Your own observation of symptoms; medical history and physical exam by a doctor; blood test to measure acetaminophen level.

POSSIBLE COMPLICATIONS

- Severe liver damage.
- Severe kidney damage.
- Low blood sugar.
- Death with fatal doses.

PROBABLE OUTCOME

Full recovery without complications with adequate treatment.

TREATMENT

FIRST AID

- After determining how much acetaminophen your child has swallowed, call your doctor or poison control center immediately!
- If recommended by your doctor or the poison control center, try to make your child vomit with syrup of ipecac. This is a non-prescription liquid that you should keep on hand when there are young children at home. Specific instructions are on the bottle. Don't give more than what is recommended on the label. Give 1/2 to 1 full glass of water immediately after the ipecac. Don't give milk or carbonated beverages.
  —Ipecac is not recommended for children under 6 months of age.
  —Children 6 to 8 months—usual dose is 1 teaspoon.
  —Children 8 months to 1 year—usual dose is 2 teaspoons.
  —Children 1 to 3 years—usual dose is 3 teaspoons.

You may repeat the dose in 30 minutes if vomiting doesn't occur.

- Whether your child does or does not vomit, call your poison control center or physician again within 30 minutes. The child's stomach may need to be pumped.

MEDICATION

- Ipecac (see above).
- Activated charcoal (sometimes) if prescribed by your physician.
- Oral antidote to acetaminophen (by prescription only).
- I.V. fluids in hospital, if needed.

ACTIVITY

Your child's activity level should return to normal only after damage to organs has been ruled out or treated and healed.

DIET & FLUIDS

Intravenous fluids, if necessary, containing glucose and potassium.

OK FOR SCHOOL, PRESCHOOL, OR NURSERY?

Only after crisis is over.

CALL YOUR DOCTOR IF

You even *suspect* that your child has taken an overdose of acetaminophen (or any other medicine). If you cannot reach your doctor, call the poison control center or go immediately to a hospital emergency room. Take the bottle with you if it is available.

ACHILLES' TENDON STRAIN

GENERAL INFORMATION

DESCRIPTION

An Achilles' tendon strain is an injury to the Achilles' tendon or its adjoining muscle or bone. These 3 parts comprise a unit. The strain occurs at the weakest part of the unit. The Achilles' tendon, the muscle attached to the Achilles' tendon, the heel bone, and the soft tissue surrounding the strain are involved.

Appropriate health care includes: doctor's diagnosis; application of tape, plaster splits, or casts (sometimes); self-care during rehabilitation; physical therapy; surgery (sometimes).

SIGNS & SYMPTOMS

- Pain when flexing or extending the foot.
- Muscle spasm at the rear of the calf.
- Swelling around the Achilles' tendon.
- Loss of strength (moderate or severe strain).
- Crepitation ("crackling") feeling and sound when the injured area is pressed with fingers.
- Calcification of the muscle or its tendon (visible with X-ray).
- Inflammation of the sheath covering the Achilles' tendon.

CAUSES

- Prolonged overuse of muscle-tendon units in the child's ankle.
- A single episode of stressful overactivity, as in hurdling, long-jumping, high-jumping, or starting a sprint.

RISK FACTORS

Contact sports; running; sports that require quick starts, such as long-jumping, hurdling, or running races; any cardiovascular medical problem that results in decreased circulation; medical history of any bleeding disorder; obesity; poor nutrition; previous Achilles' tendon injury; poor muscle conditioning.

PREVENTING COMPLICATIONS OR RECURRENCE

Your child should participate in an appropriate strengthening and conditioning program and should warm up before participating in sports. The child should tape the Achilles' area and wear proper shoes for sports.

WHAT TO EXPECT

MEDICAL TESTS

Your own observation of symptoms; medical history and physical exam by a doctor; X-rays of injured areas to rule out fractures.

POSSIBLE COMPLICATIONS

Prolonged healing time if the child resumes activity too soon; proneness to repeated injury; an unstable or arthritic ankle following repeated injury; inflammation at the attachment to bone (periostitis); prolonged disability (sometimes).

PROBABLE OUTCOME

If this is a first-time injury, proper care and sufficient healing time before the child resumes activity should prevent permanent disability. Torn ligaments and tendons require as long to heal as bone fractures. Average healing times are: mild strain—2 to 10 days; moderate strain—10 days to 6 weeks; severe strain—6 to 10 weeks. If this is a repeat injury, complications listed above are more likely to occur.

TREATMENT

FIRST AID

Follow instructions for R.I.C.E., the first letters of *rest*, *ice*, *compression*, and *elevation*. See R.I.C.E. Appendix 39 for details.

HOME CARE

If a cast or splints are used, leave the child's toes free and exercise them occasionally. If a cast or splints are not used:

- Use ice massage 3 or 4 times a day for 15 minutes at a time. See Glossary.
- After the first 24 hours, apply heat instead of ice, if it feels better to your child. Use heat lamps, hot soaks, hot showers, heating pads, or heat liniments and ointments.
- Provide the child with whirlpool treatments, if available.
- Wrap the injured ankle with an elasticized bandage between treatments. Insert a heel lift in the child's shoe.
- Massage gently and often to provide comfort and decrease swelling.

MEDICATION

- For minor discomfort use aspirin, acetaminophen, or ibuprofen; topical liniments and ointments.
- Your doctor may prescribe stronger pain relievers; injection of a long-acting local anesthetic to reduce pain (rare); injection of a corticosteroid, such as triamcinolone, to reduce inflammation (rare).

ACTIVITY

For a moderate or severe strain, your child should walk with crutches for at least 72 hours—longer with a cast or splints. See Appendix 37 (Safe Use of Crutches). The child can resume normal activities gradually after the pain has subsided.

DIET & FLUIDS

No restrictions.

OK FOR SCHOOL, PRESCHOOL, OR NURSERY?

Yes, when condition and sense of well-being will allow.

CALL YOUR DOCTOR IF

- Your child has symptoms of a moderate or severe Achilles' tendon strain, or a mild strain persists longer than 10 days.
- Pain or swelling worsens despite treatment.
- The following occurs with a cast or splint: pain, numbness, or coldness below the injury; dusky, blue, or gray toenails.

ACNE
(Acne Vulgaris)

GENERAL INFORMATION

DESCRIPTION

Acne is an inflammatory skin condition—common in adolescence—characterized by skin eruptions on the face, chest and back. It usually begins at puberty and may continue for years. Acne is more common in boys, but it can affect both sexes, all ages.

Appropriate health care includes:

- Self-care after diagnosis.
- Physician's monitoring of general condition and medications.
- Surgery (dermabrasion) to remove unsightly scars after acne heals (sometimes).

SIGNS & SYMPTOMS

- Blackheads (black spots the size of a pinhead).
- Whiteheads (white spots similar to blackheads).
- Pustules (small pus-filled lesions).
- Redness and inflammation around eruptions.

CAUSES

Oil glands in the skin become plugged for unknown reasons, but sex-hormone changes during adolescence play a role. When oil backs up, it becomes infected by bacteria normally present in glands. Contrary to myth, acne is *not* caused by dirt or masturbation. Cleanliness can lessen it, but sexual activity has no effect on it.

RISK FACTORS

- Exposure to extremely hot or cold weather.
- Stress.
- Oily skin.
- Endocrine disorders.
- Use of drugs, such as cortisone, male hormones, or oral contraceptives.
- Family history of acne.

PREVENTING COMPLICATIONS OR RECURRENCE

Cannot be prevented at present. Tendency to develop severe acne is inherited.

WHAT TO EXPECT

MEDICAL TESTS

- Your own observation of symptoms.
- Medical history and physical exam by a doctor.

POSSIBLE COMPLICATIONS

- Poor self-image and psychological distress.
- Permanent facial scars.

PROBABLE OUTCOME

Most cases respond well to treatment, and the condition tends to disappear after adolescence. Despite good treatment, acne will flare up from time to time.

ACNE
(Acne Vulgaris)

TREATMENT

HOME CARE

• If the adolescent's skin is oily, cleanse it as follows: Gently massage face with soap for 3 to 5 minutes. Don't massage sorest places. Cleanse skin gently—rough scrubbing spreads infection. Rinse soap off for 2 to 3 minutes. After cleansing, use an astringent, such as alcohol, to remove oil. Use a fresh washcloth each day. Bacteria grow in damp, wet cloths.
• Shampoo hair at least twice a week. Don't let hair hang over the face—even at night. Hair spreads oil and bacteria. Use dandruff shampoo to treat or prevent dandruff.
• After vigorous exercise, wash sweat and oil off as soon as possible.
• Don't squeeze, scratch, pick, or rub the skin. Acne heals better without damage to the skin. If you *must* squeeze pimples, blackheads or whiteheads, wash your hands first. Cleanse the area with alcohol before and after squeezing.
• Don't rest your face on your hands while reading, studying, or watching TV.

MEDICATION

• Your doctor may prescribe antibiotics to fight infection (some are taken orally, others applied to skin); cortisone injections into lesions; skin lotions with drying agents; vitamin A; medicated creams, gels, and liquids to apply to skin (one of the useful medicines included is tretinoin—brand name Retin-A).
• *Caution:* Pregnant females should not take oral medications for acne.

ACTIVITY

No restrictions.

DIET & FLUIDS

• Foods don't cause acne, but some foods may make it worse. Keep a record of the foods your child eats. To discover any food sensitivities, eliminate all the following foods from the diet: chocolate, ice cream, nuts, peanut butter, cheese, iodized salt, seafood (especially lobster, shrimp, clams and oysters), pork and bacon, carbonated and alcoholic drinks, spicy foods, cold cuts, potato chips, popcorn, and pickles. Then reintroduce them one at a time. If acne flares up 2 or 3 days after a food is eaten, leave it out of the diet. If not, it may be included again.
• Acne usually improves in the summer, so some foods that cannot be eaten in the winter may be tolerated in the summer.

OK FOR SCHOOL, PRESCHOOL, OR NURSERY?

Yes. No need to isolate when eruptions occur. Acne is *not* contagious.

CALL YOUR DOCTOR IF

• Your adolescent has acne.
• New, unexplained symptoms develop. Drugs used in treatment may produce side effects.

ADDISON'S DISEASE (Adrenal Insufficiency)

GENERAL INFORMATION

DESCRIPTION

Addison's disease is caused by underactive adrenal glands. The adrenal glands are small solid glands found just above and adjacent to the kidneys.
Appropriate health care includes:
- Physician's monitoring of general condition and medications.
- Self-care after diagnosis.
- Hospitalization for an "adrenal crisis," which may be necessary at times of physiological stress (see POSSIBLE COMPLICATIONS below).

SIGNS & SYMPTOMS

- Weakness and fatigue.
- Gastrointestinal disturbances (nausea, vomiting, abdominal pain, diarrhea, decreased appetite, and weight loss).
- Low blood pressure causing faintness and dizziness.
- Brownish skin (looks suntanned) with white patches.
- Darkening of freckles, scars, and breast nipples.
- Hair loss.
- Feeling cold all the time.
- Dramatic behavior or mood changes, including aggression or depression.

CAUSES

Low levels of cortisone-like hormones are produced by the adrenal glands. The cause of adrenal insufficiency is usually unknown but is sometimes a complication of:
- Tuberculosis.
- Cancer.
- Pituitary disease.
- Use of cortisone drugs for other conditions. When cortisone is withdrawn, normal adrenal function sometimes does not return.

RISK FACTORS

- Stress, such as broken bones, infections, surgery.
- Diabetes mellitus.
- Injury to the abdomen.

PREVENTING COMPLICATIONS OR RECURRENCE

Don't discontinue use of cortisone drugs or change the dosage without consulting your doctor.

WHAT TO EXPECT

MEDICAL TESTS

- Your own observation of symptoms. "Before and after" pictures may emphasize the gradual skin change.
- Medical history and physical exam by a doctor.
- Laboratory blood counts, blood and urine measurement of adrenal hormones, and a test of adrenal-gland function.

ADDISON'S DISEASE (Adrenal Insufficiency)

POSSIBLE COMPLICATIONS

- "Adrenal crisis" (pains, weakness, change in mental status, low blood pressure, high or low temperature, fainting) caused by any injury or illness.
- Misdiagnosis as a mental condition.

PROBABLE OUTCOME

Symptoms can usually be controlled with hormone-replacement treatment. Adrenal crisis is fatal without treatment.

TREATMENT

HOME CARE

- This is a lifelong condition. Your child must learn how to care for himself. Strict attention to medication schedules is vital.
- The child must learn about adrenal crisis and its relationship to body stress (infection, surgery or injury).
- Advise your doctor and dentist that your child has Addison's disease.
- The child should wear a Medic-Alert bracelet or pendant (see Glossary).
- Stay up-to-date on the child's immunizations.

MEDICATION

- Your doctor may prescribe a cortisone drug. Follow medication schedule. Never change or omit medication without your doctor's advice.
- See Medications section for information regarding medicines your doctor may prescribe.

ACTIVITY

No restrictions.

DIET & FLUIDS

Your child should eat a low-salt diet (see Appendix 29).

OK FOR SCHOOL, PRESCHOOL, OR NURSERY?

Yes, so long as condition is stable.

CALL YOUR DOCTOR IF

- Your child has symptoms of Addison's disease—especially an adrenal crisis. Call immediately. Adrenal crisis is an emergency!
- The following occurs after diagnosis:
  - — Any signs of infection, such as fever, chills, muscle aches, headache, and dizziness.
  - — Serious injury, such as bone fracture, dislocation, or internal injuries.
- Your child is scheduled for elective surgery or requires anesthesia for any reason.
- New, unexplained symptoms develop. Drugs used in treatment may produce side effects, such as protruding abdomen, thin extremities, puffy face and eyes, acne, and growth of facial hair.

AGRANULOCYTOSIS
(Granulocytopenia; Neutropenia)

GENERAL INFORMATION

DESCRIPTION

Agranulocytosis is a reduction in the normal number of circulating white blood cells (granulocytes or neutrophils) in the bloodstream. These cells are the first to attack bacterial infections. This condition involves the bone marrow and blood. Appropriate health care includes:

- Self-care after diagnosis.
- Physician's monitoring of general condition and medications.
- Hospitalization for intensive treatment during the active phase; strict reverse isolation techniques (see Glossary) and transfusions of white blood cells may sometimes be imperative.

SIGNS & SYMPTOMS

- Fever.
- Aching.
- Sore throat.
- Ulcers (especially in the mouth and throat), which do not produce pus.
- Any sign of infection in someone who has had agranulocytosis in the past. This may signal a recurrence.

CAUSES

Increased destruction or impaired production of granulocytes (white blood cells). The most common reason for this is an adverse reaction to medications, including anti-cancer drugs, anti-convulsants, antihistamines, anti-thyroid drugs, arsenic, chloramphenicol, dibenzapine, gold salts, indomethacin, nitrofurantoin, nitrous oxide, phenothiazines, phenylbutazone, procainamide, sulfonamides, synthetic penicillins, and thiazide diuretics.

RISK FACTORS

Genetic factors. A rare form, infantile genetic agranulocytosis, is inherited.

PREVENTING COMPLICATIONS OR RECURRENCE

Prevent recurrences by having the child avoid any suspect medicine or drug that may have triggered agranulocytosis previously.

WHAT TO EXPECT

MEDICAL TESTS

- Your own observation of symptoms.
- Medical history and physical exam by a doctor.
- Laboratory studies of blood and bone marrow, and cultures of blood, nose, throat, and urine.

POSSIBLE COMPLICATIONS

- Kidney damage.
- Dangerous, sometimes fatal infections (bacterial, fungal, viral, or others)—even with vigorous treatment.

AGRANULOCYTOSIS
(Granulocytopenia; Neutropenia)

PROBABLE OUTCOME

Usually curable within 6 weeks of intensive treatment.

TREATMENT

HOME CARE

Hospitalization may be necessary during the acute phase. The following may be helpful advice to the child after hospitalization:

- Be extra careful about personal cleanliness.
- Keep the mouth clean by rinsing frequently with warm salt water (1 teaspoon salt to 8 oz. water) or gargling with hydrogen peroxide.
- Pay particular attention to oral hygiene. Brush teeth gently with a very soft brush, avoiding irritation of the gums.
- Avoid contact with harmful materials, such as cleaning chemicals, glue, insecticide, fertilizer, paint remover, and others.

MEDICATION

Your doctor may:

- Prescribe intravenous and oral antibiotics, if the white blood cell count is very low.
- Prescribe lithium to stimulate bone marrow to produce more granulocytes.
- Stop prescribing any drug that is suspected of causing agranulocytosis.
- See Medications section for information regarding medicines your doctor may prescribe.

ACTIVITY

Your child should rest in bed during the acute stage but may resume normal activities gradually after symptoms subside.

DIET & FLUIDS

No restrictions.

OK FOR SCHOOL, PRESCHOOL, OR NURSERY?

When white count returns to normal and there is no sign of infection.

CALL YOUR DOCTOR IF

- Your child has symptoms of agranulocytosis.
- The following occurs after treatment has begun:
  - — Any sign of infection, especially fever.
  - — Swelling of the feet and ankles.
  - — Painful urination or decreased urine output during any 24-hour period.
- New, unexplained symptoms develop. Drugs used in treatment may produce side effects.

AIDS (Acquired Immunodeficiency Syndrome)

GENERAL INFORMATION

DESCRIPTION

AIDS is a major failure of the body's immune system (immunodeficiency). This decreases the body's ability to fight infection and suppress multiplication of abnormal cells, such as cancer. Body parts involved include the immune system, including special blood cells (lymphocytes) and cells of organs (bone marrow, spleen, liver, and lymph glands). These cells manufacture antibodies to protect against disease and cancer. Only about 1% of cases occur in children less than 13 years old. It is most common in adolescent or adult males, but it also occurs in infants of both sexes if born of an infected mother.

Appropriate health care includes:

- Doctor's treatment.
- Psychotherapy or counseling to help your child cope with anxiety and depression about having the disease and the likelihood of death.
- Hospitalization (medical schools may provide some free care if your child is willing to participate in research).

SIGNS & SYMPTOMS

Fatigue; fever; unexplained weight loss; recurrent respiratory and skin infections; diarrhea; swollen lymph glands throughout the body; genital changes; enlarged spleen and salivary glands; meningitis (newborn).

CAUSES

A virus called human immunodeficiency virus (HIV), which has been isolated from blood, semen, saliva, tears. Among infants, AIDS is also transmitted from an infected mother to the fetus through the placenta while the baby is still in the uterus. The virus is transmitted by:

- Homosexual activity.
- Use of contaminated needles for intravenous drug use.
- Transfusions of blood or blood products from a person with AIDS.
- Sexual contact with an affected person. Usual non-sexual contact does not transmit the disease, so a person with AIDS is not a risk to the general population.

RISK FACTORS

- Multiple homosexual sexual partners.
- Multiple heterosexual partners (less likely).
- Exposure of hospital workers and laboratory technicians to blood, feces and urine of AIDS patients.
- Being an infant born to a mother with AIDS.
- Multiple blood transfusions.

PREVENTING COMPLICATIONS OR RECURRENCE

Your child should avoid sexual contact with affected persons and should avoid intravenous self-administered drugs. Condoms should be used for sexual activity with homosexual partners. Anyone with AIDS should not donate blood to blood banks because of the danger of transmitting the disease to others.

OTHER

- By law, AIDS must be reported to public health agencies.
- For further information, call the AIDS hotline (800) 342-AIDS.

AIDS (Acquired Immunodeficiency Syndrome)

WHAT TO EXPECT

MEDICAL TESTS

- Your own observation of symptoms.
- Medical history and physical exam by a doctor.
- Laboratory blood studies of lymphocytes and HIV antibodies test (may not become positive for 6 months after contact).

POSSIBLE COMPLICATIONS

- Serious infection in various body systems; cancer.
- About half the children with AIDS die within 1 year of diagnosis.

PROBABLE OUTCOME

- This condition is currently considered incurable. However, your child's symptoms can be relieved or controlled. Scientific research into causes and treatment continues.
- AIDS may not develop for years following a positive test. Once ill, survival averages 2-1/2 years, but it may be shorter or longer.

TREATMENT

HOME CARE

- Early diagnosis is helpful. If your child is at risk, a medical evaluation should be obtained—even if your child feels well.
- Contact social agencies in your area about AIDS support groups.

MEDICATION

- Drugs are currently not effective in curing AIDS. Your doctor may prescribe antibiotics for your child to prevent infections or control them as they develop.
- See Medications section for information regarding medicines your doctor may prescribe.

ACTIVITY

No restrictions on normal activity, but your child should refrain from unprotected sexual encounters.

DIET & FLUIDS

No special diet.

OK FOR SCHOOL, PRESCHOOL, OR NURSERY?

When appetite returns and alertness, strength, and feeling of well-being will allow.

CALL YOUR DOCTOR IF

- Your child has symptoms of AIDS.
- Infection occurs after diagnosis. Symptoms include: fever; cough; diarrhea; skin rash or eruption; general ill feeling.

ALCOHOLISM

GENERAL INFORMATION

DESCRIPTION

Alcoholism means a psychological and physiological dependence on alcohol, resulting in chronic disease and disruption of interpersonal, family, and work relationships. The brain, central nervous system, liver, and heart are involved. Alcoholism occurs 4 times more often in males than females. It may develop at any age after adolescence, when drinking begins.

Appropriate health care includes:

- Self-care. The first and most difficult step of treatment is for your child to admit the problem exists.
- Doctor's treatment.
- Psychotherapy or counseling.

SIGNS & SYMPTOMS

Early stages to look for in your child:

- Low tolerance for anxiety.
- Need for alcohol at the beginning of the day, or at times of stress.
- Insomnia; nightmares.
- Habitual Monday-morning hangovers, and frequent absences from school and work.
- Preoccupation with obtaining alcohol and hiding drinking from family and friends.
- Guilt or irritability when others suggest drinking is excessive.

Late stages:

- Frequent blackouts; memory loss.
- Delirium tremens (tremors, hallucinations, confusion, sweating, rapid heartbeat). These occur most often with alcohol withdrawal.
- Liver disease (jaundice, internal bleeding, bloating).
- Neurological impairment (numbness and tingling in hands and feet, declining sexual interest and potency, confusion, coma).
- Congestive heart failure (shortness of breath, swelling of feet).

CAUSES

Not fully understood, but include:

- Personality factors, especially dependency, anger, mania, depression, or introversion.
- Family influences, especially alcoholic or divorced parents.
- Social and cultural pressure to drink.
- Body-chemistry disturbances (perhaps).

RISK FACTORS

- Genetic factors. Some ethnic groups have high alcoholism rates — either for social or biological reasons.
- Use of recreational drugs.
- Crisis situations, including frequent moves, or loss of friends or family.

PREVENTING COMPLICATIONS OR RECURRENCE

- Provide your child with a loving, stable family environment. Use alcohol in moderation — if at all — to provide a healthy role model.
- Encourage your child to admit when an alcohol problem exists, and seek professional care. Some employers and health-insurance companies pay for treatment.

WHAT TO EXPECT

MEDICAL TESTS

- Your own observation of symptoms.
- Medical history and physical exam by a doctor.
- Laboratory studies of blood and liver function.
- EEG (see Glossary).

POSSIBLE COMPLICATIONS

- Chronic liver disease.
- Gastric erosion with bleeding; stomach inflammation.
- Neuritis, tremors, seizures, and brain impairment.
- Inflammation of the pancreas.
- Inflammation of the heart.
- Mental and physical damage to the fetus if a mother drinks during pregnancy.
- Family members of alcoholics may develop psychological symptoms requiring treatment and support groups such as Al-Anon.

PROBABLE OUTCOME

- Without treatment: progressive brain and liver disease; poor school performance and possibly criminal behavior; painful, premature death.
- With treatment, alcoholism is often curable.

TREATMENT

HOME CARE

Instructions for your child:

- Keep appointments with doctors and counselors.
- Join a local Alcoholics Anonymous group and attend regularly.
- Reassess your lifestyle — friends, school, work, family — to identify and alter factors that encourage drinking.

MEDICATION

Your doctor may prescribe disulfiram (Antabuse), which causes several extremely unpleasant physical symptoms when your child consumes alcohol.

ACTIVITY

Your child should not drink and drive.

DIET & FLUIDS

Your child should have a normal, well-balanced diet. Vitamin supplements, such as thiamine and folic acid, are often necessary.

OK FOR SCHOOL, PRESCHOOL, OR NURSERY?

When appetite returns and alertness, strength, and feeling of well- being will allow.

CALL YOUR DOCTOR IF

Your child or any family member has symptoms of alcoholism.

ALOPECIA AEREATA

GENERAL INFORMATION

DESCRIPTION

Alopecia aereata is a sudden hair loss in circular patches on the scalp. The hair loss is not accompanied by other visible evidence of scalp disease. This is not contagious. Body parts involved include hair, scalp, eyebrows, eyelashes, beard, genital area, and underarm (sometimes). Alopecia aereata can affect both sexes, all ages, but is most common in children 5 to 12 years of age.

Appropriate health care includes:

- Doctor's examination for a precise diagnosis.
- Self-care after diagnosis.

SIGNS & SYMPTOMS

- Sudden hair loss in sharply defined circular patches. In rare cases, body hair loss may be total.
- No pain.
- No itch.

CAUSES

Unknown, but heredity and emotional factors, such as anxiety, may contribute to hair loss. The autoimmune system may also be involved.

RISK FACTORS

- Stress.
- Family history of alopecia aereata.

PREVENTING COMPLICATIONS OR RECURRENCE

Cannot be prevented at present.

WHAT TO EXPECT

MEDICAL TESTS

- Your own observation of symptoms.
- Medical history and physical exam by a doctor.

POSSIBLE COMPLICATIONS

- Loss of all hair.
- Slow or incomplete regrowth.

PROBABLE OUTCOME

Usually curable, with spontaneous new growth, in 18 months. Children with a few small patches are generally cured completely. The disorder recurs in 25% of cases.

TREATMENT

HOME CARE

- Consider having your child wear a hairpiece or wig during the acute phase.
- Continue to bathe and shampoo the child as usual.
- Don't tug on normal hair close to areas of hair loss.

MEDICATION

- Your doctor may prescribe topical steroids. Apply topical steroid once or twice a day unless directed otherwise. Apply immediately after bathing or shampooing for better spreading and penetration.
- For scalp and groin, use only low-potency steroid products without fluorine. In special cases, your doctor may inject steroids into affectedd areas and prescribe oral cortisone drugs to take on alternate days.
- See Medications section for information regarding medicines your doctor may prescribe.

ACTIVITY

No restrictions.

DIET & FLUIDS

No special diet.

OK FOR SCHOOL, PRESCHOOL, OR NURSERY

Yes.

CALL YOUR DOCTOR IF

- Your child has symptoms of alopecia aereata.
- The following occurs during treatment:
  —Hair loss increases.
  —Hair loss doesn't diminish in 4 weeks.
  —Areas show signs of infection (redness, swelling, tenderness, warmth) after injections.

ALTITUDE SICKNESS

GENERAL INFORMATION

DESCRIPTION

Altitude sickness refers to any of several illnesses associated with higher-than-usual altitudes. The illnesses are of several types, including acute mountain sickness (AMS), high altitude pulmonary edema (HAPE), high altitude cerebral edema (HACE), high altitude retinal hemorrhage (HARH), and subacute and chronic mountain sickness (CMS). (CMS is a complication that represents failure to recover from AMS over a long period of time.) Other altitude-related problems include frostbite, blood clots in the legs and lungs, dehydration, and swollen feet and ankles. Pre-existing illnesses that are aggravated by high altitude include sickle-cell disease or trait, chronic heart disease, and chronic lung disease. Altitude illnesses affect most body systems, especially the brain, heart, lungs, gastrointestinal tract, circulatory system, and electrolytes. Appropriate health care includes self-care and doctor's treatment; hospitalization (severe cases).

SIGNS & SYMPTOMS

- AMS: Headache, nausea, vomiting, shortness of breath, and sleep disturbances.
- HAPE: Shortness of breath, cough, weakness, headache, and coma.
- HACE: Severe headache, staggering gait, hallucinations, and stupor. These indicate swelling of the brain. Death will occur without descent.
- HARH: Visual disturbances, including spots before the eyes. Blood clots and bleeding into the retina occur in 50% of those who go above 17,000 feet.
- CMS: Shortness of breath, fatigue, bloated face and body, congestive heart failure after years of living at high altitude (rare).

CAUSES

Insufficient oxygen at high altitudes. Following are the altitudes at which each type of illness can occur in your child:

- AMS: 7,000 to 8,000 feet or higher.
- HAPE: 9,000 to 10,000 feet.
- HACE: 10,000 to 12,000 feet.
- HARH: 17,000 feet.

RISK FACTORS

Fatigue or overwork; previous episodes of altitude illness; chronic illness of any sort, particularly cardiovascular and lung diseases; obesity; excess alcohol consumption; use of mind-altering drugs, including narcotics and tranquilizers.

PREVENTING COMPLICATIONS OR RECURRENCE

Your child should avoid ascending to heights that cause symptoms. If it is necessary to climb, the child should become acclimatized gradually by a slow ascent.

WHAT TO EXPECT

MEDICAL TESTS

Your own observation of symptoms; medical history and physical exam by a doctor; laboratory studies such as EKG and chest X-ray.

POSSIBLE COMPLICATIONS

Permanent brain, eye, heart, and lung damage. The worst cases of HAPE and HACE can lead to death.

PROBABLE OUTCOME

Usually curable without residual impairment after the child returns to lower altitudes.

TREATMENT

HOME CARE

Your child should follow these instructions:

- AMS: Descend to lower altitude if illness lasts 2 or more days.
- HAPE: Oxygen, rest, and diuretics help, but rapid descent is usually necessary.
- HACE: Oxygen and corticosteroids help, but rapid descent to lower altitudes is the only certain way for the child to recover.
- HARH: No treatment except to descend.
- CMS: The child should return to lower altitudes if symptoms persist.

MEDICATION

Your doctor may prescribe:

- For AMS: diamox (carbonic anhydrase inhibitor).
- For HAPE: oxygen, furosemide (diuretic), morphine (narcotic pain reliever).
- For HACE: corticosteroids.

ACTIVITY

If any altitude illness occurs, your child should decrease activity to a level at which symptoms disappear. The child can resume activity gradually upon returning to normal altitude.

DIET & FLUIDS

No special diet.

OK FOR SCHOOL, PRESCHOOL, OR NURSERY?

Yes, when condition and sense of well-being will allow.

CALL YOUR DOCTOR IF

- Your child has symptoms of any altitude illness.
- New, unexplained symptoms develop. Drugs used in treatment may produce side effects.

AMEBIASIS
(Amebic Dysentery; Entamebiasis)

GENERAL INFORMATION

DESCRIPTION

Amebiasis is a parasitic infection of the large intestine. Body parts involved include the intestinal tract, especially the colon, and the liver (sometimes). It is contagious from one person to another, such as food handlers or family members.
Appropriate health care includes:
- Self-care after diagnosis.
- Physician's monitoring of general condition and medications.
- Hospitalization (severe cases only).

SIGNS & SYMPTOMS

- Fever.
- Intermittent diarrhea with bad-smelling stools. Diarrhea is often preceded by constipation in early stages.
- Gas and abdominal bloating.
- Abdominal cramps and tenderness.
- Mucus and blood in the stool (sometimes).
- Fatigue.
- Muscle aches.

If the liver is involved:
- Tenderness over the liver and right side of the abdomen.
- Jaundice (sometimes).

CAUSES

A microscopic parasite that is spread by flies, cockroaches and direct contact with hands or food contaminated with feces. The most common sources of infection are:
- Food handlers.
- Faulty plumbing in hotels or other places.
- Raw vegetables or fruit fertilized with human feces or washed in polluted water.

RISK FACTORS

- Crowded or unsanitary living conditions.
- Travel to a foreign country.

PREVENTING COMPLICATIONS OR RECURRENCE

- Warn your child to wash hands frequently—always before eating.
- If you or your child are in an area where food or water may be contaminated, the following measures are necessary:
  - — Boil drinking water for 5 minutes.
  - — Don't use water that may contain raw sewage for any purpose.
  - — Don't eat unpeeled fruit or vegetables and raw fish or shellfish.

OTHER

Many people—especially those who live in temperate climates—harbor the amoeba without symptoms. Symptoms occur when the parasite invades tissues of the colon. Symptoms may be very vague.

AMEBIASIS (Amebic Dysentery; Entamebiasis)

WHAT TO EXPECT

MEDICAL TESTS

- Your own observation of symptoms.
- Medical history and physical exam by a doctor.
- Laboratory studies of stool and blood serum.
- Sigmoidoscopy (see Glossary).
- X-rays of lower bowel (barium enema).

POSSIBLE COMPLICATIONS

Peritonitis; hepatitis or liver abscess; lung abscess; infection of the pericardium; brain abscess.

PROBABLE OUTCOME

In most cases without complications, amebiasis is curable in 3 weeks with treatment. In the carrier state, this disease may not cause any symptoms. In severe cases, it may cause dysentery that requires hospital treatment.

TREATMENT

HOME CARE

Be extra careful about personal cleanliness. The child should bathe frequently and wash hands with warm water and soap after each bowel movement and before handling food.

MEDICATION

- Your doctor may prescribe an anti-amoeba drug such as metronidazole, paromomycin, emetine, or diiodohydroxyquin (iodoquinol).

ACTIVITY

The child should rest in bed during an acute attack and may resume normal activities when fever disappears and diarrhea improves.

DIET & FLUIDS

Soft diet progressing to normal diet.

OK FOR SCHOOL, PRESCHOOL, OR NURSERY?

When diarrhea has stopped for 24 hours or more.

CALL YOUR DOCTOR IF

- Your child has symptoms of amebiasis.
- The following occur during treatment: abdominal cramps continue longer than 24 hours; diarrhea or blood in stool increases; vomiting begins; pain begins over liver, or jaundice occurs; a skin rash appears; irritability or a severe headache develop.

ORRHEA, PRIMARY

GENERAL INFORMATION

DESCRIPTION

Primary amenorrhea means the absence of menstruation in a young woman who has passed puberty, is at least 16 years old, and has never menstruated. The endocrine and reproductive systems are involved.

Appropriate health care includes:

- Self-care after diagnosis.
- Doctor's treatment.
- Psychotherapy or counseling, if your daughter's amenorrhea is stress-related or results from eating disorders.
- Surgery (minor) to create an opening in the hymen, if necessary.
- Surgery to correct abnormalities of your daughter's reproductive system (sometimes).

SIGNS & SYMPTOMS

Lack of menstrual periods after puberty. Most girls begin menstruating by age 14.

CAUSES

Usually unknown. Possible causes include:

- Congenital abnormalities, such as the absence or abnormal formation of female organs (vagina, uterus, ovaries).
- Intact hymen (membrane covering the vaginal opening) that has no opening to allow passage of menstrual flow.
- Disorders (tumors, infections, or lack of maturation) of the endocrine system.
- Chromosome disorders.
- Emotional distress.
- Eating disorders, including obesity, bulimia, anorexia nervosa, excessive dieting, or starvation.
- Use of certain drugs, including mind-altering drugs, sedatives, and hormones.
- Participation in highly competitive, strenuous athletic activities.
- Pregnancy following intercourse prior to the first menstrual period.

RISK FACTORS

- Stress; use of drugs, including oral contraceptives, anticancer drugs, barbiturates, narcotics, cortisone drugs, chlordiazepoxide, and reserpine.

PREVENTING COMPLICATIONS OR RECURRENCE

Instructions for your daughter:

- Don't use drugs unless prescribed for you by your doctor.
- Reduce athletic activities if they are too strenuous.
- Obtain medical treatment for any underlying disorder.

? WHAT TO EXPECT

MEDICAL TESTS

- Your own observation of symptoms.
- Medical history and physical exam by a doctor, including a pelvic exam.
- Laboratory studies, such as a buccal smear (cells scraped from inside the cheek for chromosome studies) and blood tests of hormone levels.

POSSIBLE COMPLICATIONS

Psychological distress about sexual development.

PROBABLE OUTCOME

The absence of menstruation is not a health risk. It is usually curable with hormone treatment or removal of the underlying cause. Most doctors are reluctant to begin treatment before your daughter reaches age 18 unless the cause can be identified and treated safely. Causes which sometimes cannot be corrected include chromosome disorders and abnormalities of the reproductive system.

TREATMENT

HOME CARE

Instructions for your daughter:

- If you have emotional stress or conflicts in your life, ask family, friends or competent counselors to help you resolve them.
- Don't use mood-altering, mind-altering, stimulant, or sedative drugs.

MEDICATION

- Your doctor may prescribe progesterone (hormone) treatment to induce bleeding. If bleeding begins when progesterone is withdrawn, your daughter's reproductive system is functioning. This also indicates that pituitary disease is unlikely. If progesterone withdrawal does not induce bleeding, gonad stimulants such as clomiphene or gonadotrophins may be used for the same purpose.
- See Medications section for information regarding medicines your doctor may prescribe.

ACTIVITY

No restrictions. Your daughter should exercise regularly, but not to excess. She should sleep at least 8 hours every night.

DIET & FLUIDS

Your daughter should eat 3 well-balanced meals a day. If your daughter believes she is overweight, tell your doctor. Urge her not to lose weight by crash-dieting. She should avoid alcohol and should not take vitamin and mineral supplements unless your doctor prescribes them.

OK FOR SCHOOL, PRESCHOOL, OR NURSERY?

When appetite returns and alertness, strength, and feeling of well-being will allow.

CALL YOUR DOCTOR IF

- Your daughter is 16 years old and has never had a period.
- Your daughter's periods don't begin in 6 months, despite treatment.

AMENORRHEA, SECONDARY

GENERAL INFORMATION

DESCRIPTION

Secondary amenorrhea means the cessation of menstruation for at least 3 months in a female who has previously menstruated. The condition occurs only in females from puberty to menopause. The endocrine and reproductive systems are involved. Appropriate health care includes: self-care after diagnosis; doctor's treatment; dilatation and curettage (D & C, see Glossary); psychotherapy or counseling, if the amenorrhea is stress-related.

SIGNS & SYMPTOMS

Absence of menstrual periods for 3 or more months in a female who has menstruated at least once.

CAUSES

- Pregnancy (if your daughter has had sexual intercourse).
- Breast-feeding an infant.
- Discontinuing use of birth-control pills.
- Emotional stress or psychological disorder.
- Surgical removal of the ovaries or uterus.
- Disorder of the endocrine system, including the pituitary, hypothalamus, thyroid, parathyroid, adrenal, and ovarian glands.
- Diabetes mellitus.
- Tuberculosis.
- Obesity, anorexia nervosa, or bulimia.
- Strenuous program of physical exercise, such as long-distance running.

RISK FACTORS

Stress; poor nutrition; use of certain drugs, such as narcotics, phenothiazines, reserpine, or hormones.

PREVENTING COMPLICATIONS OR RECURRENCE

- If your daughter's amenorrhea is caused by an underlying disease, such as tuberculosis, diabetes, or anorexia nervosa, obtain treatment for the primary disorder.
- If the cause of your daughter's amenorrhea is unknown, there are no specific preventive measures.

WHAT TO EXPECT

MEDICAL TESTS

- Your own observation of symptoms.
- Medical history and physical exam by a doctor.
- Laboratory studies, such as a pregnancy test, blood studies of hormone levels, and Pap smear (see Glossary).
- Surgical diagnostic procedures, such as laparoscopy or hysteroscopy (see Glossary for both).
- Therapeutic trial of progesterone. If bleeding occurs after progesterone is withdrawn, ovulation is occurring.

POSSIBLE COMPLICATIONS

None expected if no serious underlying cause can be discovered.

PROBABLE OUTCOME

Amenorrhea is not a threat to your daughter's health. Whether it can be corrected varies with the underlying cause:

- If from pregnancy or breast-feeding, menstruation will resume when these conditions cease.
- If from discontinuing use of oral contraceptives, periods should begin in 2 months to 2 years.
- If from endocrine disorders, hormone replacement usually causes periods to resume.
- If from eating disorders, successful treatment of the disorder is necessary for menstruation to resume.
- If from diabetes or tuberculosis, menstruation may never resume.
- If from strenuous exercise, periods usually resume when exercise decreases.

TREATMENT

HOME CARE

See Appendix 19 for suggestions to reduce your daughter's stress.

MEDICATION

- Your doctor may prescribe hormone replacement therapy.
- See Medications section for information regarding medicines your doctor may prescribe.

ACTIVITY

No restrictions.

DIET & FLUIDS

No special diet.

OK FOR SCHOOL, PRESCHOOL, OR NURSERY?

When appetite returns and alertness, strength, and feeling of well-being will allow.

CALL YOUR DOCTOR IF

- Your daughter's periods have ceased for 3 or more months.
- Periods don't resume in 6 months, despite treatment.
- New, unexplained symptoms develop. Hormones used in treatment may produce side effects.

ANAL FISSURE

GENERAL INFORMATION

DESCRIPTION

An anal fissure represents splitting or tearing of sensitive anal tissue. Anal fissures can affect both sexes, all ages, but are most common in infants and young children. This affects more females than males.

Appropriate health care includes:

- Home care.
- Physician's monitoring of general condition and medications.
- Surgery to remove the fissure or to alter the muscle that contracts and prevents normal healing.

SIGNS & SYMPTOMS

- Sharp pain with passage of a hard or bulky stool.
- Streaks of blood on the toilet paper, underwear, or diaper.
- Itching around the rectum.

CAUSES

Stretching of the anus from a large, hard stool.

RISK FACTORS

- Constipation.

PREVENTING COMPLICATIONS OR RECURRENCE

Your child can avoid constipation by:

- Drinking at least 8 glasses of water daily.
- Eating a diet high in fiber.
- Using stool softeners or other laxatives, if needed (rare).

WHAT TO EXPECT

MEDICAL TESTS

- Your own observation of symptoms.
- Medical history and physical exam by a doctor.
- Examination of the anus and rectum with an anoscope or sigmoidoscope to rule out other causes of anal or rectal bleeding.

POSSIBLE COMPLICATIONS

Permanent scarring that prevents normal bowel movements.

PROBABLE OUTCOME

Most infants and young children recover after the stool is softened.

TREATMENT

HOME CARE

The following should be done to prevent constipation in children until the fissure heals:

• For infants: Before bedtime, fill a rubber ear syringe with plain mineral oil. Gently insert the tip and squeeze the mineral oil into the infant's rectum. Repeat the next morning. If no bowel movement occurs, repeat at noon. After the bowel movement, clean the anus gently with cotton and water.

• For older children: Gently squeeze 4 ounces of mineral oil into the rectum. Use a sanitary napkin to catch oil that seeps out in the night.

• To relieve muscle spasms and pain around the anus, apply a warm towel to the area.

• Sitz baths also relieve pain. Use 8 inches of very warm water 2 or 3 times a day for 10 to 20 minutes. Be careful not to burn a young child.

MEDICATION

• For minor pain, use non-prescription drugs, such as acetaminophen or topical anesthetics.

• After sitz baths, apply a non-prescription ointment containing zinc oxide to help heal the fissure.

• Use mineral oil as a laxative for infants. Give the infant 1 teaspoon by mouth for each 10 pounds of body weight. Repeat each day for about 2 weeks after blood disappears from the stool.

• After giving mineral oil, wait several hours to give vitamins. Mineral oil interferes with the absorption of vitamins and other nutrients.

ACTIVITY

No restrictions. Physical activity reduces the likelihood of constipation.

DIET & FLUIDS

Encourage a high-fiber diet and extra fluids to prevent constipation.

OK FOR SCHOOL, PRESCHOOL, OR NURSERY?

Yes, unless pain is too severe during treatment.

CALL YOUR DOCTOR IF

Your child has symptoms of an anal fissure—especially pain—that persists despite treatment.

ANAPHYLAXIS (Allergic Shock)

GENERAL INFORMATION

DESCRIPTION

Anaphylaxis is a severe allergic response to medications and many other allergy-causing substances. Blood vessels throughout the body, the heart, the lungs, and the skin are involved.

Appropriate health care includes:

Doctor's treatment and hospitalization (sometimes).

SIGNS & SYMPTOMS

Any of the following may occur within seconds or a few minutes after exposure to a substance to which your child is very allergic:

- Tingling or numbness around the mouth.
- Sneezing.
- Itching all over, often accompanied by hives.
- Watery eyes.
- Tightness in the chest and difficult breathing.
- Swelling or itching in the mouth or throat.
- Pounding heart.
- Faintness.
- Loss of consciousness.

Not all symptoms occur. Seek immediate help for any.

CAUSES

Eating or receiving injections of something to which the child is sensitive. The allergic response to neutralize or get rid of the material results in a life-threatening overreaction. Things which cause reactions most often include:

- Medication of all types, especially penicillin. Injections are much riskier than oral medications.
- Stings or bites from insects, such as bees, biting ants, and some spiders.
- Injected chemicals used in some types of X-ray studies.
- Foods, especially eggs, beans, seafood, and fruit.

RISK FACTORS

- A previous mild allergic response to things listed above.
- Medical history of eczema, hay fever or asthma.

PREVENTING COMPLICATIONS OR RECURRENCE

If your child has an allergic history:

- Tell your doctor before accepting any medication. Before your child is given a shot, ask what it is.
- Keep an anaphylaxis kit, such as Ana-Kit, with you at all times. Be sure your family knows how to use the kit if anyone has a reaction.
- Have your child wear a Medic-Alert bracelet or pendant (see Glossary) warning about allergies.
- Always remain in your doctor's office 15 minutes after your child receives any injection. Report any symptoms immediately.

ANAPHYLAXIS (Allergic Shock)

WHAT TO EXPECT

MEDICAL TESTS

- Your own observation of symptoms.
- Medical history and physical exam by a doctor.
- Laboratory skin tests to determine sensitivities.
- Blood and urine tests.

POSSIBLE COMPLICATIONS

Without prompt treatment, anaphylaxis causes shock, cardiac arrest, and death.

PROBABLE OUTCOME

Full recovery with prompt treatment.

TREATMENT

HOME CARE

- If you observe signs of anaphylaxis in your child and breathing stops:
  - — Yell for help. Don't leave the victim.
  - — Begin mouth-to-mouth breathing immediately.
  - — If there is no heartbeat, give external cardiac massage.
  - — Have someone call 0 (operator) or 911 (emergency) for an ambulance or medical help.
  - — Don't stop CPR until help arrives.
- Be alert to the possibility of a reaction when taking any medicine, and be prepared to respond quickly if symptoms occur. If your child has had a previous severe allergic reaction, always carry your anaphylaxis kit.

MEDICATION

- Adrenalin by injection is the only effective immediate treatment.
- Aminophylline, cortisone drugs, or antihistamines—given after the adrenalin—help prevent the return of acute symptoms.

ACTIVITY

Your child can resume normal activities as soon as symptoms improve after an attack. Observe him for 24 hours in case symptoms recur.

DIET & FLUIDS

Have the child avoid foods to which he is allergic.

OK FOR SCHOOL, PRESCHOOL, OR NURSERY?

Not until all symptoms resolve.

CALL YOUR DOCTOR IF

- Your child has symptoms of anaphylaxis. This is an emergency!
- New, unexplained symptoms develop. Drugs used in treatment may produce side effects.

ANEMIA, APLASTIC

GENERAL INFORMATION

DESCRIPTION

Aplastic anemia is a serious disease characterized by decreased bone-marrow production of blood cells. The bone marrow, lymphatic system, and blood are involved. Appropriate health care includes:

- Physician's monitoring of general condition and medications.
- Surgery to transplant bone marrow. A bone-marrow transplant requires a donor with compatible antigens. A twin, brother or sister usually makes the best donor. Donated marrow is injected gradually into the patient's veins to try to replace poorly functioning bone marrow with normal cells.
- Hospitalization for isolation until the body can resist infection.

SIGNS & SYMPTOMS

- Paleness.
- Weakness, tiredness, faintness, and breathlessness.
- Frequent infections.
- Spontaneous bleeding from the nose, mouth, rectum, vagina, gums, and other sites—including the central nervous system.
- Red dots of bleeding under the skin.
- Unexplained bruising.
- Ulcers in the mouth, throat, and rectum.

CAUSES

- Poor bone-marrow function. Bone marrow is often infiltrated with fat cells, which supplant areas that manufacture blood cells. Infections occur because of reduced white cells, which normally protect against infection.
- Half of all cases are caused by drugs, especially immunosuppressive drugs, anti-cancer drugs, chloramphenicol, or chemicals such as benzene. Other cases probably result from immunodeficiency, severe illness, or unidentifiable causes.

RISK FACTORS

- Family history of aplastic anemia.
- Genetic factors, such as those associated with congenital hypoplastic anemia (see Glossary).
- Use of drugs listed as causes.
- Recent severe illness.

PREVENTING COMPLICATIONS OR RECURRENCE

- The child should avoid prolonged exposure to toxic compounds, such as benzene, that are used in many industrial chemicals.
- Don't use drugs that cause aplastic anemia, if substitute drugs are available.

WHAT TO EXPECT

MEDICAL TESTS

- Your own observation of symptoms.
- Medical history and physical exam by a doctor.
- Laboratory studies of blood and bone marrow.

POSSIBLE COMPLICATIONS

Poor response to treatment, resulting in uncontrollable infections and bleeding. Complications are fatal in 50% to 70% of those with severe aplastic anemia.

PROBABLE OUTCOME

If the cause can be identified and treated successfully, the disorder is curable. Anemia caused by immunosuppressive drugs usually improves spontaneously when drugs are withdrawn. Full recovery often requires 6 to 8 months.

TREATMENT

HOME CARE

- Hair loss often accompanies treatment, and may require wearing a wig temporarily.
- Keep the child's mouth scrupulously clean to decrease the chance of infection. Brush often with a soft toothbrush. Rinse the mouth with a solution of equal parts hydrogen peroxide and water, or use a medicated mouthwash, if prescribed.

MEDICATION

Your doctor may prescribe:

- Immunosuppressive drugs to prevent rejection, if a bone-marrow transplant is necessary.
- Antibiotics to prevent or treat infection.
- Medicated mouthwash to suppress fungus infections.
- See Medications section for information regarding medicines your doctor may prescribe.

ACTIVITY

The child may resume normal activities after treatment.

DIET & FLUIDS

No special diet. Your child may need iron and vitamin supplements. Ask your doctor.

OK FOR SCHOOL, PRESCHOOL, OR NURSERY?

When signs of infection have decreased, appetite returns, and alertness, strength, and feeling of well-being will allow.

CALL YOUR DOCTOR IF

- Your child has symptoms of aplastic anemia.
- The following occurs after a bone-marrow transplant:
  — Fever.
  — Any sign of infection, such as swelling anywhere on the body. Redness, tenderness or pain may not be present.
  — Skin rash.
  — Jaundice (yellow skin and eyes).
  — Joint pain.
  — Puffy feet and ankles.
  — Urinary discomfort.
  — Decreased urine during any 24-hour period.

ANEMIA, FOLIC-ACID DEFICIENCY (Megaloblastic Anemia)

GENERAL INFORMATION

DESCRIPTION

Folic-acid anemia is a deficiency in the oxygen carrying capacity of the blood. It affects the blood cells, which transport oxygen to all body parts. Folic-acid anemia affects both sexes, especially infants and adolescents.

Appropriate health care includes:

- Self-care after diagnosis.
- Physician's monitoring of general condition and medications.

SIGNS & SYMPTOMS

- Fatigue and weakness.
- Red, sore tongue.
- Paleness.
- Shortness of breath.
- Nausea, vomiting, and diarrhea.

CAUSES

- Complication of pregnancy, when the body needs 8 times more folic acid than usual.
- Inadequate intake or absorption of foods with a high folic acid content, such as meat, poultry, fish, cheese, milk, eggs, green vegetables, yeast, and mushrooms.
- Alcoholism.
- Overcooking foods, which destroys folic acid.
- Deficiency of vitamin B-12 or vitamin C.

RISK FACTORS

- Pregnancy.
- Illness, such as tropical sprue, psoriasis, acne rosacea, eczema or dermatitis herpetiformis.
- Fad diets or general poor nutrition, especially vitamin C deficiency.
- Surgical removal of the stomach.
- Smoking, which decreases vitamin C absorption. Vitamin C is necessary for folic-acid absorption.
- Use of certain drugs, such as oral contraceptives, anti-convulsants, methotrexate, or triamterene.

PREVENTING COMPLICATIONS OR RECURRENCE

Advice for your child or adolescent:

- Don't drink alcohol.
- Eat well. Include fresh vegetables, meat, and other animal proteins. Avoid fad diets. Don't overcook food.
- Don't smoke. Smoking increases vitamin requirements.
- Have regular medical checkups during pregnancy. Take prenatal vitamin supplements, if they are prescribed.

ANEMIA, FOLIC-ACID DEFICIENCY (Megaloblastic Anemia)

? WHAT TO EXPECT

MEDICAL TESTS

- Your own observation of symptoms.
- Medical history and physical exam by a doctor.
- Laboratory blood studies.

POSSIBLE COMPLICATIONS

- Increased susceptibility to infection.
- Congestive heart failure.

PROBABLE OUTCOME

Usually curable in 3 weeks with an adequate folic-acid intake.

TREATMENT

HOME CARE

- If your adolescent smokes, it is important to stop.
- If your daughter takes oral contraceptives, she should consider using another form of contraception.
- Your child's mouth should be kept scrupulously clean by using mild or diluted mouthwash and a soft toothbrush.

MEDICATION

Your doctor may prescribe:

- Folic-acid supplements. Have the child continue taking them after symptoms improve.
- Iron supplements to take orally.
- See Medications section for information regarding medicines your doctor may prescribe.

ACTIVITY

No restrictions.

DIET & FLUIDS

No special diet. The child should eat foods daily that are high in folic acid. The liver can store folic acid for a limited time only.

OK FOR SCHOOL, PRESCHOOL, OR NURSERY?

When appetite has returned and alertness, strength, and feeling of well-being will allow.

CALL YOUR DOCTOR IF

- Your child has symptoms of anemia.
- Symptoms don't improve in 2 weeks despite treatment.
- Symptoms of infection (fever, chills, and muscle aches) occur during treatment.

ANEMIA, HEMOLYTIC

GENERAL INFORMATION

DESCRIPTION

Hemolytic anemia develops due to the premature destruction of mature red blood cells. The bone marrow cannot produce red blood cells fast enough to compensate for those being destroyed. This is not contagious. The blood, bone marrow, and spleen are involved.

Appropriate health care includes:

- Physician's monitoring of general condition and medications.
- Hospitalization for transfusions during a hemolytic crisis.
- Surgery to remove an enlarged spleen (sometimes).

SIGNS & SYMPTOMS

- Fatigue.
- Shortness of breath.
- Irregular heartbeat.
- Jaundice (yellow skin and eyes, dark urine).
- Enlarged spleen.

CAUSES

- An inherited disorder, such as hereditary spherocytosis, G6PD deficiency, sickle-cell anemia, or thalassemia.
- Antibodies produced by the child's body to fight infections, which for unknown reasons attack red blood cells. This response is sometimes triggered by blood transfusions.
- Use of medications, including non-prescription drugs, that damage the child's red blood cells.

RISK FACTORS

- Family history of hemolytic anemia.
- Use of any medication.

PREVENTING COMPLICATIONS OR RECURRENCE

- Don't give your child any medicine that has previously triggered hemolytic anemia.
- Seek genetic counseling before having children if you have a family history of hemolytic anemia (inherited forms).

WHAT TO EXPECT

MEDICAL TESTS

- Your own observation of symptoms.
- Medical history and physical exam by a doctor.
- Laboratory blood studies, including a blood count, examination of bone marrow, measurement with radioactive chromium of red cell survival, and other nuclear medicine studies.

POSSIBLE COMPLICATIONS

- Excessive spleen enlargement, which increases destruction of the child's red blood cells.
- Pain, shock, and serious illness caused by hemolysis (red blood cell destruction).
- Gallstones.

PROBABLE OUTCOME

- If hemolytic anemia is acquired, it can usually be cured when the cause, such as a drug, is removed. Sometimes the child's spleen is removed surgically.
- If hemolytic anemia is inherited, it is currently considered incurable. However, the child's symptoms can be relieved or controlled.
- Scientific research into causes and treatment continues, so there is hope for increasingly effective treatment and cure.

TREATMENT

HOME CARE

If your child must have the spleen removed, your surgeon will explain the procedure and what you need to do.

MEDICATION

Your doctor may prescribe:

- Immunosuppressive drugs to control the antibody response.
- Medication to reduce pain. For minor discomfort, use non-prescription drugs such as acetaminophen.
- See Medications section for information regarding medicines your doctor may prescribe.

ACTIVITY

After treatment, your child can resume normal activities as soon as possible.

DIET & FLUIDS

No special diet.

OK FOR SCHOOL, PRESCHOOL, OR NURSERY?

Yes, when appetite has returned and alertness, strength, and feeling of well-being will allow.

CALL YOUR DOCTOR IF

- Your child has symptoms of hemolytic anemia.
- The following occurs during treatment:
  - — Fever.
  - — Cough.
  - — Sore throat.
  - — Swollen joints.
  - — Muscle aches.
  - — Bloody urine.
  - — Signs of infection in any part of the child's body (redness, pain, swelling, fever).
- New, unexplained symptoms develop. Drugs used in treatment may produce side effects.

ANEMIA, IRON-DEFICIENCY

GENERAL INFORMATION

DESCRIPTION

Iron-deficiency anemia means a decreased number of circulating blood cells, or insufficient hemoglobin in the cells due to an inadequate supply of iron for optimal formation of red blood cells. Anemia is not a disease but is a symptom (as is fever) of other disorders. For proper treatment, the cause must be found. The blood, which affects all body cells, and the bone marrow are involved. Appropriate health care includes:

- Physician's monitoring of general condition and medications.
- Self-care after diagnosis.

SIGNS & SYMPTOMS

- Signs of pronounced anemia include tiredness and weakness; paleness, especially in the hands and lining of the lower eyelids.
- Less common signs include tongue inflammation; fainting; breathlessness; rapid heartbeat; unusual quietness or withdrawal; loss of appetite; abdominal discomfort; cravings for ice, paint, or dirt; susceptibility to infection.

CAUSES

- Decreased absorption of iron or increased need for iron. Causes in infants and children include poor nutrition (between 6 months and 2 years of age, children may consume large quantities of milk, to the exclusion of iron-containing foods); premature birth (premature babies often have low stores of iron at birth).
- Causes in adolescents include rapid growth spurts; heavy menstrual bleeding; pregnancy; malabsorption of iron; gastrointestinal disease with bleeding, including cancer.

RISK FACTORS

Poverty; recent illness, such as an ulcer, diverticulitis, colitis, hemorrhoids, or gastrointestinal tumors.

PREVENTING COMPLICATIONS OR RECURRENCE

Maintain an adequate iron intake for your child through a well-balanced diet or iron supplements. Provide iron-fortified formula for bottle-fed infants. Most children under 2 should receive supplemental iron to prevent this anemia. Foods with high iron content include meat, fish, poultry, whole or enriched grain, and foods high in ascorbic acid (such as citrus).

WHAT TO EXPECT

MEDICAL TESTS

- Your own observation of symptoms.
- Medical history and physical exam by a doctor.
- Laboratory blood studies, especially of hematocrit (see Glossary), hemoglobin, and red-blood-cell counts.
- X-rays of the gastrointestinal tract.

POSSIBLE COMPLICATIONS

Failure to diagnose a bleeding malignancy.

ANEMIA, IRON-DEFICIENCY

PROBABLE OUTCOME

Usually curable with iron supplements if the underlying cause can be identified.

TREATMENT

HOME CARE

The most important part of treatment for iron-deficiency anemia is to correct the underlying cause. Iron deficiency can be treated well with iron supplements. Blood transfusions are sometimes prescribed, *but they should be unnecessary, except in rare instances.* Your child should avoid crowds and other sources of infection as much as possible.

MEDICATION

Your doctor may prescribe iron supplements. Have your child follow these instructions for best absorption:

- Take iron on an empty stomach (at least 1/2 hour before meals). If it upsets your stomach, take it with a small amount of food (except milk).
- If you take other medications, wait at least 2 hours after taking iron before taking them. Antacids and tetracyclines especially interfere with iron absorption.
- Because liquid iron supplements may discolor the teeth, drink any liquid iron preparation through a straw. Iron supplements may also cause black bowel movements, diarrhea, or constipation.

Instructions for parents:

- Continue iron supplements 2 to 3 months after blood tests are normal.
- Too much iron is dangerous. A bottle of iron tablets can poison a child. Keep iron supplements out of the reach of young children.

ACTIVITY

No restrictions.

DIET & FLUIDS

- Limit your child's milk intake to 1 pint a day (do not limit milk for infants whose diet is solely milk). Milk interferes with iron absorption.
- Encourage your child to eat protein- and iron-containing foods, including meat, beans, and leafy green vegetables.
- Increase dietary fiber to prevent constipation.
- Try to provide favorite foods and keep your child company while eating.

OK FOR SCHOOL, PRESCHOOL, OR NURSERY?

- When signs of the condition have decreased, appetite returns, and alertness, strength, and feeling of well-being will allow.
- Have your child pace activities and rest until anemia is cured.

CALL YOUR DOCTOR IF

- Your child has symptoms of anemia.
- Nausea, vomiting, severe diarrhea, or constipation occur during treatment.

ANEMIA RELATED TO EXERCISE

GENERAL INFORMATION

DESCRIPTION

Anemia related to exercise refers to a decreased number of circulating red blood cells, or insufficient hemoglobin in the cells, caused by participation in exercise. Anemia is also a symptom of other disorders and may interfere with athletic performance. For proper treatment, the cause must be found. Appropriate health care includes doctor's diagnosis and treatment.

SIGNS & SYMPTOMS

Signs of pronounced anemia:

- Decreased performance in maximum-effort activities.
- Tiredness and weakness.
- Paleness, especially in the child's hands and the lining of the lower lids.

Less common signs:

- Tongue inflammation.
- Fainting.
- Breathlessness.
- Excessively rapid heartbeat with exercise.
- Loss of appetite.

CAUSES

- Participation in exercise such as prolonged walking, running, or cross-country skiing. The forces exerted on the red blood cells in the capillaries of the feet may rupture the blood cells and lead to anemia.
- Other heavy physical exercise and exertion.

RISK FACTORS

- Heavy menstrual bleeding.
- Pregnancy.
- Rapid growth phase.
- Malabsorption of iron from food.
- Profuse sweating.
- Recent illness with bleeding, such as an ulcer, diverticulitis, colitis, hemorrhoids, or gastrointestinal tumor.

PREVENTING COMPLICATIONS OR RECURRENCE

Your child should maintain an adequate iron intake by eating a well-balanced diet or taking iron supplements.

WHAT TO EXPECT

MEDICAL TESTS

- Your own observation of symptoms.
- Medical history and physical exam by a doctor.
- Laboratory blood studies every 2 months while the child is involved in vigorous physical activity. Tests should include studies of hematocrit (see Glossary), hemoglobin, and red blood cell counts.
- X-rays of the child's gastrointestinal tract.

POSSIBLE COMPLICATIONS

- Failure to diagnose a bleeding malignancy.
- Without treatment, increasing weakness and eventual congestive heart failure.

PROBABLE OUTCOME

Usually curable with iron supplements if the underlying cause can be identified and treated. Unless anemia is severe, your child may continue training and vigorous physical activity while under treatment with iron supplements for anemia.

TREATMENT

HOME CARE

None except for the child to take iron supplements.

MEDICATION

Your doctor may prescribe iron supplements with the following instructions for your child:

- Take iron on an empty stomach (at least 1/2 hour before meals) for best absorption. If it upsets your stomach, you may take it with a small amount of food (except milk).
- If you take other medications, wait at least 2 hours after taking iron before taking them. Antacids and tetracycline especially interfere with iron absorption.
- Continue iron supplements until 2 to 3 months after blood tests return to normal.

Note: Too much iron is dangerous. A bottle of iron tablets can poison a child. Keep iron supplements out of the reach of young children.

ACTIVITY

No restrictions for your child unless the exercise-induced anemia is severe. Then the child should reduce activity level slightly while undergoing treatment and continue at a slower pace until iron levels are back to normal.

DIET & FLUIDS

- Consult your doctor about limiting your child's milk consumption. Milk interferes with iron absorption.
- Serve the child protein foods and iron-containing foods, including meat, beans, and leafy green vegetables.
- Increase fiber in the child's diet to prevent constipation (a common side effect of iron supplements).

OK FOR SCHOOL, PRESCHOOL, OR NURSERY?

Yes, when condition and sense of well-being will allow.

CALL YOUR DOCTOR IF

- Your child has symptoms of anemia.
- Nausea, vomiting, severe diarrhea, or constipation occur during treatment.

ANKLE SPRAIN

GENERAL INFORMATION

DESCRIPTION

A mild ankle sprain involves stretching and slight or partial tearing of one or more ligaments in the ankle. The ligaments that support the ankle joint; the three main bones of the ankle joint; and the blood vessels, nerves, periosteum (covering of the bone), and other soft tissue close to the injury are involved. Appropriate health care includes: doctor's care only if discomfort is great or doesn't improve in 24 hours; self-care after diagnosis; whirlpool, ultrasound, or massage.

SIGNS & SYMPTOMS

- Ankle pain at the time of injury.
- A feeling of popping or tearing in the outer part of the ankle.
- Mild tenderness at the injury site.
- Little loss of function. The injured child can bear weight and walk without help for 30 minutes or so following injury. Then, depending on the extent of injury, the joint may seem to lose some of its stability.
- Swelling in the child's ankle.
- Little or no visible bruising for several hours after injury. Then some bruising may appear.

CAUSES

Stress imposed from either side of the ankle joint, temporarily forcing or prying the ankle or heel bone out of its normal socket. The ligaments that normally hold the joint in place are stretched and sometimes torn.

RISK FACTORS

- Previous ankle injury or any sport in which sideways displacement of the ankle is likely. Runners, walkers, and participants in such sports as basketball, soccer, volleyball, skiing, distance jumping and high jumping are prone to ankle sprains. When jumping, they often accidentally land on the side of the foot.
- Poor muscle strength or conditioning and walking or running on rough surfaces, such as roads with potholes.
- Poorly fitting shoes or footwear.

PREVENTING COMPLICATIONS OR RECURRENCE

Instructions for your child:
Build your strength or conditioning; warm up before practice or competition; tape the ankle from midfoot to midcalf before practice or competition. If you cannot use tape, wrap the ankle with elastic bandages or use an elastic brace; wear proper protective shoes. Provide your ankle with substantial support during sports activities for 12 months following any significant ankle injury.

WHAT TO EXPECT

MEDICAL TESTS

X-rays of the child's ankle, foot, and knee to rule out fractures.

POSSIBLE COMPLICATIONS

Prolonged healing time if the child resumes activity too soon; proneness to repeated injury; unstable or arthritic ankle joint following repeated injury.

PROBABLE OUTCOME

The full extent of the child's injury cannot be determined for 12 to 24 hours. A mild ankle sprain usually heals enough in 5 to 7 days to allow modified activity. Complete healing requires an average of 6 weeks.

TREATMENT

FIRST AID

The goal is to prevent further injury to the child's torn ligaments. Follow instructions for R.I.C.E., the first letters of *rest*, *ice*, *compression*, and *elevation*. See Appendix 39 for details.

HOME CARE

- Continue using an ice pack on the child's ankle 3 or 4 times a day. Wrap ice chips or cubes in a plastic bag. Wrap the bag in a moist towel, and place it over the injured area. Use for 20 minutes at a time.
- Provide the child with whirlpool treatments or time in a spa, if available.
- Keep the child's foot elevated whenever possible to decrease swelling.
- Massage the child's ankle gently and often to provide comfort and decrease swelling.

MEDICATION

- For minor discomfort use non-prescription medicines such as aspirin, acetaminophen, or ibuprofen.
- Your doctor may prescribe an injection of procaine and hyaluronidase to decrease pain soon after injury or stronger medicine for pain, if needed.

ACTIVITY

Except for very minor injuries, your child should walk with crutches for about 72 hours, then resume normal activities gradually.

DIET & FLUIDS

During recovery, your child should eat a well-balanced diet.

OK FOR SCHOOL, PRESCHOOL, OR NURSERY?

Yes, when condition and sense of well-being will allow.

CALL YOUR DOCTOR IF

Your child has symptoms of an ankle sprain that does not improve within 1 week or ankle pain, swelling, or bruising increase despite treatment.

ANKYLOSING SPONDYLITIS
(Marie-Strümpell Disease)

GENERAL INFORMATION

DESCRIPTION

Ankylosing spondylitis is a chronic, progressive disease of the joints, accompanied by inflammation and stiffening. It is characterized by a "bent forward" posture caused by stiffening of the spine and support structures. Body parts involved include the sacroiliac region, the hip joints, and the lumbar, thoracic and cervical spines. Ninety percent of all cases of ankylosing spondylitis begin in males after age 10.

Appropriate health care includes:

- Self-care after diagnosis.
- Physician's monitoring of general condition and medications.
- Surgery to replace a damaged hip or to insert bone grafts in the spine (advanced stages only).

SIGNS & SYMPTOMS

- Early stages: recurrent episodes of low backache; pain can also occur along the sciatic nerve; stiffness that is worse in the morning.
- Later stages: progressive worsening of symptoms; pain spreading from the low back to the middle back or higher in the neck; joint pain in the arms, legs, feet, and hands (sometimes).
- Anemia; muscle stiffness; fatigue; weight loss.

CAUSES

Unknown, but it may be caused by genetic changes or an autoimmune disorder.

RISK FACTORS

Family history of ankylosing spondylitis.

PREVENTING COMPLICATIONS OR RECURRENCE

No specific preventive measures.

WHAT TO EXPECT

MEDICAL TESTS

Your own observation of symptoms; medical history and physical exam by a doctor; laboratory blood studies; X-rays of the spine.

POSSIBLE COMPLICATIONS

Congestive heart failure; loss of vision; amyloidosis (see Glossary); heart-valve disease; gastrointestinal disease; lung disease; permanent disability and immobilization.

PROBABLE OUTCOME

- This disease is currently considered incurable. Symptoms progress slowly and unpredictably for 10 to 20 years, but they can be relieved or controlled.
- Life expectancy is reduced by the complications—not from the disease.
- Medical literature cites instances of unexplained recovery. Scientific research continues, so there is hope for increasingly effective treatment and cure.

ANKYLOSING SPONDYLITIS (Marie-Strümpell Disease)

TREATMENT

HOME CARE

Instructions for the patient:

- Sleep on your back on a firm mattress. Use a small pillow or none at all.
- Take hot baths or use heat compresses before exercising or to relieve pain.
- Avoid excessive rest *or* exhaustion.
- Have regular massages, if possible.
- Exercise to help maintain muscle strength and prevent deformity. (See Appendix 10 for instructions).

MEDICATION

Your doctor may prescribe non-steroidal anti-inflammatory drugs. Don't give your child narcotics for pain; they are addictive.

ACTIVITY

The child should stay as active as strength allows. Instructions for the patient: Exercise to maintain good posture and retain as much upright carriage as possible—back braces don't help. Swim regularly, if possible—your buoyancy in water will allow you to move stiff, painful areas more easily. Avoid activity that puts stress on the back.

DIET & FLUIDS

No special diet.

OK FOR SCHOOL, PRESCHOOL, OR NURSERY?

When alertness, strength, and feeling of well-being will allow.

CALL YOUR DOCTOR IF

- Your child has symptoms of ankylosing spondylitis.
- The following occurs during treatment:
  - — Temperature of 101F (38.3C) or higher. This may indicate the recurrence of an acute phase.
  - — Increasing pain and disability, despite measures outlined above.

ANORExIA NERVOSA

GENERAL INFORMATION

DESCRIPTION

Anorexia nervosa is a psychological eating disorder in which a person refuses to eat adequately—in spite of hunger—and loses enough weight to become emaciated. The illness usually begins with a normal weight-loss diet. The person eats very little, and refuses to stop dieting after a reasonable weight loss. Anorexia nervosa usually affects female adolescents.

Appropriate health care includes:

- Physician's monitoring of general condition and medications.
- Psychotherapy or counseling for the patient and family.
- Hospitalization during crises for intravenous or tube feeding.
- Psychiatric hospitalization (sometimes) for at least 2 to 3 weeks. May require many months, up to 2 years.

SIGNS & SYMPTOMS

- Weight loss of at least 25% of body weight without physical illness.
- High energy level despite body wasting.
- Intense fear of obesity.
- Depression.
- Loss of appetite.
- Constipation.
- Intolerance of cold temperature.
- Refusal to maintain a minimum standard weight for age and height.
- Distorted body image. The person continues to feel fat—even when emaciated.
- Cessation of menstrual periods.

CAUSES

Unknown. However, all people have family and internal conflicts to some degree, including sexual conflicts.

RISK FACTORS

- Peer pressure to be thin.
- History of slight overweight.
- Perfectionistic, compulsive, or overachieving personalities.
- Psychological stress.

PREVENTING COMPLICATIONS OR RECURRENCE

Encourage your child to confront personal problems realistically. Try to correct or cope with problems with the help of counselors, therapists, family, and friends. See Appendix 19 for suggestions to reduce stress.

WHAT TO EXPECT

MEDICAL TESTS

- Your own observation of symptoms.
- Medical history and physical exam by a doctor.
- Laboratory blood tests for anemia and electrolyte imbalance.

POSSIBLE COMPLICATIONS

- Chronic anorexia nervosa caused by the patient's resistance to treatment.
- Electrolyte disturbances or irregular heartbeat. These may be life-threatening to your child.

PROBABLE OUTCOME

Curable if the child recognizes the emotional disturbance, wants help and cooperates in treatment. Without treatment, anorexia nervosa can cause permanent disability and death. Persons with anorexia nervosa have a high rate of attempted suicide due to low self-esteem.

TREATMENT

HOME CARE

The goal of treatment is for the child to establish healthy eating patterns to regain normal weight. The patient can accomplish this with behavior-modification training supervised by a qualified professional.

MEDICATION

- Medicine usually is not necessary for this disorder.
- See Medications section for information regarding medicines your doctor may prescribe.

ACTIVITY

No restrictions, but your child should avoid overexertion.

DIET & FLUIDS

No special diet. Your doctor may prescribe vitamin and mineral supplements for your child.

OK FOR SCHOOL, PRESCHOOL, OR NURSERY?

When appetite returns, and alertness, strength, and feeling of well-being will allow.

CALL YOUR DOCTOR IF

- Your child has symptoms of anorexia nervosa.
- Life-threatening symptoms occur, including rapid irregular heartbeat, chest pain, or loss of consciousness. Call immediately. This is an emergency!
- Weight loss continues, despite treatment.

ANXIETY

GENERAL INFORMATION

DESCRIPTION

Anxiety is a vague, uncomfortable feeling of fear, dread, or danger from an unknown source. It is characterized by a *feeling* of apprehension, uncertainty, and fear. Some children become constantly anxious about everything. The central nervous system and endocrine system are involved. Anxiety can affect all ages, and is more common in females than males.

Appropriate health care includes:

- Self-care after diagnosis.
- Physician's monitoring of general condition and medications.
- Psychotherapy or counseling.

SIGNS & SYMPTOMS

- Feeling that something undesirable or harmful is about to happen.
- Dry mouth and swallowing difficulty or hoarseness.
- Rapid breathing and heartbeat.
- Twitching or trembling.
- Muscle tension and headaches.
- Appetite changes.
- Sweating.
- Nausea, diarrhea, and weight loss.
- Sleeplessness.
- Hyperventilation.
- Irritability.
- Fatigue.
- Nightmares.
- Frequent urination.
- Memory problems.
- Constant seeking of attention and reassurance.

CAUSES

Activation of the body's defense mechanisms for fight or flight. Excess adrenalin is discharged from the adrenal glands, and adrenalin breakdown products (catecholamines) eventually affect various parts of the body.

RISK FACTORS

- Stress from any source.
- Family history of neurosis.
- Fatigue or overwork.
- Recurrence of situations that have been previously stressful or harmful.

PREVENTING COMPLICATIONS OR RECURRENCE

Determine what stressful or potentially harmful situation is causing your child to feel anxious. Deal directly with it. Consider lifestyle changes to reduce your child's stress. See Appendix 19.

WHAT TO EXPECT

MEDICAL TESTS

- Your own observation of symptoms.
- Medical history and physical exam by a doctor.
- Laboratory studies to rule out medical conditions that produce anxiety, such as hyperthyroidism.

POSSIBLE COMPLICATIONS

- Untreated anxiety may lead to neuroses, such as phobias, compulsions, or hypochondriasis.
- A sudden increase in anxiety may lead to panic and violent escape behavior.

PROBABLE OUTCOME

Anxiety can be controlled with psychological therapy. Overcoming anxiety often results in a richer, more satisfying life.

TREATMENT

HOME CARE

- Obtain therapy for your child to understand the specific but unconscious threat or source of stress.
- Learn techniques, including biofeedback and relaxation therapy, to reduce muscle tension for the anxious child or any family members.

MEDICATION

Your doctor may prescribe tranquilizers for your child. These are useful for a short time under the following circumstances:

- During periods of unusually intense anxiety.
- Until psychological insights prevent anxiety from developing.
- Until direct action solves the threatening problem.
- See Medications section for information regarding medicines your doctor may prescribe.

ACTIVITY

Your child should stay active. Physical exertion helps reduce anxiety.

DIET & FLUIDS

No special diet. The child should avoid caffeine and other stimulants and alcohol.

OK FOR SCHOOL, PRESCHOOL, OR NURSERY?

When appetite has returned and alertness, strength, and feeling of well-being will allow.

CALL YOUR DOCTOR IF

- Your child has symptoms of anxiety, and self-treatment has failed.
- Your child has a sudden feeling of panic.
- New, unexplained symptoms develop. Drugs used in treatment may produce side effects.

APC DISEASE (Pharyngoconjunctival Fever)

GENERAL INFORMATION

DESCRIPTION

APC disease is an acute, contagious viral infection that affects the eyes, throat, and central nervous system. It can occur in epidemics in children. The conjunctivae (whites of the eyes) and the throat, including tonsils and adenoids, are involved. APC disease can affect both sexes, all ages, but is most common in children and adolescents from 1 to 15 years old.

Appropriate health care includes:

- Home care after diagnosis.
- Physician's monitoring of general condition and medications.

SIGNS & SYMPTOMS

- Sore throat with redness and enlarged tonsils and adenoids.
- High fever—usually 102F (38.9C) to 105 (40.6C).
- Pain and redness in the whites of the eyes. The inflammation usually begins in one eye and spreads to the other.
- Runny nose.
- Cough and chest pain (rare).

CAUSES

A virus infection of the respiratory tract. Summer epidemics are common. They are usually associated with swimming in pools or lakes—especially in summer camps. The incubation period is 5 to 8 days.

RISK FACTORS

- Crowded or unsanitary living conditions.
- Exposure to others in swimming pools and spas.

PREVENTING COMPLICATIONS OR RECURRENCE

- You and your child should wash hands frequently to avoid spreading the virus when touching others.
- Avoid swimming pools during epidemics.

WHAT TO EXPECT

MEDICAL TESTS

- Your own observation of symptoms.
- Medical history and physical exam by a doctor.
- Laboratory blood counts.

POSSIBLE COMPLICATIONS

Secondary bacterial infection, especially pneumonia.

PROBABLE OUTCOME

Spontaneous recovery within 7 days. The eye inflammation may be slow to heal, lasting up to 10 days longer than other symptoms.

APC DISEASE
(Pharyngoconjunctival Fever)

TREATMENT

HOME CARE

• Wipe mucus away from the eyes with a cotton pad moistened with water. No other eye treatment is necessary.
• Use a cool-mist humidifier to relieve the stuffy nose.
• Don't insert cotton swabs in a child's nostrils to clear them. Instead, catch the discharge outside the nostril on a tissue.

MEDICATION

• For minor discomfort, use non-prescription drugs such as acetaminophen to reduce fever and aching; nose drops to relieve nasal stuffiness; cough medicines with decongestants.
• Your doctor may prescribe eye drops; antiviral drugs; antibiotics for secondary bacterial infections.

ACTIVITY

Keep the patient isolated as long as the eyes are red. Avoiding unnecessary contacts protects others from infection and defends the patient from further infection. Complete bed rest is not necessary, but extra rest is helpful. The child should avoid vigorous activity.

DIET & FLUIDS

Increase fluid intake, including fruit juice, water, tea and carbonated drinks. Avoid milk, which thickens nasal secretions.

OK FOR SCHOOL, PRESCHOOL, OR NURSERY?

When signs of infection have decreased, appetite returns, and alertness, strength, and feeling of well-being will allow.

CALL YOUR DOCTOR IF

• Your child has symptoms of APC disease.
• The following occurs during treatment: fever that lasts several days; increased throat pain, or white or yellow spots on the throat; cough that lasts longer than 10 days; coughing episodes that last longer than non-coughing intervals, or cough that produces thick, yellow-green or gray sputum; labored breathing between coughing bouts; shaking chills; chest pain; shortness of breath; earache, headache, or pain in the teeth or over the sinuses; skin rash; extreme lethargy; excessive irritability or delirium; enlarged, tender neck glands; bluish or gray lips, nails, or skin.

APPENDICITIS

GENERAL INFORMATION

DESCRIPTION

Appendicitis is inflammation of the vermiform appendix, a small tube that extends from the cecum, the first part of the large intestine. The appendix has no known function, but it can become diseased. Appendicitis affects 1 in 500 people each year. The appendix, cecum, and peritoneum (the membrane covering the intestinal tract) are involved. Appendicitis is rare in children under 2. The peak incidence is between ages 15 and 24.

Appropriate health care includes:

- Physician's monitoring of general condition and medications.
- Surgery to remove the appendix. Because appendicitis can be hard to diagnose, surgery is often withheld until symptoms and signs progress enough to confirm the diagnosis.

SIGNS & SYMPTOMS

- Pain that begins close to the navel and migrates toward the right lower abdomen. The pain becomes persistent and well localized. It worsens with moving, breathing deeply, coughing, sneezing, walking, or being touched.
- Nausea and vomiting (sometimes).
- Constipation and inability to pass gas.
- Diarrhea (occasionally).
- Low fever, beginning after other symptoms.
- Tenderness in the right lower abdomen, usually about a third of the distance from the navel to the top of the hip bone. (This description applies only if the appendix is in its normal position. In some cases, the tip of the appendix is located elsewhere, making diagnosis difficult.)
- Abdominal swelling (late stages).
- Increased white blood cell count.

CAUSES

Infection for unknown reason, usually with bacteria from the intestinal tract. The appendix may become obstructed from contents moving through the intestinal tract or by a constricting band of tissue. When infected, it becomes swollen, inflamed, and filled with pus.

RISK FACTORS

Recent illness, especially a roundworm infestation or gastrointestinal virus infection.

PREVENTING COMPLICATIONS OR RECURRENCE

No specific preventive measures.

WHAT TO EXPECT

MEDICAL TESTS

- Your own observation of symptoms.
- Medical history and physical exam (maybe several) by a doctor.
- Laboratory blood studies. Tests usually show higher levels of white blood cells.
- Urinalysis to rule out a urinary-tract infection, which can mimic appendicitis.
- X-ray of the abdomen.

POSSIBLE COMPLICATIONS

- Rupture of the appendix, abscess formation, and peritonitis. This is most common in older persons, not children.
- Misdiagnosis because of few or atypical symptoms—especially in the very young (or very old).

PROBABLE OUTCOME

Usually curable with surgery. If totally untreated, a ruptured appendix is fatal.

TREATMENT

HOME CARE

- While the diagnosis is uncertain, take your child's rectal temperature every 2 hours. Keep a record for your doctor. Don't let the child eat or drink until the diagnosis is certain.

MEDICATION

Don't give your child any laxatives, enemas, or medicines for pain. Laxatives may cause rupture, and pain- or fever-reducers make diagnosis more difficult.

ACTIVITY

Your child should rest in a bed or chair until surgery.

DIET & FLUIDS

Don't let the patient eat or drink anything until appendicitis has been diagnosed. Anesthesia for surgery is much safer if the stomach is empty. If your child is very thirsty, wash his mouth out with water.

OK FOR SCHOOL, PRESCHOOL, OR NURSERY?

When signs of infection have decreased, appetite returns, and alertness, strength, and feeling of well-being will allow.

CALL YOUR DOCTOR IF

- Your child has symptoms of appendicitis.
- The following occurs while surgery is pending:
  - — Fever spikes (rises suddenly) to 102F (38.9C) or over.
  - — Continued vomiting.
  - — Increased pain in the abdomen.
  - — Fainting.
  - — Blood in the stool or vomit.

ARM CONTUSION, FOREARM

GENERAL INFORMATION

DESCRIPTION

An arm contusion refers to the bruising of the skin and underlying tissues of the forearm caused by a direct blow. Contusions cause bleeding from ruptured small capillaries, allowing blood to infiltrate muscles, tendons, or other soft tissue. The tissues of the forearm, including the blood vessels, muscles, tendons, and nerves, the covering of the bone (the periosteum), and the connective tissue are involved. Appropriate health care includes a doctor's care, unless the child's contusion is quite small; self-care for minor contusions and for serious contusions during rehabilitation; physical therapy for serious contusions.

SIGNS & SYMPTOMS

- Forearm swelling—either superficial or deep.
- Pain and tenderness in the child's forearm.
- Feeling of firmness when pressure is exerted on the injured area.
- Discoloration under the child's skin, beginning with redness and progressing to the characteristic "black and blue" bruise.
- Restricted forearm activity proportional to the extent of injury.

CAUSES

Direct blow to the forearm, usually from a blunt object.

RISK FACTORS

Violent contact sports, especially when the child's forearm is not adequately protected; medical history of any bleeding disorder such as hemophilia; poor nutrition, including vitamin deficiency; use of anticoagulants or aspirin.

PREVENTING COMPLICATIONS OR RECURRENCE

Your child should wear appropriate protective gear and equipment during competition or other athletic activity if there has been a recent contusion or if the activity makes a contusion likely.

WHAT TO EXPECT

MEDICAL TESTS

Your own observation of symptoms; medical history and physical exam by a doctor for all except minor injuries; X-rays of the injured area to assess total injury to the soft tissue and to rule out the possibility of underlying fracture. (The total extent of the child's injury may not be apparent for 48 to 72 hours.)

POSSIBLE COMPLICATIONS

- Excessive bleeding, leading to disability. Infiltrative-type bleeding can sometimes lead to calcification and impaired function of injured muscles and tendons.
- Decreased blood supply to forearm muscles, causing tissue death, loss of function, and contraction of affected muscles.
- Prolonged healing time if the child's usual activities are resumed too soon.
- Possible infection if the skin is broken over the contusion.

ARM CONTUSION, FOREARM

PROBABLE OUTCOME

Healing time varies with the extent of the child's injury, but the average healing time for forearm contusions is 2 to 3 weeks.

TREATMENT

FIRST AID

Use instructions for R.I.C.E., the first letter of *rest*, *ice*, *compression*, and *elevation*. See Appendix 39 for details.

HOME CARE

- Use a sling to immobilize the child's arm.
- Wrap an elasticized bandage over a felt pad on the injured area. Keep the area compressed for about 72 hours.
- Continue ice massage. Fill a large Styrofoam cup with water and freeze. Tear a small amount of foam from the top so ice protrudes. Massage gently over the injured area in a circle about the size of a softball. Do this for 15 minutes at a time, 3 or 4 times a day, and before workouts or competition.
- Massage gently and often to provide comfort and decrease swelling.

MEDICATION

- For minor discomfort use acetaminophen or ibuprofen; topical liniments and ointments.
- Your doctor may prescribe stronger medicine for pain.

ACTIVITY

Your child should begin activities slowly and stop exercise as soon as pain begins. The child can increase activity as healing progresses.

DIET & FLUIDS

No restrictions.

OK FOR SCHOOL, PRESCHOOL, OR NURSERY?

Yes, when condition and sense of well-being will allow.

CALL YOUR DOCTOR IF

- Your child has symptoms of a forearm contusion that doesn't improve within a day or two.
- The skin is broken and signs of infection (drainage, increasing pain, fever, headache, muscle aches, dizziness, or a general ill feeling) occur.

ARM FRACTURE, FOREARM

GENERAL INFORMATION

DESCRIPTION

An arm fracture is a complete or incomplete break in one or both bones of the forearm (the radius and the ulna). Appropriate health care includes doctor's treatment; hospitalization (sometimes) to set the fracture or to insert a metal plate that immobilizes broken bones.

SIGNS & SYMPTOMS

Severe arm pain at the time of injury; swelling of the soft tissue around the fracture; visible deformity if the fracture is complete and the bone fragments separate enough to distort the child's normal arm contours; tenderness to the touch; numbness and coldness in the child's lower arm and hand if the blood supply is impaired.

CAUSES

Direct blow or indirect stress to the child's bone. Indirect stress may be caused by twisting or violent muscle contraction.

RISK FACTORS

Contact sports, especially football, soccer, or hockey; history of bone or joint disease, especially osteoporosis; poor nutrition, especially calcium deficiency.

PREVENTING COMPLICATIONS OR RECURRENCE

Your child should build strength and protective muscle mass with an appropriate conditioning program. After an arm injury, the child should use padded arm splints for contact sports.

WHAT TO EXPECT

MEDICAL TESTS

Your own observation of symptoms; medical history and physical exam by a doctor; X-rays of injured areas, including the elbow above and the wrist below the primary injury site. In young people, X-rays of the normal side should be made for comparison.

POSSIBLE COMPLICATIONS

- At the time of injury: shock; pressure on or injury to nearby nerves, ligaments, tendons, muscles, blood vessels, or connective tissues.
- After treatment or surgery: delayed union or non-union of the fracture; impaired blood supply to the fracture site; avascular necrosis (death of bone cells) due to interruption of the blood supply; death of muscle cells if the arm swells inside the cast; arrest of a child's normal bone growth; infection in open fractures (skin broken over fracture site), or at the incision if surgical setting was necessary; shortening of the injured bones; proneness to repeated injury; unstable or arthritic wrist or elbow following repeated injury; prolonged healing time if the child resumes activity too soon; problems caused by casts.

PROBABLE OUTCOME

The average healing time for this fracture is 6 to 8 weeks in adolescents and adults and 5 to 6 weeks in children. Healing is complete when there is no motion at the fracture site and when X-rays show complete bone union.

TREATMENT

FIRST AID

- Keep the child warm with blankets to decrease the possibility of shock.
- Cut away clothing, if possible, but don't move the injured arm to do so.
- Follow instructions for R.I.C.E., the first letters of *rest*, *ice*, *compression*, and *elevation*. See Appendix 39 for details.
- The doctor will manipulate and set the child's broken bones with surgery or, if possible, without. Manipulation should be done as soon as possible after injury.

HOME CARE

- Immobilization is necessary. A rigid cast of plaster splints is placed around the child's injured arm to immobilize the elbow and wrist.
- After the child's cast is removed, use frequent ice massage. See Glossary.

MEDICATION

Your doctor may prescribe:

- Narcotic or synthetic narcotic pain relievers for severe pain.
- Stool softeners to prevent constipation due to inactivity.
- Acetaminophen (available without prescription) for mild pain after initial treatment.

ACTIVITY

Your child should actively exercise all muscle groups not immobilized. These muscle contractions hasten healing. The child can resume normal activities gradually after treatment, including reconditioning the injured arm, but should not drive until healing is complete.

DIET & FLUIDS

No restrictions after surgery.

OK FOR SCHOOL, PRESCHOOL, OR NURSERY?

Yes, when condition and sense of well-being will allow.

CALL YOUR DOCTOR IF

- Your child has signs or symptoms of a forearm fracture.
- Any of the following occur after surgery or other treatment: increased pain, swelling, or drainage in the surgical area; signs of infection (headache, muscle aches, dizziness, or a general ill feeling and fever); swelling above or below the cast; blue or gray skin color beyond the cast, particularly under the fingernails; numbness or complete loss of feeling below the fracture site; nausea or vomiting; constipation.

ARTHRITIS, INFECTIOUS
(Septic Arthritis)

GENERAL INFORMATION

DESCRIPTION

Infectious arthritis is an inflammation in a joint resulting from infection. Any joint may be involved, but it is most common in larger ones, such as the hip, or those subject to trauma, such as the knee or joints in the hands.

Appropriate health care includes:

- Physician's monitoring of general condition and medications.
- Hospitalization (frequently) for complete rest and intravenous antibiotics.
- Surgery to drain fluid or remove foreign material introduced by an injury.
- Physical therapy after recovery to regain full use of the joint.

SIGNS & SYMPTOMS

- Chills and fever (sometimes high).
- Redness, swelling, tenderness, and pain (often throbbing) in the affected joint. Pain sometimes spreads to other joints. It worsens with movement.
- Pain in the buttocks, thighs, or groin (sometimes).

CAUSES

Entry into a joint by germs, usually bacteria (streptococci, staphylococci, gonococci, hemophilus, or tubercle bacillus) or fungi. Germs gain entry from:

- Infection elsewhere in the body, as with gonorrhea or tuberculosis.
- Infection next to the joint, as with skin boils, cellulitis, or bone infection.
- Injury to the joint, including puncture wounds and skin abrasions.

RISK FACTORS

- Illness that has lowered resistance.
- Sexually transmitted infections.
- Diabetes mellitus.
- Rheumatoid arthritis.
- Use of immunosuppressive drugs.
- Joint surgery.
- Injections into joints.
- Excess alcohol consumption.
- Use of mind-altering drugs, especially those that are injected.
- Poor hygiene.

PREVENTING COMPLICATIONS OR RECURRENCE

- Protect your child's exposed joints, such as the knee, during activities involving injury risks.
- Obtain prompt medical treatment for your child's infections elsewhere in the body.

OTHER

The use of aspirin and other non-steroidal anti-inflammatory drugs for other disorders may suppress signs of joint inflammation, delaying diagnosis.

ARTHRITIS, INFECTIOUS
(Septic Arthritis)

? WHAT TO EXPECT

MEDICAL TESTS

- Your own observation of symptoms.
- Medical history and physical exam by a doctor.
- Laboratory studies, such as blood counts, blood culture, and culture of fluid from the infected joint.
- X-rays of affected joints.

POSSIBLE COMPLICATIONS

Misdiagnosis as gout or another non-infectious condition, delaying antibiotic treatment; blood poisoning; permanent joint damage.

PROBABLE OUTCOME

Usually curable with early diagnosis and treatment. Recovery takes weeks or months. Treatment delay may result in a badly damaged joint and loss of movement, requiring joint replacement.

TREATMENT

HOME CARE

No specific instructions except those listed under other headings.

MEDICATION

Your doctor may prescribe:

- Antibiotics (often intravenous). Don't discontinue giving your child antibiotics until your doctor recommends it. Infection may return after symptoms disappear.
- Codeine or narcotics for a short time to relieve pain.

ACTIVITY

Splints or casts may be necessary to rest the affected joint completely. Movement delays healing. After cure, physical therapy is often necessary to restore joint function. The child can resume normal activities gradually.

DIET & FLUIDS

No special diet.

OK FOR SCHOOL, PRESCHOOL, OR NURSERY?

When signs of infection have decreased, appetite returns, and alertness, strength, and feeling of well-being will allow.

CALL YOUR DOCTOR IF

- Your child has symptoms of joint infection. Call immediately.
- The following occurs during the illness: temperature spikes to 103F (39.4C); fatigue, headache, muscle aches, and sweating.
- New, unexplained symptoms develop. Drugs used in treatment may produce side effects.

ARTHRITIS, JUVENILE RHEUMATOID

GENERAL INFORMATION

DESCRIPTION

Juvenile rheumatoid arthritis is an inflammatory disease of connective tissue—mostly joints—that affects children. The joints—usually the knees, elbows, ankles, and neck are involved. It may also involve adjacent muscles, cartilage, and membranes lining the joints. Juvenile rheumatoid arthritis starts at 2 to 5 years and usually disappears by puberty. It is 4 times more frequent in girls. Appropriate health care includes:

- Home care after diagnosis.
- Physician's monitoring of general condition and medications.
- Psychotherapy or counseling to help the family cope with the child's long-term illness. Emotional support may be the most important factor in a child's treatment.
- Surgery to correct deformed joints (sometimes).

SIGNS & SYMPTOMS

- Pain, swelling, and stiffness in the toes, knees, ankles, elbows, shoulders, or neck joints. The pain may begin suddenly or gradually, and may involve only one or many joints. The child may refuse to walk without being able to explain why.
- Daily temperature rise to about 103F (39.4C)—usually in the evening. Fever is frequently accompanied by a body rash and chills.
- Poor appetite and weight loss.
- Anemia.
- Irritability and listlessness.
- Swollen lymph glands.
- Eye pain and redness.
- Chest pain (if the disease is severe enough to affect the heart).

CAUSES

Probably caused by an autoimmune disorder, in which the body's immune system attacks its own normal tissues. The first symptoms are often associated with physical or emotional stress.

RISK FACTORS

Stress.

PREVENTING COMPLICATIONS OR RECURRENCE

Cannot be prevented at present.

WHAT TO EXPECT

MEDICAL TESTS

- Your own observation of symptoms.
- Medical history and physical exam by a doctor.
- Laboratory blood studies, including autoimmune assays (ANA tests) (see Glossary).
- X-rays of the involved joints. Changes may not appear on X-rays until the late stages.

ARTHRITIS, JUVENILE RHEUMATOID

POSSIBLE COMPLICATIONS

- Involvement of tissues other than joints, producing uveitis (an eye inflammation), an enlarged spleen, or pericarditis (inflammation of the heart muscle).
- Permanent joint deformity.

PROBABLE OUTCOME

Juvenile rheumatoid arthritis is currently considered incurable. However, in 75% to 80% of cases, the disease is in complete remission by puberty. Attacks usually last a few weeks and occur off and on throughout childhood. Symptoms can usually be controlled with treatment.

TREATMENT

HOME CARE

- If the child doesn't have a firm mattress, place a 3/4-inch plywood board between the box springs and mattress to provide better support.
- Request eye examinations at least twice a year to detect uveitis.
- Encourage the child and the family to maintain a positive outlook.

MEDICATION

Your doctor may prescribe aspirin or other non-steroidal anti-inflammatory drugs to reduce pain and inflammation.

ACTIVITY

- During an attack, keep your child in bed, except to use the bathroom, until fever and other symptoms subside. Splints may be necessary to support and protect an inflamed joint.
- After an attack passes, the child can gradually resume normal activities with rest periods during the day. The child should not become overtired and should sleep at least 10 to 12 hours each night.
- Your doctor will probably recommend exercises when the child is well enough to do them.

DIET & FLUIDS

No special diet.

OK FOR SCHOOL, PRESCHOOL, OR NURSERY?

When signs of infection have decreased, appetite returns, and alertness, strength, and feeling of well-being will allow.

CALL YOUR DOCTOR IF

- Your child has symptoms of juvenile rheumatoid arthritis.
- The following symptoms occur during treatment: chest pain; temperature of 102F (38.9C) or higher; loss of appetite.
- New, unexplained symptoms develop. Drugs used in treatment may produce side effects.

ASPIRIN POISONING

GENERAL INFORMATION

DESCRIPTION

Aspirin poisoning is an acute emergency in childhood caused by accidentally swallowing a large amount of aspirin. Adolescents may take a purposeful overdose in a suicide attempt or gesture. There are many aspirin-containing over-the-counter medicines with many different names. If you suspect a child has ingested such medicine, read the label carefully on the container to determine its exact contents.

Appropriate health care includes:

Hospitalization (sometimes) to have the child's stomach pumped out and to give other supportive treatment.

SIGNS & SYMPTOMS

- Rapid breathing.
- Rapid heartbeat.
- Fever.
- Vomiting.
- Lethargy.
- Confusion.
- Seizures and coma with severe poisoning.
- Kidney excretes excessive amounts of potassium and sodium.
- Increased metabolic rate.
- Low blood sugar.
- Laboratory signs of liver damage.
- Excessive bleeding.

CAUSES

- Swallowing more than 95 children's aspirin tablets or 20 adult aspirin tablets.
- Swallowing oil of wintergreen.

RISK FACTORS

Curious, adventurous children.

PREVENTING COMPLICATIONS OR RECURRENCE

- Keep medications out of a child's sight or reach.
- Limit the number of tablets per package.
- Use childproof caps on all medications.

WHAT TO EXPECT

MEDICAL TESTS

- Urine and blood tests.
- Electrolyte studies to test for acidosis, for sodium or potassium depletion, or for low blood sugar.
- Measurement of aspirin level in the child's blood.

POSSIBLE COMPLICATIONS

- Can lead to death if not treated quickly and competently.
- Dehydration.
- Bleeding disorders.
- Fluid accumulating in the child's brain or lungs.
- Heart and/or kidney failure.

PROBABLE OUTCOME

Complete recovery with appropriate treatment.

TREATMENT

FIRST AID

- After determining how much aspirin your child has swallowed, call your doctor or poison control center immediately!
- If recommended by your doctor or the poison control center, try to make your child vomit with syrup of ipecac. This is a non-prescription liquid that you should keep on hand when there are young children at home. Specific instructions are on the bottle. Don't give more than what is recommended on the label. Give 1/2 to 1 full glass of water immediately after the ipecac. Don't give milk or carbonated beverages.
  - —Ipecac is not recommended for children under 6 months of age.
  - —Children 6 to 8 months—usual dose is 1 teaspoon.
  - —Children 8 months to 1 year—usual dose is 2 teaspoons.
  - —Children 1 to 3 years—usual dose is 3 teaspoons.

  You may repeat the dose in 30 minutes if vomiting doesn't occur.
- Whether your child does or does not vomit, call your poison control center or physician again within 30 minutes. The child's stomach may need to be pumped.
- If none of the above works, transport the child to the nearest emergency facility to have the stomach washed out.

HOME CARE

See FIRST AID above.

MEDICATION

See FIRST AID.

ACTIVITY

Your child can resume normal activities when symptoms are clear.

DIET & FLUIDS

None until after treatment (See FIRST AID).

OK FOR SCHOOL, PRESCHOOL, OR NURSERY?

After successful treatment.

CALL YOUR DOCTOR IF

- You are suspicious of aspirin poisoning.
- Your child shows symptoms of rapid, deep breathing, confusion, or unresponsiveness despite treatment outlined in FIRST AID above.

ILLNESSES

ASTHMA

GENERAL INFORMATION

DESCRIPTION

Asthma is a chronic disorder with recurrent attacks of wheezing and shortness of breath. The lungs, bronchi, and bronchioles are involved. Asthma can affect both sexes and all ages except newborn infants. It affects more boys than girls. Appropriate health care includes:

- Self-care after diagnosis.
- Physician's monitoring of general condition and medications.
- Emergency-room care and hospitalization for severe attacks.
- Psychotherapy or counseling, if asthma is stress-related.

SIGNS & SYMPTOMS

- General symptoms: chest tightness and shortness of breath; wheezing upon breathing out; coughing, especially at night, with little sputum; rapid, shallow breathing that is easier with sitting up; breathing difficulty—neck muscles tighten; enlarged chest.
- Severe late symptoms. *This is an emergency situation.* Get the child to the hospital or treat with an emergency kit at home: bluish skin; exhaustion; grunting respiration; inability to speak; mental changes, including restlessness or confusion.

CAUSES

Spasm of air passages (bronchi and bronchioles), followed by swelling of the passages and thickening of lung secretions (sputum). This decreases or closes off air to the lungs. These changes are caused by allergens, such as pollen, dust, animal dander, molds, and some foods; lung infections, such as bronchitis; air irritants, such as smoke and odors; exercise; stress.

RISK FACTORS

Other allergic conditions, such as eczema or hay fever; family history of asthma or allergies; exposure to air pollutants; smoking; use of some drugs, such as aspirin.

PREVENTING COMPLICATIONS OR RECURRENCE

- Your child should avoid known allergens and air pollutants.
- Have the child take prescribed preventive medicines regularly—don't let him omit them when he feels well.
- See Appendix 19 for suggestions to reduce stress.

? WHAT TO EXPECT

MEDICAL TESTS

- Your own observation of symptoms.
- Medical history and physical exam by a doctor.
- Laboratory blood studies and pulmonary-function test.
- Chest X-rays.

POSSIBLE COMPLICATIONS

Respiratory failure; pneumothorax (see Glossary); lung infection; COPD (see Glossary) from recurrent attacks.

PROBABLE OUTCOME

Symptoms can be controlled with treatment and strict adherence to preventive measures. Children often outgrow asthma. Without treatment, severe attacks can be fatal.

TREATMENT

HOME CARE

- Eliminate allergens and irritants at home and at work, if possible.
- Keep regular medications with the child at all times. Ask your doctor about having emergency drugs available.
- Have the child sit upright during attacks.
- Encourage the child to practice deep breathing each morning to loosen accumulated lung secretions.

MEDICATION

Your doctor may prescribe:

- Expectorants to loosen sputum.
- Bronchodilators to open air passages.
- Intravenous cortisone drugs (emergencies only) to decrease the body's allergic response.
- Cortisone drugs by nebulizer (see Glossary), which have fewer adverse reactions than oral forms.
- Cromolyn sodium by nebulizer. This is a preventive drug.

ACTIVITY

Encourage your child to stay active but avoid sudden bursts of exercise. If an attack follows heavy exercise, the child should sit and rest and sip warm water.

DIET & FLUIDS

No special diet, but avoid serving foods to which your child is sensitive. When the child is old enough, give instructions regarding which foods to avoid when away from home. The child should drink at least 6 to 8 8-ounce glasses of liquid daily to keep secretions loose.

OK FOR SCHOOL, PRESCHOOL, OR NURSERY?

When signs of infection have decreased, appetite returns, and alertness, strength, and feeling of well-being will allow. Make every attempt to keep your child in the mainstream of peer activities. Over-protection can be harmful.

CALL YOUR DOCTOR IF

- Your child has symptoms of asthma.
- Your child has an asthma attack that doesn't respond to treatment. This is an emergency!
- New, unexplained symptoms develop. Drugs used in treatment may produce side effects.

ASTHMA AND EXERCISE-INDUCED BRONCHOSPASM (EIB)

GENERAL INFORMATION

DESCRIPTION

Asthma and exercise-induced bronchospasm is a chronic breathing disorder characterized by recurrent attacks of wheezing and shortness of breath. It affects many children and adults who exercise regularly.

Appropriate health care includes:

- Emergency-room care and hospitalization for severe attacks.
- Psychotherapy or counseling, if asthma is stress-related.

SIGNS & SYMPTOMS

- Chest tightness and shortness of breath.
- Wheezing when exhaling.
- Coughing, especially at night, with little sputum.
- Rapid, shallow breathing that is easier when the child sits up.
- Breathing difficulty—neck muscles tighten.

Severe late symptoms: (Call your doctor. This is an emergency!)

- Bluish skin.
- Exhaustion.
- Grunting respiration.
- Inability to speak.
- Mental changes, including restlessness, confusion, or delirium.

CAUSES

Spasm of air passages (bronchi and bronchioles) followed by swelling of the passages and thickening of lung secretions (sputum). This decreases or closes off air to the child's lungs.

RISK FACTORS

Allergens, such as some medications, pollen, dust, animal dander, molds, and some foods; air irritants, such as smoke, smog, and odors; exercise, especially exercise in smoggy or cold air (bronchospasm can occur within minutes while exercising in cool air—warm, humid air seldom triggers exercise-induced bronchospasm); lung infections such as bronchitis; stress; family history of asthma or allergies; smoking; use of drugs to which your child is allergic, such as aspirin.

PREVENTING COMPLICATIONS OR RECURRENCE

Instructions for your child: Avoid known allergens and air pollutants. Take prescribed preventive medicines regularly—don't omit them when you feel well. Reduce activity level (sometimes). Exercise indoors on smoggy or cold days.

WHAT TO EXPECT

MEDICAL TESTS

Your own observation of symptoms; medical history and physical exam by a doctor; laboratory blood studies and pulmonary-function test; chest X-rays.

POSSIBLE COMPLICATIONS

- Enlarged chest from repeated asthma attacks over a long period of time.
- Pneumothorax (collapsed lung).
- Repeated lung infections.
- COPD (see Glossary) from recurrent attacks.
- Respiratory failure.

PROBABLE OUTCOME

Your child's symptoms can be controlled with treatment and strict adherence to preventive measures. Children often outgrow asthma. Without treatment, severe attacks can be fatal.

TREATMENT

HOME CARE

- Eliminate allergens and irritants from your child's environment at school, at home, and at work, if possible.
- Urge the child to carry regular medications at all times. Ask your doctor about having emergency drugs available.
- Teach the child to sit upright during attacks.
- Train the child to practice deep breathing and postural drainage (see Glossary) each morning to loosen accumulated lung secretions.

MEDICATION

Your doctor may prescribe:

- Expectorants to loosen sputum.
- Bronchodilators to open the child's air passages.
- Corticosteroid drugs by nebulizer (fewer adverse reactions than oral forms).
- Cromolyn sodium by nebulizer. This is a preventive drug.

ACTIVITY

Instructions for your child:

- Stay active, but avoid sudden bursts of exercise. If an attack follows heavy exercise, sit and rest. Sip warm water.
- Continue sports activities if your symptoms can be controlled. If not, decrease exercise levels temporarily until symptoms improve.

DIET & FLUIDS

No special diet, but your child should avoid foods to which he is sensitive. Urge the child to drink at least 3 quarts of liquid daily to keep lung secretions thin and loose.

OK FOR SCHOOL, PRESCHOOL, OR NURSERY?

Yes, when condition and sense of well-being will allow.

CALL YOUR DOCTOR IF

- Your child has frequent symptoms of asthma.
- Your child has an asthma attack that doesn't respond to treatment. This is an emergency!

ATELECTASIS

GENERAL INFORMATION

DESCRIPTION

Atelectasis is a collapse of part or all of one lung, preventing normal oxygen absorption.

Appropriate health care includes:

- Physician's monitoring of general condition and medications.
- Surgery to remove tumors.
- Bronchoscopy (see Glossary) to remove foreign objects or a mucus plug.
- Self-care after diagnosis.

SIGNS & SYMPTOMS

Sudden, major collapse:

- Chest pain.
- Shortness of breath and rapid breathing.
- Shock (severe weakness, paleness of skin, rapid heartbeat).
- Dizziness.

Gradual, minor collapse:

- Cough.
- Fever.
- No other symptoms.

CAUSES

Obstruction of small or large lung air passages by:

- Thick mucus plugs from infection or other disease, including cystic fibrosis.
- Tumors in the air passages.
- Tumors or blood vessels outside the air passages, causing pressure on airways.
- Inhaled objects, such as small toys or peanuts.
- Prolonged chest or abdominal surgery with general anesthetic.
- Chest injury or fractured ribs.

RISK FACTORS

- Smoking.
- Illness that has lowered resistance or weakened the patient.
- Chronic obstructive lung disease, including emphysema and bronchiectasis.
- Use of drugs that depress alertness or consciousness, such as sedatives, barbiturates, tranquilizers, or alcohol.

PREVENTING COMPLICATIONS OR RECURRENCE

- Force your child to cough and breathe deeply every 1 to 2 hours after any surgical operation with general anesthesia. Also change the child's position often in bed, if possible.
- Increase the child's fluid intake during lung illness or after surgery—by mouth or intravenously—to keep lung secretions loose.
- Keep small objects that might be inhaled away from young children (peanuts are notorious).

WHAT TO EXPECT

MEDICAL TESTS
- Your own observation of symptoms.
- Medical history and physical exam by a doctor.
- Laboratory studies to measure oxygen and carbon dioxide in the blood.
- X-rays of the chest.

POSSIBLE COMPLICATIONS
- Pneumonia.
- Small lung abscess.
- Permanent lung scars and collapsed lung tissue.

PROBABLE OUTCOME

If atelectasis is caused by a mucus plug or inhaled foreign object, it is curable when the plug or object is removed. If it is caused by a tumor, the outcome depends on the nature of the tumor.

TREATMENT

HOME CARE
- Encourage your child to turn, cough and breathe deeply after any surgery. Hold a pillow tightly against incisions during coughing exercises.
- Your child should not smoke.
- Learn to perform postural drainage (see Glossary) on your child after hospitalization. An inhalation therapist, nurse, or doctor can demonstrate.

MEDICATION
- Your doctor may prescribe antibiotics to fight infection that inevitably accompanies atelectasis; pain relievers.
- Don't give your child sedatives. They may contribute to a recurrence.

ACTIVITY

Your child can resume normal activities as soon as symptoms improve.

DIET & FLUIDS

No special diet, but encourage your child to drink at least 8 glasses of water or other fluid daily to thin lung secretions.

OK FOR SCHOOL, PRESCHOOL, OR NURSERY?

When signs of infection have decreased, appetite returns, and alertness, strength, and feeling of well-being will allow.

CALL YOUR DOCTOR IF

- Your child has symptoms of atelectasis.
- The following occurs during treatment: distended abdomen; sudden shortness of breath; blue fingernails and lips; temperature spikes to 102F (38.9C) or higher.

ATHLETE'S FOOT
(Tinea Pedis; Ringworm of the Feet)

GENERAL INFORMATION

DESCRIPTION

Athlete's foot is a common, contagious fungus infection of the skin on the feet. The feet, especially the soles and the skin between the toes (usually the 4th and 5th toes), are involved. Athlete's foot can affect both sexes and all ages but is more common in adolescents than younger children.

Appropriate health care includes:

- Self-care after diagnosis.
- Physician's monitoring if infection is severe or persistent.

SIGNS & SYMPTOMS

- Moist, soft, gray-white or red scales on feet, especially between toes.
- Dead skin between toes.
- Itching in inflamed areas.
- Damp, musty foot odor.
- Small blisters on the feet (sometimes).

CAUSES

Infection by a trichophyton fungus.

RISK FACTORS

- Infrequent washing of the feet.
- Infrequent changes of shoes or socks.
- Use of locker rooms and public showers.
- Hot, humid weather.

PREVENTING COMPLICATIONS OR RECURRENCE

Instructions for your child:

- Bathe feet daily. Dry thoroughly and dust with talc.
- Go barefoot when possible.
- Change shoes and socks daily.
- Wear socks made of cotton, wool, or other natural, absorbent fibers. Avoid synthetics.

WHAT TO EXPECT

MEDICAL TESTS

- Your own observation of symptoms.
- Medical history and physical exam by a doctor.
- Laboratory culture and microscopic examination of scales.

POSSIBLE COMPLICATIONS

- Secondary bacterial infection in the affected area.
- Id reaction (see Glossary) on hands and face (rare).

PROBABLE OUTCOME

Usually curable in 3 weeks with treatment, but recurrence is common.

ATHLETE'S FOOT (Tinea Pedis; Ringworm of the Feet)

TREATMENT

HOME CARE

- Remove scales and material between your child's toes daily.
- Keep affected areas cool and dry. The child should go barefoot or wear sandals during treatment.

MEDICATION

- Use non-prescription anti-fungal powders, creams, or ointments after your child's daily bath.
- For severe cases, your doctor may prescribe an oral anti-fungal medication.
- See Medications section for information regarding medicines your doctor may prescribe.

ACTIVITY

No restrictions.

DIET & FLUIDS

No special diet.

OK FOR SCHOOL, PRESCHOOL, OR NURSERY?

Yes, unless the infection is so severe that the child's walking is impaired.

CALL YOUR DOCTOR IF

- Your child has severe symptoms of athlete's foot that persist, despite self-treatment.
- Your child develops a fever or the infection seems to be spreading.

BACK SPRAIN, LUMBO-DORSAL REGION

GENERAL INFORMATION

DESCRIPTION

A lumbo-dorsal back sprain is a violent overstretching of one or more ligaments in the lumbo-dorsal vertebrae of the spine. This is the most stable section of the vertebral column. Sprains involving two or more ligaments cause considerably more disability than single-ligament sprains. When the ligament is overstretched, it becomes tense and gives way at its weakest point, either where it attaches to bone or within the ligament itself. Appropriate health care includes: doctor's diagnosis; application of tape, cast (rare), or elastic bandage; self-care during rehabilitation; physical therapy (moderate or severe sprain); hospitalization (rare) for traction; surgery (severe sprain).

SIGNS & SYMPTOMS

- Severe pain at the time of injury.
- Popping or feeling of tearing in the child's back.
- Tenderness at the injury site.
- Swelling in the child's back.
- Bruising that appears soon after the child has been injured.

CAUSES

Stress on a ligament that temporarily forces the lumbo-dorsal vertebrae out of their normal location. A sprain of the lumbo-dorsal vertebrae will frequently occur when your child performs a stressful act while off-balance, or during repeated stressful activity involving muscles in the lumbo-dorsal area.

RISK FACTORS

Contact sports involving throwing and lifting; gymnastics or diving; previous spine injury; obesity; poor muscle conditioning.

PREVENTING COMPLICATIONS OR RECURRENCE

Your child should build strength with an appropriate conditioning program. The child should warm up before sports and should tape vulnerable joints before practice or competition to prevent reinjury.

WHAT TO EXPECT

MEDICAL TESTS

Your own observation of symptoms; medical history and physical exam by a doctor; X-rays of the spine to rule out fractures.

POSSIBLE COMPLICATIONS

Prolonged healing time if the child's usual activities are resumed too soon; proneness to repeated back injury; inflammation at the ligament attachment to bone (periostitis); prolonged disability (sometimes); unstable or arthritic spine following repeated injury.

BACK SPRAIN, LUMBO-DORSAL REGION

PROBABLE OUTCOME

If this is a first-time injury, proper care and sufficient healing time before your child resumes activity should prevent permanent disability. Ligaments have a poor blood supply, and torn ligaments require as much healing time as fractures. Average healing times are: mild sprains—2 to 6 weeks; moderate sprains—6 to 8 weeks; severe sprains—8 to 10 weeks.

TREATMENT

HOME CARE

If your doctor does not apply a cast, tape, or elastic bandage:
- Continue using an ice pack on the child 3 or 4 times a day. Place ice chips or cubes in a plastic bag. Wrap the bag in a moist towel, and place it over the injured area. Use for 20 minutes at a time.
- Wrap the injured area from the top of the hip to the lower rib cage with an elasticized bandage between ice treatments.
- Massage gently and often to provide comfort and decrease swelling.
- Ask your doctor about the advisability of the child using a special corset.

MEDICATION

- For minor discomfort, use aspirin, acetaminophen, or ibuprofen.
- Your doctor may prescribe stronger pain relievers; injection of a long-acting local anesthetic to reduce pain; injection of a corticosteroid, such as triamcinolone, to reduce inflammation.

ACTIVITY

Your child can resume normal activities gradually after clearance from your doctor.

DIET & FLUIDS

Increase the child's fiber and fluid intake to prevent constipation that may result from decreased activity.

OK FOR SCHOOL, PRESCHOOL, OR NURSERY?

Yes, when condition and sense of well-being will allow.

CALL YOUR DOCTOR IF

- Your child has symptoms of a moderate or severe lumbo-dorsal back sprain, or a mild sprain persists longer than 2 weeks.
- Pain, swelling, or bruising worsen despite treatment.
- Pain develops in the child's leg.
- Any of the following occur after surgery: increased pain, swelling, redness, drainage, or bleeding in the surgical area; signs of infection (headache, muscle aches, dizziness, or a general ill feeling with fever).
- New, unexplained symptoms develop. Drugs used in treatment may produce side effects.

BALANITIS

GENERAL INFORMATION

DESCRIPTION

Balanitis is inflammation of the penis of an uncircumcised male. The penis and foreskin are involved.

Appropriate health care includes:

- Physician's monitoring of general condition and medications.
- Surgery to circumcise the penis, if balanitis recurs frequently.
- Self-care after diagnosis.

SIGNS & SYMPTOMS

- Pain, redness, and swelling of the head of the penis.
- Inflammation of the foreskin.
- Chills and fever.
- Ulceration of the penis.
- Discharge from the penis.
- Burning on urination.
- Enlarged lymph glands in the groin.

CAUSES

Infection from bacteria under the foreskin of the penis that invade the head of the penis.

RISK FACTORS

- Inadequate cleansing under the foreskin.
- Trauma or minor injury to the foreskin and penis, as from excessive masturbation.

PREVENTING COMPLICATIONS OR RECURRENCE

- Have male infants circumcised.
- Wash your baby daily with soap and water. Cleanse under the foreskin.
- Stretch a tight foreskin with daily gentle retraction.
- Instruct your son to wash carefully when he is old enough to bathe himself.

WHAT TO EXPECT

MEDICAL TESTS

- Your own observation of symptoms.
- Medical history and physical exam by a doctor.
- Laboratory culture of the discharge from the infected area.

POSSIBLE COMPLICATIONS

- Ulceration of the penis.
- Spread of infection to deeper skin layers of the penis shaft.
- Blood poisoning.

PROBABLE OUTCOME

Usually curable in 1 to 2 weeks with medical treatment.

TREATMENT

HOME CARE

Use warm-water soaks to relieve pain.

MEDICATION

Your doctor may prescribe:

- Steroid creams to control swelling.
- Topical or oral antibiotics to fight infection.
- Aspirin or acetaminophen to relieve minor pain and fever.
- See Medications section for information regarding medicines your doctor may prescribe.

ACTIVITY

Your son should rest in bed if he has a fever. Allow him to read or watch TV. He can resume normal activities when the infection is cured.

DIET & FLUIDS

No special diet.

OK FOR SCHOOL, PRESCHOOL, OR NURSERY?

When signs of infection have decreased, appetite returns, and alertness, strength, and feeling of well-being will allow.

CALL YOUR DOCTOR IF

- Your son has symptoms of balinitis.
- Symptoms don't improve in 3 days, despite treatment.
- Balanitis recurs. Consider circumcision.

BAROTITIS MEDIA
(Barotrauma)

GENERAL INFORMATION

DESCRIPTION

Barotitis media is damage to the middle ear caused by pressure changes. The middle ear, eustachian tube, and nerve endings in the ear are involved.

Appropriate health care includes:

- Physician's monitoring of general condition and medications.
- Self-care after diagnosis.
- Surgery to open the eardrum and release fluid trapped in the middle ear. A plastic tube may be inserted through the surgically perforated eardrum to keep it open and equalize pressure. The tube falls out spontaneously in 9 to 12 months.

SIGNS & SYMPTOMS

- Hearing loss (to varying degrees).
- A plugged feeling in the ear.
- Severe pain.
- Dizziness.
- Ringing noises in the ear.

CAUSES

Damage caused by sudden, increased pressure in the surrounding air, such as occurs in the rapid descent of an airplane or while scuba diving. In these activities, air moves from passages in the nose into the middle ear to maintain equal pressure on both sides of the eardrum. If the tube leading from the nose to the ear (eustachian tube) doesn't function properly, pressure in the middle ear is less than outside pressure. The negative pressure in the middle ear sucks the eardrum inward. Blood and mucus may later appear in the middle ear. This damage is more likely if a person has a nose or throat infection when scuba diving or traveling by air.

RISK FACTORS

Recent respiratory-tract infection.

PREVENTING COMPLICATIONS OR RECURRENCE

- Don't allow the child to fly or scuba-dive when he has an upper-respiratory infection.
- If the child must fly anyway:

  — Use non-prescription decongestant tablets or sprays. Follow package instructions.

  — While ascending or descending, suck on hard candy or chew gum to force frequent swallowing.

  — Take a moderate-size breath, hold the nose and try to force air into the eustachian tube by gently puffing out the cheeks with the mouth closed.

  — Give an infant a bottle of water or juice while ascending or descending.

BAROTITIS MEDIA
(Barotrauma)

? WHAT TO EXPECT

MEDICAL TESTS

- Your own observation of symptoms.
- Medical history and physical exam by a doctor.

POSSIBLE COMPLICATIONS

Without treatment, fluid may accumulate, become infected and rupture the eardrum. The rupture may affect nerve endings, causing permanent hearing loss.

PROBABLE OUTCOME

With treatment, most cases of barotitis media are reversible without permanent damage or hearing loss.

TREATMENT

HOME CARE

If fluid drains from the ear, place a small piece of cotton in the outer-ear canal to absorb it.

MEDICATION

- For minor discomfort, use non-prescription decongestants and pain relievers, such as acetaminophen.
- Your doctor may prescribe:
  — Stronger prescription decongestant nasal sprays or tablets. Use for at least 2 weeks after damage.
  — Steroid nasal spray.
  — Antibiotics, if infection is present.
- See Medications section for information regarding medicines your doctor may prescribe.

ACTIVITY

Have your child resume normal activities as soon as symptoms improve, but the child should not engage in underwater activities if the eardrum has been ruptured or if the tubes have been surgically implanted.

DIET & FLUIDS

No special diet.

OK FOR SCHOOL, PRESCHOOL, OR NURSERY?

When signs of infection have decreased, appetite returns, and alertness, strength, and feeling of well-being will allow.

CALL YOUR DOCTOR IF

- Your child has symptoms of barotitis media.
- The following occurs during treatment:
  — Severe headache.
  — Fever.
  — Severe pain.
  — Dizziness.

BED-WETTING
(Enuresis)

GENERAL INFORMATION

DESCRIPTION

Bed-wetting is involuntary urination during sleep that occurs more often than once a month. Bed-wetting can affect both sexes but is more common in boys. The occurrence of bed-wetting in children is 15% at age 5, 10% at age 6, 7% at age 8, 3% at age 12, and 1% at age 18.

Appropriate health care includes:

- Self-care after diagnosis.
- Physician's monitoring of general condition and medications.
- Psychotherapy or counseling.

SIGNS & SYMPTOMS

Bed-wetting at night. This is not significant until a child is older than 6.

CAUSES

In most cases, the cause of bed-wetting is unknown. Following are the most-common causes or popular theories:

- Underlying illness, such as diabetes or a urinary-tract infection.
- A small or weak bladder that cannot hold one night's urine production.
- Psychological problems caused by stress or separation from the mother.

RISK FACTORS

- Diabetes.
- Urinary-tract infection.
- Family history of bed-wetting.

PREVENTING COMPLICATIONS OR RECURRENCE

Show your child love, support and understanding for this problem.

WHAT TO EXPECT

MEDICAL TESTS

- Your own observation of symptoms.
- Medical history and physical exam by a doctor.
- Laboratory studies of urine and blood to detect diabetes or urinary-tract infection.

POSSIBLE COMPLICATIONS

Psychological and emotional scars that may affect the child's personality for years.

PROBABLE OUTCOME

Bed-wetting may continue for several years. Your doctor will want to rule out urinary-tract infections and diabetes as causes. If these are eliminated and your child is normal in other respects, consider your child's bed-wetting a minor variation of the age at which bladder control is socially expected.

BED-WETTING (Enuresis)

TREATMENT

HOME CARE

- Prepare the bed and the child:
  - — Protect the mattress with a heavy plastic cover.
  - — Provide the child with extra-thick underwear and pajamas.
  - — Discontinue diapers or plastic pants by age 4; they inhibit the child's motivation to improve.
  - — Put an extra pair of underwear and pajama bottoms by the bed in case the child needs them during the night.
- Have the child urinate at bedtime.
- Awaken the child to urinate after he has been asleep for several hours. If the child is old enough, he may be able to set the alarm clock to awaken himself and empty his bladder during the night.
- Reward the child for staying dry. Praise him, hug him, and tell of his success to people who are important to him, such as brothers and sisters. Use gold stars or happy faces to mark dry nights on a calendar if the child likes it.
- Respond gently to accidents. Don't blame, criticize, restrict, or punish the child who has wet the bed. This can cause him to give up, or lead to emotional problems.
- Follow instructions if your doctor suggests bladder-stretching or stream-interruption exercises or behavior-modification devices.

MEDICATION

- Medicine usually is not necessary for this disorder, but your doctor may prescribe anti-depressant drugs as a last resort.
- See Medications section for information regarding medicines your doctor may prescribe.

ACTIVITY

No restrictions.

DIET & FLUIDS

No special diet. Encourage your child to drink as much fluid as possible during the day. Decrease fluid intake during the 2 hours before bedtime.

OK FOR SCHOOL, PRESCHOOL, OR NURSERY?

Yes.

CALL YOUR DOCTOR IF

- You are concerned about your child's bed-wetting, and your child is older than 6.
- The child dribbles urine, has a weak urinary stream, has pain when urinating, or must strain to urinate.
- Medication is prescribed for the child, and new, unexplained symptoms develop. Drugs used in treatment may produce side effects.

BELL'S PALSY

GENERAL INFORMATION

DESCRIPTION

Bell's palsy is paralysis on one side of the face. This is named after the physician who first described it. The 7th cranial nerve and facial muscles supplied by that nerve are involved. Bell's palsy is more common in adults, but it may also affect children.

Appropriate health care includes:

- Self-care after diagnosis.
- Physician's monitoring of general condition and medications.
- Surgery (rare).

SIGNS & SYMPTOMS

- Sudden paralysis on one side of the face, including muscles to the eyelid.
- Pain behind the ear on the affected side.
- Flat, expressionless features on one side of the face.
- Distorted smiles and frowns.
- Changes in taste, salivation, or tear formation (sometimes).

CAUSES

Unknown. The paralysis is probably caused by swelling of the facial nerve. The swelling may be caused by a virus, an autoimmune disease, or a decrease in blood flow and pressure on the facial nerve as it passes through the temporal bone of the skull.

RISK FACTORS

Unknown.

PREVENTING COMPLICATIONS OR RECURRENCE

Cannot be prevented at present.

WHAT TO EXPECT

MEDICAL TESTS

- Your own observation of symptoms.
- Medical history and physical exam by a doctor.
- CAT scan (see Glossary) to rule out other causes of pressure on the facial nerve.

POSSIBLE COMPLICATIONS

Eye irritation or injury because the eye does not close properly and is exposed to dust. If unprotected, the eye may develop ulcers on the cornea.

PROBABLE OUTCOME

- Bell's palsy is distressing, but it is not dangerous. The extent of nerve damage determines the extent of recovery. Improvement is gradual and recovery time varies, sometimes requiring many months.
- Patients with mild facial paralysis usually recover completely within several months. Patients with severe facial paralysis recover completely in 80% to 90% of cases.
- Surgery can sometimes improve facial appearance and muscle function in patients who do not recover fully.

TREATMENT

HOME CARE

- If your child has pain, apply heat to the painful area twice a day. Use an electric heating pad or wring out a towel soaked in hot water and apply for 15 minutes. Cover or close the eye during heat treatments.
- If your child cannot wink or close an eye well, buy a pair of wrap-around, plastic bubble goggles. The child should wear them to protect the eyes from dirt, dust, and dryness. You may buy goggles from a sporting goods store or optician.
- At night, apply an eye patch to shut the lid so the eye stays moist and protected.
- As muscle strength returns, use facial massage and exercises. Massage muscles of the forehead, cheek, lips and eyes using cream or oil. Exercise the weak muscles in front of a mirror. Have the child open and close the eye, wink, smile, and bare the teeth. Perform the massage and exercise for 15 to 20 minutes several times a day.
- Brush and floss teeth more often to keep the mouth healthy.

MEDICATION

Your doctor may prescribe:

- Methylcellulose eye drops for comfort and protection of the exposed eye.
- Cortisone drugs for 2 weeks to reduce swelling and inflammation of the affected nerve.
- See Medications section for information regarding medicines your doctor may prescribe.

ACTIVITY

Maintain normal activities. Rest does not help Bell's palsy.

DIET & FLUIDS

A soft diet is often necessary.

OK FOR SCHOOL, PRESCHOOL, OR NURSERY?

When signs of infection have decreased, appetite returns, and alertness, strength, and feeling of well-being will allow.

CALL YOUR DOCTOR IF

- Your child has symptoms of Bell's palsy.
- An eye becomes red or irritated, despite treatment.
- Your child cannot prevent saliva from drooling from the mouth.
- Pain worsens.
- Temperature rises to 101F (38.3C) or higher.

BLADDER INFECTION (Cystitis)

GENERAL INFORMATION

DESCRIPTION

Bladder infection is an inflammation or infection of the urinary bladder. The bladder and urethra are involved. Bladder infection can affect both sexes, all ages, but is more common in females.

Appropriate health care includes:

- Physician's monitoring of general condition and medications.
- Self-care after diagnosis.

SIGNS & SYMPTOMS

- Burning and stinging on urination.
- Frequent urination, especially at night, although the urine amount may be small.
- Increased urge to urinate.
- Pain in the abdomen over the bladder.
- Low back pain.
- Blood in the urine.
- Low fever.
- Bad-smelling urine.
- Lack of urinary control (sometimes).

CAUSES

- Bacteria that reach the bladder from another part of the body through the bloodstream.
- Bacteria that enter the urinary tract from skin around the genitals and anal area.
- Injury to the urethra.
- Use of a urinary catheter to empty the bladder, such as following surgery.

RISK FACTORS

- Infection in other parts of the genitourinary system.
- Stress.
- Illness that has lowered resistance.
- Frequent, rough, sexual intercourse.

PREVENTING COMPLICATIONS OR RECURRENCE

- Have the child take showers instead of tub baths.
- Request frequent urinalyses to monitor signs of infection.
- Encourage the child to drink 8 glasses of water every day and to avoid caffeine, which irritates the bladder.
- Avoid the use of catheters, if possible.
- Obtain prompt medical treatment for urinary-tract infections.
- Females should clean the anal area thoroughly after bowel movements. Wipe from the front to the rear—rather than rear to front—to avoid spreading fecal bacteria to the genital area.

BLADDER INFECTION (Cystitis)

WHAT TO EXPECT

MEDICAL TESTS

- Your own observation of symptoms.
- Medical history and physical exam by a doctor.
- Urinalysis and careful urine collection for bacterial culture.
- Cystoscopy (see Glossary).
- X-ray of urinary system after 2 infections have not been treated successfully.

POSSIBLE COMPLICATIONS

Inadequate treatment can cause chronic urinary-tract infections, leading to kidney failure.

PROBABLE OUTCOME

Curable in 2 weeks with prompt medical treatment. Recurrence is common.

TREATMENT

HOME CARE

Apply heat to the bladder area with a heat lamp or heating pad.

MEDICATION

Your doctor may prescribe:

- Antibiotics to fight infection.
- Antispasmodics to relieve pain.
- See Medications section for information regarding medicines your doctor may prescribe.

ACTIVITY

Resume normal activity as soon as possible.

DIET & FLUIDS

Encourage your child to do the following:

- Drink 6 to 8 glasses of water daily.
- Avoid caffeine and alcohol during treatment.

OK FOR SCHOOL, PRESCHOOL, OR NURSERY?

- When signs of infection have decreased, appetite returns, and alertness, strength, and feeling of well-being will allow.

CALL YOUR DOCTOR IF

- Your child has symptoms of cystitis.
- Fever rises to 101F (38.3C) or higher during treatment.
- Blood appears in the urine.
- Discomfort and other symptoms don't improve in 1 week.
- New, unexplained symptoms develop. Drugs used in treatment may produce side effects.
- Symptoms recur after treatment.

BLADDER OR URETHRA INJURY

GENERAL INFORMATION

DESCRIPTION

Bladder or urethra injury is damage to the urinary bladder (the organ that stores urine from the kidneys) or the urethra (the tube through which urine travels from the bladder to the outside).

Appropriate health care includes:
- Physician's monitoring of general condition and medications.
- Hospitalization; emergency care.
- Surgery to repair a punctured bladder (usually). A damaged urethra may heal without surgery.
- Self-care after diagnosis.

SIGNS & SYMPTOMS

- Severe abdominal pain.
- Shock (sweating; faintness; nausea; panting; rapid pulse; and pale, cold, moist skin).
- Painful urination or inability to urinate.
- Bloody discharge from the urethra.

CAUSES

Usually a pelvic-bone fracture that punctures the bladder or urethra.

RISK FACTORS

- Accident-proneness.
- Hazardous activities.
- Hazardous driving conditions.
- Sexual abuse of a child.

PREVENTING COMPLICATIONS OR RECURRENCE

Protect your child from injury whenever possible. Buckle automobile seat belts and shoulder harnesses to minimize internal injury in case of accident. Don't drink and drive.

WHAT TO EXPECT

MEDICAL TESTS

- Your own observation of symptoms.
- Medical history and physical exam by a doctor.
- Laboratory urine studies.
- X-rays of the urinary tract.

POSSIBLE COMPLICATIONS

- Internal bleeding.
- Urine leakage into the abdomen, causing abdominal inflammation or infection.
- Recurrent infections from scars in the urethra that narrow the urinary passage.

PROBABLE OUTCOME

A punctured bladder or urethra requires emergency hospital treatment. Most cases heal with bed rest, time, supportive treatment, or surgery.

BLADDER OR URETHRA INJURY

TREATMENT

HOME CARE

No specific instructions except those under other headings.

MEDICATION

- Your doctor may prescribe antibiotics to prevent infection.
- See Medications section for information regarding medicines your doctor may prescribe.

ACTIVITY

The child can stay as active as his strength allows. Allow 1 month for recovery.

DIET & FLUIDS

- No special diet, but exclude alcohol.
- Encourage the child to drink 6 to 8 glasses of fluid daily.

OK FOR SCHOOL, PRESCHOOL, OR NURSERY?

After healing and when signs of infection have decreased, appetite returns, and alertness, strength, and feeling of well-being will allow.

CALL YOUR DOCTOR IF

- Your child has any symptoms of bladder or urethra injury.
- During or after treatment, your child develops fever of 101F (38.3C) or higher, or chills.
- New, unexplained symptoms develop. Drugs used in treatment may produce side effects.

BLISTERS

GENERAL INFORMATION

DESCRIPTION

In the ordinary blister a patch of the outermost layer of the skin (epidermis) has separated from the under layer (dermis). Friction—from a rubbing shoe, for example—or a burn or chemical action usually causes this separation. The separated skin dies when deprived of nourishment but remains intact for several days if not disturbed. Meanwhile, the bloodstream reabsorbs the fluid in the blister and beneath the blister the dermis regenerates a new outer layer of skin. After the blister collapses, the dead skin sloughs off. Infection is the principal complication of blisters.

Appropriate health care includes:

- Home care (see below).
- Physician's care if the child's blister becomes infected.

SIGNS & SYMPTOMS

- Fluid collection under the superficial skin layer.
- Sensitivity to pressure over the blister.
- Redness and swelling around the blister.

CAUSES

- Repeated friction and pressure against the skin, especially during hot, humid weather.
- Wearing shoes that fit poorly.

RISK FACTORS

Common sites for blisters: the hands of gymnasts, the feet of runners and dancers, the fingers of baseball pitchers, and the buttocks of bicycle riders.

PREVENTING COMPLICATIONS OR RECURRENCE

Instructions for your child:

- Apply 10% tannic acid to vulnerable areas of skin once or twice daily for 2 to 3 weeks.
- Wear shoes that fit like a glove, but allow enough space for the forefoot and toes. Check for rough seams inside the shoe.
- Don't wear thick socks. Clean white cotton or cotton-wool socks are less likely to cause blisters than synthetic materials. Avoid tube socks.
- Try wearing no socks, but dust shoes with talcum powder or rub feet and shoes with petroleum jelly.
- Put tape on vulnerable areas prior to exercise.
- Don't run in shoes still wet from previous use.
- Protect your hands with gloves appropriate for your sport, if possible.

WHAT TO EXPECT

MEDICAL TESTS

- Your own observation of symptoms.
- Physical exam by a doctor if the child's blister becomes infected.

POSSIBLE COMPLICATIONS

Infection: fluid becomes pus, pain becomes worse, and red streaks develop.

PROBABLE OUTCOME

Your child's blisters usually heal in 3 to 7 days if they don't become infected.

TREATMENT

HOME CARE

No treatment is necessary for small, painless blisters (less than 1 inch across). To treat painful blisters or blisters larger than 1 inch:

- Apply ice to the child's blister for 5 minutes.
- Wash the blistered area with warm soapy water. Pat dry with a clean towel.
- Sterilize a pin or tip of a scissor by dipping it in alcohol or by holding it in the flame of a lighted match until it becomes red.
- Puncture the blister in several places around the edge.
- Apply gentle pressure to the top of the blister to squeeze out fluid. Leave the skin in place.
- Repeat all steps above once a day if the blister persists.
- Place moleskin (see Glossary) over a blister pad on top of the blister. Pad blisters on the bottoms of the child's feet with adhesive felt or foam with a hole cut slightly larger than the blister.

MEDICATION

- Use non-prescription antibiotic medicine, such as Bacitracin or Neosporin, on the skin of the child's blister.
- See Medications section for information regarding medicines your doctor may prescribe.

ACTIVITY

No restrictions unless the child's blister becomes infected.

DIET & FLUIDS

No special diet.

OK FOR SCHOOL, PRESCHOOL, OR NURSERY?

Yes, when condition and feeling of well-being will allow.

CALL YOUR DOCTOR IF

- Home treatment of the child's blisters hasn't brought relief in 1 to 3 days.
- Signs of infection occur (increased heat, redness, swelling, or pus in the blister).

BLOOD POISONING
(Septicemia)

GENERAL INFORMATION

DESCRIPTION

Blood poisoning is a bacterial infection (or toxins from bacteria) in the blood. The total body is involved.

Appropriate health care includes:

- Physician's monitoring of general condition and medications.
- Hospitalization.
- Self-care after diagnosis.

SIGNS & SYMPTOMS

- Shaking chills.
- Rapid temperature rise.
- Rapid, pounding heartbeat.
- Warm, flushed skin.
- Confusion and other symptoms of mental impairment.
- Drop in blood pressure.
- General ill feeling.

CAUSES

Infection in other body parts, such as the appendix, teeth, sinuses, pelvis, gallbladder, or urinary tract. The source may also be a burn, infected wound, or open abscess.

RISK FACTORS

- Birth through infancy.
- Illness, such as diabetes, that has lowered resistance.
- Leukemia or other cancer.
- Use of immunosuppressive drugs or self-administered intravenous drugs.

PREVENTING COMPLICATIONS OR RECURRENCE

- Obtain medical treatment for any infection.
- If dental procedures have produced blood poisoning in the past or your child has diseased heart valves, use antibiotics before any dental treatment—including simple prophylaxis by a dentist or hygienist.

WHAT TO EXPECT

MEDICAL TESTS

- Your own observation of symptoms.
- Medical history and physical exam by a doctor.
- Laboratory studies, such as culture of the blood to identify germs responsible for the illness, urinalysis, and blood count.

POSSIBLE COMPLICATIONS

- Shock, with very low blood pressure, overwhelming infection, and death.
- Persistent infection of the heart valves.

PROBABLE OUTCOME

Usually curable in 1 week with intravenous antibiotics.

TREATMENT

HOME CARE

Reduce fever if it goes over 104F (40C). See Appendix 17, How to Reduce Your Child's Fever. Don't reduce lower temperatures; a slight fever helps mobilize the body's defenses against infection.

MEDICATION

- Your doctor may prescribe antibiotics to fight infection.
- Use non-prescription drugs, such as acetaminophen, to reduce fever over 104F (40C).
- See Medications section for information regarding medicines your doctor may prescribe.

ACTIVITY

Your child may resume normal activities gradually as symptoms improve.

DIET & FLUIDS

No special diet, but increase the child's fluids during fevers to prevent dehydration.

OK FOR SCHOOL, PRESCHOOL, OR NURSERY?

When signs of infection have decreased, appetite returns, and alertness, strength, and feeling of well-being will allow.

CALL YOUR DOCTOR IF

- Your child has symptoms of blood poisoning.
- The following occurs during treatment:
  — Fever higher than 103F (39.4C).
  — Signs of infection (swelling, pain, redness) anywhere in the body.
- Your child has elective surgery or a dental procedure after an episode of blood poisoning.
- New, unexplained symptoms develop. Drugs used in treatment may produce side effects.

BLOOD-TRANSFUSION REACTION

GENERAL INFORMATION

DESCRIPTION

Blood-transfusion reaction symptoms are triggered by the body's response to a foreign substance. The blood, blood vessels, kidneys, heart, skin, central nervous system, and lungs are involved.

Appropriate health care includes:

- Physician's monitoring of general condition and medications.
- Hospitalization. Patients receiving transfusions are usually in a hospital or outpatient surgical facility, and reactions can be treated when they occur. Keep your child awake and alert during a blood transfusion, if possible, so you can notify medical personnel immediately if symptoms occur in your child.
- Self-care after diagnosis.

SIGNS & SYMPTOMS

Less serious:

- Chills and fever.
- Backache or other aches and pains.
- Hives and itching.

More serious:

- Blood-cell destruction (hemolysis), causing shortness of breath, severe headache, chest or back pain, and blood in the urine.

CAUSES

Transfusions of a different blood type than that of the patient. This may occur from errors in matching or from the use of incompletely matched blood in an emergency.

RISK FACTORS

- Blood transfusions in emergency situations, when careful typing and matching of blood must be bypassed.
- Blood transfusions from donors who carry infections.

PREVENTING COMPLICATIONS OR RECURRENCE

- Blood-bank and hospital personnel have safety procedures to prevent reactions except in situations that are uncontrollable (see CAUSES).
- Use of diphenhydramine (an antihistamine) and acetaminophen prior to transfusion may prevent minor reactions.
- If surgery is planned at least 1 month in advance, an older child's own blood may be drawn and stored for use during surgery, if necessary. Transfusion with one's own blood is least likely to produce a reaction, but your doctor will instruct you as to age and weight minimums for any blood donation.

WHAT TO EXPECT

MEDICAL TESTS

- Your own observation of symptoms.
- Medical history and physical exam by a doctor.
- Laboratory blood tests to recheck compatibility and detect complications.

POSSIBLE COMPLICATIONS

- Acute kidney failure.
- Anaphylaxis.
- Congestive heart failure from too rapid transfusion.
- Hypothermia from blood that is too cold.

PROBABLE OUTCOME

Most reactions clear gradually after the transfusion is halted. A few reactions are fatal.

TREATMENT

HOME CARE

Use cool baths if hives persist after transfusion.

MEDICATION

Your doctor may prescribe:

- Antihistamines to decrease hives and itching.
- Cortisone drugs to decrease the likelihood of acute kidney failure.
- Antihypertensives, if blood pressure rises too high, or hypertensives, such as ephedrine or epinephrine, if blood pressure drops too low.
- See Medications section for information regarding medicines your doctor may prescribe.

ACTIVITY

Your child can resume normal activities as soon as symptoms improve after transfusion.

DIET & FLUIDS

No special diet.

OK FOR SCHOOL, PRESCHOOL, OR NURSERY?

When appetite has returned and alertness, strength, and feeling of well-being will allow.

CALL YOUR DOCTOR IF

Your child has symptoms of a blood-transfusion reaction during or after a transfusion. Call immediately. This is an emergency!

BOILS (Furuncles)

GENERAL INFORMATION

DESCRIPTION

Boils are painful, deep, bacterial infections of hair follicles. Boils are common and contagious. The skin and hair follicles are involved.

Appropriate health care includes:

- Self-care after diagnosis.
- Physician's monitoring of general condition and medications, which may also include incision and drainage of the boil.

SIGNS & SYMPTOMS

- A domed nodule that is painful, tender, and red and has pus on the surface. Boils appear suddenly and ripen in 24 hours. They are usually 1-1/2cm to 3cm in diameter; some are larger.
- Fever.
- Swelling of the closest lymph glands.

CAUSES

Infection, usually from staphylococcus bacteria, that begins in the hair follicle and bores into the skin's deeper layers.

RISK FACTORS

- Poor nutrition.
- Illness that has lowered resistance.
- Diabetes mellitus.
- Use of immunosuppressive drugs.

PREVENTING COMPLICATIONS OR RECURRENCE

Keep the child's skin clean.

WHAT TO EXPECT

MEDICAL TESTS

- Your own observation of symptoms.
- Medical history and physical exam by a doctor.
- Laboratory culture of the pus to identify the germ.

POSSIBLE COMPLICATIONS

The infection may enter the bloodstream and spread to other body parts.

PROBABLE OUTCOME

Without treatment, a boil will heal in 10 to 20 days. With treatment, the boil should heal in less time, symptoms will be less severe, and new boils should not appear. The pus that drains when a boil opens spontaneously may contaminate nearby skin, causing new boils.

BOILS (Furuncles)

TREATMENT

HOME CARE

- Relieve your child's pain with gentle heat from warm-water soaks (see Glossary), a heating pad, hot-water bottle, or lamp close to the skin. Use 3 or 4 times daily for 20 minutes.
- Prevent the spread of boils by using clean towels only once, or using paper towels and discarding them.

MEDICATION

- Your doctor may prescribe a penicillin drug, such as oxacillin, dicloxacillin or nafcillin, or erythromycin antibiotics to fight infection.
- Don't use non-prescription antibiotic creams or ointments on the boil's surface. They are ineffective.
- See Medications section for information regarding medicines your doctor may prescribe.

ACTIVITY

Your child should decrease activity until the boil heals to avoid sweating.

DIET & FLUIDS

No special diet.

OK FOR SCHOOL, PRESCHOOL, OR NURSERY?

When signs of infection have decreased, appetite returns, and alertness, strength, and feeling of well-being will allow.

CALL YOUR DOCTOR IF

- Your child has a boil.
- The following occurs during treatment:
  - — Symptoms don't improve in 3 to 4 days, despite treatment.
  - — New boils appear.
  - — Fever rises above 100F (37.8C).
  - — Other family members develop boils.
- New, unexplained symptoms develop. Drugs used in treatment may produce side effects.

BONE FRACTURE

GENERAL INFORMATION

DESCRIPTION

A bone fracture is a complete or incomplete break in a bone.
Following are the different types of fractures:
- Complete fracture. The broken bone is completely separated.
- Incomplete (greenstick) fracture. The broken bone is not completely separated.
- Comminuted fracture. There are more than 2 bone fragments at the fracture site.
- Open fracture (compound). The fractured bone has broken the skin.
- Closed fracture (including stress fracture). The fractured bone has not broken the skin.
- Compression fracture. The break occurs from extreme pressure on the bone.
- Impacted fracture. The broken ends have been driven into each other.
- Avulsion fracture. Force has been applied to a strong tendon, causing it to pull on and break off a portion of bone.
- Pathologic fracture. A break that occurs from a minor injury in bone weakened or destroyed by disease.

Appropriate health care includes:
- Physician's monitoring of general condition and medications.

Almost all fractures require immobilization with casts or splints.
- Hospitalization for anesthesia and treatment of severe fractures.
- Surgery if the fracture must be repaired with rods, plates, or screws.
- Physical therapy for rehabilitation.
- Self-care after diagnosis and treatment.

SIGNS & SYMPTOMS

- Pain and swelling at the fracture site.
- Tenderness close to the fracture.
- Paleness and deformity (sometimes).
- Loss of pulse below the fracture, usually in an extremity (sometimes).
- Numbness, tingling, or paralysis below the fracture.
- Bleeding or bruising at the site.
- Weakness and inability to bear weight.

CAUSES

Injury.

RISK FACTORS

- Tumors of the bone or bone marrow.
- Activities that carry the risk of injury.
- Reckless behavior that increases the chance of an auto accident.

PREVENTING COMPLICATIONS OR RECURRENCE

- Advise your adolescent not to drink alcohol or use mind-altering drugs and drive.
- Have your child wear protective gear for sports.
- Use auto seat belts or harnesses.

BONE FRACTURE

WHAT TO EXPECT

MEDICAL TESTS

- Your own observation of symptoms.
- Medical history and physical exam by a doctor.
- Laboratory studies to determine blood loss.
- X-rays of injured parts.

POSSIBLE COMPLICATIONS

- Failure to heal (non-union).
- Shock from blood loss.
- Travel of a fat embolus (clump of fat cells) from the injury site to the lungs or brain.
- Obstruction of nearby arteries.

PROBABLE OUTCOME

Usually curable with skillful first aid and aftercare. Your child's broken bone should be manipulated, realigned, and immobilized as soon as possible. Realignment is much more difficult after 6 hours. Healing time varies. Recovery is complete when there is no bone motion at the fracture site, and X-rays show complete healing.

TREATMENT

HOME CARE

- See emergency first-aid instructions in the back of this book.
- See Care of Casts, Appendix 41.

MEDICATION

Your doctor may prescribe pain relievers or muscle relaxants.

ACTIVITY

Your child may resume normal activities as soon as symptoms improve.

DIET & FLUIDS

No special diet. Give your child vitamin C supplements to promote bone healing.

OK FOR SCHOOL, PRESCHOOL, OR NURSERY?

When doctor advises that fracture is healing and activity will not cause harm.

CALL YOUR DOCTOR IF

- Your child has symptoms of a bone fracture.
- The following occurs after immobilization or surgery:
  - — Swelling above or below the fracture site.
  - — Severe, persistent pain.
  - — Blue or gray skin below the fracture site, especially under nails.
  - — Numbness or loss of feeling below the fracture site.

Report any of the above signs immediately!

BOTULISM

GENERAL INFORMATION

DESCRIPTION

Botulism is a serious, non-contagious form of food poisoning caused by eating contaminated food containing a toxin that severely affects the nervous system. The central nervous system and the muscular system are involved.

Appropriate health care includes:

• Physician's monitoring of general condition and medications.
• Hospitalization for intensive care. A respirator may be necessary.
• Self-care after diagnosis.

SIGNS & SYMPTOMS

The following symptoms usually appear suddenly 18 to 36 hours after eating contaminated food:

• Blurred or double vision; drooping eyelids; dry mouth; slurred speech; swallowing difficulty.
• Vomiting and diarrhea.
• Weakness of the arms and legs, leading to paralysis.
• No fever; no disturbance of mental abilities.

The following symptoms appear in infants: severe constipation; feeble cry; inability to suck.

CAUSES

• Infection with bacteria, clostridium botulinum, found in contaminated or incompletely cooked, canned foods, including honey. This germ generates a powerful poison (toxin) that is absorbed from the digestive tract and spreads to the central nervous system.
• Foods likely to cause botulism include home-canned vegetables and fruits and undercooked sausage, smoked meats, and fish. In infants under 1 year, raw honey or other uncooked foods may cause botulism.
• The bacteria also may contaminate a wound and produce the toxin.

RISK FACTORS

• Infancy.
• Home-canned foods. Green beans are especially susceptible to spoilage.

PREVENTING COMPLICATIONS OR RECURRENCE

• If a can is bulging, or the contents have a peculiar color or odor, *don't even taste the food.*
• Don't eat any foods not definitely known to be properly cooked and canned.
• Don't give infants honey in foods or cough suppressants.
• Call your local home-extension service for details about canning food and cooking it safely.

OTHER

Call your local health department if you suspect botulism. The health department can notify the news media to alert others in danger and require retailers to remove contaminated food from store shelves.

? WHAT TO EXPECT

MEDICAL TESTS

- Your own observation of symptoms—especially if several persons eat the same food and become sick.
- Medical history and physical exam by a doctor.
- Laboratory blood tests.
- Laboratory analysis of suspected food.

POSSIBLE COMPLICATIONS

- Lung infections as a result of impaired swallowing and choking on food.
- Respiratory failure caused by weak breathing muscles.

PROBABLE OUTCOME

With prompt care, the outlook is good. The larger the toxin dose and the sooner symptoms begin, the more dangerous the condition. The overall death rate is 10% to 25%.

TREATMENT

HOME CARE

- Induce vomiting, if it is only a few hours since the poisoned food was eaten.
- If you suspect botulism, refrigerate some of the contaminated food for laboratory testing, if possible.

MEDICATION

Botulism antitoxin injections prevent the condition from worsening. The antitoxin is available through the Centers for Disease Control, Atlanta, Georgia. The anti-toxin is derived from horse serum. It is life-saving but has serious side effects.

ACTIVITY

Bed rest is necessary during hospitalization. After treatment, the child can resume normal activities gradually.

DIET & FLUIDS

Intravenous fluids and foods are usually necessary during hospitalization because of swallowing difficulty. After treatment, no special diet is necessary, except to avoid honey for children under 2 years of age.

OK FOR SCHOOL, PRESCHOOL, OR NURSERY?

When signs of infection have decreased, appetite returns, and alertness, strength, and feeling of well-being will allow.

☎ CALL YOUR DOCTOR IF

- Your child has symptoms of botulism. Call an ambulance immediately. This is an emergency!
- Weakness, blurred vision, or slurred speech occur after returning from intensive care. These may signal a need for additional treatment.

BOWED LEGS and BLOUNT'S DISEASE

GENERAL INFORMATION

DESCRIPTION

A child has bowed legs when the ankles touch and the knees do not touch. Bowed legs are part of a baby's normal growth and development and become easily observable at about age 2-1/2 months. The legs may remain normally bowed in appearance for several years. If a child remains bowlegged there may be an underlying disorder of bone malformation or an underlying bone disease sometimes called *Blount's disease.* Blount's disease occurs more frequently between ages 1 and 3 but may occur as late as 9 years through adolescence. Girls are more likely to be bowlegged than boys.

Appropriate health care includes:

- Doctor's diagnosis and treatment, possibly with night braces.
- Surgery to provide relief of symptoms, if simple measures don't correct the problem.

SIGNS & SYMPTOMS

- Curving or bowing of the child's legs just below the knee.
- Walking with the affected knee flexed, causing more bowing.

CAUSES

Blount's disease:

- Abnormal growth center at the upper part of the child's tibia (shin bone).
- Rickets (vitamin D deficiency).
- Bone malformations present at birth.

RISK FACTORS

- Walking earlier than average.
- Obesity.
- Short stature.

PREVENTING COMPLICATIONS OR RECURRENCE

- If the cause is *rickets,* give the child 400 units of vitamin D daily.
- Other causes: No preventive measures known.

? WHAT TO EXPECT

MEDICAL TESTS

- X-rays of the child's knees and legs to look for underlying bone deformities.
- Blood tests to rule out metabolic bone diseases.

POSSIBLE COMPLICATIONS

Severe knee-joint complications.

PROBABLE OUTCOME

- Normal bowed legs usually correct themselves by age 4 or 5 years but may persist until 8 years.
- Bowed legs caused by abnormalities can be corrected only by treating the underlying disease.

TREATMENT

HOME CARE

When indicated, your physician may recommend night braces to pull the legs slowly into a straighter position. If simple measures don't correct the problem, surgery will usually provide relief of symptoms.

MEDICATION

- Medication usually is not necessary for this disorder.
- See Medications section for information regarding medicines your doctor may prescribe.

ACTIVITY

Maintain normal activity for your child's age and size.

DIET & FLUIDS

No restrictions.

OK FOR SCHOOL, PRESCHOOL, OR NURSERY?

Yes.

CALL YOUR DOCTOR IF

Your child's legs seem unusually bowed, getting worse or persisting beyond age 3.

BRAIN OR EPIDURAL ABSCESS

GENERAL INFORMATION

DESCRIPTION

A brain or epidural abscess is a collection of pus caused by a bacterial infection in the brain or the outermost of 3 membranes that cover the brain and spinal cord. The brain, meninges (membranes that cover the brain), and the skull are all involved. Appropriate health care includes:

- Physician's monitoring of general condition and medications.
- Surgery to drain pus from the abscess.
- Self-care after diagnosis.

SIGNS & SYMPTOMS

The following symptoms usually appear gradually over several hours. They resemble symptoms of a brain tumor or stroke:

- Pain in the back, if the infection is in the covering of the spinal cord.
- Headache.
- Nausea and vomiting.
- Weakness, numbness, or paralysis of one side of the body.
- Irregular gait.
- Convulsions.
- Fever.
- Confusion or delirium.
- Speaking difficulty.

CAUSES

The primary source of bacterial infection that causes a brain or epidural abscess often cannot be found. These 3 sources are the most common:

- An infection that spreads from an infected skull, such as in osteomyelitis, mastoiditis, or sinusitis.
- An infection that is introduced by a skull injury.
- An infection that spreads through the bloodstream from other infected organs, such as the lungs, skin, or heart valves.

RISK FACTORS

- Head injury.
- Illness that has lowered resistance, especially diabetes mellitus.
- Recent infection, especially around the nose and face.

PREVENTING COMPLICATIONS OR RECURRENCE

Consult your doctor for treatment of any infection in your child's body—especially one around the nose or face—to prevent its spread.

WHAT TO EXPECT

MEDICAL TESTS

- Your own observation of symptoms.
- Medical history and physical exam by a doctor.
- Laboratory studies such as blood studies, spinal-fluid studies, EEG (see Glossary), CAT scan (see Glossary).
- X-rays of the skull.

POSSIBLE COMPLICATIONS
Seizures, coma, and death without treatment.

PROBABLE OUTCOME
Usually curable with antibiotic treatment and surgery to drain pus.

TREATMENT

HOME CARE
No specific instructions except those under other headings.

MEDICATION
Your doctor may prescribe:
- Antibiotics for 4 to 6 weeks to fight infection.
- Anticonvulsants to prevent seizures.
- See Medications section for information regarding medicines your doctor may prescribe.

ACTIVITY
While in the hospital, the patient will need bed rest. After a 2- to 3-week recovery, your child should be as active as renewed strength and a feeling of well-being allow.

DIET & FLUIDS
The child should eat a normal, well-balanced diet. Vitamin and mineral supplements should not be necessary unless there is evidence of deficiency or an inability to eat normally.

OK FOR SCHOOL, PRESCHOOL, OR NURSERY?
When signs of infection have decreased, appetite returns, and alertness, strength, and feeling of well-being will allow.

CALL YOUR DOCTOR IF

- Your child has any symptoms of a brain or epidural abscess.
- Fever rises to 101F (38.3C) or higher.
- New, unexplained symptoms develop. Drugs used in treatment may produce side effects.

BRAIN TUMOR

GENERAL INFORMATION

DESCRIPTION

A brain tumor is an abnormal growth in the brain that may be benign or malignant. A non-malignant brain tumor may cause as much disability as a malignant tumor unless it is treated appropriately. The brain and the central nervous system are involved.

Appropriate health care includes:

- Physician's monitoring of general condition and medications.
- Surgery, radiation, and chemotherapy.
- Self-care after diagnosis.

SIGNS & SYMPTOMS

- Headaches that worsen when lying down.
- Vomiting with nausea, or sudden vomiting without nausea.
- Vision disturbances, including double vision.
- Weakness on one side of the body.
- Lack of balance and dizziness.
- Loss of sense of smell.
- Memory loss.
- Personality changes.
- Seizures.

CAUSES

Some tumors begin in the brain (primary tumors), but most brain tumors have spread from other cancers—especially cancer of the breast, lungs, or intestines, or malignant melanoma of the skin. Symptoms are caused by increasing pressure in the skull as the tumor enlarges.

RISK FACTORS

The following risk factors are related to cancers in other body parts that spread to the brain:

- Poor nutrition, especially a low-fiber diet (intestinal cancer).
- Excess sun exposure (malignant melanoma).
- Previous cancer at any other body site.

PREVENTING COMPLICATIONS OR RECURRENCE

Encourage your adolescent to do the following:

- Practice breast self-exam.
- Don't smoke.
- Eat a high-fiber diet.
- Protect from excessive sun exposure by using sunscreens and protective clothing.

WHAT TO EXPECT

MEDICAL TESTS

- Your own observation of symptoms.
- Medical history and physical exam by a doctor.
- Laboratory studies of blood and cerebrospinal fluid.
- X-rays of the skull, bones, lungs, and gastrointestinal tract.
- EEG (see Glossary).
- CAT scan (see Glossary).
- Radionuclide studies (see Glossary).
- MRI (see Glossary).

POSSIBLE COMPLICATIONS

Disability and death if a tumor is inoperable because of size or location.

PROBABLE OUTCOME

- Brain tumors that are not treated lead to death or permanent brain damage. Bones of the skull restrict a tumor's outward growth, so the brain is compressed as a tumor grows.
- If a tumor is discovered and treated early with surgery or radiation therapy and chemotherapy, full recovery is often possible.

TREATMENT

HOME CARE

No specific instructions except those listed under other headings.

MEDICATION

Your doctor may prescribe:

- Cortisone drugs to diminish swelling of the brain tissue.
- Anticonvulsant drugs to control seizures.
- Pain relievers.
- Anti-cancer drugs.

ACTIVITY

Your child can stay as active as his strength allows. He should work and exercise moderately and rest when tired.

DIET & FLUIDS

Your child should eat a high-protein diet to aid healing and growth. Vitamin and mineral supplements should not be necessary unless he cannot eat normally.

OK FOR SCHOOL, PRESCHOOL, OR NURSERY?

When appetite returns and alertness, strength, and feeling of well-being will allow.

CALL YOUR DOCTOR IF

- Your child has symptoms of a brain tumor.
- New, unexplained symptoms develop. Drugs used in treatment may produce side effects.

ILLNESSES

BREAST ABSCESS

GENERAL INFORMATION

DESCRIPTION

A breast abscess is an infected area of breast tissue that becomes filled with pus when the body fights the infection. Body parts involved include breast tissue, the nipple, milk glands, and milk ducts. Breast abscesses can affect girls at puberty and, very seldom, boys.

Appropriate health care includes:

- Self-care after diagnosis.
- Physician's monitoring of general condition and medications.
- Surgery to drain the abscess.

SIGNS & SYMPTOMS

- Breast pain, tenderness, redness, or hardness.
- Fever and chills.
- A general ill feeling.
- Tender lymph glands in the child's underarm area.

CAUSES

Bacteria that enter the breast through the nipple—usually a cracked nipple during the early days of breast-feeding.

RISK FACTORS

- Post-partum pelvic infection.
- Fatigue.

PREVENTING COMPLICATIONS OR RECURRENCE

Instructions for your daughter:

- Clean the nipples and breasts thoroughly before and after nursing.
- Lubricate the nipples after nursing with lanolin or Vitamin A & D ointment.
- Avoid clothing that irritates the breasts.
- Don't allow a nursing infant to chew nipples.

WHAT TO EXPECT

MEDICAL TESTS

- Your own observation of symptoms.
- Medical history and physical exam by a doctor.
- Laboratory culture of the discharge from the abscess to identify the bacteria (usually staphylococcus).

POSSIBLE COMPLICATIONS

It may be necessary for your daughter to discontinue breast-feeding if the infection is severe enough to require extensive treatment with certain antibiotics (especially tetracycline) and pain relievers.

PROBABLE OUTCOME

Usually curable in 3 to 10 days with treatment. Draining the abscess greatly hastens healing.

TREATMENT

HOME CARE

- Use warm-water soaks to relieve pain and hasten healing.
- Your daughter should discontinue nursing the baby from the infected breast until it heals. She can use a breast pump to express milk regularly from the infected breast until she can resume nursing on that side.

MEDICATION

Your doctor may prescribe:

- Antibiotics to fight infection.
- Pain relievers.
- See Medications section for information regarding medicines your doctor may prescribe.

ACTIVITY

After treatment, your child can resume normal activity as soon as symptoms improve.

DIET & FLUIDS

No special diet.

OK FOR SCHOOL, PRESCHOOL, OR NURSERY?

When abscess has healed or drained.

CALL YOUR DOCTOR IF

- Your child has symptoms of a breast abscess.
- Any of the following occurs during treatment:
  - — Fever rises to 103F (39.4C) or higher.
  - — Pain becomes unbearable.
  - — Infection seems to be spreading, despite treatment.
  - — Symptoms don't improve in 72 hours.
- New, unexplained symptoms develop. Drugs used in treatment may produce side effects.

BREAST CONTUSION

GENERAL INFORMATION

DESCRIPTION

A breast contusion is a bruising of the skin and underlying tissues of the breast or nipple. Contusions cause bleeding from ruptured small capillaries that allow blood to infiltrate fatty tissue, muscles, tendons, nerves, or other soft tissue. The skin, nipple, subcutaneous fatty tissue, blood vessels (both large vessels and capillaries), muscles, and connective tissue of a male or female breast are involved.

Appropriate health care includes:

- Doctor's care unless the contusion is quite small.
- Self-care during recovery.

SIGNS & SYMPTOMS

- Local swelling of the breast—either superficial or deep.
- Pain in the child's breast or nipple.
- Feeling of firmness when pressure is exerted on the injury area.
- Tenderness.
- Discoloration under the child's skin, beginning with redness and progressing to the characteristic "black and blue" bruise.
- Hard, tender ring surrounding the nipple.

CAUSES

Direct blow to the child's breast, usually by a blunt object.

RISK FACTORS

- Contact sports such as wrestling, baseball, softball, or boxing, especially if the child's breast area has inadequate protection.
- Medical history of any bleeding disorder such as hemophilia.
- Poor nutrition.
- Obesity.

PREVENTING COMPLICATIONS OR RECURRENCE

- Your child should wear appropriate protective gear for the chest during competition or other athletic activity if there is risk of contusion.
- Your daughter should wear breast support—a sport brassiere, elasticized binder, or both—for participation in contact sports.

WHAT TO EXPECT

MEDICAL TESTS

- Your own observation of symptoms.
- Medical history and physical exam by a doctor for all except minor injuries. The total extent of the child's injury may not be apparent for 48 to 72 hours following injury.
- X-rays of the injured area to assess total injury to soft tissue and to rule out the possibility of an underlying fracture.
- Follow-up exam to make sure that any lumps remaining 3 months after injury do not represent possible malignancy.

POSSIBLE COMPLICATIONS
- Excessive bleeding leading to disability. Infiltrative-type bleeding can (rarely) lead to calcification.
- Prolonged healing time if the child's usual activities are resumed too soon.
- Infection if the skin over the injury is broken.

PROBABLE OUTCOME
Healing time varies from 2 to 6 weeks, depending on the extent of injury.

TREATMENT

FIRST AID
Use instructions for R.I.C.E., the first letters of *rest*, *ice*, *compression*, and *elevation*. Elevate the foot of the child's bed. See Appendix 39 for details.

HOME CARE
Instructions for your child:
- Continue to use ice massage. Fill a large Styrofoam cup with water and freeze. Tear a small amount of foam from the top so ice protrudes. Massage firmly over the injured area in a circle about the size of a softball. Do this for 15 minutes at a time, 3 or 4 times a day, and before workouts or competition.
- After 48 hours, apply heat instead of ice if it feels better. Use heat lamps, hot soaks, hot showers, heating pads, or heat liniments or ointments.
- Take whirlpool treatments, if available.
- Protect the injured area with pads or an elasticized-bandage wrap between treatments.

MEDICATION
- For minor discomfort, use non-prescription medicines such as acetaminophen or ibuprofen. Do not use aspirin for injuries involving bleeding.
- Your doctor may prescribe stronger medicine for the child's pain, if needed.

ACTIVITY
Your child should begin activities slowly and stop exercise as soon as pain begins. The child can increase activity as healing progresses.

DIET & FLUIDS
Serve the child a well-balanced diet that includes extra protein, such as meat, fish, poultry, cheese, milk, and eggs. Your child should increase fiber and fluid intake to prevent constipation that may result from decreased activity.

OK FOR SCHOOL, PRESCHOOL, OR NURSERY?
Yes, when condition and sense of well-being will allow.

CALL YOUR DOCTOR IF

- Your child's breast contusion doesn't improve within a day or two.
- Signs of infection (drainage from skin, headache, muscle aches, dizziness, fever, or a general ill feeling) occur if the skin was broken.
- Any firm nodules that may appear following the injury do not disappear in 3 months.

BRONCHIECTASIS

GENERAL INFORMATION

DESCRIPTION

Bronchiectasis is a lung disease in which the bronchial tubes become blocked and accumulate thick secretions. Frequent secondary infections occur. It is not contagious unless associated with tuberculosis. The lungs and bronchial tubes are involved.

Appropriate health care includes:

- Self-care after diagnosis.
- Physician's monitoring of general condition and medications.
- Surgery to remove isolated areas of damaged lung tissue.

SIGNS & SYMPTOMS

Frequent coughing with bad-smelling, green or yellow sputum (sometimes flecked with blood); repeated lung infections; shortness of breath; general ill feeling; frequent fatigue; anemia (frequently).

CAUSES

Damage to the small bronchial tubes, which may develop over years. Common sources of damage include repeated infections; chronic bronchitis; allergies; smoke or dust; inhalation of a foreign object; tuberculosis; fungus infection.

RISK FACTORS

Poor nutrition; repeated pneumonia; family history of tuberculosis; obesity; smoking; fatigue or overwork; exposure to allergens; cold, humid weather.

PREVENTING COMPLICATIONS OR RECURRENCE

- Obtain medical treatment for your child's lung infections.
- Have the child avoid as many risks for infection as possible.

WHAT TO EXPECT

MEDICAL TESTS

- Your own observation of symptoms.
- Medical history and physical exam by a doctor.
- X-rays of the lung, including a bronchogram (see Glossary).

POSSIBLE COMPLICATIONS

COPD (chronic obstructive pulmonary disease); repeated pneumonia; destruction of lung tissue.

PROBABLE OUTCOME

With treatment, most patients with bronchiectasis can lead nearly normal lives without major disability.

TREATMENT

HOME CARE

- Encourage your child not to smoke.
- Learn and practice postural drainage (see Glossary) on your child twice a day.
- Have the child sleep with 3- to 5-inch blocks under the foot of the bed to prevent mucus from collecting in the lower lobes of the lungs.
- If your child goes to school (or works) around heavy air pollution, do everything possible to limit exposure—including changing schools (or jobs).
- Install air conditioning with a filter and humidity control in your home.
- The child should avoid sudden temperature changes.
- Encourage your child to avoid loud talking, loud laughing, crying, exertion, or sudden temperature changes, if these trigger coughing episodes.
- Keep your child's teeth and mouth in excellent condition.
- If your child has an allergic background, avoid allergens.

MEDICATION

Your doctor may prescribe:

- Antibiotics for 10 days every month if bacterial infections have caused your child's bronchiectasis or triggered episodes of pneumonia or acute bronchitis.
- Bronchodilators to enlarge airways.
- Expectorants to loosen secretions.

ACTIVITY

The child should remain as active as possible.

DIET & FLUIDS

Encourage your child to drink a minimum of 8 glasses of fluid a day. This thins lung secretions so they can be coughed out more easily.

OK FOR SCHOOL, PRESCHOOL, OR NURSERY?

When signs of infection have decreased, appetite returns, and alertness, strength, and feeling of well-being will allow.

CALL YOUR DOCTOR IF

- Your child has symptoms of bronchiectasis.
- After diagnosis, there are symptoms of a respiratory infection or bronchitis.
- Temperature rises to 101F (38.3C).
- Blood appears in the sputum, sputum thickens despite treatment, or postural drainage reveals a change in color, amount, or character of sputum.
- Chest pain increases.
- Shortness of breath occurs without coughing or when at rest.

BRONCHIOLITIS

GENERAL INFORMATION

DESCRIPTION

Bronchiolitis is inflammation of the bronchioles, the smallest branches of the respiratory tree. These carry air from the large bronchial tubes to microscopic air sacs in the lungs. The air sacs transfer oxygen to the bloodstream. Bronchiolitis can affect children of both sexes, usually under age 6.

Appropriate health care includes:

- Self-care after diagnosis.
- Physician's monitoring of general condition and medications.
- Hospitalization for intensive care and oxygen (severe cases).

SIGNS & SYMPTOMS

Sudden breathing difficulty, usually preceded by a mild common cold and cough, and characterized by the following:

- Wheezing.
- Rapid, shallow breathing (60 to 80 times a minute).
- Retractions (see-saw movements) of the chest and abdomen.
- Fever.
- Blue skin or nails (severe cases).

CAUSES

Viral or bacterial infection, or a combination of the two. Some young children develop this disorder after every cold. Bronchiolitis is contagious and often becomes epidemic.

RISK FACTORS

- Illness that has lowered resistance, especially respiratory infection.
- Family history of allergies.
- Obesity in infancy.

PREVENTING COMPLICATIONS OR RECURRENCE

- Use a cool-mist humidifier in the child's room. Use it every night during and after a respiratory infection for a child who is subject to bronchiolitis.
- Observe and avoid any activities that seem to trigger attacks in the child, such as active play in the cool night air.
- Decrease the child's exposure to groups of people, especially other children, to avoid colds.

? WHAT TO EXPECT

MEDICAL TESTS

- Your own observation of symptoms.
- Medical history and physical exam by a doctor.
- Laboratory blood studies.
- X-rays of the lungs.

POSSIBLE COMPLICATIONS

Permanent lung damage leading to chronic bronchitis, collapse of a small portion of the lung, bronchiectasis, repeated pneumonia, and (rarely) chronic obstructive pulmonary disease (COPD).

PROBABLE OUTCOME

Usually curable in 7 days with treatment. Some studies indicate that infants who have 2 or more episodes of bronchiolitis before age 2 are more likely to develop allergies and asthma.

TREATMENT

HOME CARE

Keep the humidity in the child's room as high as possible, preferably with a cool-mist humidifier. If you don't have a humidifier, run cold or hot water in the shower with windows and doors closed to produce a high-humidity room. Hold the child in this room for 20 minutes several times a day, especially at bedtime. If the child awakens at night with wheezing or shortness of breath, repeat the process.

MEDICATION

- Your doctor may prescribe antibiotics to fight bacterial infections.
- See Medications section for information regarding medicines your doctor may prescribe.

ACTIVITY

Have the child rest until symptoms have subsided for 48 hours. Then normal activities may be resumed gradually.

DIET & FLUIDS

Offer the child clear fluids frequently. Give water, tea, carbonated drinks, lemonade, weak bouillon, diluted fruit juice, or gelatin. Don't offer milk; it may thicken mucus secretions.

OK FOR SCHOOL, PRESCHOOL, OR NURSERY?

When signs of infection have decreased, appetite returns, and alertness, strength, and feeling of well-being will allow.

CALL YOUR DOCTOR IF

- Symptoms don't improve in 4 hours, despite treatment.
- Temperature (rectal) rises to 101F (38.3C) or higher.
- Breathing becomes more difficult.
- A cough begins that produces colored phlegm.
- The skin, lips, or nails turn dark blue.
- The child becomes lethargic.

BRONCHITIS, ACUTE

GENERAL INFORMATION

DESCRIPTION

Acute bronchitis is an inflammation of the air passages of the lungs. The trachea, bronchi, and bronchioles are involved.

Appropriate health care includes:

- Self-care, if the child is in good overall health.
- Physician's monitoring of general condition and medications if the child has chronic lung disease or if complications develop.
- Hospitalization for extreme illness (rare).

SIGNS & SYMPTOMS

- Cough that produces little or no sputum.
- Low fever (usually less than 101F or 38.3C).
- Burning chest discomfort or feeling of pressure behind the breastbone.
- Wheezing or uncomfortable breathing (sometimes).

CAUSES

- Infection from one of many respiratory viruses. Most cases of acute bronchitis begin with a cold virus in the nose and throat that spreads to the airways. A secondary bacterial infection is common.
- Lung inflammation from breathing air that contains irritants, such as chemical fumes (ammonia), acid fumes, dust, or smoke.

RISK FACTORS

- Chronic obstructive pulmonary disease (COPD).
- Smoking.
- Cold, humid weather.
- Poor nutrition.
- Recent illness that has lowered resistance.

PREVENTING COMPLICATIONS OR RECURRENCE

Your child should avoid close contact with persons who have any respiratory infection.

WHAT TO EXPECT

MEDICAL TESTS

- Your own observation of symptoms.
- Medical history and physical exam by a doctor.
- Laboratory blood counts to detect complicating infections and cultures of sputum and blood to identify the bacteria.
- X-rays of the chest (for complications only).

POSSIBLE COMPLICATIONS

- Bacterial lung infection (various kinds of pneumonia).
- Chronic bronchitis from recurrent episodes of acute bronchitis.

PROBABLE OUTCOME

Usually curable with treatment in 1 week. Cases with complications are usually curable in 2 weeks with medication.

TREATMENT

HOME CARE

- If your child is a smoker, urge him not to smoke during the illness. Smoking delays recovery and makes complications more likely.
- Increase air moisture in the child's room. Give the patient frequent hot showers. Use a cool-mist humidifier by the bed.

MEDICATION

- For minor discomfort, give your child:
  - — Acetaminophen to reduce fever.
  - — Non-prescription cough suppressants. Give them to the child only if the cough is non-productive (without sputum). It may be dangerous to stop a cough entirely—this traps excess mucus and irritants in bronchial tubes, leading to pneumonia and poor oxygen exchange in the lungs.
- Your doctor may prescribe:
  - — Antibiotics to fight bacterial infections.
  - — Expectorants to thin mucus so it can be coughed up more easily.
  - — Cough suppressants.
- See Medications section for information regarding medicines your doctor may prescribe.

ACTIVITY

The child should rest in bed until his temperature returns to normal. Then he can resume normal activity gradually as symptoms improve.

DIET & FLUIDS

No special diet. The child should drink at least 8 to 10 glasses of fluid each day to help thin mucus secretions so they can be coughed up more easily.

OK FOR SCHOOL, PRESCHOOL, OR NURSERY?

When signs of infection have decreased, appetite returns, and alertness, strength, and feeling of well-being will allow.

CALL YOUR DOCTOR IF

- Your child has symptoms of bronchitis.
- The following occurs during the illness:
  - — High fever and chills.
  - — Chest pain.
  - — Thickened, discolored, or blood-streaked sputum.
  - — Shortness of breath, even when the child is at rest.
  - — Vomiting.

BRONCHITIS, CHRONIC

GENERAL INFORMATION

DESCRIPTION

Chronic bronchitis is a recurring inflammation and degeneration of the bronchial tubes, with or without active infection. This is not contagious or cancerous. The bronchial tubes (bronchi) are involved. Chronic bronchitis can affect both sexes, all ages, but is most common in boys.

Appropriate health care includes:

- Self-care after diagnosis.
- Physician's monitoring of general condition and medications. Many lung and heart disorders cause symptoms identical to those of chronic bronchitis. Your doctor must exclude these possibilities to make a diagnosis.

SIGNS & SYMPTOMS

- Frequent cough or coughing spasms.
- Shortness of breath.
- Sputum that is thick and difficult to cough up. Sputum production varies according to whether infection is present.
- Barrel chest (in the late stages).

CAUSES

Repeated irritation or infection in the bronchial tubes, causing them to thicken, narrow, and lose elasticity. Underlying irritants include allergens, air pollution, and tobacco smoke.

RISK FACTORS

Smoking (the greatest risk factor); any lung illness that has lowered resistance; family history of tuberculosis or other disease of the respiratory tract; exposure to air pollutants; poor nutrition; obesity; crowded living conditions.

PREVENTING COMPLICATIONS OR RECURRENCE

Instructions for your child or adolescent: Don't smoke. (This is the most reversible risk.) Avoid irritating fumes in the environment. Obtain prompt medical treatment for respiratory infections.

WHAT TO EXPECT

MEDICAL TESTS

- Your own observation of symptoms.
- Medical history and physical exam by a doctor.
- Laboratory studies of sputum and pulmonary function.
- X-rays of the chest.

POSSIBLE COMPLICATIONS

- Recurrent pneumonia.
- Chronic obstructive pulmonary disease (COPD). COPD is incurable. It is characterized by purple lips and nails and congestive heart failure.

PROBABLE OUTCOME

Chronic bronchitis is usually curable with treatment—if the patient is a non-smoker and doesn't have an underlying chronic disease, such as congestive heart failure, bronchiectasis, or tuberculosis. Chronic bronchitis usually reduces life expectancy if a person smokes and doesn't stop, or if there is an underlying chronic disease.

TREATMENT

HOME CARE

Instructions for a chronic bronchitis patient:

- Stop smoking.
- If you go to school or work or live in an area with heavy air pollution, do everything you can to avoid or reduce it. Consider changing schools and jobs and installing air-conditioning with a filter and humidity control in your home.
- Avoid sudden temperature changes or exposure to cold, wet weather.
- Avoid talking loudly, laughing loudly, crying and exertion, if these trigger coughing episodes.
- Practice bronchial drainage and deep-breathing techniques. Your physician will provide instructions.

MEDICATION

- Don't give your child cough suppressants; they make chronic bronchitis worse.
- Your doctor may prescribe:
  - Antibiotics to fight chronic or recurrent infection.
  - Expectorants to loosen secretions.
  - Bronchodilators to open bronchial tubes.

ACTIVITY

No restrictions. Your child should remain as active as possible.

DIET & FLUIDS

No special diet. Increase the child's fluid intake to 8 to 10 glasses a day.

OK FOR SCHOOL, PRESCHOOL, OR NURSERY?

- Yes, except during episodes of acute bronchitis with fever. In such cases, OK to return when signs of infection have decreased, appetite returns, and alertness, strength, and feeling of well-being will allow.

CALL YOUR DOCTOR IF

- Your child has symptoms of chronic bronchitis.
- Your child develops a fever of 101F (38.3C).
- Blood appears in the sputum.
- Chest pain increases.
- Shortness of breath occurs even when the child is resting or not coughing.
- Sputum thickens despite efforts to thin it.
- Vomiting occurs.

BRUCELLOSIS
(Undulant Fever; Bang's Disease)

GENERAL INFORMATION

DESCRIPTION

Brucellosis is a bacterial infection transmitted to humans from infected cows, pigs, sheep or goats. It is not contagious from person to person. The blood-producing organs, including bone marrow, lymph glands, liver, and spleen are involved.

Appropriate health care includes:

- Physician's monitoring of general condition and medications.
- Hospitalization.
- Self-care after treatment of the acute phase.

SIGNS & SYMPTOMS

The disease has an acute form and a chronic form. In the acute form, the following symptoms appear suddenly:

- Chills, intermittent fever, sweating.
- Marked fatigue.
- Tenderness along the spine.
- Headache.
- Enlarged lymph glands.

In the chronic form, the following symptoms appear suddenly:

- Fatigue.
- Muscle pain.
- Backache.
- Constipation.
- Weight loss.
- Depression.
- Abscesses in the ovaries, kidney and brain (rare).

CAUSES

Infection is caused by the bacteria brucella, which is transmitted to humans through unpasteurized milk or milk products (butter, cheese) or meat products.

RISK FACTORS

- Pernicious anemia or previous stomach surgery. These conditions result in reduced stomach acid; stomach acid decreases the chance of infection.
- Living or working around animals, such as living on a farm or working in a butcher shop.

PREVENTING COMPLICATIONS OR RECURRENCE

- Don't serve your child unpasteurized milk from any source.
- Encourage your child to use gloves and aprons when working around animals.

BRUCELLOSIS (Undulant Fever; Bang's Disease)

WHAT TO EXPECT

MEDICAL TESTS

- Your own observation of symptoms.
- Medical history and physical exam by a doctor.
- Laboratory blood studies.

POSSIBLE COMPLICATIONS

- Heart, bone, brain, or liver infection (rare).
- Chronic illness and disability from inadequate treatment and care.

PROBABLE OUTCOME

Usually curable in 3 to 4 weeks with treatment.

TREATMENT

HOME CARE

- It usually is not necessary to isolate the ill child.
- All family members who may have been exposed to the same infected milk products should have medical checkups and diagnostic tests.

MEDICATION

Your doctor may prescribe:

- Antibiotics to fight infection, such as tetracycline, for a minimum of 3 weeks.
- Cortisone drugs to reduce the inflammatory response in severe cases.
- Pain relievers for muscle pain.
- See Medications section for information regarding medicines your doctor may prescribe.

ACTIVITY

Your child should rest in bed until fever and other symptoms subside, then resume normal activities gradually.

DIET & FLUIDS

No special diet. Increase the child's calories if weight loss has been significant.

OK FOR SCHOOL, PRESCHOOL, OR NURSERY?

When appetite has returned and alertness, strength, and feeling of well-being will allow.

CALL YOUR DOCTOR IF

- Your child has symptoms of undulant fever.
- Fever or other symptoms recur after treatment.

BRUISES AND HEMATOMAS

GENERAL INFORMATION

DESCRIPTION

Bruises are purple-red stains in the skin resulting from a blow or bump that ruptures small blood vessels near the skin's surface. Children with fair skin bruise more easily than those with darker skin. Hematomas are dome-shaped collections of blood—usually clotted—under the skin and the scalp or inside the abdomen. The hematoma is formed by bleeding from a broken blood vessel. Bruises and hematomas fade from purple-red to maroon, then green or yellow. Appropriate health care includes: doctor's care unless the bruise or hematoma is very small; needle aspiration of blood from the hematoma if the hematoma is accessible; at the same time, hyaluronidase (an enzyme) can be injected into the hematoma space; self-care for minor bruises or hematomas, or during the rehabilitation phase following serious hematomas; physical therapy for serious hematomas.

SIGNS & SYMPTOMS

- Swelling over the injury site.
- Fluctuance (feeling of tenseness to the touch, like pushing on an overinflated balloon).
- Tenderness for 1 to 3 days.
- Redness that progresses through several color changes—purple, green-yellow, and yellow—before it completely heals.

CAUSES

Direct blow to the injured part, usually with a blunt object. Bleeding into the tissue causes the surrounding tissue to be pushed away.

RISK FACTORS

Contact sports, especially if the child is not adequately protected; medical history of any bleeding disorder such as hemophilia; poor nutrition, including vitamin deficiency; use of anticoagulants or aspirin.

PREVENTING COMPLICATIONS OR RECURRENCE

Protect the child's body with padding if there is a risk during participation in athletic activity. If the child must compete before healing, use tape, padding, splits, or a cast to prevent reinjury.

? WHAT TO EXPECT

MEDICAL TESTS

Your own observation of symptoms; medical history and physical exam by a doctor; X-rays of the injured area to assess the total injury and to rule out underlying bone fractures. The total extent of the child's injury may not be apparent for 48 to 72 hours.

POSSIBLE COMPLICATIONS

Infection introduced through a break in the child's skin at the time of injury, or during aspiration of the hematoma by a doctor; prolonged healing time if the child resumes activity too soon; calcification of the blood remaining in the hematoma, if blood has not been completely removed or absorbed.

BRUISES AND HEMATOMAS

PROBABLE OUTCOME

Complete resorption of blood and healing within 10 to 60 days unless blood is removed from significant hematomas with aspiration, which reduces healing time.

TREATMENT

HOME CARE

- Use instructions for R.I.C.E., the first letters of *rest*, *ice*, *compression*, and *elevation*. See Appendix 39 for details.
- Use ice soaks on the child's injury 3 or 4 times a day. Fill a bucket with ice water, and soak the injured area for 20 minutes at a time.
- After 48 hours, localized heat promotes healing.
- Don't massage the bruised area or the hematoma. You may trigger bleeding again.

MEDICATION

- For minor discomfort use non-prescription medicines such as acetaminophen or ibuprofen; topical liniments and ointments.
- Your doctor may prescribe stronger medicine for pain, if needed.

ACTIVITY

Your child can begin activities slowly and stop exercise as soon as pain begins. The child should increase activity as healing progresses. To prevent delayed healing, protect the injured part against excessive motion soon after injury. Motion breaks down the clot and causes irritation throughout, leading to possible scar formation, calcification, and limited movement after healing.

REHABILITATION

- Your child should begin daily rehabilitation exercises when able.
- Use a gentle ice massage on the child's injury for 10 minutes before and after physical activity. Fill a large Styrofoam cup with water and freeze. Tear a small amount of foam from the top so ice protrudes. Massage firmly over the injured area in a circle about the size of a softball.

DIET & FLUIDS

During recovery, your child should eat a well-balanced diet that includes extra protein, such as meat, fish, poultry, cheese, milk, and eggs.

OK FOR SCHOOL, PRESCHOOL, OR NURSERY?

Yes, when condition and sense of well-being will allow.

CALL YOUR DOCTOR IF

- Your child has signs or symptoms of a serious bruise or hematoma that doesn't begin to improve in 1 or 2 days.
- The child's skin is broken and signs of infection (drainage, increasing pain, fever, headache, muscle aches, dizziness, or a general ill feeling) occur.

BULIMIA (Binge-Eating Syndrome; Binge-Purge Syndrome; Bulimarexia)

GENERAL INFORMATION

DESCRIPTION

Bulimia is a psychological eating disorder characterized by abnormal, constant craving for food and binge eating, followed by self-induced vomiting or laxative use. The brain and central nervous system, kidneys, liver, endocrine system, and gastrointestinal tract are involved. Bulimia usually affects adolescents and young adults.

Appropriate health care includes:

- Physician's monitoring of general condition and medications.
- Psychotherapy or counseling that may include hypnosis or biofeedback training.
- Hospitalization (severe cases).
- Self-care after diagnosis.

SIGNS & SYMPTOMS

Recurrent episodes of binge eating (rapid consumption of a large amount of food in a short time, usually less than 2 hours), plus at least 3 of the following:

- Preference for high-calorie, convenience foods during a binge.
- Secretive eating during a binge. Patients are aware that the eating pattern is abnormal, and they fear being unable to stop eating.
- Termination of an eating binge with purging measures, such as laxative use or self-induced vomiting.
- Depression and guilt following an eating binge.
- Repeated attempts to lose weight with severely restrictive diets, self-induced vomiting, and use of laxatives or diuretics.
- Frequent weight fluctuations greater than 10 pounds from alternately fasting and gorging.
- No underlying physical disorder.
- Etching of teeth from stomach acid.
- Reddened and sore throat from irritation of vomiting stomach acid.

CAUSES

Unknown. The disorder often begins during or after stringent dieting and may be caused by stress related to insufficient food intake.

RISK FACTORS

- Anorexia nervosa.
- Depression.
- Stress, including lifestyle changes, such as moving or starting a new school or job.
- Neurotic preoccupation with being physically attractive.

PREVENTING COMPLICATIONS OR RECURRENCE

Raise your children in a wholesome family environment with emphasis on caring and good communication rather than on external appearances.

BULIMIA (Binge-Eating Syndrome; Binge-Purge Syndrome; Bulimarexia)

WHAT TO EXPECT

MEDICAL TESTS

- Your own observation of symptoms. Many patients are secretive, and parents may be unaware of this condition.
- Medical history and physical exam by a doctor.
- Laboratory blood studies, including measurement of electrolyte levels.

POSSIBLE COMPLICATIONS

Fluid and electrolyte imbalance from vomiting, inducing life-threatening heartbeat irregularities.

PROBABLE OUTCOME

Most patients can control the behavior with counseling, psychotherapy, biofeedback training, and individual or group psychotherapy. Without treatment, complications can be fatal.

TREATMENT

HOME CARE

See Appendix 19 for suggestions to reduce stress and improve overall health.

MEDICATION

- Medication is usually not necessary for this disorder. However, some doctors have successfully treated bulimia with anti-depressants.
- See Medications section for information regarding medicines your doctor may prescribe.

ACTIVITY

No restrictions.

DIET & FLUIDS

If hospitalization is necessary, your doctor may prescribe intravenous fluids for your child. During recovery, vitamin and mineral supplements will be necessary until signs of deficiency disappear and normal eating patterns are established.

OK FOR SCHOOL, PRESCHOOL, OR NURSERY?

When appetite has returned and alertness, strength, and feeling of well-being will allow.

CALL YOUR DOCTOR IF

- You suspect your child has bulimia.
- The following occurs during treatment:
  - — Rapid, irregular heartbeat or chest pain.
  - — Loss of consciousness.
  - — Cessation of menstrual periods.
  - — Repeated vomiting or diarrhea.
  - — Continued weight loss, despite treatment.

BUNION
(Hallux Valgus)

GENERAL INFORMATION

DESCRIPTION

Bunions are overgrowth of tissue at the base of the great (big) toe. Bunions may be congenital or hereditary. A bunion often impairs athletic performance until it is corrected with medical treatment or surgery.

Appropriate health care includes:

- Self-care for mild cases.
- Surgery for persistent or severe cases to remove the overgrown tissue and correct the position of the bones.

SIGNS & SYMPTOMS

- An inward-turned great toe that may overlap the second—and sometimes the third—toe.
- Thickened skin over the bony protrusion at the base of the great toe.
- Fluid accumulation under the thickened skin (sometimes).
- Foot pain and stiffness.
- Inflammation and swelling around the child's bunion.

CAUSES

Irritation of the bony bump when the big toe is directed toward the little toe.

RISK FACTORS

- Narrow-toed, high-heeled shoes that compress your child's toes together.
- Arthritis.
- Family history of foot disorders.

PREVENTING COMPLICATIONS OR RECURRENCE

Instructions for your child:

- Wear wide-toed, well-fitting shoes with strong arch supports.
- Don't wear high heels or shoes without room for your toes in their normal position.
- Don't wear socks or stockings that are too tight.
- After treatment, prevent a recurrence by placing a 1/4-inch thickness of foam rubber between the big toe and the second toe.

WHAT TO EXPECT

MEDICAL TESTS

- Your own observation of symptoms.
- Medical history and physical exam by a doctor or podiatrist.
- X-rays of the child's foot.

POSSIBLE COMPLICATIONS

- Infection of the bunion, especially in children with diabetes mellitus.
- Inflammation and arthritic changes in other joints caused by walking difficulty, which places abnormal stress on the child's foot, hip, and spine.
- Excessive bleeding or infection if surgery is required.

PROBABLE OUTCOME

Usually improves with treatment and preventive measures to guard against recurrence.

BUNION
(Hallux Valgus)

TREATMENT

HOME CARE

Instructions for your child:

• Before bedtime, separate the great toe from the others with a foam-rubber pad.

• When wearing shoes, place a thick, ring-shaped adhesive pad over the bunion.

• Use arch supports to relieve pressure on the bunion. These are available in shoe-repair shops.

MEDICATION

• Usually not necessary for this disorder unless infection develops.

• See Medications section for information regarding medicines your doctor may prescribe.

ACTIVITY

No restrictions as long as the child's bunion is protected from irritation. If surgery is necessary, the child can resume normal activities gradually afterward. Advise your child to walk on his heels until the surgical site heals. Elevate the foot of the child's bed to reduce swelling over the incision. Your child should avoid vigorous exercise for 6 weeks following surgery.

DIET & FLUIDS

During recovery from surgery, serve the child a well-balanced diet that includes extra protein, such as meat, fish, poultry, cheese, milk, and eggs. Your child should increase fiber and fluid intake to prevent constipation that may result from decreased activity.

OK FOR SCHOOL, PRESCHOOL, OR NURSERY?

Yes, when condition and sense of well-being will allow.

CALL YOUR DOCTOR IF

• Your child has a bunion that is interfering with normal activities.

• Signs of infection (fever, headache, heat, increased tenderness, or pain) develop during treatment or after surgery.

BURNS

GENERAL INFORMATION

DESCRIPTION

Burns are injuries to the skin, and sometimes other organs, from contact with heat, radiation, electricity, or chemicals. The skin, underlying tissue, and respiratory system (sometimes) are involved.

Appropriate health care includes:

- Self-care for most first-degree burns.
- Physician's monitoring of general condition and medications for more severe burns.
- Hospitalization for all large third-degree burns and some second-degree burns. Special burn centers exist for the worst cases.
- Surgery to graft skin over third-degree burns.

SIGNS & SYMPTOMS

Burns are of 3 types:

- First-degree burns are limited to the upper skin layer. They produce redness, tenderness, pain, swelling, and slight fever.
- Second-degree burns affect deeper skin layers. Symptoms are more severe and include blisters.
- Third-degree burns involve all skin layers. Skin is white (appears cooked), and there may be no pain in the initial stages.

CAUSES

- Rise in skin temperature from heat sources, such as fire, steam, or electricity.
- Tissue injury caused by chemicals or radiation, including sunlight.

RISK FACTORS

- Stress, carelessness, smoking in bed, or excess alcohol consumption, all of which make accidents more likely.

PREVENTING COMPLICATIONS OR RECURRENCE

- Have your child wear sun-screen lotions outdoors.
- Fireproof your home. Install smoke alarms and plan emergency exits.
- Have your child wear protective gear and observe safety precautions around heat or radiation.
- Remind your child not to touch uncovered electric wires.
- Teach children safety rules for matches, fires and electrical outlets.
- Discard extension cords with a pronged plug on one end and a bulb socket on the other. These are hazardous.
- If you have small children, put safety caps on unused outlets. Discard frayed cords.

WHAT TO EXPECT

MEDICAL TESTS

- Your own observation of symptoms.
- Medical history and physical exam by a doctor.
- Laboratory blood and urine tests, and studies of kidney and liver function (severe burns).

POSSIBLE COMPLICATIONS

- Infection at the burn site.
- Pneumonia.
- Shock due to loss of fluids and electrolytes (severe burns).
- Permanent scars.
- Vision impairment, if eyes are injured.

PROBABLE OUTCOME

Most persons recover if the extent of burns (including third-degree burns) is limited to 50% of the body surface. For less-severe burns, skin usually repairs itself in 1 to 3 weeks.

TREATMENT

HOME CARE

For severe burns, see First-aid instructions in the back of this book. For less-severe burns:

- Apply non-prescription body lotion to your child to cool first-degree burns.
- Immerse your child's small second- or third-degree burn areas in cold water for 10 minutes to reduce pain and swelling.
- Keep the child's burn area clean. Soak the child in a tub or use lukewarm compresses once a day. You may add 2 tablespoons of powdered detergent to the tub to help soak off crusting areas. Use plain water for compresses.
- Prop the child's burn area higher than the rest of the body, if possible.
- You may use dressings on the child's burn.

MEDICATION

- To treat minor burns, use non-prescription antibiotic ointments, topical anesthetics, and aspirin.
- To treat severe burns, your doctor may prescribe pain relievers, antibiotics, and a tetanus booster shot.
- See Medications section for information regarding medicines your doctor may prescribe.

ACTIVITY

Depends on location and extent of the burn. Ask your doctor.

DIET & FLUIDS

No special diet for minor burns. More severe burns require intravenous feeding.

OK FOR SCHOOL, PRESCHOOL, OR NURSERY?

When appetite has returned and alertness, strength, and feeling of well-being will allow.

CALL YOUR DOCTOR IF

- Your child has a second- or third-degree burn, or a first-degree burn over a large area.
- An infant has a burn, even if it seems minor.
- The following occurs during treatment:
  - — No healing in 6 days.
  - — Chills and fever.
  - — Increased pain, redness, swelling, or pus in the burn area.

CALCIUM IMBALANCE

GENERAL INFORMATION

DESCRIPTION

Calcium is a component of the blood that helps regulate the heartbeat, transmit nerve impulses, contract muscles, and form bones and teeth. Too much *or* too little can cause serious—sometimes life-threatening—medical problems. Body parts involved include membranes of all body cells, muscles, bones, parathyroid glands, and parathyroid hormones (these regulate calcium absorption and utilization).

Appropriate health care includes: self-care after diagnosis; physician's monitoring of general condition and medications; hospitalization (sometimes) followed by self-care at home.

SIGNS & SYMPTOMS

- Too little calcium: muscle spasms and twitching; numbness and tingling in the arms, legs, hands, and feet; seizures; irregular heartbeat; high blood pressure.
- Too much calcium: lethargy; loss of appetite; vomiting and diarrhea; dehydration and thirst; irregular heartbeat; low blood pressure; seizures or coma (worst cases only).

CAUSES

- Too little calcium: underactive parathyroid glands from disease or damage during neck surgery; inadequate dietary intake of calcium and vitamin D; malabsorption from the gastrointestinal tract (usually for unknown reasons); severe burns; severe infections; chronic pancreatitis; kidney failure; decreased blood levels of magnesium.
- Too much calcium: overactive parathyroid glands; multiple fractures and prolonged bed rest; multiple myeloma; tumors—benign or malignant—that destroy bone.

RISK FACTORS

- Too little calcium: use of certain drugs, including thiazide diuretics and calcium-channel blockers; injury, cancer, or surgery of the thyroid gland or parathyroid glands; excess alcohol consumption leading to poor nutrition.
- Too much calcium: improper diet, especially overconsumption of milk products or non-prescription antacids that contain calcium; repeated transfusions with citrated blood.
- Either too little or too much calcium: chronic kidney disease.

PREVENTING COMPLICATIONS OR RECURRENCE

Urge your child to eat a normal, balanced diet. If your child drinks alcoholic beverages, not more than 1 or 2—if any—should be consumed daily. Urge your child not to use non-prescription antacids on a regular basis.

? WHAT TO EXPECT

MEDICAL TESTS

Your own observation of symptoms; medical history and physical exam by a doctor; laboratory blood studies of calcium levels; EKG (see Glossary); X-rays of bones.

POSSIBLE COMPLICATIONS

Cardiac arrest; fractures of weak bones.

PROBABLE OUTCOME

Unless your child's calcium imbalance is caused by cancer, most cases are curable with treatment in 1 week.

TREATMENT

HOME CARE

The underlying cause must be corrected before your child can follow a treatment program to prevent a recurrence.

MEDICATION

Your doctor may prescribe: intravenous calcium gluconate or calcium carbonate for too little calcium; intravenous saline solution and loop diuretics (furosemide and ethacrynic acid) for too much calcium.

ACTIVITY

After treatment, the child can resume normal activities as symptoms improve.

DIET & FLUIDS

- For a mild low-calcium level, your child should take calcium supplements and vitamin D. Increase the child's intake of protein, milk, and milk products.
- For a mild high-calcium level, restrict your child's consumption of dairy products and calcium-containing antacids.

OK FOR SCHOOL, PRESCHOOL, OR NURSERY?

When appetite has returned and alertness, strength, and feeling of well-being will allow.

CALL YOUR DOCTOR IF

- Your child has symptoms of a calcium imbalance.
- Symptoms recur after treatment.

CANDIDIASIS OF INTERTRIGINOUS SKIN (Moniliasis)

GENERAL INFORMATION

DESCRIPTION

Candidiasis of intertriginous skin is a yeast infection in skin folds or areas of adjacent skin that come in contact with each other, such as in the diaper area of an infant, the groin or under the breasts. This is contagious from person to person and from place to place on the same person. Body parts involved include the skin of the scrotum, vagina and vaginal lips, underarm area, spaces between fingers and toes, inner thighs, under the breasts, and over the base of the spine (sacrum). Candidiasis of intertriginous skin can affect older children and adolescents.

Appropriate health care includes: self-care after diagnosis; physician's monitoring of general condition and medications (sometimes).

SIGNS & SYMPTOMS

Plaques (patches or flat areas) with the following characteristics:

- Bright red patches with poorly defined borders. They are often 6cm to 12cm in diameter or larger.
- Some plaques appear to have pus.
- Skin appears moist and crusted.
- Itching is usually severe.
- Smaller plaques sometimes surround larger plaques. Smaller plaques are less than 1mm in size. They form small pustules (small white blisters with pus inside).

CAUSES

Yeast infection of the skin caused by candida fungus (usually candida albicans). The spore form of this organism normally grows in the intestinal tract and the vagina. Skin signs do not begin until yeast changes from its spore form to another growth phase, the mycelial phase. Damaged skin, moisture, and warmth are all necessary for the infection to take over.

RISK FACTORS

Use of oral antibiotics; use of steroids (oral, injectable or topical); diabetes; obesity; poor nutrition; excessive sweating; crowded or unsanitary living conditions.

PREVENTING COMPLICATIONS OR RECURRENCE

- If your child must take antibiotics, consult your doctor about eating yogurt, buttermilk, or sour cream, or taking acidophilus tablets. These help prevent yeast infections that may result as an adverse effect of the drugs.
- Keep the child's skin cool and dry.

WHAT TO EXPECT

MEDICAL TESTS

- Your own observation of symptoms.
- Medical history and physical exam by a doctor.
- Laboratory culture to identify the yeast organism.

CANDIDIASIS OF INTERTRIGINOUS SKIN (Moniliasis)

POSSIBLE COMPLICATIONS

- Secondary bacterial infections.
- Id reactions (in Illnesses section).
- Blood poisoning.

PROBABLE OUTCOME

Usually curable in 2 weeks with treatment. Without treatment, healing may be slow (4 to 5 years). Recurrence is common.

TREATMENT

HOME CARE

- Keep your child's skin cool and dry. Expose affected areas to sunlight as much as possible.
- Let the child wear loose cotton clothing. Avoid synthetic or wool fabrics.
- Protect skin from injury.
- If your daughter has a vaginal infection as well as infection of the surrounding skin, obtain treatment for the vaginitis (see Vaginitis, Monilial).

MEDICATION

- Your doctor may prescribe anti-fungal topical medications such as nystatin, haloprigin, miconazole, or clotrimazole. Gently massage a small amount into the affected area 3 or 4 times a day. Use only enough to cover. Larger amounts don't help.
- Continue to use the medication on your child for 1 week after symptoms and signs disappear, to prevent further recurrences.
- See Medications section for information regarding medicines your doctor may prescribe.

ACTIVITY

No restrictions, except for the child to avoid heat and sweating.

DIET & FLUIDS

No special diet.

OK FOR SCHOOL, PRESCHOOL, OR NURSERY?

Yes.

CALL YOUR DOCTOR IF

- Your child has symptoms of candidiasis.
- The following occurs during treatment:
  - — Infection continues to spread, despite treatment.
  - — Your child develops signs of secondary bacterial infection (pain, tenderness, redness, warmth, oozing).
- New, unexplained symptoms develop. Drugs used in treatment may produce side effects.

CANKER SORES (Aphthous Ulcers)

GENERAL INFORMATION

DESCRIPTION

Canker sores are painful ulcers that occur in the lining of the mouth. Ulcers are not cancerous, but they may be contagious. The mouth and adjacent areas are involved. Canker sores can affect both sexes, all ages, but is more common in females.

Appropriate health care includes:

- Self-care after diagnosis.
- Physician's monitoring of general condition and medications (sometimes).

SIGNS & SYMPTOMS

Mouth ulcers with the following characteristics:

- Ulcers are small, painful, shallow, and covered by a gray membrane. Borders are surrounded by an intense red halo.
- Ulcers appear on lips, gums, inner cheeks, tongue, palate, and throat. Usually 2 or 3 ulcers appear during an attack, but 10 to 15 ulcers are not uncommon.
- Ulcers may be so painful during the first 2 or 3 days that they interfere with eating or speaking.
- Ulcers are preceded by tingling or burning for 24 hours (sometimes).

CAUSES

Unknown, but following are the most likely causes:

- Emotional or physical stress, anxiety, or premenstrual tension.
- Injury to your child's mouth lining caused by hot food, toothbrushing, or dental work.
- Irritation from foods, such as chocolate, citrus, acid foods (vinegar, pickles), salted nuts, or potato chips.
- Virus infection.

RISK FACTORS

Recent dental treatment.

PREVENTING COMPLICATIONS OR RECURRENCE

- Your child should brush teeth at least twice a day and floss regularly to keep the mouth clean and healthy.
- Your child should avoid stress if possible. See Appendix 19.
- Observe if canker sores develop after your child eats specific foods. Encourage the child not to eat foods that seem to trigger attacks.

WHAT TO EXPECT

MEDICAL TESTS

- Your own observation of symptoms.
- Medical history and physical exam by a doctor.
- Laboratory culture of the sores.

POSSIBLE COMPLICATIONS

Dehydration in severe cases where eating and drinking are limited.

CANKER SORES
(Aphthous Ulcers)

PROBABLE OUTCOME

Most ulcers heal without scarring in 2 weeks. Recurrent attacks are common. They vary from a single lesion 2 or 3 times a year to an uninterrupted succession of multiple lesions.

TREATMENT

HOME CARE

- Rinse the child's mouth 3 or more times a day with salt solution (1/2 teaspoon salt to 8 oz. water).
- Clean sores frequently with 2% hydrogen peroxide on a cotton applicator.
- If your child's canker sore is caused by a rough tooth or braces, consult your dentist. The sore won't heal until the cause is eliminated.

MEDICATION

Your doctor may prescribe:
- Topical anesthetics to relieve your child's pain.
- Antibiotics, such as tetracycline, to fight infection. Tetracycline is effective if the liquid form is held in the child's mouth for 2 to 5 minutes to coat the ulcers before swallowing. If started early, it prevents pain.
- Protective dental paste with a steroid derivative, such as Orabase with triamcinolone acetonide. If applied as soon as the ulcer begins, this prevents pain. Keep the medicine prescribed by your doctor for the child's first attack. Use it immediately at the sign of a recurrent attack. The sooner treatment starts, the milder the attack.
- See Medications section for information regarding medicines your doctor may prescribe.

ACTIVITY

No restrictions.

DIET & FLUIDS

No restrictions, except to have the child avoid foods that aggravate ulcers. Encourage your child to drink as many fluids and eat as well-balanced a diet as possible while healing. To minimize pain, let your child sip liquids through straws. Foods that cause the least pain are milk, liquid gelatin, yogurt, ice cream, and custard.

OK FOR SCHOOL, PRESCHOOL, OR NURSERY?

- When appetite has returned and alertness, strength, and feeling of well-being will allow. Keep the child's eating and drinking utensils separate until sores heal.

CALL YOUR DOCTOR IF

- Your child's temperature rises to 102F (38.9C) or higher.
- Ulcers don't improve in 3 days despite treatment.
- Pain is unbearable and isn't relieved by treatment.
- A child with canker sores loses weight.

CARDIOMYOPATHY (Hypertrophic Cardiomyopathy; Nutritional Cardiomyopathy)

GENERAL INFORMATION

DESCRIPTION

Cardiomyopathy is a disorder of the heart muscle that can be caused by many medical problems. The heart muscle is weakened and cannot pump blood efficiently. Decreasing heart function eventually affects the lungs, liver, and circulatory system. Cardiomyopathy can affect both sexes and all ages but is most common in adult males.

Appropriate health care includes:

- Self-care after diagnosis.
- Physician's monitoring of general condition and medications.

SIGNS & SYMPTOMS

If cardiomyopathy is extensive enough to cause congestive heart failure in your child, the following symptoms may occur:

- Irregular or rapid heartbeat.
- Shortness of breath with activity.
- Swelling of the child's feet and ankles.
- Fatigue.
- Cough with frothy, bloody sputum.
- Loss of appetite.

CAUSES

- Nutritional deficiency, especially of vitamin B-4 (thiamine).
- Mineral deficiency, especially of potassium.
- Fat tissue in the child's heart that replaces muscle fibers.
- Amyloid deposits (see Glossary) due to other disorders.
- Tuberous sclerosis (see Glossary).
- Hemochromatosis (see Glossary).
- Severe anemia.
- Friedreich's ataxia (see Glossary).
- Stress.
- Virus infection (rare).
- Coronary artery disease (advanced stages).
- Alcoholism.

RISK FACTORS

Obesity; family history of cardiomyopathy; use of certain drugs, such as diuretics; smoking; alcoholism.

PREVENTING COMPLICATIONS OR RECURRENCE

Your child should eat a well-balanced diet and drink alcohol moderately, if at all.

CARDIOMYOPATHY (Hypertrophic Cardiomyopathy; Nutritional Cardiomyopathy)

WHAT TO EXPECT

MEDICAL TESTS

- Your own observation of symptoms.
- Medical history and physical exam by a doctor.
- EKG (see Glossary).
- X-rays of the heart and lungs.
- Cardiac catheterization and radioactive studies to determine left ventricular ejection fraction. When the ejection fraction falls below 20% and no simpler measures exist, many prominent medical authorities recommend heart transplants.

POSSIBLE COMPLICATIONS

Congestive heart failure.

PROBABLE OUTCOME

- If the underlying disorder can be corrected, cardiomyopathy may be curable.
- If the underlying cause can't be corrected, cardiomyopathy is incurable. Some patients are candidates for a heart transplant.

TREATMENT

HOME CARE

Weigh the child daily before breakfast and record the weight. Report any marked weight change to your doctor. This may indicate excess fluid accumulation.

MEDICATION

Your doctor may prescribe:

- Digitalis to improve your child's heart function.
- Diuretics to decrease fluid retention.
- Vitamins or potassium supplements (if the disorder is caused by a deficiency).
- See Medications section for information regarding medicines your doctor may prescribe.

ACTIVITY

After treatment your child can resume normal activities gradually.

DIET & FLUIDS

Low-salt diet (see Appendix 29).

OK FOR SCHOOL, PRESCHOOL, OR NURSERY?

Only upon clearance of your doctor.

CALL YOUR DOCTOR IF

- Your child has symptoms of cardiomyopathy or symptoms recur after treatment.
- Your child has chest pain.
- New, unexplained symptoms develop. Drugs used in treatment may produce side effects.

ILLNESSES

CAT-SCRATCH FEVER

GENERAL INFORMATION

DESCRIPTION

Cat-scratch fever is a mild infectious disease of unknown cause resulting from a scratch by a cat. It is not contagious from person to person. More than one family member can be infected at one time. The skin and lymph glands are involved. Appropriate health care includes:

- Self-care after diagnosis.
- Physician's monitoring of general condition and medications.
- Surgery to drain the lymph gland, if it contains pus.

SIGNS & SYMPTOMS

- A lump, with or without pus or fluid, which starts on the scratched skin 1 to 2 weeks after the cat scratch.
- Swollen lymph glands near the affected area.
- Low fever of 99F to 101F (37.2C to 38.3C).
- Fatigue.
- Headache.

CAUSES

Infection from germs—probably viral—carried on cat's claws. The infection spreads to lymph glands near the scratch by way of lymphatic vessels.

RISK FACTORS

Owning or handling cats.

PREVENTING COMPLICATIONS OR RECURRENCE

- Have pet cats declawed by the veterinarian.
- Teach your child to respect animals and not provoke them.
- Urge your child not to pick up strange cats.

WHAT TO EXPECT

MEDICAL TESTS

- Your own observation of symptoms.
- Medical history and physical exam by a doctor. Tell your doctor of any cat scratches in the previous 2 weeks.
- Laboratory skin test to confirm the diagnosis.

POSSIBLE COMPLICATIONS

Eye inflammation (rare).

PROBABLE OUTCOME

Spontaneous recovery within 3 weeks.

TREATMENT

HOME CARE

- It is not necessary to isolate the ill child because the disease is not transmitted from person to person.
- It should not be necessary to destroy the cat. Consult your veterinarian.

MEDICATION

- Your doctor may prescribe antibiotics for your child, although their effectiveness is not proven.
- See Medications section for information regarding medicines your doctor may prescribe.

ACTIVITY

The child should rest in bed until fever subsides and energy returns, then resume normal activities gradually.

DIET & FLUIDS

No special diet.

OK FOR SCHOOL, PRESCHOOL, OR NURSERY?

When signs of infection have decreased, appetite returns, and alertness, strength, and feeling of well-being will allow.

CALL YOUR DOCTOR IF

- Your child has symptoms of cat-scratch fever.
- A swollen lymph gland becomes painful and red. This may indicate that a doctor should open and drain the infected gland.

CATARACT

GENERAL INFORMATION

DESCRIPTION

A cataract is a clouding of the lens of the eye. The lens is a crystal-clear, flexible structure near the front of the eyeball. It helps to keep vision in focus, and screens and refracts light rays. The lens has no blood supply. It is nourished by the vitreous (the watery substance that surrounds it). Cataracts may form in one or both eyes. If they form in both eyes, their growth rate may be very different. Cataracts are not cancerous. All ages are affected. Some infants are born with congenital cataracts.

Appropriate health care includes:

- Doctor's (ophthalmologist's) treatment.
- Surgery to remove the lens.

SIGNS & SYMPTOMS

- Blurred vision that may be worse in bright light. The blurring may first become apparent while driving at night, when lights seem to scatter or have halos.
- Double vision (occasionally).
- Opaque, milky-white pupil (advanced stages only).

CAUSES

- Injury to the eye.
- Illnesses associated with high blood sugar, such as diabetes mellitus.
- Inflammation, such as uveitis (see Glossary).
- Drugs, especially cortisone and its derivatives.
- Exposure to X-rays, microwaves, and infrared radiation.
- Hereditary causes, including the effect of German measles on the unborn child of a mother who contracts the disease early in her pregnancy.
- Galactosemia (see Glossary) in an infant.

RISK FACTORS

Exposure to any causes listed above.

PREVENTING COMPLICATIONS OR RECURRENCE

- Women of childbearing age should be vaccinated against German measles if they have not had the disease or been immunized.
- The use of cortisone drugs or any others that affect the eye lens should be monitored carefully by a doctor.
- Eye disorders that may cause cataract formation, such as iritis and uveitis, should receive prompt medical treatment.

WHAT TO EXPECT

MEDICAL TESTS

- Your own observation of symptoms.
- Medical history and physical exam by a doctor.

POSSIBLE COMPLICATIONS

- Loss of vision.
- Postoperative complications, including rupture of the eye, adhesions, infections, and retinal detachment.

PROBABLE OUTCOME

Usually curable with surgery. Some cataracts never impair vision enough to require surgery. During the time cataracts are forming, frequent eyeglass changes may help vision.

TREATMENT

HOME CARE

Special eyeglasses or contact lenses will be needed after surgery.

MEDICATION

- Medicine usually is not necessary for this disorder.
- See Medications section for information regarding medicines your doctor may prescribe.

ACTIVITY

No restrictions, except that your child should not drive at night if vision is poor.

DIET & FLUIDS

No special diet.

OK FOR SCHOOL, PRESCHOOL, OR NURSERY?

When appetite returns and alertness, strength, and feeling of well-being will allow.

CALL YOUR DOCTOR IF

Your newborn baby or older child has symptoms of cataracts.

CELIAC DISEASE
(Gluten Enteropathy; Non-Tropical Sprue)

GENERAL INFORMATION

DESCRIPTION

Celiac disease is an allergic condition in the small intestine, triggered by gluten, which prevents the intestine from absorbing nutrients. Most forms are inherited. Celiac disease is not contagious or cancerous. The digestive system is involved. Celiac disease usually begins during infancy or early childhood (2 weeks to 1 year). Symptoms appear when the child first begins eating food with gluten. Rarely, celiac disease may appear for the first time in adults.

Appropriate health care includes:

- Home care and self-care after diagnosis.
- Physician's monitoring of general condition and medications.

SIGNS & SYMPTOMS

- Weight loss or slowed weight gain in an infant following the introduction of cereal to the diet.
- Poor appetite.
- Loose, pale, bulky, bad-smelling stools, or frequent gas.
- Swollen abdomen or abdominal pain.
- General undernourished appearance.
- Mouth ulcers.
- Anemia or vitamin deficiency, with fatigue, paleness, skin rash, or bone pain.
- Mildly bowed legs.

CAUSES

Celiac disease is a congenital disorder caused by an intolerance for gluten, a protein present in most grains.

RISK FACTORS

- Family history of celiac disease.
- Other allergies.

PREVENTING COMPLICATIONS OR RECURRENCE

Cannot be prevented at present.

WHAT TO EXPECT

MEDICAL TESTS

- Your own observation of symptoms.
- Medical history and physical exam by a doctor.
- Laboratory studies of stool and blood.
- X-rays of the digestive system.

POSSIBLE COMPLICATIONS

In rare cases, gluten withdrawal does not bring immediate improvement.

CELIAC DISEASE
(Gluten Enteropathy; Non-Tropical Sprue)

PROBABLE OUTCOME

With a strict, gluten-free diet, most children with celiac disease can expect a normal life. Improvement begins in 2 to 3 weeks.

TREATMENT

HOME CARE

No special instructions except those listed under other headings.

MEDICATION

Your doctor may prescribe:

- Iron and folic acid for anemia.
- Calcium and multiple-vitamin supplements for deficiencies.
- Oral cortisone drugs to reduce the body's inflammatory response during a severe attack.
- See Medications section for information regarding medicines your doctor may prescribe.

ACTIVITY

No restrictions.

DIET & FLUIDS

Gluten-free diet. It is difficult to exclude gluten from the child's diet completely, so be patient while becoming familiar with the diet.

OK FOR SCHOOL, PRESCHOOL, OR NURSERY?

Yes, except during acute episodes when the disease is out of control.

CALL YOUR DOCTOR IF

- Your child has symptoms of celiac disease.
- Symptoms don't decrease within 3 weeks after beginning a gluten-free diet.
- The child fails to regain lost weight or grow and develop as expected.
- Fever develops.

CELLULITIS
(Erysipelas)

GENERAL INFORMATION

DESCRIPTION

Cellulitis is a non-contagious infection of the connective tissue beneath the skin. Skin anywhere on the body is involved, but most likely cellulitis occurs on the face or lower legs.

Appropriate health care includes:

- Self-care after diagnosis.
- Physician's monitoring of general condition and medications.

SIGNS & SYMPTOMS

- Sudden tenderness, swelling, and redness in an area of the child's skin. The area of cellulitis is initially 5cm to 20cm in diameter, and grows rapidly in the first 24 hours. A thin red line often extends from the middle of the cellulitis toward the heart. Cellulitis does not develop into a boil.
- Fever, sometimes accompanied by chills and sweats.
- General ill feelings.
- Swollen lymph glands nearest the cellulitis (sometimes).

CAUSES

Infection from staphylococcus or streptococcus bacteria.

RISK FACTORS

- Use of immunosuppresive or cortisone drugs.
- Chronic illness, such as diabetes mellitus, or a recent infection that has lowered resistance.
- Any injury that breaks the skin.

PREVENTING COMPLICATIONS OR RECURRENCE

- Your child should avoid skin damage and use protective clothing or gear when participating in strenuous work or sports.
- Keep the child's skin clean.

WHAT TO EXPECT

MEDICAL TESTS

- Your own observation of symptoms.
- Medical history and physical exam by a doctor.
- Laboratory blood culture, if blood poisoning is suspected.

POSSIBLE COMPLICATIONS

- Blood poisoning, if bacteria enter the bloodstream.
- Brain infection or meningitis, if cellulitis occurs on the central part of the face.

PROBABLE OUTCOME

Usually curable in 7 to 10 days with treatment, unless the child has a chronic disease or is receiving immunosuppressive treatment. In that case, cellulitis may lead to blood poisoning and become life-threatening.

TREATMENT

HOME CARE

Use warm-water soaks (see Glossary) to hasten healing and relieve the child's pain and inflammation.

MEDICATION

- Your doctor may prescribe a penicillin drug, such as oxacillin, dicloxacillin or nafcillin, or erythromycin to fight infection. Have the child finish the prescribed dose, even if symptoms disappear.
- See Medications section for information regarding medicines your doctor may prescribe.

ACTIVITY

Your child should rest in bed until the fever disappears and other symptoms improve. Then the child can resume normal activities.

DIET & FLUIDS

No special diet. Vitamin C supplements (250mg to 500mg daily) may hasten healing.

OK FOR SCHOOL, PRESCHOOL, OR NURSERY?

When signs of infection have decreased, appetite returns, and alertness, strength, and feeling of well-being will allow.

CALL YOUR DOCTOR IF

- Your child has symptoms of cellulitis, especially on the face.
- The following occurs during treatment:
  - — Fever of 101F (38.3C) or higher.
  - — Drowsiness and lethargy.
  - — Blister over the area of cellulitis.
  - — Red streaks that continue to extend, despite treatment.
- New, unexplained symptoms develop. Drugs used in treatment may produce side effects.

CEREBRAL PALSY (CP)

GENERAL INFORMATION

DESCRIPTION

Cerebral palsy is a group of muscular and nervous-system disorders that usually begins in infancy and remains throughout life, causing varying degrees of disability. Cerebral palsy is not inherited. The central nervous system and muscular system are involved.

Appropriate health care includes:

- Home care when possible.
- Physician's monitoring of general condition and medications.
- Psychotherapy or counseling to help the family acknowledge the condition and help the child achieve maximum potential.
- Surgery to correct muscular-system deformities (sometimes).
- Time in an extended-care facility for children with severe CP (sometimes).

SIGNS & SYMPTOMS

Number and severity of the following symptoms vary widely among children with CP:

- Early sucking difficulty with the breast or bottle.
- Lack of normal muscle tone (early); slow development (walking, talking).
- Unusual body postures; stiffness and muscle spasms (later).
- Purposeless body movements; poor coordination or balance.
- Crossed eyes; deafness; convulsions.
- Various degrees of mental retardation (sometimes). Many are *not* mentally retarded at all!

CAUSES

Defects in the brain and spinal column. The reason for these defects is often unknown. Known reasons include:

- Birth injury, including prolonged oxygen deprivation.
- Use of drugs during pregnancy that damage the fetus.
- Infections, such as German measles, in the mother during pregnancy.
- Rh incompatibility or bile blockage in the newborn.
- Meningitis or encephalitis during infancy or childhood.

RISK FACTORS

Prematurity; excess alcohol consumption during pregnancy.

PREVENTING COMPLICATIONS OR RECURRENCE

Instructions for the mother:

- Before becoming pregnant, obtain immunizations against German measles if you have never had the disease or an immunization.
- Arrange for good medical care during pregnancy, labor, and delivery.
- Eat a normal, well-balanced diet during pregnancy.
- Don't drink alcohol or use any drug, including non-prescription drugs, during pregnancy without consulting your doctor.
- Don't smoke during pregnancy. It leads to low birth-weight babies with complications.

CEREBRAL PALSY (CP)

? WHAT TO EXPECT

MEDICAL TESTS

Your own observation of symptoms; medical history and physical exam by a doctor (sometimes a neurologist). A parent's intuition is often important. Obtain a second opinion, if necessary. Laboratory blood studies; EEG (see Glossary); psychological tests.

POSSIBLE COMPLICATIONS

- Hepatitis, if the child is institutionalized.
- Pressure sores, if the child is confined to bed.
- Contractures, if the child's limbs are not properly exercised.

PROBABLE OUTCOME

Children vary widely in the severity of this condition.. A child with CP may have high intelligence despite major muscular disability. Many children can be cared for in a loving home. Those with less-severe impairment can lead near-normal, productive lives. Children with severe impairments may require special care.

TREATMENT

HOME CARE

- Because early diagnosis is important, be sure your child has regular medical checkups. Failure to diagnose CP may deny the child opportunities for special programs that maximize growth and development.
- Maintain an optimistic outlook for yourself and your child. High expectations can sometimes be met.
- Seek help and advice from other parents whose children have cerebral palsy.
- Investigate resources in your community, including educational and physical-therapy programs, to obtain treatment that maximizes your child's capabilities.

MEDICATION

Your doctor may prescribe:

- Anti-convulsants to control seizures.
- Muscle relaxants to relieve spasms.
- See Medications section for information regarding medicines your doctor may prescribe.

ACTIVITY

Encourage your child to do as much as possible.

DIET & FLUIDS

No special diet.

OK FOR SCHOOL, PRESCHOOL, OR NURSERY?

Yes, if able. The child may require special education classes.

CALL YOUR DOCTOR IF

You are concerned about your child's development or suspect CP.

CERVICAL EROSION

GENERAL INFORMATION

DESCRIPTION

Cervical erosion is a condition in which the lining of the uterus spreads to cover the tip of the cervix. This abnormally placed tissue is more likely to become inflamed or infected. It is not cancerous. The cervix and uterus lining are involved. This condition occurs only in adolescent and adult females.

Appropriate health care includes:

- Doctor's treatment.
- Minor surgery to cauterize or freeze the cervix (if a Pap smear is normal). Surgery is often done without anesthesia in the doctor's office or an out-patient surgical facility.
- Conization of the cervix (see Glossary) or hysterectomy if a Pap smear is not normal.

SIGNS & SYMPTOMS

- No symptoms (usually).
- Increased mucus discharge from the vagina (sometimes).
- Unexplained vaginal bleeding (sometimes).

CAUSES

Usually unknown, but may accompany pregnancy, childbirth, or the use of oral contraceptives.

RISK FACTORS

- Stress.
- Repeated vaginal infections.
- Obesity.

PREVENTING COMPLICATIONS OR RECURRENCE

Cannot be prevented at present.

WHAT TO EXPECT

MEDICAL TESTS

- Medical history and physical exam—including pelvic examination—by a doctor.
- Pap smear (see Glossary).

POSSIBLE COMPLICATIONS

Occasionally precedes cancer of the cervix.

PROBABLE OUTCOME

This disorder is usually curable with treatment. Allow 3 months for the cervix to return completely to normal. Cervical erosion frequently recurs.

TREATMENT

HOME CARE

- Your daughter should not douche unless instructed to by her doctor.
- Obtain medical treatment for any vaginal infection your daughter may also have.
- Encourage your daughter to use pads instead of tampons during menstruation.

MEDICATION

- Your doctor may prescribe oral antibiotics or topical antibiotics to apply to the cervix.
- See Medications section for information regarding medicines your doctor may prescribe.

ACTIVITY

After treatment (except following a hysterectomy), your daughter can resume normal activity and sexual relations immediately.

DIET & FLUIDS

No special diet.

OK FOR SCHOOL, PRESCHOOL, OR NURSERY?

When appetite returns and alertness, strength, and feeling of well-being will allow.

CALL YOUR DOCTOR IF

- Your daughter has symptoms of cervical erosion.
- The following occurs after treatment:
  —Increased discharge.
  —Pain with intercourse or bleeding afterward.
  —Vaginal bleeding between periods.
- New, unexplained symptoms develop. Drugs used in treatment may produce side effects.

CHICKENPOX
(Varicella)

GENERAL INFORMATION

DESCRIPTION

Chickenpox is a very contagious, mild disease caused by the herpes zoster virus. The skin and mucous membranes are involved.

Appropriate health care includes:
- Self-care after diagnosis.
- Physician's monitoring of general condition and medications, if complications arise.

SIGNS & SYMPTOMS

The following are usually mild in children, severe in adults:
- Fever.
- Abdominal pain or a general ill feeling that lasts 1 or 2 days.
- Skin eruptions that appear almost anywhere on the body, including the scalp and penis, and inside the mouth, nose, throat, or vagina. They may be scattered over large areas, and they occur least on the arms and legs. Blisters collapse within 24 hours and form scabs. New crops of blisters erupt every 3 to 4 days. (Adults have additional symptoms that resemble influenza.)

CAUSES
- Infection with the herpes zoster virus. Incubation after exposure is 7 to 21 days.
- A newborn is protected for several months from chickenpox if the mother had the disease prior to or during pregnancy. The immunity diminishes in 10 to 12 months.

RISK FACTORS

Use of immunosuppressive drugs.

PREVENTING COMPLICATIONS OR RECURRENCE

Cannot be prevented at present. An experimental vaccine is available for high-risk persons, such as those who take anti-cancer or immunosuppressive drugs.

WHAT TO EXPECT

MEDICAL TESTS
- Your own observation of symptoms.
- Medical history and physical exam by a doctor.

POSSIBLE COMPLICATIONS
- Secondary bacterial infection of chickenpox blisters.
- Encephalitis (rare).
- Shingles many years later in adulthood (possibly).
- Scarring (rare). This is more common if blisters become infected.

PROBABLE OUTCOME
- Spontaneous recovery. Children usually recover in 7 to 10 days. (Adults take longer and are more likely to develop complications.) After recovery, a person usually has lifelong immunity against a recurrence of chickenpox.
- After chickenpox runs its course, the virus remains dormant in the body (probably in the roots of nerves near the spinal cord). The same virus may later cause shingles.

TREATMENT

HOME CARE

- Use cool-water soaks or cool-water compresses to reduce your child's itching.
- Keep the patient as quiet and cool as possible. Heat and sweat trigger itching.
- Keep the child's nails short to discourage scratching, which can lead to secondary infection.

MEDICATION

- The following non-prescription medicines may decrease your child's itching:
  — Steroid lotion, ointment, or cream. This reduces inflammation and relieves itching in 24 to 48 hours.
  — Topical anesthetics and topical antihistamines, which provide quick, short-term relief. Preparations containing lidocaine and pramoxine are least likely to cause allergic skin reactions.
  — Lotions that contain phenol, menthol, and camphor (such as calamine lotion). These are soothing, but use with care. Large amounts may be absorbed through the skin into the bloodstream, and they can be toxic.
- If you must reduce fever, use acetaminophen instead of aspirin. Aspirin may contribute to the development of Reye's syndrome, a form of encephalitis, when given to children during a viral illness.
- See Medications section for information regarding medicines your doctor may prescribe.

ACTIVITY

Bed rest is not necessary. Allow quiet activity in a cool environment. Your child may play outdoors in the shade during nice weather. Keep an ill child away from others until all blisters have crusted.

DIET & FLUIDS

No special diet.

OK FOR SCHOOL, PRESCHOOL, OR NURSERY?

The child can return when lesions have all scabbed over, temperature is normal, and sense of well-being has returned.

CALL YOUR DOCTOR IF

- Your child has symptoms of chickenpox.
- Lethargy, headache, or sensitivity to bright light develop.
- Fever rises over 103F (39.4C).
- Chickenpox lesions contain pus or otherwise appear infected.

CHLAMYDIA INFECTION

GENERAL INFORMATION

DESCRIPTION

Chlamydia are intracellular parasites that have many of the same physical characteristics of viruses. They cause inflammation of the urethra (the anatomical tube that allows urine from the bladder to pass outside the body), vagina, cervix, uterus, Fallopian tubes, anus, ovaries, and epididymis. This is a common sexually transmitted disease. Chlamydia infection may also be transmitted to the eyes or lungs of a newborn infant. If chlamydia is found by microscopic exam and culture of discharge in any person who is sexually active, all sexual partners must be treated. Appropriate health care includes your own observation of symptoms; medical history and physical exam by a doctor; doctor's treatment.

SIGNS & SYMPTOMS

- Sometimes no symptoms at all during early stages.
- Vaginal discharge (females).
- Urethral discharge (males).
- Anal swelling, pain, or discharge.
- Reddening of the vagina or tip of the penis.
- Abdominal pain.
- Fever.
- Discomfort on urinating.
- Genital discomfort or pain.

CAUSES

- Vaginal sexual intercourse.
- Rectal sexual intercourse.
- Vaginal infection during delivery of a newborn, which may infect the baby.
- Oral sexual intercourse (fellatio or cunnilingus).

RISK FACTORS

Unprotected sexual activity, particularly in young females; diabetes mellitus; general poor health; hot weather, non-ventilating clothing—especially underwear—or any other condition that increases genital moisture, warmth, and darkness. These foster the growth of germs.

PREVENTING COMPLICATIONS OR RECURRENCE

Use of latex condoms during sexual activity; treatment of all sexual partners of any infected person (usually 2 weeks of an oral antibiotic such as tetracycline).

WHAT TO EXPECT

MEDICAL TESTS

Your own observation of symptoms; medical history and physical exam by a doctor; vaginal smear for laboratory analysis; rectal smear for laboratory analysis; urethral smear for laboratory analysis; re-exam after completing the prescribed treatment.

POSSIBLE COMPLICATIONS

Sterility in a female; infecting one's sexual partner; secondary bacterial infections in pelvic organs, genitals, or rectum.

PROBABLE OUTCOME

Complete cure with adequate antibiotic treatment.

TREATMENT

HOME CARE

Instructions for your daughter:

- Keep the genital area clean. Use plain unscented soap.
- Take showers rather than tub baths.
- Wear cotton panties or pantyhose with a cotton crotch. Avoid panties made from non-ventilating materials, such as nylon.
- Don't sit around in wet clothing—especially a wet bathing suit.
- After urination or bowel movements, cleanse by wiping or washing from front to back (vagina to anus).
- Lose weight if you are obese.
- Avoid douches.
- If you have diabetes, adhere strictly to your treatment program.
- Avoid irritating sprays.
- Avoid pants that are tight in the crotch and thighs.
- Change tampons frequently.
- If urinating causes burning:
  - — Urinate through a tubular device, such as a toilet-paper roll or plastic cup with the end cut out.
  - — Urinate while bathing.

MEDICATION

Your doctor may prescribe oral antibiotics, such as tetracycline, to take for 2 weeks.

ACTIVITY

Your child should avoid overexertion, heat, and excessive sweating and should delay sexual relations until feeling well. Allow about 3 weeks for your child's recovery.

DIET & FLUIDS

No special diet.

OK FOR SCHOOL, PRESCHOOL, OR NURSERY?

Not until treatment has removed symptoms.

CALL YOUR DOCTOR IF

- Your daughter has symptoms of vaginitis.
- Symptoms in your child persist longer than 1 week or worsen despite treatment.
- Unusual vaginal bleeding or swelling develops.

CHOLECYSTITIS OR CHOLANGITIS, ACUTE

GENERAL INFORMATION

DESCRIPTION

These acute conditions refer to infection or inflammation of the gallbladder (cholecystitis) or the ducts (cholangitis) that drain bile from the gallbladder to the small intestine. These conditions may be confused with hepatitis, pancreatitis, or duodenal ulcer. The gallbladder (located under the liver) and bile ducts in the liver leading to the gallbladder are involved. The conditions are most common in adults but may rarely occur in children or adolescents. Appropriate health care includes: doctor's treatment; surgery to remove an infected gallbladder and gallstones (surgery is rarely an emergency); hospitalization (usually).

SIGNS & SYMPTOMS

- Cramping pain in the upper right of the abdomen. Pain may also occur in the chest (imitating a heart attack), in the upper back or the right shoulder. These symptoms frequently follow a meal rich in fats.
- Tenderness in the child's upper abdomen.
- Nausea and vomiting.
- Belching.
- Slight fever. A high fever and chills indicate a bacterial infection.
- Jaundice (sometimes).
- Pale stools (sometimes).
- Skin itching (sometimes).

CAUSES

Inflammation or bacterial infection, which are usually caused by gallstone formation and blockage of bile ducts.

RISK FACTORS

Diet that is high in fat; gallstones, whether or not they have caused symptoms; chronic or acute pancreatitis; coronary-artery disease; family history of gallbladder disease.

PREVENTING COMPLICATIONS OR RECURRENCE

- Your child should avoid any food that causes indigestion.
- Your child should have surgery to remove gallstones, even if they cause no symptoms.

WHAT TO EXPECT

MEDICAL TESTS

- Your own observation of symptoms.
- Medical history and physical exam by a doctor.
- Laboratory blood studies.
- X-rays of the child's gallbladder.
- Ultrasonography (see Glossary) of the gallbladder and bile ducts.
- Radioisotope studies (see Glossary) of liver and pancreas.

POSSIBLE COMPLICATIONS

- Gallbladder rupture and peritonitis.
- Gallbladder abscess.
- Misdiagnosis as a heart attack.

PROBABLE OUTCOME

Symptoms of some mild attacks subside spontaneously in 1 to 4 days, if no complications develop. Most episodes require hospitalization and treatment. Recurrences are common. Your child's attacks will cease with surgery to remove the gallbladder.

TREATMENT

HOME CARE

After an acute attack of cholecystitis, consider elective surgery for your child to prevent a future emergency.

MEDICATION

- Don't medicate your child with non-prescription pain relievers during an attack. These may mask symptoms of a bacterial infection — allowing it to worsen — and delay treatment.
- Your doctor may prescribe analgesics, including narcotics, to relieve your child's pain.
- See Medications section for information regarding medicines your doctor may prescribe.

ACTIVITY

Your child should rest in bed until symptoms disappear or recovery from surgery is complete. While in bed, moving the legs often reduces the likelihood of deep-vein blood clotting. Your child may read or watch TV.

DIET & FLUIDS

Because of nausea and vomiting, intravenous fluids are usually necessary during attacks. Clear liquids or a non-fat diet are appropriate as soon as your child can tolerate solid foods.

OK FOR SCHOOL, PRESCHOOL, OR NURSERY?

When appetite returns and alertness, strength, and feeling of well-being will allow.

CALL YOUR DOCTOR IF

- Your child has symptoms of cholecystitis or cholangitis. If symptoms are accompanied by shortness of breath, sweating, and nausea, call immediately! This is an emergency!
- The following occurs during an attack:
  - —Fever.
  - —Jaundice.
  - —Recurrent vomiting.
  - —Intolerable pain.

ILLNESSES

CIRCUMCISION

GENERAL INFORMATION

DESCRIPTION

Circumcision is the removal of the foreskin of the penis. It is performed routinely soon after birth in many male children, although the American Academy of Pediatrics has a policy statement concluding that "there is no medical indication for routine circumcision of the newborn." If your son is not circumcised soon after birth, there is the possibility of phimosis (tightness of the foreskin, preventing it being drawn back) later. Adhesions may develop, requiring circumcision as an adult. The chart on these pages describes circumcision performed at birth and at times other than at birth or several days after birth for religious reasons.

Appropriate health care includes:

Surgery performed in a hospital or outpatient surgical facility if non-surgical treatment fails.

SIGNS & SYMPTOMS

- Inability to retract the foreskin completely after 18 months to 3 years of age.
- Infection of the penis (balanitis).

CAUSES

Poor hygiene.

RISK FACTORS

None.

PREVENTING COMPLICATIONS OR RECURRENCE

Good hygiene.

WHAT TO EXPECT

MEDICAL TESTS

- Your own observation of symptoms.
- Medical history and physical exam by a doctor.
- Before surgery: blood and urine studies.
- After surgery: blood studies.

POSSIBLE COMPLICATIONS

- Excessive bleeding.
- Surgical-wound infection.

PROBABLE OUTCOME

Expect complete healing without complications. Allow about 3 weeks for your son to recover from surgery. The average hospital stay is 0 to 1 day.

TREATMENT

HOME CARE

After surgery:

- For an infant circumcised soon after birth, protect the surgical site with petroleum jelly at the time of each diaper change.
- For an older boy, follow these suggestions:
  - — If the wound bleeds during the first 24 hours after surgery, press a clean tissue or cloth to it for 10 minutes.
  - — Use ice packs to relieve pain in the surgical area for the first 24 hours after surgery.
  - — Use an electric heating pad, a heat lamp, or a warm compress to relieve surgical-wound pain beginning 24 hours after surgery.
  - — Bathe and shower the boy as usual. The surgical wound may be washed gently with mild unscented soap.
  - — Change your son's bandage daily. Between showers, keep the wound dry for the first 2 or 3 days after surgery. If a bandage gets wet, change it promptly.
  - — Apply non-prescription antibiotic ointment to the wound before applying new bandages.

MEDICATION

- Your doctor may prescribe:
  - — Pain relievers. Don't give your son prescription pain medication longer than 4 to 7 days. He should use *only* as much as he needs.
  - — Antibiotics to fight infection.
- Use non-prescription drugs, such as acetaminophen, for minor pain.
- See Medications section for information regarding medicines your doctor may prescribe.

ACTIVITY

- Your son can resume normal activity as soon as possible.
- Your son should avoid vigorous exercise for 4 weeks after surgery.

DIET & FLUIDS

No special diet.

OK FOR SCHOOL, PRESCHOOL, OR NURSERY?

Yes, after complete healing.

CALL YOUR DOCTOR IF

- Your son experiences pain, swelling, redness, drainage, or increased bleeding in the surgical area.
- Your son develops signs of infection (headache, muscle aches, dizziness, or a general ill feeling and fever).
- Your son has difficulty urinating.
- New, unexplained symptoms develop. Drugs used in treatment may produce side effects.

CLUBFOOT (Talipes)

GENERAL INFORMATION

DESCRIPTION

Clubfoot is an inherited deformity of the foot or feet. The condition is not painful, but if uncorrected, it prevents normal walking. Clubfoot occurs more often in newborn boys than girls.

Appropriate health care includes:

- Physician's monitoring of general condition and medications.
- Surgery to correct the deformity (rare).
- Self-care after diagnosis.

SIGNS & SYMPTOMS

Foot or feet of the newborn point down, turn inward, and curl under.

CAUSES

A shortened Achilles tendon and deformed bones in the foot. This is an inherited condition or is caused by the position of the fetus in the uterus.

RISK FACTORS

Unknown.

PREVENTING COMPLICATIONS OR RECURRENCE

Cannot be prevented at present. Crippling can be prevented with early diagnosis and treatment.

WHAT TO EXPECT

MEDICAL TESTS

- Your own observation of symptoms.
- Medical history and physical exam by a doctor.
- X-rays of the feet.

POSSIBLE COMPLICATIONS

Permanent foot deformity and crippling without treatment.

PROBABLE OUTCOME

The foot can usually be restored to normal in young children with about 3 months of treatment. For older children, treatment may improve—but not completely correct—the disorder.

TREATMENT

HOME CARE

- The goal of treatment is to correct the deformity and support the correction until your child's foot muscles are strong enough to maintain it. Your doctor may prescribe stretching exercises, massage, physical therapy, various splints for day or night, casts, or surgery.
- Your child will need patience and encouragement with all these methods. Your attitude and the time you spend with the child are an important part of parent-child bonding.
- After surgery or casting, elevate the child's feet with pillows at nap or bedtime to reduce the risk of swelling and pain.
- If your child has a cast, inspect it daily for signs of infection. These include: a wet spot, bad odor or tightness, or the foot in the cast may appear blue, pale, and cold compared to the other. See Care of Casts, Appendix 41.

MEDICATION

- Medicine usually is not necessary for this disorder.
- See Medications section for information regarding medicines your doctor may prescribe.

ACTIVITY

No restrictions. Corrective shoes will be necessary following treatment with splints or casts.

DIET & FLUIDS

No special diet.

OK FOR SCHOOL, PRESCHOOL, OR NURSERY?

Yes.

CALL YOUR DOCTOR IF

- Your child has signs of a foot deformity.
- Bleeding or signs of infection occur under a cast.
- Signs of muscle pulling return after treatment.

COLD, COMMON

GENERAL INFORMATION

DESCRIPTION

The common cold is a contagious viral infection of the upper-respiratory passages. The nose, throat, sinuses, ears, eustachian tubes, trachea, larynx, and bronchial tubes are involved.

Appropriate health care includes: self-care after diagnosis; physician's monitoring of general condition and medications (for complications only).

SIGNS & SYMPTOMS

- Runny or stuffy nose. Nasal discharge is watery at first, then becomes thick and greenish yellow.
- Sore throat.
- Hoarseness.
- Cough that produces little or no sputum.
- Low fever.
- Fatigue.
- Watering eyes.
- Loss of appetite.

CAUSES

Any of at least 200 viruses. Virus particles spread through the air or from person-to-person contact, especially hand-shaking.

RISK FACTORS

Stress; fatigue or overwork; poor nutrition; smoking; exposure to cold; wet weather; crowded or unsanitary living conditions.

PREVENTING COMPLICATIONS OR RECURRENCE

- To prevent spreading a cold to others, have your child avoid unnecessary contact during the contagious phase (first 2 to 4 days).
- The child should wash his hands frequently, especially after blowing his nose or before handling food.
- Keep the child away from the risks listed above.

WHAT TO EXPECT

MEDICAL TESTS

Your own observation of symptoms; medical history and physical exam by a doctor; laboratory throat culture.

POSSIBLE COMPLICATIONS

Bacterial infections of the ears, throat, sinuses, or lungs.

PROBABLE OUTCOME

Spontaneous recovery in 7 to 14 days.

TREATMENT

HOME CARE

- To relieve your child's nasal congestion, use salt-water drops (¼ teaspoon of salt to 1 cup of water).
- Use a cool-mist humidifier to increase air moisture.
- Use Vaseline on the skin between the child's nose and lip to prevent rawness from nasal drainage.
- For a baby too young to blow his nose, use an infant nasal aspirator. If mucus is thick and sticky, loosen it by putting 2 or 3 drops of salt solution (see above) into each nostril. Don't insert cotton swabs into a child's nostrils. Instead, catch the discharge outside the nostril on a tissue or swab, roll it around and pull the discharge out of the nose.
- For an infant or very young child, lay the child on his stomach to sleep. This improves nasal drainage and breathing.

MEDICATION

- No medicine, including antibiotics, can cure the common cold. To relieve your child's symptoms, use non-prescription drugs, such as acetaminophen, nose drops or sprays, cough remedies, and throat lozenges.
- If you must reduce fever, use acetaminophen instead of aspirin. Aspirin may contribute to the development of Reye's syndrome, a form of encephalitis, when given to children during a viral illness.

ACTIVITY

Bed rest is not necessary, but have the child avoid vigorous activity, resting often.

DIET & FLUIDS

Your child should drink extra fluids, including water, fruit juice, tea, and carbonated drinks. Avoid giving the child milk because it may thicken secretions.

OK FOR SCHOOL, PRESCHOOL, OR NURSERY?

When signs of infection have decreased, appetite returns, and alertness, strength, and feeling of well-being will allow.

CALL YOUR DOCTOR IF

The following occurs during your child's illness: increased throat pain, or white or yellow spots on the tonsils or other parts of the throat; coughing episodes that last longer than intervals between coughing, cough that produces thick yellow-green or gray sputum, cough that lasts longer than 10 days, or difficult or labored breathing between coughing bouts; fever that lasts several days or rises to 101F (38.3C); shaking chills; chest pain or shortness of breath; earache or headache; skin rash; pain in the teeth or over the sinuses; unusual lethargy; unusual irritability; delirium; enlarged, tender glands in the neck; dusky blue or gray lips, skin, or nail beds; inability to bottle-feed or breast-feed in an infant.

COLD SORES
(Fever Blisters; Herpes Simplex)

GENERAL INFORMATION

DESCRIPTION

Cold sores are a common, contagious viral infection. The lips, gums, and mouth area, the cornea (rarely), and the genitals (occasionally) are involved.

Appropriate health care includes:

- Self-care after diagnosis.
- Doctor's treatment, especially if the eye is affected, in which case it requires continuing physician's monitoring of general condition and medications.

SIGNS & SYMPTOMS

- Eruptions of very small, painful blisters—usually around the mouth, but sometimes on the genitals. The blisters are grouped together and are surrounded by a red ring. They fill with fluid, then dry up and disappear.
- If the child's eye is infected: eye pain and redness, feeling that something is in the eye, sensitivity to light, and tearing.

CAUSES

- Infection with a herpes virus that invades the skin, often remaining for months or years before causing active inflammation. Most persons develop antibodies that control the virus unless risk factors (below) develop.
- The virus is transmitted by person-to-person contact or by contact with saliva, stools, urine, or discharge from an infected eye. The blisters and ulcers of herpes simplex are contagious until they heal, both in the first and in succeeding flare-ups.

RISK FACTORS

Eczema in children; physical or emotional stress; illness that has lowered resistance, including a cold, minor gastrointestinal upset, or fever from any cause; excess sun exposure; menstrual periods; dental treatment that stretches the child's mouth; use of immunosuppressive drugs.

PREVENTING COMPLICATIONS OR RECURRENCE

- Your child should avoid physical contact with others who have active lesions.
- Your child should wash hands often during a flare-up to avoid spreading the virus.

WHAT TO EXPECT

MEDICAL TESTS

- Your own observation of symptoms.
- Medical history and physical exam by a doctor.
- Laboratory virus cultures (rare).

POSSIBLE COMPLICATIONS

- Permanent vision impairment, if herpes eye infections are untreated.
- Severe, widespread infection in patients with eczema.
- Meningitis or encephalitis (rare).

COLD SORES (Fever Blisters; Herpes Simplex)

PROBABLE OUTCOME

Spontaneous recovery in a few days to a week, occasionally longer. Recurrence is common. The virus remains in the body for life, but it is usually dormant. Research continues in developing a vaccine.

TREATMENT

HOME CARE

Instructions for your child:

- Drink cool liquids or suck frozen juice bars to reduce discomfort.
- Apply an ice cube for 1 hour during the first 24 hours after a lesion appears. This may make it heal more quickly.
- Don't rub or scratch an infected eye.
- To prevent flare-ups, use zinc oxide or sun-screen preparations on your lips when you spend much time outdoors.

MEDICATION

- Use acetaminophen to relieve minor pain. Don't use aspirin, especially for children and adolescents. The use of aspirin during some viral illnesses may lead to Reye's syndrome, a form of encephalitis.
- Don't try to treat an infected eye—especially with cortisone ointments or drops—without consulting your doctor. Cortisone preparations promote growth of the herpes virus in the cornea.
- Your doctor may prescribe:
  - — Anti-viral topical or oral medication.
  - — Antibiotic ointment if lesions become infected with bacteria.
  - — Anti-cancer topical medication for eye infections.
- See Medications section for information regarding medicines your doctor may prescribe.

ACTIVITY

No restrictions, except to avoid close contact—especially kissing—until lesions heal.

DIET & FLUIDS

No special diet.

OK FOR SCHOOL, PRESCHOOL, OR NURSERY?

When appetite has returned and alertness, strength, and feeling of well-being will allow.

CALL YOUR DOCTOR IF

The following occurs with a cold sore:

- Signs of secondary bacterial infection, such as fever, pus instead of clear fluid in the lesions, headache, and muscle aches.
- Eruption of lesions on the genitals similar to those around the mouth.
- New, unexplained symptoms. Drugs used in treatment may produce side effects.

COLIC IN INFANTS

GENERAL INFORMATION

DESCRIPTION

Colic in infants means repeated episodes of excessive crying that cannot be explained. Crying ranges from fussiness to agonized screaming. Colic is not contagious. The lower intestinal tract most likely is affected. Colic in infants can affect both sexes, but it is more common in boys. Colic affects infants up to 5 months old and is most common in a first child.

Appropriate health care includes:

- Home care after diagnosis.
- Physician's monitoring of general condition and medications (sometimes).

SIGNS & SYMPTOMS

Excessive crying with the following characteristics:

- Crying bouts usually occur in late afternoon or evening.
- Crying bouts usually begin at 2 to 4 weeks and last through 3 or 4 months.
- The infant's abdomen may rumble, and the child may draw up the legs as if in pain.
- No specific disease, such as an ear infection, hernia, allergy, or urinary infection, can be discovered.

CAUSES

Unknown. Colic may be related to physical pain or emotional upset. Some likely possibilities include: hunger, insufficient sleep, milk that is too hot, overfeeding, food allergy, reactions to tension in the home, loneliness, or tiredness.

RISK FACTORS

No known risk factor.

PREVENTING COMPLICATIONS OR RECURRENCE

No specific preventive measures. Remove any causes that can be identified.

WHAT TO EXPECT

MEDICAL TESTS

- Your own observation of symptoms.
- Medical history and physical exam by a doctor.

POSSIBLE COMPLICATIONS

None expected.

PROBABLE OUTCOME

All babies cry, and many have fussy periods. Crying is an important activity and means of communication. Colic is a distressing, but not dangerous, condition. The symptoms can sometimes be relieved. When they can't, the colic *will* disappear after the 4th or 5th month.

TREATMENT

HOME CARE

- Be patient and tolerant.
- Don't feed the baby every time he cries. Look for a reason, such as a gas bubble, a cramped position, too much heat or cold, a soiled diaper, an open diaper pin, or a desire to be cuddled. If the baby stops crying when picked up, the crying is not a result of hunger or gas. If the child continues crying, offer a feeding. If the crying stops then, it is due to hunger.
- The symptoms of overfeeding can mimic gas pains. If the baby is still screaming in agony after an hour, gently insert an infant glycerine suppository into the baby's rectum as a last resort.
- During an attack of gas, hold the baby securely, and gently massage the lower abdomen. Rocking may be soothing. Apply a good heating pad, set on "low," to the abdomen; be careful not to burn.
- Offer the baby a pacifier.
- Allow the baby to cry if you are certain everything is all right (not hungry, not soiled, no fever, no open pins) and you have done all you can.
- Ask someone to take care of the baby to relieve you as often as possible.

MEDICATION

Drugs are used only as a last resort when babies and parents are both exhausted. In that event, your doctor may prescribe anti-spasmodics. If so, carefully follow instructions on the label. Don't use any medicine, including non-prescription medicine, without telling your doctor.

ACTIVITY

No restrictions.

DIET & FLUIDS

- Interrupt bottle feedings after every ounce and burp the baby. Interrupt breast feedings every 5 minutes.
- Allow at least 20 minutes to feed the baby. Don't prop the baby for feedings.
- Nipple holes should not be too large. A vigorous baby may require blind nipples in which you can make small homemade nipple holes.

OK FOR SCHOOL, PRESCHOOL, OR NURSERY?

Yes.

CALL YOUR DOCTOR IF

- The baby's rectal temperature rises to 101F (38.3C) or higher.
- You fear that you are about to lose emotional control.
- The baby is taking a prescription drug, and new, unexplained symptoms develop. The drug may produce side effects.

COLITIS, ULCERATIVE

GENERAL INFORMATION

DESCRIPTION

Ulcerative colitis is a serious chronic inflammatory disease of the colon characterized by ulceration and episodes of bloody diarrhea. The ulcerated areas are inflamed and may form abscesses in the lining of the large intestine. The rectum and large bowel are involved. Ulcerative colitis is most common in females and is unusual before puberty.

Appropriate health care includes:

- Self-care after diagnosis.
- Physician's monitoring of general condition and medications.
- Psychological counseling.
- Surgery to remove the diseased colon (sometimes). For an explanation of this surgery and postoperative care, see ileostomy in the Glossary.
- Hospitalization during worst episodes.

SIGNS & SYMPTOMS

Early symptoms include:

- Pain in the left side of the child's abdomen that improves after bowel movements.
- Episodes of bloody diarrhea with mucus, alternating with symptom-free intervals.

During an acute attack:

- Increased bloody diarrhea (up to 10 to 20 bowel movements a day).
- Severe cramps and pain around the rectum.
- Sweating.
- Nausea.
- Loss of appetite and weight loss.
- Bloated abdomen.
- Fever as high as 104F (40C).

CAUSES

Unknown.

RISK FACTORS

- Stress, anxiety or depression.
- Family history of ulcerative colitis.
- Excess alcohol consumption.

PREVENTING COMPLICATIONS OR RECURRENCE

No specific preventive measures.

WHAT TO EXPECT

MEDICAL TESTS

- Your own observation of symptoms.
- Medical history and physical exam by a doctor.
- Laboratory stool and blood studies.
- X-ray of the colon (barium enema).
- Sigmoidoscopy (see Glossary).

POSSIBLE COMPLICATIONS

- Life-threatening blood loss, ulceration through the intestinal wall, or peritonitis during acute attacks.
- Malnutrition, wasting of the child's body, or chronic disability.
- Inflammation of joints, eyes, and skin.
- Colon cancer. The risk is greater in persons with ulcerative colitis.

PROBABLE OUTCOME

Often curable with counseling and medical treatment or surgery. If not curable, the child's symptoms can be controlled with treatment.

TREATMENT

HOME CARE

- To reduce your child's cramps, apply a hot-water bottle, warm moist towels or heating pad to the abdomen.
- Try to reduce your child's stress. See Appendix 19.

MEDICATION

- Don't use aspirin. It increases the bleeding risk.
- Your doctor may prescribe:
  — Anti-diarrhea medication for minimal symptoms.
  — Sulfa drugs, such as sulfasalazine, for moderate symptoms.
  — Cortisone drugs for severe disease.
- See Medications section for information regarding medicines your doctor may prescribe.

ACTIVITY

Bed rest may be necessary during an acute attack. However, your child can resume normal activity as soon as symptoms improve.

DIET & FLUIDS

- Urge your child not to drink alcohol.
- During early treatment, the child should avoid milk and milk products.

OK FOR SCHOOL, PRESCHOOL, OR NURSERY?

When weight loss ceases, appetite returns, and alertness, strength, and feeling of well-being will allow.

CALL YOUR DOCTOR IF

- Your child has symptoms of ulcerative colitis.
- Fever and chills develop.
- Frequency of bowel movements or bleeding increases.
- Abdomen becomes distended.
- Jaundice (yellow eyes and skin and dark urine) develops.
- Vomiting begins or abdominal pain increases.

COLLARBONE (CLAVICLE) FRACTURE

GENERAL INFORMATION

DESCRIPTION

A collarbone fracture is a complete or incomplete break in the outer third of the clavicle (collarbone). Frequently, this fracture extends into the shoulder joint and is associated with rupture of the shoulder ligaments. Appropriate health care includes: doctor's treatment; hospitalization (sometimes) for anesthesia and surgery to set the fracture; special shoulder harness to promote healing (sometimes).

SIGNS & SYMPTOMS

Severe pain at the fracture site; swelling around the fracture; visible deformity if the fracture is complete and bone fragments separate enough to distort the child's normal contours; tenderness to the touch; numbness or coldness in the child's shoulder and arm on the affected side if the blood supply is impaired.

CAUSES

- A direct blow or indirect stress to the bone. Indirect stress may be caused by twisting or a violent muscle contraction.
- Falls from the top bunk of a bed are a common cause.

RISK FACTORS

Contact sports such as football or soccer; history of bone or joint disease, especially osteoporosis; obesity; poor nutrition, especially calcium deficiency.

PREVENTING COMPLICATIONS OR RECURRENCE

Your child should build strength and protective muscle mass with an appropriate long-term conditioning program. The child should use protective equipment, such as shoulder pads, when participating in sports.

WHAT TO EXPECT

MEDICAL TESTS

Your own observation of symptoms; medical history and physical exam by a doctor; X-rays of injured areas, including the child's shoulder joint and the joint between the shoulder and clavicle.

POSSIBLE COMPLICATIONS

- At the time of injury: shock; pressure on or injury to nearby nerves, ligaments, tendons, muscles, blood vessels, or connective tissues.
- After treatment or surgery: delayed union or non-union of the fracture, which happens frequently in fractures of the clavicle because of its naturally poor blood supply; avascular necrosis (death of bone cells) due to interruption of the blood supply; excessive scar tissue at the fracture site, causing compression on nerves and blood vessels in the neck; arrest of normal bone growth in young children; infection in open fractures (skin broken over the fracture site), or at the incision if surgical setting was necessary; shortening of the injured bones; proneness to repeated collarbone injury; an unstable or arthritic joint following repeated injury; prolonged healing time if the child resumes activity too soon.

COLLARBONE (CLAVICLE) FRACTURE

PROBABLE OUTCOME

Your child should try to resume full function and normal range of motion within 3 or 4 weeks. Healing is complete when there is no motion at the fracture site and when X-rays show complete bone union.

TREATMENT

FIRST AID

Keep the child warm with blankets to decrease the possibility of shock. Cut away clothing, if possible. Don't move the injured area to remove clothing, Follow instructions for *rest*, *ice*, *compression*, and *elevation* (R.I.C.E.). Raise the lower part of the bed. See Appendix 39 for details. The doctor will realign and set the broken bones with surgery or, if possible, without. Manipulation to set the break should be done as soon as possible after injury—in less than 6 hours, if possible.

HOME CARE

- Immobilization will be necessary. For this fracture, a figure-8 restraint usually works quite well.
- Use frequent ice massage (see Glossary) on the child if there is no cast.
- After 48 hours, localized heat promotes healing by increasing blood circulation in the injured area. Use a heating pad, hot soaks, hot showers, or heat liniments and ointments.

MEDICATION

Your doctor may prescribe:

General anesthesia, local anesthesia, or muscle relaxants; narcotic or synthetic narcotic pain relievers for severe pain; stool softeners to prevent constipation due to inactivity; acetaminophen or aspirin for mild pain.

ACTIVITY

Your child should actively exercise all muscle groups not immobilized. These muscle contractions promote fracture alignment and hasten healing. Normal activities can be resumed gradually after treatment. The child should not drive until healing is complete.

DIET & FLUIDS

No restrictions after surgery.

OK FOR SCHOOL, PRESCHOOL, OR NURSERY?

Yes, when condition and sense of well-being will allow.

CALL YOUR DOCTOR IF

- Your child has symptoms of a collarbone fracture.
- Any of the following occur after surgery or other treatment: increased pain, swelling, or drainage in the surgical area; signs of infection (headache, muscle aches, dizziness, or a general ill feeling and fever); blue or gray skin color beyond the sling, especially under the child's fingernails; loss of feeling below the fracture site; nausea or vomiting; constipation.

CONGESTIVE HEART FAILURE

GENERAL INFORMATION

DESCRIPTION

Congestive heart failure is a complication of many serious diseases in which the heart loses its full pumping capacity. Blood backs up into other organs, especially the lungs and liver. The heart, blood vessels, lungs, liver, and extremities are involved.

Appropriate health care includes:

- Self-care after diagnosis.
- Physician's monitoring of general condition and medications.
- Surgery to correct congenital defects.
- Hospitalization (frequently for severe cases).

SIGNS & SYMPTOMS

- Shortness of breath, especially with exertion or when lying flat in bed.
- Fatigue, weakness, or faintness.
- Cough (usually with sputum).
- Swelling of the abdomen, legs, and ankles.
- Rapid or irregular heartbeat.
- Low blood pressure.
- Distended neck veins.
- Enlarged liver.

CAUSES

- High blood pressure; heart-valve disease; heartbeat irregularities; congenital heart disease; cardiomyopathy; hyperthyroidism; severe anemia; heart tumor (rare); infections complicating underlying heart disease.

RISK FACTORS

Infections with high fever; smoking; obesity; excess alcohol consumption—alcohol depresses heart function; use of certain drugs, such as beta-adrenergic blockers or excess digitalis; diet that is high in fat and salt.

PREVENTING COMPLICATIONS OR RECURRENCE

If your child has a condition that can lead to congestive heart failure, obtain medical care and adhere to the treatment program. Your child should follow your dietary guidelines, and should not drink alcohol or smoke.

WHAT TO EXPECT

MEDICAL TESTS

- Your own observation of symptoms.
- Medical history and physical exam by a doctor.
- Laboratory blood studies and urinalysis.
- EKG (see Glossary).
- Heart-catheterization studies.
- X-rays of the heart, lungs, and blood vessels (angiography).
- Echocardiogram (see Glossary).

POSSIBLE COMPLICATIONS

Pulmonary edema.

PROBABLE OUTCOME

Life expectancy is reduced, but many forms are well-controlled for a while with medication and sometimes surgery. Other forms cause chronic illness. Any infection may worsen the condition.

TREATMENT

HOME CARE

- Weigh your child daily and keep a record.
- Don't allow the patient to smoke.

MEDICATION

Your doctor may prescribe:

- Diuretics to decrease fluid retention and swelling.
- Digitalis to strengthen and regulate heartbeat.
- Anti-arrhythmic drugs to stabilize heartbeat.
- Anti-coagulants to reduce blood clotting.
- Potassium replacements, if your child takes diuretics or digitalis.

ACTIVITY

In early stages, bed rest with the upper body elevated is as important as medication. Your child should avoid unnecessary exertion (such as climbing stairs) until the condition is under control. Then consult your doctor about acceptable activity.

DIET & FLUIDS

- Your child should achieve the ideal weight to reduce the heart's workload.
- Encourage your child to eat a low-salt, low-fat, high-fiber diet (see Appendices 29 and 28).
- Urge your child not to drink alcohol.

OK FOR SCHOOL, PRESCHOOL, OR NURSERY?

When appetite has returned and alertness, strength, and feeling of well-being will allow.

CALL YOUR DOCTOR IF

- Your child has symptoms of congestive heart failure.
- The following occurs during treatment: symptoms of infection, such as fever, muscle aches, headache, and dizziness; worsening of symptoms, especially rapid or irregular heartbeat or wheezing at night; cough with increased sputum or blood; weight gain of 3 or 4 pounds in 1 or 2 days.
- New, unexplained symptoms develop. Drugs used in treatment may produce side effects.

CONJUNCTIVITIS (Pinkeye)

GENERAL INFORMATION

DESCRIPTION

Conjunctivitis is an inflammation of the eyelid's underside and the white part of the eye. Appropriate health care includes:

- Self-care after diagnosis.
- Physician's monitoring of general condition and medications.

SIGNS & SYMPTOMS

The following symptoms may affect one or both eyes:

- Clear, green, or yellow discharge from your child's eye.
- After sleeping, crusts on lashes that cause eyelids to stick together.
- Eye pain.
- Swollen eyelids.
- Sensitivity to bright light.
- Redness and gritty feeling in the eye.
- Intense itching (allergic conjunctivitis only).

CAUSES

- Viral infection. Conjunctivitis may accompany colds or childhood diseases such as measles.
- Bacterial infection. Infants up to 3 days old can be infected with pinkeye from a gonococcus bacteria present in the mother's birth canal.
- Chemical irritation or wind, dust, smoke, and other types of air pollution.
- Allergies caused by cosmetics, pollen, or other allergens.
- A partially closed tear duct.
- Intense light, such as from sunlamps, snow reflection, or electric arcs in welding.

RISK FACTORS

- Newborns of mothers who are carriers of gonorrhea.
- Crowded or unsanitary living conditions.
- Exposure to others in public places.

PREVENTING COMPLICATIONS OR RECURRENCE

- Your child should wash hands frequently with soap and warm water.
- Your child should avoid exposure to eye irritants.
- Newborns in hospital deliveries are routinely given antibiotic eye drops.

WHAT TO EXPECT

MEDICAL TESTS

- Your own observation of symptoms.
- Medical history and physical exam by a doctor.
- Laboratory culture of the discharge from your child's eye.

POSSIBLE COMPLICATIONS

If untreated, pinkeye may spread and damage the cornea, permanently impairing your child's vision.

PROBABLE OUTCOME

- Allergic conjunctivitis can be cured if the allergen is removed. It is likely to recur.
- Other forms are curable in 1 to 2 weeks with treatment.

TREATMENT

HOME CARE

- Wash your child's hands often with antiseptic soap, and use paper towels to dry. Don't touch eyes. Gently wipe the discharge from your child's eye, using disposable tissues. Infections are frequently spread by contaminated fingers, towels, handkerchiefs, or wash cloths that have touched the infected eye.
- Use warm-water soaks to reduce discomfort.
- Your child should not use eye makeup.

MEDICATION

- Your doctor may prescribe antibiotic eye drops, sulfa eye drops, steroid eye drops or antibiotic ointment to fight infection. Use 3 times daily. If the infection does not improve in 2 or 3 days, it may be caused by an insensitive bacteria, virus, or allergy. At this point, an ophthalmologist may need to culture the conjunctivae or make special studies to determine the cause of the conjunctivitis.
- Most ophthalmologists believe steroid eyedrops should not be used until a diagnosis is definite. If the infection is caused by the herpes simplex virus, steroids may spread it from the conjunctiva to the cornea, damaging the eye.
- See Medications section for information regarding medicines your doctor may prescribe.

ACTIVITY

Your child can resume normal activities as soon as symptoms improve.

DIET & FLUIDS

No special diet.

OK FOR SCHOOL, PRESCHOOL, OR NURSERY?

When eye is no longer red or drains.

CALL YOUR DOCTOR IF

- Your child has symptoms of conjunctivitis.
- The infection does not improve in 48 hours, despite treatment.
- Fever occurs.
- Pain increases.
- Vision is affected.

CONSTIPATION

GENERAL INFORMATION

DESCRIPTION

Constipation means difficult or uncomfortable bowel movements. The colon and the entire intestinal tract are involved.
Appropriate health care includes: self-care after diagnosis; physician's monitoring of general condition and medications (occasionally).

SIGNS & SYMPTOMS

Children vary widely in bowel activity. Any of the following may be a sign of constipation:

- Infrequent bowel movements, sometimes accompanied by abdominal swelling.
- Hard feces.
- Straining during bowel movements.
- Pain or bleeding with bowel movements.
- Sensation of continuing fullness after a bowel movement.

CAUSES

- Inadequate fluid intake.
- Insufficient fiber in the diet. Fiber adds bulk, holds water, and creates easily passed, soft feces.
- Inactivity.
- Hypothyroidism.
- Hypercalcemia.
- Anal fissure.
- Depression.
- Chronic kidney failure.
- Back pain.

RISK FACTORS

Stress; illness requiring complete bed rest; use of certain drugs, including belladonna, calcium-channel blockers, beta-adrenergic blockers, atropine, aspirin, or anti-convulsant drugs.

PREVENTING COMPLICATIONS OR RECURRENCE

- Your child should eat a well-balanced, high-fiber diet.
- Encourage the child to exercise regularly.
- Urge the child to drink at least 8 glasses of water a day.

WHAT TO EXPECT

MEDICAL TESTS

- Your own observation of symptoms. Tell your doctor of any major change in your child's bowel pattern that lasts longer than 1 week. It may be a sign of cancer.
- Medical history and physical exam by a doctor; laboratory tests of blood and stool to detect internal bleeding; sigmoidoscopy (see Glossary).

POSSIBLE COMPLICATIONS

Hemorrhoids; laxative dependency; hernia from excessive straining; uterine or rectal prolapse; spastic colitis.

PROBABLE OUTCOME

Usually curable with exercise, diet, and adequate fluids.

TREATMENT

HOME CARE

• Set aside a regular time each day for your child's bowel movements. The best time is often within 1 hour after breakfast. Don't try to hurry the child. Encourage the child to sit at least 10 minutes, whether or not a bowel movement occurs.

• If constipation persists for 3 or 4 days, use a non-prescription, disposable enema for temporary relief. If you prefer not to use a commercial enema preparation, you may give your child an enema as follows:

— Spread a bath mat on the bathroom floor or in the tub.

— Fill an enema bag with lukewarm water.

— Hang the enema bag no higher than 30 inches from the floor.

— Have the child lie on the left side on the mat.

— Insert the lubricated nozzle gently inside the child's rectum.

— Let the water flow in slowly, a little at a time. If it hurts, stop the water flow until the pain subsides. Then start the flow again.

— Use the entire quart of water.

— Encourage your child to hold the fluid inside until the child feels uncomfortable. Then the child can sit on the toilet for a bowel movement.

MEDICATION

For occasional constipation, give your child stool softeners, mild non-prescription laxatives, or enemas. Don't give the child laxatives or enemas regularly—this can cause dependency. Avoid harsh laxatives and cathartics, such as epsom salts.

ACTIVITY

Exercise and good physical fitness help maintain healthy bowel patterns. See Appendix 36 for exercise suggestions.

DIET & FLUIDS

Encourage your child to drink at least 8 glasses of water each day. Include bulk foods, such as bran and raw fruits and vegetables, in the family's diet. Avoid serving refined cereals and breads, pastries, and sugar.

OK FOR SCHOOL, PRESCHOOL, OR NURSERY?

Yes.

CALL YOUR DOCTOR IF

• Your child has constipation that persists, despite self-care—especially if the constipation represents a change in the child's normal bowel patterns.

• Your child's constipation is accompanied by fever and severe abdominal pain.

CONVULSION, FEBRILE

GENERAL INFORMATION

DESCRIPTION

A febrile convulsion is a seizure triggered by fever and characterized by altered consciousness and uncontrolled muscle spasms. The central nervous system and the musculo-skeletal system are involved. Febrile convulsions usually affect infants and children (ages 6 months to 4 years).

Appropriate health care includes:

- Physician's diagnosis and treatment of the underlying cause and monitoring of general condition and medications.
- Home care after the seizure has subsided and after diagnosis.

SIGNS & SYMPTOMS

An infection with fever usually precedes the convulsions, but sometimes convulsions may be the first sign of fever. Symptoms include:

- Unconsciousness.
- Jerking or twitching of the child's arms, legs, or face that lasts 2 to 3 minutes.
- Loss of bladder or bowel control.
- Irritability upon regaining consciousness, followed by sleep for several hours.

CAUSES

Sudden high fever from any cause, plus an unexplained irritability of the central nervous system in some children.

RISK FACTORS

Repeated infections.

PREVENTING COMPLICATIONS OR RECURRENCE

When fever begins in a child who has had a febrile convulsion in the past, immediately begin measures to reduce the fever (See HOME CARE).

? WHAT TO EXPECT

MEDICAL TESTS

- Your own observation of symptoms.
- Medical history and physical exam by a doctor.
- Laboratory studies of blood and spinal fluid.
- EEG (see Glossary).

POSSIBLE COMPLICATIONS

- Body injury during seizure.
- Brain injury with repeated seizures.

PROBABLE OUTCOME

- Despite its frightening appearance, a convulsion caused solely by fever in a child between 6 months and 4 years of age is usually not serious.
- If the first convulsion occurs with fever in a child older than 4, it is probably caused by the fever. However, other causes should be investigated.
- If the first convulsion with fever occurs in a child younger than 6 months, a neurological examination and other studies may be necessary.

TREATMENT

HOME CARE

• During the convulsion, place the child on his side or turn his head to the side, and move potentially dangerous objects away.

• Write down details of the child's convulsion and report them to your doctor. Information should include the following:

— When did it begin?

— How soon did the seizure occur after the child's fever rose?

— Were the limb movements equal on both sides or was one side twitching more than the other?

— How long did the child's seizure last?

— Did the child sleep afterward? If so, how long?

The answers will help your doctor decide whether the child's seizure was a febrile convulsion or an epileptic seizure triggered by fever.

• After the convulsion, try to reduce fever. See How to Reduce Your Child's Fever, Appendix 17.

MEDICATION

• Your doctor may prescribe anti-convulsant drugs, such as phenobarbital, to prevent a recurrence of seizures. Some doctors recommend medication after the first convulsion; others wait to see if convulsions recur. Anti-convulsant drugs are effective only if taken daily during the susceptible years (up to age 4).

• See Medications section for information regarding medicines your doctor may prescribe.

ACTIVITY

Keep the child resting quietly in bed until fever and the underlying illness are gone. Then allow activity to return gradually to normal.

DIET & FLUIDS

After the seizure ends, encourage the child to drink extra liquids, including water, tea, cola, and fruit juice.

OK FOR SCHOOL, PRESCHOOL, OR NURSERY?

When signs of infection have decreased, appetite returns, and alertness, strength, and feeling of well-being will allow.

CALL YOUR DOCTOR IF

• Your child has a seizure with fever. Call your doctor *immediately.*

• An injury occurs during a seizure.

• The underlying illness does not improve in 3 days.

COR PULMONALE (Pulmonary Hypertension)

GENERAL INFORMATION

DESCRIPTION

Cor pulmonale is congestive heart failure resulting from raised blood pressure in the lungs. This is a complication of disorders that slow or block blood flow in the lungs. The lungs, heart, and blood vessels are involved.

Appropriate health care includes:

- Physician's monitoring of general condition and medications.
- Surgery to correct problems caused by congenital or acquired disorders, such as replacing damaged heart valves (sometimes).

SIGNS & SYMPTOMS

Early stages:

- No symptoms (usually).

Later stages:

- Weakness and fatigue.
- Shortness of breath with exertion.
- Frequent fainting.
- Swelling of the ankles and feet caused by fluid retention.
- Distended neck veins.
- Bluish skin.
- Chest pain.
- Enlarged liver and swollen abdomen.

CAUSES

- Severe chronic obstructive lung disease, such as emphysema, recurrent pneumonia, bronchiectasis, silicosis, lung cancer, tuberculosis, or collagen diseases.
- Blood clots that travel to the lung from another body site—usually a deep vein in the calf of the leg—and obstruct lung blood vessels.
- Primary diseases of the heart, including rheumatic heart disease and congenital heart disease.

RISK FACTORS

Prolonged bed rest for any illness which increases the chance of blood-clot formation; smoking.

PREVENTING COMPLICATIONS OR RECURRENCE

- Encourage your child not to smoke.
- Obtain regular medical treatment for your child for any underlying disorder that can be corrected with surgery or medical treatment.

WHAT TO EXPECT

MEDICAL TESTS

Your own observation of symptoms; medical history and physical exam by a doctor; laboratory studies of blood and lung function; X-rays of lungs; special studies that may include ultrasonography, CAT or CT scan, MRI, and radionuclide scan (see Glossary for all).

POSSIBLE COMPLICATIONS

Irreversible congestive heart failure and death.

PROBABLE OUTCOME

This condition is currently considered incurable. Many persons live 10 or 15 years after diagnosis, but disability will slowly increase. However, symptoms can be relieved or controlled. Scientific research into causes and treatment continues, so there is hope for increasingly effective treatment and cure.

TREATMENT

HOME CARE

- Your child may need oxygen. Your doctor or an oxygen therapist can arrange for the type of oxygen that allows your child to be up and about.
- Weigh the child daily and keep a record. Any sudden increase may indicate increased fluid retention.

MEDICATION

Your doctor may prescribe:

- Diuretics to prevent fluid accumulation.
- Digitalis to strengthen the force of heart-muscle contractions.
- Antibiotics for recurrent infections.
- See Medications section for information regarding medicines your doctor may prescribe.

ACTIVITY

No restrictions. Your child can be as active as the condition allows, but overexertion should be avoided. Rest between activities is advised.

DIET & FLUIDS

Your child should eat a diet that is low in salt (see Appendix 29).

OK FOR SCHOOL, PRESCHOOL, OR NURSERY?

Yes, except when ill with fever.

CALL YOUR DOCTOR IF

- Your child has symptoms of cor pulmonale.
- The following occurs during treatment:
  - — Temperature of 101F (38.3C) or higher.
  - — Weight gain of 3 to 4 pounds in 1 or 2 days.
  - — Increased shortness of breath.
  - — Increased swelling of ankles.
  - — Cough with sputum that is discolored or tinged with blood.

CORN OR CALLUS

GENERAL INFORMATION

DESCRIPTION

A corn is a painful thickening (bump) of the outer skin layer, usually over bony areas such as toe joints. A callus is a painless thickening of skin caused by repeated pressure or irritation. Corns appear on toe joints and the skin between toes; calluses appear on any part of the body—especially the hands, feet, or knees—that endures repeated pressure or irritation. Corns and calluses can affect both sexes, all ages, except infants.

Appropriate health care includes:

- Self-care after diagnosis.
- Physician's monitoring of general condition and medications (sometimes).

SIGNS & SYMPTOMS

- Corn: A small, painful, raised bump on the side or over the joint of a toe. Corns are usually 3mm to 10mm in diameter and have a hard center.
- Callus: A rough, thickened area of skin that appears after repeated pressure or irritation.

CAUSES

Corns and calluses form to protect a skin area from injury caused by repeated irritation (rubbing or squeezing). Pressure causes cells in the irritated area to grow at a faster rate, leading to overgrowth.

RISK FACTORS

- Shoes that fit poorly.
- Activities that involve pressure on the hands or knees, such as carpentry, writing, or guitar playing.

PREVENTING COMPLICATIONS OR RECURRENCE

- Your child should not wear shoes that fit poorly.
- Your child should avoid activities that create constant pressure on specific skin areas.
- When possible, the child should wear protective gear, such as gloves or knee pads.

WHAT TO EXPECT

MEDICAL TESTS

- Your own observation of symptoms.
- Medical history and physical exam by a doctor of medicine or podiatrist.

POSSIBLE COMPLICATIONS

Back, hip, knee, or ankle pain caused by a change in one's gait due to severe discomfort.

PROBABLE OUTCOME

Usually curable if the underlying cause can be removed. Allow 3 weeks for recovery. Recurrence is likely—even with treatment—if the cause is not removed.

TREATMENT

HOME CARE

- Remove the source of pressure, if possible. Discard ill-fitting shoes.
- Use corn and callus pads on your child's feet to reduce pressure on irritated areas.
- Peel or rub the thickened area with a pumice stone to remove it. Don't cut it with a razor. Soak the area in warm water to soften it before peeling.
- Ask the shoe repairman to sew a metatarsal bar onto your child's shoe to use while a corn is healing.
- Avoid surgery. It does not remove the cause. Post-surgical scarring is painful and may complicate healing.

MEDICATION

- After peeling the upper layers of the child's corn once or twice a day, apply ointment. Use a non-prescription 5% or 10% salicylic ointment. Cover with adhesive tape.
- Your doctor may inject your child's corn or callus with cortisone medicine to suppress inflammation or pain.
- See Medications section for information regarding medicines your doctor may prescribe.

ACTIVITY

Your child can resume normal activities as soon as symptoms improve.

DIET & FLUIDS

No special diet.

OK FOR SCHOOL, PRESCHOOL, OR NURSERY?

Yes.

CALL YOUR DOCTOR IF

- Your child has corns or calluses that persist despite self-treatment.
- Any signs of infection, such as redness, swelling, pain, heat, or tenderness, develop around a corn or callus.

CORNEAL ULCER

GENERAL INFORMATION

DESCRIPTION

A corneal ulcer is an open sore in the thin transparent layers that cover the eye. The parts of the eye involved include the cornea (covering), conjunctiva (white of the eye), iris (colored part of the eye), and aqueous humour (fluid in the eyeball).

Appropriate health care includes:

- Self-care after diagnosis.
- Skillful exams and continuing care from an eye specialist (M.D. ophthalmologist).

SIGNS & SYMPTOMS

- Eye pain.
- Sensitivity to bright light.
- Eyelid spasm.
- Tearing.
- Blurred vision.
- Redness in the white of the eye.

CAUSES

- Injury to the cornea or the embedding in the cornea of a foreign body, such as a small piece of steel, sand or glass. A bacterial infection—usually pneumococcal, streptococcal, or staphylococcal—may follow the injury.
- Complications of the virus, herpes simplex, that produces cold sores on the mouth.
- Infections of the eyelids and conjunctiva.
- Defective closure of the lid.

All the above infections are contagious from person to person or from one part of the body to another—especially finger-to-eye contact after touching cold sores on the mouth.

RISK FACTORS

- Recent infection or eye injury.
- Smoking or other environmental eye irritants.

PREVENTING COMPLICATIONS OR RECURRENCE

- Your child should wash hands frequently.
- Your child should avoid injury. Encourage your child to wear safety goggles to protect eyes when exposed to flying wood shavings or splinters, or metal or stone bits.
- Urge your child not to touch the eyes if there are cold sores present.

? WHAT TO EXPECT

MEDICAL TESTS

- Your own observation of symptoms.
- Medical history and physical exam by a doctor (ophthalmologist).
- Laboratory studies to identify the bacterium, virus, or fungus responsible for the infection and ulcer.

POSSIBLE COMPLICATIONS

Neglected corneal ulcers may penetrate the cornea, allowing infection to enter the eyeball. This can cause permanent vision loss.

PROBABLE OUTCOME

- A corneal ulcer is a serious eye problem. It is usually curable in 2 to 3 weeks if treated by an ophthalmologist.
- If scars from previous corneal ulcers impair your child's vision significantly, a corneal transplant (grafting a new cornea onto the eye) may make vision nearly normal.

TREATMENT

HOME CARE

Apply cool-water compresses to the child's eye as often as they feel good.

MEDICATION

- Your doctor may prescribe antibiotic eye drops, ointments, or oral antibiotics for bacterial infections. Your doctor will administer medication for viral and fungus infections.
- For minor pain, use non-prescription drugs such as acetaminophen.
- See Medications section for information regarding medicines your doctor may prescribe.

ACTIVITY

After treatment, your child can resume normal activity as soon as possible.

DIET & FLUIDS

No special diet.

OK FOR SCHOOL, PRESCHOOL, OR NURSERY?

Yes, when eye specialist suggests.

CALL YOUR DOCTOR IF

- Your child has symptoms of a corneal ulcer.
- The following occurs during treatment:
  - — Fever over 101F (38.3C).
  - — Pain that is not relieved by acetaminophen.
  - — Changed vision.
- New, unexplained symptoms develop. Drugs used in treatment may produce side effects.

CRADLE CAP

GENERAL INFORMATION

DESCRIPTION

Cradle cap causes the scalp of an infant or a child up to age 3 to have a thick yellow encrustation. It is *not* caused by poor hygiene. It is one of the manifestations of seborrheic dermatitis. (See Dermatitis, Seborrheic for treatment of older children).

Appropriate health care includes:

Self-care after diagnosis.

SIGNS & SYMPTOMS

- Thick, yellow scales over part or all of the child's scalp. Sometimes the base of these scales is red.
- Discomfort or itching (rare).

CAUSES

Overproduction of oil glands in the child's skin and scalp.

RISK FACTORS

- Hot, humid weather or cold, dry weather.
- Infrequent shampoos.
- Oily skin.
- Other skin disorders, such as psoriasis.
- Use of drying lotions that contain alcohol.

PREVENTING COMPLICATIONS OR RECURRENCE

- Brush the child's hair daily with a soft-bristled brush.
- Don't scrub hard while washing the child's hair. Bring the shampoo to a lather and quickly rinse thoroughly.

WHAT TO EXPECT

MEDICAL TESTS

Your own observation of symptoms.

POSSIBLE COMPLICATIONS

Secondary bacterial infection, causing crusts, oozing, fever, and swollen lymph glands in the child's neck.

PROBABLE OUTCOME

Curable quickly with appropriate treatment.

TREATMENT

HOME CARE

• Gently scrub the child's scalp, massaging with your fingers or a soft brush. Use soap and water or a mild shampoo every day until the scaling is controlled, then continue to shampoo twice weekly. Be sure to cleanse over the baby's "soft spot," which is really well protected. Often when the scalp is cleared, any accompanying rash elsewhere on the child's body will clear. Keep shampoos and skin products out of reach of infants.

• If the crusts are thick and will not come off with gentle scrubbing, keep applying mineral oil and warm wet cloths around the child's head for a few hours before shampooing to loosen the crusts.

• In severe cases, your doctor may prescribe a cream or lotion to be used on the child's scalp four times a day. This cream or lotion should be used only on a small area for the first few days to be sure the child's skin will tolerate it. Then it can be applied more liberally.

• The hair on many infants will fall out at 3 to 4 months of age. This is not due to the rash or the treatment.

• After shampooing, comb and brush the child's hair thoroughly. Use a fine comb. Rinse the comb in an antiseptic or in scalding water after each use.

MEDICATION

• For severe problems, your doctor may prescribe shampoos that contain coal tar, or scalp creams that contain cortisone. To apply medication to the child's scalp, part the hair a few strands at a time and rub the ointment or lotion vigorously into the scalp.

• See Medications section for information regarding medicines your doctor may prescribe.

ACTIVITY

No restrictions.

DIET & FLUIDS

No restrictions.

OK FOR SCHOOL, PRESCHOOL, OR NURSERY?

Yes.

CALL YOUR DOCTOR IF

• Your baby has symptoms of cradle cap that don't respond to self-care.

• Patches ooze, form crusts, or drain pus.

• Your baby develops fever and/or enlarged glands at the back of the scalp or in the neck.

CROUP
(Laryngo-Tracheo-Bronchitis)

GENERAL INFORMATION

DESCRIPTION

Croup is infection, inflammation, and swelling of the larynx (vocal cords) and surrounding tissue including the throat and bronchial tubes (windpipe). Croup may occur in older children but is most common in children under age 6. It may require emergency care if the windpipe is blocked. This blockage causes labored breathing and a characteristic "barking" noise with each inhalation or cough.

SIGNS & SYMPTOMS

- Fever (sometimes).
- Hoarseness.
- Barking cough and difficult breathing, especially at night.
- Chest or throat discomfort or pain.

CAUSES

Contagious viral or bacterial infection.

RISK FACTORS

Allergies.

PREVENTING COMPLICATIONS OR RECURRENCE

- To prevent recurrent attacks, run the humidifier at the child's bedside for several nights after the first attack.
- If croup is a recurring problem in your family, consider adding a humidifier to your home's heating and air-conditioning system.

WHAT TO EXPECT

MEDICAL TESTS

- Your own observation of symptoms.
- Medical history and physical exam by a doctor.
- X-rays of the chest.
- Blood counts.

POSSIBLE COMPLICATIONS

Airway obstruction and death (rare).

PROBABLE OUTCOME

Croup can be frightening, because attacks usually happen at night and the child has trouble breathing. In most cases, croup is not serious, and symptoms can be relieved. If attacks happen during the day and are accompanied by fever, the illness is more serious.

TREATMENT

HOME CARE

- Stay calm. Anxiety increases the child's breathing difficulty.
- Take the child into the bathroom and close the door.
- Turn on the hot water full force in the sink and shower to saturate the air with moisture. Open the windows to let in cold air.
- Allow 10 minutes for the steam and cold air to relieve symptoms. If severe symptoms don't improve in 10 minutes, take the child to the nearest emergency room.
- Stay in the steamed bathroom until you are ready to leave. Don't be afraid to take the child out in the cold night air—it may lessen breathing difficulty.
- If breathing improves in 10 minutes, take the child with you while you call the doctor or wait for a return call. While waiting, use a cool-mist humidifier in the room.
- Keep the child comfortable in a semiseated position. Use TV, radio, or a story to distract the child so he can relax.
- If breathing worsens again, return to the steam-filled bathroom.
- Run the humidifier by the child's bed for several nights after an attack—even if the child appears well. Simple croup often recurs.

MEDICATION

- If croup is caused by a bacterial infection, your doctor may prescribe antibiotics. However, most cases are viral, so antibiotics are ineffective.
- See Medications section for information regarding medicines your doctor may prescribe.

ACTIVITY

Decrease the child's activity and encourage rest as long as croup attacks are occurring. Don't allow the child to play outside in cool night air—this may trigger attacks (although cool air can help relieve symptoms *during* an attack).

DIET & FLUIDS

Croup usually depresses appetite. Offer frequent small amounts of fluid, such as water, ginger ale, tea, juice, or cola—not milk. Coughing may cause vomiting, so don't give the child solids during an attack.

OK FOR SCHOOL, PRESCHOOL, OR NURSERY?

When fever disappears, appetite and activity at home return to normal. Approximately 1 week.

CALL YOUR DOCTOR IF

- Your child is having trouble breathing and cannot swallow saliva or water. This is an emergency! Call and ask your doctor to meet you at the nearest emergency room.
- Breathing rate increases to 80 breaths a minute.
- Breathing is labored, and retraction (the drawing in of neck and chest with each inhalation) is pronounced.
- Nails or lips become dark or blue.
- Mild croup symptoms don't improve with 30 to 60 minutes of cool-mist treatment.

ILLNESSES

CUSHING'S SYNDROME

GENERAL INFORMATION

DESCRIPTION

Cushing's syndrome is an endocrine disorder caused by excess adrenal hormones. Children who have been treated for *any* problem necessitating prolonged use of cortisone drugs will develop a form of Cushing's syndrome. These children require greatly increased cortisone treatment during any physiological crisis, such as serious injury or severe infection. The adrenal gland (located over the kidney) and pituitary gland (at the base of the brain) are involved. Cushing's syndrome is more common in adults than children and more common in females than males.

Appropriate health care includes: physician's monitoring of general condition and medications, including consultation with an endocrinologist; surgery (sometimes) to remove ACTH-producing tumors from the pituitary or to remove adrenal-gland tumors; hospitalization for high-voltage radiation treatment of the pituitary gland (sometimes); hospitalization following *any* crisis such as a broken bone or severe infection.

SIGNS & SYMPTOMS

Round face and puffy eyes; ruddy red complexion; growth of facial hair in females; fat accumulation over the upper back and trunk, accompanied by red "stretch marks"; high blood pressure; mental and emotional changes, including psychosis; menstrual changes, including cessation of, increased, or irregular periods; enlarged clitoris; diabetes mellitus; peptic ulcers; osteoporosis; low resistance to infection.

CAUSES

Symptoms and signs result from overproduction of the cortisone-like hormone produced by the adrenal glands. The overproduction may result from: a tumor in the adrenal glands; a pituitary tumor, causing production of excessive ACTH (adreno-cortico-tropic-hormone), which the pituitary gland produces to stimulate adrenal glands to secrete hormones; prolonged use of cortisone drugs.

RISK FACTORS

Prolonged use of ACTH for treatment of pituitary cancer.

PREVENTING COMPLICATIONS OR RECURRENCE

If use of ACTH or cortisone is necessary for other disorders, such as asthma, arthritis, kidney disease, or Addison's disease, your child should take the lowest dose possible for the shortest time. Consult your doctor.

WHAT TO EXPECT

MEDICAL TESTS

- Pictures taken before symptoms begin are helpful in noting changes in appearance; medical history and physical exam by a doctor; laboratory blood and urine studies of white-blood-cell counts, pituitary and adrenal-gland function and hormone levels; X-rays of the pituitary and adrenal glands.
- Special studies that may include ultrasonography, CAT or CT scan, MRI, and radionuclide scan (see Glossary for all).

POSSIBLE COMPLICATIONS

Bone fractures due to osteoporosis; pituitary tumor, if adrenal glands are removed (rare); emergencies caused by injury, such as a broken bone or severe infection.

PROBABLE OUTCOME

- If caused by an adrenal-gland tumor, the disorder is curable with removal of the tumor or glands. Lifelong, carefully monitored drug therapy is essential if the glands are removed.
- If caused by a pituitary tumor, the disorder is curable with removal of the tumor, but tumors may recur.
- If caused by prolonged use of cortisone drugs or ACTH, the condition may improve if these are withdrawn *gradually under medical supervision.*

TREATMENT

HOME CARE

- Learn all you can about this condition and its treatment. You must often monitor your child's reactions to medications. Discontinuing drugs suddenly is dangerous.
- Have your child wear a Medic-Alert bracelet or pendant (see Glossary).
- Protect your child from fractures. Accident-proof your home. Urge your child to wear seat belts in autos and not to take risks.

MEDICATION

Your doctor may prescribe: drugs, such as aminoglutethimide or mitotane, to suppress adrenal-gland function; cortisone drugs, if adrenal glands must be removed surgically; drugs to replace pituitary hormones (sometimes); anti-hypertensive drugs to lower blood pressure; calcium supplements to treat osteoporosis.

ACTIVITY

No restrictions. The child's energy will increase once treatment begins.

DIET & FLUIDS

A low-salt diet (see Appendix 29) is sometimes necessary. Consult your doctor.

OK FOR SCHOOL, PRESCHOOL, OR NURSERY?

Yes, when condition is stable.

CALL YOUR DOCTOR IF

- Your child has symptoms of Cushing's syndrome.
- Your child has signs of infection, such as fever, chills, muscle aches, headache, and dizziness.

CYSTIC FIBROSIS (CF)

GENERAL INFORMATION

DESCRIPTION

Cystic fibrosis is an inherited disease in which mucus-producing glands throughout the body—especially in the pancreas and lung—fail to produce normal enzymes and overproduce mucus. The pancreas, lungs, sweat glands of the skin, and gastrointestinal tract are involved. Cystic fibrosis affects children of both sexes. It develops soon after birth.

Appropriate health care includes: home care after diagnosis; physician's monitoring of general condition and medications; psychotherapy or counseling to help parents and children adjust; surgery to relieve intestinal obstruction (sometimes); hospitalization to control serious infections, which occur frequently.

SIGNS & SYMPTOMS

Newborn period:

- Thick, sticky stools (meconium), which may cause intestinal obstruction.

Later:

- Poor weight gain despite good appetite.
- Bad-smelling, large, fatty stools.
- Chronic cough.
- Frequent, severe respiratory infections with sticky, hard-to-cough-up sputum.
- Salty sweat.
- Enlarged liver and spleen.

CAUSES

Genetic factors. Many people carry the genes for cystic fibrosis, and 1 in 2000 newborns is born with it. The genes cause abnormal mucus in the respiratory and gastrointestinal tracts and sweat glands. This causes lung obstruction and infection, poor digestion, and poor food absorption.

RISK FACTORS

Family history of cystic fibrosis. If both parents come from families with cystic fibrosis, the changes are 1 in 4 that each child will have the disease.

PREVENTING COMPLICATIONS OR RECURRENCE

If you have a family history of cystic fibrosis, seek genetic counseling before starting a family.

WHAT TO EXPECT

MEDICAL TESTS

- Your own observation of symptoms. Sometimes a parent notes a salty taste when kissing a child.
- Medical history and physical exam by a doctor; laboratory studies to analyze sweat, stools, and digestive juices.

POSSIBLE COMPLICATIONS

Pneumonia; chronic bronchitis; bronchiectasis; fluid and electrolyte imbalance—especially in hot weather; malnutrition; nasal polyps; rectal prolapse.

PROBABLE OUTCOME

This condition is currently considered incurable and is often fatal in childhood. Careful long-term care by parents and professionals can help children lead reasonably comfortable lives. Children with milder forms may live to adulthood, especially if the disorder is detected early.

TREATMENT

HOME CARE

- Learn as much as possible about this condition. Diet, medication, and early recognition of infection are very important.
- You will need to perform daily postural drainage to drain mucus from the child's lungs, and chest pounding to shake loose sticky mucus plugs. Ask your doctor for instructions.
- Use a cool-mist humidifier in your child's room whenever there are respiratory symptoms. Moisture helps thin mucus so it can be coughed up more easily.
- Keep your child's immunizations, including pneumonia and influenza vaccines, up to date. An immunization schedule appears in Appendix 1.
- Join a support group for parents of children with cystic fibrosis.
- Encourage your child to lead as normal and active a life as possible.

MEDICATION

Your doctor may prescribe:

- Digestive enzymes.
- Antibiotics when lung infections occur.
- Enzymes by nebulizer to help loosen lung secretions.

ACTIVITY

As much as the condition permits.

DIET & FLUIDS

Your child should eat a low-fat diet with adequate protein. Consult a dietitian for specific instructions. Vitamin and mineral supplements may be necessary. Encourage intake of liquids, which helps thin mucus.

OK FOR SCHOOL, PRESCHOOL, OR NURSERY?

Yes, during periods when signs of infection have decreased, appetite returns, and alertness, strength, and feeling of well-being will allow.

CALL YOUR DOCTOR IF

- You suspect your child has cystic fibrosis.
- After diagnosis, your child develops fever, a worsening cough, and muscle aches.

DECOMPRESSION SICKNESS (Caisson Disease; "The Bends")

GENERAL INFORMATION

DESCRIPTION

Decompression sickness is a painful, sometimes life-threatening condition of blood gases. It is caused by a sudden drop in environmental pressure. Blood throughout the body is involved.

Appropriate health care includes:

- Physician's monitoring of general condition and medications.
- Hospitalization in a decompression chamber to force nitrogen bubbles to dissolve into the blood.
- Self-care after diagnosis.

SIGNS & SYMPTOMS

The following may occur immediately or up to 24 hours after the pressure change:

- Mild to severe joint pain, especially in your child's shoulders, elbows, hips, and knees.
- Chest pain, shortness of breath, "chokes" (see Glossary), coughing, and a burning sensation behind the breastbone.
- Weakness, loss of normal sensation, paralysis, loss of consciousness, and coma (rare).
- Inability to speak, blindness, and deafness.
- Abdominal pain.
- Difficult urination.

CAUSES

Formation of nitrogen bubbles in the blood. Nitrogen is a normal blood component. If the pressure around your child's body drops rapidly—as in surfacing too quickly while scuba diving, or climbing too rapidly in a non-pressurized aircraft—the nitrogen collects in bubbles in the blood vessels, blocking them and depriving the body of essential blood nutrients.

RISK FACTORS

- Recreational scuba diving or commercial diving. Repeated dives in one day increase the risk.
- Some kinds of high-performance aircraft.

PREVENTING COMPLICATIONS OR RECURRENCE

Instructions for your child:

- Obtain professional instruction before scuba diving.
- Don't dive if you are not in good general health. You are at risk if you are obese or have a medical history of:
  - — Lung conditions, such as asthma.
  - — Spontaneous pneumothorax.
  - — Heart disease.
  - — Chronic sinusitis.
  - — Emotional instability.
  - — Alcoholism.
- Allow for a slow, gradual change to normal air pressure in situations listed above. (The U.S. Navy has tested and established guidelines.)
- Avoid air travel for 24 hours after diving.

DECOMPRESSION SICKNESS
(Caisson Disease; "The Bends")

WHAT TO EXPECT

MEDICAL TESTS
- Your own observation of symptoms.
- Medical history and physical exam by a doctor.

POSSIBLE COMPLICATIONS
- Permanent brain damage.
- Permanent bone destruction caused by inadequate nourishment from the blood.

PROBABLE OUTCOME
Complete recovery with treatment.

TREATMENT

HOME CARE
Self-care is impossible for this condition. If you observe your child with symptoms of decompression sickness, obtain emergency medical care immediately.

MEDICATION
- Medicine usually is not necessary for this disorder. Don't give your child pain relievers. These may further decrease normal breathing efficiency.
- See Medications section for information regarding medicines your doctor may prescribe.

ACTIVITY
Your child can resume normal activities as soon as symptoms improve after treatment.

DIET & FLUIDS
No special diet.

OK FOR SCHOOL, PRESCHOOL, OR NURSERY?
When appetite has returned and alertness, strength, and feeling of well-being will allow.

CALL YOUR DOCTOR IF

Your child develops any symptoms of decompression sickness within 24 hours after scuba diving or rapid ascent without pressurization.

ILLNESSES

DEHYDRATION

GENERAL INFORMATION

DESCRIPTION

Dehydration means loss of water and essential body salts. The blood, gastrointestinal tract, and kidneys are involved. Dehydration can affect both sexes, all ages, but is most dangerous in newborns and infants.

Appropriate health care includes:

- Physician's monitoring of general condition and medications.
- Self-care after diagnosis.
- Hospitalization for intravenous fluids (severe or prolonged illness only).

SIGNS & SYMPTOMS

- Dry mouth.
- Decreased or absent urination.
- Sunken eyes.
- Wrinkled skin.
- Confusion and coma.
- Low blood pressure.
- Severely sunken fontanel (soft spot in scalp) in an infant.

CAUSES

- Persistent vomiting or diarrhea from any cause.
- Heavy sweating.
- Use of drugs that deplete your child's fluids and electrolytes, such as diuretics ("water pills").
- Overexposure to sun or heat.

RISK FACTORS

- Infancy.
- Recent illness with high fever.
- Diabetes mellitus.
- Chronic kidney disease.

PREVENTING COMPLICATIONS OR RECURRENCE

- Obtain medical treatment for underlying causes of dehydration.
- If your child is vomiting or has diarrhea, give small amounts of liquid with nonprescription electrolyte supplements—or drinks such as Gatorade—every 30 to 60 minutes.
- If your child uses diuretics, weigh daily. Report to your doctor a weight loss of more than 3 pounds in 1 day or 5 pounds in 1 week.

? WHAT TO EXPECT

MEDICAL TESTS

- Your own observation of symptoms.
- Medical history and physical exam by a doctor.
- Laboratory blood studies, including blood counts and electrolyte measurement (see Glossary).

POSSIBLE COMPLICATIONS

Blood-pressure drop, shock, and death from prolonged severe dehydration.

PROBABLE OUTCOME

Curable with control of the underlying cause and replacement of necessary fluids.

TREATMENT

HOME CARE

- Weigh your child daily on an accurate home scale and record the weight so you can be aware of fluid loss.
- If your child is vomiting or has diarrhea, keep a record of the number of episodes so you can estimate fluid loss.
- For minor dehydration, give the child frequent small amounts of clear liquids. Large amounts may trigger vomiting.

MEDICATION

- Your doctor may prescribe intravenous fluids to replace lost water.
- See Medications section for information regarding medicines your doctor may prescribe.

ACTIVITY

Your child should rest in bed until symptoms are relieved. Reading or watching TV are acceptable activities.

DIET & FLUIDS

Depends on the underlying disorder. Salty foods decrease the effect of dehydration.

OK FOR SCHOOL, PRESCHOOL, OR NURSERY?

When appetite has returned and alertness, strength, and feeling of well-being will allow.

CALL YOUR DOCTOR IF

Your child has symptoms of dehydration.

DEPRESSION

GENERAL INFORMATION

DESCRIPTION

Depression is a feeling of continuing sadness, despondency, or hopelessness. The central nervous system is involved.

Appropriate health care includes:

- Self-care for mild depression.
- Physician's monitoring of general condition and medications (sometimes).
- Psychotherapy or counseling.
- Hospitalization for severe depression.

SIGNS & SYMPTOMS

- Loss of interest in life, or boredom.
- Listlessness and fatigue.
- Insomnia or excessive sleeping.
- Social isolation.
- Appetite loss or overeating.
- Constipation.
- Concentration difficulty.
- Unexplained crying bouts.
- Intense guilt feelings over minor or imaginary misdeeds.
- Difficulty making decisions.
- Irritability.
- Various pains, such as headache or chest pain, without evidence of disease.

CAUSES

- Failure in school, work, or interpersonal relationships.
- Death of a loved one.
- Loss of something important (school, home, pet).
- School or job change or move to a new area.
- Disfiguring accident or surgery.
- Major illness or disability.
- Passing from one life stage to another, such as puberty or adolescence.
- Use of some drugs, such as reserpine, beta-adrenergic blockers or benzodiazepines.
- Withdrawal from mood-altering drugs, such as narcotics, amphetamines, or caffeine.
- Some diseases, including diabetes mellitus, and hormonal abnormalities.

RISK FACTORS

Unexpressed anger or other emotion; compulsive, rigid, perfectionist, or highly dependent personalities; family history of depression; alcoholism.

PREVENTING COMPLICATIONS OR RECURRENCE

- Maintain good communication with your child.
- Raise children with love and reasonable expectations in school and home.

WHAT TO EXPECT

MEDICAL TESTS

Your own observation of symptoms; medical history and physical exam by a doctor (sometimes a psychiatrist); psychological testing.

POSSIBLE COMPLICATIONS

- Suicide. Warning signs to look for in your child include: withdrawal from family and friends; neglect of personal appearance; mention of wanting "to end it all" or being "a burden to others"; evidence of a suicide plan, such as buying or cleaning a gun or giving away possessions.
- Hallucinations or psychotic behavior.
- Manic behavior, characterized by inappropriate overactivity and comic or irresponsible behavior.

PROBABLE OUTCOME

Spontaneous recovery in many cases, but professional help can shorten the duration and help your child learn to cope in the future. Recurrence is common. The recovery rate is high, despite one's pessimism while depressed.

TREATMENT

HOME CARE

- Seek support groups or therapy for your child and your family. Contact social agencies or churches for help.
- Call your local suicide-prevention hot line if you think your child might be feeling suicidal.

MEDICATION

Your doctor may prescribe: antidepressant drugs (often tricyclics) to accompany therapy; lithium for alternating mania and depression.

ACTIVITY

No restrictions. Encourage your child to maintain daily activities and interests—even if there is no enthusiam present. Encourage your child to attend school and social functions, concerts, athletic events, plays, and movies and to keep in touch with friends and loved ones. Your child will benefit from regular, strenuous exercise, which helps relieve depression.

DIET & FLUIDS

Encourage your child to eat a normal, well-balanced diet—even if there is no appetite. Vitamin and mineral supplements may be necessary.

OK FOR SCHOOL, PRESCHOOL, OR NURSERY?

When appetite has returned and alertness, strength, and feeling of well-being will allow.

CALL YOUR DOCTOR IF

- Your child has symptoms of depression.
- You think that your child feels suicidal or hopeless.

DERMATITIS, ATOPIC

GENERAL INFORMATION

DESCRIPTION

Atopic dermatitis is a chronic inflammatory disease of the skin that is often associated with other allergic disorders that affect the respiratory system, such as asthma or hay fever. Atopic dermatitis affects children and adolescents. In young children, this problem is frequently called eczema.

Appropriate health care includes:

- Self-care after diagnosis.
- Physician's monitoring of general condition and medications.

SIGNS & SYMPTOMS

- Itching rash in areas of your child's body where heat and moisture are retained, such as skin creases of elbows, knees, neck, face, hands, feet, groin, genitals, and around the anus.
- Dry, thickened skin in affected areas.
- Uncontrolled scratching (frequently unconscious).
- Chronic fatigue from loss of sleep due to severe itching.

CAUSES

Unknown, but probably inherited and probably related to immune-system deficiency.

RISK FACTORS

- Hay fever or asthma.
- Food allergy.
- Family history of atopic dermatitis or other allergic disorders.
- Stress. The rash and itching increase during stressful periods.
- Use of immunosuppressive drugs.

PREVENTING COMPLICATIONS OR RECURRENCE

Cannot be prevented at present.

WHAT TO EXPECT

MEDICAL TESTS

Laboratory blood studies and patch tests to identify allergies.

POSSIBLE COMPLICATIONS

- Secondary bacterial infection in the affected area.
- Increased susceptibility to adverse drug reactions.
- Decreased resistance to fungal and viral infections.
- Permanent scarring from scratching.

PROBABLE OUTCOME

Unpredictable. Flare-ups and remissions may occur throughout your child's life.

TREATMENT

HOME CARE

- Use cool-water soaks for crusting, oozing lesions. These soaks decrease your child's itching and remove crusts.
- Bathe your child in cool water with cleansing agents other than soap.
- Encourage your child to wear loose-fitting, cotton clothing—avoid wool and synthetics.
- Don't allow your child to be vaccinated against smallpox. It can cause a life-threatening reaction.
- Reduce stress in your child's life, if possible. See Appendix 19 for suggestions.

MEDICATION

- To relieve your child's minor itching, use non-prescription topical steroids or coal-tar preparations.
- For severe itching, your doctor may prescribe:
  - — More potent topical steroids.
  - — Oral cortisone drugs (rarely, and for short periods only).
  - — Antihistamines or mild tranquilizers.
  - — Lubricating ointments for the child's hands.
  - — Antibiotics (sometimes) to fight secondary infections.
- See Medications section for information regarding medicines your doctor may prescribe.

ACTIVITY

No restrictions except to keep your child cool and to avoid prolonged exposure to heat.

DIET & FLUIDS

An allergy diet (see Appendix 26) may be necessary, if food allergy is suspected.

OK FOR SCHOOL, PRESCHOOL, OR NURSERY?

Yes.

CALL YOUR DOCTOR IF

- Your child has symptoms of atopic dermatitis.
- Your child develops fever or uncontrolled itching during a flare-up.

DERMATITIS, CONTACT

GENERAL INFORMATION

DESCRIPTION

Contact dermatitis is a skin inflammation caused by contact with an irritating substance. Contact dermatitis is not contagious nor malignant. The skin, especially of the hands, feet, and groin, is involved. Contact dermatitis can affect both sexes, all ages, but is more common in girls than boys.

Appropriate health care includes:

- Self-care after diagnosis.
- Physician's monitoring of general condition and medications.

SIGNS & SYMPTOMS

- Itching (sometimes).
- Slight redness.
- Cracks and fissures in the skin.
- Bright red, weeping areas (severe cases).

CAUSES

Contact with irritants, such as metals in jewelry or belt buckles, acids or solvents. (Hot water and detergent are the most common irritants.) The irritant removes the fatty layer of skin. This causes dehydration and shrinking of surface cells.

RISK FACTORS

- Constant exposure to hot water, detergents, or any irritant that changes the moisture content of skin.
- Burns from hot water or sunburn.

PREVENTING COMPLICATIONS OR RECURRENCE

- Your child should avoid contact with any irritant which has caused dermatitis in the past.
- Protect the child's skin from sunburn and other burns.

WHAT TO EXPECT

MEDICAL TESTS

- Your own observation of symptoms.
- Medical history and physical exam by a doctor.

POSSIBLE COMPLICATIONS

Pain and disfigurement of the child's hands from constant lesions.

PROBABLE OUTCOME

Your child's symptoms can be controlled with treatment and avoidance of the irritant. Recurrence is common, so treatment may be necessary for years.

TREATMENT

HOME CARE

Instructions for your child:

- Avoid the chemical or material causing the skin eruption.
- Use bath oil instead of soap for bathing.
- Pat skin dry rather than rubbing it.
- Reduce water temperature to lukewarm for bathing or other uses.
- Use only cream, lotion or ointment prescribed for the condition. Other commercial products may aggravate the condition. Apply ointment or cream to hands 6 or 7 times a day. For other body parts, lubricate twice a day, especially after bathing.
- Minimize the use of solvents, and wear heavy-duty vinyl gloves to prevent contact with irritating substances, such as water, soap, detergent, metal scouring pads, scouring powder, paint, paint thinner, turpentine, and polish for cars, floors, shoes, furniture, or metal.
- Dry the insides of vinyl gloves after use. Discard gloves if they develop a hole.
- Wear vinyl gloves when you peel or squeeze lemons, oranges, grapefruit, tomatoes, or potatoes.
- Wear leather or heavy-duty fabric gloves for household chores or gardening.
- Use a dishwashing machine to wash dishes or ask someone else to do it.
- Remove rings before washing hands or doing chores.

MEDICATION

- Your doctor may prescribe topical creams, ointments or lotions. These may include steroid preparations to reduce inflammation or lubricants to preserve moisture.
- See Medications section for information regarding medicines your doctor may prescribe.

ACTIVITY

Your child can resume normal activities gradually as irritation subsides.

DIET & FLUIDS

No special diet.

OK FOR SCHOOL, PRESCHOOL, OR NURSERY?

Yes, because it is not contagious to others.

CALL YOUR DOCTOR IF

- Your child develops a fever.
- Signs of infection (swelling, tenderness, redness, warmth) develop at the site of irritation.
- Treatment does not relieve the child's symptoms in 1 week.

DERMATITIS HERPETIFORMIS

GENERAL INFORMATION

DESCRIPTION

Dermatitis herpetiformis is a chronic skin inflammation characterized by clusters of small itching blisters. The disorder is hereditary. It is not contagious or cancerous. The skin of the elbows, knees, shoulders, arms, legs, and over the bottom of the spine (sacrum) is involved. Dermatitis herpetiformis can affect both sexes, beginning at puberty.

Appropriate health care includes:

- Self-care after diagnosis.
- Physician's monitoring of general condition and medications.

SIGNS & SYMPTOMS

Lesions with the following characteristics:

- Lesions are small clusters of 5 to 20 blisters. Blisters usually measure 2mm to 6mm in diameter.
- Clusters appear on both sides of the body in the same places.
- Lesions itch, but they are not usually painful if there are no complications.

CAUSES

Unknown, but it may be a disorder of the autoimmune system.

RISK FACTORS

Exposure to heat and humidity.

PREVENTING COMPLICATIONS OR RECURRENCE

Cannot be prevented at present. To prevent a recurrence of symptoms, your child should continue to take medication as directed and prevent injury to normal skin.

WHAT TO EXPECT

MEDICAL TESTS

- Your own observation of symptoms.
- Medical history and physical exam by a doctor.
- Biopsy (see Glossary).

POSSIBLE COMPLICATIONS

Children with dermatitis herpetiformis also may have disease of the small bowel (without symptoms), which pathologically resembles that of patients who are intolerant to gluten. The only way to diagnose this is with a biopsy.

PROBABLE OUTCOME

This is a chronic disease. Treatment can control your child's symptoms—including itching—but it will not cure the disease.

TREATMENT

HOME CARE

Your child can soak in cool water or use cool-water compresses to reduce itching.

MEDICATION

• For the child's itching, use non-prescription drugs such as:
— Low-dose steroid lotion, ointment, and cream. These reduce inflammation and itching in 24 to 48 hours.
— Topical anesthetics and topical antihistamines. These provide quick, short-term relief. Many cause skin sensitivity, but lidocaine and pramoxine usually do not.
— Lotions containing phenol, menthol, and camphor (such as calamine lotion). These are soothing, but use with care. Large amounts may be absorbed through the child's skin into the bloodstream, and they can be toxic.

• To control blistering, your doctor may prescribe 2 oral medications, sulfapyridine or dapsone. If either one is needed, it will be required indefinitely.

• See Medications section for information regarding medicines your doctor may prescribe.

ACTIVITY

No restrictions, except your child should avoid overheating and moisture.

DIET & FLUIDS

Restricting gluten in the child's diet will reduce the amount of medicine needed.

OK FOR SCHOOL, PRESCHOOL, OR NURSERY?

Yes.

CALL YOUR DOCTOR IF

• Your child has symptoms of dermatitis herpetiformis.

• New, unexplained symptoms develop. Drugs used in treatment may produce side effects.

DERMATITIS, INTERTRIGINOUS

GENERAL INFORMATION

DESCRIPTION

Intertriginous dermatitus is an inflammation of the skin in areas where two surfaces rub together, such as the underarm area, the groin, beneath the breasts, and between the buttocks. Children and adults with diabetes are particularly susceptible.

Appropriate health care includes:

- Self-care.
- Physician's monitoring of general condition and medications.

SIGNS & SYMPTOMS

- Flaking white scales over reddish patches on the child's skin.
- Itching (sometimes).
- No pain.

CAUSES

Unknown but aggravated by:

- Obesity.
- Sweating in hot weather.
- Infections caused by bacteria and fungus.

RISK FACTORS

- Stress.
- Hot, humid weather or cold, dry weather.
- Infrequent shampoos and baths.
- Oily skin.
- Other skin disorders, such as acne rosacea, acne, or psoriasis.
- Use of drying lotions that contain alcohol.
- Lack of sunlight.

PREVENTING COMPLICATIONS OR RECURRENCE

Cannot be prevented. To minimize severity or frequency of flare-ups, your child should:

- Shampoo frequently.
- Dry skin folds thoroughly after bathing.
- Wear loose, ventilating clothing.

WHAT TO EXPECT

MEDICAL TESTS

- Your own observation of symptoms.
- Medical history and physical exam by a doctor.
- Diagnostic measures including cultures of skin from involved areas.

POSSIBLE COMPLICATIONS

- Embarrassment and social discomfort.
- Secondary bacterial infection in affected areas.

PROBABLE OUTCOME

This is a chronic condition, but it is often characterized by long periods of inactivity. During active phases, your child's symptoms can be controlled with treatment.

TREATMENT

HOME CARE

Instructions for your child:

- Keep cool and dry.
- If the problem is on the skin under the breasts, wear supportive bras made of non-irritating material, such as cotton.
- Expose involved areas to sunlight as much as possible.
- Bathe frequently with non-irritating soap or plain water. Don't scrub the involved areas vigorously.
- Apply compresses dipped in Burrow's solution (1 tablet of Domeboro dissolved in 1 pint of cool water). Make compresses by dipping clean cloths folded into several layers into the solution. Apply the compresses to the involved areas for 20 minutes 6 times daily until improvement begins.
- Discontinue the use of all skin preparations other than the ones prescribed by your physician.

MEDICATION

- Medicines must be fitted to your child's own particular needs. Do not give any medicine (not even medicine you buy without prescription) without telling your doctor. If your doctor prescribes any drugs, carefully follow the instructions on the label.
- See Medications section for information regarding medicines your doctor may prescribe.

ACTIVITY

Your child should decrease activity that causes sweating, if possible, until the skin is healed.

DIET & FLUIDS

No special diet.

OK FOR SCHOOL, PRESCHOOL, OR NURSERY?

Yes.

CALL YOUR DOCTOR IF

- The Involved skin becomes infected, as evidenced by a fever over 100F, along with oozing or seepage from the inflamed area.
- The program prescribed by your child's doctor doesn't bring relief in a few days.

ILLNESSES

DERMATITIS, SEBORRHEIC

GENERAL INFORMATION

DESCRIPTION

Seborrheic dermatitis is a skin condition characterized by greasy or dry white scales. Dandruff and cradle cap are both forms of seborrheic dermatitis. This is not contagious. The skin of the scalp, eyebrows, forehead, face, and folds around the nose is involved; also the skin behind the ears, the external ear canal, and the skin of the trunk, especially over the breastbone (sternum) or in skin folds.

Appropriate health care includes:

- Self-care after diagnosis.
- Physician's monitoring of general condition and medications.

SIGNS & SYMPTOMS

Flaking white scales over reddish patches on your child's skin. Scales anchor to hair shafts. They may itch, but they are usually painless unless complicated by infection.

CAUSES

Unknown.

RISK FACTORS

- Stress.
- Hot, humid weather or cold, dry weather.
- Infrequent shampoos.
- Oily skin.
- Other skin disorders, such as acne rosacea, acne vulgaris, or psoriasis.
- Obesity.
- Parkinson's disease.
- Use of drying lotions that contain alcohol.
- Inadequate rest.

PREVENTING COMPLICATIONS OR RECURRENCE

Cannot be prevented. To minimize severity or frequency of flare-ups, your child should:

- Shampoo frequently.
- Dry skin folds thoroughly after bathing.
- Wear loose, ventilating clothing.
- Reduce stress.

WHAT TO EXPECT

MEDICAL TESTS

- Your own observation of symptoms.
- Medical history and physical exam by a doctor.

POSSIBLE COMPLICATIONS

- Embarrassment and social discomfort.
- Secondary bacterial infection in affected areas.

PROBABLE OUTCOME

This is a chronic condition, but it is often characterized by long periods of inactivity. During active phases, your child's symptoms can be controlled with treatment.

TREATMENT

HOME CARE

You or your child should shampoo the child's hair vigorously and as often as once a day. The shampoo you use is not as important as the way you scrub the scalp. Loosen scales with the fingernails while shampooing, and scrub at least 5 minutes.

MEDICATION

- For minor dandruff, use non-prescription dandruff shampoos and lubricating skin lotion.
- For severe problems, your doctor may prescribe:
  - Shampoos that contain coal tar, or scalp creams that contain cortisone. To apply medication to the scalp, the hair should be parted a few strands at a time and the ointment or lotion rubbed vigorously into the scalp.
  - Topical steroids for other affected parts.
- See Medications section for information regarding medicines your doctor may prescribe.

ACTIVITY

No restrictions. Outdoor activities in summer may help.

DIET & FLUIDS

No special diet. Your child should avoid foods that seem to worsen the condition.

OK FOR SCHOOL, PRESCHOOL, OR NURSERY?

Yes.

CALL YOUR DOCTOR IF

- Your child has symptoms of seborrheic dermatitis that don't respond to self-care.
- Patches of seborrheic dermatitis ooze, form crusts, or drain pus.

DES (Diethylstilbestrol) EXPOSURE

GENERAL INFORMATION

DESCRIPTION

Between 1946 and 1971, Diethylstilbestrol (DES), a synthetic form of estrogen, was prescribed for many pregnant women whose doctors hoped it would prevent repeated miscarriages, stillbirths, and premature births. It was also prescribed for women with diabetes and for some women who experienced abnormal bleeding during pregnancy. Beginning about 1968, physicians began discovering a benign form of tumor and a few rare instances of cancer (clear-cell carcinoma) in the vagina and cervix of daughters born of mothers who took DES during pregnancy. Sons of mothers who took DES may also have inherited abnormalities.

Appropriate health care includes:

- Physician's history and physical examination.
- Office treatments after diagnosis has been established.

SIGNS & SYMPTOMS

Girls: Abnormal vaginal discharge or bleeding (sometimes) beginning at about age 14 or at the start of menstruation.

Boys: Narrowed urethra, hypospadias (urethra opens on the underside of the penis), abnormally small penis, cysts in the testicles, undescended testicles, varicoceles, fewer sperm than normal, less than normal activity of sperm, and decreased volume of semen.

CAUSES

Taking DES during pregnancy.

RISK FACTORS

None other than the reasons DES was commonly prescribed for during 1946-1971.

PREVENTING COMPLICATIONS OR RECURRENCE

- Don't take estrogen or any other drug (if possible) during pregnancy.
- Daughters of DES mothers should not use estrogen for any purpose.
- Daughters of DES mothers should have pelvic exams performed annually or more frequently.

WHAT TO EXPECT

MEDICAL TESTS

- Obtain a record of mother's pregnancy.
- Your daughter should get pelvic exams on a regular basis beginning at age 14.
- Colposcopy (vaginal walls are spread with a speculum and tissue is viewed with a binocular microscope).
- Biopsy of abnormal tissue.

POSSIBLE COMPLICATIONS

- Difficulty in becoming pregnant.
- Higher risk of miscarriages, stillbirth, and prematurity.
- Vaginal cancer.

DES (Diethylstilbestrol) EXPOSURE

PROBABLE OUTCOME

Condition is simply and successfully treated. A very small percentage of girls with DES exposure will have cancerous changes that require additional treatment.

TREATMENT

HOME CARE

None, unless prescribed by your doctor.

MEDICATION

- Local treatment in doctor's office.
- See Medications section for information regarding medicines your doctor may prescribe.

ACTIVITY

No restrictions.

DIET & FLUIDS

No restrictions.

OK FOR SCHOOL, PRESCHOOL, OR NURSERY?

Yes.

CALL YOUR DOCTOR IF

Your daughter or son develops any of the symptoms of DES exposure.

ILLNESSES

DIABETES INSIPIDUS

GENERAL INFORMATION

DESCRIPTION

Diabetes insipidus is a temporary disorder of the hormone system, centered in the pituitary gland. The pituitary gland and the endocrine system are involved. Appropriate health care includes:

- Physician's monitoring of general condition and medications.
- Self-care after diagnosis.
- Surgery if a tumor or aneurysm is present.
- If brain surgery is necessary, see craniotomy (in Glossary) for an explanation of surgery and postoperative care.

SIGNS & SYMPTOMS

- Excessive thirst that is difficult to satisfy.
- Passage of large amounts (up to 15 quarts a day) of diluted, colorless urine.
- Dry hands.
- Constipation.

CAUSES

Deficiency of an anti-diuretic hormone (ADH) normally secreted by the pituitary gland. The deficiency may result from the following:

- Head injury, with damage to the pituitary gland.
- Tumor of the pituitary gland.
- Another type of brain tumor that applies pressure to the pituitary gland.
- Infection in the brain, such as encephalitis or meningitis.
- Bleeding inside the skull.
- Aneurysm.
- Kidney disease.

RISK FACTORS

- Preceding illness or injury in the brain.
- Atherosclerosis (hardening of the arteries).
- Family history of diabetes insipidus.

PREVENTING COMPLICATIONS OR RECURRENCE

No specific preventive measures.

WHAT TO EXPECT

MEDICAL TESTS

- Your own observation of symptoms.
- Medical history and physical exam by a doctor.
- Laboratory studies, such as water-deprivation tests to determine levels of ADH.

POSSIBLE COMPLICATIONS

Electrolyte imbalance, especially increased sodium or potassium deficiency. Either of these can cause heartbeat irregularity, fatigue, and congestive heart failure.

PROBABLE OUTCOME

- If the child's disorder is caused by a tumor or aneurysm, it can be cured by surgery.
- If the disorder is caused by a head injury, spontaneous recovery is likely within a year.
- If the disorder is caused by a preceding brain infection, symptoms may persist indefinitely.

TREATMENT

HOME CARE

Follow physician's advice.

MEDICATION

- Your doctor may prescribe synthetic ADH in nose drops, powder or injection form.
- See Medications section for information regarding medicines your doctor may prescribe.

ACTIVITY

No restrictions.

DIET & FLUIDS

No special diet. Your child should drink as much water as needed.

OK FOR SCHOOL, PRESCHOOL, OR NURSERY?

When appetite has returned and alertness, strength, and feeling of well-being will allow.

CALL YOUR DOCTOR IF

- Your child has symptoms of diabetes insipidus.
- Symptoms don't improve, despite treatment.
- New, unexplained symptoms develop. Drugs used in treatment may produce side effects.

DIABETES MELLITUS, INSULIN-DEPENDENT

GENERAL INFORMATION

DESCRIPTION

Insulin-dependent diabetes mellitus is a chronic disease of the body's metabolism characterized by an inability to produce enough insulin to process carbohydrates, fat, and protein efficiently. Treatment requires injections of insulin. Insulin-dependent diabetes is often called *ketosis-prone diabetes* if it begins in adulthood and *juvenile diabetes* if it begins in childhood. Body parts involved include islet cells of the pancreas that produce insulin and all body cells that need insulin to convert food into chemicals the body can use.

Appropriate health care includes:

- Self-care after diagnosis. Self-care is by far the most important part of your child's treatment.
- Physician's monitoring of general condition and medications.
- Hospitalization for severe complications.
- Surgery for treatment of some complications, such as failing eyesight or gangrene.

SIGNS & SYMPTOMS

- Fatigue.
- Excess thirst.
- Increased appetite *and* weight loss.
- Frequent urination, especially noted at night.
- Itching around the genitals.
- Increased susceptibility to infections, especially urinary-tract infections and yeast infections of the skin, mouth, or vagina.
- Deterioration of vision (advanced stages).

CAUSES

- Too little insulin produced by the islet cells of the pancreas for unknown reasons.
- Interference with insulin use in the body cells for unknown reasons.
- Virus infection of the pancreas.

RISK FACTORS

- Family history of diabetes mellitus. It often skips one generation.
- Pregnancy.

PREVENTING COMPLICATIONS OR RECURRENCE

Cannot be prevented.

WHAT TO EXPECT

MEDICAL TESTS

- Your own observation of symptoms.
- Medical history and physical exam by a doctor.
- Laboratory urine and blood studies to measure glucose, cholesterol, and insulin.

DIABETES MELLITUS, INSULIN-DEPENDENT

POSSIBLE COMPLICATIONS

- Cardiovascular disease, especially stroke, atherosclerosis, and coronary-artery disease.
- Kidney failure.
- Blindness.
- Peripheral vascular disease, with gangrene in legs and feet.
- Life-threatening hypoglycemia (low blood sugar) if too much insulin is used.
- Life-threatening ketoacidosis (very high blood sugar) with breakdown of body cells.

PROBABLE OUTCOME

This disease is presently considered incurable, but symptoms and progress of the disease can be controlled with rigid adherence to a treatment program. Life expectancy is somewhat reduced, but many children with diabetes have a nearly normal life span.

TREATMENT

HOME CARE

- Learn all you can about controlling your child's diabetes and recognizing signs and symptoms of ketoacidosis or hypoglycemia.
- Keep a vial of glucagon available at all times to use if hypoglycemia occurs.
- Learn to give your child insulin injections. At an appropriate time, your doctor will give the child instructions for self-injections. They will be necessary every day for life.
- Encourage your child to wear a Medic-Alert bracelet or pendant (see Glossary).
- Seek medical treatment for any infection.

MEDICATION

Your doctor will prescribe insulin by injection. The dosage must be individualized and occasionally adjusted.

ACTIVITY

No restrictions. Regular daily exercise for your child is an important part of controlling diabetes. Consult your doctor.

DIET & FLUIDS

A special diet will be prescribed by your doctor.

OK FOR SCHOOL, PRESCHOOL, OR NURSERY?

Yes, when diabetes is under control.

CALL YOUR DOCTOR IF

- Your child has symptoms of diabetes mellitus.
- The following occurs during the child's treatment:
  — Inability to think clearly, weakness, sweating, paleness, rapid heartbeat, seizures, or coma (may indicate hypoglycemia).
  — Orange odor on the breath, changes in breathing pattern, or stupor (may indicate ketoacidosis).
  — Several days of illness or weakness.
  — Numbness, tingling, or pain in the feet or hands.
  — Chest pain.

DIAPER RASH

GENERAL INFORMATION

DESCRIPTION

Diaper rash is a form of contact dermatitis that causes skin irritation in the area covered by a wet diaper. The skin around the genitals, rectum, and abdomen is involved. Diaper rash can affect any infant or young child who wears diapers. Appropriate health care includes:

- Self-care after diagnosis.
- Physician's monitoring of general condition and medications, if home treatment fails to cure the rash.

SIGNS & SYMPTOMS

- Moist, painful, red, spotty, and itchy (sometimes) skin in the diaper area. The skin may be cracked and fissured.
- In male infants, a red, raw, and occasionally bloody area may appear around the meatus (the opening at the tip of the penis).
- In female infants, a thin adhesive membrane may form between the vaginal lips.

CAUSES

- Excessive ammonia on the wet diaper and skin caused by bacterial action. (Urine does not naturally contain ammonia.)
- Monilia fungus infection—the same fungus that causes thrush.
- Allergy to soap, detergent, fabric softener, lotion, powder, or other chemicals.

RISK FACTORS

- Infrequent diaper changes.
- Improper laundering of diapers.
- Family history of skin allergies.
- Hot, humid weather.

PREVENTING COMPLICATIONS OR RECURRENCE

- Change your baby's diapers frequently.
- Don't use waterproof diapers or pants at night.
- Keep cloth diapers clean. After washing, rinse them twice to remove detergents and other chemicals.

WHAT TO EXPECT

MEDICAL TESTS

- Your own observation of symptoms.
- Medical history and physical exam by a doctor.
- Urinalysis to rule out urinary-tract infection, which may complicate healing.

POSSIBLE COMPLICATIONS

Secondary bacterial infection in the rash area.

PROBABLE OUTCOME

Usually curable with treatment. Recurrence is common.

TREATMENT

HOME CARE

- Expose the baby's buttocks to air as much as possible.
- Don't use waterproof pants during treatment—either in the day or at night. They keep skin wet and subject to rash or infection.
- Change diapers frequently—even at night if the rash is extensive.
- Don't use soap or boric acid to wash the baby's rash area. Cleanse with cotton dipped in mineral oil.
- Discontinue using baby lotion, powder, ointment, or baby oil (except zinc oxide) unless prescribed by your doctor.
- Apply small amounts of non-prescription zinc-oxide ointment to the baby's rash at the earliest sign of diaper rash, and 2 or 3 times a day thereafter.
- If you wash your own diapers, add 1 cup of vinegar to the washing machine when it is half-full of rinse water. This neutralizes detergent residue.
- If you use a diaper service, rinse the laundered diapers in 1 ounce of vinegar added to each gallon of water and dry before using.

MEDICATION

- Your doctor may prescribe medicated anti-inflammatory ointments or creams, such as hydrocortisone, nystatin, or miconazole, to apply to the baby's skin.
- See Medications section for information regarding medicines your doctor may prescribe.

ACTIVITY

No restrictions.

DIET & FLUIDS

No special diet.

OK FOR SCHOOL, PRESCHOOL, OR NURSERY?

Yes. Keep diapers separate.

CALL YOUR DOCTOR IF

- Home treatment doesn't cure the rash in 1 week.
- The following occurs during treatment:
  - — Fever.
  - — Pustules in the rash area.
  - — Male infant has a weak urinary stream.
  - — Female infant develops adhesions of the vaginal lips.
- New, unexplained symptoms develop. Medicine used in treatment may produce side effects.

DIARRHEA, ACUTE

GENERAL INFORMATION

DESCRIPTION

Acute diarrhea is the passage of many loose, watery, or unformed bowel movements. This is a symptom, not a disease. The colon, small intestine, rectum, and skin around the rectum are involved.

Appropriate health care includes:

• Self-care after diagnosis.

• Physician's monitoring of general condition and medications (if symptoms persist longer than 2 to 3 days).

SIGNS & SYMPTOMS

- Cramping abdominal pain.
- Loose, watery, or unformed bowel movements.
- Lack of bowel control (sometimes).
- Fever (sometimes).

CAUSES

- Emotional upsets.
- Food poisoning.
- Infections (viral, parasitic or bacterial).
- Regional enteritis (see Glossary).
- Malabsorption syndromes.
- Disease or tumor of the pancreas (malignant or benign).
- Diverticulitis.
- Foods, such as prunes or beans.
- Excess alcohol consumption.
- Use of drugs, such as laxatives, antacids, antibiotics, quinine, or anti-cancer drugs.
- Food allergy.
- Radiation treatments for cancer.

RISK FACTORS

- Stress.
- Recent illness.
- Excess alcohol consumption.
- Crowded or unsanitary living conditions.

PREVENTING COMPLICATIONS OR RECURRENCE

If diarrhea recurs in your child and a cause can be identified, treatment or avoidance of the cause should prevent recurrence.

OTHER

Every child is likely to have bouts of diarrhea occasionally from insignificant causes that disappear and leave no lasting effects. Most cases of acute diarrhea last a short time, and a search for the cause may not be necessary.

DIARRHEA, ACUTE

? WHAT TO EXPECT

MEDICAL TESTS

- Your own observation of symptoms.
- Medical history and physical exam by a doctor.
- Laboratory stool studies (for prolonged diarrhea).

POSSIBLE COMPLICATIONS

Dehydration if diarrhea is prolonged, especially in infants.

PROBABLE OUTCOME

Spontaneous recovery in 24 to 48 hours.

TREATMENT

HOME CARE

If cramps are present, place hot compresses, a hot-water bottle, or an electric heating pad on the abdomen.

MEDICATION

- For minor discomfort, use non-prescription drugs such as Pepto-Bismol or Kaopectate.
- See Medications section for information regarding medicines your doctor may prescribe.

ACTIVITY

Decrease your child's activity until diarrhea stops.

DIET & FLUIDS

- If diarrhea is accompanied by nausea, your child should suck ice chips only.
- If your child is not nauseated, drinking small amounts of clear liquid, such as herbal tea, ginger ale, broth, or gelatin is helpful until diarrhea stops.
- After symptoms disappear, serve the child soft foods, such as cooked cereal, rice, eggs, custard, baked potato, and yogurt, for 1 or 2 days.
- Your child can resume a normal diet 2 or 3 days after the diarrhea stops, but fruit, alcohol, and highly seasoned foods should be avoided for several more days.

OK FOR SCHOOL, PRESCHOOL, OR NURSERY?

When signs of infection have decreased, appetite returns, and alertness, strength, and feeling of well-being will allow.

CALL YOUR DOCTOR IF

- Diarrhea lasts more than 48 hours.
- Mucus, blood, or worms appear in the stool.
- Fever rises to 101F (38.3C) or higher.
- Severe pain develops in the child's abdomen or rectum.
- Dehydration develops. Signs include: dry mouth, wrinkled skin, excess thirst, and little or no urination.

ILLNESSES

DIARRHEA, CHRONIC, NON-SPECIFIC, OF CHILDHOOD

GENERAL INFORMATION

DESCRIPTION

Chronic, non-specific diarrhea of childhood means that a healthy child is having more than 5 watery or loose stools a day. Only the colon is involved. This condition usually affects young children (1 to 3-1/2 years).

Appropriate health care includes:

- Physician's monitoring of general condition and medications.
- Self-care after diagnosis.

SIGNS & SYMPTOMS

- Frequent, loose stools that often contain undigested vegetable fibers or mucus and occur primarily during the morning.
- Occasional irritation of the child's anal area caused by frequency of bowel movements.

CAUSES

Unknown.

RISK FACTORS

Family history of intestinal problems.

PREVENTING COMPLICATIONS OR RECURRENCE

Cannot be prevented at present.

WHAT TO EXPECT

MEDICAL TESTS

- Your own observation of symptoms.
- Medical history and physical exam by a doctor.
- Laboratory stool studies.

POSSIBLE COMPLICATIONS

Possible psychological fixation on bowel function because of excessive parental attention to the child's bowel habits.

PROBABLE OUTCOME

Despite the chronic diarrhea, affected children develop normally and show no signs of malnutrition. The frequent stools have no special significance. Bowel movements eventually become normal, but it may take 2 to 3 years.

DIARRHEA, CHRONIC, NON-SPECIFIC, OF CHILDHOOD

TREATMENT

HOME CARE

Don't blame or criticize your child for this problem. Don't expect toilet training to be successful as soon as with other children. Treat your child as normal and try to ignore the problem. Avoid tension. If the child becomes anxious about diarrhea, the problem may become worse or psychological problems may arise.

MEDICATION

- Medicine usually is not necessary for this disorder. Don't give your child any non-prescription anti-diarrheal drugs. Side effects may be harmful.
- See Medications section for information regarding medicines your doctor may prescribe.

ACTIVITY

No restrictions. Encourage full participation in all activities normal for your child's age group.

DIET & FLUIDS

- No special diet, but vitamin and mineral supplements may be helpful.
- The child should drink at least 6 to 8 glasses of fluid each day to replace fluid lost in stools.

OK FOR SCHOOL, PRESCHOOL, OR NURSERY?

When appetite has returned and alertness, strength, and feeling of well-being will allow.

CALL YOUR DOCTOR IF

- Your child has chronic diarrhea or stools with mucus that haven't been diagnosed.
- There is blood in the child's stool.
- Your child's rectal temperature is 102F (38.9C) or higher.
- Your child becomes listless, refuses to eat, or cries loudly and persistently even when picked up.
- Your child's growth and development are not normal.

DIC (Disseminated Intravascular Coagulation; Defibrinogenation Syndrome; Coagulopathy)

GENERAL INFORMATION

DESCRIPTION

Disseminated intravascular coagulation is a serious disruption of blood-clotting mechanisms, resulting in hemorrhaging or internal bleeding. This disorder is a complication of an underlying disorder. Blood vessels and blood in all parts of the body are involved.

Appropriate health care includes:

- Hospitalization.
- Physician's monitoring of general condition and medications.
- Surgery to correct the underlying disorder (sometimes).
- Self-care after diagnosis.

SIGNS & SYMPTOMS

- Bleeding and hemorrhaging from any or several body parts. Bleeding may be heavy. Common signs of bleeding include:
  - — Bloody vomit or red or black stools.
  - — Vaginal bleeding.
  - — Red or cloudy urine.
  - — Unexplained bruising.
- Severe abdominal or back pain caused by bleeding into body organs.
- Convulsions (rare).
- Coma (rare).

CAUSES

Depletion of blood-clotting components, causing widespread bleeding. This condition can be the result of:

- Pregnancy abnormalities, such as placenta previa, abruptio placenta, or toxemia.
- Widespread or major infection.
- Widespread cancer.
- Some kinds of surgery.
- Widespread tissue destruction, as with extensive burns.
- Poisonous snakebite.
- Transfusion of mismatched blood.

RISK FACTORS

- Poor nutrition.
- Illness that has lowered resistance.

PREVENTING COMPLICATIONS OR RECURRENCE

Obtain prompt medical treatment for the underlying causes.

WHAT TO EXPECT

MEDICAL TESTS

- Your own observation of symptoms.
- Medical history and physical exam by a doctor.
- Laboratory blood tests, especially of the blood-clotting mechanism.

DIC (Disseminated Intravascular Coagulation; Defibrinogenation Syndrome; Coagulopathy)

POSSIBLE COMPLICATIONS

- Kidney failure.
- Brain damage, with seizures or coma.
- Shock.
- Death.

PROBABLE OUTCOME

Depends on the severity. If the underlying cause of the child's DIC is treated promptly, full recovery is likely.

TREATMENT

HOME CARE

- Children with this condition are often desperately ill and require intensive hospital care. Family members can help by maintaining a positive, hopeful attitude.
- During your child's recovery, don't scrub or take scabs off sores. This may trigger new bleeding.

MEDICATION

Your doctor may prescribe:

- Blood transfusions or blood-component infusions.
- Heparin (an anticoagulant administered by injection).
- See Medications section for information regarding medicines your doctor may prescribe.

ACTIVITY

Your child should rest in bed until your doctor approves a return to normal activity. The child may read or watch TV.

DIET & FLUIDS

No special diet.

OK FOR SCHOOL, PRESCHOOL, OR NURSERY?

When signs of infection have decreased, appetite returns, and alertness, strength, and feeling of well-being will allow.

CALL YOUR DOCTOR IF

- Your child has symptoms of DIC.
- Any bleeding recurs or the child's abdomen swells rapidly during treatment.

DIPHTHERIA

GENERAL INFORMATION

DESCRIPTION

Diphtheria is a highly contagious throat infection. The throat, skin, heart, and central nervous system are involved. Diphtheria can affect older children (5 years and up), adolescents, and adults.

Appropriate health care includes:

• Physician's monitoring of general condition and medications. This is a medical emergency.

• Hospitalization.

SIGNS & SYMPTOMS

Early stages:

• Sore throat.

• Low fever.

• Swollen neck glands.

Late stages:

• Airway obstruction and breathing difficulty.

• Shock (low blood pressure, rapid heartbeat, paleness, cold skin, sweating, and anxious appearance).

CAUSES

A bacterial germ, corynebacterium diphtheriae, infects the child's throat and sometimes the skin. The incubation period is 5 to 9 days following exposure. The germ produces poisons that spread to the child's heart, central nervous system, and other organs.

RISK FACTORS

• Poor nutrition.

• Outbreak in the community.

• Crowded or unsanitary living conditions.

• Lack of up-to-date immunizations.

PREVENTING COMPLICATIONS OR RECURRENCE

• Immunization with diphtheria vaccine. See Appendix 1 for an immunization schedule.

• Improved nutrition and standard of living.

OTHER

Notify the local health department of any case of diphtheria. Anyone having contact with your child must be examined and treated.

WHAT TO EXPECT

MEDICAL TESTS

• Your own observation of symptoms.

• Medical history and physical exam by a doctor.

• Laboratory studies, such as throat culture and blood counts.

POSSIBLE COMPLICATIONS

- Heart inflammation and heart failure.
- Suffocation.
- Nerve inflammation.
- Misdiagnosis as a less-serious infection, resulting in dangerous delay of treatment.

PROBABLE OUTCOME

Usually curable in 1 week, followed by slow recovery for several weeks. A delay in treatment may result in death or long-term heart disease for your child.

TREATMENT

HOME CARE

- Quarantine your child until fully recovered. Protect susceptible individuals (the non-immunized, very young, or elderly) from exposure.
- Dispose of all the child's secretions (nose and mouth) and excretions (urine and feces) in an acceptable manner. Call the local health department for instructions.

MEDICATION

Your doctor may prescribe:

- Diphtheria antitoxin to neutralize the diphtheria toxin.
- Antibiotics to fight the remaining diphtheria germs.
- See Medications section for information regarding medicines your doctor may prescribe.

ACTIVITY

Prolonged bed rest (2 to 3 months or until fully recovered), especially if the child's heart is involved. The child may watch TV or read.

DIET & FLUIDS

No special diet, except to encourage your child to eat heartily.

OK FOR SCHOOL, PRESCHOOL, OR NURSERY?

When appetite has returned and alertness, strength, and feeling of well-being will allow.

CALL YOUR DOCTOR IF

- Your child has symptoms of diphtheria or you observe them in someone else.
- Anyone in your family is exposed to diphtheria.
- The following occurs during treatment:
  - — Temperature spikes to 102F (38.9C).
  - — Increasing breathing difficulty.
  - — Increasing shortness of breath.
  - — Confusion.

DISLOCATION OR SUBLUXATION

GENERAL INFORMATION

DESCRIPTION

Dislocation is injury to a joint so that adjoining bones no longer touch each other. Subluxation is a minor dislocation. Joint surfaces still touch, but not in a normal relation to each other. The bones in the joints, especially the jaw, elbow, shoulder, knee and spine, are involved. Some infants are born with a hip dislocation.

Appropriate health care includes:

- Physician's monitoring of general condition and medications. This may include manipulating your child's joint to reposition the bones.
- Surgery to restore the joint to its normal position (sometimes). Recurring dislocation may require surgical reconstruction or replacement of the joint.
- Self-care after the dislocation has been reduced.

SIGNS & SYMPTOMS

- Sudden joint pain, swelling, or deformity after an injury.
- Limited or absent movement around a joint.

CAUSES

- Jerking a child sharply by the hand or arm.
- Injury that stretches or tears ligaments that surround a joint and hold the bones together.
- Shallow or abnormally formed joint surfaces (congenital).
- Rheumatoid arthritis or other diseases of ligaments and tissue around a joint.

RISK FACTORS

- Rheumatoid arthritis.
- Family history of congenital hip dislocation.
- Repeated injury to a joint.

PREVENTING COMPLICATIONS OR RECURRENCE

Advise a child who is involved in strenuous sports or heavy work to protect the involved joints and to use protective devices, such as wrapped elastic bandages, tape wraps, knee or shoulder pads, and special support stockings.

WHAT TO EXPECT

MEDICAL TESTS

- Your own observation of symptoms.
- Medical history and physical exam by a doctor. (Infants should be examined for congenital hip dislocation at birth and at "well-baby" checkups.)
- X-rays of the joint and adjacent bones.

POSSIBLE COMPLICATIONS

Damage to nearby nerves or major blood vessels, causing numbness, coldness, and paleness.

PROBABLE OUTCOME

Usually curable with prompt treatment. After the dislocation has been corrected, the joint may require immobilization with a cast or sling for 2 to 8 weeks.

TREATMENT

HOME CARE

Immediately after injury:
- Apply ice packs to the involved joint to prevent swelling.
- Use a splint or sling to prevent movement while transporting the injured child to the doctor.
- If your doctor puts a cast on the joint, see Appendix 41 (Care of Casts).

MEDICATION

Your doctor may prescribe:
- General anesthesia or muscle relaxants to make joint manipulation possible.
- Acetaminophen or aspirin to relieve moderate pain.
- Narcotic pain relievers for severe pain.
- See Medications section for information regarding medicines your doctor may prescribe.

ACTIVITY

Your child can resume normal activities gradually after treatment.

DIET & FLUIDS

Your child should drink only water before manipulation or surgery to correct the dislocation. Solid food makes general anesthesia more hazardous.

OK FOR SCHOOL, PRESCHOOL, OR NURSERY?

When your child is comfortable enough to last through the day.

CALL YOUR DOCTOR IF

- Your child has difficulty moving a joint after injury.
- Any extremity becomes numb, pale, or cold after injury. This is an emergency!
- Dislocations occur repeatedly that you can "pop" back into normal position.

DOWN SYNDROME
(Mongolism; Trisomy 21)

GENERAL INFORMATION

DESCRIPTION

Down syndrome is retardation and abnormalities in many organs caused by a major chromosome abnormality that is inherited. The central nervous system, heart, and skeletal system are involved. Down syndrome affects newborns. Normal life span is shortened on average, but many children with Down syndrome survive happily for many years.

Appropriate health care includes:

- Physician's monitoring of general condition and medications.
- Psychotherapy or counseling for the parents. Many parents blame themselves and need help to cope with unnecessary, harmful guilt.
- Surgery to correct congenital heart or intestinal disorders.
- Nursing-home or group-home care, if parental-home care is not feasible.

SIGNS & SYMPTOMS

Shortly after birth:

- Lack of normal muscle tone. The baby seems "floppy."
- Head and face abnormalities, including a small or odd-shaped skull, slanting almond-shaped eyes, a small mouth, and a protruding tongue.
- Broad hands with large, unusual palm creases. The little finger curves inward (sometimes).
- Heart murmur.

Later:

- Retarded growth and development. The child never reaches full stature.
- Mental retardation. The IQ is significantly below normal.

CAUSES

An extra chromosome in the fertilized egg creates abnormalities as the fetus develops. In a third of cases, the extra chromosome comes from the father.

RISK FACTORS

- Pregnancy in females under age 16 or over 35.
- Family history of Down syndrome.
- Mother's exposure to drugs, radiation, chemicals, or infections before pregnancy.

PREVENTING COMPLICATIONS OR RECURRENCE

- If you are pregnant and over age 35, or you or your partner have a family history of Down syndrome, request amniocentesis (see Glossary). This procedure can detect whether the fetus has Down syndrome.
- If you or your partner have a family history of Down syndrome, obtain genetic counseling before starting a family.

DOWN SYNDROME
(Mongolism; Trisomy 21)

? WHAT TO EXPECT

MEDICAL TESTS

- Your own observation of symptoms.
- Medical history and physical exam by a doctor.
- Laboratory studies of your child's chromosomes.

POSSIBLE COMPLICATIONS

- Increased susceptibility to leukemia.
- Increased susceptibility to infections.
- Chronic ear infections.
- Hearing loss.
- Visual problems.
- Skin disorders.
- Congestive heart failure caused by congenital heart abnormalities.

PROBABLE OUTCOME

Special education and training allow many children with Down syndrome to lead happy, loving, and useful lives. Life expectancy is reduced for most, although a few live to retirement age.

TREATMENT

HOME CARE

Learn all you can about programs and resources in your community to help children with Down syndrome.

MEDICATION

- Your doctor may prescribe antibiotics for frequent, complicating infections. There is no medication to cure Down syndrome.
- See Medications section for information regarding medicines your doctor may prescribe.

ACTIVITY

Encourage your child to be as active as possible in a protected environment.

DIET & FLUIDS

No special diet. Extra patience may be necessary in feeding an infant with Down syndrome. Some have difficulty sucking or are not eager to eat.

OK FOR SCHOOL, PRESCHOOL, OR NURSERY?

Yes, but probably requires a special school or special care.

CALL YOUR DOCTOR IF

- Your infant seems "floppy" or does not seem to be developing normally.
- A child with Down syndrome develops signs of infection (fever, warmth, or pain).

DROWNING, NEAR-

GENERAL INFORMATION

DESCRIPTION

Near-drowning refers to the immediate aftereffects of prolonged submersion under water. The lungs, blood, and heart are involved.

Appropriate health care includes:

- Immediate cardiopulmonary resuscitation (CPR).
- Hospitalization for observation for delayed serious reactions to being submerged or severely chilled.

SIGNS & SYMPTOMS

- Confusion or unconsciousness.
- Little or no breathing or heartbeat.
- Bluish-white paleness.

CAUSES

Submersion under water results in either of the following:

- Spasm of your child's larynx (the tube from the throat to the lungs). After rescue, this spasm prevents oxygen from reaching the lungs.
- Water in the child's lungs, causing life-threatening changes in the circulating blood.

RISK FACTORS

- An accident—especially head injury—while swimming.
- Suicidal feelings.
- Excess alcohol consumption.

PREVENTING COMPLICATIONS OR RECURRENCE

- Learn cardiopulmonary resuscitation (CPR).
- Encourage all family members—including infants—to learn to swim.
- Install a fence around your home swimming pool.
- Never swim alone.
- Don't drink alcohol and swim.

WHAT TO EXPECT

MEDICAL TESTS

- Your own observation of symptoms.
- Medical history and physical exam by a doctor.
- Laboratory blood tests.

POSSIBLE COMPLICATIONS

- Pulmonary edema (body fluid in the lungs).
- Permanent brain damage.
- Heart irregularities, including cardiac arrest and death.
- Lung infection.

PROBABLE OUTCOME

Depends on the length of time your child was under water. With early rescue and treatment, full recovery is possible. Special body mechanisms may permit full recovery from near-drowning in icy water.

TREATMENT

HOME CARE

- If the child is unconscious and not breathing, yell for help. Don't leave the victim.
- Begin mouth-to-mouth breathing immediately.
- If the child has no heartbeat, give external cardiac massage.
- Have someone call 0 (operator) or 911 (emergency) for an ambulance or medical help.
- Don't stop CPR until help arrives.
- The near-drowning child should be taken to the nearest hospital for intensive care—even if the child has regained consciousness. Complications or death may occur 24 to 48 hours after the accident due to heart-rhythm disturbances.
- Remain with a recovering child to provide support and reassurance. Near-drowning is a traumatic experience.

MEDICATION

The doctor may prescribe:

- Oxygen.
- Cortisone drugs to prevent or treat lung inflammation.
- Antibiotics to prevent lung infection.
- Bronchodilators to enable oxygen to enter the lungs.
- See Medications section for information regarding medicines your doctor may prescribe.

ACTIVITY

Complete bed rest until activity is permitted by the doctor.

DIET & FLUIDS

Intravenous nutrients, if the child is unconscious upon hospitalization. After recovery, no special diet is necessary.

OK FOR SCHOOL, PRESCHOOL, OR NURSERY?

When appetite has returned and alertness, strength, and feeling of well-being will allow.

CALL YOUR DOCTOR IF

- Someone appears to have drowned. Call for emergency help immediately! See HOME CARE for additional emergency information.
- Signs of infection (fever, cough, muscle aches, and fatigue) appear after apparent recovery.

DRUG ABUSE & ADDICTION

GENERAL INFORMATION

DESCRIPTION

Drug abuse and addiction is a psychological or physiological need for chemical substances that produce temporary pleasant mood changes. The central nervous system, liver, kidneys, and blood are involved. Drug abuse and addiction can affect both sexes, all ages, but it rarely occurs in early childhood, except in newborns of addicted mothers.

Appropriate health care includes:

- Physician's monitoring of general condition and medications.
- Psychotherapy or counseling.
- Hospitalization for drug-withdrawal symptoms.
- Self-care after diagnosis. (The most important part of your child's treatment.)

SIGNS & SYMPTOMS

Depends on the substance of abuse. Most produce a temporary pleasant mood; relief from anxiety; false feelings of self-confidence; increased sensitivity to sights and sounds (including hallucinations); altered activity levels—either stupor and sleeplike states *or* frenzies; unpleasant or painful symptoms when the abused substance is withdrawn.

CAUSES

Substances of abuse may produce in your child addiction (a physiological need) or dependence (a psychological need). The most common substances of abuse include: nicotine; alcohol (has greatest number of addicts); marijuana; amphetamines; barbiturates; cocaine; opiates, including codeine, heroin, methadone, morphine, and opium; psychedelic drugs, including PCP ("angel dust"), mescaline, and LSD; volatile substances, such as glue, solvents, and paints.

RISK FACTORS

- Illness that requires prescription pain relievers or tranquilizers, family history of drug abuse, and genetic factors (possibly). Some children and adolescents may be more susceptible to addiction.
- Alcohol consumption, fatigue or overwork, poverty, and psychological problems, including depression, dependency, or poor self-esteem.

PREVENTING COMPLICATIONS OR RECURRENCE

Instructions for your child: Don't socialize with persons who use and abuse drugs; seek counseling for mental-health problems, such as depression or chronic anxiety, before they lead to drug problems; develop wholesome interests and leisure activities; after surgery, illness, or injury, discontinue the use of prescription pain relievers and tranquilizers as soon as possible. Don't use more than you need.

WHAT TO EXPECT

MEDICAL TESTS

Medical history and physical exam by a doctor, and laboratory blood tests for liver, kidney, and brain function.

POSSIBLE COMPLICATIONS

AIDS; sexually transmitted diseases, which are more likely among addicts; severe infections, such as endocarditis, hepatitis, or blood poisoning, from intravenous infections with non-sterile needles; malnutrition; accidental injury to oneself or others while in a drug-induced state; loss of job or family; irreversible damage to body organs; death caused by overdose.

PROBABLE OUTCOME

Curable with strong motivation, good medical care, and support from family and friends.

TREATMENT

HOME CARE

Encourage your child to do the following: admit you have a problem; seek professional help; be open and honest with your family and good friends, and ask their help; avoid friends who tempt you to resume your habit; join self-help groups.

MEDICATION

Your doctor may prescribe:

- Disulfiram (Antabuse) for alcoholism. This drug produces severe illness when alcohol is consumed.
- Methadone for narcotic abuse. This drug is a less-potent narcotic used to decrease the severity of physical withdrawal symptoms.

ACTIVITY

No restrictions.

DIET & FLUIDS

Urge your child to eat a normal, well-balanced diet that is high in protein. Vitamin supplements may be necessary if your child suffers from malnutrition.

OK FOR SCHOOL, PRESCHOOL, OR NURSERY?

After addiction is broken.

CALL YOUR DOCTOR IF

- Your child abuses or is addicted to drugs and wants help.
- New, unexplained symptoms develop. Drugs in treatment may produce side effects.

DRUG HYPERSENSITIVITY

GENERAL INFORMATION

DESCRIPTION

Drug hypersensitivity is a variety of allergic responses caused by medication. The skin, blood vessels, and lungs are involved.

Appropriate health care includes:

- Self-care after diagnosis.
- Physician's monitoring of general condition and medications.

SIGNS & SYMPTOMS

- Rash, itching, or hives.
- Flushed skin.
- Anxiety.
- Serum sickness (fever, rash, joint pain, and nerve damage).
- Anaphylaxis (wheezing and breathing difficulty). For signs and symptoms, see Anaphylaxis (in Illnesses section).
- Various blood disorders, such as hemolytic anemia.
- Peripheral neuropathy (nerve damage).
- Vasculitis (blood vessel inflammation).

The following reactions to medications are usually *not* the result of allergy:

— Vomiting or diarrhea.
— Fever.
— Photosensitivity (a skin reaction to sunlight).

CAUSES

Medications or drugs are "foreign" materials. When injected—or less often, when taken orally—the body develops antibodies to the medication or drug. Subsequent exposure causes an allergic reaction in the body.

RISK FACTORS

- Use of the following drugs:
  — Penicillin and cephalosporin antibiotics.
  — Sulfa drugs.
  — Animal serums.
  — Vaccines.
  — Local anesthetics.
  — Allergy extracts.
  — Iodine-containing compounds, such as those used in some X-rays.
- Injected medications, especially in high doses.
- Medical history of a child's other allergies, such as hay fever, asthma, or eczema.
- Current infectious illness (probably because infection increases immune-system functions).

PREVENTING COMPLICATIONS OR RECURRENCE

- Tell your doctor about any drug reactions your child has had.
- Learn the name of any medication your child is given. If it causes a reaction, the child must avoid it in the future.
- Encourage your child *not* to take medication—including non-prescription drugs—for minor illness, if possible.

WHAT TO EXPECT

MEDICAL TESTS
- Your own observation of symptoms.
- Medical history and physical exam by a doctor.

POSSIBLE COMPLICATIONS
- Death from severe anaphylaxis reactions.
- Disability for many months from serum sickness.

PROBABLE OUTCOME
Most of the child's reactions disappear once the medication is permanently discontinued.

TREATMENT

HOME CARE
- Learn how to treat anaphylaxis (see Illnesses section).
- Encourage your child to wear a Medic-Alert pendant or bracelet (see Glossary) if there is drug hypersensitivity.
- Keep an anaphylaxis kit at home for emergency use if anyone in the family has ever had a severe drug reaction. Ask your doctor how to obtain one.

MEDICATION
Your doctor may prescribe:
- Cortisone drugs to decrease the inflammatory reaction.
- Antihistamines to decrease the body's allergic response.
- See Medications section for information regarding medicines your doctor may prescribe.

ACTIVITY
Your child can resume normal activities as soon as symptoms improve.

DIET & FLUIDS
No special diet.

OK FOR SCHOOL, PRESCHOOL, OR NURSERY?
When appetite has returned and alertness, strength, and feeling of well-being will allow.

CALL YOUR DOCTOR IF

Your child has symptoms of drug hypersensitivity or you observe them in someone else.

DYSENTERY, BACILLARY (Shigellosis)

GENERAL INFORMATION

DESCRIPTION

Bacillary dysentery is a bacterial infection of the surface layers of the intestinal tract. This is contagious with close personal contact and occurs in epidemics. It has a 1- to 3-day incubation period. The lower small intestine (ileum) and large intestine (colon) are involved.

Appropriate health care includes:

- Home care.
- Physician's monitoring of general condition and medications.
- Hospitalization of persons (especially small children with dehydration) who are severely ill. Hospital care will include isolation and intravenous fluid supplements.

SIGNS & SYMPTOMS

- Abdominal cramps.
- Fever.
- Diarrhea (up to 20 or 30 watery bowel movements in 1 day).
- Blood, mucus, or pus in the stool.
- Nausea or vomiting.
- Muscle aches or pain.
- White blood cell count lower than normal at the onset (sometimes).

CAUSES

Bacteria called shigella bacillus, a germ that invades the lining of the colon. It spreads from person to person, usually from contaminated hands to mouth.

RISK FACTORS

- Travel to foreign countries.
- Crowded or unsanitary living conditions.

PREVENTING COMPLICATIONS OR RECURRENCE

- Urge your child to wash hands after bowel movements and before handling food.
- Isolate your child with symptoms of bacillary dysentery.
- Immerse your child's soiled clothes and bedclothes in covered buckets of soap and water until they can be boiled.

WHAT TO EXPECT

MEDICAL TESTS

Your own observation of symptoms; medical history and physical exam by a doctor; laboratory stool culture; blood counts.

POSSIBLE COMPLICATIONS

- Dangerous dehydration, especially in children.
- In rare cases, the bacteria may enter the child's bloodstream from the digestive tract and infect other body organs, such as the kidneys, gallbladder, liver, or heart, and the joints. This may cause shock and death.

DYSENTERY, BACILLARY (Shigellosis)

PROBABLE OUTCOME

Usually curable in 7 days with treatment. Most shigella infections are mild and don't require drastic treatment. However, in a severe attack, excessive dehydration can be fatal (especially in infants and young children) if treatment is unsuccessful.

TREATMENT

HOME CARE

Isolate your child from other people; use a heating pad or hot-water bottle on the child's abdomen to relieve pain.

MEDICATION

- Your doctor may prescribe antibiotics, such as ampicillin or trimethoprim with sulfamethoxazole.
- Don't give your child paregoric preparations or other anti-diarrhea drugs unless your doctor prescribes them. These may prolong the illness. If they must be used, discontinue them as soon as possible.

ACTIVITY

Your child must rest in bed, except for trips to the bathroom, until fever, diarrhea, and other symptoms have been gone for at least 3 days. The child's legs should be exercised regularly in bed.

DIET & FLUIDS

Your child should be on a liquid or soft diet until the diarrhea stops, then return to a normal diet. For infants and children, see diet instructions in Gastroenteritis in Infants & Children (in Illnesses section).

OK FOR SCHOOL, PRESCHOOL, OR NURSERY?

When signs of infection have decreased, appetite returns, and alertness, strength, and feeling of well-being will allow.

CALL YOUR DOCTOR IF

- Your child has symptoms of bacillary dysentery.
- The following occurs during treatment: fever of 102F (38.9C) or more; sore throat, headache, or earache; shortness of breath or severe cough; traces of blood in the child's sputum; severe abdominal pain or abdominal swelling; rectal bleeding; pain in the child's calf or leg; swollen joints; signs of dehydration (lethargy, sunken eyes, rapid weight loss or dry skin) appear in your child.

DYSHIDROSIS

GENERAL INFORMATION

DESCRIPTION

Dyshidrosis is a skin condition that is characterized by small blisters on the hands or feet—apparently related to stress. The tips and sides of the fingers, toes, palms, and soles are involved.

Appropriate health care includes:

- Self-care after diagnosis.
- Physician's monitoring of general condition and medications.
- Psychotherapy or counseling to help your child learn to cope with stress more effectively.

SIGNS & SYMPTOMS

Small blisters with the following characteristics:

- Blisters are very small (1mm or less in diameter). They appear on the tips and sides of the child's fingers, toes, palms, and soles.
- Blisters are opaque and deep-seated; they are either flush with the child's skin or slightly elevated. They don't break easily. Eventually, small blisters come together and form large blisters.
- Blisters may itch, cause pain, or produce no symptoms in your child. They worsen after contact with soap, water, or irritating substances.

CAUSES

- Unknown, but they are probably related to periods of anxiety, stress, and frustration in children who internalize their emotions. Children with dyshidrosis have difficulty relaxing—even during non-stressful periods.
- This problem is not caused by sweat retention, as was once believed.

RISK FACTORS

- Stress and internalized frustration or irritation.
- Obsessive-compulsive personality.

PREVENTING COMPLICATIONS OR RECURRENCE

Follow instructions under HOME CARE. These are helpful in preventing recurrences, as well as in treating active episodes.

WHAT TO EXPECT

MEDICAL TESTS

- Your own observation of symptoms.
- Medical history and physical exam by a doctor.

POSSIBLE COMPLICATIONS

Secondary bacterial infection (sometimes).

PROBABLE OUTCOME

Your child's symptoms can be controlled with treatment, but recurrence is common. Children with mild dyshidrosis have occasional attacks, and the skin returns to normal between episodes. Children with severe dyshidrosis have more severe symptoms—sometimes with persistent peeling and fissuring of the involved skin.

TREATMENT

HOME CARE

Instructions for your child to keep heat and moisture away from the affected areas:

- Wear cotton socks and leather-soled shoes. Don't wear tennis shoes or other footwear made of man-made materials.
- Remove shoes and socks frequently to allow sweat to evaporate.
- Wear heavy-duty vinyl gloves to prevent contact with irritating substances, such as water, soap, detergent, metal scrubbing pads, scouring powder, and other chemicals.
- Dry insides of gloves after use. Discard a glove if it develops a hole.
- Wear gloves when you peel or squeeze acid fruits and vegetables.
- Wear leather or heavy-duty fabric gloves for household chores or gardening.
- Use a dishwashing machine to wash dishes if possible. If not, ask someone else to wash them.
- Avoid contact with irritating chemicals, such as paint and paint thinner and polish for cars, floors, shoes, furniture, and metal.
- Remove rings before doing housework or washing hands.
- Use lukewarm water and very little mild soap to shower or bathe.

MEDICATION

- Use non-prescription topical steroid preparations to reduce inflammation and decrease the child's itching. Apply once or twice a day to the child after bathing, unless directed otherwise. If these are not effective, your doctor may prescribe stronger steroid preparations.
- See Medications section for information regarding medicines your doctor may prescribe.

ACTIVITY

No restrictions.

DIET & FLUIDS

No special diet.

OK FOR SCHOOL, PRESCHOOL, OR NURSERY?

Yes. This condition is not contagious to others.

CALL YOUR DOCTOR IF

- Your child has symptoms of dyshidrosis.
- Signs of infection (swelling, redness, tenderness, or warmth) appear around blisters.
- Symptoms don't improve after a week, despite treatment.
- Improvement begins, and then symptoms recur.

DYSMENORRHEA
(Menstrual Cramps)

GENERAL INFORMATION

DESCRIPTION

Dysmenorrhea refers to severe, painful cramps during menstruation. Primary dysmenorrhea means pain has recurred regularly since periods began. Secondary dysmenorrhea means pain began years after periods started. Females with dysmenorrhea are generally fertile—cramps indicate that ovulation occurred 12 to 14 days earlier. Dysmenorrhea usually is less severe after a woman has a baby. The female reproductive system, especially the uterus is involved. Dysmenorrhea can affect females after puberty.

Appropriate health care includes:

- Self-care after diagnosis.
- Physician's monitoring of general condition and medications.
- Psychotherapy or counseling, if your daughter's dysmenorrhea is stress-related.

SIGNS & SYMPTOMS

- Cramping and sometimes sharp pains in the lower abdomen, lower back, and thighs.
- Nausea and vomiting (sometimes).
- Diarrhea (occasionally).
- Sweating.
- Lack of energy.

Severity of symptoms varies greatly from one female to another, and from one time to the next in the same person.

CAUSES

- Strong or prolonged contractions of the muscular wall of the uterus. These may be caused by concentration of prostaglandins (hormones manufactured by the body). Research shows that females with dysmenorrhea produce and excrete more prostaglandins than those who don't have as much discomfort.
- Dilation of the cervix to allow passage of blood clots from the uterus to the vagina.
- Organic causes include:
  - — Pelvic infections.
  - — Endometriosis, especially if dysmenorrhea begins after age 20.
  - — Benign tumors of the uterus.
  - — Poor posture.
  - — An underdeveloped uterus.

RISK FACTORS

- Use of caffeine.
- Stress. The degree of dysmenorrhea may vary according to your daughter's general health or mental state. While emotional or psychological factors don't *cause* the pain, they can worsen pain or cause some females to be less responsive to treatment.

PREVENTING COMPLICATIONS OR RECURRENCE

Your daughter can take female hormones that prevent ovulation, such as oral contraceptives.

DYSMENORRHEA
(Menstrual Cramps)

? WHAT TO EXPECT

MEDICAL TESTS

- Your own observation of symptoms.
- Medical history and physical exam—including a pelvic examination—by a doctor.

POSSIBLE COMPLICATIONS

Severe pain that regularly interferes with your daughter's normal activities.

PROBABLE OUTCOME

Your daughter's symptoms can be controlled with treatment.

TREATMENT

HOME CARE

- Heat helps relieve pain. Your daughter should use a heating pad or hot-water bottle on her abdomen or back, or she should take hot baths. She can sit in a tub of hot water for 10 to 15 minutes as often as necessary.
- See Appendix 19 for suggestions to help your daughter reduce stress.

MEDICATION

- For minor discomfort, use non-prescription drugs such as acetaminophen.
- Your doctor may prescribe:
  - — Anti-prostaglandins, including non-steroidal, anti-inflammatory drugs.
  - — Oral contraceptives, which prohibit ovulation.
- See Medications section for information regarding medicines your doctor may prescribe.

ACTIVITY

No restrictions. When resting in bed, your daughter should elevate her feet or bend her knees and lie on her side if it makes her feel more comfortable.

DIET & FLUIDS

No special diet. Your doctor may prescribe vitamin B supplements for your daughter. These help relieve symptoms sometimes.

OK FOR SCHOOL, PRESCHOOL, OR NURSERY?

Yes.

CALL YOUR DOCTOR IF

- Your daughter has symptoms of dysmenorrhea that she cannot control by herself.
- Your daughter's menstrual bleeding becomes excessive (she saturates a pad or tampon more frequently than once each hour).
- Your daughter develops signs of infection, such as fever, a general ill feeling, headache, dizziness, or muscle aches.
- New, unexplained symptoms develop. Drugs used in treatment may produce side effects.

EAR INFECTION, MIDDLE-
(Otitis Media)

GENERAL INFORMATION

DESCRIPTION

Middle-ear infection means inflammation or infection in the middle ear. This is not contagious from person to person, but the preceding respiratory infection causing it may be infectious. The middle-ear space where nerves and small bones connect to the eardrum on one side and the eustachian tube on the other side is involved. Middle-ear infections can affect all ages but is most common in infants and children.

Appropriate health care includes:

• Physician's monitoring of general condition and medications.
• Home care after diagnosis.
• Surgery to insert plastic tubes through the child's eardrum to drain pus or fluid from the middle ear (rare).

SIGNS & SYMPTOMS

• Irritability.
• Earache.
• Feeling of fullness in the child's ear.
• Hearing loss.
• Fever.
• Discharge or leakage from the ear.
• Diarrhea (sometimes).
• Pulling at the ear (small children).

CAUSES

• Bacterial or viral infections which spread to the middle ear by way of the eustachian tube. These are usually upper-respiratory virus infections in the child's nose or throat.
• Sinus and eustachian-tube blockage caused by nasal allergies or enlarged adenoids in your child.
• A ruptured eardrum.

RISK FACTORS

• Recent illness, such as a respiratory infection, that has lowered your child's resistance.
• Crowded or unsanitary living conditions.
• Genetic factors. Some American Indians—especially the Navajo—seem more susceptible.
• High altitude.
• Cold climate.
• Taking a bottle to bed. Fluid pools in the child's throat near the eustachian tube.

PREVENTING COMPLICATIONS OR RECURRENCE

• If your child has an ear infection followed by a hearing loss or enlarged adenoids, ask your doctor about using a steroid nasal spray, preventive antibiotics, or decongestants during future respiratory infections. This may prevent fluid accumulation.
• Bottle-feed your infant in a sitting position—never lying down.

EAR INFECTION, MIDDLE-
(Otitis Media)

? WHAT TO EXPECT

MEDICAL TESTS

- Your own observation of symptoms.
- Medical history and physical exam by a doctor.

POSSIBLE COMPLICATIONS

- Eardrum rupture.
- Hearing impairment—usually temporary, but sometimes permanent—leading to delay of normal language development in children.
- Enlarged adenoids in children from chronic middle-ear infections.
- Mastoiditis.
- Meningitis.

PROBABLE OUTCOME

Usually curable with treatment.

TREATMENT

HOME CARE

Apply heat to the area around the child's ears to relieve pain.

MEDICATION

- Use ear drops to relieve the child's pain. You may use non-prescription drops or those prescribed for a previous infection. They will not cure the infection.
- Use non-prescription nasal sprays or drops to help open the eustachian tube and relieve pressure in the child's middle ear.
- Use non-prescription drugs, such as acetaminophen, to reduce the child's pain and fever.
- Your doctor may prescribe antibiotics if the infection appears to be bacterial rather than viral. Have your child finish the medication. The infection may remain active for several days after symptoms disappear.
- See Medications section for information regarding medicines your doctor may prescribe.

ACTIVITY

Your child should rest in bed or reduce activity until fever and pain subside.

DIET & FLUIDS

No special diet.

OK FOR SCHOOL, PRESCHOOL, OR NURSERY?

When signs of infection have decreased, appetite returns, and alertness, strength, and feeling of well-being will allow.

CALL YOUR DOCTOR IF

- Your child has symptoms of a middle-ear infection.
- The following occurs during treatment: fever above 102F (38.9C), despite treatment; severe headache; earache that persists longer than 2 days, despite treatment; swelling around the child's ear; convulsions; twitching of the child's face muscles; dizziness.

EAR INFECTION, OUTER-
(Otitis Externa; Swimmer's Ear)

GENERAL INFORMATION

DESCRIPTION

Outer-ear infection is inflammation or infection of the ear canal that extends from the eardrum to the outside. The skin of the ear canal is involved.

Appropriate health care includes:
- Self-care after diagnosis.
- Physician's monitoring of general condition and medications. Severe cases may require treatment by an ear, nose and throat specialist.

SIGNS & SYMPTOMS

- Ear pain that worsens when the child's earlobe is pulled.
- Slight fever (sometimes).
- Discharge of pus from the child's ear.
- Temporary loss of hearing on the affected side.

CAUSES

Bacterial or fungal infection of the delicate skin lining of the child's ear canal. Infection may develop because of:
- Swimming in dirty, polluted water.
- Excessive swimming in chlorinated pools. Chlorinated water dries out the ear canal, allowing bacteria or fungi to enter the skin.
- Excess moisture from any cause.
- Irritation from swabs, metal objects (such as bobby pins), or ear plugs, especially if they are left in a long time.
- Inadequate production of protective ear wax (cerumen).

RISK FACTORS

- Previous ear infections.
- Skin allergies.
- Diabetes mellitus or other disorders that predispose your child to infection.

PREVENTING COMPLICATIONS OR RECURRENCE

- Don't clean your child's ears with any object or chemical.
- Don't use ear plugs, alcohol in the ears, lamb's wool, or anything else to keep the child's ears dry. These are not only useless—they may be harmful.

? WHAT TO EXPECT

MEDICAL TESTS

- Your own observation of symptoms.
- Medical history and physical exam by a doctor.

POSSIBLE COMPLICATIONS

- Severe pain.
- Chronic inflammation that is difficult to cure.
- A boil in the child's ear canal.
- Cellulitis (deep-tissue infection).

EAR INFECTION, OUTER- (Otitis Externa; Swimmer's Ear)

PROBABLE OUTCOME

Usually curable with treatment in 7 to 10 days.

TREATMENT

HOME CARE

- Your doctor will probably cleanse the child's ear canal and insert a cotton wick. The wick allows the medication to reach all infected parts.
- Moisten the wick with medication every hour for the first 24 hours. Continue to use drops according to your doctor's instructions after the wick is removed from your child's ear.
- Clean the tip of the dropper with alcohol after each use. Don't let anyone other than your child use the medicine.
- After your child has had otitis externa, keep the prescription ear drops on hand. If the child's ear canals get wet for any reason, such as swimming or shampooing, put drops in both ears at bedtime.

MEDICATION

- Use non-prescription drugs, such as acetaminophen or aspirin, for minor pain.
- Your doctor may prescribe:
  — Ear drops that contain antibiotics and cortisone drugs to control inflammation and fight infection.
  — Oral antibiotics for severe infection.
  — Codeine or narcotics for a short time to relieve severe pain.
- See Medications section for information regarding medicines your doctor may prescribe.

ACTIVITY

Your child can resume normal activities as soon as symptoms improve. The child should avoid getting water in the ears for 3 weeks after all symptoms disappear. Any moisture—even from showering or washing hair—can trigger a recurrence.

DIET & FLUIDS

No special diet.

OK FOR SCHOOL, PRESCHOOL, OR NURSERY?

Yes, if comfort permits. This problem is not contagious to other children.

CALL YOUR DOCTOR IF

- Your child has symptoms of otitis externa.
- The following occurs during treatment:
  — Pain persists, despite treatment.
  — You feel your child's ears need cleaning. Remember that a small amount of ear wax helps protect against infection.

ILLNESSES

EAR INJURY

GENERAL INFORMATION

DESCRIPTION

Ears are easily injured because they are so exposed. The injuries may be serious and painful and may lead to disfigurement unless you follow a careful treatment plan for your child. The skin and cartilage of the external ear, the perichondrium (the thin membrane layer between the cartilage and the skin), the nerves, blood vessels, connective tissue, and parts of the internal ear (the ear drum, middle ear, and inner ear) are involved. Appropriate health care includes: self-care after diagnosis; physician's monitoring of general condition and medications.

SIGNS & SYMPTOMS

- Contusion or laceration: Pain, swelling, bleeding, and bruising of skin around the child's ear.
- Internal injury: loss of hearing, ringing in the ear, loss of equilibrium, or bleeding from a ruptured eardrum.

CAUSES

- Direct blow to the child's ear.
- Accidental insertion of a sharp object into the ear.
- Sudden, excessive changes in pressure.

RISK FACTORS

Contact sports, especially wrestling or boxing; diving.

PREVENTING COMPLICATIONS OR RECURRENCE

Your child should wear protective headgear for contact sports. Some injuries cannot be prevented.

WHAT TO EXPECT

MEDICAL TESTS

Your own observation of symptoms; medical history and physical exam by a doctor, including consultation with an ear specialist or plastic surgeon if necessary; X-rays of the skull to detect an accompanying skull fracture.

POSSIBLE COMPLICATIONS

- Chronic infection of the injured ear if the skin is broken from laceration or contusion.
- "Cauliflower ear," resulting from repeated contusions with bleeding through soft tissues. The tissues under the skin and the lining of the child's ear cartilage thicken permanently. (There is no treatment for this condition—only prevention.)
- Infection from contusion, laceration, or other injury to the child's eardrum or other internal ear structures.
- Temporary or permanent hearing loss.

PROBABLE OUTCOME

Your child's contusions and lacerations may require 10 to 14 days to heal. Sutures from lacerations are usually removed in about 10 days.

TREATMENT

FIRST AID

- Don't try to stop bleeding from inside the child's ear.
- Don't allow the injured child to hit or thump the head to try to restore hearing.
- Cover the child's external ear with a clean cloth or sterile bandage.
- Apply an ice pack of ice cubes or chips in a plastic bag or moist towel.
- Compress the area loosely with an elastic wrap. Don't wrap too tightly.
- Keep the injured child in a partial reclining position while transporting to an emergency facility.

CONTINUING CARE

- For contusions: The doctor will aspirate blood between the child's skin and ear cartilage if needed. If swelling persists, multiple small incisions may prevent a cauliflower ear from developing. The child should sleep with the head elevated with 2 pillows until symptoms subside. Change bulky bandages on your child's ear often to keep them soft and protective.
- For lacerations: Your doctor must carefully repair the child's cut to prevent deformity. Keep the wound dry and covered for 48 hours. After 48 hours, replace the bandage when it gets wet. When you change the child's bandage, apply a small amount of petroleum jelly or non-prescription antibiotic ointment to the bandage. Ignore small amounts of bleeding but control heavier bleeding by firmly pressing a facial tissue or clean cloth to the bleeding spot for 10 minutes.

MEDICATION

Your doctor may prescribe:

- Antibiotics to treat infection.
- Pain relievers.

ACTIVITY

Your child can resume normal activities as soon as possible.

DIET & FLUIDS

No restrictions.

OK FOR SCHOOL, PRESCHOOL, OR NURSERY?

When strength and feeling of well-being will allow.

CALL YOUR DOCTOR IF

- Your child has an ear injury.
- Any of the following occur after treatment: increased pain or pain that persists longer than 2 days; hearing loss; increased bleeding or swelling; signs of infection (headache, muscle aches, dizziness, fever, general ill feeling).
- New, unexplained symptoms develop. Drugs used in treatment may produce side effects.

EARDRUM, RUPTURED (Tympanic-Membrane Perforation)

GENERAL INFORMATION

DESCRIPTION

A ruptured eardrum refers to a perforation of the thin membrane (tympanic membrane) that separates the inner ear from the outer ear. The eardrum (tympanic membrane) and the middle ear are involved.

Appropriate health care includes:
- Self-care.
- Physician's monitoring of general condition and medications.
- Microsurgery to repair the perforation (rare).

SIGNS & SYMPTOMS
- Sudden pain in the child's ear.
- Partial hearing loss.
- Bleeding or discharge from the child's ear. The discharge may resemble pus within 24 to 48 hours after the rupture.
- Ringing in the child's ear.
- Dizziness.

CAUSES
- Perforation of the eardrum when a sharp object is inserted in the ear, such as a cotton swab to clean the ear or relieve an itch or an unseen twig on a tree.
- Sudden inward pressure in the child's ear, such as with a slap, a swimming or diving accident, or a nearby explosion.
- Sudden outward pressure or suction, such as with a kiss over the ear.
- Severe middle-ear infection.

RISK FACTORS
- Recent middle-ear infection.
- Head injury.

PREVENTING COMPLICATIONS OR RECURRENCE
- Don't put any object into the child's ear canal.
- Your child should try to avoid injuries that may cause a rupture (see CAUSES).
- Obtain prompt medical treatment for your child's middle-ear infections.

? WHAT TO EXPECT

MEDICAL TESTS
- Your own observation of symptoms.
- Medical history and physical exam by a doctor. When the child's eardrum ruptures, contents of the middle ear (primarily bones) can be seen with a special instrument called an otoscope. A healthy eardrum is almost transparent.

EARDRUM, RUPTURED (Tympanic-Membrane Perforation)

POSSIBLE COMPLICATIONS

- Ear infection with fever, vomiting, and diarrhea.
- Significant blood loss (rare).
- Meningitis.
- Mastoiditis (see Glossary).
- Permanent hearing loss (rare).

PROBABLE OUTCOME

If your child's ruptured eardrum does not become infected, it will usually repair itself in 2 months. If it does become infected, the infection is curable with treatment, and your child's hearing is usually not affected permanently.

TREATMENT

HOME CARE

Instructions for your child:

- Don't blow your nose, if possible. If you must, blow gently.
- Keep the ear canal dry. Don't swim, take showers, or get caught in the rain. Insert a wisp of cotton in the ear canal to keep moisture out of it when bathing.

MEDICATION

Your doctor may prescribe:

- Antibiotics to prevent or treat infections.
- Sedatives or tranquilizers to reduce your child's apprehension.
- Pain relievers. For minor pain, use non-prescription drugs such as acetaminophen.
- See Medications section for information regarding medicines your doctor may prescribe.

ACTIVITY

Your child can resume normal activities as soon as symptoms improve.

DIET & FLUIDS

No special diet.

OK FOR SCHOOL, PRESCHOOL, OR NURSERY?

Yes. This condition is not contagious to others.

CALL YOUR DOCTOR IF

- Your child has symptoms of a ruptured eardrum, especially a pus-like discharge.
- The following occurs during treatment:
  - — Fever.
  - — Pain that persists, despite treatment.
  - — Dizziness that continues longer than 12 to 24 hours.
- New, unexplained symptoms develop. Drugs used in treatment may produce side effects.

ILLNESSES

EARWAX BLOCKAGE
(Cerumen Impaction)

GENERAL INFORMATION

DESCRIPTION

Earwax blockage refers to an overproduction of earwax, causing blockage of the external ear canal. Wax is produced by the ear to protect the canal leading from the eardrum to the outside. The external ear canal on one or both sides is involved.

Appropriate health care includes:

- Self-care. Sometimes your child's earwax can be removed easily at home with ear drops and irrigation of the ear canal.
- Doctor's treatment if the wax is difficult to remove.

SIGNS & SYMPTOMS

- Decreased hearing.
- Ear pain.
- Plugged feeling in the ear.
- Ringing in the ear.

CAUSES

Overproduction of wax by glands in the child's external ear canal.

RISK FACTORS

- Exposure to dust or debris.
- Family history of overproduction of earwax.

PREVENTING COMPLICATIONS OR RECURRENCE

Your child should avoid areas where the air is dusty or filled with debris. This stimulates overproduction of earwax.

WHAT TO EXPECT

MEDICAL TESTS

- Your own observation of symptoms.
- Medical history and physical exam by a doctor.

POSSIBLE COMPLICATIONS

- Ear infection.
- Eardrum damage.

PROBABLE OUTCOME

Earwax can be removed, but stubborn cases require patience.

EARWAX BLOCKAGE (Cerumen Impaction)

TREATMENT

HOME CARE

To remove earwax from your child's ear at home:

- Buy non-prescription wax-softening ear drops.
- Have the child lie down with the affected ear toward the ceiling.
- Pull the top of the child's ear gently up and back toward the back of the head.
- Instill the ear drops in the child's ear; use the amount given in the package directions.
- Leave the drops in the child's ear for 20 minutes. The child should continue to lie down, if possible. Plug the ear with cotton.
- Then the child can sit up, leaning a little toward the affected side.
- Use a soft rubber bulb syringe to irrigate the child's ear canal gently with plain warm water or equal parts warm water and hydrogen peroxide.
- Repeat irrigations until the child's ear feels clear. If the ear doesn't clear, consult your doctor.
- Don't try to remove wax with a stick or cotton swab. You may damage the child's eardrum or cause infection in the ear canal.

MEDICATION

- For minor pain, use non-prescription drugs such as acetaminophen.
- After treatment, your doctor may prescribe wax-softening ear drops to use when needed.
- See Medications section for information regarding medicines your doctor may prescribe.

ACTIVITY

No restrictions.

DIET & FLUIDS

No special diet.

OK FOR SCHOOL, PRESCHOOL, OR NURSERY?

Yes. This condition is not contagious to others.

CALL YOUR DOCTOR IF

- Your child has symptoms of an earwax blockage that does not clear, despite treatment describe above.
- A child younger than 4 has an earwax blockage.
- Fever and ear pain accompany an earwax blockage. Do *not* irrigate the ear in this case.

ECTOPIC PREGNANCY

GENERAL INFORMATION

DESCRIPTION

An ectopic pregnancy is a pregnancy that develops outside the uterus. The most common site is in one of the narrow tubes (the Fallopian tubes) that connect the ovaries to the uterus. Other sites include the ovary itself or the area outside the reproductive organs in the abdominal cavity. The female reproductive system and abdominal cavity are involved. Ectopic pregnancies can affect women of childbearing age. Appropriate health care includes: physician's monitoring of general condition and medications; surgery (exploratory laparotomy) to remove the growing fertilized ovum and control internal bleeding; colposcopy; ultrasound examination; laparoscopy.

SIGNS & SYMPTOMS

Early stages:

- Missed menstrual period or a heavy, painful period.
- Unexplained vaginal spotting or bleeding.
- Lower abdominal pain and cramps.
- Pain in the shoulder.

Late stages:

- Sudden, sharp, severe abdominal pain caused by the rupture of a Fallopian tube.
- Dizziness, fainting, and shock (paleness, rapid heartbeat, drop in blood pressure, and cold sweats). These may precede or accompany pain (sometimes).

CAUSES

An egg from the ovary is fertilized and becomes implanted outside the uterus—usually in the Fallopian tube. As the fertilized egg enlarges, the Fallopian tube stretches and ruptures, causing life-threatening internal bleeding.

RISK FACTORS

- Use of an intrauterine device (IUD) for contraception.
- Previous pelvic infections.
- Adhesions (bands of scar tissue) from previous abdominal surgery.

PREVENTING COMPLICATIONS OR RECURRENCE

Instructions for your sexually active daughter:

- Use a contraceptive method other than an IUD.
- Obtain prompt treatment for any pelvic infection.

? WHAT TO EXPECT

MEDICAL TESTS

- Your own observation of symptoms.
- Medical history and physical exam by a doctor.
- Laboratory studies, such as a pregnancy test and blood count.
- Surgical diagnostic procedures, such as laparoscopy and culdocentesis (see Glossary for both).
- Ultrasound to outline the fetus (see Glossary).

POSSIBLE COMPLICATIONS

Shock and death from internal bleeding.

PROBABLE OUTCOME

An ectopic pregnancy cannot progress to full term or produce a viable fetus. Rupture of an ectopic pregnancy is an emergency requiring *immediate* hospitalization and surgery. Full recovery is likely with early diagnosis and surgery. Subsequent pregnancies are usually normal.

TREATMENT

HOME CARE

Instructions for your daughter after surgery:

- You may wash normally over the stitches in your incision.
- Use heat to relieve pain. Apply a heating pad or hot-water bottle to your abdomen or back.
- Hot baths also relieve discomfort and relax muscles. Sit in a tub of hot water (106F to 110F or 41.1C to 43.3C) for 10 to 15 minutes. Repeat as often as needed.

MEDICATION

- Medicine usually is not necessary for this disorder.
- See Medications section for information regarding medicines your doctor may prescribe.

ACTIVITY

Your daughter can resume normal activities, including sexual relations, as soon as possible.

DIET & FLUIDS

No special diet.

OK FOR SCHOOL, PRESCHOOL, OR NURSERY?

After recovery from surgery.

CALL YOUR DOCTOR IF

- Your daughter has symptoms of an ectopic pregnancy, especially a rupture. Call immediately. This is an emergency!
- The following occurs after surgery:
  — Excessive vaginal bleeding (soaking a pad or tampon every hour).
  — Signs of infection, such as fever, chills, headache, dizziness, or muscle aches.
  — Increased urinary frequency that lasts longer than a month. This may be a sign of bladder irritation or infection resulting from the surgery.

ECZEMA (Atopic Dermatitis; Infantile Eczema; Neurodermatitis)

GENERAL INFORMATION

DESCRIPTION

Eczema is a chronic allergic skin disorder of childhood. The skin—especially of the scalp, face, and back of the neck—and skin creases of the elbows and knees are involved. Eczema may begin between 1 month and 1 year. It usually subsides somewhat by age 3, but it may flare again at ages 10 to 12 and last through puberty.

Appropriate health care includes:

- Home care.
- Physician's monitoring of general condition and medications.
- Hospitalization (rare).

SIGNS & SYMPTOMS

Skin affected by eczema has the following characteristics:

- Itching (sometimes severe).
- Small blisters with oozing.
- Thickening and scaling from chronic inflammation.

CAUSES

An allergic reaction to a wide variety of things, including:

- Foods, such as eggs, wheat, milk, or seafood.
- Wool clothing.
- Skin lotions and ointments.

RISK FACTORS

- Stress.
- Medical history of other allergic conditions in your child, such as hay fever, asthma, or sensitivity to certain drugs.
- Clothing made of synthetic fabric, which traps perspiration.
- Weather extremes, including humidity, severe cold, and severe heat (especially with increased sweating).

PREVENTING COMPLICATIONS OR RECURRENCE

No specific preventive measures.

WHAT TO EXPECT

MEDICAL TESTS

- Your own observation of symptoms.
- Medical history and physical exam by a doctor.
- Laboratory studies, such as blood and skin tests to identify your child's allergies.

POSSIBLE COMPLICATIONS

- Bacterial infections caused by injury to the child's skin.
- Life-threatening infection from a smallpox vaccination—not usually given to children anymore since since smallpox has virtually been eradicated.
- Cataracts (for unknown reason).

ECZEMA (Atopic Dermatitis; Infantile Eczema; Neurodermatitis)

PROBABLE OUTCOME

• Variable. Some children outgrow eczema. Others are resistant to treatment, and eczema may persist through puberty. However, symptoms can usually be controlled with treatment.
• Skin irritation from any other cause can trigger a flare-up or aggravate existing eczema.

TREATMENT

HOME CARE

• Provide loose cotton clothing to help absorb your child's perspiration.
• Minimize stress in the child's life whenever possible.
• Don't allow the child to have a smallpox vaccination or to be exposed to someone who has recently had one.
• Keep the child's fingernails short and put soft gloves on at night to minimize scratching. Scratching worsens eczema.
• Bathe the child less frequently to avoid excessive skin dryness. Soap and water may trigger flare-ups. When bathing, use special non-fat soaps and tepid water. Use *no* soap on inflamed areas.
• Lubricate the child's skin after bathing.
• Protect the child from extreme temperature changes.
• Avoid anything that has previously worsened the condition.

MEDICATION

Your doctor may prescribe:
• Ointments containing coal tar or cortisone drugs to decrease inflammation. These may help your child more if used at night under a lightly applied plastic wrap. Ask your doctor.
• Antihistamines to decrease itching.
• Antibiotics for complicating infections, If they occur.
• Sedatives or tranquilizers to calm the child.
• See Medications section for information regarding medicines your doctor may prescribe.

ACTIVITY

No restrictions.

DIET & FLUIDS

No special diet. Eliminate any foods known to cause flare-ups of your child's eczema.

OK FOR SCHOOL, PRESCHOOL, OR NURSERY?

Yes. This condition is not contagious to others.

CALL YOUR DOCTOR IF

• Your child has symptoms of eczema.
• New, unexplained symptoms develop. Drugs used in treatment may produce side effects. Excessive use of cortisone drugs is dangerous, and antihistamines frequently cause drowsiness.

ELBOW CONTUSION, ULNAR NERVE
("Crazybone" or "Crazy Nerve" Contusion)

GENERAL INFORMATION

DESCRIPTION

An ulnar nerve elbow contusion is a bruising injury from a direct blow to the ulnar nerve where it lies close to the surface at the elbow. Contusions cause bleeding from ruptured small capillaries that allow blood to infiltrate the nerve. Direct injury to the nerve causes damage even if bleeding of capillaries is not a factor. The ulnar nerve and the ulnar groove in the elbow portion of the humerus (bone of the upper arm) are involved.

Appropriate health care includes:

- Doctor's care unless the contusion is quite small.
- Surgery to treat the contused nerve (usually involves transferring and transplanting the nerve into muscle, where it is sutured in place).
- Self-care for minor contusions or during rehabilitation following surgery for serious ulnar nerve contusions.
- Physical therapy following surgery.

SIGNS & SYMPTOMS

- Swelling in the child's elbow—either superficial or deep.
- Immediate pain in the elbow.
- Shocking, electric sensations extending down to the ring fingers and little fingers.
- Gradually increasing numbness and pain along the route of the ulnar nerve in the forearm and hand.
- Atrophy of muscles in the hand.

CAUSES

- Direct blow to the elbow area from a blunt object.
- Falling on the elbow.

RISK FACTORS

Contact sports such as football, soccer, or hockey, especially when the child's elbows are not adequately protected; medical history of any bleeding disorder such as hemophilia; poor nutrition, including vitamin deficiency.

PREVENTING COMPLICATIONS OR RECURRENCE

Your child should wear appropriate protective gear, such as elbow pads, while participating in sports if there is risk of elbow injury.

WHAT TO EXPECT

MEDICAL TESTS

Your own observation of symptoms; medical history and physical exam by a doctor for all except minor injuries; X-rays of the child's elbow to assess total injury to soft tissue and to rule out the possibility of underlying fractures. The total extent of injury may not be apparent for 48 to 72 hours.

ELBOW CONTUSION, ULNAR NERVE
("Crazybone" or "Crazy Nerve" Contusion)

POSSIBLE COMPLICATIONS

Permanent damage to the ulnar nerve, leading to disability in the forearm and hand; prolonged healing time if the child's usual activities are resumed too soon; infection if the skin over the contusion is broken.

PROBABLE OUTCOME

Healing time varies from 2 to 6 weeks, depending on the extent of the child's injury and whether surgery is required or not. In a few cases, some symptoms may be permanent.

TREATMENT

FIRST AID

Use instructions for R.I.C.E., the first letters of *rest*, *ice*, *compression*, and *elevation*. See Appendix 39 for details.

HOME CARE

- Wrap an elasticized bandage over a felt pad on the child's injured area. Keep the area compressed for about 72 hours.
- Immobilize the child's arm in a sling.
- Use ice soaks 3 or 4 times a day. Fill a bucket with ice water and soak the injured area for 20 minutes at a time.
- Massage gently and often from the child's fingers upward to the shoulder to provide comfort and decrease swelling.

MEDICATION

- For minor discomfort, use acetaminophen or ibuprofen; topical liniments and ointments.
- Your doctor may prescribe stronger medicine for pain.

ACTIVITY

Your child should begin activities slowly and stop exercise as soon as pain begins. The child can increase activity as healing progresses.

DIET & FLUIDS

No restrictions.

OK FOR SCHOOL, PRESCHOOL, OR NURSERY?

Yes, when condition and sense of well-being will allow.

CALL YOUR DOCTOR IF

- Your child has symptoms of an elbow or ulnar nerve contusion.
- Any of the following occur after surgery: increasing pain, swelling, redness, drainage, or bleeding in the surgical area; signs of infection (headache, muscle aches, dizziness, fever, or a general ill feeling); nausea or vomiting; constipation.
- New, unexplained symptoms develop. Drugs used in treatment may produce side effects.

ELBOW TENDINITIS OR EPICONDYLITIS (Tennis Elbow)

GENERAL INFORMATION

DESCRIPTION

Elbow tendinitis is an inflammation of muscles, tendons, bursa, or covering of the bones (periosteum) at the elbow. The elbow muscles, tendons, and one or both of the epicondyles (bony prominences on the sides of the elbow where the muscles of the forearm attach to the bone of the upper arm) are involved.

Appropriate health care includes:

- Self-care after diagnosis.
- Doctor's treatment.
- Physical therapy.
- Surgery (rare).

SIGNS & SYMPTOMS

- Pain and tenderness over the epicondyles. Pain worsens with gripping or rotation of the child's forearm.
- Weak grip.
- Pain when twisting the hand and arm, as when playing tennis, throwing a ball with a twist, bowling, golfing, pushing off while skiing, or using a screwdriver.

CAUSES

Partial tear of the tendon and the attached covering of the bone caused by:

- Chronic stress on tissues that attach forearm muscles to the elbow area.
- Sudden stress on the child's forearm.
- Wrist snap when serving balls in racket sports.
- Incorrect grip.
- Incorrect hitting position.
- Using a racket or club that is too heavy for the child.
- Using an oversize grip.

RISK FACTORS

- Participation in sports that require strenuous forearm movement, such as tennis and racquetball.
- Poor conditioning of forearm muscles prior to vigorous exercise.
- Inadequate warmup before competing.
- Returning to activity before healing is complete.

PREVENTING COMPLICATIONS OR RECURRENCE

Instructions for your child:

- Don't play sports, such as tennis, for long periods until your forearm muscles are strong and limber. Take frequent rest periods.
- Do forearm conditioning exercises to build your strength gradually.
- Warm up slowly and completely before participating in sports—especially before competition.
- Get lessons from a professional if you are a novice.
- Use a tennis-elbow strap when you resume normal activity after treatment.

ELBOW TENDINITIS OR EPICONDYLITIS (Tennis Elbow)

WHAT TO EXPECT

MEDICAL TESTS

Your own observation of symptoms; medical history and physical exam by a doctor; X-rays of the child's elbow.

POSSIBLE COMPLICATIONS

- Complete ligament tear, requiring surgery to repair.
- Slow healing.
- Frequent recurrences.

PROBABLE OUTCOME

Tennis elbow usually heals with heat treatments, corticosteroid injections and resting the child's elbow. Treatment may require 3 to 6 months.

TREATMENT

HOME CARE

- Use heat to relieve the child's pain. Use warm soaks, a heating pad, or a heat lamp. Your child may receive diathermy or ultrasound (see Glossary), whirlpool, or massage treatments in the doctor's office or a physical-therapy facility. These may bring quicker symptom relief and healing.
- Your child may need to wear a forearm splint to immobilize the elbow.

MEDICATION

Your doctor may prescribe:

- Non-steroidal anti-inflammatory drugs to reduce inflammation.
- Injections of anesthetics to temporarily relieve the child's pain.
- Injections of corticosteroids to reduce inflammation. *Caution*: Repeated injections may weaken the muscle tendon.

ACTIVITY

Your child should not repeat the activity that caused tennis elbow until symptoms disappear. Then normal activities can be resumed gradually after proper conditioning.

DIET & FLUIDS

No restrictions.

OK FOR SCHOOL, PRESCHOOL, OR NURSERY?

Yes, when condition and sense of well-being will allow.

CALL YOUR DOCTOR IF

- Your child has symptoms of tennis elbow.
- Symptoms don't improve in 2 weeks, despite treatment.

ELECTRIC SHOCK

GENERAL INFORMATION

DESCRIPTION

Electric shock is an injury caused by electricity passing through the body. An electric shock can affect the entire body.

Appropriate health care includes:

- Self-care after diagnosis (minor burns only).
- Emergency cardiopulmonary resuscitation (CPR) at the time of injury, if the victim is unconscious and not breathing. See HOME CARE.
- Physician's monitoring of general condition and medications.
- Hospitalization.

SIGNS & SYMPTOMS

Depends on where the current enters your child's body and the kind of electrical current. Following are the most common:

- Burns at areas of contact. The burns are often deep.
- Heart damage, including cardiac arrest.
- Severe muscle spasms that may cause fractures.
- Breathing paralysis.

CAUSES

Contact with electricity from downed power lines, exposed appliance wires, faulty electrical equipment, lightning strikes, or other electrical sources.

RISK FACTORS

- Standing on wet ground or under a tree during an electrical storm.
- Mishandling of electrical equipment.
- Activities that involve electrical machinery or lines.

PREVENTING COMPLICATIONS OR RECURRENCE

- Inspect your house, especially the kitchen, bathroom, and workshop, for hazards.
- Use safety plugs in empty electrical outlets to prevent children from inserting metal objects.
- Replace worn cords or wiring at home.
- Don't let your children use hair dryers or radios in the bathroom where they can fall into a tub or sink.
- Don't let your children repair electrical equipment unless they know how.
- Urge your children to wear protective gloves and clothing for activities that involve exposure to electricity.
- Get your family indoors during electrical storms.

WHAT TO EXPECT

MEDICAL TESTS

Diagnosis is usually obvious from the circumstances.

POSSIBLE COMPLICATIONS

- Pneumonia.
- Permanent brain damage.
- Severe burns of the child's skin and underlying muscle.
- Death from heart damage.

PROBABLE OUTCOME

Depends on the extent of your child's injury. Full recovery is likely if major brain or heart damage does not occur.

TREATMENT

HOME CARE

- If your child has received an electric shock by touching live electrical wires, shut off the power or remove the wires with a non-metal object before giving aid. Don't electrocute yourself trying to help your child.
- If your child is unconscious and not breathing:
  — Yell for help. Don't leave the victim.
  — Begin mouth-to-mouth breathing immediately.
  — If there is no heartbeat, give your child external cardiac massage.
  — Have someone call 0 (operator) or 911 (emergency) for an ambulance or medical help.
  — Don't stop cardiopulmonary resuscitation (CPR) until help arrives.

MEDICATION

- Medicine usually is not necessary for electric shock.
- See Medications section for information regarding medicines your doctor may prescribe.

ACTIVITY

No restrictions, if the shock is mild. If the shock is severe, the child may resume activities gradually as injuries heal.

DIET & FLUIDS

No special diet following electric shock.

OK FOR SCHOOL, PRESCHOOL, OR NURSERY?

When appetite has returned and alertness, strength, and feeling of well-being will allow.

CALL YOUR DOCTOR IF

- Your child receives an electric shock severe enough to cause injury.
- The following occurs during convalescence:
  — Irregular heartbeat.
  — Fever.
  — Cough with sputum.

EMPYEMA

GENERAL INFORMATION

DESCRIPTION

Empyema is an accumulation of pus between layers of the infected pleura (thin membranes that cover the lung). The lungs and pleura are involved.

Appropriate health care includes:

- Self-care after diagnosis.
- Physician's monitoring of general condition and medications.
- Hospitalization to remove fluid from chest.

SIGNS & SYMPTOMS

- Chest pain. Pain varies from vague discomfort to stabbing pain. It is often worse when your child coughs or breathes. Pain may extend to the lower chest wall or abdomen.
- Rapid, shallow breathing.
- Chills.
- Fever.
- Extreme fatigue.
- Bad breath.
- Weight loss.

CAUSES

A complication of:

- Lung or chest infections, such as pneumonia or tuberculosis.
- A collapsed lung or chest injury.
- Malignancy in other parts of the child's body.
- Collagen vascular disease, such as systemic lupus erythematosus.
- Infection in another part of the child's body that has spread to the chest.
- Congestive heart failure.
- Kidney disorders.
- Liver disorders.

RISK FACTORS

Poor nutrition; recent illness (see CAUSES); smoking; fatigue or overwork; wet, cold climates; crowded or unsanitary living conditions.

PREVENTING COMPLICATIONS OR RECURRENCE

Obtain medical treatment for your child for any serious disorder or infection that may cause empyema.

WHAT TO EXPECT

MEDICAL TESTS

- Your own observation of symptoms.
- Medical history and physical exam by a doctor.
- Laboratory culture of pus from the empyema cavity.
- X-ray of the child's chest.

POSSIBLE COMPLICATIONS

Meningitis; pericarditis; endocarditis; brain abscess.

PROBABLE OUTCOME

Successful treatment depends on discovery and treatment of the child's underlying disorder. Draining the pus from the infected space hastens healing. High doses of antibiotics are needed, and hospitalization is usually required.

TREATMENT

HOME CARE

- To reduce your child's chest pain, wrap the entire chest *loosely* with 2 or 3 non-adhesive 6-inch elastic bandages.
- Use a cool-mist humidifier to loosen bronchial secretions so your child can cough them up more easily.
- Urge your child to practice these breathing exercises:
  — Purse your lips and breathe forcefully against resistance (as if blowing out a candle) 10 times. Repeat every hour.
  — Take 10 deep breaths every hour.
- Urge your child not to smoke.

MEDICATION

- Your doctor may prescribe antibiotics to fight infection. The type of antibiotic will depend on the type of germ responsible for your child's illness and the results of sensitivity studies (see Glossary).
- For minor pain, use non-prescription drugs such as acetaminophen.

ACTIVITY

Your child should reduce activity until the pain and fever are gone. The child can gradually return to normal activity. Allow 2 months for recovery.

DIET & FLUIDS

No special diet. Give the child vitamin supplements. Encourage increased fluid intake.

OK FOR SCHOOL, PRESCHOOL, OR NURSERY?

When signs of infection have decreased, appetite returns, and alertness, strength, and feeling of well-being will allow.

CALL YOUR DOCTOR IF

- Your child has symptoms of empyema.
- The following occurs during treatment: fever rises rapidly over 101F (38.3C); pain increases; breathlessness worsens; cough becomes dry and non-productive; fingernails or toenails turn blue or dark; blood appears in the sputum.

ENCEPHALITIS, VIRAL OR ASEPTIC
(Acute Viral Encephalitis; Aseptic Encephalitis)

GENERAL INFORMATION

DESCRIPTION

Viral encephalitis is an acute inflammation in the brain caused by a contagious viral infection. The brain and sometimes the meninges (membranes that cover the brain) are involved.

Appropriate health care includes:

- Physician's monitoring of general condition and medications.
- Hospitalization (more severe cases only).
- Self-care after diagnosis or hospitalization.

SIGNS & SYMPTOMS

Mild cases:

- No symptoms (sometimes).
- Fever.
- General ill feeling.

Severe cases:

- Vomiting.
- Headache.
- Stiff neck.
- Pupils of different size.
- Unconsciousness.
- Personality changes.
- Seizures.
- Occasional weakness or paralysis of an arm or leg.
- Double vision.
- Speech impairment.
- Hearing loss.
- Drowsiness that progresses to coma.

CAUSES

- Viruses that cause other illnesses, including polio, herpes, measles, mumps, chickenpox, infectious mononucleosis, infectious hepatitis, German measles, smallpox, Coxsackie virus, echovirus diseases, and Eastern and Western equine virus.
- Viruses carried by mosquitoes or other insects.
- Lead poisoning.
- Vaccine reactions.
- Leukemia.

RISK FACTORS

- Infancy.
- Illness that has lowered your child's resistance.
- Crowded or unsanitary living conditions.

PREVENTING COMPLICATIONS OR RECURRENCE

- Urge your child to avoid contact with anyone who has encephalitis.
- Consult your doctor for treatment of any infection in your child's body—especially those mentioned as causes—to attempt to prevent the spread of infection.

ENCEPHALITIS, VIRAL OR ASEPTIC
(Acute Viral Encephalitis; Aseptic Encephalitis)

? WHAT TO EXPECT

MEDICAL TESTS
- Your own observation of symptoms.
- Medical history and physical exam by a doctor.
- Laboratory studies of your child's blood and cerebrospinal fluid.

POSSIBLE COMPLICATIONS
A very small percentage of patients suffer permanent brain damage that impairs mental or muscle functions.

PROBABLE OUTCOME
- Mild viral encephalitis is common and may go unnoticed. A severe case usually requires hospitalization for your child.
- Complications and fatalities from encephalitis are most common in infants (and the elderly). People in other age groups usually recover completely. Unless the attack is severe, you can expect your child to recover fully within 2 to 3 weeks.

TREATMENT

HOME CARE
No specific instructions except those listed under other headings.

MEDICATION
Antibiotics are not helpful with viral diseases such as this. Your doctor may prescribe:
- Anti-viral drugs, such as amantadine.
- Cortisone drugs to suppress inflammation (rare).
- See Medications section for information regarding medicines your doctor may prescribe.

ACTIVITY
Your child will need bed rest in a darkened room. After a 2- to 3-week recovery, the child should be as active as strength and feeling of well-being allow.

DIET & FLUIDS
No special diet.

OK FOR SCHOOL, PRESCHOOL, OR NURSERY?
When signs of infection have decreased, appetite returns, and alertness, strength, and feeling of well-being will allow.

CALL YOUR DOCTOR IF
- Your child has any symptoms of encephalitis.
- Temperature rises to 101F (38.3C) or higher.
- New, unexplained symptoms develop. Drugs used in treatment may produce side effects.

ENCOPRESIS

GENERAL INFORMATION

DESCRIPTION

Encopresis means lack of bowel control in a child who has previously been toilet-trained and does not have diarrhea or constipation. A child cannot be expected to have complete bowel control until at least 2-1/2 years of age. The bowels, particularly the colon and rectum, are involved. Encopresis can affect children over age 2-1/2.

Appropriate health care includes:

- Home care.
- Physician's monitoring of general condition and medications, if home care fails.
- Psychotherapy or counseling (sometimes).

SIGNS & SYMPTOMS

Bowel movements in underwear.

CAUSES

- Physical or emotional crisis in your child's life, such as the birth of a sibling or a recent illness with diarrhea.
- Resistance to using the toilet because of too much pressure to do so.
- If the problem is long-term, the original cause may be forgotten, and the child's behavior may persist as a habit.

RISK FACTORS

- Stress.
- Recent illness that brought the child increased attention.

PREVENTING COMPLICATIONS OR RECURRENCE

- Don't lavish attention on a child for being ill.
- Avoid undue emphasis on toilet-training. Approach it calmly with realistic expectations. Don't shame or blame the child for accidents.
- Be sensitive to stressful situations your child faces. Talk together about the child's feelings.

WHAT TO EXPECT

MEDICAL TESTS

- Your own observation of symptoms.
- Medical history and physical exam by a doctor, if necessary.

POSSIBLE COMPLICATIONS

None expected. The symptoms frequently trigger more emotional difficulties than the initial cause.

PROBABLE OUTCOME

Usually curable, unless there is a serious underlying physical problem.

TREATMENT

HOME CARE

- Let your child decide when it is time to go to the bathroom. Don't remind him or make him sit on the toilet against his will. This fosters a negative attitude.
- Praise your child for having bowel movements in the toilet—he deserves positive reinforcement for success. Other family members may also praise the child.
- Provide a prearranged reward if your child stays clean all day. The favorite reward of many children is 30 minutes of free time with either parent, doing whatever the child chooses. Incentives build motivation to succeed.
- Respond gently to accidents. When your child is soiled, he should clean himself and change into clean underwear. For younger children (under age 5), the parent will probably have to do this.
- Don't blame, criticize, restrict, or punish your child for accidents. This may cause him to give up, as well as lead to secondary emotional problems.
- Don't allow siblings or others to tease the child.
- Never put your child back in diapers.
- Ask for the school's cooperation. The child needs quick access to the bathroom at school, especially if he is shy or new at school. Remind him that there should be nothing embarrassing about leaving the classroom to go to the bathroom.

MEDICATION

Don't use:

- Laxatives and stool softeners. These will probably cause diarrhea in addition to the original problem.
- Enemas and suppositories. These may make the child resistant and uncooperative.
- See Medications section for information regarding medicines your doctor may prescribe.

ACTIVITY

No restrictions.

DIET & FLUIDS

No special diet.

OK FOR SCHOOL, PRESCHOOL, OR NURSERY?

Yes. It is important to encourage normal childhood activities.

CALL YOUR DOCTOR IF

Your child has encopresis, and it persists longer than 2 months despite your efforts.

ENDOCARDITIS
(Bacterial Endocarditis; Infective Endocarditis)

GENERAL INFORMATION

DESCRIPTION

Endocarditis is a severe and sometimes life-threatening non-contagious infection of the valves or lining of the heart. The heart muscle, heart valves, and endocardium (lining of the heart chambers and valves) are involved.

Appropriate health care includes:
- Physician's monitoring of general condition and medications.
- Hospitalization until the acute illness subsides.
- Self-care after the acute illness.

SIGNS & SYMPTOMS

Early symptoms:
- Fatigue and weakness.
- Intermittent fever, chills, and excessive sweating, especially at night.
- Weight loss.
- Vague aches and pains.
- Heart murmur.

Late symptoms:
- Severe chills and high fever.
- Shortness of breath on exertion.
- Swelling of the child's feet, legs, and abdomen.
- Rapid or irregular heartbeat.

CAUSES

Bacteria or fungi that enter your child's blood and infect the valves and heart lining of a damaged heart (see RISK FACTORS). Bacteria or fungi further damage the heart valves, muscles, and linings.

RISK FACTORS

Risk of heart-valve damage increases with:
- Rheumatic fever.
- Congenital heart disease.

Risk of endocarditis following heart-valve damage increases with:
- Pregnancy.
- Injections of contaminated materials into the child's bloodstream, such as with self-administered intravenous drugs.
- Use of immunosuppressive drugs.
- Artificial heart valves.
- Excess alcohol consumption.

PREVENTING COMPLICATIONS OR RECURRENCE

Instructions for a child who has heart-valve damage or a heart murmur:
- Request antibiotics prior to medical procedures that may introduce bacteria into the blood. These include dental work, childbirth, and surgery of the urinary or gastrointestinal tract.
- Consult your doctor before becoming pregnant.
- Don't use mind-altering drugs.
- Don't drink more than 1 or 2—if any—alcoholic drinks a day.

ENDOCARDITIS
(Bacterial Endocarditis; Infective Endocarditis)

? WHAT TO EXPECT

MEDICAL TESTS

Your own observation of symptoms; medical history and physical exam by a doctor; laboratory blood counts and blood cultures; EKG (see Glossary); X-rays of the child's heart and lungs, including echocardiogram (see Glossary).

POSSIBLE COMPLICATIONS

- Blood clots that may travel to the brain, kidneys, or abdominal organs, causing infections, abscesses, or stroke.
- Heart-rhythm disturbances (atrial fibrillation is most common).

PROBABLE OUTCOME

Usually curable with early diagnosis and treatment. If treatment is delayed, your child's heart function may deteriorate, resulting in congestive heart failure and death.

+ TREATMENT

HOME CARE

- If your child has damaged valves, tell your doctor and dentist before treatment.
- After having endocarditis, your child should stay under a doctor's care to prevent a relapse.

MEDICATION

Your doctor may prescribe antibiotics for your child for many weeks to fight infection. Antibiotic treatment is often intravenous.

ACTIVITY

- Your child should rest in bed until fully recovered. While in bed, flexing the legs often helps prevent clots from forming in deep veins.
- Your child can resume normal activities when strength allows.

DIET & FLUIDS

No special diet, unless your child has an underlying heart disorder. In that case, the child should follow a low-salt diet (see Appendix 29).

OK FOR SCHOOL, PRESCHOOL, OR NURSERY?

When signs of infection have decreased, appetite returns, and alertness, strength, and feeling of well-being will allow.

☎ CALL YOUR DOCTOR IF

- Your child has symptoms of endocarditis.
- The following occurs during or after treatment: weight gain without diet changes; blood in the child's urine; chest pain; sudden weakness or numbness in the muscles of the child's face, trunk, or limbs.

EPIDIDYMITIS

GENERAL INFORMATION

DESCRIPTION

Epididymitis is an inflammation and infection of the epididymis, an oblong structure attached to the upper part of each testis. Epididymitis can affect males beginning at puberty.

Appropriate health care includes:

- Self-care after diagnosis.
- Physician's monitoring of general condition and medications.

SIGNS & SYMPTOMS

- Enlarged, hardened testicle.
- Fever.
- Tender scrotal contents.
- Tenderness of the second testicle (sometimes).
- Acute urethritis (often).

CAUSES

- Usually a complication of a bacterial infection elsewhere in your son's body, such as gonococcal infection of the urethra, prostate infection, or bladder or kidney infection.
- Epididymitis may also complicate an infection of the scrotum or be caused by scrotal injury.

RISK FACTORS

Your son's recent illness, especially acute or chronic prostatitis, urethritis, or urinary-tract infection.

PREVENTING COMPLICATIONS OR RECURRENCE

Instructions for your son:

- Avoid urethral catheters if possible.
- Use rubber condoms during intercourse to protect from venereal disease. Don't engage in sexual activity with persons who have venereal disease.

WHAT TO EXPECT

MEDICAL TESTS

- Your own observation of symptoms.
- Medical history and physical exam by a doctor.
- Laboratory studies, such as urinalysis and culture of prostate secretions, to identify the germ responsible for your son's illness.

POSSIBLE COMPLICATIONS

- Constipation (sometimes) because bowel movements aggravate pain.
- Sterility or narrowing and blockage of the urethra if the epididymitis involves both testicles. This requires your son to have surgery.

PROBABLE OUTCOME

Usually curable with treatment.

TREATMENT

HOME CARE

Instructions for your son:

- Support the weight of the scrotum and tender testicles. Roll a soft bath towel and place it between your legs under the inflamed area.
- Apply either an ice bag or warm compresses, electric heating pad, or hot water bottle to the inflamed parts. Use whichever relieves pain best.
- Wear an athletic supporter or two pairs of athletic briefs when you resume normal activity.

MEDICATION

Your doctor may prescribe:

- Antibiotics to fight infection.
- Pain relievers.
- Stool softeners.
- Hormones to decrease sexual tension, if necessary.
- See Medications section for information regarding medicines your doctor may prescribe.

ACTIVITY

Instructions for your son:

Rest in bed until fever, pain, and swelling improve. Don't engage in sexual intercourse. If sexual desire and erections become a problem, consult your doctor for medication. Wait at least a month after *all* symptoms disappear before resuming sexual relations.

DIET & FLUIDS

- Urge your son not to drink alcohol, tea, coffee, or carbonated beverages. These irritate the urinary system.
- Encourage your son to eat natural laxative foods, such as prunes, fresh fruit, whole-grain cereals, and nuts, to prevent constipation.

OK FOR SCHOOL, PRESCHOOL, OR NURSERY?

When signs of infection have decreased, appetite returns, and alertness, strength, and feeling of well-being will allow.

CALL YOUR DOCTOR IF

- Your son has symptoms of epididymitis.
- His pain is not relieved by measures outlined above.
- His temperature reaches 103F (39.4C).
- He becomes constipated.
- His symptoms don't improve within 4 days after treatment begins.

EPIGLOTTITIS, ACUTE

GENERAL INFORMATION

DESCRIPTION

Acute epiglottitis is a sudden, life-threatening childhood infection of the epiglottis (a small flap of tissue in the back of the throat that guards the airway entrance to the lung). Epiglottitis is contagious. The epiglottis and surrounding tissue are involved. Acute epiglottitis can affect children from ages 2 to 12 years.

Appropriate health care includes:

- Physician's monitoring of general condition and medications.
- Hospitalization for oxygen and other intensive care.
- Surgery to make an opening in the child's windpipe (trachea) or to place a tube in the trachea to permit breathing. Usually the tube is withdrawn or the opening is closed in 4 to 7 days. This procedure is frequently needed for severe infections of the epiglottis. The surgery can be life-saving.

SIGNS & SYMPTOMS

Sudden onset of the following:

- Sore throat.
- Fever.
- Hoarseness.
- Drooling caused by difficulty swallowing saliva.
- Increasing breathing difficulty.
- Noisy, high-pitched, squeaky inhalations.
- Purple skin and nails.
- Odd head posture. The child tilts the neck back and leans forward with the tongue stuck out and the nostrils flared, trying to inhale more air.

CAUSES

Infection of the epiglottis by a bacteria (usually hemophilus influenza, pneumococcus, or streptococcus). The child's swollen epiglottis blocks the trachea (the main lung airway).

RISK FACTORS

- Illness that has lowered your child's resistance.
- Crowded or unsanitary living conditions.

PREVENTING COMPLICATIONS OR RECURRENCE

If your child has had epiglottitis previously, treat all respiratory infections early and with medical supervision.

WHAT TO EXPECT

MEDICAL TESTS

- Your own observation of symptoms.
- Medical history and physical exam by a doctor.
- Laboratory studies, such as blood counts and a throat culture.
- X-rays of the child's throat to determine the amount of airway obstruction.

POSSIBLE COMPLICATIONS

Without treatment, complete airway obstruction and death within hours.

PROBABLE OUTCOME

Full recovery with prompt diagnosis and treatment of your child.

TREATMENT

HOME CARE

- Have the child sit up rather than lie down.
- Keep the child calm and still until you reach the hospital. Panic increases the child's breathing difficulty.
- After hospitalization, use a cool-mist humidifier at night in the child's room for 2 to 3 weeks.

MEDICATION

- Your doctor may prescribe antibiotics to control infection. Continue for a minimum of 10 days.
- See Medications section for information regarding medicines your doctor may prescribe.

ACTIVITY

Bed rest is necessary for your child until all symptoms disappear. Activities may then be resumed gradually.

DIET & FLUIDS

Fluids only (usually intravenous) until the child can swallow. After hospitalization, encourage extra fluids and provide your child with a normal diet.

OK FOR SCHOOL, PRESCHOOL, OR NURSERY?

When signs of infection have decreased, appetite returns, and alertness, strength, and feeling of well-being will allow.

CALL YOUR DOCTOR IF

- Your child has symptoms of epiglottitis, especially signs of breathing difficulty. This is an emergency!
- Your child has had epiglottitis in the past, and symptoms of respiratory infection appear.

EPILEPSY

GENERAL INFORMATION

DESCRIPTION

Epilepsy is a disorder of brain function characterized by sudden seizures, brief attacks of inappropriate behavior, a change in one's state of consciousness, or bizarre movements. Seizures—also called fits or convulsions—are a symptom, not a disease. Epilepsy is not contagious. Epilepsy can affect both sexes, all ages. Seizures usually begin between ages 2 and 14.

Appropriate health care includes: self-care after diagnosis; physician's monitoring of general condition and medications; surgery to remove any tumor, scar, or abscess, if one is causing convulsions in your child; psychotherapy or counseling to help you and your child learn to understand and cope with the disorder.

SIGNS & SYMPTOMS

There are several forms of epilepsy (listed below), each with its own characteristics:

- Petit mal epilepsy, which mostly affects children. The child stops activity and stares blankly for a minute or so—unaware of what is happening.
- Grand mal epilepsy, which affects all ages. The person loses consciousness, stiffens, then twitches and jerks uncontrollably. The person suffering the seizure may lose bladder control. The seizure lasts several minutes and is often followed by deep sleep or mental confusion. Prior to the seizure, the person may have warning signals: a tense feeling, visual disturbances, smelling a bad odor, or hearing strange noises.
- Focal epilepsy, in which a small part of the body begins twitching uncontrollably. The twitching spreads until it may involve the whole body. The person does not lose consciousness.
- Temporal-lobe epilepsy, in which the person suddenly behaves out of character or inappropriately, such as becoming suddenly violent or angry, laughing for no reason, or making agitated or bizarre body movements, including odd chewing movements.

CAUSES

More than 50 brain disorders, but the organic cause can be determined in only 25% of cases. Common causes include:

- Brain damage at birth.
- Drug or alcohol abuse.
- Severe head injury.
- Brain infection.
- Brain tumor or an expanding lesion that compresses the brain (occasionally).

RISK FACTORS

Family history of seizure disorders; use of mind-altering drugs; exposure to toxic fumes; low blood sugar; excess alcohol consumption.

PREVENTING COMPLICATIONS OR RECURRENCE

No specific preventive measures.

WHAT TO EXPECT

MEDICAL TESTS

Your own observation of symptoms; medical history and physical exam by a doctor; laboratory blood studies, EEG (see Glossary); X-rays of the child's head; CAT or CT scan (see Glossary).

POSSIBLE COMPLICATIONS

Continuing seizures (despite treatment), and mental deterioration (rare).

PROBABLE OUTCOME

Epilepsy is incurable, except in relatively rare cases where epilepsy is caused by treatable brain damage, tumors, or infection. However, anti-convulsant drugs can prevent most seizures and allow your child to lead a near-normal life.

TREATMENT

HOME CARE

- Your child should carry a Medic-Alert bracelet or pendant that mentions epilepsy in case the child has a seizure.
- Your child should avoid any circumstance that has triggered a seizure previously, if possible.

MEDICATION

- Your doctor will prescribe anti-convulsant drugs. Your child's response to the treatment will be monitored. Medication changes or adjustments are often necessary.
- Learn as much as you can about your child's medication. The drugs used cause significant side effects, in addition to suppressing seizures.
- See Medications section for information regarding medicines your doctor may prescribe.

ACTIVITY

No restrictions. Most states allow persons with epilepsy to drive a vehicle after being seizure-free for a year.

DIET & FLUIDS

No special diet. Urge your child not to drink alcohol. It may decrease the effectiveness of the medication and provoke seizures.

OK FOR SCHOOL, PRESCHOOL, OR NURSERY?

Yes. Make every attempt to provide your child with normal childhood opportunities for growth, learning, and development.

CALL YOUR DOCTOR IF

- Your child has a seizure.
- New, unexplained symptoms develop during treatment for epilepsy. Drugs used in treatment may produce side effects.

ERYTHEMA NODOSUM

GENERAL INFORMATION

DESCRIPTION

Erythema nodosum is an inflammatory disease of the skin and tissue under the skin, characterized primarily by painful red nodules on the legs. It is not contagious. The skin of the legs, especially the areas over the large bone in the lower leg, is involved. The disease occasionally involves the arms or other areas. Erythema nodosum is most likely in females beginning at age 12.

Appropriate health care includes:

- Physician's monitoring of general condition and medications.
- Self-care after diagnosis.

SIGNS & SYMPTOMS

Nodules with the following characteristics:

- Nodules are red, painful or tender, and warm.
- Nodules are large (4cm to 10cm). Usually no more than 6 nodules appear on your child at a time.
- Nodules usually occur on the front of the child's lower legs. They appear on one side and then the other.
- Nodules usually appear suddenly. They are often accompanied by fever and swollen, red, tender ankles and knees.
- Nodules change color from pink to red to blue to brown over 7 to 10 days.

CAUSES

Sometimes unknown. Known causes include:

- Use of drugs, such as birth-control pills (especially those high in estrogen), sulfonamides, iodides, and bromides.
- Preceding infection, including streptococcus (most common), coccidioidomycosis, histoplasmosis, sarcoidosis, blastomycosis, tuberculosis, and yersinia infections (see Glossary).
- Autoimmune disease.
- Chronic bowel inflammation.
- Dysproteinemia (see Glossary).
- Consumption of foods with food dyes or preservatives.

RISK FACTORS

Pregnancy.

PREVENTING COMPLICATIONS OR RECURRENCE

Remove or treat the cause of your child's illness, if it can be identified.

WHAT TO EXPECT

MEDICAL TESTS

- Your own observation of symptoms.
- Medical history and physical exam by a doctor.
- Laboratory studies, such as anti-streptococcal titre (see Glossary).
- X-rays of the child's chest to detect sarcoidosis or tuberculosis.

POSSIBLE COMPLICATIONS

Rarely, erythema nodosum can indicate a hidden malignancy in the child's gastrointestinal tract, liver, or lung.

PROBABLE OUTCOME

Individual nodules on your child diminish in size and tenderness and heal in 10 to 20 days. However, others may begin. The disease may last several months. Once it disappears, erythema nodosum probably will not return. Treatment hastens recovery.

TREATMENT

HOME CARE

- Elevate the child's legs whenever possible.
- Use elastic wrap or support stockings on your child's leg.
- Use wrapped or immersion soaks to hasten healing and relieve your child's discomfort. Warm-water soaks are usually more soothing for pain or inflammation. Cool-water soaks feel better for itching.

MEDICATION

- For minor discomfort, use non-prescription drugs such as acetaminophen.
- Your doctor may prescribe a non-steroidal anti-inflammatory drug or cortisone drugs to reduce inflammation.
- See Medications section for information regarding medicines your doctor may prescribe.

ACTIVITY

Your child should rest in bed as much as possible with the legs elevated. Overexertion will cause lesions to recur. When symptoms subside, the child can resume normal activity slowly. Allow 3 weeks for recovery.

DIET & FLUIDS

No special diet.

OK FOR SCHOOL, PRESCHOOL, OR NURSERY?

Yes. This condition is not contagious to others.

CALL YOUR DOCTOR IF

- Your child has symptoms of erythema nodosum.
- The following occurs during treatment:
  - — Symptoms don't improve after 3 days of treatment.
  - — Temperature rises to 101F (38.3C).
- Any new symptoms arise which you think may be due to the disorder or the medications prescribed.

ESOPHAGEAL STRICTURE or CORROSIVE ESOPHAGITIS

GENERAL INFORMATION

DESCRIPTION

Esophageal stricture refers to a narrowing of the esophagus (the tube connecting the mouth to the stomach) caused by inflammation. The narrowing interferes with swallowing. Corrosive esophagitis refers to a narrowing of the esophagus caused by chemical damage.

Appropriate health care includes:

- Physician's monitoring of general condition and medications.
- Hospitalization for supportive care and intravenous nutrition.
- Surgery to remove stricture if other measures fails.
- Psychotherapy or counseling if your child feels suicidal.

SIGNS & SYMPTOMS

- Sudden or gradual decrease in your child's ability to swallow. This gradual swallowing difficulty affects solid foods first, then liquids.
- Pain in the child's mouth and chest after eating.
- Increased salivation.
- Rapid breathing.
- Vomiting, sometimes with mucus or blood. Cancer of the esophagus often causes similar symptoms.

CAUSES

Scarring of the child's esophagus following inflammation or damage caused by:

- Chronic heartburn or hiatal hernia.
- Prolonged use of feeding tubes.
- Accidental swallowing of lye or other corrosive chemicals by a child who is ignorant of the danger.
- Deliberate swallowing of lye or other corrosive chemicals by a child who is suicidal.

RISK FACTORS

Careless storage of corrosive chemicals, such as lye, kerosene, harsh detergent, or bleach.

PREVENTING COMPLICATIONS OR RECURRENCE

- Store all chemicals out of the reach of young children.
- Avoid prolonged use of a feeding tube in your child.

WHAT TO EXPECT

MEDICAL TESTS

- Your own observation of symptoms.
- Medical history and physical exam by a doctor.
- Surgical diagnostic procedures such as endoscopy (see Glossary).
- X-rays of the child's esophagus (barium swallow).

ESOPHAGEAL STRICTURE or CORROSIVE ESOPHAGITIS

POSSIBLE COMPLICATIONS

- Malnutrition from your child's inability to eat normally.
- Perforation of the damaged esophagus. This may be life-threatening.

PROBABLE OUTCOME

Usually curable with treatment. Your child's normal swallowing can be maintained with regular treatment to stretch the stricture.

TREATMENT

HOME CARE

The child's stricture must be stretched regularly (about once a month) with large, heavy dilators. Your doctor will provide specific instructions. The stricture will eventually return if regular treatments are not continued.

MEDICATION

Your doctor may prescribe:

- Cortisone drugs to reduce the child's inflammation and diminish the possibility of scarring.
- Antibiotics to prevent infection.
- See Medications section for information regarding medicines your doctor may prescribe.

ACTIVITY

Your child can resume normal activities gradually.

DIET & FLUIDS

- Provide a soft or liquid diet for your child to eat after treatment until normal swallowing is possible. Avoid serving spicy foods that irritate the esophagus.
- Urge your child not to drink alcohol.

OK FOR SCHOOL, PRESCHOOL, OR NURSERY?

When appetite has returned and alertness, strength, and feeling of well-being will allow.

CALL YOUR DOCTOR IF

- Your child has symptoms of esophageal stricture or corrosive esophagitis.
- The following occurs during treatment:
  - — Chest pain.
  - — Fever.
  - — Inability to speak.
  - — Feeling of air bubbles under the skin of the child's chest.

EXOPHTHALMOS
(Proptosis)

GENERAL INFORMATION

DESCRIPTION

Exophthalmos is a protrusion or bulging of one or both eyes. The eyes and surrounding tissue are involved. Appropriate health care includes: physician's monitoring of general condition and medications; surgery to remove a tumor, blood clot, or aneurysm, or to return the child's eyes to their normal position, if necessary, after the underlying cause (such as an overactive thyroid gland) is corrected, or to correct congenital abnormalities.

SIGNS & SYMPTOMS

Bulging eyes, which creates a staring or frightened look; double vision; pain (sometimes); infrequent blinking (sometimes).

CAUSES

Swelling of the tissues behind the child's eye. Swelling may be caused by an overactive thyroid gland (most common cause); an infection or tumor in the supportive tissues behind the child's eye; an aneurysm, blood clot, or hemorrhage in the veins or arteries behind the child's eye; an injury to the eye or face; a congenital deformity of the head.

RISK FACTORS

Unknown.

PREVENTING COMPLICATIONS OR RECURRENCE

Obtain prompt medical treatment for your child for the underlying disorder.

WHAT TO EXPECT

MEDICAL TESTS

- Your own observation of symptoms; medical history and physical exam by a doctor; biopsy (see Glossary) of tissue behind the child's eyes; blood and other laboratory studies, particularly studies of your child's thyroid gland function; X-rays of the child's head.
- Special studies that may include:

  — Ultrasonography: A non-invasive technique that translates sound waves into images displayed on a screen and photographed (see Glossary).

  — CAT or CT Scan (computerized axial tomography): Non-invasive computerized X-ray images that show sections (or "slices") of an organ or region of the body clearly and precisely (see Glossary).

  — MRI (magnetic resonance imaging): A non-invasive (non-X-ray) computerized test that uses radio frequency energy and a powerful magnetic field to produce images with excellent detail (see Glossary).

  — Radionuclide Scan: A nuclear medicine procedure that uses radioactive isotopes injected into a patient. The isotope tracers are absorbed in various concentrations by targeted organs, which are then photographed (see Glossary).

POSSIBLE COMPLICATIONS

Injury to the child's eye and impaired vision.

PROBABLE OUTCOME

Spontaneous recovery in most cases after the underlying cause is treated. If not, surgery can often correct any remaining protrusion in your child's eye.

TREATMENT

HOME CARE

- If the disorder is caused by an injury to your child, see a doctor immediately.
- If your child's vision is affected, don't let the child drive or engage in dangerous activity.
- If your child's eyelids don't blink properly, wearing goggles to protect the eyes from wind or dust is necessary.

MEDICATION

- If the child's lids don't blink properly, use non-prescription lubricating eye drops.
- Your doctor may prescribe drugs to treat the underlying cause, such as:
  - — Anti-thyroid drugs for hyperthyroidism.
  - — Antibiotics to fight infection.
  - — Cortisone drugs to reduce inflammation.
- See Medications section for information regarding medicines your doctor may prescribe.

ACTIVITY

No restrictions.

DIET & FLUIDS

No special diet.

OK FOR SCHOOL, PRESCHOOL, OR NURSERY?

Yes, after treatment.

CALL YOUR DOCTOR IF

- Your child has symptoms of exophthalmos.
- Symptoms don't improve within 5 days after treatment begins.
- New, unexplained symptoms develop. Drugs used in treatment may produce side effects.

EXTRADURAL HEMORRHAGE
(Epidural Hemorrhage)

GENERAL INFORMATION

DESCRIPTION

An extradural hemorrhage is bleeding between the skull and the outermost of 3 membranes that cover the brain (meninges). The skull, meninges, and brain are involved.

Appropriate health care includes:

- Physician's monitoring of general condition, medications, and treatment. An extradural hemorrhage is an emergency that requires rapid treatment to prevent permanent brain damage or death.
- Surgery to stop your child's bleeding and remove blood clots.
- Home care after surgery.

SIGNS & SYMPTOMS

These symptoms develop within 24 to 96 hours after a head injury:

- Headache that steadily worsens.
- Drowsiness or unconsciousness.
- Nausea or vomiting.
- Inability to move arms and legs.
- Change in the size of eye pupils.

CAUSES

Head injury.

RISK FACTORS

- Use of anticoagulant drugs.
- Bleeding disorders, such as hemophilia or aplastic anemia.
- Injuries. These occur more often after excess alcohol consumption or use of mind-altering drugs.

PREVENTING COMPLICATIONS OR RECURRENCE

Attempt to avoid head injury in the following ways:

- Insist that your children use seat belts or infant seat restraints in cars.
- Urge your child to wear protective head gear during contact sports or while riding a bicycle or motorcycle.
- Urge your child not to drink alcohol or use mind-altering drugs and drive.

WHAT TO EXPECT

MEDICAL TESTS

- Your own observation of symptoms.
- Medical history and physical exam by a doctor.
- Laboratory studies of the child's blood and cerebrospinal fluid.
- Sophisticated hospital diagnostic tests, such as X-rays of the head, arteriography, radioscopic scan, MRI, and CAT scan (see Glossary for all).

POSSIBLE COMPLICATIONS

Fatal compression of the child's brain if bleeding lasts longer than 24 hours.

EXTRADURAL HEMORRHAGE (Epidural Hemorrhage)

PROBABLE OUTCOME

Quick diagnosis and prompt surgery usually bring your child to complete recovery.

TREATMENT

HOME CARE

No specific instructions except those under other headings.

MEDICATION

- Your doctor may prescribe cortisone drugs to reduce the swelling inside the child's skull.
- See Medications section for information regarding medicines your doctor may prescribe.

ACTIVITY

Your child should stay as active as strength allows, resting when tired. Moderate work and exercise is allowed. If speech or muscle control has been damaged, your child may need physical therapy or speech therapy.

DIET & FLUIDS

Your child should eat a normal, well-balanced diet. Vitamin and mineral supplements should not be necessary unless your child cannot eat normally.

OK FOR SCHOOL, PRESCHOOL, OR NURSERY?

Yes, after full recovery.

CALL YOUR DOCTOR IF

- Your child has had a head injury—even if it seems minor—and symptoms of extradural hemorrhage develop.
- The following occurs during treatment:
  - — Temperature rises to 101F (38.3C) or higher.
  - — Surgical wound becomes red, swollen, or tender.
  - — Headache worsens.

EYE CONTUSION OR LACERATION

GENERAL INFORMATION

DESCRIPTION

Eye contusions or lacerations are injuries to the eye, including blunt injuries (contusions) or cuts (lacerations). The eyeball, eyelid, bones around the eyeball (eye socket), and muscles attached to the eyeball are involved.

Appropriate health care includes:

- Physician's monitoring of general condition, medications, and treatment, which may include suturing a laceration.
- Self-care after treatment.

SIGNS & SYMPTOMS

- Swelling, redness, tenderness, pain, bleeding, or bruising ("black eye") in or around the child's eye.
- Change in ability to see clearly.

CAUSES

A blunt or sharp blow or cut to the child's eye or surrounding structures.

RISK FACTORS

- Activities that expose your child's eye to injury, such as athletics or carpentry.
- Eye injuries often occur in fights. Fights are more likely with alcohol consumption or in hostile environments that foster aggression.

PREVENTING COMPLICATIONS OR RECURRENCE

Your child should wear protective eye coverings, if possible, for any exposure to eye injury.

WHAT TO EXPECT

MEDICAL TESTS

- Your own observation of symptoms.
- Medical history and physical exam by a doctor.
- X-rays of bone surrounding the child's eye.

POSSIBLE COMPLICATIONS

- Permanent vision loss.
- Infection.

PROBABLE OUTCOME

Usually curable with treatment to prevent infection. Suturing of lacerations in and around the child's eye is often necessary. Sutures are usually removed in about 7 days. Allow 2 weeks for complete healing.

TREATMENT

HOME CARE

Instructions for your child:

- Protect your eyes from bright light or sunlight by wearing dark glasses temporarily.
- Use ice packs or warm moist compresses to relieve discomfort. Prepare a compress by folding a clean cloth in several layers. Dip in warm water, wring out slightly, and apply to the eye. Dip the compress often to keep it moist. Keep applying the compress for an hour, rest an hour and repeat.
- Sleep with your head elevated with 2 pillows until symptoms subside.

MEDICATION

Your doctor may prescribe:

- Antibiotic eye drops or ointments to prevent infection.
- Pain relievers.
- Eye drops to dilate the eye pupil and rest the eye muscles (sometimes).
- See Medications section for information regarding medicines your doctor may prescribe.

ACTIVITY

Your child can resume normal activities gradually after treatment.

DIET & FLUIDS

No special diet.

OK FOR SCHOOL, PRESCHOOL, OR NURSERY?

Yes, after your child's healing has progressed enough to permit normal activity.

CALL YOUR DOCTOR IF

- Your child has a cut or other eye injury.
- The following occurs after an eye injury:
  - — Fever.
  - — Severe eye pain that persists, despite treatment.
  - — Vision changes.

EYE, FOREIGN BODY IN

GENERAL INFORMATION

DESCRIPTION

A foreign body in the eye is an embedding of a small speck of metal, wood, stone, sand, paint, or other foreign material in the eye. The eye, usually only the conjunctiva (outer eye covering) is involved.

Appropriate health care includes:

- Physician's monitoring of general condition and medications.
- Emergency-room care (sometimes).
- Self-care after removal of the particle.

SIGNS & SYMPTOMS

- Severe pain, irritation, and redness in the child's eye.
- Foreign body visible with the naked eye (usually). Sometimes the foreign body is very small, trapped under the child's eyelid and invisible except with medical examination.

CAUSES

Accident.

RISK FACTORS

- Windy weather.
- Certain activities, such as carpentry, in which fine particles of wood or other material fly loose in the air.

PREVENTING COMPLICATIONS OR RECURRENCE

Your child should wear protective eye coverings if activities or hobbies involve the risk of eye injury.

WHAT TO EXPECT

MEDICAL TESTS

- Your own observation of symptoms.
- Medical history and physical exam by a doctor. This may include staining the child's eye with a harmless substance (fluorescein) to outline the object and examine the eye through a magnifying lens.

POSSIBLE COMPLICATIONS

- Infection, especially if the foreign body is not removed completely.
- Severe, permanent vision damage caused by penetration of deeper eye layers.

PROBABLE OUTCOME

Most objects can be removed simply from your child's eye under local anesthesia in a doctor's office or emergency room.

TREATMENT

HOME CARE

Instructions for your child:

- Ask someone else to drive you to the doctor's office. Don't try to drive yourself.
- Don't rub the eye.
- Keep the eye closed, if possible, until you are examined.
- Wear an eye patch to keep the eye closed, or dark glasses, for 24 hours after removal to protect your eye from bright light.
- Use moist compresses to relieve discomfort after removal. Prepare by folding a clean cloth in several layers. Dip in warm water, wring out slightly and apply to the eye. Dip the compress often to keep it moist. Keep applying the compress for an hour, rest an hour, and repeat.

MEDICATION

Your doctor may prescribe:

- Antibiotic eye drops or ointment to prevent infection.
- Pain relievers.
- Local anesthetic eye drops.
- See Medications section for information regarding medicines your doctor may prescribe.

ACTIVITY

Your child should resume normal activities gradually after removal of the foreign body and the patch, if one is applied.

DIET & FLUIDS

No special diet.

OK FOR SCHOOL, PRESCHOOL, OR NURSERY?

Yes, when pain or discomfort are not severe.

CALL YOUR DOCTOR IF

- Your child has a foreign body in the eye.
- The following occurs after removal:
  - — Pain increases or does not disappear in 2 days.
  - — Your child develops a fever.
  - — Your child's vision changes.

EYE INJURY

GENERAL INFORMATION

DESCRIPTION

Injuries to the eye include contusions and fractures of bones that form the eye socket or orbit, contusions and lacerations of the eyelids, and abrasions of the cornea (the transparent covering of the pupil of the eye) or other injury to the eyeball. The bones that form the orbit; the eyelids; the eyeball including the cornea, conjunctiva (white of the eye), iris (colored part of the eye), and aqueous humor (fluid in the eyeball); and the muscles, tendons, periosteum (covering of the bone), nerves, blood vessels, skin, and connective tissue in the vicinity of the eye are also involved. Appropriate health care includes doctor's treatment; emergency room care; hospitalization for repair of facial bones (sometimes).

SIGNS & SYMPTOMS

- Injury to the orbit: pain; swollen lids; protruding eyeball if bleeding occurs in back of the child's eye; numbness around the eye; inability to move the eye normally; decreased vision.
- Injury to the lids: pain; a cut, laceration, or contusion with swelling, redness, tenderness, pain, bleeding, or bruising (''black eye'') in or around the child's eye; a change in the child's ability to see clearly.
- Injury to the eyeball: eye pain; sensitivity to bright light; eyelid spasm; tearing; blurred vision; redness in the white of the eye; irregular size of the pupils.

CAUSES

Direct blow in the vicinity of the child's eye; irritation from many different materials, such as pesticides on plants or gravel or dust; a foreign body imbedded in the eye; scratching of the cornea.

RISK FACTORS

Contact sports such as football or soccer; racket sports; windy weather; rough terrain for workouts or competition.

PREVENTING COMPLICATIONS OR RECURRENCE

Your child should wear a face mask or protective glasses for sports and should avoid allergens, if possible.

WHAT TO EXPECT

MEDICAL TESTS

- Medical history and physical exam by an ophthalmologist or cosmetic surgeon.
- X-rays of the child's skull and facial bones to detect possible fractures.

POSSIBLE COMPLICATIONS

Infection, especially when imbedded foreign bodies are not completely removed from the child's cornea; permanent (sometimes total) loss of vision if infection penetrates the eyeball from the cornea; bleeding into the eye as a result of a blunt injury; scarring if eyelid lacerations are unattended.

PROBABLE OUTCOME

Cornea injury with infection: This serious eye problem is usually curable in 2 to 3 weeks with special care from an ophthalmologist. *Eyelid injury:* Eyelid lacerations usually heal in 1 to 2 weeks if they are carefully closed surgically by a specialist in plastic surgery. *Orbit (bone) injury:* Facial surgery by a cosmetic surgeon usually improves appearance. Bones require 6 to 8 weeks to heal. *Injuries due to foreign bodies:* These injuries heal easily if the foreign body is removed and antibiotic medication is used to fight infection.

TREATMENT

FIRST AID

Don't try to remove the child's contact lenses. Don't rub the eye. Don't wash the eye. Cover both eyes with loose cloth pads. (Both eyes must be covered to prevent movement of the injured eye.) Apply crushed ice in a soft cloth bag or a towel—not a heavy ice bag. Avoid any pressure on the eye.

HOME CARE

- After emergency treatment: Protect eyes from bright light or sunlight by having the child wear dark glasses. Use ice packs or warm water compresses, wrung out slightly, to relieve discomfort. The child should sleep with the head elevated with 2 pillows until symptoms subside. Urge the child not to rub the eye.
- For lacerations after suturing: Keep the child's wound dry and covered for 48 hours. If you change the bandage, apply a small amount of petroleum jelly or non-prescription antibiotic ointment to each new bandage. After 48 hours, replace the bandage if it gets wet. Ignore small amounts of bleeding. Control heavier bleeding by firmly pressing a facial tissue or clean cloth to the bleeding spot, avoiding pressure on the eyeball itself.

MEDICATION

Your doctor may prescribe antibiotic eyedrops or ointment to prevent infection; pain relievers; local anesthetic eyedrops or drops to dilate the pupil and rest the eye muscle.

ACTIVITY

Your child can resume normal activities gradually after treatment.

DIET & FLUIDS

No restrictions.

OK FOR SCHOOL, PRESCHOOL, OR NURSERY?

Yes, when condition and sense of well-being will allow.

CALL YOUR DOCTOR IF

Your child has a foreign body in the eye or a cut or other eye injury; the following occurs during or after treatment: pain increases or does not disappear in 2 days; the child's vision changes; the eye does not move up and down normally; there is a fever over 101F (38.3C); the child experiences pain that is not relieved by acetaminophen.

EYE TUMOR

GENERAL INFORMATION

DESCRIPTION

An eye tumor is a growth in the eye in which cell multiplication is uncontrolled and progressive. Eye tumors are of 3 types: retinoblastoma, malignant melanoma, or secondary tumors that have spread from other parts of the body. Usually only one eye is involved. Retinoblastoma invades both eyes in 25% of cases. Retinoblastoma affects young children between ages 1 and 5, melanoma affects adults over 60, and secondary tumors affect all ages.

Appropriate health care includes one of the following:

- Surgery to remove the tumor.
- Radiation therapy.
- Cryotherapy (see Glossary).
- Treatment with laser beams.

SIGNS & SYMPTOMS

The following are characteristic of all 3 types:

- Possibly no signs in the early stages.
- Gradual loss of vision.
- Bulging eyes (sometimes).

Retinoblastoma may have the following additional signs:

- Crossed eyes.
- A tumor that is visible through the pupil.

CAUSES

- Melanoma and secondary tumors: Unknown.
- Retinoblastoma: Inherited tendency.

RISK FACTORS

Family history of retinoblastoma. The genetic trait is dominant, but it does not affect all the children of the family.

PREVENTING COMPLICATIONS OR RECURRENCE

Cannot be prevented at present. If your family has a history of retinoblastoma, obtain genetic counseling before having children.

WHAT TO EXPECT

MEDICAL TESTS

- Your own observation of symptoms.
- Medical history and physical exam by a doctor.
- Echography (see Glossary).
- Fluorescein dye tests (see Glossary) to outline blood vessels in the child's eye.
- X-rays of the child's skull.
- Radionuclide Scan: A nuclear medicine procedure that uses radioactive isotope injected into a patient. The isotope tracers are absorbed in various concentrations by targeted organs, which are then photographed (see Glossary).
- MRI (magnetic resonance imaging): A non-invasive (non-X-ray) computerized test that uses radio frequency energy and a powerful magnetic field to produce images with excellent detail (see Glossary).

POSSIBLE COMPLICATIONS

- Spread to other parts of the child's body.
- Partial or complete loss of the child's vision.

PROBABLE OUTCOME

- Some eye tumors are curable in 6 months with medical treatment.
- Other eye tumors are considered incurable. A fatal spread to other body parts usually occurs rapidly. However, medical literature cites a few instances of unexplained recovery. Scientific research into causes and treatment continues, so there is hope for increasingly effective treatment and cure.

TREATMENT

HOME CARE

The surgeon will provide instructions for postoperative care for your child.

MEDICATION

Your doctor may prescribe:

- Pain relievers.
- Anti-cancer drugs.
- See Medications section for information regarding medicines your doctor may prescribe.

ACTIVITY

After treatment, your child can resume normal activities as soon as possible.

DIET & FLUIDS

No special diet.

OK FOR SCHOOL, PRESCHOOL, OR NURSERY?

Yes, after treatment is complete.

CALL YOUR DOCTOR IF

- Your child has symptoms of an eye tumor.
- Pain becomes intolerable during treatment.
- New, unexplained symptoms develop that may indicate the malignancy has spread to other body parts.

FACIAL BONES, FRACTURE OF

GENERAL INFORMATION

DESCRIPTION

Fracture of facial bones means, simply, broken bones in the face. The facial nerves, blood vessels, skin, and bones are involved. The facial bones include those of the upper jaw (maxilla), of the lower jaw (mandible), of the cheek (zygoma), and around the eyes (orbital), as well as the nose (see Nose Fracture in Illnesses section).

Appropriate health care includes:

- Physician's monitoring of general condition, medications, and treatment. A plastic surgeon, oral surgeon, ophthalmologist, or ear, nose and throat specialist may be consulted.
- Surgery to realign fractured bones and reconstruct normal facial contours.
- Self-care after diagnosis and treatment.

SIGNS & SYMPTOMS

The following apply to the site of your child's injury:

- Swelling.
- Tenderness, crepitation (a crackly feeling upon touching), or pain.
- Redness that becomes multicolored soon after injury.
- Loss of sensation in the lips and nose from nerve damage.
- Double or blurred vision.

CAUSES

Injury, especially from auto or bicycle accidents, sports injuries, and fist fights.

RISK FACTORS

- Hostile, aggressive personalities.
- Participation in contact sports.
- Excess alcohol consumption.

PREVENTING COMPLICATIONS OR RECURRENCE

Instructions for your child:

Avoid injury whenever possible. Wear protective headgear for contact sports or when riding motorcycles or bicycles. Use auto seat belts. Don't drink or use mind-altering drugs and drive.

WHAT TO EXPECT

MEDICAL TESTS

- Your own observation of symptoms.
- Medical history and physical exam by a doctor.
- Laboratory blood studies to measure blood loss.
- X-rays of the child's skull and facial bones.
- Special studies that may include ultrasonography, CAT or CT scan, MRI, and radionuclide scan (see Glossary for all).

POSSIBLE COMPLICATIONS

- Infection in the injured area.
- Permanent disfigurement.

PROBABLE OUTCOME

• Surgery usually produces good cosmetic results and a return to normal function. It should be done as soon as possible after your child has been injured.

• Teeth that have been knocked out can sometimes be replanted. A broken jaw is corrected by securing the teeth with wire or plastic splints so the jaw heals in its proper position. Your child's speech will be changed while the wires are in place, but it should return to normal when they are removed. Normal vision should return if the child's eye is not injured.

• Allow about 6 weeks for recovery.

TREATMENT

HOME CARE

Instructions for your child:

• Don't exercise to the point that you must pant for breath, because breathing may be difficult for a while.

• Protect your face from pressure. Sleep on your back.

• Don't blow your nose hard or use makeup until healing is complete.

• If your jaws are wired, learn how to release them quickly in case of emergency, such as severe coughing or vomiting.

MEDICATION

Your doctor may prescribe:

• Pain relievers.

• Antibiotics to fight infection, if necessary.

ACTIVITY

Your child should rest quietly for about 2 days, then resume normal activities as strength returns.

DIET & FLUIDS

Your child should eat a high-protein, liquid diet for several days. If the child's jaw is wired, the liquid diet will be necessary for up to 8 weeks. Add soft solid foods when the child is able to eat them. Give the child vitamin and mineral supplements to hasten healing.

OK FOR SCHOOL, PRESCHOOL, OR NURSERY?

Yes, when general health and state of well-being permit.

CALL YOUR DOCTOR IF

• Your child has a facial-bone fracture.

• The following occurs during treatment: fever; impaired vision; severe headache; loss of sensation in the child's face; intolerable pain; illness of any kind during healing; loosening of wires or splints.

• New, unexplained symptoms develop. Drugs used in treatment may produce side effects.

FAILURE TO THRIVE

GENERAL INFORMATION

DESCRIPTION

Failure to thrive means the failure of infants, children, and adolescents to grow and develop normally. This is different from marasmus, in which infants in emotionally deprived environments become listless, weaken, and sometimes die. Failure to thrive affects young children (1 to 5 years) of both sexes.

Appropriate health care includes:

- Physician's monitoring of general condition and medications.
- Psychotherapy or counseling, if the parents have emotional problems that prevent a healthy relationship with the child.
- Hospitalization (short-term), if complicated diagnostic procedures are necessary or the child's food intake must be verified.
- Home care.

SIGNS & SYMPTOMS

- Persistent vomiting in an infant between 0 and 6 months.
- Height, weight, and head circumference do not progress normally, as measured on doctors' growth charts.
- Physical skills are slow to develop. Such skills include:
  - — Turning over in bed.
  - — Sitting.
  - — Standing and walking.
- Mental and social skills are delayed. These skills include:
  - — Talking.
  - — Social interaction.
  - — Self-feeding.
  - — Toilet training.

Normal growth and development vary widely. The *rate of change*—as measured at regular medical checkups—is more significant.

CAUSES

- Parental inexperience.
- A negative emotional environment (neglect, abuse, or rejection).
- Malnutrition.
- Chronic disease, such as kidney failure or chronic infection.
- Genetic disorders, such as Down syndrome or cystic fibrosis.
- Endocrine diseases, including disorders of the thyroid, pituitary, adrenal, pancreas, and sexual glands.

RISK FACTORS

Poverty; parents who were raised in a negative emotional environment or are poorly educated; crowded or unsanitary living conditions.

PREVENTING COMPLICATIONS OR RECURRENCE

- Arrange for parenting classes if you are an expectant mother or father.
- Take your child regularly to the doctor for "well-baby" checkups.

WHAT TO EXPECT

MEDICAL TESTS

- Your own observation of symptoms.
- Medical history and physical exam by a doctor.
- Tests, such as the Denver Developmental Test, which measures the child's growth and development.
- Laboratory blood tests, including hormone studies.
- X-rays of the child's hands, which provide a good measure of body growth.

POSSIBLE COMPLICATIONS

Permanent mental, emotional, or physical disability.

PROBABLE OUTCOME

- If a child's failure to thrive is caused by parental inexperience or psychological problems, recovery is possible with education and counseling for the parents.
- If a child's failure to thrive is caused by an underlying physical illness or disorder, including malnutrition, recovery depends on whether the condition can be corrected.

TREATMENT

HOME CARE

- Read books and pamphlets on child-rearing, or attend parenting classes.
- Ask a visiting nurse to visit your home for guidance.
- Provide as much love and support as possible for your child. Examine your feelings and behavior toward your child. If you don't think they are what they should be, arrange for psychological counseling.

MEDICATION

If an underlying disorder is causing failure to thrive, your doctor may prescribe medication to treat the child's condition.

ACTIVITY

No restrictions.

DIET & FLUIDS

- Provide your child with an adequate, well-balanced diet. See Appendix 24.
- If malnutrition is causing your child's failure to thrive, your doctor may prescribe a special diet.

OK FOR SCHOOL, PRESCHOOL, OR NURSERY?

Yes. Make every attempt to keep activities normal for your child's age.

CALL YOUR DOCTOR IF

You are concerned that your child is not developing properly. Trust your instincts—obtain a second doctor's opinion, if necessary.

FAINTING
(Blackout; Syncope)

GENERAL INFORMATION

DESCRIPTION

Fainting is a sudden, temporary loss of consciousness. The circulatory system (heart and blood vessels) and brain are involved.

Appropriate health care includes:

- Care from bystanders.
- Self-care after regaining consciousness.
- Physician's monitoring of general condition and medications, if fainting is caused by other conditions (see CAUSES).

SIGNS & SYMPTOMS

- Sudden lightheadedness.
- Blurred vision (sometimes).
- Nausea (sometimes).
- General weakness, then falling.
- Paleness and sweating.
- Rapid heartbeat and rapid breathing. If your child's heartbeat or breathing is not present, this may be cardiac arrest rather than fainting.

CAUSES

A sudden decrease in blood pressure, which temporarily deprives the brain of blood. The drop in blood pressure may result from:

- Heartbeat abnormalities—too fast, too slow, or irregular.
- Prolonged straining, such as from severe coughing or attempted bowel movements when constipated.
- Prolonged standing in unusually hot weather.
- Standing for unusually long periods with the knees locked (any temperature).
- Sudden emotional stress.
- Heart diseases that limit the amount of blood the child's heart pumps.
- Getting out of bed or a chair suddenly (orthostatic hypotension).
- Epilepsy.
- Low blood sugar.
- Heart attack (rare).
- Anemia (rare).

RISK FACTORS

- Stress.
- Heart disease.
- Use of certain drugs, such as heart medications that slow the heartbeat. These include digitalis, beta-adrenergic blockers, and other anti-hypertensive drugs.
- Hot, humid weather.

PREVENTING COMPLICATIONS OR RECURRENCE

- Your child should avoid sudden changes in physical activity.
- If your child's fainting episodes are caused by medication, consult your doctor about changing drugs.

FAINTING
(Blackout; Syncope)

? WHAT TO EXPECT

MEDICAL TESTS
- Your own observation of symptoms.
- Medical history and physical exam by a doctor.

POSSIBLE COMPLICATIONS
- Injury while fainting.
- Mistaking cardiac arrest for fainting.

PROBABLE OUTCOME

Simple fainting disappears in 1 or 2 minutes.

TREATMENT

HOME CARE
- If your child faints, check for breathing and a neck pulse. If neither is present:
  — Dial 0 (operator) or 911 (emergency) for an ambulance or medical help. Then give first aid immediately.
  — Begin cardiac massage and mouth-to-mouth breathing (CPR). Don't stop until help arrives.
- If your child faints, is breathing, and has a pulse, leave the child on the ground and elevate both legs. This helps return blood to the heart.
- If your child feels faint, urge the child to sit down immediately and bend over, or lie down.
- If your child is subject to frequent fainting spells, urge the child to avoid activities in which fainting may endanger life, such as climbing to high places, driving vehicles, or operating dangerous machinery.

MEDICATION

Medication usually is not necessary for fainting. Medication may be necessary to treat the child's underlying disorders.

ACTIVITY

Your child can resume normal activities upon regaining consciousness.

DIET & FLUIDS

No special diet unless your child's fainting episodes are caused by low blood sugar. If so, your child should eat 5 or 6 small meals a day. The meals should be high in protein, high in complex carbohydrates, and low in simple carbohydrates (sugar).

OK FOR SCHOOL, PRESCHOOL, OR NURSERY?

Yes, when underlying cause is under control.

CALL YOUR DOCTOR IF

- Your unconscious child has no pulse and is not breathing. Give CPR immediately and have someone else call. This is an emergency!
- Your child faints and does not regain consciousness in 2 minutes.
- Fainting is a symptom of another condition (see CAUSES).

FECAL IMPACTION

GENERAL INFORMATION

DESCRIPTION

Fecal impaction is a severe form of constipation in which a large mass of feces cannot be passed. Fecal impaction is not a serious condition, but it complicates other illnesses. The lower colon and rectum are involved.

Appropriate health care includes:

- Self-care.
- Doctor's or nurse's treatment to remove feces manually or by enema.

SIGNS & SYMPTOMS

- Absence of normal bowel movements.
- Thin, watery discharge from the child's rectum.
- Sense of fullness in the rectum, but inability to pass stool.
- Lack of urinary control.
- A firm mass in the lower left abdomen (sometimes).
- Pain or cramps (sometimes). Impaction often develops slowly without discomfort.
- Low fever (sometimes).

CAUSES

- Rectal disorders that make your child's normal bowel movements uncomfortable, such as painful hemorrhoids or anal fissure.
- Rectal or colon tumors.
- Barium that is swallowed for X-rays of the intestinal tract.
- Loss of nerve supply to the colon or rectum, as with a spinal-cord injury.
- Insufficient fiber and liquid in the child's diet.

RISK FACTORS

- Prolonged bed rest for any condition, such as surgery or fracture.
- Back disorders with nerve pressure.
- Decreased fluid and fiber intake.
- Use of some drugs, such as narcotic pain killers, atropine, phenothiazines, or tricyclic anti-depressants.

PREVENTING COMPLICATIONS OR RECURRENCE

- If confined to bed, your child should drink extra fluids and increase consumption of dietary fiber.
- If simple constipation develops, the child can use a mild laxative, such as milk of magnesia, or a stool softener, or an enema.

WHAT TO EXPECT

MEDICAL TESTS
- Your own observation of symptoms.
- Medical history and physical exam, including a rectal exam, by a doctor.

POSSIBLE COMPLICATIONS
- A child who has a serious congenital heart disease may suffer fatal rupture of the heart muscle while straining to pass a fecal impaction.
- Rectal prolapse (protrusion outside the body).
- Aggravation of hemorrhoids.

PROBABLE OUTCOME
Usually curable with treatment, but recurrence is common unless the underlying cause is removed.

TREATMENT

HOME CARE
- If your doctor prescribes it, use an oil-retention enema on the child before and after manual removal of the impaction. Follow instructions on the package.
- See Constipation (in Illnesses section) for suggestions to improve bowel habits.

MEDICATION
- After removal of the impaction, your doctor may prescribe laxatives or stool softeners for your child.
- See Medications section for information regarding medicines your doctor may prescribe.

ACTIVITY
No restrictions. Your child should be as active as possible. Good physical fitness improves bowel function.

DIET & FLUIDS
- Urge your child to eat a normal, well-balanced diet high in fiber.
- Encourage your child to drink at least 8 glasses of fluid each day.

OK FOR SCHOOL, PRESCHOOL, OR NURSERY?
Yes.

CALL YOUR DOCTOR IF
- Your child has symptoms of a fecal impaction.
- Your child's normal bowel pattern changes.
- Your child cannot pass feces while under treatment for other conditions.

FEVER OF UNDETERMINED ORIGIN (FUO)

GENERAL INFORMATION

DESCRIPTION

Fever of undetermined origen is a prolonged (2 to 3 weeks) temperature above normal for which no cause is evident. Any body organs or system which may be the source of a fever-producing condition may be involved.

Appropriate health care includes:

- Self-care after diagnosis.
- Physician's monitoring of general condition and medications.

SIGNS & SYMPTOMS

Fever (measured rectally) for at least 2 weeks. Fever may be intermittent.

CAUSES

- Infections.
- Collagen or autoimmune diseases.
- Tumors and cancer, especially kidney cancer and leukemia.
- Self-induced in some psychologically unstable children.

RISK FACTORS

- Poor nutrition.
- Illness that has lowered your child's resistance.
- Chemical or environmental exposure to polluted water or air.
- Travel in areas with unsanitary conditions.
- Exposure to others with contagious diseases.

PREVENTING COMPLICATIONS OR RECURRENCE

No specific preventive measures.

WHAT TO EXPECT

MEDICAL TESTS

- Your own observation of symptoms.
- Medical history and physical exam by a doctor. Because fever may be the first evidence of a serious condition in an early stage, your doctor may recommend thorough diagnostic testing for your child.
- Laboratory studies, such as blood studies and a urine culture (see Glossary).
- X-rays.
- Special studies that may include:

  — MRI (magnetic resonance imaging): A non-invasive (non-X-ray) computerized test that uses radio frequency energy and a powerful magnetic field to produce images with excellent detail (see Glossary).

  — Radionuclide Scan: A nuclear medicine procedure that uses radioactive isotopes injected into a patient. The isotope tracers are absorbed in various concentrations by targeted organs, which are then photographed (see Glossary).

POSSIBLE COMPLICATIONS

Depends on the underlying condition causing the child's fever.

FEVER OF UNDETERMINED ORIGIN (FUO)

PROBABLE OUTCOME

Spontaneous recovery in about 10% of cases. In other cases, the outcome depends on successful detection and treatment of the child's underlying disorder.

TREATMENT

HOME CARE

Until the cause of your child's fever has been diagnosed, keep a daily temperature chart.

MEDICATION

- For minor discomfort, use non-prescription drugs such as acetaminophen. Until the underlying cause is determined, your doctor may withhold prescription drugs to avoid masking symptoms of the underlying disorder. Occasionally, in a critically ill child awaiting results of laboratory studies, the doctor may recommend a therapeutic trial of antibiotics or other drugs.
- See Medications section for information regarding medicines your doctor may prescribe.

ACTIVITY

Bed rest may be advisable for your child.

DIET & FLUIDS

No special diet.

OK FOR SCHOOL, PRESCHOOL, OR NURSERY?

When signs of infection have decreased, appetite returns, and alertness, strength, and feeling of well-being will allow.

CALL YOUR DOCTOR IF

- Your child has an unexplained fever that lasts longer than 24 hours.
- New symptoms develop. They may provide a clue about the underlying cause of the child's fever.

FINGER DISLOCATION

GENERAL INFORMATION

DESCRIPTION

A finger dislocation is an injury to any finger joint causing adjoining finger bones to be displaced from their normal position so they no longer touch each other. Fractures and ligament sprains frequently accompany this dislocation. Any of the many finger bones, ligaments that hold the finger bones in place, and the soft tissue surrounding the dislocation site, including the periosteum (covering of the bone), nerves, tendons, blood vessels, and connective tissue, are involved. Appropriate health care includes manipulating the joint by a trained professional to reposition the child's bones; surgery (sometimes) to restore the joint to its normal position and repair the child's torn ligaments and tendons. Acute or recurring dislocations may require surgical reconstruction or eventual replacement of the joint.

SIGNS & SYMPTOMS

- Excruciating pain in the child's finger at the time of injury.
- Loss of function in the dislocated joint.
- Severe pain when the child attempts to move the injured finger.
- Visible deformity if the dislocated finger has locked in the dislocated position. The child's bones may spontaneously reposition themselves and leave no deformity, but the damage is the same.
- Tenderness over the dislocation.
- Swelling and bruising at the injury site.
- Numbness or paralysis beyond the dislocation from pinching, cutting, or pressure on the child's blood vessels or nerves.

CAUSES

- Direct or indirect blow to the child's hand, finger, or thumb.
- End result of a severe finger sprain.

RISK FACTORS

- Contact sports, especially basketball, baseball, and soccer.
- Previous finger or hand dislocation or sprain.
- Arthritis of any type (rheumatoid, gout).
- Poor muscle conditioning in the child's hand.

PREVENTING COMPLICATIONS OR RECURRENCE

Your child should protect vulnerable joints with protective devices or tape and should condition the hand muscles.

WHAT TO EXPECT

MEDICAL TESTS

Your own observation of symptoms. X-rays of the child's hand and wrist.

POSSIBLE COMPLICATIONS

- At the time of injury: shock; pressure on or injury to nearby nerves, ligaments, tendons, muscles, blood vessels, and connective tissue.
- After treatment or surgery: impaired blood supply to the dislocated area; death of bone cells due to interruption of the blood supply; infection introduced during surgical treatment; excessive bleeding around the dislocation site; continuing recurrent dislocations with progressively less severe injuries; prolonged healing if activity is resumed too soon; an unstable or arthritic joint following repeated injury or surgery.

PROBABLE OUTCOME

Complete healing of a child's injured ligaments requires a minimum of 6 weeks.

TREATMENT

FIRST AID

Use instructions for R.I.C.E., the first letters of *rest*, *ice*, *compression*, and *elevation*. See Appendix 39 for details.

HOME CARE

- After removal of the child's splint or cast, begin daily rehabilitation exercises.
- Tape the child's injured finger to adjacent fingers, if instructed to do so by your doctor.

MEDICATION

Your doctor may prescribe general anesthesia or local anesthesia to make joint manipulation possible during surgery; acetaminophen or aspirin to relieve moderate pain; narcotic pain relievers for severe pain; antibiotics to fight infection, if surgery is necessary.

ACTIVITY

If surgery is not necessary, your child does not have to restrict activity except for the limitations imposed by immobilization of the hand. If surgery is necessary, the child can resume normal activities gradually.

DIET & FLUIDS

No restrictions.

OK FOR SCHOOL, PRESCHOOL, OR NURSERY?

Yes, when condition and sense of well-being will allow.

CALL YOUR DOCTOR IF

- Your child has signs or symptoms of a dislocated finger.
- Any of the following occur after treatment: numbness, paleness, or coldness in the child's finger—*this is an emergency*; swelling above or below the splint or cast; blue or gray skin color, particularly under the fingernails.
- Any of the following occur after surgery: increased pain, swelling, or drainage in the surgical area; signs of infection, including headache, muscle aches, dizziness, or a general ill feeling and fever.
- Finger dislocations that can be "popped" back into normal position occur repeatedly.

FLUID & ELECTROLYTE DISORDERS
(Fluid & Electrolyte Imbalance)

GENERAL INFORMATION

DESCRIPTION

Fluid and electrolyte disorders refer to an imbalance in the mixture of water and salts (electrolytes) needed for normal body function. Necessary salts contain sodium, potassium, calcium, bicarbonate, and phosphate. All body parts—even hard bone—are bathed in a precise blend of water and natural salts.

Appropriate health care includes:

- Physician's monitoring of general condition and medications.
- Self-care after diagnosis of a minor imbalance.
- Hospitalization for intravenous fluids and treatment of a serious imbalance, including the underlying cause. This is especially important in infants.

Dehydration with fluid and electrolyte imbalance can be life-threatening in the very young.

SIGNS & SYMPTOMS

Depends on whether water or salts are out of proportion. The following may indicate either imbalance problem:

- Dry mouth.
- Wrinkled skin.
- Increased, decreased, or absent urination.
- Fatigue.
- Puffy legs, hands, face, or abdomen.
- Lung congestion.
- Weakness and confusion.
- Heartbeat irregularities.

CAUSES

Fluid and salts may be *lost* by:

- Vomiting.
- Diarrhea.
- Heavy perspiration.
- Some medications, such as diuretics.
- Nasogastric tubes during hospitalization.

Fluid and salts may *accumulate* from:

- Congestive heart failure.
- Excess intravenous fluids.
- Acute or chronic kidney failure.
- Diabetes insipidus.
- Adrenal disease.
- Chronic lung disease.
- Use of cortisone drugs, female hormones, or sodium bicarbonate.

RISK FACTORS

Fever; kidney disease; diabetes mellitus; heart disease; anorexia nervosa or bulimia; use of diuretics; infancy and early childhood—infants and young children lose fluid very quickly when sick; alcoholism.

FLUID & ELECTROLYTE DISORDERS
(Fluid & Electrolyte Imbalance)

PREVENTING COMPLICATIONS OR RECURRENCE

For vomiting or diarrhea, give the child small amounts of clear liquids every 30 minutes; during serious illness, keep a fluid-balance record (see HOME CARE).

? WHAT TO EXPECT

MEDICAL TESTS

Your own observation of symptoms; medical history and physical exam by a doctor; laboratory studies of the child's urine, stool, blood, and electrolytes—especially sodium, chloride, and potassium; radioactive studies of the child's total body water.

POSSIBLE COMPLICATIONS

Dehydration; heartbeat irregularities; cardiac arrest; death.

PROBABLE OUTCOME

Usually curable in 24 to 48 hours with early treatment of your child, depending on the underlying cause.

TREATMENT

HOME CARE

- Keep a fluid-balance record during a child's serious illness at home. Record liquids taken in each day; use a measuring cup to estimate. Measure and record how much urine is passed each day. Ask your doctor if you need to save a specimen for testing.
- Weigh your child daily on an accurate home scale. Any sudden weight increase or decrease may indicate fluid changes.

MEDICATION

- For fluid loss in your child, your doctor may prescribe:
  - — Salt-containing drinks to make at home.
  - — Intravenous fluids during hospitalization.
- For fluid accumulation and sodium overload in your child, your doctor may prescribe diuretics and potassium supplements.

ACTIVITY

Your child should rest in bed until strength returns.

DIET & FLUIDS

For a serious fluid imbalance, your doctor may withhold solid food from the child until the fluid imbalance returns to normal.

OK FOR SCHOOL, PRESCHOOL, OR NURSERY?

Yes, after imbalanced fluids and electrolytes have returned to normal and sense of well-being will allow.

CALL YOUR DOCTOR IF

- Your child has symptoms of a fluid and electrolyte imbalance.
- Your child's weight increases or decreases 4 or more pounds in 1 day.

FOLLICULITIS, BACTERIAL

GENERAL INFORMATION

DESCRIPTION

Bacterial folliculitis is a superficial or deep bacterial irritation and infection of hair follicles of the skin. This is contagious. The skin anywhere on the body can be involved, but usually the condition affects the exposed areas of the arms, legs, and face.

Appropriate health care includes:

- Self-care after diagnosis.
- Physician's monitoring of general condition and medications.

SIGNS & SYMPTOMS

Pustules (small white blisters with pus inside) with the following characteristics:

- Pustules are yellow-white and surrounded by narrow red rings.
- Pustules are 1mm to 2mm in size; there may be few or many.
- Pustules discharge a blood-stained pus made from dead cells.
- Some pustules are pierced by hair; others may be adjacent to hair follicles.

CAUSES

- Infection of the hair follicles with staphylococcus bacteria, usually after a minor skin injury. Infection spreads to other parts of the child's body by fingernails, frequently from staphylococcus in the nose.
- Infection with pseudomonas bacteria following the use of contaminated hot tubs or spas. This is rare but increasing.

RISK FACTORS

- Recent illness such as a nose infection.
- Diabetes.
- Eczema or dermatitis.
- Crowded or unsanitary living conditions.

PREVENTING COMPLICATIONS OR RECURRENCE

- Keep the child's skin clean.
- Avoid hot, humid environments, which foster bacterial growth.

WHAT TO EXPECT

MEDICAL TESTS

- Your own observation of symptoms.
- Medical history and physical exam by a doctor.
- Laboratory culture of the discharge from the pustule.

POSSIBLE COMPLICATIONS

The infection may enter the child's bloodstream and spread to other body parts.

PROBABLE OUTCOME

Without treatment, an individual pustule heals in 7 days—but as some heal, new ones appear. Without treatment, boils or deep skin infections may develop. Treatment will shorten the course of your child's infection. Healing should be complete in 2 weeks. Recurrence is common.

TREATMENT

HOME CARE

- Urge your child not to scratch pustules. The germs that cause them can be transferred from under the fingernails to other parts of the body.
- Use warm-water soaks to relieve the child's itching and hasten healing.

MEDICATION

- If there are only a few pustules on your child, use non-prescription antibiotics, such as bacitracin, mycitracin, or neomycin. Apply and gently massage a small amount into the affected areas 3 or 4 times a day. Use only the small amount needed to cover—larger quantities don't help.
- If there are many pustules on your child, your doctor may prescribe injections or oral antibiotics, such as erythromycin or dicloxacillin, to fight infection.
- See Medications section for information regarding medicines your doctor may prescribe.

ACTIVITY

Your child can resume normal activities as soon as symptoms improve.

DIET & FLUIDS

No special diet.

OK FOR SCHOOL, PRESCHOOL, OR NURSERY?

Yes, but only after pustules have healed. This problem may be contagious to others, particularly young children.

CALL YOUR DOCTOR IF

- The pustules spread, despite treatment.
- Your child's temperature rises to 101F (38.3C).
- Your child's ankles swell.
- Your child develops a boil or signs of spreading infection.
- Symptoms of bacterial folliculitis recur after treatment.

FOLLICULITIS, FUNGAL

GENERAL INFORMATION

DESCRIPTION

Fungal folliculitis is a superficial or deep fungal irritation and infection of hair follicles of the skin. It is contagious. The skin on the hands, arms, legs, face, and scalp is involved.

Appropriate health care includes:

- Self-care after diagnosis.
- Physician's monitoring of general condition and medications (sometimes).

SIGNS & SYMPTOMS

Plaques (patches or flat areas) with clearly defined borders and pustules (small white blisters with pus inside) on top. Pustules are 1mm to 2mm in diameter and frequently appear in clusters.

CAUSES

A fungus infection that causes a small abscess next to the hair follicle.

RISK FACTORS

- Illness that has lowered your child's resistance.
- Diabetes.
- Eczema or dermatitis.
- Exposure to heat and high humidity.

PREVENTING COMPLICATIONS OR RECURRENCE

- Your child should protect the skin as much as possible from minor injury.
- Your child should avoid hot, humid environments.

WHAT TO EXPECT

MEDICAL TESTS

- Your own observation of symptoms.
- Medical history and physical exam by a doctor.
- Laboratory culture of the pustule.

POSSIBLE COMPLICATIONS

Bacterial folliculitis and fungal folliculitis are difficult to differentiate. Fungal folliculitis may be misdiagnosed in your child and treated with steroid creams, which aggravate the disorder.

PROBABLE OUTCOME

Usually curable in 6 weeks with treatment.

TREATMENT

HOME CARE

- Your child should avoid injury to the skin.
- Females should use depilatory creams instead of razors.
- Males should not shave during treatment until lesions on the face heal.

MEDICATION

- Your doctor may prescribe griseofulvin (an oral anti-fungal medication) and topical anti-fungal agents. Follow directions on the label.
- These medications may cause side effects or adverse reactions. Side effects usually disappear when your child's body adjusts to the drug or the drug is discontinued.
- Don't let the child use any medicine, including non-prescription medicine, without telling your doctor.
- See Medications section for information regarding medicines your doctor may prescribe.

ACTIVITY

No restrictions.

DIET & FLUIDS

No special diet.

OK FOR SCHOOL, PRESCHOOL, OR NURSERY?

Yes, after skin has healed.

CALL YOUR DOCTOR IF

- Your child has symptoms of fungal folliculitis.
- The following occurs during treatment:
  - — Signs of spreading infection (redness, swelling, warmth, pain).
  - — Fever over 101F (38.3C).
- New, unexplained symptoms develop. Drugs used in treatment may produce side effects.

FOOD ALLERGY

GENERAL INFORMATION

DESCRIPTION

Food allergy is a disorder caused by a hypersensitivity to a food.
Appropriate health care includes:

- Diagnostic measures including skin tests and elimination diets.
- Physician's monitoring of general condition and medications.

SIGNS & SYMPTOMS

Irregular but sometimes includes:

- Irritability.
- "Colic."
- Diarrhea.
- Eczema.
- Skin eruptions around the rectum.
- Stuffy nose.
- Vomiting.
- Asthma.
- Headache.
- Fatigue.
- Personality difficulties.

CAUSES

The most likely causes of food allergy are cow's milk, wheat, eggs, chocolate, peas, beans, tomatoes, nuts, spices, fresh fruit, and seafood. There are many other single causes, as well as the possibility that a particular combination of two or more foods may be the offender.

RISK FACTORS

Food allergy is more frequent in children from families in which other members have allergy problems.

PREVENTING COMPLICATIONS OR RECURRENCE

No preventive measures known. Recurrences may be prevented by your child avoiding foods that cause symptoms.

WHAT TO EXPECT

MEDICAL TESTS

- Your own observation of symptoms.
- Medical history and physical exam by a doctor.
- Trial of allergy elimination diet.

POSSIBLE COMPLICATIONS

None expected.

PROBABLE OUTCOME

Your child's food allergy can be controlled with diet. Complete cure may come after several symptom-free years. Some children never overcome allergies to some foods.

TREATMENT

HOME CARE

If your child has a skin rash due to food allergy, limit the number of baths as much as you can and do not allow the child to soak or play in the water. Children with eczema usually have very dry skin. Bathing causes further drying.

MEDICATION

- Medicines must be fitted to your child's own particular needs. Do not give any medicine (not even medicine you buy without a prescription) without telling your doctor. Doctors sometimes prescribe antihistamines, sympathomimetic drugs, or corticosteroids. If drugs are prescribed, carefully follow the instructions on the label.
- See Medications section for information regarding medicines your doctor may prescribe.

ACTIVITY

There should be no restrictions on your child's usual activities.

DIET & FLUIDS

- If your child is in early infancy, your doctor may prescribe discontinuing use of a cow's milk formula and substituting a milk-free formula or a meat-base formula.
- In later years, your doctor may prescribe having the child's total diet consist only of meat, cooked or canned fruit, potatoes, rice, and gelatin for a period of two weeks. Symptoms due to allergy should be relieved during this time. After the trial period of two weeks, carefully add other foods to the child's diet one at a time. Do not add more than one new food a week. If symptoms recur after adding a new food, eliminate it for at least a year.

OK FOR SCHOOL, PRESCHOOL, OR NURSERY?

Yes. If your child is not old enough to understand which foods are allergenic, make sure the teacher has a list—in writing—of foods the child should avoid.

CALL YOUR DOCTOR IF

- Your child's symptoms have not improved in two weeks.
- New symptoms develop.

FOOT STRESS-FRACTURE (March Fracture; Fatigue Fracture)

GENERAL INFORMATION

DESCRIPTION

A foot stress-fracture is a complete or incomplete hairline break in a foot (metatarsal) bone. This type of fracture may look similar to a bone tumor on an X-ray. Stress fractures may not become apparent for several weeks after pain begins in the foot. The metatarsal bones of the foot, the metatarsal joints, and the soft tissue around the fracture site, including muscles, nerves, tendons, ligaments, periosteum (covering of the bone), blood vessels, and connective tissue, are involved.

Appropriate health care includes:

- Physician's monitoring of general condition and medications.
- Physical therapy and rehabilitation.
- Self-care during rehabilitation.

SIGNS & SYMPTOMS

- Pain in the foot when the child is walking or running. Pain diminishes or disappears when the load is taken off the child's feet.
- Tenderness to the touch in the fracture area.

CAUSES

Fatigue of the child's foot bones caused by repeated overload, as with marching, walking, running, or jogging.

RISK FACTORS

- Walking, running, jogging, or standing for prolonged periods.
- History of bone or joint disease, especially osteoporosis.
- Obesity.
- Poor nutrition, especially calcium deficiency.

PREVENTING COMPLICATIONS OR RECURRENCE

Heed early warnings of an impending stress fracture, such as your child's complaining of foot pain after extended standing or walking. Adjust the child's activities before a fracture occurs. Ensure an adequate calcium intake (1000mg to 1500mg a day) with milk and milk products or calcium supplements.

WHAT TO EXPECT

MEDICAL TESTS

Your own observation of symptoms; medical history and physical exam by a doctor; X-rays of both feet and ankles (X-rays are often normal for the first 10 to 24 days after symptoms begin); radioactive technetium 99 scan (see Glossary), if symptoms are typical but the child's X-rays are negative.

POSSIBLE COMPLICATIONS

Complete fracture from continued stress on the child's foot after symptoms begin; pressure on or injury to nearby nerves, ligaments, tendons, blood vessels, or connective tissues; problems arising from plaster casts, splints, or other immobilizing materials (See Appendix 41, Care of Casts); an unstable or arthritic joint following repeated injury.

FOOT STRESS-FRACTURE (March Fracture; Fatigue Fracture)

PROBABLE OUTCOME

The average healing time for this fracture is 6 to 8 weeks with adequate treatment. Healing is considered complete when there is no pain at the fracture site and when X-rays show complete bone union.

TREATMENT

HOME CARE

Your doctor will probably apply a short, weight-bearing cast to your child's leg. For care of casts see Appendix 41.

MEDICATION

Your doctor may prescribe:
- Narcotic or synthetic narcotic pain relievers for severe pain.
- Stool softeners to prevent constipation due to inactivity.
- Acetaminophen or ibuprofen (available without prescription) for mild pain after initial treatment.
- See Medications section for information regarding medicines your doctor may prescribe.

ACTIVITY

Instructions for your child:
- Don't bear weight on the injured foot. Learn to walk with crutches, and use them through the first week with your walking cast. See Appendix 37 (Safe Use of Crutches). Prop your foot up whenever possible.
- Begin reconditioning and rehabilitation exercises as prescribed by your doctor.
- Resume normal daily activities gradually after treatment.

DIET & FLUIDS

No restrictions.

OK FOR SCHOOL, PRESCHOOL, OR NURSERY?

Yes, when condition and sense of well-being will allow.

CALL YOUR DOCTOR IF

- Your child has unexplained foot pain.
- Your child's toes become dark, blue, cold, or numb while the cast is on.

FROSTBITE

GENERAL INFORMATION

DESCRIPTION

Frostbite is temporary or permanent tissue damage from exposure to subfreezing temperature. The arms and legs (especially the fingers and toes) and the face (especially the nose and ears) are involved.

Appropriate health care includes:

- Self-care until medical help is available.
- Physician's monitoring of general condition and medications.
- Hospitalization (sometimes).
- Surgery to remove permanently damaged (gangrenous) tissue (sometimes).

SIGNS & SYMPTOMS

During exposure:

- Gradual numbness, hardness, and paleness in the affected area.

Upon rewarming:

- Pain and tingling or burning (sometimes severe) in the affected area, with color change from white to red, then purple.
- Blisters (severe cases).
- Shivering.
- Slurred speech.
- Memory loss.

CAUSES

Formation of ice crystals in the child's skin and blood vessels, leading to tissue injury or tissue death, depending on temperature and length of exposure.

RISK FACTORS

Diabetes mellitus; blood-vessel disease such as Raynaud's phenomenon (see Illnesses section); peripheral neuropathy (see Glossary); windy weather, which increases the chill factor; smoking; excess alcohol consumption.

PREVENTING COMPLICATIONS OR RECURRENCE

- Anticipate sudden temperature changes and encourage your child to carry a jacket, gloves, socks, hat, and scarf.
- Urge your child not to drink or smoke prior to anticipated exposure.

WHAT TO EXPECT

MEDICAL TESTS

- Your own observation of symptoms.
- Medical history and physical exam by a doctor.
- X-rays of the child's damaged areas.

POSSIBLE COMPLICATIONS

- Amputation of dead or infected tissue, especially fingers, toes, nose, or ears, following severe exposure.
- Cardiac arrest, if frostbite is accompanied by total body hypothermia.

PROBABLE OUTCOME

For mild cases, full recovery is possible with treatment for your child. Severe cases usually require amputation of the affected part.

TREATMENT

HOME CARE

The following instructions apply to emergency care for your child until medical care is available:

- Upon reaching shelter, remove clothing from the child's frostbitten parts.
- *Never* massage damaged tissue.
- Immerse the affected parts in warm water (about 100F or 37.8C). Use a thermometer, if available. Higher temperatures may cause further injury.
- Your child should drink warm fluids with a high sugar content, if available.
- Your child should not smoke.
- After rewarming, cover the affected areas on your child with soft cloth bandages.
- Don't let the child use affected limbs until there has been medical attention. If feet are involved, don't let the child walk.

MEDICATION

- Your doctor may prescribe:
  - — Analgesics, including narcotics, to relieve severe pain. Don't give the child strong pain killers longer than 4 to 7 days.
  - — Antibiotics to fight infection.
- Use non-prescription drugs, such as acetaminophen, for minor pain.
- See Medications section for information regarding medicines your doctor may prescribe.

ACTIVITY

Your child can resume normal activities after treatment.

DIET & FLUIDS

No special diet.

OK FOR SCHOOL, PRESCHOOL, OR NURSERY?

When appetite has returned and alertness, strength, and feeling of well-being will allow.

CALL YOUR DOCTOR IF

- Your child has symptoms of frostbite or you observe them in someone else.
- The following occurs during treatment: increased pain, swelling, redness, or drainage at the site of injury; fever, muscle aches, dizziness, or a general ill feeling.
- New, unexplained symptoms develop. Drugs used in treatment may produce side effects.

GALLSTONES (Cholelithiasis)

GENERAL INFORMATION

DESCRIPTION

Gallstones are in the gallbladder (the organ under the liver that stores bile). Most gallstones are composed primarily of cholesterol. They are not cancerous. The gallbladder and bile ducts are involved. They are more common in women, but adolescents and adults of both sexes can be affected. 10% of the U.S. population—and 20% of those over 40—have gallstones.

Appropriate health care includes:

- Self-care.
- Doctor's treatment.
- Surgery to remove the gallbladder and stones in the bile ducts.
- Medications and lithotripsy (shockwave treatment) can sometimes remove gallstones.

SIGNS & SYMPTOMS

- Colicky pain in the upper right abdomen or between the child's shoulder blades.
- Nausea and vomiting.
- Bloating or belching.
- Intolerance for fatty foods (indigestion, bloating, and belching).
- Jaundice.
- No symptoms in about 40% of cases.

CAUSES

Unknown, but following are the most common theories:

- Failure of the child's gallbladder to empty competently.
- Alterations in bile mucus.
- Increased bilirubin (see Glossary) concentration in bile.
- Infection in the tubes that carry bile out of the child's liver.

RISK FACTORS

- Recent illness, such as coronary-artery disease, cirrhosis of the liver, or disorder of the small intestine.
- Family history of gallstones.
- Genetic factors. Some ethnic groups are more susceptible. About 70% of Native Americans have gallstones.
- Obesity.
- Excess alcohol consumption.

PREVENTING COMPLICATIONS OR RECURRENCE

No specific preventive measures, except for your child to eat a low-fat diet (see Appendix 28).

GALLSTONES
(Cholelithiasis)

? WHAT TO EXPECT

MEDICAL TESTS

- Your own observation of symptoms.
- Medical history and physical exam by a doctor.
- Laboratory studies, such as blood count; blood chemistry; CAT or CT scan (see Glossary); and ultrasound (see Glossary).
- X-rays of the child's gallbladder.

POSSIBLE COMPLICATIONS

Infection or rupture of the gallbladder.

PROBABLE OUTCOME

Many children with gallstones have no symptoms. For those who do, the disorder is curable with surgery.

TREATMENT

HOME CARE

If your child has gallstones and experiences pain in the upper right abdomen, apply heat to the area. If the child's pain worsens or continues more than 3 hours, call your doctor.

MEDICATION

- For minor discomfort, use non-prescription drugs such as acetaminophen.
- Your doctor may prescribe oral medication to try to dissolve the child's stones. This treatment is still experimental.
- See Medications section for information regarding medicines your doctor may prescribe.

ACTIVITY

No restrictions, except for your child to rest during attacks of gallbladder colic.

DIET & FLUIDS

- During an attack, your child can sip water occasionally, but should not eat.
- At other times, the child should eat a low-fat diet (see Appendix 28).

OK FOR SCHOOL, PRESCHOOL, OR NURSERY?

When appetite returns and alertness, strength, and feeling of well-being will allow.

CALL YOUR DOCTOR IF

- Your child has symptoms of gallstones.
- Your child's temperature rises to 101F (38.3C) or higher.

GANGRENE

GENERAL INFORMATION

DESCRIPTION

Gangrene is dead tissue. Gangrene develops when a wound becomes infected or tissue is destroyed by an accident. Any body part can be affected, but the most common sites are the toes, feet, legs, fingers, hands, and arms. The most dangerous sites are abdominal organs.

Appropriate health care includes:

- Physician's monitoring of general condition and medications.
- Time in a decompression chamber to halt the progress of gangrene.
- Surgery to remove dead tissue, sometimes by amputation.
- Physical therapy, if amputation is necessary.
- Self-care during convalescence.

SIGNS & SYMPTOMS

- Black skin with dead underlying muscle and bone.
- Crepitation of the skin. This feels like pressing on air bubbles under the skin.
- Swelling.
- Pain.
- Bad-smelling discharge from ulcers in dead tissue.
- Moderate fever up to 101F (38.3C).

CAUSES

Gangrene occurs when blood flow to a body part is blocked or severely reduced. The following may interrupt your child's blood flow and cause gangrene:

- Infection with clostridia perfringens germs.
- Tissue injury caused by accidents, surgery, or deep puncture wounds.
- Crushing injury that cuts off the blood supply.
- Blood clot in an artery.
- Hardening of the arteries.
- Prolonged frostbite.

RISK FACTORS

Diabetes mellitus; smoking, which impairs blood circulation; excess alcohol consumption, which interferes with blood-vessel function.

PREVENTING COMPLICATIONS OR RECURRENCE

- If your child has diabetes, it is important to adhere closely to the treatment program to control diabetes. Examine the child's feet often for signs of unhealthy tissue. Keep your child's nails trimmed. The child should wear comfortable, well-fitting shoes.
- Consult your doctor if there are signs of infection (warmth, swelling, redness, pain, or tenderness) in your child's skin injury.

WHAT TO EXPECT

MEDICAL TESTS
- Your own observation of symptoms.
- Medical history and physical exam by a doctor.
- Laboratory blood cultures from the gangrene site.
- X-rays of any suspicious area to detect gas in tissues.

POSSIBLE COMPLICATIONS
Blood poisoning; shock; DIC (disseminated intravascular coagulation), a blood-clotting disorder; limb amputation to prevent death.

PROBABLE OUTCOME
Usually curable in the early stages with antibiotic treatment and surgery to remove dead tissue. Without treatment, gangrene is fatal.

TREATMENT

HOME CARE
After surgery or intensive hospital care:
- Wear sterile gloves to change your child's dressings.
- Place any material that touches ulcerated areas in double plastic bags and burn it.
- Whirlpool treatments and massages help increase your child's circulation.
- Your child should not smoke!

MEDICATION
Your doctor may prescribe: antibiotics—usually intravenously in the early stages—to fight infection; pain relievers; anticoagulants to prevent blood clotting.

ACTIVITY
Your child should rest in bed until gangrene stops progressing and healing begins. Then the child can resume activity gradually. Moving the legs frequently while in bed helps prevent blood clots in deep veins. The child may read or watch TV.

DIET & FLUIDS
- Serve a high-protein, high-calorie diet while your child's body is repairing damaged tissue.
- Give your child vitamin and mineral supplements, including zinc. The child should take 220mg of zinc orally twice a day.
- Encourage your child to drink adequate fluids (6 to 8 glasses daily).

OK FOR SCHOOL, PRESCHOOL, OR NURSERY?
Yes, after treatment is complete.

CALL YOUR DOCTOR IF
- Your child has symptoms of gangrene.
- Your child has persistent pain, despite medication and treatment.
- During convalescence, your child's temperature rises to 102F (38.9C) or higher.

GASTRIC EROSION

GENERAL INFORMATION

DESCRIPTION

Gastric erosion is a slight ulceration of the stomach lining. This is not contagious or cancerous. Gastric erosion affects all ages, but it occurs mostly in males. Appropriate health care includes:

- Self-care after diagnosis.
- Physician's monitoring of general condition and medications.

SIGNS & SYMPTOMS

- Vomiting blood. Blood may be bright red or resemble black coffee grounds.
- Blood in the child's stool. Blood will appear black or "tarry."

CAUSES

Probably caused by drugs that irritate the child's stomach lining. Most likely drugs are alcohol, caffeine, tobacco, aspirin, non-steroidal anti-inflammatory drugs used to treat arthritis and gout, and cortisone drugs used to treat asthma, Addison's disease, or other conditions.

RISK FACTORS

- Stress.
- Use of any oral medication.

PREVENTING COMPLICATIONS OR RECURRENCE

- Your child should not take medicines without enteric (protective) coatings.
- Your child should not drink alcohol if there has been gastric erosion. It may trigger bleeding.

WHAT TO EXPECT

MEDICAL TESTS

- Your own observation of symptoms.
- Medical history and physical exam by a doctor.
- Laboratory studies of the child's stool and blood tests for anemia.
- X-rays of the upper digestive tract.

POSSIBLE COMPLICATIONS

Bleeding is an uncommon but dangerous complication. Another major complication is perforation, in which the erosion penetrates the child's stomach wall. Surgery is necessary to correct either complication.

PROBABLE OUTCOME

Curable in 2 weeks with treatment if the cause is eliminated. Recurrence is common.

TREATMENT

HOME CARE

- Check your child's stool every day for signs of bleeding. If the stool is black, remove a stool portion from the toilet bowl and take it to your doctor's office for examination.
- Help your child avoid stressful situations (see Appendix 19).
- Urge your child not to smoke or drink alcoholic beverages.

MEDICATION

- Your doctor may prescribe H-2 blockers for your child to reduce production of stomach acid.
- For minor pain, use non-prescription antacids.
- See Medications section for information regarding medicines your doctor may prescribe.

ACTIVITY

Your child can resume normal activities as soon as symptoms improve.

DIET & FLUIDS

Your child should avoid hot and spicy foods. The child should eat small frequent meals for 2 weeks. Urge your child not to drink alcohol.

OK FOR SCHOOL, PRESCHOOL, OR NURSERY?

Not until symptoms subside and strength and sense of well-being will allow.

CALL YOUR DOCTOR IF

- Your child has signs of bleeding described in SIGNS & SYMPTOMS.
- Your child develops diarrhea. This may represent an adverse reaction to drugs used in treatment. The prescription may need adjustment.
- Your child has severe pain that is not relieved by treatment.
- Your child is unusually weak, pale, or lightheaded.
- Symptoms of gastric erosion recur after treatment.

GASTRITIS

GENERAL INFORMATION

DESCRIPTION

Gastritis is irritation, inflammation, or infection of the stomach lining. Appropriate health care includes:

- Self-care after diagnosis.
- Physician's monitoring of general condition and medications.
- Hospitalization (if bleeding with bright blood or coffee ground-looking material appears in vomitus, or the child's stools become black or tarry).

SIGNS & SYMPTOMS

- Mild nausea and diarrhea.
- Vomiting (occasionally).
- Abdominal pain and cramps.
- Loss of appetite.
- Fever.
- Weakness.
- Swollen abdomen.
- Sharp, dull, or annoying pain in the chest.
- Acid taste in the mouth.
- Belching or gas.

CAUSES

- Excess stomach acid caused by heavy drinking, smoking, or overeating (especially foods not easily digested).
- Food allergy.
- Virus infection. This form may be contagious.
- Adverse reaction to alcohol, caffeine, or drugs.
- Unknown (sometimes).

RISK FACTORS

- Stress.
- Improper diet.
- Illness that has lowered your child's resistance.
- Use of drugs, such as aspirin, non-steroidal anti-inflammatories, cortisone, caffeine, and many more.
- Fatigue or overwork.
- Excess alcohol consumption.
- Smoking.

PREVENTING COMPLICATIONS OR RECURRENCE

Instructions for your child:

- Eat and drink moderately.
- Avoid foods you find hard to digest.
- Don't smoke.
- Discuss with your doctor any medicines you take. Avoid medicines that irritate your stomach, if possible.

? WHAT TO EXPECT

MEDICAL TESTS

- Your own observation of symptoms.
- Medical history and physical exam by a doctor.
- Laboratory studies to measure your child's stomach acid.

POSSIBLE COMPLICATIONS

Bleeding is an uncommon but dangerous complication. Another major complication is ulceration or perforation, in which stomach acid erodes into or through the child's stomach wall. Surgery is necessary to correct either complication.

PROBABLE OUTCOME

Usually curable in a week if the cause is eliminated.

TREATMENT

HOME CARE

Consider lifestyle changes for your child (see Appendix 19).

MEDICATION

- For minor discomfort, use non-prescription antacids.
- Your doctor may prescribe additional medication, depending on the cause of your child's gastritis.
- See Medications section for information regarding medicines your doctor may prescribe.

ACTIVITY

Your child can resume normal activities as soon as symptoms improve.

DIET & FLUIDS

Instructions for your child:
Don't eat solid food on the first day of the attack. Drink liquids frequently, preferably milk or water. Resume a normal diet slowly, but avoid hot and spicy foods until symptoms disappear. For a well-balanced diet, see Appendix 24.

OK FOR SCHOOL, PRESCHOOL, OR NURSERY?

When appetite has returned and alertness, strength, and feeling of well-being will allow.

CALL YOUR DOCTOR IF

- Your child vomits blood.
- Your child's bowel movements become black or tarry.
- Pain becomes severe.
- Signs of dehydration, such as a dry mouth, wrinkled skin, excess thirst, or decreased urination, develop.

GASTROENTERITIS

GENERAL INFORMATION

DESCRIPTION

Gastroenteritis is irritation or infection of the digestive tract. Sometimes it is contagious to others. The stomach, small intestine, and large intestine are involved. Gastroenteritis can affect both sexes of newborns, infants, and children (0 to 5 years).

Appropriate health care includes:

- Home care.
- Physician's monitoring of general condition and medications.
- Hospitalization if your child has severe dehydration and needs intravenous fluids.

SIGNS & SYMPTOMS

- Vomiting.
- Diarrhea.
- Irritability.
- Poor appetite.
- Fever.

CAUSES

- Virus.
- Bacterial infection.
- Intestinal parasites.

RISK FACTORS

- Poor or improper diet.
- Illness that has lowered your child's resistance.
- Crowded or unsanitary living conditions.

PREVENTING COMPLICATIONS OR RECURRENCE

Wash your hands often with warm water and soap, especially before eating or handling your child, to avoid passing germs from hand to mouth.

WHAT TO EXPECT

MEDICAL TESTS

- Your own observation of symptoms.
- Medical history and physical exam by a doctor.
- Laboratory stool and blood studies.

POSSIBLE COMPLICATIONS

Possible dehydration with 10 or more liquid bowel movements in 1 day. Signs of dehydration in your child may include lethargy, sunken eyes, dry mouth, sunken fontanels (soft spots on a baby's head), wrinkled skin, and little or no urination.

PROBABLE OUTCOME

The child's condition should improve in 48 hours if the bowel is allowed to rest. If diarrhea or vomiting is so severe that the child cannot retain fluids, serious dehydration can occur.

TREATMENT

HOME CARE

- Check the child's rectal temperature once or twice a day. Don't check more often, to avoid stimulating diarrhea.
- Observe the child for signs of dehydration.
- Wash your hands after handling the child or before preparing food.

MEDICATION

- Don't use *any* non-prescription anti-diarrhea drugs without consulting your doctor. They can harm the child.
- See Medications section for information regarding medicines your doctor may prescribe.

ACTIVITY

Reduce the child's activity until the illness improves. The child may resume normal activity 24 hours after vomiting stops.

DIET & FLUIDS

Fluids are necessary, but the child's bowel needs rest.

- For a bottle-fed infant, prepare a mixture of 16 oz. (1 pint) water, 1/4 teaspoon salt, and 1 tablespoon sugar.
- For a breast-fed infant, consult your doctor for diet instructions.
- For an older child, offer the following clear liquids: apple, grape, or cranberry juice; sweetened herbal tea; "flat" cola or lemon-lime soda; gelatin and gelatin water; and bouillon.
- For an infant under 1 year, give 1/2 oz. of fluid every 20 minutes. For a child over 1 year, give 1 oz. every 30 minutes. Don't exceed these amounts during the first day or two, even if the child is not satisfied. Offer only as much as you intend the child to have. Don't supplement clear fluids with milk or solid food.
- When the child has been free of diarrhea for 1 day, offer one of the following low-residue foods: applesauce, banana, bread, cooked carrots, cooked cherries, eggs, ground meat, melon, noodles, cooked peaches, cooked pears, cooked peas, potatoes, rice, and sugar cookies.
- If diarrhea doesn't recur within 2 hours after the solid feeding, continue feeding the child from the preceding list for 24 hours. Gradually work back to a normal diet.

OK FOR SCHOOL, PRESCHOOL, OR NURSERY?

Only after all symptoms subside. Some forms of gastroenteritis are contagious to others.

CALL YOUR DOCTOR IF

- Your child's rectal temperature rises to 103F (39.4C) or higher.
- Your child shows signs of dehydration listed under POSSIBLE COMPLICATIONS.
- Your child doesn't improve in 48 hours despite treatment.
- An infant under 2 months old has symptoms of gastroenteritis.

GIARDIASIS

GENERAL INFORMATION

DESCRIPTION

Giardiasis is bowel inflammation caused by a parasite found in contaminated water. The gastrointestinal tract, especially the small bowel, is involved.
Giardiasis can affect both sexes, all ages, but is more common in children than in adolescents or adults.
Appropriate health care includes:
- Self-care after diagnosis.
- Physician's monitoring of general condition and medications.

SIGNS & SYMPTOMS

- Sudden diarrhea and abdominal cramping. Some children have only mild diarrhea and indigestion.
- Loose, bulky, bad-smelling stools.
- Slight fever.

CAUSES

Infestation of a microscopic parasite, giardia lamblia. Giardia parasites enter the child's body through food or water, and multiply in the small intestine. Local inflammation, causing diarrhea and other symptoms, occurs in 1 to 3 weeks.

RISK FACTORS

- Crowded or unsanitary living conditions, especially a substandard water supply and poor sanitation system.
- Drinking stream water while camping.
- Previous stomach surgery. Stomach acid normally provides some protection against this infection.

PREVENTING COMPLICATIONS OR RECURRENCE

- Boil water that is not known to be safe, or treat it with commercial chemical purifiers.
- Avoid serving your family uncooked foods that may have been rinsed in contaminated water.
- Wash your hands often, especially before meals, and teach your child to wash hands, to avoid catching infection from other persons.

WHAT TO EXPECT

MEDICAL TESTS

- Your own observation of symptoms.
- Medical history and physical exam by a doctor. Tell your doctor if your child has been traveling or camping in the previous month.
- Laboratory stool studies to detect parasites.

POSSIBLE COMPLICATIONS

- Chronic bowel inflammation.
- Malabsorption and weight loss.
- Dehydration.

PROBABLE OUTCOME

Spontaneous recovery in about a month for most children. Medication hastens recovery.

TREATMENT

HOME CARE

- Prevention is the best treatment. Urge your child to be cautious when away from normal water supplies.
- Your child should practice careful personal hygiene during an episode of diarrhea or if around someone who has diarrhea.

MEDICATION

- Don't give your child non-prescription drugs for gastrointestinal problems. These can mask symptoms.
- Your doctor may prescribe an anti-parasite drug, metronidazole, which is very effective. Alcohol interacts with metronidazole to cause abdominal cramps and nausea, so your child should not drink alcohol during treatment.
- See Medications section for information regarding medicines your doctor may prescribe.

ACTIVITY

No restrictions.

DIET & FLUIDS

Your child should maintain an adequate fluid intake (at least 8 glasses of water or liquid a day).

OK FOR SCHOOL, PRESCHOOL, OR NURSERY?

Yes, after all symptoms subside.

CALL YOUR DOCTOR IF

- Your child has symptoms of giardiasis.
- New, unexplained symptoms develop. Drugs used in treatment may produce side effects.

GILBERT'S SYNDROME (Hyperbilirubinemia)

GENERAL INFORMATION

DESCRIPTION

Gilbert's syndrome refers to increased blood levels of bilirubin (a yellow chemical byproduct of red blood cell breakdown). This condition is not contagious or malignant. It is probably inherited. The blood and liver are involved.

Appropriate health care includes:

- Doctor's diagnosis.
- No care necessary after an accurate diagnosis has been established.

SIGNS & SYMPTOMS

- Slight jaundice (yellow skin and eyes).
- No other symptoms (usually).

CAUSES

The liver is inefficient in changing bilirubin to bile, leaving above-normal levels of bilirubin in the child's blood. This causes jaundice. Any liver abnormality associated with this disorder is minor.

RISK FACTORS

- Stress.
- Poor nutrition, especially fasting.
- Genetic factors. This disorder is probably inherited.

PREVENTING COMPLICATIONS OR RECURRENCE

No specific preventive measures.

WHAT TO EXPECT

MEDICAL TESTS

- Your own observation of symptoms (sometimes). The minor jaundice may be unnoticeable.
- Medical history and physical exam by a doctor.
- Laboratory blood studies of bilirubin, liver function, bone marrow (sometimes), and liver biopsy (sometimes).

POSSIBLE COMPLICATIONS

Misdiagnosis of a serious liver disease as Gilbert's syndrome.

PROBABLE OUTCOME

The condition is harmless to your child.

GILBERT'S SYNDROME (Hyperbilirubinemia)

TREATMENT

HOME CARE

If you or others notice a yellowing of your child's eyes or skin—it may seem like a good suntan—see your doctor for a diagnosis. Some more serious conditions also begin with mild jaundice.

MEDICATION

- Medicine is not necessary for this disorder.

ACTIVITY

No restrictions.

DIET & FLUIDS

No special diet.

OK FOR SCHOOL, PRESCHOOL, OR NURSERY?

Yes.

CALL YOUR DOCTOR IF

Your child's skin looks a bit yellow.

GINGIVITIS

GENERAL INFORMATION

DESCRIPTION

Gingivitis is inflammation or infection of the gums. The gum tissue around the teeth is involved.

Appropriate health care includes:

- Self-care after diagnosis.
- Doctor's or dentist's treatment.
- Surgery to remove infected gum tissue, if other treatment fails.

SIGNS & SYMPTOMS

- Gums that are swollen, red, and soft around the child's teeth.
- Gums that bleed easily.
- Bad breath.
- Fever (sometimes).
- No pain.

CAUSES

- Poor nutrition, especially vitamin deficiencies that cause diseases such as scurvy or pellagra.
- Plaque (food particles, germs, and mucus at the base of the child's teeth).
- Blood disorders, including leukemia.
- Adverse reactions to drugs, such as anti-convulsants (primarily phenytoin and barbiturates).
- Exposure to lead and bismuth.

RISK FACTORS

- Diabetes.
- Poor nutrition, especially vitamin deficiency.
- Infections.
- Pregnancy.

PREVENTING COMPLICATIONS OR RECURRENCE

Instructions for your child:

- Practice good oral hygiene (see HOME CARE) to prevent plaque formation.
- Have regular dental checkups twice a year.
- Eat a well-balanced diet. Take vitamin supplements if you cannot eat well-balanced meals.

WHAT TO EXPECT

MEDICAL TESTS

- Your own observation of symptoms.
- Medical history and physical exam by a doctor.
- Laboratory culture of the plaque to identify the bacteria responsible for the child's infection.

POSSIBLE COMPLICATIONS

Extensive involvement may require painful, prolonged gum surgery for your child.

PROBABLE OUTCOME

Usually curable in 2 weeks with treatment.

TREATMENT

HOME CARE

Instructions for your child:

• Brush your teeth properly. Scrub clear, sticky plaque off the teeth daily with a soft toothbrush. Place the brush at the gum line and gently rotate it, pointing bristles toward the gum. Brush one section of teeth at a time. A soft brush is less likely to damage teeth and gums than a hard brush.

• Floss your teeth at least once a day. Use waxed or unwaxed dental floss. Wind most of it around the middle finger of each hand. Use index fingers as guides to force the floss between the teeth gently. Gently clean adjacent tooth surfaces with a back-and-forth sawing motion at the gum line. Floss between all upper teeth, using the thumbs as guides.

• Use a fluoride toothpaste.

• Make regular appointments with your dentist for cleaning and treatment of cavities.

MEDICATION

Your doctor or dentist may prescribe:

• Antibiotics to fight infection.

• Fluoride mouthwash.

• Vitamins, if your child has a deficiency.

• See Medications section for information regarding medicines your doctor may prescribe.

ACTIVITY

No restrictions.

DIET & FLUIDS

No special diet. Your child should avoid candy, sweet drinks, or sweet snacks. Sugar stimulates the production of acid, which attacks normal teeth. The best desserts are fruit and cheese, rather than ice cream or other high-sugar desserts.

OK FOR SCHOOL, PRESCHOOL, OR NURSERY?

Yes.

CALL YOUR DOCTOR IF

• Your child has symptoms of gingivitis.

• The following occurs during treatment:

— Bleeding increases.

— Pain becomes intolerable.

— Temperature rises to 101F (38.3C) or higher.

— Neck or face becomes swollen.

— Swallowing becomes difficult.

• New, unexplained symptoms develop. Drugs used in treatment may produce side effects.

GLAUCOMA, ACUTE INFANTILE

GENERAL INFORMATION

DESCRIPTION

Acute infantile glaucoma is a condition of a child's eye in which the fluid that normally drains into and out of the eye is suddenly obstructed. The obstruction causes the child severe pain and loss of vision. Glaucoma may develop soon after birth, or during infancy and adolescence.

Appropriate health care includes:

- Doctor's treatment. Call immediately. This is an emergency!
- Hospitalization during the attack until pressure in the child's eye decreases.
- Surgery (iredectomy with laser beam) to prevent further attacks—if other treatment is unsuccessful.

SIGNS & SYMPTOMS

- Extreme sensitivity to light.
- Severe, throbbing eye pain and headache.
- Redness in the child's eye.
- Blurred vision or halos around lights.
- Vomiting and weakness.
- Tender, firm eyeball.
- Dilated, fixed pupil.
- Swollen upper eyelid.
- Enlargement and clouding of the child's cornea.

CAUSES

Unknown.

RISK FACTORS

Family history of glaucoma or farsightedness.

PREVENTING COMPLICATIONS OR RECURRENCE

No known prevention measures for acute infantile glaucoma.

WHAT TO EXPECT

MEDICAL TESTS

- Medical history and physical exam by a doctor.
- Laboratory studies such as tonometry (measurement of pressure within the eyeball).

POSSIBLE COMPLICATIONS

Total blindness in the child's affected eye, if treatment is delayed or unsuccessful.

PROBABLE OUTCOME

Your child's symptoms can be controlled and infantile glaucoma can sometimes be cured if treatment begins quickly.

TREATMENT

HOME CARE

Follow post-operative instructions of your eye surgeon (ophthalmologist) if hospitalization was required, or your doctor's general instructions if hospitalization was not required.

MEDICATION

Your doctor may prescribe:

- Eye drops to lower pressure inside the child's eye. Follow the instructions and schedule carefully, even if your child's symptoms subside or the eye drops are occasionally uncomfortable.
- Diuretics to decrease fluid pressure in the child's eye.
- Pain relievers.
- See Medications section for information regarding medicines your doctor may prescribe.

ACTIVITY

After treatment, your child can resume normal activities gradually, but the child should avoid fatigue.

DIET & FLUIDS

Your child should adhere to a low-salt diet.

OK FOR SCHOOL, PRESCHOOL, OR NURSERY?

Yes, after successful treatment.

CALL YOUR DOCTOR IF

- Your child has symptoms of acute glaucoma. This is an emergency!
- New, unexplained symptoms develop. Drugs used in treatment may produce side effects.

GLOMERULONEPHRITIS (Post-Infectious, Acute or Chronic Glomerulonephritis)

GENERAL INFORMATION

DESCRIPTION

Glomerulonephritis is an inflammation of the glomeruli (small, round filters in the kidney). Damaged glomeruli cannot effectively filter waste products from the bloodstream. The kidneys are involved. Glomerulonephritis can affect both sexes, all ages, but is most common in children 1 to 11 years of age.

Appropriate health care includes:

- Self-care after diagnosis.
- Physician's monitoring of general condition and medications.
- Hospitalization (severe cases).

SIGNS & SYMPTOMS

Mild glomerulonephritis produces no symptoms. Diagnosis is possible only with urine studies. Severe glomerulonephritis produces the following: smoky or slightly red urine; general ill feeling; drowsiness; nausea or vomiting; headaches; fever (sometimes); loss of appetite; decreased urination; fluid accumulation in the child's body, especially puffy eyes and ankles; shortness of breath; high blood pressure; protein in the child's urine; disturbed vision.

CAUSES

- Classic acute glomerulonephritis follows a streptococcal infection. The most common infection sites are the throat and skin. Kidney symptoms usually begin 2 or 3 weeks after the child's strep infection.
- Chronic glomerulonephritis is rare and may have different causes than acute glomerulonephritis.

RISK FACTORS

Exposure to people in public places where strep infections can be transmitted to your child.

PREVENTING COMPLICATIONS OR RECURRENCE

- Your child should avoid exposure to people with strep infection.
- Consult your doctor for antibiotic treatment for your child of any infection that may be strep.

WHAT TO EXPECT

MEDICAL TESTS

- Your own observation of symptoms.
- Medical history and physical exam by a doctor.
- Laboratory studies, such as blood counts, repeated urinalyses to determine the presence of protein or other abnormal elements, and streptococcal antibody titer (a sophisticated blood study).
- Kidney-function tests.
- Radionuclide scan and MRI (see Glossary for all).

POSSIBLE COMPLICATIONS

Kidney failure, which may require dialysis or other dramatic treatment.

GLOMERULONEPHRITIS (Post-Infectious, Acute or Chronic Glomerulonephritis)

PROBABLE OUTCOME

Symptoms subside in 2 weeks to several months. Over 90% of children recover without complications. (Adults recover also—but more slowly).

TREATMENT

HOME CARE

- Record your child's temperature 3 times a day.
- Collect and record the amount of urine your child passes in each 24-hour period. Some of this collection will be analyzed in the doctor's office.

MEDICATION

Your doctor may prescribe:

- Cortisone or cytotoxic drugs, if the child's illness is severe.
- Diuretics to increase urination.
- Anti-hypertensives, if high blood pressure accompanies the illness.
- Iron and vitamin supplements, if anemia develops.

ACTIVITY

- Your child should stay in bed, except to go to the bathroom, until all signs of illness have passed. This may be several weeks or months. Bed rest ensures an adequate blood flow to the kidney; blood flow is best when lying down. The child may read or watch TV.
- Your child can resume normal activities after recovery. Your doctor will determine when all signs and symptoms have disappeared.

DIET & FLUIDS

As long as your child's kidneys function properly, the child may eat a normal, well-balanced diet. Greatly decrease the sodium in your diet.

OK FOR SCHOOL, PRESCHOOL, OR NURSERY?

Not until your physician clears your child for normal activities.

CALL YOUR DOCTOR IF

- Your child has symptoms of glomerulonephritis.
- The following occur during treatment: severe headache or convulsion; failure to pass at least 22 ounces of urine in a 24-hour period; fever; skin rash; increased fluid retention; increased nausea, vomiting, or diarrhea.

GONORRHEA

GENERAL INFORMATION

DESCRIPTION

Gonorrhea is an infectious disease of the reproductive organs that is sexually transmitted (venereal disease). The urethra in males, the urethra and reproductive system in females, and the rectum, throat, joints, and eyes (sometimes) in both sexes are involved. Gonorrhea can affect both sexes and all ages—even young children—of persons who have sexual contact with infected persons. Appropriate health care includes: physician's monitoring of general condition and medications; hospitalization for complications; self-care after diagnosis.

SIGNS & SYMPTOMS

- Burning urination.
- Thick green-yellow discharge from the penis or vagina.
- Little or no fever.
- Pain or tenderness with sexual intercourse (sometimes).
- Rectal discomfort and discharge (sometimes).
- Mild sore throat (sometimes).

Females often have few or no symptoms. Males usually have more pronounced symptoms.

CAUSES

Infection from gonococcus bacteria that grow well on delicate, moist tissue. The bacteria are usually transmitted sexually, but some cases are of unknown origin. Sexual activity involving the rectum or mouth may transmit infection to those areas if either partner is infected.

RISK FACTORS

Child sexual abuse; many sexual partners, whether heterosexual or homosexual; prostitution.

PREVENTING COMPLICATIONS OR RECURRENCE

- Your sexually active child should avoid sexual partners whose health practices and status are uncertain.
- Using a rubber condom during sexual intercourse is a good practice.
- Females should never use someone else's douche equipment.

OTHER

This condition must be reported to the local health department to prevent its spread. It sometimes occurs simultaneously with syphilis. Your cooperation is important, and your child's confidentiality will be maintained.

WHAT TO EXPECT

MEDICAL TESTS

Your own observation of symptoms; medical history and physical exam by a doctor; blood studies; laboratory culture and microscopic analysis of the discharge from the reproductive organs, rectum, or throat.

POSSIBLE COMPLICATIONS

- Gonococcal eye infection. This may cause blindness in children born of mothers who have gonorrhea.
- Blood poisoning (gonococcal septicemia).
- Infectious arthritis.
- Pelvic inflammatory disease.
- Epididymitis.
- Endocarditis.
- Sexual impotence in males, if untreated (sometimes).

PROBABLE OUTCOME

Usually curable in 1 to 2 weeks with treatment.

TREATMENT

HOME CARE

Instructions for your child:

- Use separate linens and disposable eating utensils during treatment.
- Wash hands frequently—especially after urination and bowel movements.
- Don't touch eyes with hands.
- Inform all sexual contacts so they can seek treatment.

MEDICATION

- Your doctor will prescribe antibiotics to fight the infection.
- Your child can take non-prescription drugs, such as acetaminophen or aspirin, to reduce discomfort—but not in place of antibiotics. Home remedies or folk-medicine treatments are ineffective.
- See Medications section for information regarding medicines your doctor may prescribe.

ACTIVITY

No restrictions, except not to resume sexual activity until a follow-up culture shows the infection is cured.

DIET & FLUIDS

No special diet. Your child should reduce consumption of caffeine and alcohol during treatment. These irritate the urethra.

OK FOR SCHOOL, PRESCHOOL, OR NURSERY?

When signs of infection have decreased, appetite returns, and alertness, strength, and feeling of well-being will allow.

CALL YOUR DOCTOR IF

- Your child develops symptoms of gonorrhea.
- Your child develops chills, fever, abdominal pain, swelling of the testicles, genital sores, or joint pain—either before or during treatment.
- New, unexplained symptoms develop. Drugs used in treatment may produce side effects.

GRANULOMA ANNULARE

GENERAL INFORMATION

DESCRIPTION

Granuloma annulare is a chronic skin disorder characterized by lesions that appear in the shape of a ring. This is not malignant or contagious. The skin on the bottoms of feet and backs of fingers, and on the hands, arms, elbows, legs, and knees is involved. Granuloma annulare can affect all ages but is most common in children (4 to 12 years).

Appropriate health care includes:

- Self-care after diagnosis.
- Physician's monitoring of general condition and medications, which may include injections of steroid medications into lesions.

SIGNS & SYMPTOMS

Papules (small raised bumps on the child's skin) with the following characteristics:

- Papules have a domed or slightly flat shape, 3mm to 6mm in diameter.
- Papules are non-scaling.
- Papules are pink or violet. Those on the lower extremities are darker than ones on other parts of the child's body.
- Papules don't itch or hurt the child.
- Multiple papules cluster in a ring. Ring diameters range from 1cm to 10cm.

Papules around the ring border are close but don't grow completely together. This gives the border a beaded appearance. The ring's center is often darker than the edge. Ringed lesions change in size and shape over a period of several weeks to 6 months.

CAUSES

Unknown.

RISK FACTORS

Injury to the child's skin, including sunburn.

PREVENTING COMPLICATIONS OR RECURRENCE

Your child should avoid injury to the skin. Protect the child's skin from sunburn with sunscreen or clothing.

WHAT TO EXPECT

MEDICAL TESTS

- Your own observation of symptoms.
- Medical history and physical exam by a doctor.
- Biopsy (see Glossary) to confirm diagnosis.

POSSIBLE COMPLICATIONS

- Papules and nodules occasionally ulcerate.
- Body temperature may rise if a large part of the child's body is covered with plastic dressing (see TREATMENT). If fever occurs, stop treatment.

PROBABLE OUTCOME
Spontaneous recovery within 2 years, but therapy hastens recovery.

TREATMENT

HOME CARE
Protect involved areas from injury.

MEDICATION
Your doctor may prescribe topical steroids with occlusion to hasten your child's healing. To use steroids:
- Gently rub a small amount of the steroid drug into the affected area.
- Reapply a small amount.
- Cover the affected area with clear kitchen plastic wrap. If your child's skin becomes dry and itchy, provide additional moisture by covering the affected area with a damp, clean cloth before applying the plastic wrap. You may also soak the affected area briefly in water after applying medicine to the child.
- Ask your doctor how often to change the plastic dressing.
- Reapply medicine every time you change the plastic dressing.
- See Medications section for information regarding medicines your doctor may prescribe.

ACTIVITY
No restrictions.

DIET & FLUIDS
No special diet.

OK FOR SCHOOL, PRESCHOOL, OR NURSERY?
Yes.

CALL YOUR DOCTOR IF
- Your child has symptoms of granuloma annulare.
- Lesions ulcerate.
- New lesions occur during treatment.
- Signs of infection, such as redness, swelling, pain, or tenderness, develop around the child's lesions.
- Your child becomes sensitive to the occlusive plastic dressing.
- New, unexplained symptoms develop. Steroid drugs used in treatment may produce side effects.

GRANULOMA, PYOGENIC

GENERAL INFORMATION

DESCRIPTION

Pyogenic granuloma refers to skin lesions composed of small blood vessels. These are not contagious or cancerous. The skin anywhere on the body, but most commonly on the face and shoulder, is involved. Pyogenic granuloma can affect children of both sexes (ages 5-15) and women during pregnancy.

Appropriate health care includes:

- Physician's monitoring of general condition and medications.
- Surgery or cryotherapy (see Glossary) to remove papules.
- Self-care after surgery.

SIGNS & SYMPTOMS

Papules (small raised bumps on the child's skin) with the following characteristics:

- Papules appear first as pinhead-sized but grow rapidly within weeks to full size (2mm to 20mm).
- Papules bleed easily when injured.
- Papules don't hurt or itch.

CAUSES

Unknown. Pyogenic refers to an infectious process, but these lesions are misnamed. Because they frequently appear in late childhood or pregnancy, hormonal changes may be a factor in their development.

RISK FACTORS

Pregnancy.

PREVENTING COMPLICATIONS OR RECURRENCE

Cannot be prevented at present.

OTHER

Because pyogenic granuloma resembles melanoma (skin cancer), medical diagnosis is important for your child.

WHAT TO EXPECT

MEDICAL TESTS

- Your own observation of symptoms.
- Medical history and physical exam by a doctor.
- Biopsy (see Glossary).

POSSIBLE COMPLICATIONS

None expected.

PROBABLE OUTCOME

Spontaneous recovery, usually within 2 to 6 months. Recurrence is common.

TREATMENT

HOME CARE

After your child's surgery:

- Apply rubbing alcohol to the scab twice a day.
- Apply an adhesive bandage to the scab during the day. Leave it uncovered at night.
- Wash the wound as usual. Dry gently and completely after the child bathes or swims.

MEDICATION

- For minor pain, use non-prescription drugs, such as acetaminophen or aspirin.
- If the child's scab cracks or oozes, apply a non-prescription antibiotic ointment several times a day.
- See Medications section for information regarding medicines your doctor may prescribe.

ACTIVITY

No restrictions.

DIET & FLUIDS

No special diet.

OK FOR SCHOOL, PRESCHOOL, OR NURSERY?

Yes. Not contagious to others.

CALL YOUR DOCTOR IF

- Your child has symptoms of pyogenic granuloma.
- The child's wound bleeds after surgery, and bleeding cannot be stopped by applying pressure for 10 minutes.
- The child's wound shows signs of infection, such as redness, swelling, pain, or increased tenderness.

GROIN STRAIN

GENERAL INFORMATION

DESCRIPTION

A groin strain is injury to the muscles or tendons in the area of the groin where the abdomen meets the thigh. Muscles, tendons, and bones comprise units. These units stabilize the pelvis and allow its motion. A strain occurs at a unit's weakest part. This injury occurs mainly in older adolescents and adults; it rarely affects younger children. Appropriate health care includes doctor's diagnosis; self-care; physical therapy (moderate or severe strain); surgery (severe strain).

SIGNS & SYMPTOMS

- Pain in the child's groin with motion or stretching the leg at the hip joint.
- Muscle spasm in the abdomen or thigh.
- Swelling in the child's groin.
- Loss of strength (moderate or severe strain).
- Crepitation ("crackling") feeling and sound when the child's injured area is pressed with fingers.
- Calcification of a muscle or its tendon (visible with X-ray).

CAUSES

- Prolonged overuse of muscle-tendon units in the groin.
- A single violent injury, or force applied to a groin muscle-tendon unit.

RISK FACTORS

Contact sports; sports that require quick starts, such as the beginning of a race; any cardiovascular medical problem that results in decreased circulation; medical history of any bleeding disorder; obesity; poor nutrition; previous groin injury; poor muscle conditioning.

PREVENTING COMPLICATIONS OR RECURRENCE

Your child should participate in a strengthening and conditioning program appropriate for each sport. Warming up before each practice or competition is important.

WHAT TO EXPECT

MEDICAL TESTS

Your own observation of symptoms; medical history and physical exam by a doctor; X-rays of the child's injured hip, thigh, and pelvis to rule out possible fractures.

POSSIBLE COMPLICATIONS

Prolonged healing time if activity is resumed too soon; proneness to repeated injury; an unstable or arthritic hip following repeated injury; inflammation at the attachment to the child's bone (periostitis); prolonged disability (sometimes).

PROBABLE OUTCOME

If this is a first-time injury, proper care and sufficient healing time before your child resumes activity should prevent permanent disability. Average times are: mild strain—2 to 10 days; moderate strain—10 days to 6 weeks; severe strain—6 to 10 weeks. If this is a repeat injury, the complications listed above are more likely to occur.

TREATMENT

FIRST AID

Use instructions for R.I.C.E., the first letters of *rest*, *ice*, *compression*, and *elevation*. Raise the foot of the bed on blocks. See Appendix 39 for details.

HOME CARE

- Use ice massage 3 or 4 times a day for 15 minutes at a time. Fill a large Styrofoam cup with water and freeze. Tear a small amount of foam from the top so ice protrudes. Massage firmly over the injured area in a circle about the size of a softball.
- After the first 24 hours, apply heat instead of ice, if it feels better to the child. Use heat lamps, hot soaks, hot showers, heating pads, or heat liniments and ointments.
- Support the injured groin area with an elasticized bandage between treatments.
- Begin rehabilitation exercises for the child, as prescribed by your doctor.

MEDICATION

- For minor discomfort, use aspirin, acetaminophen, or ibuprofen; topical liniments and ointments.
- Your doctor may prescribe stronger pain relievers; injection of a long-acting local anesthetic to reduce pain; injection of a corticosteroid, such as triamcinolone, to reduce inflammation.

ACTIVITY

- For a moderate or severe strain, the child should walk with crutches for at least 72 hours. See Appendix 37 (Safe Use of Crutches).
- The child can resume normal activities gradually.

DIET & FLUIDS

Your child should eat a well-balanced diet that includes extra protein, such as meat, fish, poultry, cheese, milk, and eggs. Increase the child's fiber and fluid intake to prevent constipation that may result from decreased activity.

OK FOR SCHOOL, PRESCHOOL, OR NURSERY?

Yes, when condition and well-being will allow.

CALL YOUR DOCTOR IF

- Your child has symptoms of a groin strain.
- Pain or swelling worsens despite treatment.

GUILLAIN-BARRÉ SYNDROME (Infectious Polyneuritis; Acute Idiopathic Polyneuritis)

GENERAL INFORMATION

DESCRIPTION

Guillain-Barré syndrome is an inflammatory condition of nerves and muscles that causes rapid weakness and loss of sensation. The central nervous system—including the brain, the coverings of the brain (meninges), and the spinal cord—and peripheral nerves and muscles are involved. Guillain-Barré syndrome can affect both sexes, all ages, but occurs far more commonly in adults than children.

Appropriate health care includes:

- Physician's monitoring of general condition and medications.
- Hospitalization.
- Self-care after diagnosis.

SIGNS & SYMPTOMS

Early stages:

- Muscle weakness in hands and feet, arms and legs, abdomen and chest. The weakness spreads within 72 hours; it may create life-threatening breathing difficulty for your child.
- Shock (weakness, faintness, cold hands and feet, rapid heartbeat, sweating).

Later stages:

- Complete paralysis (sometimes) for weeks or months.

CAUSES

Unknown, but it may be an autoimmune disorder. It sometimes follows an immunization or minor surgery.

RISK FACTORS

- Recent surgery.
- Recent immunization.
- Recent illness, such as a minor respiratory infection, gastroenteritis, Hodgkin's disease, or lupus erythematosus.

PREVENTING COMPLICATIONS OR RECURRENCE

Cannot be prevented at present.

WHAT TO EXPECT

MEDICAL TESTS

- Your own observation of symptoms.
- Medical history and physical exam by a doctor.
- Laboratory study of spinal fluid.

POSSIBLE COMPLICATIONS

- Paralysis of eyelid muscles, resulting in eye damage.
- Thrombophlebitis.
- Pneumonia.
- Respiratory failure.
- Pressure sores, if the child is immobilized.
- Constipation or fecal impaction.

GUILLAIN-BARRÉ SYNDROME (Infectious Polyneuritis; Acute Idiopathic Polyneuritis)

PROBABLE OUTCOME

Complete recovery without residual effects in most cases. Some persons recover in 15 to 20 days, while others require a year or more. Many mechanical devices can aid mobility until your child recovers.

TREATMENT

HOME CARE

- Urge your child to remain mentally and socially active during recovery.
- Encourage coughing to rid the child's lungs of mucus.

MEDICATION

Your doctor may prescribe:

- Laxatives to prevent constipation.
- Cortisone drugs, although they are not always effective.
- See Medications section for information regarding medicines your doctor may prescribe.

ACTIVITY

Your child should remain as active as muscle strength permits. Have a family member or visiting nurse passively move and stretch the child's muscles.

DIET & FLUIDS

No special diet. Your child should drink at least 8 glasses of fluid a day to prevent constipation.

OK FOR SCHOOL, PRESCHOOL, OR NURSERY?

No, not until the illness has run its course and the child's strength returns to normal.

CALL YOUR DOCTOR IF

- Your child has symptoms of Guillain-Barré syndrome.
- The following occurs during treatment:
  - — Fever.
  - — Breathing difficulty.
  - — Sores on the child's skin.
  - — Vision changes.
  - — Swollen or tender calves.
  - — Constipation.
- New, unexplained symptoms develop. Drugs used in treatment may produce side effects.

GYNECOMASTIA

GENERAL INFORMATION

DESCRIPTION

Gynecomastia means development of breast tissue in males. Boys have mammary glands just as girls do. Normally, all males have a low grade of female hormones (estrogens) as well as male hormones (testosterones or androgens) in their bodies. If the balance becomes disrupted, gynecomastia can result—some degree of gynecomastia may develop in as many as half of all boys. Appropriate health care includes:

- Evaluation by your son's personal physician.
- Surgery (rarely) for cosmetic purposes.

SIGNS & SYMPTOMS

- Slight swelling of the dark brown area surrounding both nipples (areola), beginning at puberty (usually between 10 and 16 years for boys).
- Swelling increases in warm weather.
- Rare, minor pain in enlarged area—worse when participating in sports activities.
- Size can vary from a barely noticeable "button" to a significantly enlarged breast, similar to a woman's.

CAUSES

- Sensitivity to normal hormonal changes in early puberty—the only common cause.
- *Rare causes:*
  —Mistakenly taking pills with estrogen (such as birth-control pills).
  —Testicular tumors.
  —Adrenal tumors.
  —Inherited factors.
  —Brain tumor.
  —Alcohol and other drug abuse, particularly marijuana.

RISK FACTORS

Inherited tendency toward gynecomastia.

PREVENTING COMPLICATIONS OR RECURRENCE

Keep substances containing estrogen away from children.

WHAT TO EXPECT

MEDICAL TESTS

- Physical exam and family history by a physician.
- Blood tests, radioactive tests, and X-rays to rule out rare causes (rarely needed).

POSSIBLE COMPLICATIONS

- Emotional and behavioral problems.
- Anxiety regarding not being a "male."
- Worry about possible tumors.

PROBABLE OUTCOME

As normal hormonal activity subsides at puberty (usually 12 to 18 months after the onset of gynecomastia), the condition disappears.

TREATMENT

HOME CARE

None, except providing your son with accurate information and offering emotional support.

MEDICATION

None.

ACTIVITY

No restrictions.

DIET & FLUIDS

No restrictions.

OK FOR SCHOOL, PRESCHOOL, OR NURSERY?

Yes.

CALL YOUR DOCTOR IF

- Your son's breasts become quite large at puberty and don't change in a reasonable time.
- Fluid seeps from the nipple of an enlarged male breast. (This may indicate a brain tumor.)

HAND, FOOT & MOUTH DISEASE

GENERAL INFORMATION

DESCRIPTION

Hand, foot and mouth disease is a virus infection that begins in the throat. The throat, tonsils, skin, gastrointestinal tract and central nervous system—including the brain, the coverings of the brain (meninges), and the spinal cord—and peripheral nerves are involved. Hand, foot and mouth disease is most prevalent in infants and young children (2 weeks to 3 years).

Appropriate health care includes:

- Home care.
- Physician's monitoring of general condition and medications.

SIGNS & SYMPTOMS

- Sudden fever.
- Sore throat with blisters and ulcers in the child's mouth and throat lining.
- Headache.
- Rash with blisters on the child's hands, feet, and groin.
- Loss of appetite.
- Abdominal pain (sometimes).

CAUSES

Infection from the Coxsackie virus A-16, which is transmitted from person to person.

RISK FACTORS

Summer and fall seasons.

PREVENTING COMPLICATIONS OR RECURRENCE

Prevent exposure of infants and young children to anyone with a respiratory illness.

WHAT TO EXPECT

MEDICAL TESTS

- Your own observation of symptoms.
- Medical history and physical exam by a doctor.

POSSIBLE COMPLICATIONS

- Convulsions with high fever (sometimes, especially in infants).
- Permanent brain damage caused by spread of infection to the child's central nervous system.

PROBABLE OUTCOME

Spontaneous recovery in 4 to 5 days.

TREATMENT

HOME CARE

- Dip a cotton applicator in 2% hydrogen peroxide, and apply to the blisters in the child's mouth.
- Rinse the child's mouth with salt water (1/2 teaspoon salt to 1 cup water) after eating, if the child is old enough to rinse without swallowing.
- Boil eating utensils and other items that touch the child's mouth or saliva—or use disposable utensils—to avoid transmitting the disease.
- Boil bottle nipples separately for 20 minutes before sterilizing a baby's formula in the bottles.

MEDICATION

- To reduce high fever, use non-prescription drugs such as acetaminophen. Antibiotics are not effective against this disease.
- See Medications section for information regarding medicines your doctor may prescribe.

ACTIVITY

Keep your child in bed until fever and other symptoms disappear. Normal activities may be resumed gradually.

DIET & FLUIDS

Encourage your child to increase fluid intake, including milk, liquid gelatin, ice cream, custard, or drinks made with syrup of wild cherry (available from your druggist). If drinking is painful, older children may use a straw.

OK FOR SCHOOL, PRESCHOOL, OR NURSERY?

When signs of infection have decreased, appetite returns, and alertness, strength, and feeling of well-being will allow.

CALL YOUR DOCTOR IF

- Your child has symptoms of hand, foot and mouth disease.
- The following occurs during treatment:
  — Fever of 101F (38.3C) or higher.
  — Skin lesions.
  — Significant weight loss (10% of body weight).
  — Signs of dehydration (wrinkled skin, weight loss, irritability, lethargy, and dry-looking tongue).
  — Pain in the child's neck or extremities.
  — Convulsion.
  — Decreased urination or dark urine.

HAND OR WRIST GANGLION
(Synovial Hernia; Synovial Cyst)

GENERAL INFORMATION

DESCRIPTION

A hand or wrist ganglion is a small, usually hard nodule lying directly over a tendon or a joint capsule on the back or palm of the hand or on the back of the wrist. Occasionally the nodule may become quite large. The back or palm of the hand, the tendon sheath (a thin membranous covering to the tendon), and any of the joint spaces in the hand are involved.

Appropriate health care includes:

• Doctor's care for diagnosis and possible injections of local anesthetic or cortisone.

• Surgery (usually). Surgery will be conducted under local or general anesthesia in an outpatient surgical facility or hospital operating room.

SIGNS & SYMPTOMS

• A hard lump over a tendon or joint capsule in the child's hand or wrist. The nodule "yields" to heavy pressure because it is not solid.

• No pain usually, but overuse of the hand may cause mild pain and aching.

• Tenderness if the lump is pressed hard.

• Discomfort with extremes of motion (flexing or extending) and with repetition of the exercise that produced the ganglion.

CAUSES

• Mild sprains and chronic sprains to a child's hand joint, causing weakness of the joint capsule.

• A defect in the fibrous sheath of the joint or tendon that permits a segment of underlying synovium (the thin membrane that lines the tendon sheath) to herniate through it.

• Irritation accompanying the herniated synovium, causing continued secretion of fluid. The sac gradually fills, enlarges, and becomes hard, forming the ganglion.

RISK FACTORS

• Repeated injury, especially mild sprains. Hand and wrist ganglions frequently occur in bowlers and tennis players and handball, racquetball, and squash players.

• Inadequate warmup prior to practice or competition.

PREVENTING COMPLICATIONS OR RECURRENCE

Your child should build strength with an appropriate conditioning program and should warm up before sports.

WHAT TO EXPECT

MEDICAL TESTS

• Your own observation of symptoms.

• Medical history and physical exam by a doctor.

• X-rays of the child's hand and wrist.

POSSIBLE COMPLICATIONS

- After surgery: excessive bleeding; surgical-wound infection; recurrence if surgical removal is incomplete.
- Calcification of the ganglion (rare).

PROBABLE OUTCOME

Ganglions sometimes disappear spontaneously, only to recur later. Surgery is often the only treatment to guarantee cure. After surgery, allow about 3 weeks for your child's recovery if no complications occur.

TREATMENT

HOME CARE

Immediately after surgery:

- If the child's wound bleeds during the first 24 hours after surgery, press a clean tissue or cloth to it for 10 minutes.
- Your child can bathe and shower as usual, washing the incision gently with mild unscented soap.
- Between baths, the child should keep the wound dry with a bandage for the first 2 or 3 days after surgery. If a bandage gets wet, change it promptly.
- The child can take whirlpool treatments, if available, after the wound heals.

MEDICATION

- Your doctor may prescribe pain relievers. Your child should not take prescription pain medication longer than 4 to 7 days. The child should use the minimum needed to control pain.
- Use non-prescription drugs, such as acetaminophen, for minor pain.

ACTIVITY

- The child can return to normal activity as soon as possible.
- The child should avoid vigorous exercise for 3 weeks after surgery.

DIET & FLUIDS

No restrictions.

OK FOR SCHOOL, PRESCHOOL, OR NURSERY?

Yes, when condition and sense of well-being will allow.

CALL YOUR DOCTOR IF

- Your child has signs or symptoms of a hand or wrist ganglion.
- Any of the following occur after surgery:
  — Increased pain, swelling, redness, drainage, or bleeding in the surgical area.
  — Signs of infection (headache, muscle aches, dizziness, or a general ill feeling, and fever).
- New, unexplained symptoms develop. Drugs used in treatment may produce side effects.

HAY FEVER
(Allergic Rhinitis)

GENERAL INFORMATION

DESCRIPTION

Hay fever is an allergic response to airborne allergens that affects the eyes and upper respiratory tract. The nose, eyes, sinuses, throat, mouth, and lungs are involved.

Appropriate health care includes:

- Self-care.
- Physician's monitoring of general condition, medications, and treatment for complications or severe illness.

SIGNS & SYMPTOMS

- Itching, watery eyes.
- Frequent sneezing; stuffy nose with a clear discharge.
- Itching in the roof of the child's mouth.
- Wheezing (sometimes).
- Cough (sometimes).

CAUSES

An allergic sensitivity in your child to airborne allergens such as:

- Pollen from weeds, flowers, grasses, and trees.
- Mold.
- Dust.
- Mites.
- Tobacco smoke and other air pollutants.

RISK FACTORS

- Medical history of allergic reactions, such as eczema or asthma.
- Smoking.
- Spring and autumn. Most plants produce pollen during these seasons.

PREVENTING COMPLICATIONS OR RECURRENCE

- Change furnace or air-conditioner filters often.
- Encourage your child to wear a filter face mask during exposure to allergens.
- Install an air-purification unit in your home's heating and air-conditioning system.

WHAT TO EXPECT

MEDICAL TESTS

- Your own observation of symptoms.
- Medical history and physical exam by a doctor.
- Laboratory tests such as a blood count and allergy skin tests (see Glossary).

POSSIBLE COMPLICATIONS

- Sleeping difficulty and chronic fatigue.
- Sinus infection.

PROBABLE OUTCOME

Symptoms can be controlled with treatment.

HAY FEVER (Allergic Rhinitis)

TREATMENT

HOME CARE

Eliminate as many allergens in your child's environment as possible. Prepare your child's bedroom as follows:

- Empty the room of furniture, rugs, or carpet, and drapes or curtains.
- Clean the walls, woodwork, and floors with a damp mop. Wax the floor.
- Take the mattress and box springs outside and vacuum or clean them.
- Cover the box springs, mattress, and pillows with plastic covers.
- Use only rugs that can be washed once a week.
- Use bedclothes that can be washed often, such as cotton sheets, washable mattress pads, and synthetic fiber blankets. Don't use chenille bedspreads, quilts, or comforters.
- Use wood or plastic chairs. Don't used stuffed chairs.
- Use plastic curtains, if possible. Dust them daily.
- Use a vacuum cleaner, damp rags, and a damp or oiled mop to clean the child's bedroom thoroughly once a week.
- Keep windows and doors closed as much as possible.
- Don't let the child handle objects that are very dusty, such as books or stored clothing.
- Don't keep stuffed animals or toys in the house.
- Remove *all* pets (except fish) from the house.

MEDICATION

To reduce the child's allergic response, your doctor may prescribe:

- Antihistamines, decongestants, cortisone eye drops or nasal spray, cortisone tablets (severe cases only), or cromolyn nasal spray. These medications relieve the child's symptoms, but they don't cure hay fever.
- Desensitization injections for known allergens.
- See Medications section for information regarding medicines your doctor may prescribe.

ACTIVITY

No restrictions.

DIET & FLUIDS

Your child should avoid foods that cause allergic reactions.

OK FOR SCHOOL, PRESCHOOL, OR NURSERY?

Yes. This condition is not contagious.

CALL YOUR DOCTOR IF

- Your child has severe symptoms of hay fever that are interfering with normal activities.
- Signs of infection appear, such as fever, headache, muscle aches, or thick, discolored nasal discharge. A sinus infection may be complicating the child's allergy.
- New, unexplained symptoms develop. Drugs used in treatment may produce side effects.

HEAD INJURY

GENERAL INFORMATION

DESCRIPTION

A head injury can occur with or without unconsciousness or other visible signs. Appropriate health care includes:

- Home care.
- Physician's monitoring of general condition and medications.
- Hospitalization for observation, if signs and symptoms are severe.

SIGNS & SYMPTOMS

Depends on the extent of your child's injury. The presence or absence of swelling at the injury site is not related to the seriousness of the injury. See also Head Injury, Skull Fracture in Illnesses section. Signs and symptoms include any or all of the following:

- Drowsiness or confusion.
- Vomiting and nausea.
- Blurred vision.
- Pupils of different size.
- Loss of consciousness—either temporarily or for long periods.
- Amnesia or memory lapses.
- Irritability.
- Headache.
- Bleeding of the child's scalp, if the skin is broken.

CAUSES

Injury. The worst injuries usually result from motor-vehicle accidents.

RISK FACTORS

- Contact sports, especially football or boxing.
- Seizure disorders.
- Excess alcohol consumption.

PREVENTING COMPLICATIONS OR RECURRENCE

- Urge your child not to drink or use mind-altering drugs and drive.
- Encourage your child to wear protective headgear for contact sports and cycling.
- Use your auto seat belt or shoulder harness and encourage everyone in the family to do the same. Place young children in safety car seats.

WHAT TO EXPECT

MEDICAL TESTS

- Your own observation of symptoms.
- Medical history and physical exam by a doctor.
- Laboratory studies of your child's blood and cerebrospinal fluid.
- X-rays of the child's skull and neck.
- CAT or CT Scan (computerized axial tomography) of the head: Non-invasive computerized X-ray images that show sections (or "slices") of an organ or region of the body clearly and precisely (see Glossary).

POSSIBLE COMPLICATIONS

- Bleeding under the skull (subdural hemorrhage and hematoma).
- Bleeding into the brain.

PROBABLE OUTCOME

Usually curable with early recognition of danger signs and medical treatment. Complications can be life-threatening to your child or cause permanent disability.

TREATMENT

HOME CARE

- The extent of injury can be determined only with careful examination and observation. After a doctor's examination, your injured child may be sent home—but a responsible person must stay and watch the child for serious symptoms. The first 24 hours after injury are critical, although serious aftereffects can appear later.
- If you are watching the patient, it is important to awaken the child every hour for 24 hours. Report to the doctor immediately if you can't awaken or arouse the child. Report also any of the following:
  - — Vomiting.
  - — Inability to move arms and legs equally well on both sides.
  - — Temperature above 100F (37.8C).
  - — Stiff neck.
  - — Pupils of unequal size or shape.
  - — Convulsions.
  - — Noticeable restlessness.
  - — Severe headache that persists longer than 4 hours after injury.
  - — Confusion.

MEDICATION

- Don't give *any* medicine—including non-prescription acetaminophen or aspirin—until the diagnosis is certain.
- See Medications section for information regarding medicines your doctor may prescribe.

ACTIVITY

Your child should rest in bed until the doctor determines the danger is over. Normal activity may then be resumed as symptoms improve.

DIET & FLUIDS

Full liquid diet for the child until the danger passes.

OK FOR SCHOOL, PRESCHOOL, OR NURSERY?

When appetite has returned and alertness, strength, and feeling of well-being will allow.

CALL YOUR DOCTOR IF

Your child has symptoms of a head injury or you observe them in someone else.

ILLNESSES

HEAD INJURY, SKULL FRACTURE

GENERAL INFORMATION

DESCRIPTION

A skull fracture may be either a closed, or simple, break in the bone, leaving the skin or bone covering (periosteum) intact, or an open, or compound, break that breaks the skin and periosteum.

Appropriate health care includes: doctor's diagnosis and care; hospitalization (serious skull fractures); home care if hospitalization is not necessary.

SIGNS AND SYMPTOMS

- Pain and swelling over the skull fracture.
- Bruising over the fracture and around the child's eyes and nose.
- Profuse bleeding from the scalp if the skin is broken.
- Leakage of clear fluid (cerebrospinal fluid) into the ear or nose.
- Additional signs, if brain damage accompanies the skull fracture: drowsiness or confusion; vomiting and nausea; blurred vision; loss of consciousness—either temporarily or for long periods; amnesia or memory lapses; irritability; headache.

CAUSES

A direct blow to the child's head.

RISK FACTORS

- Contact sports, especially if the child's head is not protected adequately.
- Sports that involve heavy equipment such as baseball bats or golf clubs, or sports in which falling on the head is possible, such as basketball, gymnastics, diving, or cycling.

PREVENTING COMPLICATIONS OR RECURRENCE

Your child should wear a protective helmet or other appropriate headgear during athletic activity in which head injury is possible.

WHAT TO EXPECT

MEDICAL TESTS

Your own observation of symptoms; physical exam by a doctor (the total extent of injury may not be apparent for 48 to 72 hours); X-rays and CAT scan of the head and neck; laboratory studies of blood and cerebrospinal fluid.

POSSIBLE COMPLICATIONS

- Hematoma (a collection of blood) that creates pressure on the brain. This can cause permanent brain damage or death, depending on the extent of injury.
- Infection if skin over the skull fracture is broken.

PROBABLE OUTCOME

Most skull fractures without complications heal within 4 to 6 weeks.

Complications can be life-threatening or cause permanent brain damage (see HOME CARE below).

TREATMENT

FIRST AID

Use instructions for R.I.C.E. See Appendix 39 for details. This is critical to minimize bleeding and swelling!

HOME CARE

After a doctor's examination, the injured child may be sent home—but a responsible person must watch for symptoms. The first 24 hours are critical, but serious aftereffects can appear later. Awaken the child every hour for 24 hours. Report to the doctor immediately if you can't arouse the child of if there is vomiting, inability to move arms and legs equally well on both sides, temperature above 100F (37.8C), stiff neck, pupils of unequal size or shape, convulsions, noticeable restlessness, severe headache that persists longer than 4 hours after injury, or confusion.

MEDICATION

Don't give *any* medicine—including non-prescription acetaminophen or aspirin—until the extent of the child's injury is certain.

ACTIVITY

The child should rest in bed until the doctor determines that the danger of complications—especially hematomas—is over. Normal activity may then be resumed as symptoms improve.

DIET & FLUIDS

Your child should have only liquids until the danger of complications passes.

OK FOR SCHOOL, PRESCHOOL, OR NURSERY?

Yes, when condition and sense of well-being will allow.

CALL YOUR DOCTOR IF

- Your child has signs of a skull fracture after a blow to the head.
- After returning home, any symptoms appear that are listed under HOME CARE.

HEADACHE, MIGRAINE

GENERAL INFORMATION

DESCRIPTION

A migraine headache is an intense, incapacitating headache, accompanied by other symptoms, that occurs repeatedly in some children and adults. The blood vessels leading to the scalp and brain plus pain receptors in the brain are involved. Migraine headaches can affect both sexes but are more common in adolescent and adult females.

Appropriate health care includes:

- Self-care after diagnosis.
- Physician's monitoring of general condition and medications.

SIGNS & SYMPTOMS

The nature of attacks varies between children and from time to time in the same person. Symptoms of a classic migraine attack appear in the following sequence:

- Inability to see clearly, followed by seeing bright spots and zig-zag patterns. Visual disturbances may last several minutes or several hours, but they disappear once the headache begins.
- Dull, boring pain in the temple that spreads to the entire side of the child's head. Pain becomes intense and throbbing.
- Nausea and vomiting.

In other types of migraine attack, the above symptoms (vision disturbances, headache, or vomiting) may be absent, or other symptoms may be present. Some children become pale, with bloodshot eyes and a runny nose or eyes.

CAUSES

Constriction, then dilation and inflammation of blood vessels that go to the child's scalp and brain. Vision disturbances occur when blood vessels narrow. Headache begins when they widen again. Attacks may be triggered by:

- Tension. Emotional problems are probably the most common reason for migraine attacks, but headaches don't necessarily coincide with emotional upset. They often occur on weekends, when a child's stress is decreased.
- Menstruation.
- Fatigue.
- Use of contraceptives.
- Consumption of alcohol or certain foods.

RISK FACTORS

Stress; family history of migraines; use of many prescription and non-prescription drugs; smoking; excess alcohol consumption.

PREVENTING COMPLICATIONS OR RECURRENCE

- See Appendix 19 for suggestions to reduce your child's stress.
- An aspirin a day may prevent migraine attacks in older children and adults.
- Use of the drug propranolol prevents attacks in some children.

? WHAT TO EXPECT

MEDICAL TESTS

- Your own observation of symptoms.
- Medical history and physical exam by a doctor.
- Laboratory blood studies.
- CAT scan (see Glossary) of the head.

POSSIBLE COMPLICATIONS

None expected.

PROBABLE OUTCOME

Your child's symptoms can be controlled with treatment.

TREATMENT

HOME CARE

At the first sign of a migraine attack:

- Apply a cold cloth or ice pack to your child's head or splash the child's face with cold water.
- Give the child a non-prescription pain reliever, such as aspirin or acetaminophen.
- Urge your child to lie down in a quiet, dark room for several hours. The child should try to relax. Listening to music, sleeping, or meditating are suitable activities.

MEDICATION

Your doctor may prescribe:

- Antihistamines to expand the child's blood vessels.
- Anti-emetics to decrease nausea and vomiting.
- Vasoconstrictors to narrow the child's blood vessels.
- Pain relievers.
- Beta-adrenergic blockers to prevent attacks, if headaches are so frequent or severe that the child can't function normally. The medication may have undesirable side effects and it does not help everyone.

ACTIVITY

Your child should rest during attacks. Between attacks, exercise is desirable to achieve maximum fitness.

DIET & FLUIDS

Because some attacks are caused by foods, such as cheese or chocolate, keep a record of what your child ate before each attack. Your child should avoid foods that seem to trigger migraine attacks. Otherwise, no special diet is necessary.

OK FOR SCHOOL, PRESCHOOL, OR NURSERY?

When appetite has returned and alertness, strength, and feeling of well-being will allow.

CALL YOUR DOCTOR IF

- Your child has a migraine attack that persists longer than 24 hours, despite treatment.
- Frequent migraine attacks interfere with the child's normal life.

HEADACHE, TENSION OR VASCULAR

GENERAL INFORMATION

DESCRIPTION

Simple tension or vascular headaches include 3 types of pain: from muscle strain in the scalp, neck, and face; from constricted blood vessels in the head that cause pressure on blood-vessel walls; and from dilated blood vessels in the brain. Sensory nerves in the skin, scalp, blood vessels, and muscles of the head are involved.

Appropriate health care includes: self-care; physician's monitoring of general condition and medications, if headache persists or worsens despite self-care; biofeedback training or counseling for chronic headaches caused by stress.

SIGNS & SYMPTOMS

Any of the following:

- Moderate pain in the front or back of the head, accompanied by tight muscles in the neck or scalp.
- Constant pain over the temples, accompanied by the feeling that a vise is over the back of the head.
- Throbbing pain all over the head.

CAUSES

Tension, producing strain on muscles of the neck, scalp, face, and jaw; sleep disturbances; excessive eating or drinking; physically exhausting work; anxiety or depression; eye strain, including sun glare; use of drugs or alcohol; low blood sugar; hormone changes during the menstrual cycle; allergic reactions; maligned teeth.

RISK FACTORS

Stress, either mental or physical; environments that are noisy, stuffy, hot, poorly lit, or have irritating odors; exposure to or consumption of nitrites, sulfites, monosodium glutamate or other food additives.

PREVENTING COMPLICATIONS OR RECURRENCE

Instructions for your child: get enough sleep—an average of 8 hours for males and 7 hours for females; don't skip meals, especially breakfast; don't overeat; exercise regularly (see Appendix 19) to reduce tension and improve circulation; drink alcohol moderately—no more than 1 or 2 drinks a day, if at all; don't smoke cigarettes, and avoid smoky environments; don't use mood-altering, mind-altering, stimulant, or sedative drugs; avoid foods that contain nitrites or other additives to which you are sensitive.

WHAT TO EXPECT

MEDICAL TESTS

- Your own observation of symptoms.
- Medical history and physical exam by a doctor.
- Special studies that may include ultrasonography, CAT or CT scan, MRI, and radionuclide scan (see Glossary for all).

POSSIBLE COMPLICATIONS

None expected for a simple headache.

PROBABLE OUTCOME

Most tension or vascular headaches can be relieved with simple treatment (see below).

TREATMENT

HOME CARE

Urge your child to stop any activity and try to relax:

- Massage the child's shoulders, neck, jaw, and scalp.
- Give your child a hot bath.
- Encourage the child to lie down. Place a warm or cold cloth, whichever feels better, over the aching area.

MEDICATION

Give your child acetaminophen or aspirin to relieve pain. Your child should try not to get dependent on stronger, prescription-type pain killers, sedatives, or tranquilizers.

ACTIVITY

Your child should rest in a quiet room.

DIET & FLUIDS

- Most children feel better if they don't eat, unless the headache is from low blood sugar.
- Urge your child not to drink alcohol.

OK FOR SCHOOL, PRESCHOOL, OR NURSERY?

When appetite has returned and alertness, strength, and feeling of well-being will allow.

CALL YOUR DOCTOR IF

Your child has a headache and any of the following:

- Fever of 101F (38.3C) or higher.
- Recent head injury.
- Drowsiness.
- Nausea and vomiting.
- Pain in one eye.
- Blurred vision.
- High blood pressure.
- Pain and tenderness around the eyes and cheekbones that worsens when the child leans forward.
- Vision disturbances and vomiting prior to the headache.
- Persistent headache pain for longer than 24 hours without other symptoms.
- Suspicion that a prescription or non-prescription drug caused the headache.

HEARING IMPAIRMENT OR LOSS

GENERAL INFORMATION

DESCRIPTION

Hearing impairment or loss means a decreased ability or complete inability to hear. Classifications include the following: *conductive loss,* in which middle-ear bones degenerate and don't transmit sound waves (see Otosclerosis in Illnesses section); *sensorineural loss,* in which the 8th cranial nerve (the acoustic nerve) is damaged—often for unknown reasons; and *mixed loss,* involving both conductive and sensorineural disabilities. The middle-ear bones that conduct sound are involved, as are branches of the 9th cranial nerve that transmit sound to the brain.

Appropriate health care includes:

- Physician's monitoring of general condition and medications.
- Surgery for conductive-type deafness (sometimes).
- Speech therapy and rehabilitation, if necessary.

SIGNS & SYMPTOMS

In an infant:

- Lack of response to environmental sounds—especially startling sounds.

In an older child:

- Difficulty in discriminating (listening selectively) to environmental sounds.
- Ringing in the ears.
- Lack of speech or inarticulate speech.

CAUSES

- Drugs taken during the mother's pregnancy.
- Congenital, transmitted as a dominant or recessive genetic trait.
- Chronic middle-ear infections or spread of infection to the inner ear.
- Blood-vessel disorders, including hypertension.
- Head injury.
- Brain tumor.
- Blood clot that travels to the acoustic nerve.
- Multiple sclerosis.
- Syphilis.
- Blood-coagulation disorders.
- Prolonged exposure to sound levels of 85 decibels or above.

RISK FACTORS

- Family history of congenital or acquired deafness.
- Use of drugs, such as streptomycin, tobramycin, quinine, furosemide, ethacrynic acid, or heavy doses of aspirin.
- Children with hobbies or occupations involving high noise levels, such as rock musicians.

PREVENTING COMPLICATIONS OR RECURRENCE

- Your child should avoid prolonged use or overdosage of drugs that cause hearing loss.
- Obtain medical treatment for underlying disorders that cause hearing loss.
- Urge your child to avoid prolonged exposure to loud noise. If exposure is unavoidable, the ears can be protected with ear plugs.

HEARING IMPAIRMENT OR LOSS

WHAT TO EXPECT

MEDICAL TESTS

- Your own observation of symptoms.
- Medical history and physical exam by a doctor.
- Laboratory studies, such as blood studies, audiogram, Weber test, Rinne test, skull X-rays (see Glossary for all).

POSSIBLE COMPLICATIONS

- Permanent deafness.
- Delayed language development in a child.

PROBABLE OUTCOME

Some conductive hearing loss is curable with surgery. Hearing loss caused by prolonged exposure to loud noise sometimes disappears when the noise is eliminated. Other types of hearing loss are usually permanent.

TREATMENT

HOME CARE

- Contact local rehabilitation facilities for your child to learn sign-language and lip-reading skills.
- Encourage your child to learn to use and wear a hearing aid, if one is prescribed.
- Consult your phone company about special audio equipment for your phone.
- Urge your child to resist the temptation to withdraw socially because of hearing difficulty. Isolation will increase communication problems and frustration, and will make adjustment more difficult.

MEDICATION

- Medicine usually is not necessary for this disorder.
- See Medications section for information regarding medicines your doctor may prescribe.

ACTIVITY

No restrictions.

DIET & FLUIDS

No special diet.

OK FOR SCHOOL, PRESCHOOL, OR NURSERY?

When appetite has returned and alertness, strength, and feeling of well-being will allow.

CALL YOUR DOCTOR IF

- Your child shows signs of hearing impairment.
- You suspect your child has a hearing loss, especially if the child does not respond to loud noises or direct conversation or if the child must ask others often to repeat themselves or if family members frequently ask if your child's hearing is all right.

HEART BLOCK (Atrioventricular Block)

GENERAL INFORMATION

DESCRIPTION

A heart block is a persistent disruption (either mild or major) in transmission of electrical signals between the heart's upper and lower chambers. Contractions of the atria (upper heart chambers) lose synchronization with those of the ventricles (lower heart chambers). The heartbeat is no longer regulated normally to quicken under exertion or stress and slow down at other times. The heart's electrical-transmission system that coordinates contractions of heart-muscle cells are involved. The heart's natural pacemaker initiates the electrical system.

Appropriate health care includes:

- Self-care after diagnosis.
- Doctor's treatment.
- Surgery to implant an artificial pacemaker (sometimes).

SIGNS & SYMPTOMS

- No symptoms (sometimes) for less-severe forms.
- Slow, irregular heartbeat.
- Sudden loss of consciousness.
- Convulsions (sometimes).

CAUSES

- Coronary-artery disease, a sign of arteriosclerosis (hardening of the arteries).
- Congenital heart abnormalities.
- Excessive digitalis and some other medications.

RISK FACTORS

- Stress.
- Improper diet that is high in fat and salt.
- Obesity.
- Smoking.
- Diabetes mellitus.
- Heart disease, including atherosclerosis, congestive heart failure or heart-valve disease.
- High blood pressure.
- Previous electrolyte imbalance.
- Use of some drugs, such as digitalis, quinidine, or beta-adrenergic blockers.
- Sick-sinus syndrome (see Glossary).

PREVENTING COMPLICATIONS OR RECURRENCE

- Obtain medical treatment for any underlying disease in your child.
- Urge your child not to smoke.
- Encourage your child to exercise regularly (see Appendix 36).
- Provide your child with a diet that is low in fat (see Appendix 28) and low in salt (see Appendix 29).

HEART BLOCK (Atrioventricular Block)

WHAT TO EXPECT

MEDICAL TESTS

- Your own observation of symptoms.
- Medical history and physical exam by a doctor.
- EKG (see Glossary).
- Holter monitor, a 12- or 24-hour continuous EKG monitor (see Glossary).

POSSIBLE COMPLICATIONS

Uncontrolled slow, rapid or irregular heartbeat and cardiac arrest.

PROBABLE OUTCOME

Symptoms can be controlled with surgery to implant a pacemaker.

TREATMENT

HOME CARE

- Your child should wear a Medic-Alert bracelet or pendant (see Glossary) in case of a sudden loss of consciousness.
- Your child should not smoke.

MEDICATION

- There are no medications that cure heart block, but there are some that make it worse. Your child should not take medications to relieve allergy or nasal congestion, including antihistamines, or any stimulant, including caffeine, cocaine, or marijuana.
- See Medications section for information regarding medicines your doctor may prescribe.

ACTIVITY

Don't think of your child as an invalid. Unless your doctor advises against it, mild exercise is helpful and not to be feared. Your child should begin a regular exercise program—walking is ideal—and increase the amount daily.

DIET & FLUIDS

Instructions for your child:

- Lose weight if you are overweight. A reducing diet appears in Appendix 31. Don't use amphetamines or other appetite suppressants to curb your appetite.
- Avoid excessive use of alcoholic beverages. Alcohol depresses the heartbeat.
- Avoid caffeine in all forms. It is in coffee, tea, cocoa, cola drinks, and chocolate.

OK FOR SCHOOL, PRESCHOOL, OR NURSERY?

When appetite returns and alertness, strength, and feeling of well-being will allow.

CALL YOUR DOCTOR IF

- Your child has symptoms of heart block, especially an episode with loss of consciousness.
- After diagnosis, stress increases in your child's life.

HEART-RHYTHM IRREGULARITY (Arrhythmia)

GENERAL INFORMATION

DESCRIPTION

Heart-rhythm irregularities indicate abnormalities in the rhythm of the heartbeat. The heart and nerves that transmit impulses to coordinate heart-muscle contractions are involved.

Appropriate health care includes:

- Doctor's treatment.
- Psychotherapy or counseling, if stress is a major factor.
- DC cardioversion (see Glossary) in a hospital or outpatient surgical facility.
- Surgery to correct some heart problems (coronary-artery bypass, damaged valve replacement, or insertion of a pacemaker).

SIGNS & SYMPTOMS

- Awareness of one's own heartbeat, including whether it skips, is always fast, slow, irregular, or suddenly changes rhythm.
- Shortness of breath.
- Sudden faintness or weakness.
- No symptoms (frequently).

CAUSES

- Heart diseases, such as rheumatic fever, congenital heart disease, cardiomyopathy, previous heart attack, or heart-muscle inflammation.
- Endocrine disorders, especially thyroid and adrenal-gland diseases.
- Fluid and electrolyte imbalance, especially too little or too much potassium.
- Side effects of certain drugs, especially digitalis, beta-adrenergic blockers, stimulants, and diuretics.
- Overdose of certain drugs, including antidepressants, marijuana, and cocaine.
- Postoperative effects following chest or heart surgery.

RISK FACTORS

- Stress.
- Chronic kidney disease.
- Hypertension.
- Use of certain drugs, such as caffeine, alcohol, amphetamines, and many non-prescription cough and cold remedies.
- Smoking.
- Fatigue, overwork, or sleep deprivation.

PREVENTING COMPLICATIONS OR RECURRENCE

If your child has any disorders listed as causes or risks, follow the treatment program carefully to control the disease. If medication is part of your child's treatment, consult your doctor about having blood levels monitored and electrolytes measured periodically.

HEART-RHYTHM IRREGULARITY
(Arrhythmia)

WHAT TO EXPECT

MEDICAL TESTS

- Your own observation of symptoms.
- Medical history and physical exam by a doctor (sometimes a cardiologist).
- Laboratory blood studies.
- EKG and 24-hour Holter monitor (see Glossary for both).
- X-rays of the heart, including echocardiogram (see Glossary).

POSSIBLE COMPLICATIONS

- Fainting.
- Congestive heart failure.
- Death from prolonged (more than 3 to 6 minutes) cardiac arrest.

PROBABLE OUTCOME

Most rhythm disturbances can be controlled with treatment. Very occasional, irregular heartbeats are harmless and require no treatment for your child.

TREATMENT

HOME CARE

- Consider lifestyle changes for your child. See Appendix 19.
- Urge your child to wear a Medic-Alert bracelet or pendant (see Glossary) showing the name of the condition.
- A few arrhythmias are fatal unless cardiopulmonary resuscitation (CPR) is performed immediately. Take a course to learn CPR, especially if someone in your home or neighborhood has heart disease.

MEDICATION

Your doctor may prescribe antiarrhythmic medications. You may need to try several to find the most effective one.

ACTIVITY

Your child can resume most normal activities as soon as symptoms improve. Consult your doctor about exercise.

DIET & FLUIDS

- Some heart medicines require extra potassium, found mostly in citrus fruits, bananas, dried apricots or peaches, raisins, lentils, and whole-grain cereals. Ask your doctor if your child needs to eat more of these.
- Urge your child not to drink caffeine-containing beverages, such as coffee, tea, cola, or chocolate.

OK FOR SCHOOL, PRESCHOOL, OR NURSERY?

When appetite returns and alertness, strength, and feeling of well-being will allow.

CALL YOUR DOCTOR IF

Your child has symptoms of heart-rhythm irregularity.

HEART-VALVE DISEASE
(Valvular Heart Disease)

GENERAL INFORMATION

DESCRIPTION

Valvular heart disease is a complication of disorders that distort or destroy the valves of the heart. The aortic, mitral, tricuspid, and pulmonic heart valves are involved.

Appropriate health care includes: self-care after diagnosis; physician's monitoring of general condition and medications; hospitalization for precise diagnosis; surgery to replace or open defective valves (sometimes).

SIGNS & SYMPTOMS

- No symptoms (sometimes).
- Fatigue and weakness.
- Dizziness or fainting.
- Chest pain.
- Shortness of breath.
- Lung congestion.
- Heart-rhythm irregularities.
- Heart murmurs (abnormal heart sounds heard by the doctor through a stethoscope).
- Abnormal blood pressure (high or low).

CAUSES

The heart has 4 valves. The mitral and tricuspid valves (main heart valves) control blood flow into the ventricles. The aortic and pulmonic valves control blood flow out of the heart. Heart-valve disease can be either narrowed valves (stenosis), which obstructs blood flow, or widened or scarred valves, which allow blood to leak backward into the heart (insufficiency). The disorder may be inherited or caused by any of the following:

- Rheumatic fever.
- Atherosclerosis.
- High blood pressure.
- Congenital heart defects.
- Endocarditis.
- Syphilis (rare).

RISK FACTORS

Family history of heart-valve disease; pregnancy; fatigue or overwork.

PREVENTING COMPLICATIONS OR RECURRENCE

- Obtain medical treatment for your child for conditions and diseases that cause heart-valve damage, such as high blood pressure, endocarditis, and syphilis.
- Give the child antibiotics prescribed for streptococcal infections to prevent rheumatic fever.
- If you have a family history of congenital heart disease, obtain genetic counseling before starting a family.

HEART-VALVE DISEASE
(Valvular Heart Disease)

WHAT TO EXPECT

MEDICAL TESTS

- Your own observation of symptoms.
- Medical history and physical exam by a doctor.
- Laboratory blood tests.
- EKG (see Glossary).
- Heart catheterization (see Glossary).
- X-rays of the heart, lungs and blood flow (angiography).
- Special studies that may include ultrasonography, CAT or CT scan, MRI, radionuclide scan and echocardiogram (see Glossary for all).

POSSIBLE COMPLICATIONS

Infection of the valves; congestive heart failure.

PROBABLE OUTCOME

Depends on the underlying condition. Many complications of valvular disease can be controlled with medication or cured with surgery.

TREATMENT

HOME CARE

Tell any doctor, dentist or anesthesiologist who treats your child that the child has heart-valve disease. Remind those involved, even if you think they know the details of your child's medical history.

MEDICATION

Your doctor may prescribe:

- Antibiotics to treat or prevent bacterial infection of abnormal heart valves.
- Anti-arrhythmic drugs to stabilize heartbeat irregularities.
- Digitalis medication to strengthen or regulate the heartbeat.
- See Medications section for information regarding medicines your doctor may prescribe.

ACTIVITY

As much as your child can tolerate. No restrictions are necessary with some forms of heart-valve disease.

DIET & FLUIDS

Your child should eat a low-fat, low-salt diet (see Appendices 28 and 29).

OK FOR SCHOOL, PRESCHOOL, OR NURSERY?

When appetite has returned and alertness, strength, and feeling of well-being will allow.

CALL YOUR DOCTOR IF

- Your child has symptoms of heart-valve disease.
- During treatment, the child develops signs of infection, such as fever, chills, muscle aches, headache, fatigue, and a general ill feeling.

HEARTBEAT, RAPID
(Tachycardia; Paroxysmal Tachycardia)

GENERAL INFORMATION

DESCRIPTION

Paroxysmal tachycardia is a heartbeat that is much more rapid than usual and is not caused by overexertion. Normal heartbeat ranges are 80 to 100 beats per minute in children and 70 to 90 beats per minute in adults. Tachycardia ranges from 150 to 300 beats per minute. A child with no heart disease may exercise and raise the heartbeat to 160 or more. This type of tachycardia is normal and is not a medical problem. The heart muscle and the electrical system of the heart are involved.

Appropriate health care includes:

- Physician's monitoring of general condition and medications.
- Self-care after diagnosis.
- Hospitalization if the attack persists despite treatment.
- DC electrocardioversion, a controlled electric shock (rarely necessary).
- Studies to discover underlying cause *after* treating any life-threatening tachycardia.

SIGNS & SYMPTOMS

- Heart pounding or palpitations. The pulse at the child's wrist or neck will be 110 to 180 beats per minute, which is much faster than normal.
- Faintness or a feeling of impending death.
- Increased urination; chest pain; involuntary cough; breathlessness.

CAUSES

Unknown. This usually occurs in young persons with no evidence of disease, but it may also occur in older patients who have coronary-artery disease.

RISK FACTORS

- Heart disease; stress; smoking; use of some drugs, such as caffeine, ephedrine, or other sympathomimetic drugs; fatigue or overwork.

PREVENTING COMPLICATIONS OR RECURRENCE

- Urge your child not to smoke.
- Reduce the child's stress, if possible. See Appendix 19.

WHAT TO EXPECT

MEDICAL TESTS

- Your own observation of symptoms.
- Medical history and physical exam by a doctor.
- EKG (see Glossary).
- Special studies that may include ultrasonography, CAT or CT scan, MRI, and radionuclide scan (see Glossary for all).

HEARTBEAT, RAPID (Tachycardia; Paroxysmal Tachycardia)

POSSIBLE COMPLICATIONS
Uninterrupted tachycardia can lead to life-threatening congestive heart failure, heart attack, or cardiac arrest.

PROBABLE OUTCOME
Rapid heartbeat can usually be controlled with treatment.

TREATMENT

HOME CARE
Instructions for your child that sometimes reduce heartbeat:
- Hold your breath briefly.
- Pinch the skin on your arm enough to cause pain.
- Bathe your face in cold water, submerge your head briefly in a sink of cool water, or take a cool shower and let the water beat on your head.
- Hold your nostrils closed and blow gently through the nose, making the eardrums pop.
- Massage the carotid area in the neck, *if you have been taught to do this safely.* Ask your doctor for instructions.

MEDICATION
- For repeated attacks, your doctor may prescribe medication to control your child's heart rhythm. These include digitalis, quinidine, calcium-channel blockers, procainamide, beta-adrenergic blockers, and others.
- See Medications section for information regarding medicines your doctor may prescribe.

ACTIVITY
Your child should lie down during an attack until the heartbeat returns to normal, then resume regular activities. Between attacks, encourage the child to exercise regularly (see Appendix 36) with the doctor's approval. Physical fitness helps prevent tachycardia.

DIET & FLUIDS
No special diet, but your child should avoid caffeinated beverages.

OK FOR SCHOOL, PRESCHOOL, OR NURSERY?
When appetite has returned and alertness, strength, and feeling of well-being will allow.

CALL YOUR DOCTOR IF

- Your child has an episode of rapid, irregular heartbeat that does not end in 4 or 5 minutes.
- Your child develops shortness of breath.
- Your child has chest pain.

ILLNESSES

HEARTBURN
(Esophageal Reflux)

GENERAL INFORMATION

DESCRIPTION

Heartburn is discomfort in the upper digestive tract. Heartburn is a symptom—not a disease—and has nothing to do with the heart. The stomach and lower esophagus are involved. Heartburn is more common in adults, but it does occur in children and adolescents.

Appropriate health care includes:

- Self-care.
- Physician's monitoring of general condition and medications.
- Hospitalization for special studies or surgery (rarely).

SIGNS & SYMPTOMS

The following signs are worse at night:

- Belching or slight regurgitation of stomach contents into the mouth, producing an acid taste.
- Heavy, uncomfortable sensation in the chest.
- Swallowing difficulty.
- Mild abdominal pain.
- Vomiting (rarely).

RISK FACTORS

- Stress.
- Improper diet.
- Obesity.
- Smoking.
- Excess alcohol consumption.
- Use of drugs, such as aspirin, arthritis medicine, or cortisone.

PREVENTING COMPLICATIONS OR RECURRENCE

No specific preventive measures. Consider lifestyle changes (see Appendices 19 and 48).

WHAT TO EXPECT

MEDICAL TESTS

- Your own observation of symptoms.
- Medical history and physical exam by a doctor.
- Laboratory studies, such as blood studies, EKG (see Glossary) to exclude chance of heart disease, esophagoscopy (see Glossary), or gastroscopy (see Glossary).
- X-rays of the upper digestive tract (sometimes).

POSSIBLE COMPLICATIONS

- Misdiagnosis of a heart attack with symptoms similar to heartburn (rare).
- If heartburn is caused by a large hiatal hernia, surgery may be necessary to repair the hernia (rare).
- If heartburn is caused by ulcers in the esophagus, surgery may be necessary to remove scar tissue. Scar tissue forms with repeated ulceration and healing and may interfere with swallowing.

HEARTBURN (Esophageal Reflux)

PROBABLE OUTCOME

Symptoms can be controlled with treatment, but recurrence is common.

TREATMENT

HOME CARE

Instructions for your child:

- Elevate the head of the bed 4 to 6 inches with blocks.
- Don't smoke.
- Lose weight if you are overweight.
- Don't bend over, lie down, or exercise immediately after eating.
- Don't wear tight pantyhose, girdles, belts, or pants.

MEDICATION

- For minor discomfort, give the child non-prescription liquid antacids. These preparations coat the inside of the child's esophagus and neutralize stomach acid. Follow instructions on the bottle. The usual dose is 1 tablespoon taken 1 hour after meals and at bedtime.
- See Medications section for information regarding medicines your doctor may prescribe.

ACTIVITY

Your child can resume normal activities as soon as symptoms subside.

DIET & FLUIDS

Your child should avoid foods and beverages that stimulate heavy stomach-acid secretion, such as spicy dishes, coffee, acid fruit juice, or alcohol. Urge the child to avoid chocolate and reduce consumption of fatty foods.

OK FOR SCHOOL, PRESCHOOL, OR NURSERY?

When appetite has returned and alertness, strength, and feeling of well-being will allow.

CALL YOUR DOCTOR IF

- Swallowing becomes more difficult for your child.
- Your child regurgitates blood with the heartburn.
- The following symptoms accompany the child's heartburn:
  - — Shortness of breath.
  - — Sweating.
  - — Pain in the jaw, neck, and arm.
  - — Nausea.

HEATSTROKE; HEAT EXHAUSTION; HEAT CRAMPS (Sunstroke or Heat Prostration)

GENERAL INFORMATION

DESCRIPTION

Heatstroke is an illness caused by prolonged exposure to hot temperatures. The total body is involved. Appropriate health care includes: self-care after diagnosis (mild cases); physician's monitoring of general condition and medications; hospitalization to lower body temperature and provide intravenous fluids.

SIGNS & SYMPTOMS

Heatstroke:

- Sudden dizziness, weakness, faintness, and headache.
- Skin that is hot and dry.
- No sweating.
- High body temperature—frequently 102F (38.9C) or higher.
- Rapid heartbeat.
- Muscle cramps.

Heat exhaustion:

- Skin that is cool and moist.
- Pale or gray skin color.
- Slow pulse.
- Confusion.
- Muscle cramps.
- Low or normal body temperature.
- Dark yellow or orange urine.

CAUSES

- *Heatstroke*: Failure of the body's heat-regulating mechanisms, leading to a heat buildup in the child's body. The failure may be a result of chronic illness; diabetes; blood-vessel disease; alcoholism.
- *Heat exhaustion*: Loss of body fluids from the child sweating and failing to drink enough replacement fluid.

RISK FACTORS

Sweating and inadequate fluid intake; recent illness involving fluid loss from vomiting or diarrhea; hot humid weather; working or exercising in a hot environment.

PREVENTING COMPLICATIONS OR RECURRENCE

Instructions for your child:

- Wear light, loose-fitting clothing in hot weather.
- Drink extra iced water if you sweat heavily. Be guided by your urine output. If the output decreases, increase your water intake.
- If you become overheated, improve your ventilation. Open a window or use a fan or air conditioner. This promotes sweat evaporation, which cools the skin.
- Don't take salt tablets.
- Recognize early symptoms of heat illness. Reduce exercise until the symptoms disappear.

HEATSTROKE; HEAT EXHAUSTION; HEAT CRAMPS (Sunstroke or Heat Prostration)

? WHAT TO EXPECT

MEDICAL TESTS

Your own observation of symptoms; medical history and physical exam by a doctor; laboratory studies of the child's blood and urine to measure electrolyte levels.

POSSIBLE COMPLICATIONS

Shock; brain damage caused by prolonged, high body temperature (106F or 41.1C).

PROBABLE OUTCOME

Prompt treatment usually brings full recovery in 1 to 2 days.

TREATMENT

HOME CARE

- If your child has symptoms and is very hot and *not sweating:*
  — Cool the child rapidly. Use a cold-water bath or wrap the child in wet sheets.
  — Arrange for transportation to the nearest hospital. This is an emergency!
- If your child is faint *but sweating:*
  — Give the child cold or iced liquids (water, soft drinks, or fruit juice). Don't give salt pills.
  — Arrange for transportation to the hospital, except in mild cases. Call your doctor for advice.

MEDICATION

Medicine usually is not necessary for this disorder.

ACTIVITY

Your child can resume normal activity as soon as symptoms improve.

DIET & FLUIDS

Your child should drink extra fluids and eat foods high in potassium (orange juice, bananas) or take potassium supplements.

OK FOR SCHOOL, PRESCHOOL, OR NURSERY?

Yes, when appetite has returned and alertness, strength, and feeling of well-being will allow.

☎ CALL YOUR DOCTOR IF

Your child has symptoms of heatstroke or heat exhaustion, or you observe them in someone else. Call immediately! These conditions may be serious or fatal.

HEEL PAIN
(Heel Spur; Calcaneal Bursitis or Neuritis)

GENERAL INFORMATION

DESCRIPTION
Heel pain involves discomfort of the following types: *Contusion or bone bruise*—inflammation of the tissue that covers bone (periosteum). *Heel spur*—a hard bony shelf as wide as the width of the heelbone caused by repeated pulling away of periosteum from the heelbone (calcaneus). The repeated stress or injury causes inflammation and calcification of tendons and ligaments in the foot. *Plantar fasciitis*—inflammation of the fibrous band that originates at the bottom of the calcaneus. This hurts worse when running faster or when weight is on the ball of the foot. *Heel bursitis*—formation in the heel area of an irritated or inflamed protective sac of fluid due to irritation caused by a heel spur.
Appropriate health care includes self-care; doctor's diagnosis and treatment.

SIGNS & SYMPTOMS
- Deep discomfort under the heel while the child is walking, running, or at rest.
- Redness.
- Tenderness.
- Increased heat.

CAUSES
Running, jogging, or fast walking.

RISK FACTORS
Previous serious foot, ankle, or heel injury; repeated heel injury from any cause; prolonged standing; obesity.

PREVENTING COMPLICATIONS OR RECURRENCE
Instructions for your child:
- Avoid activities that cause constant foot strain.
- Wear athletic shoes with good shock absorption in the heel, good flexibility, and good support to control side-to-side motion.
- Don't wear everyday shoes with more than 1-1/2-inch heels.

WHAT TO EXPECT

MEDICAL TESTS
- Your own observation of symptoms.
- Medical history and physical exam by a doctor.
- X-rays of the heel.

POSSIBLE COMPLICATIONS
Inflammation and arthritic changes in the child's heel that place abnormal stress on previously pain-free joints, such as those in the knee, hip, and spine.

PROBABLE OUTCOME
Usually curable with conservative treatment (See TREATMENT).

HEEL PAIN (Heel Spur; Calcaneal Bursitis or Neuritis)

TREATMENT

HOME CARE

Instructions for your child:

- Use ice massage. Fill a large Styrofoam cup with water and freeze. Tear a small amount of foam from the top so ice protrudes. Massage firmly over the heel in a circle. Do this for 15 minutes at a time, 3 or 4 times a day.
- Elevate your foot above the level of your heart to reduce swelling and prevent accumulation of fluid. Use pillows for propping, or elevate the foot of the bed.
- Use doughnutlike or horseshoelike padding in your shoes, such as cushion pads, homemade felt inlays, sponge-rubber heel pads, or shaped pieces of indoor-outdoor carpeting. Put in both shoes, even if only one heel hurts. Otherwise, the normal mechanics of standing and moving will be altered and may cause pain in other areas.
- Try a plastic or rubber heel cup (available at sporting-goods stores and drug stores).
- Don't walk on your toes while treating heel pain.
- Do this stretch exercise:
  - — Sit on the floor with your legs straight.
  - — Grasp your toes with your hands.
  - — Pull your toes slowly toward you for 30 seconds.
  - — Repeat several times for 5 to 10 minutes.
- When returning to athletics or exercise, use ice massage for 10 minutes before warmup and after exercise.

MEDICATION

To relieve minor pain, use non-prescription drugs, such as ibuprofen, acetaminophen, or aspirin.

ACTIVITY

Your child should stay off his feet as much as possible, especially at the beginning of treatment.

DIET & FLUIDS

No special diet, unless your child is overweight. If so, the child should lose weight to reduce stress on the foot.

OK FOR SCHOOL, PRESCHOOL, OR NURSERY?

Yes, when condition and sense of well-being will allow.

CALL YOUR DOCTOR IF

- Your child has persistent heel pain, despite treatment.
- Any of the following occur after surgery:
  - — Pain, swelling, redness, drainage, or bleeding increases in the surgical area.
  - — Your child develops signs of infection (headache, muscle aches, dizziness, or a general ill feeling and fever).

HEMATURIA

GENERAL INFORMATION

DESCRIPTION

Hematuria is blood in the urine. This may or may not be visible with the naked eye. It is a common occurrence in children and adults who exercise strenuously. Hematuria following vigorous physical exercise does not necessarily represent any disease of the kidney or other parts of the urinary tract.

Appropriate health care includes:

- Doctor's diagnosis and treatment if an underlying urinary-tract disorder is present.
- Self-care after diagnosis.

SIGNS & SYMPTOMS

- Bloody urine with many red blood cells present (gross hematuria).
- "Smoky" colored urine. Red blood cells are visible in large quantities when the child's urine is examined under the microscope (microscopic hematuria). Clear urine may also contain some red blood cells that are visible under the microscope.

Additional symptoms in athletes that indicate the need for laboratory studies of the kidneys:

- Discomfort, frequency, or urgency in urinating (may represent infection).
- Colicky pain in either flank (area on the side of the abdomen under the last rib).
- Hematuria lasting longer than 48 hours after your child exercises.
- Decreased urine output for 12 hours after prolonged, strenuous exercise.

CAUSES

Prolonged exercise, such as running a marathon, with no underlying disease (benign hematuria).

RISK FACTORS

- Kidney disease.
- Kidney, ureter, bladder, or urethral injury.
- Stone in the child's ureter, kidney, or bladder.
- Infection.
- Tumor of the urinary tract.

PREVENTING COMPLICATIONS OR RECURRENCE

Instructions for your child:

- Obtain treatment for any illness of the kidney or urinary tract.
- Don't get dehydrated. Drink lots of water—a minimum of 8 glasses per day—and much more during hot weather and prolonged exercise.
- Include urine studies in your routine checkups every 2 to 3 months during periods of vigorous activity, such as participation in sports.

WHAT TO EXPECT

MEDICAL TESTS

- Your own observation of symptoms.
- Medical history and physical exam by a doctor.
- Laboratory studies such as urinalysis, urine culture, blood studies, intravenous pyelogram (special kidney X-rays), cystoscopy, angiography, or sonogram (see Glossary for these).

POSSIBLE COMPLICATIONS

Anemia due to blood loss.

PROBABLE OUTCOME

If there is no underlying disease of the child's urinary tract, benign hematuria usually clears spontaneously with 24 to 48 hours.

TREATMENT

HOME CARE

Your child should drink extra water, particularly during hot weather and prolonged, strenuous exercise.

MEDICATION

- Medicine usually is not necessary unless the blood in the child's urine is caused by illness. If so, your doctor may prescribe antibiotics for infection or medicine appropriate for other forms of kidney disease.
- See Medications section for information regarding medicines your doctor may prescribe.

ACTIVITY

No restrictions.

DIET & FLUIDS

No special diet.

OK FOR SCHOOL, PRESCHOOL, OR NURSERY?

Yes, when condition and sense of well-being will allow.

CALL YOUR DOCTOR IF

Your child has signs or symptoms of hematuria.

HEMIPLEGIA

GENERAL INFORMATION

DESCRIPTION

Hemiplegia means partial or complete paralysis of one side of the body. The central nervous system—including the brain, the coverings of the brain (meninges), and the spinal cord—and peripheral nerves are involved.

Appropriate health care includes: physician's monitoring of general condition and medications; hospitalization; psychotherapy or counseling for depression, and learning to cope with disability; physical therapy; long-term nursing-home care (sometimes).

SIGNS & SYMPTOMS

Because of the anatomy of the brain and spinal cord, injury to one side of the brain affects the opposite side of the body. The following signs and symptoms vary greatly between individuals:

- Weakness or paralysis of the arm and leg on the affected side.
- Difficulty speaking, understanding, or recognizing words.
- Altered or lost sensation on the affected side.
- Difficulty with self-feeding.
- Urinary incontinence.
- Blurred, double or decreased vision.

CAUSES

Brain injury in an area that controls one side of the body. Injury may result from:

- Stroke (the most common). Stroke may be caused by bleeding in the brain or by a blood clot or other obstruction of a blood vessel to the brain.
- Brain tumor.
- Head injury.
- Multiple sclerosis.

RISK FACTORS

Hypertension; diabetes.

PREVENTING COMPLICATIONS OR RECURRENCE

- Obtain medical treatment to control your child's hypertension or diabetes.
- Protect your child from head injury:
  - — Use seat belts in cars.
  - — Urge your child to wear protective headgear during contact sports or while riding a bicycle or motorcycle.
  - — Urge your child not to drink alcohol or use mind-altering drugs and drive.

WHAT TO EXPECT

MEDICAL TESTS

Your own observation of symptoms; medical history and physical exam by a doctor; laboratory studies of blood, urine, and cerebrospinal fluid; EKG (see Glossary); X-rays of the brain and neck; special studies that may include ultrasonography, CAT or CT scan, MRI, and radionuclide scan (see Glossary for all).

POSSIBLE COMPLICATIONS

- Pressure sores.
- Shortening of the muscles (contractures).
- Slow deterioration of the musculo-skeletal system.
- Injury or burns due to reduced mobility and decrease of pain responses.

PROBABLE OUTCOME

Depends on the extent of the child's injury. Brain tissue does not repair itself, but other parts of the brain can take over lost functions.

TREATMENT

HOME CARE

- Ask family and friends for support, and obtain professional help in readjusting your life.
- Let the child sleep on an egg-crate foam mattress or a waterbed to prevent pressure sores.

MEDICATION

No medication can repair damaged brain tissue, but your doctor may prescribe:

- Medications to control hypertension, diabetes, or other underlying disorders.
- Anti-coagulants to prevent blood-clot formation, if a stroke resulting from a clot caused the paralysis.

ACTIVITY

Your child can resume normal activities gradually. With rehabilitation, many lost functions can be compensated for or restored. Passive exercise for paralyzed or partially paralyzed muscles prevents contractures.

DIET & FLUIDS

No special diet for hemiplegia, but diabetes or hypertension may require special diets. Consult your doctor.

OK FOR SCHOOL, PRESCHOOL, OR NURSERY?

Yes, only when strength and sense of well-being will allow.

CALL YOUR DOCTOR IF

- Your child has symptoms of hemiplegia.
- The following occurs during treatment: signs of infection, such as fever, muscle aches, chills, and headache; difficulty in emptying the bladder.
- New, unexplained symptoms develop. Drugs used in treatment may produce side effects.

HEMOPHILIA

GENERAL INFORMATION

DESCRIPTION

Hemophilia is an inherited deficiency of a blood-clotting factor that results in dangerous bleeding. Primarily blood and bone marrow throughout the body are involved. Hemophilia affects 1 in 10,000 males, and appears early in childhood. Females carry the disease but do not exhibit symptoms.

Appropriate health care includes:

- Physician's monitoring of general condition and medications. Doctor should be a qualified hematologist (blood specialist).
- Hospitalization or care in an outpatient facility for transfusions of plasma and various blood factors when needed.
- Self-care.

SIGNS & SYMPTOMS

- Painful, swollen joints or swelling in the leg or arm (especially the knee or elbow) when bleeding occurs.
- Frequent bruises.
- Excessive bleeding from minor cuts.
- Spontaneous nosebleeds.
- Blood in the urine.

CAUSES

The deficiency of a coagulation factor passed by a female carrier to male children in an X-linked recessive gene.

RISK FACTORS

No known risk factor.

PREVENTING COMPLICATIONS OR RECURRENCE

Cannot be prevented at present. If your family has a history of hemophilia, obtain genetic counseling before having children.

WHAT TO EXPECT

MEDICAL TESTS

- Your own observation of symptoms.
- Medical history and physical exam by a doctor.
- Laboratory blood studies.

POSSIBLE COMPLICATIONS

- Dangerous bleeding episodes requiring emergency treatment.
- Permanent joint disability caused by persistent bleeding.
- Hepatitis or AIDS from blood transfusions.

PROBABLE OUTCOME

This condition is currently considered incurable but not fatal. If bleeding can be controlled, patients can expect a nearly normal life span. Scientific research into causes and treatment continues, so there is hope for increasingly effective treatment and cure.

TREATMENT

HOME CARE

- For bleeding at any accessible site, apply direct pressure by hand or elastic bandage or apply ice and elevate the child's limb. Call your doctor immediately.
- In case of emergency, your child should wear a bracelet or pendant mentioning hemophilia.

MEDICATION

- Your doctor may prescribe:
  - Medication to reduce joint pain.
  - Transfusions of plasma or clotting factors.
- Your child should not take aspirin. It may increase bleeding.
- See Medications section for information regarding medicines your doctor may prescribe.

ACTIVITY

Your child should avoid activities that can cause injury, such as contact sports. Urge the child to swim, bicycle, or walk instead. Otherwise, no restrictions.

DIET & FLUIDS

No special diet.

OK FOR SCHOOL, PRESCHOOL, OR NURSERY?

When appetite has returned and alertness, strength, and feeling of well-being will allow.

CALL YOUR DOCTOR IF

- Your child has symptoms of hemophilia.
- The following occurs after diagnosis:
  - Injury with swelling. This may indicate bleeding under the skin.
  - Bleeding that isn't quickly controlled.
  - Tender, painful, swollen joint.

HEPATITIS, ACUTE VIRAL

GENERAL INFORMATION

DESCRIPTION

Acute viral hepatitis is inflammation of the liver caused by a virus. Liver cells and bile ducts are involved.

Appropriate health care includes: Self-care after diagnosis (mild cases); physician's monitoring of general condition and medications; and hospitalization (severe cases).

SIGNS & SYMPTOMS

Symptoms vary greatly between children.

- *Early symptoms are non-specific and include:* flu-like symptoms, such as fever, headache, muscle aches, fatigue, nausea, vomiting, diarrhea, loss of appetite, and general ill feeling.
- *Later symptoms include:* abdominal pain; foul breath with a bitter taste; jaundice (yellow eyes and skin) caused by a buildup of bile in the blood; dark urine from bile spilling over into the urine; light, "clay-colored" or whitish stools; swollen, tender liver (sometimes) and spleen (sometimes).

CAUSES

Any of 3 different but related viruses that may infect the liver. All are contagious.

- Type A (infectious hepatitis): Usually is spread by person-to-person contact. It also enters the body through water or food, especially raw shellfish, that has been contaminated by sewage.
- Type B (serum hepatitis): Usually enters the body through inoculations of serum or blood transfusions contaminated with the virus or from infections with non-sterile needles (frequently used by IV drug abusers) or syringes or from sexual activities with an infected person. Blood-sucking insects are also suspected as sources of Type B.
- Type Non-A, Non-B: Usually enters the body by contaminated blood transfusions.

RISK FACTORS

Crowded or unsanitary living conditions or travel to areas with poor sanitation; oral-anal sexual practices; use of intravenous, mind-altering drugs; alcoholism; blood transfusions; volunteering or working in a hospital; kidney-dialysis treatment; homosexual practices; poor nutrition; illness that has lowered resistance; exposure to others in public places.

PREVENTING COMPLICATIONS OR RECURRENCE

Instructions for your child: Avoid risks listed above. Don't eat shellfish from areas with poor sanitation systems. If you are exposed to someone with hepatitis, consult your doctor about receiving gamma-globulin (GG) injections to decrease the risk of hepatitis. (GG can suppress—but not prevent—infectious hepatitis after exposure.) If you are in a high-risk group, such as hospital workers or volunteers, or male homosexuals, consult your doctor about a vaccine for Type-B hepatitis. (Vaccines are not available for other forms.) If you are traveling where hepatitis is endemic (constantly present), consult your doctor about a vaccine or gamma globulin injection.

HEPATITIS, ACUTE VIRAL

WHAT TO EXPECT

MEDICAL TESTS

Medical history and physical exam by a doctor; laboratory studies of blood, stool, and liver function; urinalysis; special nuclear medicine studies and ultrasonography (see Glossary for all).

POSSIBLE COMPLICATIONS

Liver failure in severe cases (very rare).

PROBABLE OUTCOME

In younger children, this is a common infection that is usually mild. It is usually curable in 2 to 3 weeks, but wait 2 more weeks before sending your child to school or other public places. In older children and adolescents, jaundice and other symptoms peak and then gradually disappear over 3 to 16 weeks. Most children in good general health recover fully in 1 to 4 months. A small percentage (1% to 2%) may proceed to chronic hepatitis. Recovery from viral hepatitis usually provides permanent immunity against it.

TREATMENT

HOME CARE

See Appendix 12, Care of the Sick Child at Home.

MEDICATION

Your doctor may prescribe cortisone drugs for severe cases to reduce liver inflammation.

ACTIVITY

Bed rest is necessary, except to use the bathroom, until fever is gone, jaundice disappears, and appetite returns. Your child can then sit in a chair, read, or watch TV. Children differ widely in the rate at which they can return to normal activity.

DIET & FLUIDS

Encourage your child to eat, despite a poor appetite, small well-balanced meals to help promote recovery. At least 8 glasses of water are necessary each day. Hard candy may taste good and be nourishing to the liver. Urge your child not to drink alcohol.

OK FOR SCHOOL, PRESCHOOL, OR NURSERY?

When your doctor determines that your child is no longer contagious.

CALL YOUR DOCTOR IF

- Your child has symptoms of hepatitis or has been exposed to someone who has it.
- The following occurs during treatment: increasing loss of appetite; excessive drowsiness or mental confusion; vomiting, diarrhea, or abdominal pain; deepening jaundice; skin rash or itching.

HERNIA

GENERAL INFORMATION

DESCRIPTION

A hernia is a protrusion of an internal organ through a weakness or abnormal opening in the muscle around it. The most-common types include inguinal hernia, incisional hernia, femoral hernia, umbilical hernia, and hiatal hernia. Each type of hernia involves the following body parts: *umbilical*—muscles around the navel; *inguinal* or *femoral*—connective tissue in the groin; and *incisional*—muscles at the site of previous surgery.

Appropriate health care includes:

- Physician's monitoring of general condition and medications.
- Surgery to repair the opening caused by weakened muscle or connective tissue.

SIGNS & SYMPTOMS

- A lump that usually returns to its normal position with gentle pressure or by lying down.
- Mild discomfort or pain at the site of the lump (sometimes).
- Scrotal swelling, with or without pain.
- Vomiting in young infants.

CAUSES

Weakness in connective tissue or a muscle wall. This may be present at birth or acquired later in life. Incisional hernias result from previous surgery.

RISK FACTORS

- Prematurity in infants.
- Obesity.
- Pregnancy.
- Straining.

PREVENTING COMPLICATIONS OR RECURRENCE

- A weak area may not herniate until it ruptures with heavy lifting or straining. If your child must lift something, these are instructions on how to lift properly: Bend your knees, lift the object, and rise using your leg muscles. Keep the object close to your body. Don't lift by bending from the waist and using your back muscles to lift.
- If constipation is a problem, see Constipation (in Illnesses section) for treatment.

WHAT TO EXPECT

MEDICAL TESTS

- Your own observation of symptoms.
- Medical history and physical exam by a doctor.
- Laboratory blood studies.
- X-rays of the abdomen (sometimes).

POSSIBLE COMPLICATIONS

If your child's hernia becomes strangulated (loses its blood supply), the protruding part may cause intestinal obstruction with fever, severe pain, and shock, and may require emergency surgery.

PROBABLE OUTCOME

Umbilical hernias usually heal spontaneously by age 4 and rarely require surgery. Other hernias are usually curable with surgery.

TREATMENT

HOME CARE

- For an explanation of surgery and postoperative care, see Hernia (in Illnesses section).
- Whenever your child lies down prior to surgery, push the hernia gently into place if it protrudes visibly.
- Don't have your child wear a hernia truss. It injures or weakens tissues, making surgery difficult or impossible.

MEDICATION

- For minor discomfort, use non-prescription drugs such as acetaminophen.
- See Medications section for information regarding medicines your doctor may prescribe.

ACTIVITY

Your child should avoid heavy lifting—either before or after surgery.

DIET & FLUIDS

No special diet.

OK FOR SCHOOL, PRESCHOOL, OR NURSERY?

When surgery has healed and appetite has returned and alertness, strength, and feeling of well-being will allow.

CALL YOUR DOCTOR IF

Your child has symptoms of a hernia. If the child has fever or severe pain, call immediately!

HERPANGINA

GENERAL INFORMATION

DESCRIPTION

Herpangina is a viral inflammation of the mouth and throat. The soft palate (back of the mouth and tonsil area) is involved. Herpangina usually affects young children (1 to 10 years).

Appropriate health care includes:

- Home care.
- Physician's monitoring of general condition and medications.

SIGNS & SYMPTOMS

- Fever.
- Sudden sore throat, with redness, inflammation, and painful swallowing.
- General ill feeling.
- Vomiting and abdominal pain (sometimes).
- Tiny blisters (vesicles) in the affected areas. The blisters become small ulcers.

CAUSES

Infection from a virus (Coxsackie virus) that is spread from person to person.

RISK FACTORS

Summer and early fall seasons.

PREVENTING COMPLICATIONS OR RECURRENCE

Cannot be prevented at present, but washing hands carefully prevents its spread.

WHAT TO EXPECT

MEDICAL TESTS

- Your own observation of symptoms.
- Medical history and physical exam by a doctor.
- Throat culture to rule out possible streptococcal infections.

POSSIBLE COMPLICATIONS

Febrile convulsions (caused by fever).

PROBABLE OUTCOME

Spontaneous recovery in a few days to a week.

TREATMENT

HOME CARE

Try to reduce your child's fever if it rises above 105F (40.6C) rectally. See How to Reduce Your Child's Fever, Appendix 17.

MEDICATION

- Medicine usually is not necessary for this disorder. Use non-prescription drugs, such as acetaminophen, to relieve pain and fever.
- See Medications section for information regarding medicines your doctor may prescribe.

ACTIVITY

Bed rest is necessary until the fever and sore throat disappear.

DIET & FLUIDS

No special diet. Encourage your child to drink extra fluids, such as water, fruit ices, ice chips, or cool-gelatin solutions. Avoid acid fruit juices, which irritate inflamed tissues.

OK FOR SCHOOL, PRESCHOOL, OR NURSERY?

When signs of infection have decreased, appetite returns, and alertness, strength, and feeling of well-being will allow.

CALL YOUR DOCTOR IF

Your child has symptoms of herpangina.

HERPES, GENITAL

GENERAL INFORMATION

DESCRIPTION

Genital herpes is a virus infection of the genitals transmitted by sexual relations (intercourse or oral sex). Genital herpes may increase the risk of cervical cancer. The penis, vagina, cervix, thighs, and buttocks (sometimes) are involved. Genital herpes can affect sexually active persons of both sexes and all ages. Appropriate health care includes: self-care after diagnosis; physician's monitoring of general condition and medications.

SIGNS & SYMPTOMS

- Painful blisters, preceded by itching and irritation, on the vaginal lips or the penis. In females, the blisters may extend into the vagina to the cervix and urethra. After a few days, the blisters rupture and leave painful, shallow ulcers which last 1 to 3 weeks.
- Difficult, painful urination; enlarged lymph glands; fever; feeling ill.

CAUSES

- Herpes Type 2 virus (HSV-2). (Herpes Type 1 virus causes common cold sores, which appear around the mouth.) Genital herpes is transmitted by a sexual partner who has active herpes lesions. Lesions may be on the genitals, hands, lips, or mouth (including Type 1 virus). The virus lies dormant inside the infected cells until conditions for multiplication are right; then the infected cells grow.
- A generalized form of herpes that can be fatal can be transmitted from an actively infected mother to the newborn. Infection takes place as the fetus passes through the mother's birth canal.

RISK FACTORS

- Serious illness that has lowered resistance.
- Use of immunosuppressive or anti-cancer drugs.
- Stress (increases susceptibility to a primary infection or a recurrence). Stress may lead to diminished efficiency of the immune responses that usually suppress growth of the virus.

PREVENTING COMPLICATIONS OR RECURRENCE

Instructions for a child who is sexually active: avoid sexual intercourse if either partner has blisters or sores; use a latex condom during intercourse if either sex partner has inactive genital herpes; avoid oral sex with a partner who has cold sores on the mouth; if you are pregnant, tell your doctor if you have had herpes or any genital lesions in the past. Precautions should be taken to prevent infection of the baby.

WHAT TO EXPECT

MEDICAL TESTS

Your own observation of symptoms; medical history and physical exam by a doctor; smear of lesions on glass slide to study microscopically; viral or tissue culture.

POSSIBLE COMPLICATIONS

- Generalized disease and death in persons of any age who must take anti-cancer drugs or immunosuppressive drugs.
- Transmittal of life-threatening systemic herpes to a newborn infant from an infected mother.
- Secondary bacterial infection.

PROBABLE OUTCOME

- Genital herpes is currently considered incurable, but symptoms can be relieved with treatment.
- During symptom-free periods, the virus returns to its dormant state. Symptoms recur when the virus is reactivated. Recurrent symptoms are not new infections.
- The discomfort varies from person to person and from time to time in the same person. Usually, the first herpes infection is much more uncomfortable than following ones.

TREATMENT

HOME CARE

- Females should wear cotton panties or pantyhose with a cotton crotch—not panties made from non-ventilating materials.
- Females should not douche unless told to by a doctor.
- To reduce pain during urination, females may urinate in a bath or shower, or urinate through a tubular device, such as a toilet-paper roll or plastic cup with the end cut out.

MEDICATION

Your child's doctor may prescribe an anti-viral drug, such as acyclovir, in oral or topical form. This drug reduces the intensity and duration of the first attack. It does not prevent recurrent attacks.

ACTIVITY

Your child should reduce normal activities until fever diminishes and feeling of well-being returns. Your child should not resume sexual relations until at least 1 month after full recovery.

DIET & FLUIDS

No special diet.

OK FOR SCHOOL, PRESCHOOL, OR NURSERY?

When signs of infection have decreased, appetite returns, and alertness, strength, and feeling of well-being will allow.

CALL YOUR DOCTOR IF

- Your child has symptoms of genital herpes.
- Symptoms don't improve in 1 week, despite treatment.
- Unusual vaginal bleeding or swelling occurs.
- Fever returns during treatment or the child becomes generally ill.
- Symptoms of herpes recur after treatment.

HERPETIC WHITLOW

GENERAL INFORMATION

DESCRIPTION

Herpetic whitlow is an inflammation of skin folds around the fingernails caused by a contagious herpes virus. Fingernails or toenail beds are involved. Herpetic whitlow is more common in adults than children.

Appropriate health care includes:

- Self-care after diagnosis.
- Physician's monitoring of general condition, medications, and treatment, which may include minor surgery to relieve pressure of pus pockets under the skin.

SIGNS & SYMPTOMS

- Sudden pain around the nail.
- Redness, swelling, and warmth around the nail.
- Swelling of the lymph glands nearby, such as in the elbow or armpit.
- Groupings of tiny blisters that are barely visible around the nail.

CAUSES

Herpes virus hominus, Type 1 or Type 2. Herpetic whitlow is often transmitted to the fingers from cold sores (herpes simplex) on the mouth.

RISK FACTORS

- Occupational exposure to constant wetness, such as with dishwashers or maintenance personnel.
- Occupational exposure to herpes infection, such as with nurses, dentists, or dental assistants who provide mouth care.

PREVENTING COMPLICATIONS OR RECURRENCE

- Your child should avoid exposure to people who have active herpes infections.
- Your child should keep hands warm and dry.

WHAT TO EXPECT

MEDICAL TESTS

- Your own observation of symptoms.
- Medical history and physical exam by a doctor.
- Laboratory culture of discharge from the infected area.

POSSIBLE COMPLICATIONS

Spread of herpes infection to other body parts, such as the lips or genitals.

PROBABLE OUTCOME

The first episode is usually curable in 2 months with treatment. However, recurrent attacks are common.

TREATMENT

HOME CARE

• Encourage your child to protect hands to prevent further injury or spread of the infection to others. The child should wear heavy-duty vinyl gloves to avoid contact with irritating substances, such as water, soap, detergent, metal scrubbing pads, scouring pads, scouring powder, and other chemicals.
• Urge your child not to touch other persons until inflammation clears.

MEDICATION

Your doctor may prescribe:
• Topical steroid preparations to reduce inflammation. They include creams, ointments, and lotions. Your child should apply the topical steroid only once or twice a day unless directed otherwise. Apply it immediately after bathing to aid penetration.
• Oral anti-viral medications (not always effective, but safe enough for a trial in severe cases that do not respond to traditional treatment).
• See Medications section for information regarding medicines your doctor may prescribe.

ACTIVITY

No restrictions.

DIET & FLUIDS

No special diet.

OK FOR SCHOOL, PRESCHOOL, OR NURSERY?

When appetite has returned and alertness, strength, and feeling of well-being will allow.

CALL YOUR DOCTOR IF

• Your child has symptoms of herpetic whitlow.
• Temperature rises over 101F (38.3C).
• Symptoms don't improve in 3 days, despite treatment.
• Herpes lesions appear elsewhere on the child's body.

HIATAL HERNIA

GENERAL INFORMATION

DESCRIPTION

A hiatal hernia is an abnormal weakness or opening in the diaphragm, which is the big, thin muscle that separates the chest cavity from the abdominal cavity. The esophagus, stomach, and diaphragm are involved.

Appropriate health care includes:

- Self-care after diagnosis.
- Physician's monitoring of general condition and medications.
- Surgery to close the weakness in the diaphragm and keep the stomach in its natural place (rare).

SIGNS & SYMPTOMS

The following symptoms usually develop within 1 hour or more after eating:

- "Heartburn" (a burning sensation in the area of the heart and behind the breastbone).
- Belching.
- Swallowing difficulty (rare).

CAUSES

- Congenital weakness in the muscular ring of the diaphragm through which the esophagus passes and empties into the stomach.
- Abdominal injury, causing tremendous pressure that tears a hole in some part of the diaphragm.
- Either of the above can allow gastric (stomach) acid to flow backward from the stomach into the esophagus, irritating the esophagus. The hernia weakens the sphincter that controls the opening between the two—the stomach may even protrude into the lower chest. Lying flat or exerting abdominal pressure (like straining) may push the stomach upward.

RISK FACTORS

Chronic constipation and straining during bowel movements; obesity; pregnancy; constant straining or lifting with tightening of the abdominal muscles; smoking.

PREVENTING COMPLICATIONS OR RECURRENCE

No specific preventive measures.

WHAT TO EXPECT

MEDICAL TESTS

- Your own observation of symptoms.
- Medical history and physical exam by a doctor.
- X-rays of the esophagus and stomach.
- Gastroscopy with a flexible gastroscope (see Glossary) to view the esophagus and stomach.

POSSIBLE COMPLICATIONS

- Bleeding from the esophagus. This can be excessive, leading to shock.
- Misdiagnosis as a heart attack.

PROBABLE OUTCOME

Your child's symptoms can usually be controlled with the suggestions listed below. If symptoms cannot be controlled and it appears that irritation of the esophagus is causing scarring and ulceration, the condition can be corrected with surgery.

TREATMENT

HOME CARE

Instructions for your child:

- Raise the head of your bed 4 to 6 inches. This allows gravity to keep stomach acid away from the hernia.
- Avoid large meals. Eat 4 or 5 small meals a day instead. Don't eat anything for at least 2 hours before bedtime.
- Lose weight if you are overweight. A reducing diet appears in Appendix 31.
- Don't smoke.
- Don't wear tight pantyhose, girdles, belts, or pants.
- Don't strain during bowel movements, urination, or lifting.

MEDICATION

Your doctor may prescribe:

- Antacids. These are most effective for some children when they take them 1 hour before meals and at bedtime. Others find them more helpful 1 to 2 hours after meals and at bedtime. Your child can try both ways to find the best schedule.
- Stool softeners.

ACTIVITY

No restrictions.

DIET & FLUIDS

Your child should avoid alcoholic beverages, caffeine-containing beverages (coffee, tea, cocoa, cola drinks), and any other food, juice, or spice that aggravates symptoms. Urge the child to eat slowly and chew food thoroughly (35 to 50 chews for each mouthful).

OK FOR SCHOOL, PRESCHOOL, OR NURSERY?

When appetite has returned and alertness, strength, and feeling of well-being will allow.

CALL YOUR DOCTOR IF

- Your child has symptoms of a hiatal hernia, especially the sensation that food stops beneath the breastbone. Call immediately if pain is accompanied by shortness of breath, sweating, or nausea.
- Your child vomits blood or has recurrent vomiting.
- Temperature rises over 100F (37.8C).
- Symptoms don't improve with treatment in 1 month.

HICCUP
(Hiccough; Singultus)

GENERAL INFORMATION

DESCRIPTION

Hiccups are repeated involuntary spasmodic contractions of the diaphragm. Hiccups are a symptom—not a disease. The diaphragm (the big, thin muscle which separates the chest from the abdomen) and the phrenic nerve (the nerve that connects the diaphragm to the brain) are involved.

Appropriate health care includes:

- Self-care.
- Physician's monitoring of general condition and medications (prolonged hiccups).
- Surgery to cut phrenic nerve (only severe, prolonged cases that have not responded to simpler measures).

SIGNS & SYMPTOMS

A sharp, quick sound produced from the mouth by a spasm of the diaphragm. The spasm closes muscles in the back of the throat during inhalation.

CAUSES

Irritation of nerves from the brain that control breathing muscles, especially the diaphragm. The cause of short hiccup episodes is usually unknown. Prolonged or recurrent hiccup episodes may be caused by:

- Swallowing hot or irritating substances.
- Diseases of the pleura (thin membrane layers that cover the lung).
- Pneumonia.
- Uremia.
- Alcoholism.
- Use of certain prescription or non-prescription drugs.
- Disorders of the stomach, esophagus, bowel, or pancreas.
- Pregnancy.
- Bladder irritation.
- Hepatitis.
- Spread of cancer from another part of the body to the liver or part of the pleura.
- Peritonitis.
- Recent surgery, especially abdominal surgery.
- Emotional causes.

RISK FACTORS

- Illness that has diminished health.
- Recent abdominal surgery.
- Use of drugs, especially those that irritate the stomach.

PREVENTING COMPLICATIONS OR RECURRENCE

Cannot be prevented at present.

HICCUP
(Hiccough; Singultus)

WHAT TO EXPECT

MEDICAL TESTS

- Your own observation of symptoms.
- Medical history and physical exam by a doctor.

POSSIBLE COMPLICATIONS

None unless your child's hiccups are prolonged, which may indicate serious disease.

PROBABLE OUTCOME

Short hiccup episodes usually don't indicate disease. They will subside with the treatment discussed below. Continued hiccups can be debilitating and require medical attention to determine the cause.

TREATMENT

HOME CARE

These instructions for your child are for short hiccup episodes. Prolonged hiccups require medical care.

- Hold your breath and count to 10.
- Breathe into a paper bag, and rebreathe air in the bag. Don't use a plastic bag because it may cling to nostrils.
- Insert your thumb between your teeth and upper lip; press the upper lip with your index finger just below the right nostril.
- Drink a glass of water rapidly.
- Swallow dry bread or crushed ice.
- Pull gently on the tongue.
- Close eyelids and apply gentle pressure to the eyeballs.
- Swallow a teaspoon of dry sugar.

MEDICATION

- For prolonged or recurrent hiccups, your doctor may prescribe a mild tranquilizer or sedative.
- See Medications section for information regarding medicines your doctor may prescribe.

ACTIVITY

No restrictions.

DIET & FLUIDS

No special diet.

OK FOR SCHOOL, PRESCHOOL, OR NURSERY?

Yes.

CALL YOUR DOCTOR IF

- Your child's hiccups persist longer than 8 hours.
- You suspect a prescription drug may be causing the child's hiccups.

HIDRADENITIS SUPPURATIVA

GENERAL INFORMATION

DESCRIPTION

Hidradenitis suppurativa is a skin disorder characterized by nodules in the armpit. It appears rarely on the buttocks or groin or under the breasts. It is most common in females 13 to 15 years old, but it can occur in both sexes.

Appropriate health care includes:

- Self-care after diagnosis.
- Doctor's treatment.
- Surgery to open and drain abscesses or to remove involved skin (severe cases only).

SIGNS & SYMPTOMS

Nodules with the following characteristics:

- Nodules are firm, tender, and domed.
- Nodules are 1cm to 3cm in diameter.
- Larger nodules soften in the center and become painful. When pressed, they feel like an overfilled inner tube.
- Nodules open and drain pus spontaneously.
- Individual nodules (with or without drainage) heal slowly over 10 to 30 days.
- Nodules leave scars.
- Severity of the disorder varies from a few lesions per year to a constant succession of lesions that form as old ones heal. Lesions frequently recur at the same site.

CAUSES

Hormonal influences that activate the apocrine glands under the arms. Secretions in these glands enlarge the gland. The outlets become blocked, probably by heat, sweat, or incomplete gland development. The secretions that are dammed in the glands force sweat and bacteria into surrounding tissue, which becomes infected.

RISK FACTORS

- Obesity.
- Exposure to environmental heat and moisture.
- Genetic factors. This disorder is most common in black females.

PREVENTING COMPLICATIONS OR RECURRENCE

No specific preventive measures.

WHAT TO EXPECT

MEDICAL TESTS

- Your own observation of symptoms.
- Medical history and physical exam by a doctor.
- Laboratory culture of the discharge from the child's draining abscess.

POSSIBLE COMPLICATIONS

Scarring.

PROBABLE OUTCOME

This disorder may last many years—from puberty through the following 10 to 20 years. Your child's symptoms can be controlled with treatment.

TREATMENT

HOME CARE

Instructions for your child:

- Don't use commercial underarm deodorants.
- Minimize heat and sweating.
- Avoid constrictive clothing and clothing made of synthetic fibers.
- Lose weight if you are overweight.
- Wash with antibacterial soaps.
- Use soaks to relieve itching and hasten healing. Warm-water soaks are usually more soothing for pain or inflammation. Cool-water soaks feel better for itching.
- Discontinue underarm shaving.

MEDICATION

- Your doctor may do any of the following for your child:
  —Inject cortisone drugs directly into the lesions.
  —Prescribe antibiotics to fight infection.
  —Prescribe hormones to help subdue inflammation.
  —Provide instructions for acceptable deodorant protection.
  —Prescribe pain medication. For minor discomfort, use non-prescription drugs such as acetaminophen.
- See Medications section for information regarding medicines your doctor may prescribe.

ACTIVITY

Your child should restrict activity in hot weather, and should avoid hot jobs if possible. Swimming is excellent, especially swimming in the ocean.

DIET & FLUIDS

No special diet unless your child needs to lose weight. See Appendix 31 for a reducing diet.

OK FOR SCHOOL, PRESCHOOL, OR NURSERY?

When appetite returns and alertness, strength, and feeling of well-being will allow.

CALL YOUR DOCTOR IF

- Your child has symptoms of hidradenitis suppurativa.
- Lesions don't improve after 5 days of treatment.
- Your child's temperature rises to 101F (38.3C).
- Lesions appear that become soft and seem to have pus, but don't drain spontaneously.
- New, unexplained symptoms develop. Drugs used in treatment may produce side effects.

HIP DISLOCATION, CONGENITAL

GENERAL INFORMATION

DESCRIPTION

Congenital hip dislocation is a disorder in which the head of the thigh bone doesn't fit properly into, or is outside of, the hip socket. One or both hip joints may be involved. Congenital hip dislocations are present at birth. About 1 in every 60 newborns has a possible hip dislocation. About 85% are girls.

Appropriate health care includes:

- Home care after diagnosis.
- Physician's monitoring of general condition and medications.
- Surgery (sometimes).

SIGNS & SYMPTOMS

- The earliest symptom may be a clicking sound in a newborn when the legs are pulled apart. However, this symptom is not always present.
- After the newborn period, partial dislocation may become full dislocation. Then the thigh bone (femur) rides up behind or to the side of its hip socket. The limb will appear shorter than its mate. Skin folds of the buttocks will not be symmetrical; the side with the dislocated hip will have more creases than the other.
- A child old enough to walk may limp or favor one side.

CAUSES

Unknown. Congenital hip dislocations seem more common after breech deliveries than after head-first or Cesarean deliveries. Theories about the reasons include hormonal changes in the mother during pregnancy, abnormal fetal position in the uterus, or birth injury.

RISK FACTORS

Unknown.

PREVENTING COMPLICATIONS OR RECURRENCE

Cannot be prevented at present.

WHAT TO EXPECT

MEDICAL TESTS

Your own observation of symptoms; medical history and physical exam by a doctor; X-rays of the hip.

POSSIBLE COMPLICATIONS

Late detection and treatment can lead to permanent crippling.

PROBABLE OUTCOME

If congenital hip dislocation is detected early, it can often be cured. Surgery is used only when conservative treatment fails or the disorder has not been discovered until late in childhood.

TREATMENT

HOME CARE

• To correct the dislocation, the head of the thigh bone must be returned to its socket in the pelvic bone and held firmly in place.
— For mild forms, use triple diapers to immobilize the child, and arrange for frequent medical exams.
— For more severe forms, splints, casts, or traction are used to immobilize the ball and socket until it heals. Plaster casts may be necessary for several months. They must be replaced every 1-1/2 to 2 months. See Care of Casts, Appendix 41.

• While an infant or young child is immobilized, the child will require more physical care than normal. Soiled diapers, especially, should not be left on the child for any length of time.

• During the first few days that your child is in a cast, splints, or traction, stay as close by as possible to give reassurance and love.

• Remove braces or splints for bathing, but replace them immediately afterward.

• Turn the child in bed at least every 2 hours during the day and every 4 hours at night.

MEDICATION

Medicine usually is not necessary for this disorder.

ACTIVITY

• If traction is required, your child must stay in bed until the dislocation is corrected. The child may read or watch TV.

• If a cast or splints are used and the child's condition allows it, put the child on the floor for short play periods—either alone or with other children. Car rides are acceptable.

DIET & FLUIDS

No special diet.

OK FOR SCHOOL, PRESCHOOL, OR NURSERY?

Yes. Try to keep activity as normal as possible.

CALL YOUR DOCTOR IF

• Your child has signs of a congenital hip dislocation.
• The following occurs during treatment:
— Rectal temperature rises to 101F (38.3C) or higher, which may indicate infection of the skin or urinary tract.
— The cast, bar, or other immobilization device does not seem to hold the child's hip in position.
— A dent appears in the cast, which might cause a pressure sore.
— The child shows signs of severe pain.
— Color or mobility of the child's legs and feet change.
— The child loses appetite.

HISTOPLASMOSIS

GENERAL INFORMATION

DESCRIPTION

Histoplasmosis is a fungus infection confined mostly to people who live in eastern and midwestern parts of the U.S. The lungs, the central nervous system—including the brain, the coverings of the brain (meninges), and the spinal cord—and peripheral nerves, as well as the gastrointestinal system are involved.

Appropriate health care includes:

- Self-care after diagnosis.
- Physician's monitoring of general condition and medications.
- Hospitalization for complications.

SIGNS & SYMPTOMS

- Cough and other symptoms similar to a cold.
- Loss of appetite, diarrhea, and weight loss.
- Fever.
- Headache.
- Irritability.
- Paleness.
- Abdominal swelling.
- Breathing difficulty (rare).

CAUSES

Infection by the fungus histoplasma capsulatum. People become infected by breathing dust that contains fungus spores. The fungus is found in soil contaminated by feces of birds and bats that carry the fungus. Contaminated soil is most often in pigeon lofts, barns, chicken houses, damp areas under bridges, along streams, and in caves.

RISK FACTORS

- Recent severe illness, especially uremia, diabetes mellitus, chronic lung disease, cancer, or severe burns.
- Geographic location. The disease occurs most often in the western Appalachian slopes and the Mississippi, Missouri and Ohio River valleys.
- Use of immunosuppressive, anti-cancer or cortisone drugs.

PREVENTING COMPLICATIONS OR RECURRENCE

Your child should avoid areas where the soil is likely to be infected with histoplasma spores.

WHAT TO EXPECT

MEDICAL TESTS

- Your own observation of symptoms.
- Medical history and physical exam by a doctor.
- Laboratory studies, such as a sputum culture, blood studies for rising and falling titers (see Glossary), and skin tests.

POSSIBLE COMPLICATIONS

Spread of infection to the child's heart, spleen, adrenal glands, and meninges (membranes that cover the brain). This is rare, but it can be fatal.

PROBABLE OUTCOME

Usually curable—even with complications—with intensive care and 10 to 12 weeks of treatment with anti-fungal drugs. Most children only feel tired or "bad" for several weeks.

TREATMENT

HOME CARE

- Isolation is not necessary. The disease is not transmitted from person to person.
- Use a cool-mist humidifier with pure water and no medicine in it to increase air moisture near your child. This helps thin lung secretions so they can be coughed up more easily.
- Urge your child not to smoke.
- Use a heating pad on the child's chest to relieve pain.
- Weigh your child daily and keep a record.

MEDICATION

- Your doctor may prescribe anti-fungal drugs that must be given intravenously in a hospital.
- Don't suppress the child's cough with cough medicine if it produces sputum. Coughing rids the lungs of mucus. If the cough is painful and non-productive, consult your doctor about a prescription cough suppressant.
- Use acetaminophen or aspirin to relieve your child's pain.

ACTIVITY

Your child should stay in bed until the fever, pain, and shortness of breath disappear for at least 48 hours. Then normal activities can be resumed gradually. Many children are fatigued and weak after recovery. Don't expect too much too soon.

DIET & FLUIDS

No special diet.

OK FOR SCHOOL, PRESCHOOL, OR NURSERY?

When signs of infection have decreased, appetite returns, and alertness, strength, and feeling of well-being will allow.

CALL YOUR DOCTOR IF

- Your child has symptoms of histoplasmosis.
- The following occurs during treatment:
  - — Weight loss continues.
  - — Fever rises to 101F (38.3C) orally.
  - — Diarrhea is uncontrollable.
  - — Severe headache and stiff neck begin.

HIVES
(Urticaria; Giant Urticaria; Angioneurotic Edema)

GENERAL INFORMATION

DESCRIPTION

Hives are an allergic disorder characterized by skin changes with raised areas, redness, and itching. The skin anywhere on the body is involved, including the scalp, lips, palms, and soles.

Appropriate health care includes: self-care after diagnosis; physician's monitoring of general condition and medications; emergency-room care for life-threatening reactions that include wheezing, shortness of breath, and fainting.

SIGNS & SYMPTOMS

Itchy skin papules (small, raised bumps) with the following characteristics:

- They swell and produce pink or red lesions called wheals. Wheals have clearly defined edges and flat tops. They measure 1cm to 5cm in diameter.
- Wheals join together quickly and form large, flat plaques (larger areas of raised, skin-colored lesions).
- Wheals and plaques change shape, resolve, and reappear in minutes or hours. This rapid change is unique to hives.

CAUSES

Release of histamines, sometimes for unknown reason. Following are the most common causes:

- Medications. Nearly every drug causes hives in some children.
- Insect bites.
- Viral infections.
- Auto-immune disease.
- Dysproteinemias.
- Exposure to cold, heat, water, or sunlight.
- Cancer, especially leukemia.
- Exposure to animals, especially cats.
- Eating eggs, fruits, nuts, and shellfish. Other foods sometimes cause hives in infants but not in adults.
- Food dyes and preservatives (possibly).

RISK FACTORS

Stress; other allergies or a family history of allergies.

PREVENTING COMPLICATIONS OR RECURRENCE

If your child has had hives and you have identified the cause, avoid the source.

WHAT TO EXPECT

MEDICAL TESTS

Your own observation of symptoms; medical history and physical exam by a doctor; allergy skin tests and desensitization injections (sometimes).

POSSIBLE COMPLICATIONS

- Swelling of the child's larynx and inability to breathe.
- Hives may be the first sign of life-threatening anaphylaxis. If so, it will be followed by itching, a runny nose, wheezing, paleness, cold sweats, and low blood pressure. Without prompt treatment, coma and cardiac arrest can occur.

PROBABLE OUTCOME

Unpredictable, depending on the cause. If a medication or acute viral infection is responsible, hives usually disappear within hours or days. Some cases become chronic and last for months or years. Most eventually go into spontaneous remission—even if the cause is not identified.

TREATMENT

HOME CARE

Instructions for your child:

- Don't take drugs (including aspirin, laxatives, sedatives, vitamins, antacids, pain killers, or cough syrups) not prescribed for you.
- Don't wear tight underwear or foundation garments. Any skin irritation may trigger new outbreaks.
- Don't take hot baths or showers.
- Apply cold-water compresses or soaks to relieve itching.

MEDICATION

Your doctor may prescribe:

- Antihistamines, ephedrine, terbutaline, or cortisone drugs to relieve itching and rash.
- Sedatives or tranquilizers for anxiety.
- Epinephrine by injection for severe symptoms.

ACTIVITY

Your child should decrease activities until several days after hives disappear and should avoid getting hot, sweaty, or excited.

DIET & FLUIDS

- If foods are suspected as a cause, keep a food diary for your child to help identify the offending food.
- Urge your child to avoid alcohol and coffee or other caffeine-containing beverages. These may trigger outbreaks.

OK FOR SCHOOL, PRESCHOOL, OR NURSERY?

When appetite has returned and alertness, strength, and feeling of well-being will allow.

CALL YOUR DOCTOR IF

- The following *emergency symptoms* occur during an episode of hives: swollen lips; shortness of breath or wheezing; a tight or constricted feeling in the throat.
- New, unexplained symptoms develop. Drugs used in treatment may produce side effects.

HODGKIN'S DISEASE

GENERAL INFORMATION

DESCRIPTION

Hodgkin's disease is a malignant tumor of the lymph glands. This is less common than lymphoma (non-Hodgkin's disease). The lymphocytes (white blood cells), lymph glands (glands which check infection and produce immune substances), and spleen (a large lymph gland located high in the left side of the abdomen just below the ribs) are involved. Hodgkin's disease may affect all ages but is rare in children under 10.

Appropriate health care:

- Physician's monitoring of general condition and medications.
- Hospitalization for short periods of treatment.
- Surgery to discover the extent of disease (called "staging").
- Radiation therapy.

SIGNS & SYMPTOMS

- Itching all over the body.
- Swollen, non-tender, rubbery, distinct lymph glands anywhere in the body—but most commonly in the armpit or groin.
- Intermittent fever.
- Pain in the diseased area after drinking alcohol.
- Weight loss.
- Jaundice (yellow skin and eyes).
- General ill feeling.
- Anemia.
- Bleeding from the gastrointestinal tract.

CAUSES

Unknown, but research suggests a virus infection may be a factor.

RISK FACTORS

No known risk factor.

PREVENTING COMPLICATIONS OR RECURRENCE

No specific preventive measures.

WHAT TO EXPECT

MEDICAL TESTS

- Your own observation of symptoms.
- Medical history and physical exam by a doctor.
- Laboratory studies of blood and bone marrow.
- Lymphangiogram (see Glossary).
- Biopsy (see Glossary) of lymph node.
- X-rays of various body parts that may be involved.

POSSIBLE COMPLICATIONS

Spread of malignancy to other parts of the body.

PROBABLE OUTCOME

Usually curable with radiation therapy and anti-cancer drugs. With treatment, the 10-year survival rate is about 80%. The potential for cure varies according to the cell type discovered from biopsy of the lymph node.

TREATMENT

HOME CARE

Try to remain optimistic about your child's treatment and chances for cure. A good mental attitude is a powerful ally for the child as well as the rest of the family.

MEDICATION

- Your doctor may prescribe anti-cancer drugs. Medication may cause side effects or adverse reactions in some children. New symptoms may be caused by the medicine, by the original disorder, or by a new illness. Side effects caused by medicine usually disappear when the body adjusts to the drug or when the drug is discontinued.
- See Medications section for information regarding medicines your doctor may prescribe.

ACTIVITY

Urge your child to remain as active as possible.

DIET & FLUIDS

No special diet.

OK FOR SCHOOL, PRESCHOOL, OR NURSERY?

When appetite has returned and alertness, strength, and feeling of well-being will allow.

CALL YOUR DOCTOR IF

- Your child has symptoms of Hodgkin's disease.
- The following occurs during treatment:
  - — Fever.
  - — Signs of infection (redness, swelling, pain, or tenderness) anywhere in the body.
  - — Swelling of the feet and ankles.
  - — Discomfort when urinating or decreased urination during any 24-hour period.
- You think your child's medicine is causing symptoms.

HYPERALDOSTERONISM

GENERAL INFORMATION

DESCRIPTION

Hyperaldosteronism is an endocrine disease caused by overproduction of aldosterone, a hormone manufactured by the adrenal glands. Excess aldosterone causes the kidneys to absorb too much sodium and water and to eliminate too much potassium. The adrenal glands (which are attached at the upper part of the kidneys), the kidneys, the fluids and electrolytes in the bloodstream, and other body cells are involved. Appropriate health care includes: self-care after diagnosis; physician's monitoring of general condition and medications; hospitalization; surgery to examine the adrenal glands and remove any tumors.

SIGNS & SYMPTOMS

- General symptoms: fatigue and weakness; temporary paralysis (sometimes); tingling sensations in the arms, legs, hands, and feet; frequent urination, especially at night; thirst; severe muscle spasms; vision disturbances.
- The following are apparent with diagnostic tests: low blood levels of potassium; high blood levels of sodium; high blood pressure.

CAUSES

Increased adrenal secretion of aldosterone. This is caused by the following:

- A tumor of the adrenal gland.
- High blood pressure or kidney disease, causing increased production in the kidneys of a hormone (renin) that controls aldosterone levels.

RISK FACTORS

A diet that contains large amounts of licorice; kidney disease; congestive heart failure; cirrhosis of the liver; use of oral contraceptives; use of diuretic drugs that cause potassium loss; pregnancy.

PREVENTING COMPLICATIONS OR RECURRENCE

A child who has kidney disease or high blood pressure should remain under a doctor's care and adhere strictly to the treatment program—even if there are no symptoms.

WHAT TO EXPECT

MEDICAL TESTS

- Your own observation of symptoms.
- Medical history and physical exam by a doctor.
- Laboratory blood studies of electrolyte levels.
- EKG (see Glossary).
- Surgical diagnostic procedures such as laparoscopy (see Glossary).
- X-rays of the kidneys.
- Special studies that may include ultrasonography, CAT or CT scan, MRI, and radionuclide scan (see Glossary for all).

POSSIBLE COMPLICATIONS

- Congestive heart failure.
- Atherosclerosis.
- Kidney failure.

PROBABLE OUTCOME

If your child's disorder is caused by an adrenal tumor, it is usually curable with surgery. If it is caused by kidney disease or high blood pressure, medical treatment for these disorders will control symptoms of hyperaldosteronism.

TREATMENT

HOME CARE

- Weigh your child daily and keep a record. Report a gain of 3 or more pounds in a 24-hour period.
- Encourage your child to wear a Medic-Alert bracelet or pendant (see Glossary).

MEDICATION

Your doctor may prescribe:

- Cortisone drugs to replace adrenal hormones, if the adrenal gland is removed. This is essential for life. Don't let your child discontinue or change the dose without consulting your doctor.
- Spironolactone to decrease the aldosterone effect if surgery is not performed. This drug may cause breast enlargement and sexual impotence in males.
- See Medications section for information regarding medicines your doctor may prescribe.

ACTIVITY

No restrictions if surgery is not necessary. If it is, your child can resume normal activities gradually.

DIET & FLUIDS

Encourage your child to eat a diet that is low in sodium (see Appendix 29) and high in potassium. Foods rich in potassium include dried apricots and peaches, raisins, citrus fruits, lentils, and whole-grain cereals. Urge the child not to eat licorice.

OK FOR SCHOOL, PRESCHOOL, OR NURSERY?

When appetite has returned and alertness, strength, and feeling of well-being will allow.

CALL YOUR DOCTOR IF

- Your child has symptoms of hyperaldosteronism.
- New, unexplained symptoms develop. Drugs used in treatment may produce side effects.

HYPERHIDROSIS

GENERAL INFORMATION

DESCRIPTION

Hyperhidrosis means excessive sweating. Sweating is a normal body function that helps maintain even body temperature. Excess sweat serves no purpose and often creates social embarrassment because of odor or stained clothes. In extreme cases, excess sweat can ruin clothes and shoes. The skin, especially of the underarms, genital area, palms, and soles, is involved. Hyperhidrosis can affect older children but not infants.

Appropriate health care includes:

- Self-care.
- Physician's monitoring of general condition and medications for underlying conditions, or if self-care is unsuccessful.
- Psychotherapy or counseling, if stress is a major factor.
- Surgery to remove sweat glands or sever nerves to major sweat areas (rare).

SIGNS & SYMPTOMS

- Heavy perspiration from underarm area, soles, and palms—and to a lesser degree, from other body parts.
- Unpleasant odor, which is caused by bacteria in sweat.

CAUSES

- Stress or chronic anxiety.
- Fever and infection.
- Malignancy, such as lymphoma.
- Hyperthyroidism.
- Heart attack.
- Some drugs and medicines, such as narcotics.
- Withdrawal from addicting drugs.
- Unknown in some cases.

RISK FACTORS

- Stress.
- Strenuous activity.
- Hot weather.

PREVENTING COMPLICATIONS OR RECURRENCE

Encourage your child to resolve tension-causing conditions. See Appendix 19.

WHAT TO EXPECT

MEDICAL TESTS

- Your own observation of symptoms.
- Medical history and physical exam by a doctor.

POSSIBLE COMPLICATIONS

- Psychological distress caused by social embarrassment.
- Rashes from deodorants or antiperspirants.
- Dehydration if water intake is insufficient to replace water lost in sweat.

PROBABLE OUTCOME

Your child's symptoms can be controlled with treatment.

TREATMENT

HOME CARE

Instructions for your child:

- Bathe frequently.
- Change clothes frequently.
- Wear loose-fitting clothes of natural fibers, such as cotton.
- Use underarm sweat shields.
- Use antiperspirants and deodorants.
- Use drying powders.
- Wear cotton socks.
- Wear leather shoes or sandals. Don't use man-made materials.

MEDICATION

Your doctor may prescribe:

- Tranquilizers or anti-cholinergics to reduce activity of the central nervous system.
- Special solutions to reduce sweating, such as topical applications of aluminum chloride.
- See Medications section for information regarding medicines your doctor may prescribe.

ACTIVITY

No restrictions.

DIET & FLUIDS

No special diet. Urge your child to drink at least 8 glasses of water a day—more in hot weather.

OK FOR SCHOOL, PRESCHOOL, OR NURSERY?

Yes.

CALL YOUR DOCTOR IF

Excessive sweating is causing your child problems at school or work or in social situations.

HYPERLIPIDEMIA, TYPES I, II, III, IV, V (Hyperlipoproteinemia)

GENERAL INFORMATION

DESCRIPTION

Hyperlipidemia means above-normal levels of fat in the blood. The blood and arteries are involved. Different types of hyperlipidemia appear at different ages. Appropriate health care includes:

- Self-care after diagnosis.
- Physician's monitoring of general condition and medications.
- Surgery to remove fat deposits in the skin and tendons.

SIGNS & SYMPTOMS

- Yellowish nodules of fat in the skin beneath eyes, elbows, and knees, and in tendons.
- Enlarged spleen and liver (some types).
- Whitish ring around the eye pupil (some types).

CAUSES

The blood contains a variety of fats (lipids) joined to blood proteins, forming lipoproteins. These include cholesterol, triglycerides, and high-density lipoproteins (HDL). They provide energy and are "building blocks" for some tissues and hormones. In excess, they filter out and are deposited in blood vessels, tendons, and other tissues, where they cause symptoms and disease.

RISK FACTORS

- Improper diet that is high in fat and cholesterol.
- Family history of hyperlipidemia.
- Use of oral contraceptives or estrogen.
- Diabetes mellitus.
- Hypothyroidism.
- Nephrosis.
- Alcoholism.

PREVENTING COMPLICATIONS OR RECURRENCE

- Your child should eat a diet that is low in fat. See Appendix 28.
- If your child has diabetes, adhere closely to the treatment program.

WHAT TO EXPECT

MEDICAL TESTS

- Medical history and physical exam by a doctor.
- Laboratory blood studies to measure blood lipids.
- Radionuclide Scan: A nuclear medicine procedure that uses radioactive isotopes injected into a patient. The isotope tracers are absorbed in various concentrations by targeted organs, which are then photographed (see Glossary).

POSSIBLE COMPLICATIONS

- Heart attack.
- Stroke.
- Acute pancreatitis.

HYPERLIPIDEMIA, TYPES I, II, III, IV, V (Hyperlipoproteinemia)

PROBABLE OUTCOME

Usually curable with lifelong dietary control and medication.

TREATMENT

HOME CARE

See Appendix 19 for suggestions to reduce stress and improve the health of your child. Stress increases the risk of heart disease, a major complication of hyperlipidemia.

MEDICATION

- Your doctor may prescribe:
  - — Medications to control blood lipids, such as niacin, clofibrate, or cholestyramine.
  - — Medications to treat underlying diseases, such as diabetes or thyroid conditions.
- Advise your daughter not to take oral contraceptives, but use other forms of birth control instead.
- See Medications section for information regarding medicines your doctor may prescribe.

ACTIVITY

No restrictions unless the child's tendons are weakened by fat deposits.

DIET & FLUIDS

- Urge your child to eat a diet that is low in fat. See Appendix 28.
- Encourage your child to lose weight if overweight. See Appendix 31 for a reducing diet.
- Advise your child not to drink alcohol.

OK FOR SCHOOL, PRESCHOOL, OR NURSERY?

When appetite has returned and alertness, strength, and feeling of well-being will allow.

CALL YOUR DOCTOR IF

- Your child has symptoms or there is a family history of hyperlipidemia.
- New, unexplained symptoms develop. Drugs used in treatment may produce side effects.

ILLNESSES

HYPERPARATHYROIDISM

GENERAL INFORMATION

DESCRIPTION

Hyperparathyroidism is excess parathyroid hormone circulating in the blood. The excess amounts increase blood levels of calcium (hypercalcemia) and decrease blood levels of phosphorous (hypophosphatemia). Body parts involved include the parathyroid glands in the neck, as well as the teeth and the blood, which affects all body tissues—especially the heart, blood vessels, bones, kidneys, gastrointestinal tract, central nervous system, and skin. Hyperparathyroidism is more common in adults than children.

Appropriate health care includes:

- Physician's monitoring of general condition and medications.
- Surgery to remove parathyroid tumors, if they are present.
- Self-care after treatment or surgery.

SIGNS & SYMPTOMS

- Severe flank pain caused by kidney stones.
- Chronic low-back pain caused by bone softening.
- Easy bone fractures caused by decreased calcium in the bones.
- Upper abdominal pain caused by a peptic ulcer or pancreatitis.
- Depression.

CAUSES

Benign tumors of the parathyroid glands, which are located next to the thyroid gland in the neck.

RISK FACTORS

- Recent illness, especially endocrine disorders.
- Medical history of rickets or vitamin D deficiency.
- Kidney failure.
- Use of laxatives.
- Use of digitalis.

PREVENTING COMPLICATIONS OR RECURRENCE

No specific preventive measures.

WHAT TO EXPECT

MEDICAL TESTS

- Your own observation of symptoms.
- Medical history and physical exam by a doctor.
- Laboratory studies of blood and urine.
- X-rays of bones.
- Special studies that may include ultrasonography, CAT or CT scan, MRI, and radionuclide scan (see Glossary for all).

POSSIBLE COMPLICATIONS

- Cataracts.
- Kidney damage.
- Psychosis.
- Hypoparathyroidism caused by removal of too much parathyroid tissue during surgery.
- Hypothyroidism if the thyroid gland is injured inadvertently during surgery on the parathyroid glands.

PROBABLE OUTCOME

Curable with surgery.

TREATMENT

HOME CARE

To prevent fractures:

- Encourage your child to use a walker or cane until blood studies return to normal. This may take up to 6 months.
- Install safety rails near the tub, shower, and toilet.
- Tape rugs down around the edges.
- Keep the house—especially stairs—brightly lit to avoid stumbling.

MEDICATION

- Your doctor may prescribe:
  - — Diuretics to force sodium and calcium excretion.
  - — Vitamin D.
- Don't give your child antacids that contain calcium.
- See Medications section for information regarding medicines your doctor may prescribe.

ACTIVITY

No restrictions.

DIET & FLUIDS

- Encourage your child to limit calcium-containing foods, such as milk and cheese.
- Urge your child to avoid highly seasoned or spicy foods, especially if there is an ulcer present.

OK FOR SCHOOL, PRESCHOOL, OR NURSERY?

When appetite has returned and alertness, strength, and feeling of well-being will allow.

CALL YOUR DOCTOR IF

- Your child has symptoms of hyperparathyroidism.
- The following occurs during treatment:
  - — Muscle cramps, numbness, or weakness.
  - — Breathing difficulty.
  - — Persistent heartburn or pain in the upper abdomen.
  - — Drastic mood or behavior changes.

HYPERTENSION (High Blood Pressure)

GENERAL INFORMATION

DESCRIPTION

Hypertension is an increase in the force against arteries (blood vessels) as blood circulates through them. Hypertension is sometimes called "the silent killer" because it often has no symptoms in the early stages. The heart, blood vessels, kidneys, and eyes (advanced stages) are involved. Hypertension is more common in adults than children.

Appropriate health care includes:

- Self-care after diagnosis.
- Physician's monitoring of general condition and medications.
- Surgery (sometimes for rare, curable forms of hypertension).

SIGNS & SYMPTOMS

Usually no symptoms unless the condition is severe. Following are symptoms of a hypertensive crisis:

- Headache.
- Drowsiness.
- Confusion.
- Numbness and tingling in the hands and feet.
- Coughing blood.
- Severe shortness of breath.

CAUSES

Usually unknown. A small number of cases result from the following:

- Chronic kidney disease.
- Severe narrowing of the aorta (major artery of the heart).
- Tumors of the adrenal gland.
- Hardening of the arteries.

RISK FACTORS

- Obesity.
- Smoking.
- Stress.
- Diet that is high in salt or saturated fat.
- Sedentary lifestyle.
- Genetic factors. Hypertension is most common among blacks.
- Family history of hypertension, stroke, heart attack, or kidney failure.
- Use of contraceptive pills.

PREVENTING COMPLICATIONS OR RECURRENCE

Essential hypertension (from unknown causes) cannot be prevented at present. If there is a family history of hypertension, obtain frequent blood-pressure checks. If hypertension is detected early, treatment that includes diet, exercise, stress management, and medication can usually prevent complications.

HYPERTENSION (High Blood Pressure)

? WHAT TO EXPECT

MEDICAL TESTS

- Your own observation of symptoms.
- Medical history and physical exam by a doctor.
- Laboratory studies such as blood studies of kidney function, urinalysis, and EKG (see Glossary).
- X-rays of the chest and kidneys.
- Special studies that may include ultrasonography, CAT or CT scan, MRI, and radionuclide scan (see Glossary for all).

POSSIBLE COMPLICATIONS

Stroke; heart attack; congestive heart failure and pulmonary edema; kidney failure; blindness caused by ruptured blood vessels.

PROBABLE OUTCOME

- With treatment, complications are preventable (except for possible side effects of drugs). Life expectancy is normal.
- Without treatment, life expectancy is reduced because of the likelihood of heart attack or stroke.

TREATMENT

HOME CARE

- Consider lifestyle changes for your child to reduce stress. See Appendix 19.
- Learn to take your child's blood pressure. Your doctor or nurse can teach you.

MEDICATION

- Many anti-hypertensive medications can reduce blood pressure. Your doctor will prescribe the type appropriate for your child. Don't stop giving them without consulting your doctor.
- Don't give your child non-prescription cold and sinus remedies. These contain chemicals, such as ephedrine and pseudoephedrine, that raise blood pressure.

ACTIVITY

Your child should exercise at least 3 times a week. This helps reduce stress and maintain normal body weight; it may lower blood pressure. See Appendix 36.

DIET & FLUIDS

- Low-salt diet (see Appendix 29).
- Reducing diet if overweight (see Appendix 31).

OK FOR SCHOOL, PRESCHOOL, OR NURSERY?

Yes. Your child should try to stay as active as feeling of well-being will allow.

CALL YOUR DOCTOR IF

- Your child has symptoms of a hypertensive crisis.
- Chest pain occurs.

HYPERVENTILATION SYNDROME (Panic Attack)

GENERAL INFORMATION

DESCRIPTION

Hyperventilation syndrome is breathing so fast that carbon-dioxide levels in the blood are decreased, temporarily upsetting normal blood chemistry. The central nervous system—including the brain, the coverings of the brain (meninges), and the spinal cord—and peripheral nerves, lungs, skin, hands, and feet are involved. Hyperventilation syndrome is more common in young adults than in children, but it can affect all ages.

Appropriate health care includes:

- Self-care.
- Physician's monitoring of general condition and medications, if the cause is organic or symptoms are prolonged.
- Psychotherapy or counseling, if hyperventilation occurs often and is caused by anxiety.

SIGNS & SYMPTOMS

- Rapid breathing.
- Numbness and tingling around the mouth, hands, and feet.
- Weakness or faintness.
- Muscle spasm or contractions in the hands and feet.
- Fainting (occasionally).

CAUSES

A change in the normal ratio of acid to other elements in the blood caused by breathing out too much carbon dioxide. Hyperventilation can accompany fever, diseases of the heart and lungs, or severe injury. If disease or injury is not present, hyperventilation is caused by anxiety.

RISK FACTORS

- Stress.
- Feelings of guilt.
- Fatigue or overwork.
- Illness, such as those listed above.
- Smoking.
- Excess alcohol consumption.

PREVENTING COMPLICATIONS OR RECURRENCE

- Encourage your child to avoid anxiety-producing situations.
- See Appendix 19 for suggestions to reduce the child's stress.

WHAT TO EXPECT

MEDICAL TESTS

- Your own observation of symptoms.
- Medical history and physical exam by a doctor.
- Appropriate laboratory studies to help establish a precise diagnosis.

POSSIBLE COMPLICATIONS

- Seizures.
- Fainting.

PROBABLE OUTCOME

Symptoms can be controlled with the following instructions:

- If hyperventilation is caused by a disease, it will stop when the disease is cured.
- Recurrent attacks caused by anxiety should stop if underlying stress can be eliminated.

TREATMENT

HOME CARE

During an attack, your child should follow these instructions to increase carbon dioxide in the blood and relieve symptoms:

- Cover your mouth and nose completely with a paper bag.
- Breathe slowly into the bag and rebreathe the air. The air in the bag contains additional carbon dioxide.
- Breathe slowly in and out of the bag at least 10 times.
- Put the bag aside and breathe normally a few minutes.
- Repeat the process until the symptoms diminish or disappear.
- If symptoms return, repeat the process as often as needed.

MEDICATION

- Medicine usually is not necessary for this disorder.
- See Medications section for information regarding medicines your doctor may prescribe.

ACTIVITY

After treatment, your child can resume normal activity as soon as possible.

DIET & FLUIDS

No special diet.

OK FOR SCHOOL, PRESCHOOL, OR NURSERY?

When appetite has returned and alertness, strength, and feeling of well-being will allow.

CALL YOUR DOCTOR IF

- Your child has symptoms of hyperventilation that don't diminish with self-treatment.
- The following occurs during an attack:
  - — Fainting.
  - — Seizure.
  - — Sudden fever.

HYPOCHONDRIASIS

GENERAL INFORMATION

DESCRIPTION

Hypochondriasis is a person's conviction that he or she has a serious or fatal disease, despite evidence to the contrary from medical examinations and tests. The brain and other parts of the central nervous system are involved.

Appropriate health care includes:

- Physician's monitoring of general condition and medications.
- Psychotherapy or counseling. This offers the best hope for cure. However, few children (or adults) with hypochondriasis accept the conclusion that their health problem is psychological.

SIGNS & SYMPTOMS

Anxiety and persistent reports of symptoms involving any body part. Concern about heart disease or cancer is common. Symptoms may change, but the child's belief that a serious condition exists does not. Frequently reported symptoms include insomnia, sexual dysfunction, and gastrointestinal discomfort, such as bloating, belching, and cramps.

CAUSES

- Overly protective parents in early childhood.
- Lack of social outlets and contacts.
- Guilt feelings and an imagined need for punishment.
- Extreme need for attention.

RISK FACTORS

- Stress.
- Major life changes, such as the parents' divorce, a school or job change, a parent's remarriage, a move, or the loss of a valued person or object.
- Depression.
- Psychosis.

PREVENTING COMPLICATIONS OR RECURRENCE

Don't reward illness by giving your child special privileges and undue attention for being sick. Provide adequate love and support during healthy periods.

WHAT TO EXPECT

MEDICAL TESTS

- Your own observation of symptoms.
- Medical history and physical exam by a doctor. After a thorough medical evaluation, repeat testing should be avoided.

POSSIBLE COMPLICATIONS

- Wasting money on unnecessary—and sometimes dangerous—medical care.
- Insisting on unnecessary surgical procedures or medications.
- Failure of a doctor to take symptoms of real disease seriously when they do develop.

PROBABLE OUTCOME

Generally resistant to treatment. Most children with hypochondriasis maintain a lifelong belief that they have a serious disease, and as adults they change doctors frequently.

TREATMENT

HOME CARE

Children with hypochondriasis are often difficult to live with because of their constant worry and demands for attention. Realize that the child really suffers, and try to be supportive. Reward positive behavior that is not related to physical complaints. Don't encourage the "sick role."

MEDICATION

- Medicine usually is not necessary for this disorder. Your doctor may prescribe mild tranquilizers for a short time while therapy is being arranged.
- See Medications section for information regarding medicines your doctor may prescribe.

ACTIVITY

No restrictions.

DIET & FLUIDS

No special diet.

OK FOR SCHOOL, PRESCHOOL, OR NURSERY?

Yes.

CALL YOUR DOCTOR IF

- Your child has symptoms of hypochondriasis and you or your child want professional help to overcome the problem.
- New, unexplained symptoms develop. Tranquilizers used in treatment may produce side effects or dependence.

HYPOGLYCEMIA, FUNCTIONAL

GENERAL INFORMATION

DESCRIPTION

Functional hypoglycemia is low blood sugar caused by abnormal function—not disease—of the pancreas. The pancreas, pancreatic islet-cell secretions (mostly *insulin*), and eventually all body cells are involved.

Appropriate health care includes:

- Self-care after diagnosis.
- Physician's monitoring of general condition and medications.
- Psychotherapy or counseling to learn to cope with stress.

SIGNS & SYMPTOMS

The following vary greatly among children in frequency and severity:

- Weakness or faintness.
- Sweating.
- Excessive hunger.
- Nervousness and trembling hands.
- Heartbeat irregularities.
- Headache.
- Confusion.
- Personality changes.
- Loss of consciousness.
- Seizures (sometimes).

CAUSES

- Functional hypoglycemia probably results when the pancreas produces too much insulin in response to sugars and other carbohydrates, heavy exercise, pregnancy, or unknown causes.
- The following drugs decrease blood-sugar levels in some children: tobacco, caffeine, alcohol, aspirin, sulfonurea medications, phenformin, haloperidol, propoxyphene, and chlorpromazine.
- Some doctors believe functional hypoglycemia may be the first indication that diabetes mellitus is developing.

RISK FACTORS

- Stress.
- Improper diet.
- Smoking.
- Use of drugs, such as those listed above.
- Fatigue or overwork.

PREVENTING COMPLICATIONS OR RECURRENCE

Instructions for your child:

- Follow instructions under DIET & FLUIDS (opposite page). Don't skip meals.
- Avoid stress.
- Don't smoke.
- Don't drink alcohol.

WHAT TO EXPECT

MEDICAL TESTS

- Your own observation of symptoms.
- Medical history and physical exam by a doctor.
- Laboratory studies, such as blood-sugar and glucose-tolerance tests.
- Special studies that may include:

— Ultrasonography: A non-invasive technique that translates sound waves into images displayed on a screen and photographed (see Glossary).

— CAT or CT Scan (computerized axial tomography): Non-invasive computerized X-ray images that show sections (or "slices") of an organ or region of the body clearly and precisely (see Glossary).

— MRI (magnetic resonance imaging): A non-invasive (non-X-ray) computerized test that uses radio frequency energy and a powerful magnetic field to produce images with excellent detail (see Glossary).

— Radionuclide Scan: A nuclear medicine procedure that uses radioactive isotopes injected into a patient. The isotope tracers are absorbed in various concentrations by targeted organs, which are then photographed (see Glossary).

POSSIBLE COMPLICATIONS

Repeated attacks can cause personality changes.

PROBABLE OUTCOME

Symptoms can be controlled with treatment.

TREATMENT

HOME CARE

Consider lifestyle changes for your child. See Appendices 19 and 48.

MEDICATION

- Medicine usually is not helpful for this disorder.
- See Medications section for information regarding medicines your doctor may prescribe.

ACTIVITY

No restrictions.

DIET & FLUIDS

Encourage your child to eat 5 or 6 small meals a day that are low in simple carbohydrates, moderate in fats, and high in protein. Between-meals snacks should include protein, such as chicken, eggs, cheese, or skim milk, rather than carbohydrates. The child should avoid highly concentrated sweets, such as candy.

OK FOR SCHOOL, PRESCHOOL, OR NURSERY?

Yes. Your child should stay active.

CALL YOUR DOCTOR IF

Your child has symptoms of functional hypoglycemia.

HYPOGLYCEMIA OF DIABETES

GENERAL INFORMATION

DESCRIPTION

Diabetic hypoglycemia is low blood sugar in a child taking medication, such as insulin or oral anti-diabetic drugs, for diabetes. The brain quickly stimulates electrical and chemical messages to all body cells, both on a conscious and unconscious level.

Appropriate health care includes: self-care (early stages) and physician's monitoring of general condition and medications.

SIGNS & SYMPTOMS

- *Mild hypoglycemic reaction:* excessive hunger; weakness; nervousness; emotional instability; difficulty concentrating; sweating; headache.
- *Moderate hypoglycemic reaction:* increased weakness; excessive sweating; cold, clammy skin; numbness around the mouth or fingers; pounding heartbeat; memory loss; double vision; staring expression; difficulty walking; unawareness of surroundings.
- *Severe hypoglycemic reaction:* muscle twitching; unconsciousness; convulsions; lack of urinary control.

CAUSES

Too much insulin or oral anti-diabetic drug or not enough food for the condition the child's body is in. Factors which affect this include: more exercise than usual; irregular meals, skipped meals, or partial meals; loose bowel movements, diarrhea, or vomiting of the last meal; infection; anger or excitement.

RISK FACTORS

Stress; illness with fever; smoking, which decreases blood sugar; use of other drugs, which may also reduce blood sugar, such as diuretics, caffeine, or alcohol; liver or pancreas disorder.

PREVENTING COMPLICATIONS OR RECURRENCE

Urge your child to follow a diabetic diet and exercise and medication instructions carefully; keep hard candy available for your child's early symptoms; request glucagon and an injection kit from your doctor to keep on hand for your child.

WHAT TO EXPECT

MEDICAL TESTS

Your own observation of symptoms; medical history and physical exam by a doctor; laboratory studies of blood sugar; home studies for blood sugar, urine sugar, and urine acetone (reagent strip tests, which are available for home use without a doctor's prescription).

POSSIBLE COMPLICATIONS

Repeated attacks can cause permanent brain damage.

PROBABLE OUTCOME

The disorder is curable in 10 to 15 minutes if glucose can be given orally or by injection.

TREATMENT

HOME CARE

- Encourage your child to wear a Medic-Alert bracelet or pendant (see Glossary).
- For a mild hypoglycemic reaction: Give the child 1/2 cup of orange juice or a non-dietetic soft drink, or 1/2 candy bar, 6 or 7 hard candies, or 2 teaspoons of honey, syrup or sugar. Repeat, if necessary, in 10 to 15 minutes.
- For moderate hypoglycemic reaction: Give the child something sugary to eat or drink as above, but follow it with a carbohydrate that is absorbed more slowly, such as a banana, apple, cereal, bread, or crackers.
- For a severe hypoglycemic reaction: If the child is unconscious, inject glucagon (1/2cc to 1cc) deeply into a muscle and at right angles to the big muscle in the arm or leg. After the child regains consciousness, give sweet foods as above. Prop the child in a sitting position as soon as possible. Call the doctor.

MEDICATION

- Urge your child always to carry hard candy. Your doctor may prescribe glucagon to have available for emergencies.
- See Medications sections for information regarding medicines your doctor may prescribe.

ACTIVITY

After treatment, your child can resume normal activity as soon as possible.

DIET & FLUIDS

Ask your doctor if the child's basic diet plan needs changing.

OK FOR SCHOOL, PRESCHOOL, OR NURSERY?

When alertness, strength, and feeling of well-being will allow.

CALL YOUR DOCTOR IF

- Your child has diabetes, takes medication, and has symptoms of hypoglycemia—especially severe symptoms.
- Symptoms don't disappear with treatment above.
- Hypoglycemic reactions occur frequently.

HYPOPARATHYROIDISM

GENERAL INFORMATION

DESCRIPTION

Hypoparathyroidism is decreased production of hormones by the parathyroid glands, causing a low level of calcium in the blood. Body parts involved include the parathyroid glands in the neck, as well as the teeth and the blood (the blood affects all body tissues, especially the heart, blood vessels, bones, kidneys, gastrointestinal tract, skin, and the central nervous system—including the brain, the coverings of the brain (meninges), and the spinal cord—and peripheral nerves).

Appropriate health care includes:

- Physician's monitoring of general condition and medications during the acute stage.
- Self-care after diagnosis during the chronic stage.
- Hospitalization for severe muscle spasms (occasional).

SIGNS & SYMPTOMS

Acute phase:

- Tingling fingertips.
- Muscle tension and spasms in the hands and feet.
- Spasms of the larynx and throat muscles, causing breathing difficulty.
- Scaling skin.
- Splitting nails.

Chronic phase:

- Poor tooth development.
- Seizures.
- Mental retardation in children.
- Psychosis in adults.

CAUSES

- Complication of surgery on the parathyroid glands, the thyroid glands, or other neck tissues.
- Genetic autoimmune disorder (possibly).
- Radiation of the thyroid gland.
- Hemochromatosis (see Glossary).
- Tuberculosis.
- Neck injury.

RISK FACTORS

Recent infection of any kind.

- Pregnancy.
- Use of diuretic drugs.

PREVENTING COMPLICATIONS OR RECURRENCE

No specific preventive measures.

HYPOPARATHYROIDISM

WHAT TO EXPECT

MEDICAL TESTS

- Your own observation of symptoms.
- Medical history and physical exam by a doctor.
- Laboratory blood and urine studies.
- EKG (see Glossary).
- X-rays of bones to detect increased bone density.
- Special studies that may include ultrasonography, CAT or CT scan, MRI, and radionuclide scan (see Glossary for all).

POSSIBLE COMPLICATIONS

Cataracts; brain damage; heartbeat abnormalities; congestive heart failure.

PROBABLE OUTCOME

This condition is currently considered incurable. It requires lifelong replacement therapy to control symptoms. Without treatment, it is fatal. Scientific research continues, so there is hope for increasingly effective treatment and cure.

TREATMENT

HOME CARE

- If muscle cramps start, place a paper bag over your child's mouth. The child should blow into it and rebreathe the air in the bag. This will raise carbon-dioxide levels in the blood and decrease muscle spasms.
- Your child should apply lubricating creams or ointments to dry, scaling skin.
- Keep the child's nails trimmed to prevent splitting.

MEDICATION

Your doctor may prescribe:

- Vitamin D and calcium supplements in high doses.
- Intravenous calcium supplements during hospitalization for severe muscle spasms.
- Sedatives and anti-convulsants for frequent muscle spasms.

ACTIVITY

No restrictions.

DIET & FLUIDS

High calcium, low-phosphorous diet. Your doctor or dietitian will provide specific instructions.

OK FOR SCHOOL, PRESCHOOL, OR NURSERY?

When appetite has returned and alertness, strength, and feeling of well-being will allow.

CALL YOUR DOCTOR IF

- Your child has unexplained muscle spasms of the hands, feet, or throat, or numbness or tingling in the hands or feet.
- Muscle spasms don't decrease in 1 week, despite treatment.

HYPOTHERMIA

GENERAL INFORMATION

DESCRIPTION

Hypothermia is a dangerous cooling of the body from exposure to cold air or water. All major organ systems are involved, including decreased blood flow through the kidneys and brain. Hypothermia can affect all ages but is more common in the elderly than in children. (Also see DROWNING, NEAR-, in Illnesses section.)

Appropriate health care includes:

- Physician's monitoring of general condition and medications.
- Hospitalization. Arrange transportation to the nearest emergency center immediately.

SIGNS & SYMPTOMS

Early symptoms:

- Poor muscle coordination.
- Mental confusion and amnesia.
- Shivering and low body temperature (95F to 98F or 35C to 36.7C) rectally.
- Slow pulse.

Late symptoms:

- Rigid muscles.
- Temperature drop to 77F to 84F (25C to 28.9C).
- Purple fingers, toes, and nail beds.
- Loss of consciousness.

CAUSES

Prolonged exposure to cold temperatures, especially outdoors with a high wind-chill factor.

RISK FACTORS

- Thin or wet clothing.
- Slender body size. Slender children lose heat more rapidly than obese children.
- Smoking, which decreases circulation to extremities.
- Excess alcohol consumption.
- Mental impairment.

PREVENTING COMPLICATIONS OR RECURRENCE

- Obtain warm housing and adequate clothing for your child before winter.
- In cold weather, encourage the child to wear windproof clothing in many layers, including a scarf, hat, and mittens.
- Urge your child not to leave home during a severe winter storm.
- Instruct your child not to skate or fish on ice before determining that the ice is safe.
- Children who are unable to care for themselves fully, such as the mentally impaired, should be supervised during cold weather.

WHAT TO EXPECT

MEDICAL TESTS
- Your own observation of symptoms.
- Medical history and physical exam by a doctor.
- Laboratory studies, such as kidney-function studies.

POSSIBLE COMPLICATIONS
- Shock.
- Pneumonia.
- Death.

PROBABLE OUTCOME
Sometimes fatal, depending on the length and amount of temperature loss. Chances of survival are excellent if the patient is conscious on arrival at the emergency center. Sometimes, with continued resuscitative efforts, there can be remarkable or miraculous recovery.

TREATMENT

HOME CARE
The following may be helpful while waiting for emergency help:
- Place the child in bed and cover with a blanket or electric blanket at normal body temperature.
- A warm (not hot) bath may be helpful—but call the nearest emergency center for advice.
- If the child is outdoors, cover with blankets or shield from the wind.

MEDICATION
- The doctor may prescribe medicine to support blood pressure if the child's condition is critical.
- See Medications section for information regarding medicines your doctor may prescribe.

ACTIVITY
After treatment, normal activity should be resumed gradually.

DIET & FLUIDS
Don't give alcohol to a child with hypothermia. It is of no help and may be harmful.

OK FOR SCHOOL, PRESCHOOL, OR NURSERY?
When appetite has returned and alertness, strength, and feeling of well-being will allow.

CALL YOUR DOCTOR IF

You observe symptoms of hypothermia in your child.

ID REACTION
(Autoeczematization; Autosensitization)

GENERAL INFORMATION

DESCRIPTION

An id reaction is an allergic response to a skin disorder of the feet, groin, or other area, producing an itching rash somewhere else in the body. Body parts with the original disorder include the groin, ears, hands, and feet; body parts with the allergic response include the hands, feet, arms, legs, or trunk.

Appropriate health care includes:

- Physician's monitoring of general condition and medications.
- Self-care after diagnosis.

SIGNS & SYMPTOMS

- Itching (often severe).
- Vesicles (fluid-filled, small blisters) of varying size on the skin.

CAUSES

Unknown. An id reaction may be a disorder of the body's immunological response to the original ailment. It occurs most often with some forms of dermatitis, outer-ear infections, and eczema of the hand or foot.

RISK FACTORS

- Recent skin rash anywhere.
- Stress.
- Medical history of allergies.

PREVENTING COMPLICATIONS OR RECURRENCE

Treat all your child's skin disorders thoroughly until they disappear.

WHAT TO EXPECT

MEDICAL TESTS

- Your own observation of symptoms.
- Medical history and physical exam by a doctor.
- Laboratory culture of the original skin disorder.

POSSIBLE COMPLICATIONS

Adverse reaction to medication used in treatment.

PROBABLE OUTCOME

Usually curable in 2 weeks. Recurrence is rapid if treatment is discontinued before the id reaction and the original disorder are completely gone.

ID REACTION (Autoeczematization; Autosensitization)

TREATMENT

HOME CARE

• Treat the child's original skin disorder until it heals completely to prevent a recurrence of the id reaction. For instructions, consult your doctor or refer to the disorder in this book.
• Minimize your child's stress, if possible. (See Appendix 19).

MEDICATION

• Your doctor may prescribe topical or oral cortisone drugs. Oral steroids quickly control the id reaction, but they slow healing of the underlying disorder.
• See Medications section for information regarding medicines your doctor may prescribe.

ACTIVITY

No restrictions.

DIET & FLUIDS

No special diet.

OK FOR SCHOOL, PRESCHOOL, OR NURSERY?

When appetite has returned and alertness, strength, and feeling of well-being will allow.

CALL YOUR DOCTOR IF

• Your child has symptoms of an id reaction.
• The following occurs during treatment:
— Fever higher than 101F (38.3C).
— Heat, redness, pain, or tenderness in any of the lesions. This indicates infection.
• New, unexplained symptoms develop. Drugs used in treatment may produce side effects.

IDIOPATHIC HYPERTROPHIC SUBAORTIC STENOSIS (IHSS)

GENERAL INFORMATION

DESCRIPTION

Idiopathic hypertrophic subaortic stenosis is a chronic heart condition that produces an enlarged heart muscle, restricting the amount of blood the heart pumps. Only the heart is involved.

Appropriate health care includes:

- Physician's monitoring of general condition and medications, including consultation with a cardiologist.
- Surgery to reduce the obstruction, if medication does not control the problem.
- DC electrocardioversion (electric shock to the heart) for treatment of life-threatening heartbeat irregularities.

SIGNS & SYMPTOMS

- Chest pain (angina pectoris).
- Heart-rhythm irregularity.
- Fainting.
- Shortness of breath.
- Swollen feet and ankles.
- Distended neck veins.
- Enlarged and tender liver (under the rib cage).
- Heart murmur (see Glossary).

CAUSES

The underlying cause is unknown. The effects cause thickening of the left chamber (ventricle) of the heart. This obstructs the flow of blood, and the heart may be unable to pump enough blood during exertion. In some cases, this condition may be inherited as a dominant genetic trait.

RISK FACTORS

Family history of IHSS.

PREVENTING COMPLICATIONS OR RECURRENCE

If you have a family history of IHSS, obtain genetic counseling before starting a family.

WHAT TO EXPECT

MEDICAL TESTS

- Your own observation of symptoms.
- Medical history and physical exam by a doctor.
- Laboratory studies, such as cardiac catheterization to measure blood flow through the heart chambers.
- X-rays of the heart.
- EKG and echocardiogram (see Glossary for both) of the heart.
- Special studies that may include ultrasonography, CAT or CT scan, MRI, and radionuclide scan (see Glossary for all).

IDIOPATHIC HYPERTROPHIC SUBAORTIC STENOSIS (IHSS)

POSSIBLE COMPLICATIONS

Fatal heartbeat irregularity.

PROBABLE OUTCOME

Usually controllable with medication or surgery.

TREATMENT

HOME CARE

- Keep your child under close medical supervision.
- Urge your child to wear a Medic-Alert bracelet or pendant (see Glossary).
- Family members, close friends, and business acquaintances should learn cardiopulmonary resuscitation (CPR), in case cardiac arrest occurs.

MEDICATION

Your doctor may prescribe:

- Beta-adrenergic blockers or calcium-channel blockers to prevent heartbeat irregularities.
- Don't give your child nitroglycerin for angina pain. It dilates arteries, which may be harmful.
- If digitalis is prescribed for your child, discuss the risks with your doctor. It may trigger heartbeat irregularities.
- See Medications section for information regarding medicines your doctor may prescribe.

ACTIVITY

Your doctor should guide you and your child about how much physical activity is ideal. The ability to increase activity is dependent on the response to therapy. Don't regard your child as an invalid.

DIET & FLUIDS

A low-salt diet (see Appendix 29) may be necessary, if your child has fluid accumulation (a possible sign of congestive heart failure).

OK FOR SCHOOL, PRESCHOOL, OR NURSERY?

When appetite has returned and alertness, strength, and feeling of well-being will allow.

CALL YOUR DOCTOR IF

- Your child has symptoms of IHSS, or symptoms worsen during treatment.
- New, unexplained symptoms develop. Drugs used in treatment may produce side effects.

IMMUNODEFICIENCY DISEASE, Including AIDS (Acquired Immunodeficiency Syndrome)

GENERAL INFORMATION

DESCRIPTION

Immunodeficiency disease is a defect in the body's immune system. A healthy immune system protects the body against germs (bacteria, viruses, and fungi), cancer (partial protection) and any foreign material that enters the body. When the system fails, the body becomes susceptible to infection and cancer. The immune system (blood, bone marrow, lymph tissue, liver, spleen, and thymus gland) is involved.

Appropriate health care includes:

- Physician's monitoring of general condition and medications.
- Surgery to transplant bone marrow or the thymus gland (occasionally).
- Hospitalization for treatment of serious infection.

SIGNS & SYMPTOMS

Recurrent, severe infections and illnesses. The most common include:

- Ear or respiratory infections, such as otitis media and pneumonia.
- Yeast infections, especially candidiasis.
- Cancer, especially leukemia and lymphoma.
- Bleeding disorders.
- Eczema.
- Meningitis or encephalitis.

CAUSES

- Birth defects that involve an incomplete or absent immune system.
- Surgical removal of the spleen before age 2.
- Use of immunosuppressive drugs.
- Radiation treatment.
- Some cancers, such as Hodgkin's disease.
- Hypogammaglobulinemia (see Glossary).
- Viral infections, such as AIDS (acquired immunodeficiency syndrome).

RISK FACTORS

- Poor nutrition.
- Male homosexual activity, blood transfusions, or intravenous drug use (AIDS only).
- Family history of immunodeficiency disease.

PREVENTING COMPLICATIONS OR RECURRENCE

- If you have a family history of immunodeficiency disease, seek genetic counseling before starting a family.
- If you are a practicing homosexual, become celibate or practice "safe sex." See special entry on AIDS.

IMMUNODEFICIENCY DISEASE, Including AIDS (Acquired Immunodeficiency Syndrome)

WHAT TO EXPECT

MEDICAL TESTS

- Your own observation of symptoms, especially repeated infections in your child.
- Medical history and physical exam by a doctor.
- Laboratory blood studies of antibodies, microscopic examination of blood and tissue cells, and skin tests.
- X-rays of the thymus gland.
- Radioactive studies of immune function.
- Special studies that may include ultrasonography, CAT or CT scan, MRI, radionuclide scan (see Glossary for all).

POSSIBLE COMPLICATIONS

Uncontrolled bacterial, viral or fungal infections that don't respond to treatment; cancer; infectious arthritis.

PROBABLE OUTCOME

Severe forms of immunodeficiency are usually fatal. Minor forms can be treated successfully.

TREATMENT

HOME CARE

- Your child should avoid exposure to persons with contagious illnesses.
- Your child should not take *any* type of vaccine without medical advice.
- Your child should not take prescribed cortisone or immunosuppressive drugs without getting a second medical opinion.

MEDICATION

Your doctor may prescribe antibiotics to fight infections; injections of antibodies; transfusions of blood components; injections of gamma globulin (sometimes).

ACTIVITY

Bed rest is usually necessary for your child during acute illnesses. Otherwise, there are no restrictions on activity.

DIET & FLUIDS

No special diet.

OK FOR SCHOOL, PRESCHOOL, OR NURSERY?

When appetite has returned and alertness, strength, and feeling of well-being will allow.

CALL YOUR DOCTOR IF

- Your child has symptoms of immunodeficiency disease.
- After diagnosis, your child has signs of infection, such as chills, fever, muscle aches, headache, dizziness, and cough with thick, discolored or blood-streaked sputum.

IMPETIGO
(Pyoderma)

GENERAL INFORMATION

DESCRIPTION

Impetigo is a contagious, common bacterial skin infection that affects the superficial layers of the skin. The skin of the face, arms, and legs is involved. Impetigo is most common in infants and children.

Appropriate health care includes:
- Home care after diagnosis.
- Physician's monitoring of general condition and medications.

SIGNS & SYMPTOMS

- A red rash with many small blisters. Some blisters contain pus, and yellow crusts form when they break. The blisters don't hurt, but they may itch.
- Slight fever (sometimes).

CAUSES

Staphylococci or streptococci bacteria growing in the upper skin layers.

RISK FACTORS

- Fair complexion.
- Skin that is sensitive to sun and irritants, such as soap and makeup.
- Poor nutrition.
- Illness that has lowered resistance.
- Warm, moist weather.
- Crowded or unsanitary living conditions.
- Poor hygiene.

PREVENTING COMPLICATIONS OR RECURRENCE

- Your child should bathe daily with soap and water.
- Keep the child's fingernails short. Urge the child not to scratch impetigo blisters.
- If there is an outbreak in the family, urge all members to use anti-bacterial soap.
- Use separate towels for each family member, or substitute paper towels temporarily.

WHAT TO EXPECT

MEDICAL TESTS

- Your own observation of symptoms.
- Medical history and physical exam by a doctor.
- Laboratory skin culture to identify the germ causing the infection.

POSSIBLE COMPLICATIONS

- Penetration of the infection to deeper skin layers (ecthyma or cellulitis). This may cause scarring. Treatment is the same as for impetigo.
- Acute glomerulonephritis.

PROBABLE OUTCOME

Curable in 10 days with treatment.

IMPETIGO (Pyoderma)

TREATMENT

HOME CARE

- Follow the suggestions listed under PREVENTING COMPLICATIONS OR RECURRENCE.
- Scrub lesions with gauze and antiseptic soap. Break any pustules. Remove all crusts, and expose and cleanse all lesions. If crusts are difficult to remove, soak them in warm soapy water and scrub gently.
- Cover impetigo sores with gauze and tape to keep the child's hands away from them.
- Treat new lesions the same way, even if you are not sure they are impetigo.
- Separate and boil bed linen, if possible, as well as towels, clothes, and other items that have touched sores.
- Males who shave should do so around sores on the face, not over them, using an aerosol shaving cream and changing razor blades each day. They should not use a shaving brush—it may harbor germs.

MEDICATION

Your doctor may prescribe:

- Oral antibiotics, such as dicloxacillin or erythromycin. To avoid complications, your child should take antibiotics for 10 days even if symptoms disappear.
- Antibiotic ointments for very small areas of infection. Rub antibiotic ointment into the child's lesions for 60 seconds at least 4 times a day. If your doctor has not prescribed an ointment, you may use a non-prescription ointment containing neomycin and bacitracin.
- See Medications section for information regarding medicines your doctor may prescribe.

ACTIVITY

No restrictions.

DIET & FLUIDS

No special diet.

OK FOR SCHOOL, PRESCHOOL, OR NURSERY?

When signs of infection have decreased, appetite returns, and alertness, strength, and feeling of well-being will allow.

CALL YOUR DOCTOR IF

- Your child has symptoms of impetigo.
- Fever of 101F (38.3C) or higher orally develops.
- The sores continue to spread or don't begin to heal in 3 days, despite treatment.

ILLNESSES

INCONTINENCE, STRESS

GENERAL INFORMATION

DESCRIPTION

Stress incontinence is an involuntary loss of urine in females that accompanies any action that suddenly increases pressure in the abdomen. The urinary bladder and urethra are involved. Females of all ages can be affected.

Appropriate health care includes:
- Self-care.
- Doctor's treatment.
- Surgery to tighten relaxed or damaged muscles that support the bladder.

SIGNS & SYMPTOMS

Unintentional loss of urine with lifting, sneezing, singing, coughing, laughing, crying, or straining to have a bowel movement.

CAUSES

Shortening of the urethra and loss of the normal muscular support for the bladder and floor of the pelvis. These changes occur during pregnancy and after childbirth, particularly repeated childbirth. They may also occur as a natural consequence of aging.

RISK FACTORS
- Repeated childbirth.
- Obesity.
- Chronic lung disease with a cough.

PREVENTING COMPLICATIONS OR RECURRENCE

Instructions for your daughter:
- Eat a normal, well-balanced diet and exercise regularly to build and maintain muscle strength.
- Learn and practice Kegel exercises (see HOME CARE) after childbirth, before symptoms of stress incontinence begin.

WHAT TO EXPECT

MEDICAL TESTS
- Your own observation of symptoms.
- Medical history and physical exam by a doctor.
- Urinalysis to determine if a urinary-tract infection is causing your daughter's symptoms.

POSSIBLE COMPLICATIONS
- Complete loss of urinary control. This requires surgery.
- Urinary-tract infections.
- Social isolation due to concern about embarrassment.

PROBABLE OUTCOME

If the stress incontinence is not severe enough to require surgery, exercise can improve your daughter's muscle function. If it is severe, it can be cured with surgery.

TREATMENT

HOME CARE

Instructions for your daughter:

• Learn to recognize, control, and develop the muscles of the pelvic floor. These are the ones you use to interrupt urination in mid-stream. The following exercises (Kegel exercises) strengthen these muscles so you can control or relax them completely:

• To identify which muscles are involved, alternately start and stop urinating when using the toilet.

• Practice tightening and releasing these muscles while sitting, standing, walking, driving, watching TV, or listening to music.

• Tighten the muscles a small amount at a time, "like an elevator going up to the 10th floor." Then release very slowly, "one floor at a time."

• Tighten the muscles from front to back, including the anus, as in the previous exercise.

• Practice exercises every morning, afternoon, and evening. Start with 5 times each, and gradually work up to 20 or 30 each time.

• Wear absorbent underpants.

MEDICATION

• Medicine usually is not necessary for this disorder, but your doctor may prescribe:

—Antibiotics if your daughter has a complicating urinary-tract infection.

—A pessary (support device) made of rubber or other material to fit inside the vagina to support the uterus and lower muscular layer of the bladder.

• See Medications section for information regarding medicines your doctor may prescribe.

ACTIVITY

No restrictions.

DIET & FLUIDS

Your daughter should lose weight if she is obese. A reducing diet appears in Appendix 31.

OK FOR SCHOOL, PRESCHOOL, OR NURSERY?

When signs of infection have decreased, appetite returns and alertness, strength, and feeling of well-being will allow.

CALL YOUR DOCTOR IF

• Your daughter has symptoms of stress incontinence.

• Any sign of infection develops, such as fever, pain on urination, frequent urination, or a general ill feeling.

• Symptoms don't improve after 3 months of Kegel exercises, or symptoms become intolerable and your daughter wishes to consider surgery.

INDIGESTION (Dyspepsia)

GENERAL INFORMATION

DESCRIPTION

Indigestion is a vague chest or abdominal discomfort—with no apparent organic cause—that occurs during or soon after eating or drinking. The stomach, esophagus, and small intestine are involved.

Appropriate health care includes:

- Self-care.
- Physician's monitoring of general condition and medications (severe, recurrent indigestion only).

SIGNS & SYMPTOMS

- Mild nausea; heartburn; upper abdominal pain; gas or belching; bloated or full feeling; acid taste.

CAUSES

Symptoms seem related to eating, drinking, or swallowing air while talking or chewing gum. They occur often with emotional upset while eating, excessive smoking, constipation, eating improperly cooked food, eating high-fat food, poor digestion of gas-forming foods (such as beans, cucumbers, cabbage, turnips, and onions), food allergy, or overindulgence in alcohol.

RISK FACTORS

Stress, smoking, excess alcohol consumption, use of drugs that may irritate the stomach, and fatigue or overwork.

PREVENTING COMPLICATIONS OR RECURRENCE

Instructions for your child: Avoid foods you don't digest well, don't smoke, relax after meals, avoid emotional situations during meals, and don't eat fast.

OTHER

Persistent symptoms can indicate disease in the digestive tract or other body parts. Occasionally, symptoms occur in children with no apparent disease. This indicates an abnormal function in a normal part of the body.

WHAT TO EXPECT

MEDICAL TESTS

- Your own observation of symptoms.
- Medical history and physical exam by a doctor.
- X-rays of the upper digestive tract.
- Gastroscopy (see Glossary).

POSSIBLE COMPLICATIONS

Indigestion may mimic signs of a heart attack or serious disease of the esophagus or stomach, causing the serious disorder to be ignored.

INDIGESTION (Dyspepsia)

PROBABLE OUTCOME

Symptoms can be controlled with treatment, but recurrence is likely.

TREATMENT

HOME CARE

Treatment and prevention are similar. Instructions for your child:

- Allow time for leisurely meals. Chew food carefully and thoroughly. Avoid conflicts during meals.
- Don't smoke immediately before a meal.
- Avoid excitement or exercise immediately after a meal.
- Avoid situations that make you swallow air, such as chewing gum.
- Observe episodes of indigestion for changes in symptoms. If character, timing, frequency, or severity changes, a more serious disorder may be responsible. These include heartburn from irritation of the lower esophagus, gallbladder disease, ulcers, or stomach cancer.

MEDICATION

- For minor discomfort, use non-prescription antacids.
- For serious discomfort, your doctor may prescribe H-2 blockers, anti-spasmodics or tranquilizers to relieve your child's tension.

ACTIVITY

No restrictions.

DIET & FLUIDS

No special diet. Your child should avoid foods—especially those listed under causes—that cause discomfort.

OK FOR SCHOOL, PRESCHOOL, OR NURSERY?

When appetite has returned and alertness, strength, and feeling of well-being will allow.

CALL YOUR DOCTOR IF

- The pattern of indigestion symptoms changes markedly.
- Your child develops the following:
  - Vomiting, weight loss or loss of appetite.
  - Black, tarry stool or vomiting of blood.
  - Fever.
  - Severe pain in the upper right abdomen.
  - Discomfort that continues unrelated to meals, eating, or chewing gum.
- Indigestion is accompanied by:
  - Shortness of breath.
  - Sweating.
  - Pain radiating to the jaw, neck, or arm.

ILLNESSES

INFLUENZA
(Flu; Grippe)

GENERAL INFORMATION

DESCRIPTION

Influenza is a common, contagious respiratory infection caused by a virus. Incubation after exposure is 24 to 48 hours. All parts of the respiratory system—nose, sinuses, throat, trachea, bronchial tubes, and lungs—are involved. Influenza can affect both sexes, all ages, but it is unusual in infants. Appropriate health care includes:

- Self-care after diagnosis.
- Physician's monitoring of general condition and medications (sometimes).

SIGNS & SYMPTOMS

- Chills and moderate to high fever.
- Muscle aches, including backache.
- Cough, usually with little or no sputum.
- Sore throat.
- Hoarseness.
- Runny nose.
- Headache.
- Fatigue.

CAUSES

Infection by viruses of the myxovirus class. The viruses are spread by personal contact.

RISK FACTORS

Stress; fatigue or overwork; poor nutrition; recent illness that has lowered resistance; chronic illness, especially chronic lung disease.

PREVENTING COMPLICATIONS OR RECURRENCE

- Your child should avoid risks listed above.
- Your child should avoid unnecessary contact with persons who have upper-respiratory infections during the flu season (winter).
- A child with chronic heart or lung disease should have a yearly influenza vaccine injection. A vaccine protects against only a few—not all—types of flu.

WHAT TO EXPECT

MEDICAL TESTS

- Your own observation of symptoms.
- Medical history and physical exam by a doctor.
- Laboratory studies, such as blood tests and sputum culture (only for complications).
- X-rays of the chest.

POSSIBLE COMPLICATIONS

Bacterial infections, including middle-ear infection, sinusitis, throat infections, bronchitis, or pneumonia. These can be especially dangerous for very young children.

INFLUENZA (Flu; Grippe)

PROBABLE OUTCOME

Spontaneous recovery in 7 to 14 days if no complications occur. If complications arise, treatment with antibiotics is usually necessary, and recovery may take 3 to 6 weeks.

TREATMENT

HOME CARE

- To relieve nasal congestion, use salt-water drops (¼ teaspoon of salt to 1 cup of water).
- To relieve a sore throat, the child can gargle often with warm or cold double-strength tea.
- Use a cool-mist humidifier to increase air moisture around the child. This thins lung secretions so they can be coughed up more easily. Don't put medicine in the humidifier; it does not help.
- To avoid spreading germs to others, urge your child to wash hands frequently—especially after blowing the nose or before handling food.

MEDICATION

- For minor discomfort, use non-prescription drugs, such as acetaminophen, cough syrups, nasal sprays, or decongestants.
- Don't give aspirin to a child younger than 16. Some research shows a link between the use of aspirin in children during a virus illness and the development of Reye's syndrome (a type of encephalitis).
- Your doctor may prescribe an anti-viral drug, amantadine, for seriously ill children or for those at greatest risk from complications.

ACTIVITY

Rest is the best medicine. If your child is in good general health, rest helps the body fight the virus.

DIET & FLUIDS

No special diet. If your child has a high fever, encourage extra fluids—at least 8 glasses of water a day. Extra fluids, including fruit juice, tea, and carbonated drinks, also help thin lung secretions. The child should avoid milk because it thickens secretions in some children.

OK FOR SCHOOL, PRESCHOOL, OR NURSERY?

When signs of infection have decreased, appetite returns, and alertness, strength, and feeling of well-being will allow.

CALL YOUR DOCTOR IF

- Your child has symptoms of influenza.
- The following occurs during treatment: increased fever or cough; blood in the sputum; earache; shortness of breath or chest pain; thick discharge from the nose, sinuses, or ears; sinus pain; neck pain or stiffness.
- New, unexplained symptoms develop. Drugs used in treatment may produce side effects.

INNER EAR DISORDERS
(Including Meniere's Disease and Labyrinthitis)

GENERAL INFORMATION

DESCRIPTION

The inner ear houses two main structures: a part of the eighth cranial nerve, which is important in hearing, and another part to help maintain balance. When your child's inner ear is disturbed or diseased, both hearing and balance may be altered. Many of the same symptoms experienced with seasickness and motion sickness may occur. Labyrinthitis is a disorder accompanied by inflammation of the semicircular canals in the inner ear (the labyrinth). Meniere's disease is a disorder accompanied by fluid in the inner ear's semicircular canals. All disorders of the inner ear may be accompanied by the same or similar symptoms. Appropriate health care includes hospitalization for the worst cases. If deafness accompanies other symptoms, see an ear specialist immediately!

SIGNS & SYMPTOMS

- For Meniere's disease: severe dizziness; noises in the affected ear, such as ringing or buzzing; hearing loss that increases with each attack. Possible accompanying symptoms: vomiting; sweating; jerky eye movements; loss of balance.
- For labyrinthitis: extreme dizziness—especially with head movement—that begins gradually and peaks in 48 hours; involuntary eye movement; nausea and vomiting; loss of balance, especially falling toward the affected side; temporary hearing loss.

CAUSES

- For Meniere's: unknown.
- For labyrinthitis: virus infection (usually in the inner ear); bacterial infection in the inner ear; spread of a chronic middle-ear infection; ingestion of toxic drugs; allergy; cholesteatoma (an accumulation of debris covered by skin in the outer-ear canal).

RISK FACTORS

- Stress.
- Recent viral illness, especially respiratory infection; family history of allergies.
- Smoking.
- Excess alcohol consumption.
- Use of some prescription or non-prescription drugs, especially aspirin.
- Fatigue or overwork.

PREVENTING COMPLICATIONS OR RECURRENCE

Obtain prompt medical treatment for your child's ear infections.

WHAT TO EXPECT

MEDICAL TESTS

- Your own observation of symptoms.
- Medical history and physical exam by a doctor.
- Diagnostic measures including audiometry and ice-water tests.

INNER EAR DISORDERS (Including Meniere's Disease and Labyrinthitis)

POSSIBLE COMPLICATIONS

Permanent hearing loss on the side affected (rare).

PROBABLE OUTCOME

Recovery—either spontaneous or with treatment—in 1 to 6 weeks.

TREATMENT

HOME CARE

Instructions for your child:

- Avoid glaring light and don't read during attacks.
- Rest quietly in bed until dizziness and nausea disappear.
- Don't walk without assistance.
- Avoid sudden changes in position.

MEDICATION

Your doctor may prescribe:

- Anti-nausea drugs.
- Tranquilizers to reduce the child's dizziness.
- Antihistamines, which sometime lessen symptoms.
- Diuretics to decrease fluid in the inner ear.

ACTIVITY

Keep the child's head as still as possible. Your child should rest in bed until the dizziness subsides. Then normal activities may be resumed gradually. Urge the child to avoid hazardous activities, such as driving, climbing, or working around dangerous machinery, until 1 week after symptoms disappear.

DIET & FLUIDS

Temporarily decrease the child's salt and fluid intake.

OK FOR SCHOOL, PRESCHOOL, OR NURSERY?

Yes, when condition and sense of well-being will allow.

CALL YOUR DOCTOR IF

- Your child has symptoms of labyrinthitis or Meniere's disease. If deafness occurs, call immediately!
- The following occurs during treatment: decreased hearing in either ear; persistent vomiting; convulsions; fainting; fever of 101F (38.3C) or higher.
- New, unexplained symptoms develop. Drugs used in treatment may produce side effects.

INSECT BITES & STINGS

GENERAL INFORMATION

DESCRIPTION

Insect bites and stings cause skin eruptions and other symptoms. The victim often doesn't remember being bitten or stung. The skin on any part of the body and the lymph glands in the neck, armpit, groin, or elbow are involved.

Appropriate health care includes:
- Self-care.
- Physician's monitoring of general condition and medications (sometimes).

SIGNS & SYMPTOMS

Red lumps in the skin. The lumps usually appear within minutes after the bite or sting, but some don't appear for 6 to 12 hours. Skin reactions fall into 2 categories:
- A toxic reaction with pain, such as from bee stings.
- A toxic reaction with itching due to the body's release of histamine at the bite site, such as from mosquitoes.

CAUSES

Bites or stings from mosquitoes, fleas, chiggers, bedbugs, ants, spiders, bees, and other insects.

RISK FACTORS
- Areas with heavy insect infestations.
- Warm weather in spring and summer.

PREVENTING COMPLICATIONS OR RECURRENCE
- After identifying the cause, remove it if possible. Treat animals for fleas and exterminate the house or kennel.
- If your child cannot avoid exposure to biting insects, apply insect repellents with diethyltoluamide (DEET).
- Recent evidence indicates that vitamins in the B-vitamin group may be a deterrent to insect bites.

WHAT TO EXPECT

MEDICAL TESTS
- Your own observation of symptoms.
- Medical history and physical exam by a doctor.

POSSIBLE COMPLICATIONS
- Anaphylaxis (for hypersensitive children). This is an emergency! See Anaphylaxis (in Illnesses section).
- Secondary bacterial infection at the site of the bite. This may cause swollen lymph glands in the neck, armpit, groin, or elbow.

PROBABLE OUTCOME

Most troublesome symptoms disappear in 2 to 3 days, but scratching may prolong your child's symptoms for several weeks. Treatment helps, but it doesn't cure quickly.

TREATMENT

HOME CARE

- Use immersion or wrapped soaks to relieve your child's itching and hasten healing. Warm-water soaks are usually more soothing for pain and inflammation. Cool-water soaks feel better for itching.
- If your child has had anaphylaxis (severe allergic reaction) following an insect bite, ask your doctor for an anaphylaxis kit to treat it in the future.

MEDICATION

- For minor discomfort, you may use the following for your child:
  — Non-prescription oral antihistamines to decrease itching.
  — Non-prescription topical steroid preparations to reduce inflammation and decrease itching. Use according to label directions. For face and groin, use only low-potency steroid products without fluorine.
- For serious symptoms, your doctor may:
  — Prescribe stronger topical steroids or oral steroids if the reaction is severe.
  — Inject epinephrine or cortisone to prevent or diminish anaphylaxis symptoms.
- See Medications section for information regarding medicines your doctor may prescribe.

ACTIVITY

No restrictions.

DIET & FLUIDS

No special diet.

OK FOR SCHOOL, PRESCHOOL, OR NURSERY?

When appetite has returned and alertness, strength, and feeling of well-being will allow.

CALL YOUR DOCTOR IF

- Your child has symptoms of anaphylaxis. This is an emergency!
- Self-care does not relieve symptoms, or symptoms don't improve after 2 to 3 days of medical treatment.
- A bitten area becomes red, swollen, warm, and tender, indicating infection.
- Temperature rises to 101F (38.3C).

INSOMNIA

GENERAL INFORMATION

DESCRIPTION

Insomnia is a sleep disturbance—difficulty either falling asleep or remaining asleep. All body cells, especially the central nervous system—including the brain, the coverings of the brain (meninges), and the spinal cord—and peripheral nerves are involved.

Appropriate health care includes:
- Self-care after diagnosis.
- Physician's monitoring of general condition and medications.
- Psychotherapy or counseling, if the cause is psychological.

SIGNS & SYMPTOMS

- Restlessness when trying to fall asleep.
- Brief sleep followed by wakefulness.
- Normal sleep until very early in the morning (3 a.m. or 4 a.m.), then wakefulness (often with frightening thoughts).
- Periods of sleeplessness, alternating with periods of excessive sleep or sleepiness at inconvenient times.

CAUSES

- Depression. This is usually characterized by early-morning wakefulness.
- Overactivity of the thyroid gland.
- Anxiety caused by stress.
- Noisy environment (including a snoring sleeper sharing the room).
- Allergies and early-morning wheezing.
- Heart or lung conditions that cause shortness of breath when lying down.
- Painful disorders, such as fibromyositis or arthritis.
- Urinary or gastrointestinal problems that require urination or bowel movements during the night.
- Consumption of stimulants, such as coffee, tea, or cola drinks.
- Use of some medications, including dextroamphetamines or cortisone drugs.
- Erratic work hours.
- New environment or location.
- Jet lag after travel.
- Lack of physical exercise.
- Alcoholism.
- Drug abuse, including overuse of sleep-inducing drugs.
- Withdrawal from addictive substances.

RISK FACTORS

Stress; obesity; smoking.

PREVENTING COMPLICATIONS OR RECURRENCE

Encourage your child to establish a lifestyle that fosters healthy sleep patterns (see HOME CARE).

WHAT TO EXPECT

MEDICAL TESTS

Your own observation of symptoms; medical history and physical exam by a doctor; laboratory thyroid studies; EEG (see Glossary); tests in a sleep-study laboratory.

POSSIBLE COMPLICATIONS

Impaired relationships; poor school work performance; lower resistance to disease; injury from falling asleep around machinery or while driving.

PROBABLE OUTCOME

Most children can establish good sleep patterns if the underlying cause of insomnia is treated or eliminated.

TREATMENT

HOME CARE

- Seek ways to minimize stress in your child's life. See Appendix 19.
- Obtain medical treatment for any underlying medical disorder.
- Urge your child not to use stimulants for several hours before bedtime.
- Encourage the child to relax in a warm bath before bedtime.

MEDICATION

Your doctor may prescribe sleep-inducing drugs for a short time if:

- Temporary insomnia is interfering with your child's daily activities.
- Your child has a medical disorder that regularly disturbs sleep.
- Your child needs to establish regular sleep patterns.

Long-term use of sleep inducers may be counter-productive or addictive. Urge your child not to use sleeping pills given by friends, and not to take non-prescription sleeping pills.

ACTIVITY

Your child should exercise regularly (see Appendix 36) to create healthy fatigue.

DIET & FLUIDS

No special diet, but your child should not eat within 3 hours of bedtime if indigestion has previously disturbed sleep. Drinking a glass of warm milk before bedtime helps some children.

OK FOR SCHOOL, PRESCHOOL, OR NURSERY?

When appetite has returned and alertness, strength, and feeling of well-being will allow.

CALL YOUR DOCTOR IF

- Your child has insomnia.
- New, unexplained symptoms develop. Drugs used in treatment may produce side effects.

INTESTINAL OBSTRUCTION

GENERAL INFORMATION

DESCRIPTION

Intestinal obstruction is a partial or complete blockage of the intestines. Both the small and large intestines are involved.

Appropriate health care includes:

- Physician's monitoring of general condition and medications.
- Surgery to remove the obstruction (usually).
- Hospitalization for diagnosis and replacement of lost fluids prior to surgery.

SIGNS & SYMPTOMS

- Abdominal pain and cramps.
- Nausea and vomiting. In the advanced stage, vomit resembles feces.
- Weakness, dizziness, or fainting.
- Little or no urine, due to fluid loss.
- Audible noises from the abdomen in early stages. Later, *no* sounds are audible.
- Abdominal bloating, swelling, and gas.
- Fever (sometimes).
- Diarrhea (partial obstruction only).
- Rectal bleeding (sometimes).

CAUSES

- Adhesions (constricting bands of fibrous tissue that result from previous surgery).
- Intestinal hernias.
- Intestinal inflammation or tumors—either benign or cancerous.
- Tumors in adjacent organs that cause pressure on the intestines.
- Foreign objects inside the intestines (swallowed objects, or parasites such as worms).
- Twisted bowel (volvulus, see Glossary).
- Severe constipation (fecal impaction).

RISK FACTORS

Previous abdominal surgery.

PREVENTING COMPLICATIONS OR RECURRENCE

- Encourage your child to eat a diet high in fiber and to drink at least 6 to 8 glasses of liquid a day to avoid constipation or fecal impaction.
- Obtain prompt medical treatment for repair of hernias.
- See your doctor if your child's bowel habits change significantly for longer than 7 days. This may be an early symptom of bowel cancer.

? WHAT TO EXPECT

MEDICAL TESTS

- Your own observation of symptoms.
- Medical history and physical exam by a doctor.
- Laboratory blood studies to measure fluids and electrolytes and to detect bleeding or infection.
- X-rays of the intestinal tract and abdomen (upper and lower GI series).

POSSIBLE COMPLICATIONS

- Dehydration and shock.
- Bowel gangrene.
- Peritonitis.

PROBABLE OUTCOME

Surgery can usually correct the obstruction, but it may not correct the underlying cause, such as cancer. Without treatment, complications can be fatal.

TREATMENT

HOME CARE

Intestinal obstruction usually develops rapidly into an emergency. Home remedies are of no value and some—such as enemas or laxatives—may be harmful to your child.

MEDICATION

- Medication is not helpful for intestinal obstruction. However, your doctor may prescribe medication appropriate for the underlying disorder.
- See Medications section for information regarding medicines your doctor may prescribe.

ACTIVITY

Your child should rest in bed until the obstruction is corrected. If surgery is necessary, the child can resume normal activities gradually.

DIET & FLUIDS

Don't give the child anything to eat until the obstruction is corrected. There will probably be intravenous nourishment given until then.

OK FOR SCHOOL, PRESCHOOL, OR NURSERY?

When appetite has returned and alertness, strength, and feeling of well-being will allow.

CALL YOUR DOCTOR IF

- Your child's bowel habits change.
- Your child has early symptoms of intestinal obstruction.

INTUSSUSCEPTION

GENERAL INFORMATION

DESCRIPTION

Intussusception is an intestinal obstruction in which the bowel telescopes (folds back on itself). The intestine (usually the large intestine) is involved. Intussusception can affect children of all ages but is most common in infants and children between 2 months and 6 years. It is more common in boys for unknown reasons.

Appropriate health care includes:

- Physician's monitoring of general condition, medications, and treatment.
- Special X-ray studies (barium enema) rarely may reduce the intussusception and avoid further treatment.
- Surgery to remove the strangulated bowel and rejoin healthy sections.
- Hospitalization until the obstruction is corrected.
- Home care during convalescence.

SIGNS & SYMPTOMS

Early stages:

- Cramping abdominal pain. Infants cry out, bring the legs up to the abdomen, and become pale and sweaty during an attack.
- Vomiting.

Later stages:

- Rectal bleeding. This may be dark red material that resembles jelly.
- Swollen abdomen.
- Mass in the abdomen that can be felt.

CAUSES

Unknown factors cause a loop of bowel to turn in on itself. This blocks the bowel's blood supply, causing gangrene and peritonitis. The disorder may be caused by a virus infection, but that is unproven.

RISK FACTORS

- Family history of intussusception.
- The seasons (for unknown reasons). It is most common in late spring, early summer, and midwinter.

PREVENTING COMPLICATIONS OR RECURRENCE

No specific preventive measures.

WHAT TO EXPECT

MEDICAL TESTS

- Your own observation of symptoms.
- Medical history and physical exam by a doctor.
- Laboratory blood tests.
- X-rays of the abdomen and intestinal tract (barium enema, see Glossary). The radiologist may manipulate the barium and clear the obstruction.

POSSIBLE COMPLICATIONS

- Dehydration and shock.
- Intestinal perforation and peritonitis.
- Gangrene.

PROBABLE OUTCOME

Spontaneous recovery in 24 hours (sometimes). If not, this is curable with early diagnosis and surgery or barium treatment. Without treatment, complications are life-threatening. The disorder sometimes recurs.

TREATMENT

HOME CARE

Observe your child carefully if symptoms develop. Prevent complications by seeking medical treatment during early stages.

MEDICATION

- Medicine usually is not necessary for this disorder unless infection develops. Then your doctor may prescribe antibiotics.
- Don't use home remedies or non-prescription drugs, such as laxatives, for this condition. They may be dangerous.
- See Medications section for information regarding medicines your doctor may prescribe.

ACTIVITY

Your child should rest in bed until the obstruction is cleared. The child may then resume activities gradually.

DIET & FLUIDS

Don't feed a child with signs of intestinal obstruction. Intravenous fluids are necessary until the obstruction is removed. No special diet is required then.

OK FOR SCHOOL, PRESCHOOL, OR NURSERY?

When intussusception has been relieved, appetite has returned and alertness, strength, and feeling of well-being will allow.

CALL YOUR DOCTOR IF

Your child has signs or symptoms of intestinal obstruction. This condition changes quickly from a curable one to a life-threatening one.

IRRITABLE COLON (Spastic Colitis; Mucous Colitis; Irritable Bowel Syndrome)

GENERAL INFORMATION

DESCRIPTION

Spastic colon is an irritative and inflammatory disorder of both the small and large intestine. It is not contagious, inherited, or cancerous. This condition usually affects older adolescents or young adults. Appropriate health care includes: self-care after diagnosis; physician's monitoring of general condition and medications.

SIGNS & SYMPTOMS

The following symptoms usually begin in early adult life. Episodes may last for days, weeks, or months.

- Cramp-like pain in the middle or to one side of the lower abdomen. Pain is usually relieved with bowel movements.
- Nausea.
- Bloating and gas.
- Occasional loss of appetite that may lead to weight loss.
- Diarrhea or constipation, usually alternating.
- Fatigue.
- Depression.
- Anxiety.
- Difficulty in concentrating.

CAUSES

- Stress and emotional conflict resulting in your child feeling anxious or depressed.Situations that often precede an attack include:
  - — Obsessive worry about everyday problems.
  - — Marital tension.
  - — Fear of loss of a beloved person or object.
  - — Death of a loved one.
- Symptoms may also be triggered by eating, though no specific food has been identified as responsible.

RISK FACTORS

Stress; improper diet; fatigue or overwork; poor physical fitness; smoking; excess alcohol consumption; use of drugs.

PREVENTING COMPLICATIONS OR RECURRENCE

Your child should try to reduce stress or modify the response to it.

WHAT TO EXPECT

MEDICAL TESTS

- Your own observation of symptoms.
- Medical history and physical exam by a doctor.
- Laboratory studies, including stool studies, to exclude other disorders such as lactose intolerance, ulcers, parasites, enzyme deficiency, and ulcerative colitis.
- X-ray of the colon (barium enema).

IRRITABLE COLON (Spastic Colitis; Mucous Colitis; Irritable Bowel Syndrome)

POSSIBLE COMPLICATIONS

- Poor nutrition caused by malabsorption.
- Psychological fixation on bowel function, leading to neurosis.
- Increased risk of colon cancer later in life.

PROBABLE OUTCOME

Curable if the underlying causes can be eliminated or modified. If not, your child's symptoms can be controlled with treatment.

TREATMENT

HOME CARE

Medication, diet changes, and adequate rest can help, but the cure is more dependant on defining, confronting, and solving conflicts in the child's day-to-day living. See Appendix 19 (How to Help Your Child Cope with Stress and Psychosomatic Illness).

MEDICATIONS

Medication may help your child, but it will not cure this disorder. Your doctor may prescribe:

- Antispasmodics to relieve the child's severe abdominal cramps.
- Tranquilizers to reduce anxiety.
- See Medications section for information regarding medicines your doctor may prescribe.

ACTIVITY

No restrictions. Good physical fitness improves bowel function.

DIET & FLUIDS

- Increase fiber in the child's diet to promote good bowel function. See Appendix 24 (Well-Balanced Diet).
- Your child should not eat foods that aggravate symptoms.

OK FOR SCHOOL, PRESCHOOL, OR NURSERY?

Yes, when condition and sense of well-being will allow.

CALL YOUR DOCTOR IF

- Your child develops a fever.
- Your child's stool is black or tarry-looking.
- Your child begins vomiting.
- An unexplained weight loss of 5 pounds or more occurs.
- Your child's symptoms don't improve despite treatment.

JAW DISLOCATION
(Temporo-Mandibular Joint Dislocation)

GENERAL INFORMATION

DESCRIPTION

Temporo-mandibular joints connect the lower jaw (mandible) with the skull. They are just forward of the ears. With dislocation, the mouth cannot be closed because the head of the mandible (the condyle) slides backward into a depression in the skull. The jaw is involved.

Appropriate health care includes:

• Doctor's or dentist's treatment. Muscles tighten and pain increases within 15 to 30 minutes after dislocation, so a dislocated jaw should be treated quickly.

• Self-care after diagnosis and treatment.

• Hospitalization for anesthesia and reduction if simpler measures don't remedy the problem.

SIGNS & SYMPTOMS

• Inability to close the mouth.
• Pain and swelling in the jaw.
• Bleeding under the skin of the jaw.
• Obvious asymmetry of the face.
• Numbness of the chin and lower lip (sometimes).

CAUSES

• Injury inflicted in a fight, auto accident, or contact sports.

• Some persons dislocate mandibles with little provocation, as with yawning, yelling, biting large pieces of food, or opening the mouth very wide for any reason.

RISK FACTORS

Injuries are most often associated with:
• Accident-proneness.
• Excess alcohol consumption or use of mind-altering drugs.
• Non-use of seat belts.

PREVENTING COMPLICATIONS OR RECURRENCE

Instructions for your child:

• Avoid opening your mouth widely, if possible, when you yawn, bite large pieces of food, yell or scream during excitement, call out loudly, or sing.

• Use seat belts and shoulder harnesses in vehicles. Don't drink alcohol or use mind-altering drugs and drive.

WHAT TO EXPECT

MEDICAL TESTS

• Your own observation of symptoms.
• Medical history and physical exam by a doctor.
• X-rays of the jaw.

JAW DISLOCATION
(Temporo-Mandibular Joint Dislocation)

POSSIBLE COMPLICATIONS

Obstruction of the airway and inhalation of mucus and blood into the lungs, leading to pneumonia. This occurs most often with dislocation accompanied by fractures.

PROBABLE OUTCOME

Usually curable with treatment.

TREATMENT

HOME CARE

- Make sure an injured child with a fractured or dislocated jaw has no breathing obstruction. If there is an obstruction, seek emergency help immediately.
- If your child's jaw is injured, don't panic. Stay calm. Go to the nearest dental office or emergency facility for help.
- Tell your child not to try to talk with a dislocated jaw—write messages instead. Don't try to push or force your child's mouth closed. The mouth cannot close normally until the dislocation is corrected.

MEDICATION

Your doctor may prescribe:

- Pain relievers.
- Muscle relaxants.
- See Medications section for information regarding medicines your doctor may prescribe.

ACTIVITY

Your child should rest in bed with the head turned to one side. The child may read or watch TV. Normal activities may be resumed in 2 to 3 days. Allow 6 weeks for muscles and tendons attached to the joint to heal.

DIET & FLUIDS

A liquid diet may be necessary for up to 4 weeks. Start with clear liquids, then go on to serving the child a full liquid diet, including blenderized foods, milk shakes, and juices. The child should not chew solid foods without the doctor's or dentist's permission.

OK FOR SCHOOL, PRESCHOOL, OR NURSERY?

When appetite has returned and alertness, strength, and feeling of well-being will allow.

CALL YOUR DOCTOR IF

- Your child has symptoms of a dislocated jaw.
- Pain is intolerable.

JAW (MANDIBLE) FRACTURE

GENERAL INFORMATION

DESCRIPTION

A jaw fracture is a complete or incomplete break in the lower jaw (the mandible). Appropriate health care includes: doctor's or dentist's treatment to manipulate and set the broken bone; hospitalization (sometimes) for anesthesia and surgery to set the fracture and wire the child's jaw together.

SIGNS & SYMPTOMS

- Severe pain at the fracture site.
- Swelling of soft tissue surrounding the fracture.
- Blood at the base of the child's teeth near the fracture site.
- Visible deformity if the fracture is complete and bone fragments separate enough to distort the child's normal facial contours.
- Tenderness to the touch.
- Numbness around the fracture site (sometimes).

CAUSES

Direct blow (usually) or indirect stress to the bone. Indirect stress may be caused by violent muscle contraction.

RISK FACTORS

Contact sports, especially boxing; history of bone or joint disease; poor nutrition, especially calcium deficiency.

PREVENTING COMPLICATIONS OR RECURRENCE

Your child should use appropriate protective equipment, such as a face mask or mouthpiece, when participating in contact sports.

WHAT TO EXPECT

MEDICAL TESTS

Your own observation of symptoms; medical history and physical exam by a doctor; X-rays of injured area.

POSSIBLE COMPLICATIONS

At the time of injury:

- Shock.
- Pressure on or injury to nearby nerves, ligaments, tendons, muscles, blood vessels, or connective tissues.

After treatment or surgery:

- Delayed union or non-union of the fracture (rare).
- Impaired blood supply to the fracture site.
- Infection in open fractures (skin broken over fracture site), or at the incision if surgical setting was necessary.
- Proneness to repeated jaw injury.
- An unstable or arthritic jaw following repeated injury.
- Prolonged healing time if activity is resumed too soon.
- Nutritional problems arising because the child's jaw is wired closed.

JAW (MANDIBLE) FRACTURE

PROBABLE OUTCOME

The average healing time for this fracture is 6 to 8 weeks.

TREATMENT

FIRST AID

- Use instructions for R.I.C.E., the first letters of *rest*, *ice*, *compression*, and *elevation*. See Appendix 39 for details.
- The doctor will realign and set the broken bones either with surgery or, if possible, without. Manipulation should be done as soon as possible after injury.

HOME CARE

- Immobilization will be necessary. Mandible fractures usually require wiring the child's jaw together.
- Use an ice pack on the child's jaw 3 or 4 times a day. Wrap ice chips or cubes in a plastic bag, and wrap the bag in a moist towel. Place it over the injured area for 20 minutes at a time.
- After 72 hours, apply heat instead of ice if it feels better. Use heat lamps, hot soaks, hot showers, or a heating pad.
- Your child should learn how to "quick-release" the wired teeth for any emergency such as severe coughing or vomiting.

MEDICATION

- General anesthesia, local anesthesia, or muscle relaxants to make bone manipulation and fixation of bone fragments possible.
- Narcotic or synthetic narcotic pain relievers in liquid form for severe pain.
- Stool softeners in liquid form to prevent constipation due to a liquid diet.
- Liquid acetaminophen (non-prescription) for mild pain after initial treatment.

ACTIVITY

Your child should rest quietly for 2 days, then resume normal activities gradually. The child should not exercise to the point of panting for breath, because breathing may be difficult for a while.

DIET & FLUIDS

During recovery, the child should follow a high-protein liquid diet such as malted milk and eggnog. Add soft foods as the child is able. Most children can handle rich soups, ground meat, whipped potatoes, and gravy.

OK FOR SCHOOL, PRESCHOOL, OR NURSERY?

Yes, when condition and sense of well-being will allow.

CALL YOUR DOCTOR IF

- Your child has signs or symptoms of a jaw fracture.
- Any of the following occur after surgery or other treatment: increased pain, swelling, or drainage in the surgical area; signs of infection (headache, muscle aches, dizziness, or a general ill feeling, and fever; nausea or vomiting; numbness or complete loss of feeling around the jaw; constipation.

JOCK ITCH
(Tinea Cruris)

GENERAL INFORMATION

DESCRIPTION

Jock itch is an infection of the skin in the groin with one of several fungus germs. These fungi thrive in the groin, where darkness, warmth, and moisture stimulate their growth. Jock itch is more likely to occur in males than females. It is contagious from person to person.

Appropriate health care includes:

- Diagnosis and prescription of medications by a doctor.
- Self-care after diagnosis.

SIGNS & SYMPTOMS

- Scaling patches on the skin of the child's groin, thighs, and buttocks. The patches have well-defined edges. Occasionally small, pus-filled blisters appear.
- Itching of involved areas.
- Pain (if the child's skin becomes secondarily infected with bacteria).

CAUSES

- Athlete's foot, a fungus infection of the feet that can spread to the groin area.
- Other fungus infections that spread to the groin.

RISK FACTORS

- Contact with infected surfaces, such as towels or benches.
- Hot, humid weather.
- Excessive sweating.
- Obesity, which fosters sweating.
- Friction of skin against skin from constant movement.

PREVENTING COMPLICATIONS OR RECURRENCE

Instructions for your child:

- Dry thoroughly after bathing.
- Don't sit around in a wet bathing suit.
- Wear absorbent, loose, cotton underwear.
- Wear clean, dry athletic supporters and underwear for each workout.
- Use non-prescription tolnafate (Tinactin) after bathing if you have had jock itch. This powder discourages recurrence.

WHAT TO EXPECT

MEDICAL TESTS

- Your own observation of symptoms.
- Medical history and physical exam by a doctor.
- Laboratory studies, including microscopic examination of scraped-off scales suspended in potassium hydroxide liquid.

JOCK ITCH
(Tinea Cruris)

POSSIBLE COMPLICATIONS

- Contact or allergic dermatitis accompanying jock itch that requires additional treatment, usually with steroid topical applications.
- Slow healing.
- Secondary bacterial infection in the affected area.
- Rash from an "id reaction" (allergic immunological response to the disorder) on the hands and face (rare).

PROBABLE OUTCOME

Your child's symptoms can be controlled in 2 to 3 weeks with treatment. Recurrences are common.

TREATMENT

HOME CARE

Instructions for your child:

- Bathe with clear water only. Don't use soaps until the skin clears completely. Soap irritates infected skin.
- Wear loose cotton underwear.
- Change to dry clothes immediately after swimming.
- If you have an athlete's foot infection also, treat both areas with equal care.

MEDICATION

Your doctor may prescribe:

- Topical treatment with anti-fungal medicines such as clotrimazole, haloprigin, or miconazole.
- Oral anti-fungal medication, such as griseofulvin, if topical medication doesn't bring relief in 7 to 10 days.

ACTIVITY

No restrictions.

DIET & FLUIDS

No special diet.

OK FOR SCHOOL, PRESCHOOL, OR NURSERY?

Yes, when condition and sense of well-being will allow.

CALL YOUR DOCTOR IF

- Your child has symptoms of jock itch that doesn't clear spontaneously in 5 days.
- New, unexplained symptoms develop. Drugs used in treatment may produce side effects.

ILLNESSES

KERATITIS

GENERAL INFORMATION

DESCRIPTION

Keratitis is an inflammation of the cornea (the clear central portion of the eye that covers the pupil).

Appropriate health care includes:

• Physician's (ophthalmologist's) monitoring of general condition, medications, and treatment.

• Surgery to replace the cornea with a transplanted cornea from a donor (severe cases only).

SIGNS & SYMPTOMS

• Eye pain.
• Photophobia (sensitivity to light).
• Tears.

CAUSES

• Bacterial, viral or fungal infections. The most common is the herpes simplex virus, Type I.
• Drying of the eye caused by an eyelid disorder or insufficient tear formation.
• Foreign object in the eye.
• Intense light, such as from welding arcs or the reflection of intense sunlight from snow or water. (Symptoms may not appear for 24 hours after exposure.)
• Vitamin A deficiency.
• Allergy or sensitivity to eye cosmetics, air pollution, airborne particles (pollen, dust, mold, or yeasts) and other allergens.

RISK FACTORS

• Poor nutrition, especially insufficient vitamin A.
• Illness that has lowered resistance.
• Crowded or unsanitary living conditions.
• Viral infections elsewhere in the body, especially cold sores or genital herpes.

PREVENTING COMPLICATIONS OR RECURRENCE

• Urge your child to wear protective glasses during activities that involve eye hazards.
• Encourage your child to eat a well-balanced diet that contains sufficient vitamin A, or to take multiple-vitamin supplements containing vitamin A.

WHAT TO EXPECT

MEDICAL TESTS

• Your own observation of symptoms.
• Medical history and physical exam by a doctor.
• Laboratory culture of the discharge from the eye.

POSSIBLE COMPLICATIONS

• Glaucoma.
• Ulceration of the cornea.
• Permanent scarring in the eye.
• Vision loss.

PROBABLE OUTCOME

Depends on the cause. With early treatment, most types of keratitis are curable.

TREATMENT

HOME CARE

A temporary eye patch is often necessary. It may limit your child's ability to take care of himself.

MEDICATION

- Your doctor may prescribe:
  - — Antibiotic or anti-viral eye drops and ointments.
  - — Artificial tears.
- Don't treat any eye inflammation without consulting your doctor. *Don't use non-prescription eye drops containing topical corticosteroids. These may worsen the condition or cause eyeball perforation.*
- See Medications section for information regarding medicines your doctor may prescribe.

ACTIVITY

Eye patching will restrict activity. Your child can resume normal activities gradually.

DIET & FLUIDS

No special diet.

OK FOR SCHOOL, PRESCHOOL, OR NURSERY?

When treatment is complete and no symptoms persist.

CALL YOUR DOCTOR IF

- Your child has symptoms of keratitis.
- Your child's vision diminishes in any way.

KERATOSIS PILARIS

GENERAL INFORMATION

DESCRIPTION

Keratosis pilaris is a common skin disorder in which the openings of the hair follicles become filled with hard plugs. These are not contagious. The skin on the back of the upper arms and the front of the thighs or buttocks is involved. Keratosis pilaris affects children and young adults.

Appropriate health care includes:

- Self-care.
- Physician's monitoring of general condition and medications.

SIGNS & SYMPTOMS

Papules (small raised bumps) with the following characteristics:

- Papules are small, firm, and white, with a dry "sandpaper" feeling.
- Papules are clustered. Each one is about 1mm in size.
- Papules are at the openings of hair follicles. They can be scooped out with the fingernails.
- When scooped out, a papule usually contains a coiled hair inside of white, semisolid material.
- Papules don't itch or hurt.

CAUSES

- Unknown, but it may be hereditary. Papules commonly occur in association with allergic dermatitis and several types of ichthyosis, both of which have strong hereditary links.
- Lesions similar—possibly identical—to those of keratosis pilaris appear in persons with vitamin A deficiency.

RISK FACTORS

- History of skin allergies.
- Family history of keratosis pilaris.
- Poor nutrition, especially vitamin A deficiency.

PREVENTING COMPLICATIONS OR RECURRENCE

Cannot be prevented at present.

WHAT TO EXPECT

MEDICAL TESTS

- Your own observation of symptoms.
- Medical history and physical exam by a doctor.
- Biopsy (see Glossary).

POSSIBLE COMPLICATIONS

Secondary infection of papules.

PROBABLE OUTCOME

Keratosis pilaris is a chronic, harmless skin problem with no permanent cure. Individual papules may come and go over a matter of weeks. All gradually disappear by age 30.

TREATMENT

HOME CARE

Instructions for your child:

- Take long soaking tub baths.
- Use mild, unscented soap.
- Scrub gently with a stiff brush to remove the plugs in the follicles temporarily.
- Apply lubricating ointments or creams to the affected areas 6 or 7 times a day. The most useful time is immediately after bathing, when lubrication helps the skin retain moisture.

MEDICATION

- Medicine usually is not necessary for this disorder.
- See Medications section for information regarding medicines your doctor may prescribe.

ACTIVITY

No restrictions.

DIET & FLUIDS

No special diet.

OK FOR SCHOOL, PRESCHOOL, OR NURSERY?

Yes.

CALL YOUR DOCTOR IF

Signs of infection develop around the keratoses pilaris. Signs include pain or tenderness, redness, swelling, and fever of 101F (38.3C) or higher.

KIDNEY FAILURE, ACUTE

GENERAL INFORMATION

DESCRIPTION

Acute kidney failure is the sudden failure of the kidneys to function. This usually has a short, relatively severe course, but it is curable.

Appropriate health care includes:

- Physician's monitoring of general condition, medications and treatment.
- Surgery, if the cause can be corrected by surgery.
- Hospitalization for fluid and electrolyte therapy and kidney dialysis (sometimes).

SIGNS & SYMPTOMS

Early stages:

- Little or no urine output.

Later stages:

- Nausea, vomiting, diarrhea, and appetite loss.
- Mental changes, including irritability, drowsiness, stupor, or coma.
- Convulsions.
- Severe itching.
- High or low blood pressure.
- Unexplained bruising, bleeding spots under the skin, or spontaneous bleeding.

The symptoms of the underlying cause (see below) will also be present.

CAUSES

Conditions in the kidney, or in other areas of the body, that cause your child's kidneys to stop functioning. This leads to a buildup of waste products in the blood and tissues. Underlying conditions include:

- Shock with very low blood pressure.
- Blood poisoning (septicemia).
- Congestive heart failure.
- Fluid and electrolyte imbalance.
- Blood-transfusion reaction.
- Severe accident with extensive muscle injury.
- Acute glomerulonephritis.
- Multiple myeloma.
- Obstruction of blood vessels that supply the kidney.
- Kidney stones that obstruct both ureters or the urethra.
- Prostate enlargement.
- Use of certain medications, including anti-cancer drugs, kanamycin, amphotericin B, anti-convulsants, or excessive vitamin D.
- Overdose of many poisons or drugs, especially mind-altering drugs.

RISK FACTORS

Having only one kidney; recent surgery; accidents with severe injuries; medical history of conditions affecting the kidney, such as diabetes or gout.

PREVENTING COMPLICATIONS OR RECURRENCE

No specific preventive measures. Your child should avoid causes and risk factors when possible.

KIDNEY FAILURE, ACUTE

WHAT TO EXPECT

MEDICAL TESTS

- Your own observation of symptoms.
- Medical history and physical exam by a doctor.
- Laboratory blood counts, and blood and urine tests that measure kidney function and fluid and electrolyte balance.
- EKG (see Glossary).
- Needle biopsy (see Glossary) of kidneys.
- X-rays of the abdomen, kidneys, ureters, and bladder to detect kidney stones.

POSSIBLE COMPLICATIONS

Congestive heart failure; increased risk of infections; chronic kidney failure.

PROBABLE OUTCOME

If your child's underlying condition can be controlled and the kidney failure can be treated promptly, complete recovery is likely. If not, the disorder can lead to chronic kidney failure or death.

TREATMENT

HOME CARE

No specific instructions except those listed under other headings.

MEDICATION

Your doctor may prescribe:

- Medications appropriate to control the underlying condition.
- Antibiotics if infection develops.

ACTIVITY

Your child should rest in bed until the condition is cured. Then the child can resume normal activities as soon as symptoms improve.

DIET & FLUIDS

Your child's food and water intake must be rigorously controlled to prevent fluid and electrolyte imbalance, and to minimize buildup of body wastes.

OK FOR SCHOOL, PRESCHOOL, OR NURSERY?

Yes. This should not be a disabling or infectious disorder.

CALL YOUR DOCTOR IF

- Your child has symptoms of kidney failure.
- The following occurs during treatment:
  - — Chills, fever, headache, or muscle aches.
  - — Shortness of breath.
  - — Unexpected bleeding from any body opening.

KIDNEY FAILURE, CHRONIC (Uremia)

GENERAL INFORMATION

DESCRIPTION

Chronic kidney failure is the inability of the kidneys to eliminate the body's nitrogen waste products. Uremia usually develops gradually. Poor kidney function eventually affects all body systems.

Appropriate health care includes:

- Physician's monitoring of general condition and medications.
- Kidney transplant, if possible.
- Kidney dialysis (see Glossary), if available.
- Hospitalization for complications and care in final stages.

SIGNS & SYMPTOMS

None or few symptoms until 60% to 75% of kidney filtration fails. Then, one or more of the following:

- Listlessness, mental confusion, and drowsiness.
- High blood pressure.
- Shortness of breath.
- Bad breath.
- Inflamed, bleeding gums and mouth ulcers.
- Abdominal pain.
- Itching skin.
- Numbness, tingling, and burning in the legs and feet.
- Muscle cramps.
- Decreased sex drive.
- Cessation of menstruation.
- Anemia, with paleness and fatigue.
- Unusual bleeding.
- Muscle and bone pain. Bones break easily.

CAUSES

- Collagen diseases, such as systemic lupus erythematosus.
- Chronic glomerulonephritis.
- Chronic urinary-tract infections.
- Congenital kidney abnormalities, such as polycystic kidney disease.
- Kidney damage due to diabetes mellitus.
- Urinary-tract obstruction.
- Overdose of many drugs and chemicals, especially phenacetin or streptomycin.
- Blood-vessel diseases, such as hardening of the arteries in, or leading to, the kidney.

RISK FACTORS

Use of mind-altering drugs.

PREVENTING COMPLICATIONS OR RECURRENCE

Obtain medical treatment for underlying diseases that lead to uremia *before* uremia results.

KIDNEY FAILURE, CHRONIC (Uremia)

WHAT TO EXPECT

MEDICAL TESTS

Laboratory blood and urine studies of kidney function; X-rays of kidneys; kidney biopsy (see Glossary).

POSSIBLE COMPLICATIONS

Pericarditis; myocarditis; pneumonia; pancreatitis; hormone deficiencies; fluid and electrolyte imbalance; gastrointestinal ulcers.

PROBABLE OUTCOME

Kidney transplants can sometimes cure younger patients. Otherwise, kidney failure is a condition that worsens gradually and causes death. Kidney dialysis treatment can improve the quality of life and prolong life for several years.

TREATMENT

HOME CARE

Instructions for your child:

- To decrease itching, add 1 cup of oatmeal to your daily bath.
- Brush teeth and use mouthwash often to minimize gum and mouth problems.
- Weigh daily and keep a record.
- Measure the fluids you drink and the urine you pass each day. Keep a record and take it with you to doctor visits. You should pass about 2500cc or more of urine a day. If you pass less, decrease fluid intake so intake does not exceed output by more than 800cc a day. For example, if you pass 2000cc in 24 hours, don't drink more than 2800cc in the next 24 hours.

MEDICATION

Your doctor may prescribe: diuretics to reduce fluid accumulation; iron and folic-acid supplements for anemia; stool softeners to prevent constipation; digitalis for congestive heart failure.

ACTIVITY

Your child must reduce activity, being careful not to become overheated or fatigued. The child should sleep more at night and take rests during the day. If your child is confined to bed, encourage flexing the legs often to reduce the chance of blood clots in leg veins.

DIET & FLUIDS

Urge your child to eat a low-salt, low-potassium, low-protein diet with added fiber. Serve the child frequent small, high-calorie meals.

OK FOR SCHOOL, PRESCHOOL, OR NURSERY?

Not until kidney function returns to normal.

CALL YOUR DOCTOR IF

- Your child has symptoms of uremia.
- The following occurs during treatment: fever, vomiting or diarrhea, urine output of less than 2000cc, severe headache, and convulsion.

ILLNESSES

KIDNEY INFECTION, ACUTE (Acute Pyelonephritis)

GENERAL INFORMATION

DESCRIPTION

Acute kidney infection is a non-contagious bacterial infection of the kidneys. The kidneys and urinary tract are involved. Acute kidney infection can affect both sexes but is more common in females of all ages.

Appropriate health care includes:

- Self-care after diagnosis.
- Physician's monitoring of general condition and medications.

SIGNS & SYMPTOMS

Sudden onset of:

- Fever and shaking chills.
- Burning, frequent urination.
- Cloudy urine or blood in the urine.
- Aching (sometimes severe) in one or both sides of the lower back.
- Abdominal pain.
- Marked fatigue.

Note: Young children may not have typical symptoms or signs. Sometimes the only symptom may be fever, fatigue, or headache without discomfort with urinating.

CAUSES

Bacteria (most commonly escherichia coli) invade one or both kidneys. The infection may begin in the bladder. The most common sources of bacterial infection are:

- Infections elsewhere in the body that travel to the kidneys through the bloodstream or lymph glands.
- Blockage or abnormality of the urinary system, caused by stones, obstructions, bladder dysfunction from nerve diseases, tumors, or congenital abnormalities.
- Catheters, tubes, or surgical procedures used for other medical conditions.

RISK FACTORS

Diabetes mellitus; chronic urinary-bladder infection or tumor; paralysis from spinal-cord injury or tumor; pregnancy.

PREVENTING COMPLICATIONS OR RECURRENCE

No specific preventive measures for males. For females:

- After bowel movements, always wipe from the vaginal area toward the rectum.
- Avoid prolonged moistness around the urethra, such as that caused by nylon underpants or wet swim suits.

OTHER

Acute kidney infections in males of any age may indicate a serious underlying disease, such as a tumor or obstruction. Consult your doctor even if your child's symptoms disappear spontaneously.

KIDNEY INFECTION, ACUTE (Acute Pyelonephritis)

WHAT TO EXPECT

MEDICAL TESTS

Your own observation of symptoms; medical history and physical exam by a doctor; special X-rays; urinalysis and urine culture (see Glossary).

POSSIBLE COMPLICATIONS

Chronic kidney infection and hypertension.

PROBABLE OUTCOME

Usually curable in 10 to 14 days with treatment. Your child should return to the doctor to assure complete cure.

TREATMENT

HOME CARE

To collect urine for urinalysis or culture:

- Females: Clean the vaginal area with warm, soapy water; sponge dry. Spread the vaginal lips with one hand and urinate briefly into the toilet bowl. Then urinate into the container.
- Males: Pull back the foreskin of the penis if you are not circumcised. Clean the end of the penis with soapy water. Urinate briefly into the toilet bowl, then into the special container.

MEDICATION

Your doctor may prescribe:

- Oral antibiotics. Your child should take all the antibiotics prescribed, even if symptoms disappear.
- Intravenous or injected antibiotics, if oral antibiotics don't cure the infection.
- Urinary analgesics to relieve pain.

ACTIVITY

Your child should rest in bed until high fever and discomfort subside.

DIET & FLUIDS

No special diet. Encourage the child to drink at least 2 quarts of liquid daily; include cranberry juice to acidify the urine.

OK FOR SCHOOL, PRESCHOOL, OR NURSERY?

When signs of infection have decreased, appetite returns, and alertness, strength, and feeling of well-being will allow.

CALL YOUR DOCTOR IF

- Your child has symptoms of a kidney infection.
- The following occurs during treatment:
  - — Symptoms and fever persist after 48 hours of antibiotic treatment. Occasionally a different antibiotic is needed.
  - — Symptoms return (especially if accompanied by fever) after antibiotic treatment.
- New, unexplained symptoms develop. Drugs used in treatment may produce side effects.

KIDNEY INFECTION, CHRONIC (Chronic Pyelonephritis)

GENERAL INFORMATION

DESCRIPTION

Chronic kidney infection develops slowly and lasts for months or years. It leads to scarring and eventual loss of kidney function. The kidneys and other parts of the urinary system (ureter, bladder, and urethra) are involved. Chronic kidney infection can affect both sexes, all ages, but is more common in females.

Appropriate health care includes:

- Self-care after diagnosis.
- Physician's monitoring of general condition and medications.
- Surgery to relieve obstruction in the urinary tract, if one exists.

SIGNS & SYMPTOMS

Usually no signs or symptoms, unlike acute kidney infection. The following occur if chronic kidney failure develops:

- Anemia.
- Weakness.
- Loss of appetite.
- Hypertension.
- Pain in one or both sides of the lower back.
- Protein and blood in the urine.

CAUSES

Frequent, acute bacterial kidney infections.

RISK FACTORS

- History of diabetes mellitus.
- Urinary obstruction, such as stones or tumors.
- Long-term use of catheters.

PREVENTING COMPLICATIONS OR RECURRENCE

- Obtain prompt medical treatment for acute kidney infections, including 2 or more weeks of antibiotic treatment. Don't let your child discontinue prescribed medication even if symptoms disappear after a few days of treatment.
- Obtain treatment for any abnormality of the urinary tract that causes infection.

WHAT TO EXPECT

MEDICAL TESTS

- Medical history and physical exam by a doctor.
- Laboratory blood studies of kidney function, urinalysis and urine culture (see Glossary).
- X-rays of kidneys.
- Special studies that may include ultrasonography, CAT or CT scan; MRI, and radionuclide scan (see Glossary for all).

KIDNEY INFECTION, CHRONIC (Chronic Pyelonephritis)

POSSIBLE COMPLICATIONS

- Kidney-caused hypertension.
- Chronic kidney failure.

PROBABLE OUTCOME

Symptoms can be controlled with treatment:

- If only one kidney is chronically infected and antibiotic treatment is unsuccessful, surgical removal of the affected kidney may prevent complications.
- If chronic kidney failure develops in both kidneys, a kidney transplant or kidney dialysis (see Glossary) can be life-saving.

TREATMENT

HOME CARE

Follow your child's treatment plan carefully. This may not be easy for an illness that causes few symptoms in the early stages.

MEDICATION

Your doctor may prescribe:

- Antibiotics for months or years.
- Drugs to keep the child's urine slightly acid.
- See Medications section for information regarding medicines your doctor may prescribe.

ACTIVITY

No restrictions.

DIET & FLUIDS

No special diet. Urge your child to drink 2 quarts of liquid daily; include cranberry juice to acidify the urine.

OK FOR SCHOOL, PRESCHOOL, OR NURSERY?

When signs of infection have decreased, appetite returns, and alertness, strength, and feeling of well-being will allow.

CALL YOUR DOCTOR IF

- Your child has symptoms of chronic kidney failure.
- Your child has symptoms of an acute kidney infection, such as urgent, frequent or burning urination, fever and chills, fatigue, and cloudy urine.

KIDNEY OR URETER INJURY

GENERAL INFORMATION

DESCRIPTION

Kidney or ureter injury involves bruising or tearing of the kidney or ureter. Kidneys filter waste material from the bloodstream and produce urine. Ureters are the tubes that carry urine from the kidneys to the bladder.

Appropriate health care includes:

- Physician's monitoring of general condition and medications.
- Hospitalization for shock or internal bleeding.
- Surgery to repair the ureter or remove the kidney, if other treatment fails.

SIGNS & SYMPTOMS

- Pain or tenderness in the back, just below the ribs on the injured side.
- Fever less than 101F (38.3C).
- Blood in the urine.

If your child has severe pain with large amounts of blood in the urine, one or both kidneys may be seriously injured.

CAUSES

A blow or penetrating wound to the side of the body under the ribs.

RISK FACTORS

Accident-proneness; hazardous activities; hazardous driving conditions; excess alcohol consumption.

PREVENTING COMPLICATIONS OR RECURRENCE

Protect your child from injury whenever possible. Require that all automobile passengers buckle their seat belts and shoulder harnesses to minimize internal injury in case of accident. Don't drink and drive.

WHAT TO EXPECT

MEDICAL TESTS

- Your own observation of symptoms.
- Medical history and physical exam by a doctor.
- Laboratory urine studies.
- X-rays of the urinary tract.
- Special studies that may include:

  — Ultrasonography: A non-invasive technique that translates sound waves into images displayed on a screen and photographed (see Glossary).

  — CAT or CT Scan (computerized axial tomography): Non-invasive computerized X-ray images that show sections (or "slices") of an organ or region of the body clearly and precisely (see Glossary).

  — MRI (magnetic resonance imaging): A non-invasive (non-X-ray) computerized test that uses radio frequency energy and a powerful magnetic field to produce images with excellent detail (see Glossary).

  — Radionuclide Scan: A nuclear medicine procedure that uses radioactive isotopes injected into a patient. The isotope tracers are absorbed in various concentrations by targeted organs, which are then photographed (see Glossary).

KIDNEY OR URETER INJURY

POSSIBLE COMPLICATIONS

- Internal bleeding.
- Shock (sweating, faintness, nausea, panting, rapid pulse, and pale, cold, moist skin).
- Urine leakage into the abdomen, causing abdominal inflammation or infection.
- Scarring and narrowing of the injured ureter.

PROBABLE OUTCOME

Usually curable with time, bed rest, and surgery or protection against infection. The surgery to remove an injured kidney (if it does not heal with other measures) is not complicated. After recovery, your child can lead a normal life with one kidney.

TREATMENT

HOME CARE

No special instructions except those listed under other headings.

MEDICATION

Your doctor may prescribe:

- Pain relievers.
- Antibiotics to treat or protect against infection.
- See Medications section for information regarding medicines your doctor may prescribe.

ACTIVITY

Your child will need bed rest for 1 to 2 weeks after the injury. After recovery, the child can resume normal activities gradually.

DIET & FLUIDS

- No special diet.
- Encourage your child to drink 6 to 8 glasses of fluid daily.
- Urge your child not to drink alcohol.

OK FOR SCHOOL, PRESCHOOL, OR NURSERY?

When appetite has returned and alertness, strength, and feeling of well-being will allow.

CALL YOUR DOCTOR IF

- Your child has symptoms of a kidney or ureter injury.
- Symptoms recur after treatment, especially blood in the urine.
- New, unexplained symptoms develop. Drugs used in treatment may produce side effects.

KIDNEY, POLYCYSTIC

GENERAL INFORMATION

DESCRIPTION

Polycystic kidney disease is an inherited kidney disorder in which cysts develop in the kidneys. The cysts enlarge the kidney and reduce its function. This is not cancerous. Most cases show no symptoms until adulthood. Then symptoms progress slowly for up to 20 years.

Appropriate health care includes:

- Self-care after diagnosis.
- Physician's monitoring of general condition and medications.
- Surgery to perform a kidney transplant (rare).
- Hospitalization for dialysis (rare).

SIGNS & SYMPTOMS

- Early stages: blood in the urine that may be visible only by microscopic examination; repeated kidney infections; a mass in the abdomen; no symptoms (frequently) until the cysts replace so much normal kidney structure that kidney failure occurs.
- Symptoms of kidney failure: pain in the lower back; frequent urination; increasing fatigue and weakness; headache; bad breath; hypertension; nausea, vomiting, or diarrhea; fluid retention, especially swelling around the ankles or eyes; shortness of breath; chest pain; itching skin; cessation of menstruation in females of childbearing age.

CAUSES

This disease is inherited; the cause is unknown.

RISK FACTORS

Family history of polycystic disease.

PREVENTING COMPLICATIONS OR RECURRENCE

Cannot be prevented at present. If polycystic kidney disease runs in your family, consult your doctor for tests to discover if your child has kidney cysts. Even if your child feels well and doesn't have the disease, schedule regular checkups. If you have a family history of polycystic kidney disease, seek genetic counseling before starting a family.

WHAT TO EXPECT

MEDICAL TESTS

- Your own observation of symptoms.
- Medical history and physical exam by a doctor.
- X-rays and ultrasonography of kidneys and other parts of the urinary tract.
- Special studies that may include ultrasonography, CAT or CT scan, MRI, and radionuclide scan (see Glossary for all).

POSSIBLE COMPLICATIONS

- Urinary-tract infections.
- Chronic kidney failure.

PROBABLE OUTCOME

Polycystic kidney disease is currently considered incurable, but persons with it have a normal life expectancy. Your doctor may slow the progressive kidney damage by treating complications as they arise. Scientific research into causes and treatment continues. This offers hope for increasingly effective treatment and eventual cure.

TREATMENT

HOME CARE

There is no specific treatment for polycystic kidney disease. The treatment described below applies primarily to patients with polycystic disease who have chronic kidney failure.

MEDICATION

- Without complications, medicine usually is not necessary for this disorder.
- If necessary, your doctor may prescribe antibiotics for infection or antihypertensives to control high blood pressure.
- Most drugs are excreted by the kidney. If your child has chronic kidney failure and takes prescription drugs, the dose may need adjustment because of this disorder.

ACTIVITY

Your child should take short, frequent rest periods during the day. Otherwise, advise your child to stay as active as strength allows.

DIET & FLUIDS

- Encourage your child to eat a low-salt (see Appendix 29), low-protein diet.
- Urge your child to drink at least 8 glasses of fluid every day.
- Iron and multiple-vitamin supplements may be necessary to ensure good nutrition because of the dietary restrictions. Your doctor may also prescribe calcium and vitamin D supplements for your child to prevent softening of the bones (osteoporosis) that may occur later in life.

OK FOR SCHOOL, PRESCHOOL, OR NURSERY?

Yes.

CALL YOUR DOCTOR IF

- Your child has symptoms of polycystic kidney disease.
- Your child has symptoms of kidney failure.
- Your child has fever or other signs of infection.
- Urination decreases.

KNEE-CARTILAGE INJURY (Meniscus Injury)

GENERAL INFORMATION

DESCRIPTION

A knee-cartilage injury is damage to cartilage in the knee at the top of the lower leg bone (tibia). Knee-cartilage injuries frequently accompany dislocations of the kneecap or ligament sprains in the knee. This is sometimes a vaguely diagnosed knee injury that resists conservative treatment. The cartilage at the top of the tibia that normally cushions the force to the knee, the knee joint, the ligaments that lend stability to the knee, and the soft tissue that includes nerves, synovial membranes, periosteum (covering of the bone), blood vessels, lymph vessels, and bursae of the knee joint are involved.

Appropriate health care includes:

- Doctor's care.
- Surgery to remove the damaged meniscus. This is usually done with arthroscopy, which is visual examination of a joint using an arthroscope, a fiber-optic instrument with a lighted tip.
- Self-care during recovery following surgery.
- Physical therapy and rehabilitation after surgery.

SIGNS & SYMPTOMS

- Pain and tenderness in the child's knee, especially when bearing weight.
- Locking of the knee joint.
- "Giving way" of the knee.
- "Water" on the knee (sometimes).

CAUSES

- A direct blow to the child's knee.
- Prolonged overuse of an injured knee.
- Twisting or violent muscle contraction.

RISK FACTORS

Contact sports, especially football; obesity; poor nutrition; previous knee injury; poor muscle conditioning.

PREVENTING COMPLICATIONS OR RECURRENCE

Your child should do the following: engage in vigorous pre-sport strengthening and conditioning; avoid concrete or asphalt surfaces and other rigid surfaces for continuous conditioning exercises; warm up adequately and tape a previously injured knee before practice or competition.

WHAT TO EXPECT

MEDICAL TESTS

Your own observation of symptoms; medical history and physical exam by a doctor; X-rays of the child's knee to rule out fracture; arthroscopy for knee injuries that have some, but not all, signs of cartilage injury (this instrument is also used for surgery on the knee).

POSSIBLE COMPLICATIONS

- Prolonged disability, knee instability, and pain without surgery.
- Arthritic changes in later years whether surgery was performed or not.
- Proneness to repeated knee injury.
- Postoperative complications, including bleeding into the child's knee joint, surgical-wound infection, and slow healing.

PROBABLE OUTCOME

Surgery is the only definitive treatment for knee-cartilage injuries. With surgery, expect complete healing if no complications occur. Allow 6 weeks for full recovery from surgery.

TREATMENT

HOME CARE

Instructions for your child during the postoperative phase:

- Walk on crutches until your surgeon instructs otherwise.
- After the cast is removed, use an electric heating pad, heat lamp, or a warm compress to relieve incisional pain.
- Take whirlpool treatments, if available.
- Wrap the injured knee with an elasticized bandage between treatments.
- Massage gently and often to provide comfort and decrease swelling.
- On follow-up visits, your surgeon may aspirate fluid that has accumulated in the knee joint.

MEDICATION

- For minor discomfort, use non-prescription medicines such as aspirin, acetaminophen, or ibuprofen.
- Your doctor may prescribe stronger medicine for pain, if needed.

ACTIVITY

Your child can return gradually to full activity as the range of motion and strength in the injured leg becomes equal to the normal leg.

DIET & FLUIDS

Increase the child's fiber and fluid intake to prevent constipation that may result from decreased activity.

OK FOR SCHOOL, PRESCHOOL, OR NURSERY?

Yes, when condition and sense of well-being will allow.

CALL YOUR DOCTOR IF

- Your child has symptoms of a knee-cartilage injury.
- Any of the following occurs after surgery: increased pain, swelling, redness, drainage, or bleeding in the surgical area; signs of infection (headache, muscle aches, dizziness, or a general ill feeling, and fever); nausea or vomiting.

KNEE SPRAIN and TORN KNEE LIGAMENTS

GENERAL INFORMATION

DESCRIPTION

Knee sprain is the violent stretching of one or more ligaments in the knee. Sprains involving two or more ligaments cause considerably more disability than single-ligament sprains. When the ligament is overstretched, it becomes tense and gives way at its weakest point, either where it attaches to bone or within the ligament itself. If the ligament pulls loose a fragment of bone, it is called a *sprain-fracture*. A severe sprain may lead to complete rupture of a knee ligament and total loss of function. A severe sprain requires surgery for treatment. Appropriate health care includes physical therapy and surgery (sometimes).

SIGNS & SYMPTOMS

Severe pain at the time of injury; feeling of popping or tearing inside the child's knee; tenderness at the injury site; swelling in the knee; bruising that appears soon after injury.

CAUSES

Stress on a ligament that temporarily forces or pries the child's knee out of its normal location. Sprains occur frequently in runners, walkers, and those who jump in such sports as basketball, soccer, volleyball, skiing, and distance- or high-jumping. These athletes often accidentally land on the side of the foot.

RISK FACTORS

Contact, running and jumping sports; previous knee injury; obesity; poor muscle conditioning; inadequate protection from equipment.

PREVENTING COMPLICATIONS OR RECURRENCE

Instructions for your child: Build your strength with a conditioning program appropriate for your sport; warm up before practice or competition; tape vulnerable joints before practice or competition; wear proper protective shoes—a twist or injury to the foot can affect the knee.

WHAT TO EXPECT

MEDICAL TESTS

X-rays of the child's knee, hip, and ankle to rule out fractures.

POSSIBLE COMPLICATIONS

Prolonged healing time if the child's usual activities are resumed too soon; proneness to repeated injury; inflammation at the ligament attachment to the bone (periostitis); prolonged disability (sometimes); an unstable or arthritic knee following repeated injury.

PROBABLE OUTCOME

If this is a first-time injury, proper care and sufficient healing time before your child resumes activity should prevent permanent disability. Ligaments have a poor blood supply, and torn ligaments require as much healing time as fractures. Average healing times are: mild sprains—2 to 6 weeks; moderate sprains—6 to 8 weeks; severe sprains—8 weeks to 10 months.

KNEE SPRAIN and TORN KNEE LIGAMENTS

TREATMENT

HOME CARE

Your child should use crutches with tops just below the armpits. The doctor usually applies a splint from the ankle to the groin to immobilize the sprained knee. If the doctor does not apply a cast, tape, or elastic bandage:

• Continue using an ice pack on the child's knee 3 or 4 times a day. Place ice chips or cubes in a plastic bag. Wrap the bag in a moist towel and place it over the injured knee. Use for 20 minutes at a time.

• Wrap the child's injured knee with an elasticized bandage.

• Provide the child with whirlpool treatments, if available.

• Massage gently and often to provide comfort and decrease swelling.

MEDICATION

• For minor discomfort, use aspirin, acetaminophen, or ibuprofen; topical liniments and ointments.

• Your doctor may prescribe stronger pain relievers; injection of a long-acting local anesthetic to reduce the child's pain; injection of a corticosteroid, such as triamcinolone, to reduce inflammation; general anesthetic for surgery or arthroscopy (see Glossary) of the knee joint.

ACTIVITY

Your child can resume normal activities gradually after clearance from your doctor.

DIET & FLUIDS

No restrictions.

REHABILITATION

Instructions for your child:

• Begin daily rehabilitation exercises when the cast or supportive wrapping is no longer necessary.

• Use ice massage for 10 minutes before and after exercise.

OK FOR SCHOOL, PRESCHOOL, OR NURSERY?

Yes, when condition and sense of well-being will allow.

CALL YOUR DOCTOR IF

• Your child has symptoms of a moderate or severe knee sprain, or a mild sprain persists longer than 2 weeks.

• Pain, swelling, or bruising worsens despite treatment.

• Any of the following occur after casting or splinting: pain, numbness, or coldness below the cast or splint; blue, gray, or dusky toenails.

• Any of the following occur after surgery, if it was required: increased pain, swelling, redness, drainage, or bleeding in the surgical area; signs of infection (headache, muscle aches, dizziness, or a general ill feeling with fever).

• New, unexplained symptoms develop. Drugs used in treatment may produce side effects.

KNEE SYNOVITIS WITH EFFUSION
("Water on the Knee")

GENERAL INFORMATION

DESCRIPTION

Knee synovitis with effusion is inflammation of the synovium, the smooth, lubricated lining of the knee. The synovium's lubricating fluid helps the knee move freely and prevents bone surfaces from rubbing against each other. Inflammation triggers an excess of fluid production and accumulation in the knee. Synovitis with effusion is often a complication of a knee injury or of collagen diseases, such as gout or rheumatoid arthritis.

Appropriate health care includes:

- Doctor's care, including aspiration of fluid from the knee. Because most knee synovitis with effusion is caused by injury to some part of the knee, treating the underlying injury is as important as treating the effusion.
- Self-care during rehabilitation.
- Physical therapy.

SIGNS & SYMPTOMS

- Pain in the child's knee (sometimes).
- Swelling and heat above the kneecap.
- Generalized swelling and redness if the inflammation is caused from infection or joint disease, such as gout, rather than from athletic injury.

CAUSES

- Single injury or repeated injury that damages any part of the knee.
- Bacterial infection (frequently gonorrhea).
- Metabolic disturbance, such as an acute attack of gout or rheumatoid arthritis.

RISK FACTORS

Participation in contact sports such as football, baseball, soccer, or rugby; repeated knee injury; poor muscle strength or conditioning, which makes knee injury more likely; medical history of gout, rheumatoid arthritis, or other inflammatory joint diseases; infection in another joint; vitamin or mineral deficiency, which makes complications following injury more likely.

PREVENTING COMPLICATIONS OR RECURRENCE

- Your child should engage in a vigorous muscle strengthening and conditioning program prior to beginning regular sports participation. The child should warm up adequately before workouts or competition.
- Your child should wear protective knee pads during participation in contact sports.

? WHAT TO EXPECT

MEDICAL TESTS

Your own observation of symptoms; medical history and physical exam by a doctor; X-rays of the knee joint; laboratory examination of fluid removed from the knee.

KNEE SYNOVITIS WITH EFFUSION ("Water on the Knee")

POSSIBLE COMPLICATIONS

Prolonged healing time if activity is resumed too soon; proneness to repeated knee injury; unstable or arthritic knee following repeated bouts of synovitis; chronic synovitis that may prevent athletic participation.

PROBABLE OUTCOME

Knee synovitis with effusion can usually be cured completely in 2 to 4 weeks with heat and corticosteroid injections. However, recurrences are common following minor knee injuries.

TREATMENT

HOME CARE

- Use an elastic bandage to compress the child's knee after fluid has been removed and between physical-therapy sessions.
- Apply heat frequently. Use heat lamps, hot soaks, hot showers, heating pads, or heat liniments and ointments.
- The child can take whirlpool treatments, if available.
- Massage gently and often to provide comfort and decrease swelling.

MEDICATION

- Your doctor may prescribe antibiotics if infection is present; non-steroidal anti-inflammatory drugs or anti-gout medicine; injection of a long-acting local anesthetic mixed with a corticosteroid to help reduce pain and inflammation.
- Give the child aspirin or ibuprofen for minor discomfort.

ACTIVITY

- Your child can continue the usual activities during treatment if there is no pain, but protect the knee with tape and an elastic bandage during competitive sports. If there is pain, your child should reduce activities until the pain subsides.
- Use ice massage on the child for 10 minutes before and after exercise. Fill a large Styrofoam cup with water and freeze. Tear a small amount of foam from the top so ice protrudes. Massage firmly over the injured area in a circle about the size of a softball.

DIET & FLUIDS

No restrictions.

OK FOR SCHOOL, PRESCHOOL, OR NURSERY?

Yes, when condition and sense of well-being will allow.

CALL YOUR DOCTOR IF

- Your child's knee becomes red, hot, swollen, or painful.
- After aspiration of fluid from the knee, your child develops signs of infection (headache, fever, muscle aches, dizziness, or a general ill feeling).

LACERATIONS (CUTS) OF THE SKIN

GENERAL INFORMATION

DESCRIPTION

Lacerations are open wounds in the skin. The wounds sometimes extend to underlying tissue and muscle. Appropriate health care includes closure of large and bleeding lacerations by a physician. Most cuts and scrapes heal well without sutures.

SIGNS & SYMPTOMS

- Pain at the lacerated site.
- Heavy bleeding in lacerations of the child's scalp and forehead.
- Swelling, redness, and tenderness around the laceration (sometimes).

CAUSES

Direct blow with a sharp or blunt object (knife, athletic equipment, stick, etc.).

RISK FACTORS

Contact sports; auto, motorcycle, or bicycle racing; uneven terrain for a playing field.

PREVENTING COMPLICATIONS OR RECURRENCE

Your child should wear protective padding and equipment appropriate for a sport.

WHAT TO EXPECT

MEDICAL TESTS

X-rays of bones adjacent to severe lacerations to rule out fractures.

POSSIBLE COMPLICATIONS

Excessive bleeding; allergy to local anesthetics; wound infection due to bacterial contamination of the child's laceration. If infection complicates healing, fever, pain, and edema (collection of fluid) around the incision will occur. The edema may cause the child's sutures to become tighter and break; scarring and disfigurement (sometimes).

PROBABLE OUTCOME

Lacerations usually heal in 2 weeks if they are sutured properly and do not become infected.

TREATMENT

HOME CARE

For your child's minor cuts:

- Hold the wounded area under running water and clean with mild soap.
- Pat the skin dry.
- Hold the edges of a shallow straight cut together with tape stretched across the laceration.
- Apply a sterile dressing.

LACERATIONS (CUTS) OF THE SKIN

For your child's serious cuts and brisk bleeding:
- Cover the injured area with a cloth or your bare hands, if no cloth is available.
- Apply strong pressure directly to the laceration for 10 minutes while awaiting an ambulance or transportation to an emergency room.
- If direct pressure doesn't control extremely heavy bleeding and bleeding is from an arm or leg, use a light tourniquet. Make a tourniquet from a length of cloth or similar material. Note how long the tourniquet is in place so emergency medical personnel will know. Don't leave the tourniquet on longer than 20 minutes.

For wound care without brisk bleeding:
- Clean the child's wound carefully with soap and water.
- The wound will be cleaned again and sutured in the doctor's office or an emergency medical facility, usually under local anesthesia.
- Keep the wound covered with a bandage and moderate compression for 2 days to help prevent fluid collection under the sutures.
- If the bandage gets wet, replace it and apply non-prescription antibiotic ointment.
- If bleeding occurs after suturing, control it by applying firm pressure to the child's wound with a facial tissue or clean cloth. Hold the pressure for 10 minutes.
- Prevent tetanus by having the child get a booster dose of tetanus toxoid or human antitetanic serum.
- Protect a child's laceration with extra padding during contact sports until it heals.

MEDICATION

- Inquire regarding the need of a tetanus booster for your child.
- Your doctor may prescribe:
  — Pain relievers. Don't give your child prescription pain medication longer than 4 to 7 days. The child should use only as much as needed.
  — Antibiotics to fight infection.
- Use non-prescription drugs, such as acetaminophen, to relieve minor pain.

ACTIVITY

Your child should avoid vigorous exercise for 1 to 6 weeks after suturing.

DIET & FLUIDS

No special diet.

OK FOR SCHOOL, PRESCHOOL, OR NURSERY?

Yes, after treatment is complete.

CALL YOUR DOCTOR IF

- Pain, swelling, redness, drainage, or bleeding increases in the child's wound area.
- Your child develops signs of infection: headache, muscle aches, dizziness, or a general ill feeling and fever.

LACTOSE INTOLERANCE
(Milk Intolerance; Lactase Deficiency)

GENERAL INFORMATION

DESCRIPTION

Lactose intolerance is a disorder characterized by difficulty in digesting cow's milk. Lactose intolerance occurs—with varying severity—in 75% of the black population, 90% of Orientals and American Indians, and less than 20% of Caucasians of northwest European origin. It is not contagious or cancerous. The digestive system is involved.

Appropriate health care includes:

- Self-care after diagnosis, including dietary adjustments.
- Physician's monitoring of general condition and medications.

SIGNS & SYMPTOMS

In infants and children:

- Foamy diarrhea with diaper rash.
- Vomiting.
- Slow weight gain, growth, and development.

In adolescents and adults:

- Rumbling abdominal sounds, abdominal cramps, and diarrhea.
- Gas and bloating.
- Nausea.

CAUSES

- Deficiency or absence of the enzyme lactase. Lactase is necessary to digest all milk except mother's milk. Without it, sugars in milk absorb fluid and cause diarrhea. Although some infants are born with the disorder, lactose intolerance usually develops in adulthood.
- Temporary lactose intolerance can occur in an infant after a severe bout of gastroenteritis that damages the intestinal lining.

RISK FACTORS

Family history of enzyme-lactase deficiency.

PREVENTING COMPLICATIONS OR RECURRENCE

Cannot be prevented at present. If you are pregnant and there is a history of lactose intolerance in your family, consider breast-feeding your baby. If not, you may need an alternate non-milk formula for your infant.

WHAT TO EXPECT

MEDICAL TESTS

- Your own observation of symptoms.
- Medical history and physical exam by a doctor.
- Laboratory studies, such as a stool exam and lactose-tolerance test.
- X-rays of the child's lower intestinal tract.
- Therapeutic trial with a milk-free diet.

POSSIBLE COMPLICATIONS

Infants with an inherited deficiency will not thrive without treatment.

LACTOSE INTOLERANCE (Milk Intolerance; Lactase Deficiency)

PROBABLE OUTCOME

This condition is currently considered incurable. However, your child's symptoms can be relieved or controlled with a diet free of milk and milk products. Symptoms worsen at times for unexplained reasons.

TREATMENT

HOME CARE

No special instructions except those listed under other headings.

MEDICATION

- Your doctor may prescribe a supplement for your child to neutralize lactose in milk.
- See Medications section for information regarding medicines your doctor may prescribe.

ACTIVITY

No restrictions.

DIET & FLUIDS

- If the condition is present at birth, your doctor will probably prescribe an infant formula that contains little or no lactose, such as a soybean-based formula.
- If the lactose intolerance is temporary and caused by gastroenteritis, the substitute formula should be necessary for a short time only. Cow's milk can be introduced again later.
- Older children and adolescents with lactose intolerance should avoid milk and milk products, such as cheese and ice cream.

OK FOR SCHOOL, PRESCHOOL, OR NURSERY?

Yes. This is not contagious.

CALL YOUR DOCTOR IF

- Your child has symptoms of lactose intolerance.
- Your child's temperature rises to 101F (38.3C) or higher.
- Your infant fails to gain weight.
- Your infant refuses food or formula.
- Vomiting or diarrhea reappears in a child who has previously had a temporary intolerance to milk or milk products.
- A milk-free diet doesn't relieve your child's symptoms.

LARVA MIGRANS, CUTANEOUS (Creeping Eruption)

GENERAL INFORMATION

DESCRIPTION

Creeping eruption is a skin infestation of hookworm or roundworm larvae. These parasites usually infect dogs and cats. The skin areas that come in contact with the ground—usually the feet, legs, or buttocks—are involved.

Appropriate health care includes:

- Home care after diagnosis.
- Physician's monitoring of general condition and medications.

SIGNS & SYMPTOMS

Skin rash or small blisters, progressing to thin raised lines on the child's skin leading from the parasite's entry point. The random lines create tunnel-like lesions that lengthen up to 1cm a day. Most children have several tracks simultaneously, each of a different length and pattern.

CAUSES

Infestation by larvae of hookworms and roundworms found in the intestinal tracts of dogs and cats.

RISK FACTORS

- Play in warm, moist sand in which cats or dogs have defecated.
- Work or play that involves crawling in confined spaces and contact with infected soil, as under a house.

PREVENTING COMPLICATIONS OR RECURRENCE

- Teach your child to handle cat litter carefully and to avoid touching soil outside.
- Urge your child not to play in soil used by cats and dogs for elimination.
- Have pets treated for worms.

WHAT TO EXPECT

MEDICAL TESTS

- Your own observation of symptoms.
- Medical history and physical exam by a doctor.

POSSIBLE COMPLICATIONS

Secondary bacterial infection of affected skin.

PROBABLE OUTCOME

Usually curable in 1 to 2 weeks with treatment.

LARVA MIGRANS, CUTANEOUS
(Creeping Eruption)

TREATMENT

HOME CARE

No specific instructions except those listed under other headings.

MEDICATION

Your doctor may prescribe:

- Topical thiabendazole for local application in a 2% solution with dimethyl sulfoxide (DMSO). Follow instructions carefully. Apply it to the end of the track (farthest from the point of entry).
- Oral thiabendazole for serious infestations by many larvae. This form causes your child to suffer adverse reactions and side effects.
- See Medications section for information regarding medicines your doctor may prescribe.

ACTIVITY

No restrictions.

DIET & FLUIDS

No special diet.

OK FOR SCHOOL, PRESCHOOL, OR NURSERY?

Yes. This is not contagious.

CALL YOUR DOCTOR IF

- Your child has symptoms of larva migrans.
- Skin lesions on your child develop pus, indicating secondary infection.
- Your child takes oral thiabendazole and new, unexplained symptoms develop.

LARYNGITIS

GENERAL INFORMATION

DESCRIPTION

Laryngitis is a minor inflammation of the larynx (voice box) and surrounding tissues, causing temporary hoarseness. The larynx (voice box) and the upper part of the neck, behind the Adam's apple, are involved.

Appropriate health care includes:

- Self-care after diagnosis.
- Physician's monitoring of general condition and medications.

SIGNS & SYMPTOMS

- Hoarseness or loss of voice.
- Sore throat or tickling in the back of the throat.
- Sensation of a lump in the throat.
- Slight fever (sometimes).
- Swallowing difficulty.

CAUSES

Inflammation of the vocal cords and surrounding area caused by:

- Viruses.
- Bacteria.
- Allergies.
- Excessive use of the voice.
- Electrolyte-balance disturbances, especially low potassium, that cause muscle weakness.
- Tumor (rare).

RISK FACTORS

- Exposure to irritants distributed by air-conditioning systems, such as mold, pollen, and pollutants.
- Extremely cold weather.
- Recent respiratory illness, such as bronchitis or pneumonia.
- Smoking.
- Excess alcohol consumption.

PREVENTING COMPLICATIONS OR RECURRENCE

- Urge your child to avoid yelling or straining the voice.
- Treat your child's respiratory infections carefully.

WHAT TO EXPECT

MEDICAL TESTS

- Your own observation of symptoms.
- Medical history and physical exam by a doctor. Treatment by an ear, nose and throat specialist might be helpful for persistent cases.

POSSIBLE COMPLICATIONS

Total breathing obstruction, if laryngitis is part of a serious infection of the child's respiratory system, such as epiglottitis.

PROBABLE OUTCOME

Spontaneous recovery for viral laryngitis in 10 to 14 days. Bacterial infections are usually curable in 7 to 10 days with antibiotic treatment.

TREATMENT

HOME CARE

- Urge your child not to use the voice—to whisper or write notes instead. For most cases, resting the voice for a few days is all that is needed.
- Use a cool-mist humidifier around the child to increase air moisture and ease the constricted feeling in the throat. Hot, steamy showers also help.

MEDICATION

- For minor discomfort, use non-prescription drugs, such as acetaminophen, aspirin, or cough syrup.
- See Medications section for information regarding medicines your doctor may prescribe.

ACTIVITY

Your child should rest more frequently.

DIET & FLUIDS

No special diet.

OK FOR SCHOOL, PRESCHOOL, OR NURSERY?

When signs of infection have decreased, appetite returns, and alertness, strength, and feeling of well-being will allow.

CALL YOUR DOCTOR IF

- Your child has hoarseness or other symptoms of laryngitis that last longer than 2 weeks. This may be an early sign of cancer.
- Your child feels very ill or has a high fever or breathing difficulty. If these symptoms develop, call your doctor immediately.

LEAD POISONING

GENERAL INFORMATION

DESCRIPTION

Lead is everywhere—in food, soil, and air, and in human bodies. It serves no useful biological purpose, but an excess can cause illness and disability. The body absorbs up to 10% of the lead it takes in. In iron-deficient children, 50% of ingested lead may be absorbed. Lead poisoning is more likely in children 6 months to 6 years who live in homes built before the 1960s.

Appropriate health care includes:

- Hospitalization for severe cases.
- Home care with special attention to prevent further exposure to lead.
- Possible long-term pediatric convalescent center after rigorous treatment.

SIGNS & SYMPTOMS

- Anemia (inhibits production of *heme*, the iron-carrying component of hemoglobin).
- Early: Fatigue, paleness, constipation, appetite loss, irritability, behavioral changes, short-memory loss, sleep disorders, slowing of the child's mental development.
- More severe: Vomiting, abdominal pain, headache, clumsiness, weakness, confusion, seizures.

CAUSES

- Chewing objects with lead, such as paint.
- Swallowing contaminated dust or soil.
- Inhaling dust with lead.

RISK FACTORS

- Living in heavily industrialized and urban areas.
- Iron deficiency that causes lead to be more easily absorbed by a child.
- Being 6 months to 6 years of age.
- Underlying illness (such as sickle cell anemia).

PREVENTING COMPLICATIONS OR RECURRENCE

- Use lead-free paint throughout your home so children won't be exposed.
- Educate children not to put foreign objects of any kind in their mouths.

WHAT TO EXPECT

MEDICAL TESTS

- Medical history and physical exam by a doctor.
- Urine and blood tests for lead.
- Laboratory analysis of household samples of paint, dust, soil, air.
- X-rays to study the extent of the deposit of lead in the child's bones.

POSSIBLE COMPLICATIONS

Permanent problem with seizures, mental retardation, cerebral palsy, severe kidney damage.

PROBABLE OUTCOME

If treatment begins before the child's brain and nervous system are involved, the outlook is good for a normal life and life-span, but eliminating lead from a child's body can be a very slow process.

TREATMENT

HOME CARE

- Discover sources of exposure to lead and remove them, or remove the child from the environment.
- Discuss with your physician or social worker ways and means to increase mental stimulation for the child.
- Provide strong family support.
- Get frequent follow-up exams to monitor the child's progress.

MEDICATION

- Medicine to increase urine flow through the child's kidney.
- Chelation therapy intravenously or intramuscularly in a physician's office, the out-patient section of a hospital, or in the hospital. This treatment may last 3 days to 3 months.
- Side effects of chelation treatment can include nausea, vomiting, bruising, skin rash, heartbeat irregularities. These are reversible upon cessation of chelation treatment.

ACTIVITY

Your child can increase slowly to normal activity.

DIET & FLUIDS

No special diet.

OK FOR SCHOOL, PRESCHOOL, OR NURSERY?

When strength and sense of well-being will allow.

CALL YOUR DOCTOR IF

Your child develops any new symptoms after treatment. Medications used can cause side effects.

LEG FRACTURE, FIBULA

GENERAL INFORMATION

DESCRIPTION

A leg fracture of the fibula is a complete or incomplete break in the smaller of the two bones of the lower leg. Fractures of the fibula are not uncommon, and displacement is seldom severe. These fractures sometimes accompany severe ankle sprains. See also Leg Fracture, Tibia.

Appropriate health care includes:

Doctor's diagnosis. Setting of the fracture is usually not necessary.

SIGNS & SYMPTOMS

- Severe pain at the fracture site.
- Swelling of soft tissue surrounding the fracture.
- Visible deformity if the fracture is complete and bone fragments separate enough to distort the child's normal leg contours.
- Tenderness to the touch.
- Numbness or coldness in the child's foot if the blood supply is impaired.

CAUSES

Direct blow or indirect stress to the bone. Indirect stress may be caused by the child twisting or turning quickly, or by a violent muscle contraction.

RISK FACTORS

- Contact sports such as football, soccer, or hockey.
- History of bone or joint disease.

PREVENTING COMPLICATIONS OR RECURRENCE

Your child should build adequate muscle strength and achieve good conditioning prior to exercise, athletic practice, or competition. Increased muscle mass helps protect a child's bones and underlying tissue.

WHAT TO EXPECT

MEDICAL TESTS

X-rays of injured areas, including the knee and ankle.

POSSIBLE COMPLICATIONS

- Pressure on or injury to nearby nerves, ligaments, tendons, muscles, blood vessels, or connective tissues.
- Delayed union or non-union of the fracture.
- Impaired blood supply to the fracture site.
- Arrest of normal bone growth in a child.
- Shortening of the child's injured bones.
- Prolonged healing time if the child resumes activity too soon.
- Proneness to repeated injury.

PROBABLE OUTCOME

The average healing time for this fracture is 4 to 6 weeks.

TREATMENT

FIRST AID

- Keep the child warm with blankets to decrease the possibility of shock.
- Cut away clothing, if possible. Don't move the injured area to remove clothing.
- Follow instructions for R.I.C.E., the first letters of *rest*, *ice*, *compression, and elevation*. See Appendix 39 for details.

HOME CARE

- Setting the broken bone for a fibula fracture is usually not necessary. The tibia (the big bone adjacent to the fibula) provides immobilization. A fibula fracture usually requires only a snug, toe-to-knee cotton elastic bandage. If pain is severe, a walking plaster cast below the child's knee may be necessary for about 5 weeks.
- After the bandage or cast is removed, use frequent ice massage.
- Provide the child with whirlpool treatments, if available.

MEDICATION

Your doctor may prescribe:

- Narcotic or synthetic narcotic pain relievers for severe pain.
- Stool softeners to prevent constipation due to inactivity.
- Acetaminophen (available without prescription) for mild pain after initial treatment.
- See Medications section for information regarding medicines your doctor may prescribe.

ACTIVITY

Instructions for your child:

- Actively exercise all muscle groups not immobilized. These muscle contractions promote fracture alignment and hasten healing. Use ice massage for 10 minutes before and after workouts.
- Begin walking and light running when there is no pain or tenderness.
- Resume normal activities gradually after treatment.

DIET & FLUIDS

Your child should eat a well-balanced diet.

OK FOR SCHOOL, PRESCHOOL, OR NURSERY?

Yes, when condition and sense of well-being allow.

CALL YOUR DOCTOR IF

- Your child has signs or symptoms of a leg fracture.
- Any of the following occur after surgery or other treatment:
  - Signs of infection (headache, muscle aches, dizziness, or a general ill feeling and fever).
  - Swelling above or below the bandage or cast.
  - Change in the child's skin color to blue or gray beyond the cast, particularly under the toenails.
  - Numbness or complete loss of feeling below the fracture site.
  - Nausea or vomiting.
  - Constipation.

LEG FRACTURE, TIBIA

GENERAL INFORMATION

DESCRIPTION

A leg fracture of the tibia is a complete or incomplete break in the large bone of the leg between the knee and ankle. See also Leg Fracture, Fibula.
Appropriate health care includes:
Hospitalization (sometimes) to set the fracture.

SIGNS & SYMPTOMS

- Severe pain at the fracture site.
- Swelling of soft tissue surrounding the fracture.
- Visible deformity if the fracture is complete and bone fragments separate enough to distort the child's normal leg contours.
- Numbness or coldness in the child's foot if the blood supply is impaired.

CAUSES

- Direct blow to the child's leg.
- Weakening of the bone from repeated stress, resulting in a stress fracture that progresses to a complete fracture. This is especially common in joggers, marathon runners, and walkers.
- Indirect stress caused by twisting or violent muscle contraction.

RISK FACTORS

Contact sports; history of bone or joint disease; obesity; poor nutrition, especially calcium deficiency.

PREVENTING COMPLICATIONS OR RECURRENCE

Your child should build strength with a good conditioning program and should use appropriate protective equipment, including good shoes for running and shin guards for participation in contact sports.

WHAT TO EXPECT

MEDICAL TESTS

X-rays of the injured area, from the knee joint above to the ankle joint below.

POSSIBLE COMPLICATIONS

- At the time of the child's injury: shock; pressure on or injury to nearby nerves, ligaments, tendons, muscles, blood vessels, or connective tissues.
- After treatment or surgery: delayed union or non-union of the fracture; impaired blood supply to the fracture site; avascular necrosis (death of bone cells) due to interruption of the blood supply; shortening of the child's injured bones; arrest of normal bone growth in a child; infection in open fractures (skin broken over fracture site), or at the incision if surgical setting was necessary; an unstable or arthritic ankle or knee joint if the fracture is close to either; prolonged healing time if activity is resumed too soon; proneness to repeated leg injury; problems caused by casts. See Appendix 41 (Care of Casts).

LEG FRACTURE, TIBIA

PROBABLE OUTCOME

The average healing time for this fracture if 6 to 8 weeks.

TREATMENT

FIRST AID

- Follow instructions for R.I.C.E., the first letters of *rest*, *ice*, *compression*, and *elevation*. See Appendix 39 for details.
- The doctor will set (realign) the broken bones with surgery or, if possible, without.

HOME CARE

Immobilization will be necessary. A rigid cast is placed around the injured leg to immobilize the child's knee and ankle.

MEDICATION

Your doctor may prescribe:

- General anesthesia, local anesthesia, or muscle relaxants to make bone manipulation and fixation of bone fragments possible.
- Narcotic or synthetic narcotic pain relievers for severe pain.
- Stool softeners to prevent constipation due to inactivity.
- Acetaminophen for mild pain.

ACTIVITY

Your child will have to learn to walk with crutches. See Appendix 37. The child can resume normal activities gradually after treatment but should not drive until healing is complete.

DIET & FLUIDS

Give the child only water before manipulation or surgery to treat the fracture. Solid food in the stomach makes vomiting while under anesthesia more hazardous.

OK FOR SCHOOL, PRESCHOOL, OR NURSERY?

Yes, when condition and sense of well-being will allow.

CALL YOUR DOCTOR IF

- Your child has signs or symptoms of a tibia fracture.
- Any of the following occur after surgery or other treatment:
  — Increased pain, swelling, or drainage in the surgical area.
  — Signs of infection (headache, muscle aches, dizziness, or a general ill feeling and fever).
  — Swelling above or below the child's cast.
  — Blue or gray skin color beyond the cast, especially under the toenails.
  — Loss of feeling below the fracture site.
  — Nausea or vomiting.
  — Constipation.

LEGG-PERTHES DISEASE
(Slipped Femoral Epiphysis; Coxa Plana)

GENERAL INFORMATION

DESCRIPTION

Legg-Perthes disease is a gradual weakening of the upper end of the thigh bone where it meets the pelvis. Either leg at the hip joint (occasionally both) is involved. Legg-Perthes disease usually affects older children (5 to 11 years) of both sexes, but it is more common in boys.

Appropriate health care includes:

- Physician's monitoring of general condition, medications, and treatment, including consultation with an orthopedist.
- Surgery to reinforce the bone's attachment to the joint and prevent further deformity (sometimes).
- Hospitalization (sometimes) for traction (a steady pull on the leg).
- Home care after diagnosis or hospitalization.

SIGNS & SYMPTOMS

- Pain and stiffness in the child's hip and thigh.
- Pain in the leg—often the *knee*—even though the disorder is in the hip.
- Limping.

CAUSES

Unknown. Injury is usually not a factor.

RISK FACTORS

Family history of hip disorders; use of cortisone drugs for other disorders; overweight; periods of rapid growth.

PREVENTING COMPLICATIONS OR RECURRENCE

Help an overweight child lose weight. A reducing diet appears in Appendix 31.

WHAT TO EXPECT

MEDICAL TESTS

- Your own observation of symptoms.
- Medical history and physical exam by a doctor.
- X-ray of the hip.
- Special studies that may include:

  — Ultrasonography: A non-invasive technique that translates sound waves into images displayed on a screen and photographed (see Glossary).

  — CAT or CT Scan (computerized axial tomography): Non-invasive computerized X-ray images that show sections (or "slices") of an organ or region of the body clearly and precisely (see Glossary).

  — MRI (magnetic resonance imaging): A non-invasive (non-X-ray) computerized test that uses radio frequency energy and a powerful magnetic field to produce images with excellent detail (see Glossary).

  — Radionuclide Scan: A nuclear medicine procedure that uses radioactive isotopes injected into a patient. The isotope tracers are absorbed in various concentrations by targeted organs, which are then photographed (see Glossary).

LEGG-PERTHES DISEASE
(Slipped Femoral Epiphysis; Coxa Plana)

POSSIBLE COMPLICATIONS

- Bone infection.
- Permanent damage to the thigh bone and hip joint.

PROBABLE OUTCOME

Often curable in 3 to 4 years with early treatment. Delayed treatment may cause permanent bone injury and require surgery to replace the hip.

TREATMENT

HOME CARE

- Children often have difficulty accepting the need for bed rest, casts, braces, or other treatment. Enlist the help of your doctor, a counselor, a school nurse, or other significant persons, if necessary, to discuss the situation with your child.
- Help your child find activities and interests that don't involve athletics.
- Use heat to relieve pain. Warm compresses, heating pads, whirlpool baths, heat lamps, diathermy, and ultrasound are effective.

MEDICATION

- For minor discomfort, use non-prescription drugs, such as aspirin, acetaminophen, or ibuprofen.
- See Medications section for information regarding medicines your doctor may prescribe.

ACTIVITY

Bed rest may be necessary for 6 months to 1 year until the condition improves, or until after surgery. When the bones can bear weight, crutches, braces or casts are usually necessary. After that, the child may resume activities gradually. See Appendix 41, Care of Casts.

DIET & FLUIDS

No special diet, unless the child is overweight. See Appendix 31, Obesity: Guidelines for Losing Weight.

OK FOR SCHOOL, PRESCHOOL, OR NURSERY?

Yes, when strength and feeling of well-being allows.

CALL YOUR DOCTOR IF

- Your child has hip pain, knee pain, stiffness, or a limp.
- The following occurs during treatment:
  - — Symptoms don't improve in 4 weeks, despite treatment.
  - — Pain increases.
  - — Temperature rises to 101F (38.3C).

LEUKEMIA, ACUTE

GENERAL INFORMATION

DESCRIPTION

Acute leukemia is a malignant overgrowth of white blood cells in bone marrow or tissues that are part of the lymphatic system (lymph glands, spleen, liver). These excess cells accumulate and spill into the bloodstream, eventually involving other tissues. Common forms of leukemia include acute lymphocytic leukemia (especially prevalent in children), acute myelogenous leukemia, and acute monocytic leukemia. Acute leukemia is the most common form of cancer in children. The bone marrow and lymph tissue are involved in the early stages. The disease eventually affects all body tissues. Acute leukemia can affect both sexes, all ages, but is more common in males. Acute lymphocytic leukemia has a peak incidence between ages 2 and 5.

Appropriate health care includes:

- Physician's monitoring of general condition and medications.
- Home care after diagnosis and treatment and during remission.
- Hospitalization for treatment in the initial stage or for relapse.

SIGNS & SYMPTOMS

- Low fever.
- Tiredness.
- Anemia.
- Increasing paleness.
- General ill feeling.
- Easy bruising and spontaneous bleeding (nosebleeds, bleeding from the gums, or prolonged menstruation).
- Enlarged spleen and abdominal pain.
- Susceptibility to infection, especially pneumonia.
- Mouth infections with ulcers and sores.
- Headache and lethargy, if your child's meninges (brain membranes) are affected.

CAUSES

Unknown, but there are many suspected predisposing factors—especially viruses and radiation.

RISK FACTORS

- Family history of leukemia.
- Excess exposure to X-rays.
- Congenital disorders, especially Down syndrome.
- Being identical twins.
- Exposure to benzenes, which are used in many industrial chemicals.
- Use of cytotoxic drugs.

PREVENTING COMPLICATIONS OR RECURRENCE

Cannot be prevented. If you have a family history of leukemia, obtain genetic counseling before starting a family.

WHAT TO EXPECT

MEDICAL TESTS

- Your own observation of symptoms.
- Medical history and physical exam by a doctor.
- Laboratory studies of the child's blood, bone marrow, and cerebrospinal fluid.

POSSIBLE COMPLICATIONS

- Hemorrhage.
- Death from destruction of the body's defenses against infection.

PROBABLE OUTCOME

Treatment brings remission in 90% of children and cure in 50% for some forms of leukemia. Other forms are eventually fatal.

TREATMENT

HOME CARE

- A child with leukemia should avoid ill persons and crowds to prevent dangerous exposure to infection.
- The child should rinse the mouth often with a warm salt-water solution to decrease mouth ulcers. Use 1 tablespoon salt in 8 oz. water.
- Encourage your child to use a soft toothbrush to prevent gum abrasion.

MEDICATION

Your doctor may prescribe anti-cancer drugs; cortisone drugs; pain relievers; antibiotics to fight infection; uricosuric drugs to increase excretion of uric acid that may accumulate as a side effect of anti-cancer drugs.

ACTIVITY

No restrictions for your child during remissions. Bed rest is usually necessary during active phases of the disease.

DIET & FLUIDS

Encourage your child to drink extra fluids. Older children and adults should drink 8 to 10 glasses of fluid daily, and younger children should drink 4 to 6 glasses of fluid. During chemotherapy, urge your child to eat and drink high-calorie foods and beverages, such as milkshakes or eggnog.

OK FOR SCHOOL, PRESCHOOL, OR NURSERY?

Yes, during remission or when appetite has returned and alertness, strength, and feeling of well-being will allow.

CALL YOUR DOCTOR IF

- Your child has symptoms of leukemia.
- The following occurs during active stages *or* remissions:
  - — Fever, chills, cough, or sore throat.
  - — Abnormal bleeding. Apply pressure and ice while awaiting your doctor's return call.
  - — Constipation.

LICE
(Pediculosis; Head Lice; Body Lice; "Crabs")

GENERAL INFORMATION

DESCRIPTION

Pediculosis is a skin inflammation caused by tiny parasites (lice) that live on the body or in clothing. Body parts involved include hairy areas anywhere—especially the scalp, eyebrows, or genital area—and skin—especially areas in which clothing is in close contact with skin, such as the shoulders, waist, genital area, or buttocks.

Appropriate health care includes:
- Self-care after diagnosis.
- Physician's monitoring of general condition and medications.

SIGNS & SYMPTOMS

- Itching and scratching, sometimes intense and usually in your child's hair-covered areas.
- Eggs ("nits") on hair shafts.
- Scalp inflammation and matted hair.
- Enlarged lymph glands at the back of the scalp or in the groin (sometimes).
- Red bite marks and hives.

CAUSES

Tiny (3mm to 4mm) parasites that bite through your child's skin to obtain nourishment (blood). The bites cause itching and inflammation. Some lice live on skin, although they are difficult to see. Others live in clothing near skin. Eggs (nits) adhere to hairs.

RISK FACTORS

- Crowded or unsanitary living conditions.
- Family history of lice.
- Sexual intercourse with an infected person.

PREVENTING COMPLICATIONS OR RECURRENCE

Instructions for your child:
- Bathe and shampoo often.
- Avoid wearing the same clothing more than a day or two.
- Change bed linens often.
- Don't share combs, brushes, or hats with others.

WHAT TO EXPECT

MEDICAL TESTS

- Your own observation of symptoms. You may see nits (like tiny footballs) on the side of your child's hairs.
- Medical history and physical exam by a doctor.

POSSIBLE COMPLICATIONS

Infection at the site of deep scratching may cause diseases such as typhus (rare).

LICE
(Pediculosis; Head Lice; Body Lice; "Crabs")

PROBABLE OUTCOME

Usually curable with medicated creams, lotions, and shampoos. Allow 5 days after treatment for your child's symptoms to disappear. Lice often recur.

TREATMENT

HOME CARE

The following measures apply to *all* members of the household:

- Use medicated shampoo, cream, or lotion prescribed by your doctor.
- Machine-wash *all* clothing and linen in hot water. Dry in the dryer's hot-air cycle. Iron the clothing and linen, if possible. Washing removes the lice, and ironing destroys nits.
- If you don't have a washing machine, iron the clothes and linen, or seal for 10 days in a plastic bag to kill lice and nits.
- Dry-clean non-washable items or seal in a plastic bag for 10 days.
- Boil articles such as combs, curlers, hairbrushes, and barrettes.
- Hair does not have to be shaved.

MEDICATION

Your doctor may prescribe anti-lice (pediculocide) cream, lotion, or shampoo. Apply creams or lotions to your child's infected body parts according to instructions. To use the shampoo:

- Wet the child's hair. Apply 1 tablespoon of shampoo. Lather for 4 minutes, working the lather well into the scalp.
- If shampoo gets in the child's eyes, wash out immediately with water.
- Rinse the child's hair thoroughly and towel dry. Don't use this towel again without laundering.
- Comb the child's hair with a fine comb dipped in hot vinegar to remove the lice. The comb must run through the hair repeatedly from the scalp outward until the hair is completely free of nits.
- A single application of shampoo is effective in more than 90% of cases. Don't use more frequently than recommended, because the shampoo may cause skin irritation or be absorbed into the body.
- If the lice infect eyelashes, they must be removed carefully by your doctor. The prescribed medications should *not* go into the eye or on the eyelashes. You may apply petroleum jelly to the child's eyelashes for 7 or 8 days after removal of the lice.

ACTIVITY

No restrictions.

DIET & FLUIDS

No special diet.

OK FOR SCHOOL, PRESCHOOL, OR NURSERY?

Yes, after treatment has been completed.

CALL YOUR DOCTOR IF

Your child, or anyone in your household, has symptoms of lice—or if symptoms recur after treatment.

LICHEN PLANUS

GENERAL INFORMATION

DESCRIPTION

Lichen planus is a chronic skin eruption that is not cancerous or contagious. The skin of the legs, trunk, arms, wrists, scalp, or penis may be involved, as well as the lining of the mouth or vagina or the toenails and fingernails (around or partially under the nailbed). Appropriate health care includes:

- Self-care after diagnosis.
- Doctor's treatment.

SIGNS & SYMPTOMS

- Small, slightly raised bumps that itch. The bumps are purplish with a whitish surface.
- An irregular whitish line inside the mouth or vagina.
- Sudden hair loss in patches on the child's head.

CAUSES

Unknown, but may be caused by a virus. In a few cases, lichen planus may be an adverse reaction to certain drugs.

RISK FACTORS

- Stress.
- Fatigue or overwork.

PREVENTING COMPLICATIONS OR RECURRENCE

Cannot be prevented at present.

WHAT TO EXPECT

MEDICAL TESTS

- Your own observation of symptoms.
- Medical history and physical exam by a doctor.
- Biopsy of questionable papules (raised bumps).

POSSIBLE COMPLICATIONS

None expected.

PROBABLE OUTCOME

Symptoms can be controlled with treatment, but the disorder lasts months or years. Urge your child to be patient and persist with the treatment, even if results are disappointing or slow.

TREATMENT

HOME CARE

Use cool-water soaks to relieve itching.

MEDICATION

- Your doctor may prescribe:
  —Antihistamines for their sedative effect to control itching.
  —Cortisone creams or ointments to reduce inflammation and decrease itching. Your child should use these only once or twice a day unless directed otherwise. Immediately after bathing is the best time to apply for better spreading and penetration. For the face and groin, your child should use only low-potency steroid products without fluorine.
  —Cortisone tablets for severe cases.
- See Medications section for information regarding medicines your doctor may prescribe.

ACTIVITY

No restrictions.

DIET & FLUIDS

No special diet.

OK FOR SCHOOL, PRESCHOOL, OR NURSERY?

When appetite returns and alertness, strength, and feeling of well-being will allow.

CALL YOUR DOCTOR IF

- Your child has symptoms of lichen planus.
- New, unexplained symptoms develop. Drugs used in treatment may produce side effects.

LIPOMAS

GENERAL INFORMATION

DESCRIPTION

Lipomas are benign tumors of fat cells. The trunk, neck, back, upper thighs, and arms are involved. These are common in both sexes from puberty to old age.

Appropriate health care includes:

- Doctor's treatment.
- Surgery to remove the lipoma (sometimes).

SIGNS & SYMPTOMS

Nodules under the skin with the following characteristics:

- Nodules are dome-shaped and about 2cm to 10cm in diameter. Some grow larger.
- Nodules feel "doughy," smooth, and easily movable.
- Only one—or many—lipomas may occur at one time.

CAUSES

Unknown, but the tendency is probably inherited. Minor injury may trigger growth.

RISK FACTORS

Family history of lipomas.

PREVENTING COMPLICATIONS OR RECURRENCE

Cannot be prevented at present. If your child is obese, losing weight helps reduce the size of lipomas.

WHAT TO EXPECT

MEDICAL TESTS

- Your own observation of symptoms.
- Medical history and physical exam by a doctor.

POSSIBLE COMPLICATIONS

Large lipomas may interfere with muscle function.

PROBABLE OUTCOME

These tumors are benign in children (but may be malignant in adults) and require no treatment, but they may be removed if they are unsightly or interfere with your child's muscle function. Surgical removal is usually done in a doctor's office.

TREATMENT

HOME CARE

After surgical removal of your child's lipoma:

- Apply rubbing alcohol to the scab twice a day.
- Apply an adhesive bandage to the scab during the day. Leave it uncovered at night.
- Wash the wound as usual. Dry gently and completely after the child bathes or swims.
- If the scab cracks or oozes, apply non-prescription antibiotic ointment several times a day.
- Return to your doctor for removal of the child's sutures in 5 to 10 days.

MEDICATION

- Medication usually is not necessary for this disorder.
- See Medications section for information regarding medicines your doctor may prescribe.

ACTIVITY

After surgical removal, your child can resume normal activities gradually. Allow 1 month for complete healing.

DIET & FLUIDS

No special diet.

OK FOR SCHOOL, PRESCHOOL, OR NURSERY?

When appetite returns and alertness, strength, and feeling of well-being will allow.

CALL YOUR DOCTOR IF

The following occurs after your child's surgery:

- Fever.
- Bleeding that does not respond to moderate pressure.
- Signs of infection (warmth, swelling, or redness) at the surgical site.

LIVER CANCER

GENERAL INFORMATION

DESCRIPTION

Liver cancer is the uncontrolled growth of malignant cells in the liver. Liver cancer may be primary—resulting from abnormal liver or bile-duct cells—or it may result from the spread of cancer from another site. The most common sources are cancers of the rectum, colon, lung, breast, pancreas, esophagus, or skin (malignant melanoma). The liver and bile ducts are involved.

Appropriate health care includes:

- Self-care after diagnosis.
- Doctor's treatment.
- Surgery to confirm the diagnosis.
- Radiation therapy.
- Liver transplant. These are available at a few medical centers in the U.S.

SIGNS & SYMPTOMS

- Loss of appetite and weight loss.
- Tender mass in the right upper abdomen.
- Pain in the upper abdomen.
- Low fever, usually less than 101F (38.3C).
- Yellow eyes and skin (sometimes).
- Swollen abdomen from fluid retention (sometimes).

CAUSES

Unknown.

RISK FACTORS

- Cirrhosis of the liver.
- Use of anabolic steroids.
- Excess alcohol consumption.
- Previous hepatitis B infection.

PREVENTING COMPLICATIONS OR RECURRENCE

No specific preventive measures.

WHAT TO EXPECT

MEDICAL TESTS

- Your own observation of symptoms.
- Medical history and physical exam by a doctor.
- Laboratory blood studies.
- CAT or CT scan (see Glossary).
- X-rays of the child's chest.

POSSIBLE COMPLICATIONS

- Sodium retention, leading to life-threatening fluid accumulation in the abdomen and lower body parts.
- Kidney failure.
- Death from loss of liver function.

PROBABLE OUTCOME

This condition is currently considered incurable and fatal within a short time. However, pain can be controlled. Treatment is usually attempted, although it is not likely to be successful. Scientific research into causes and treatment continues, so there is hope for increasingly effective treatment and cure for your child.

TREATMENT

HOME CARE

The only appropriate home care consists of keeping your child comfortable and maintaining as high a level of nutrition as possible, in consultation with your doctor.

MEDICATION

- Your doctor may prescribe:
  - —Anticancer drugs.
  - —Pain relievers.
- See Medications section for information regarding medicines your doctor may prescribe.

ACTIVITY

No restrictions. Your child should stay as active as strength allows.

DIET & FLUIDS

Low-salt diet (see Appendix 29).

OK FOR SCHOOL, PRESCHOOL, OR NURSERY?

When appetite returns and alertness, strength, and feeling of well-being will allow.

CALL YOUR DOCTOR IF

- Your child has symptoms of liver cancer, especially unexplained weight loss, low fever, or a mass in the abdomen.
- Your child develops a swollen abdomen during treatment.
- New, unexplained symptoms develop. Drugs used in treatment may produce side effects.

LUNG ABSCESS

GENERAL INFORMATION

DESCRIPTION

A lung abscess is an infected area of lung tissue, surrounded by lung inflammation. The infected lung tissue dies and is replaced with pus. The infection is not contagious from person to person. The lung and bronchial tubes are involved.

Appropriate health care includes:

- Physician's monitoring of general condition and medications.
- Surgery (sometimes) to aspirate pus from the abscess or to remove the abscess and part of the lung, if the abscess does not heal.
- Self-care during convalescence.

SIGNS & SYMPTOMS

- Cough with sputum. The sputum is puslike, is often blood-streaked, and sometimes smells bad.
- Bad breath.
- Sweating.
- Fever to 101F (38.3C) or higher.
- Chills.
- Weight loss.
- Chest pain (sometimes).

CAUSES

Usually a complication of pneumonia. A lung abscess sometimes occurs when an unconscious or sedated child inhales infected material from the upper-breathing passages. The patient may be unconscious from a head injury or an anesthetic (including dental anesthesia) or may be intoxicated from alcohol or heavily sedated. Lung abscesses are generally caused by virulent bacteria, such as klebsiella, pseudomonas; staphylococcus, or beta-hemolytic streptococcus.

RISK FACTORS

- Recent illness, especially pneumonia that has been slow to heal.
- Alcoholism.
- Recent general anesthesia or injury causing unconsciousness.

PREVENTING COMPLICATIONS OR RECURRENCE

- Obtain prompt medical treatment for your child's respiratory infections, especially pneumonia.
- Keep the child's teeth and mouth in good condition to prevent oral infections that could result in a lung abscess.

WHAT TO EXPECT

MEDICAL TESTS

- Your own observation of symptoms.
- Medical history and physical exam by a doctor.
- Laboratory blood tests and a culture of pus from the child's abscess to determine what antibiotic to use.
- X-rays of the lung.

POSSIBLE COMPLICATIONS

- Chronic abscess, leading to weight loss, anemia, bronchiectasis, or chronic lung disease, if the child's abscess does not respond well to antibiotic treatment.
- Rupture of the abscess, causing empyema or massive bleeding in the lung.
- Spread of infection to other body parts, especially the brain.

PROBABLE OUTCOME

Usually curable with prolonged antibiotic treatment (up to 6 months).

TREATMENT

HOME CARE

Instructions for your child:

- Don't smoke.
- Practice deep-breathing exercises as often as possible.
- Learn postural drainage to help rid the lung of bronchial secretions. Lie on the bed on your stomach with your head and chest hanging over the edge. Force yourself to cough. Continue until you cannot raise any more sputum. Practice this twice a day for 5 to 10 minutes.

MEDICATION

- Your doctor may prescribe antibiotics for prolonged periods to fight infection and prevent recurrence.
- See Medications section for information regarding medicines your doctor may prescribe.

ACTIVITY

No restrictions.

DIET & FLUIDS

No special diet. Encourage your child to increase fluid intake to at least 8 glasses a day. By drinking extra liquids, the body is forced to eliminate part of the fluid through the lungs. This makes thick lung secretions thinner, so they can be coughed up more easily.

OK FOR SCHOOL, PRESCHOOL, OR NURSERY?

Yes, but only when signs of infection have decreased, appetite returns, and alertness, strength, and feeling of well-being will allow.

CALL YOUR DOCTOR IF

- Your child has symptoms of a lung abscess.
- The following occurs during treatment:
  — Fever rises to 101F (38.3C) or higher.
  — Sputum thickens, despite treatment.
  — Postural drainage reveals a change in color, amount, or consistency of the sputum.
- Symptoms of a lung infection recur after treatment, especially a sputum-producing cough, fever, or general ill feeling.

LUPUS ERYTHEMATOSUS, DISCOID

GENERAL INFORMATION

DESCRIPTION

Discoid lupus erythematosus is a skin disorder. This is different from systemic lupus erythematosus, a connective-tissue disease that affects many different organs. About 1 in 20 persons with discoid lupus progresses to systemic lupus. Only the skin of the face, scalp, ears, neck, and arms is involved.

Appropriate health care includes:

- Self-care after diagnosis.
- Doctor's treatment.

SIGNS & SYMPTOMS

Plaques (red, raised skin lesions) with the following characteristics:

- Plaques are 1cm to 4cm in diameter and have clearly defined borders.
- They may appear anywhere on the child's face, but the cheeks and jawline are the most common sites. Some people describe them as "butterfly" lesions when two lesions of unequal size appear on both sides of the nose.
- Lesions sometimes appear on the child's scalp with localized patches of hair loss.
- Lesions scar as they heal.

CAUSES

Unknown, but probably an autoimmune disorder.

RISK FACTORS

Exposure to sunlight.

PREVENTING COMPLICATIONS OR RECURRENCE

No specific preventive measures. Protection from sunlight decreases the severity.

WHAT TO EXPECT

MEDICAL TESTS

- Your own observation of symptoms.
- Medical history and physical exam by a doctor.
- Laboratory blood studies and biopsy of your child's skin lesions to rule out systemic lupus erythematosus.

TREATMENT

HOME CARE

Instructions for your child:

- Don't go outdoors between 10 a.m. and 2 p.m., when the sun's ultraviolet light is strongest. If you can't avoid exposure to bright sunlight, wear protective clothing and maximum-protection sun-screen products. Avoid fluorescent lighting, if possible.
- See your doctor for regular checkups, even when in remission.

MEDICATION

- Your doctor may prescribe:
  —Injections of triamcinolone into lesions or hydroxychloroquine by mouth to shrink lesions.
  —Topical steroids (occasionally) to decrease redness of your child's lesions.
- See Medications section for information regarding medicines your doctor may prescribe.

ACTIVITY

No restrictions.

DIET & FLUIDS

No special diet.

OK FOR SCHOOL, PRESCHOOL, OR NURSERY?

When appetite returns and alertness, strength, and feeling of well-being will allow.

CALL YOUR DOCTOR IF

- Your child has symptoms of discoid lupus erythematosus.
- The following occurs during treatment:
  —Lesions on the child's hands.
  —Swelling, redness, pain in joints.

LUPUS ERYTHEMATOSUS, SYSTEMIC

GENERAL INFORMATION

DESCRIPTION

Systemic lupus erythematosus is an inflammatory disease of connective tissue. Lupus is not inherited or cancerous. The connective tissue (collagen) is involved. Many body systems are affected, including the joints, skin, kidneys, brain, heart, and lungs. Appropriate health care includes: self-care after diagnosis; doctor's treatment.

SIGNS & SYMPTOMS

Lupus symptoms frequently flare up and then subside. Episodes generally include fever and fatigue, plus any 4 of the following:

- Rash, usually on the cheeks.
- Ulcers in the child's mouth.
- Red palms and hands.
- Joint pain with redness, swelling, and tenderness—but no deformity.
- Swelling of the child's face and legs.
- Shortness of breath.
- Rapid or irregular heartbeat.
- Chest pain.
- Hair loss.
- Swelling of the lymph glands.
- Protein in the child's urine.
- Increased sensitivity to the sun.
- Anemia.
- Mental changes, including psychosis.

CAUSES

Unknown, but lupus is probably an autoimmune disorder. In an autoimmune disorder, the body's immune system functions abnormally and attacks its own normal tissue—usually connective tissue.

RISK FACTORS

- Stress.
- Use of drugs, such as hydralazine, procainamide, methyldopa, and chlorpromazine.
- Genetic factors. The incidence is higher among blacks.

PREVENTING COMPLICATIONS OR RECURRENCE

Cannot be prevented at present.

WHAT TO EXPECT

MEDICAL TESTS

- Your own observation of symptoms.
- Medical history and physical exam by a doctor. A child with vague, recurrent symptoms may require long-term observation before a final diagnosis can be made.
- Laboratory studies of antinuclear antibodies, blood count and sedimentation rate (see Glossary).

POSSIBLE COMPLICATIONS

- Bacterial or viral pneumonia.
- Impaired kidney function.
- Pericarditis.
- Seizures.
- Hypertension.

PROBABLE OUTCOME

Lupus is currently considered incurable. The disease is characterized by remissions and relapses. Life expectancy is reduced, but your child's symptoms can be relieved or controlled for many years. Medical literature cites instances of unexplained recovery. Scientific research into causes and treatment continues, so there is hope for increasingly effective treatment and cure.

TREATMENT

HOME CARE

- Obtain prompt medical treatment for any infection in your child.
- Your child should not take any immunizations or drugs without consulting the doctor. Immunizations and some drugs may cause relapses or worsen the child's current symptoms.
- A woman with lupus should not become pregnant without consulting the doctor. Pregnancy may overload the kidneys and cause death.

MEDICATION

Your doctor may prescribe immunosuppressive, steroid, and non-steroidal anti-inflammatory drugs or anti-malarial drugs. These relieve the child's symptoms but don't cure the disease.

ACTIVITY

Your child should remain as active as possible.

DIET & FLUIDS

If your child's kidneys or heart are affected, restrict salt intake. Otherwise, no special diet is necessary.

OK FOR SCHOOL, PRESCHOOL, OR NURSERY?

When appetite returns and alertness, strength, and feeling of well-being will allow.

CALL YOUR DOCTOR IF

- Your child has symptoms of systemic lupus erythematosus.
- Any of the following occurs after diagnosis: fever of 101F (38.3C) or higher; blood in the urine; shortness of breath; chest pain; bloody stool; severe abdominal pain; any illness with fever.

LYME DISEASE
(LD; Lyme Arthritis)

GENERAL INFORMATION

DESCRIPTION

Lyme disease is an inflammatory disorder characterized by a skin rash, followed in weeks to months by symptoms in the central nervous system (brain and spinal cord), cardiovascular system, and joints. This is named for Lyme, Connecticut, where it was first described. Body parts involved include the skin of the thighs, buttocks, or underarms; the central nervous system—including the brain, the coverings of the brain (meninges), and the spinal cord—and peripheral nerves; the heart and blood vessels; and any joint, especially in the neck and back.

Appropriate health care includes:

- Self-care after diagnosis during treatment and convalescence.
- Physician's monitoring of general condition and medications.

SIGNS & SYMPTOMS

First stage:

- A red papule (small, raised bump) on the skin of the thighs, buttocks, or armpits that grows as large as 5cm.

Later stages—any of the following:

- Muscle aches and pains.
- Fatigue.
- Chills and fever.
- Stiff neck with headache.
- Backache.
- Nausea and vomiting.
- Sore throat.
- Enlargement of the child's spleen and lymph glands.
- Migrating joint pain, eventually accompanied by redness and warmth.
- Enlarged heart and heart-rhythm disturbances.

CAUSES

Unknown, but evidence suggests it is transmitted by the bite of a tiny tick, ixodes dammini. Many children report a tick bite at the site of the skin lesion 3 days to 3 weeks prior to the skin rash.

RISK FACTORS

Areas where ticks are numerous.

PREVENTING COMPLICATIONS OR RECURRENCE

Your child should wear protective clothing and use insect repellents in areas with ticks.

WHAT TO EXPECT

MEDICAL TESTS

- Your own observation of symptoms.
- Medical history and physical exam by a doctor.
- Laboratory blood studies.

LYME DISEASE
(LD; Lyme Arthritis)

POSSIBLE COMPLICATIONS

- Congestive heart failure.
- Permanent joint deformity.
- Permanent brain damage.

PROBABLE OUTCOME

The skin rash is curable in some children in 10 days with treatment, and this may prevent development of other symptoms. If not, symptoms in the joints, central nervous system, and cardiovascular system usually subside slowly over 2 to 3 years. Symptoms often recur after several years—without another tick bite.

TREATMENT

HOME CARE

- Urge your child to use crutches to keep weight off affected joints, if necessary.
- Heat relieves joint pain. Encourage the child to take hot baths or use heating pads, heat lamps, or whirlpool treatments.

MEDICATION

Your doctor may prescribe:

- Penicillin or another antibiotic for at least 10 days, if a secondary bacterial infection develops in the affected skin.
- Non-steroidal anti-inflammatory drugs.
- Cortisone drugs to reduce the inflammatory response in the child's heart or central nervous system.
- See Medications section for information regarding medicines your doctor may prescribe.

ACTIVITY

Your child should rest in bed until symptoms of active inflammation subside. The child may read or watch TV and may resume normal activities gradually.

DIET & FLUIDS

No special diet.

OK FOR SCHOOL, PRESCHOOL, OR NURSERY?

Yes, but only when signs of infection have decreased, appetite returns, and alertness, strength, and feeling of well-being will allow.

CALL YOUR DOCTOR IF

- Your child has symptoms of Lyme disease.
- New, unexplained symptoms develop. Drugs used in treatment may produce side effects.

ILLNESSES

LYMPHOMA, NON-HODGKIN'S (Lymphosarcoma; Reticulum Cell Sarcoma)

GENERAL INFORMATION

DESCRIPTION

Non-Hodgkin's lymphoma is a malignant tumor of the lymph glands. This is more common than Hodgkin's disease. The lymphocytes (white blood cells), the lymph glands (glands which check infection and produce immune substances), and the spleen (a large lymph gland) are involved.

Appropriate health care includes:

- Physician's monitoring of general condition and medications.
- Hospitalization for short periods of treatment.
- Surgery to discover the extent of disease.
- Radiation therapy.
- Chemotherapy.

SIGNS & SYMPTOMS

- Swollen, non-tender, rubbery, distinct lymph glands anywhere in the child's body—but most commonly in the armpit, neck, or groin.
- Weight loss.
- General ill feeling.
- Anemia.
- Bleeding from the gastrointestinal tract.
- Jaundice (yellow skin and eyes).

CAUSES

Unknown, but research suggests a virus infection may be a factor.

RISK FACTORS

Family history of lymphoma.

PREVENTING COMPLICATIONS OR RECURRENCE

No specific preventive measures.

WHAT TO EXPECT

MEDICAL TESTS

- Your own observation of symptoms.
- Medical history and physical exam by a doctor.
- Laboratory studies of blood and bone marrow.
- Lymphangiogram (see Glossary).
- Biopsy (see Glossary) of lymph node.
- X-rays of various body parts that may be involved.
- CAT or CT scan (see Glossary).

POSSIBLE COMPLICATIONS

Spread of cancer to other parts of the body.

PROBABLE OUTCOME

Usually curable with radiation therapy and anti-cancer drugs. If cured, your child's life expectancy is normal. The potential for cure varies according to the cell type discovered from biopsy of the lymph node. Consult your doctor.

LYMPHOMA, NON-HODGKIN'S
(Lymphosarcoma; Reticulum Cell Sarcoma)

TREATMENT

HOME CARE

Try to remain optimistic about the treatment and chances for cure. A good mental attitude is a powerful ally to you and your child.

MEDICATION

- Your doctor may prescribe anti-cancer drugs. Medication may cause side effects or adverse reactions in some children. New symptoms may be caused by the medicine, by the original disorder, or by a new illness. Side effects caused by medicine usually disappear when the child's body adjusts to the drug or when the drug is discontinued.
- See Medications section for information regarding medicines your doctor may prescribe.

ACTIVITY

Your child should remain as active as strength allows.

DIET & FLUIDS

No special diet.

OK FOR SCHOOL, PRESCHOOL, OR NURSERY?

Yes, during remission and when appetite has returned and alertness, strength, and feeling of well-being will allow.

CALL YOUR DOCTOR IF

- Your child has symptoms of lymphoma.
- The following occurs during treatment:
  - — Fever.
  - — Signs of infection (redness, swelling, pain, or tenderness) anywhere in the body.
  - — Swelling of the feet and ankles.
  - — Discomfort when urinating or decreased urination in any 24-hour period.
- You think the medicine is causing your child's symptoms.

ILLNESSES

MALABSORPTION
(Malabsorptive Syndrome)

GENERAL INFORMATION

DESCRIPTION

Malabsorption means poor absorption of nutrients from the intestinal tract into the bloodstream. The intestinal tract, liver, and pancreas are involved.

Appropriate health care includes:

- Self-care after diagnosis.
- Physician's monitoring of general condition and medications.

SIGNS & SYMPTOMS

- Diarrhea.
- Weakness.
- Weight loss.
- Gas and vague abdominal discomfort.
- Bad-smelling, copious stools.
- Mild anemia (sometimes).

CAUSES

- Deficiency of intestinal enzymes.
- Inadequate digestion caused by disease of the pancreas (such as cystic fibrosis), gallbladder, or liver.
- Change in bacteria that normally live in your child's intestinal tract.
- Disease of the intestinal walls, including worms or parasites, tropical sprue, and celiac disease.
- Surgery that reduces the intestinal tract, decreasing the area for absorption.

RISK FACTORS

- Family history of malabsorption or cystic fibrosis.
- Use of drugs, such as mineral oil and other laxatives.
- Travel to foreign countries.
- Intestinal surgery.
- Excess alcohol consumption.

PREVENTING COMPLICATIONS OR RECURRENCE

- Your child should avoid prolonged dependence on mineral oil and other laxatives.
- Your child should avoid excess alcohol consumption.

WHAT TO EXPECT

MEDICAL TESTS

- Your own observation of symptoms.
- Medical history and physical exam by a doctor.
- Laboratory studies of stool, chromosomes, and blood.
- X-rays of the intestinal tract.
- Special studies that may include ultrasonography, CAT or CT scan, MRI, and radionuclide scan (see Glossary for all).

POSSIBLE COMPLICATIONS

- Prolonged illness.
- Failure to thrive in infants.
- Additional illness caused by nutritional, vitamin or mineral deficiency.

PROBABLE OUTCOME

The degree to which your child's symptoms can be controlled depends on the cause, but many things are common to all malabsorptive disorders. The onset is usually slow and difficult to diagnose. Disorders may be present for months or years before being recognized. Treatment is long and complicated and may need to be changed often. Patience and a positive attitude are important in effecting a cure.

TREATMENT

HOME CARE

Your child may need injections of vitamin B-12 and iron because neither is absorbed well with any malabsorptive disorder.

MEDICATION

Your doctor may prescribe:

- Enzymes to replace missing intestinal enzymes.
- Anti-spasmodics to reduce discomfort.
- See Medications section for information regarding medicines your doctor may prescribe.

ACTIVITY

No restrictions. Your child can resume normal activities as soon as symptoms improve.

DIET & FLUIDS

Your child will need a special diet, depending on the cause of the illness. Your doctor or nutritionist will provide specific information. For a milk-free diet for lactase deficiency, see Appendix 30.

OK FOR SCHOOL, PRESCHOOL, OR NURSERY?

Yes, when appetite has returned and alertness, strength, and feeling of well-being will allow.

CALL YOUR DOCTOR IF

Your child has symptoms of malabsorption or any of the following:

- Tarry bowel movements.
- Fever of 101F (38.3C) or higher.
- Severe abdominal pain.
- Muscle cramps.

MALARIA

GENERAL INFORMATION

DESCRIPTION

Malaria is an infection caused by a single-cell parasite, which is transmitted by the bite of an anopheles mosquito. Body parts involved include the blood cells, the blood vessels, the liver, and the central nervous system—including the brain, the coverings of the brain (meninges), and the spinal cord—and peripheral nerves.

Appropriate health care includes:
- Self-care after diagnosis.
- Physician's monitoring of general condition and medications.
- Hospitalization (severe cases).

SIGNS & SYMPTOMS

The first episode of the following symptoms usually occurs about 8 to 30 days after the mosquito bite:
- Headache.
- Fatigue.
- Nausea.
- Hard, shaking chills with fever for 12 to 24 hours.
- Rapid breathing.
- Heavy sweating, accompanied by a drop in the child's body temperature.

Episodes may recur every 2 or 3 days until the disease is treated. Without treatment, the disease can continue for years.

CAUSES

- There are 4 types of malarial parasites; they are transferred from person to person by a mosquito bite. The mosquito becomes infected with malaria after biting a person with the disease. The organisms multiply in the mosquito, then enter the bloodstream of the next person the mosquito bites.
- Once in a person's bloodstream, the parasites travel to the liver, where they thrive and multiply rapidly. After several days, thousands re-enter the bloodstream and destroy red-blood cells. Some parasites remain in the liver, continue to multiply, and are released again at intervals into the bloodstream.

RISK FACTORS

- Crowded or unsanitary living conditions.
- Hot, humid climates.
- Geographic locations, such as Latin America, Asia, and Africa. Malaria is uncommon in the U.S., but it often affects travelers or military personnel and their families stationed in foreign countries.

PREVENTING COMPLICATIONS OR RECURRENCE

- Urge your child to take anti-malaria drugs before visiting an area where malaria is prevalent and to continue to take the drugs after returning. The public health department or your doctor can give you instructions.
- If you live in a mosquito-infected area, destroy mosquito breeding areas, install window screens and mosquito nets over beds, and use insect repellents.

? WHAT TO EXPECT

MEDICAL TESTS

- Your own observation of symptoms.
- Medical history and physical exam by a doctor. Tell your doctor of your child's recent travel.
- Laboratory studies, such as studies of blood smears to identify the parasite.

POSSIBLE COMPLICATIONS

- Anemia caused by blood-cell destruction.
- Clumping of blood cells, which may cause brain or kidney damage.

PROBABLE OUTCOME

Usually curable in 2 weeks with treatment. Malaria can be fatal without treatment in children (or adults) who don't receive adequate nourishment or have low resistance to disease.

TREATMENT

HOME CARE

- Protect your child from secondary bacterial infection while ill with malaria. Urge your child to wash hands and bathe often.
- Make your environment mosquito-free so the infection cannot be transmitted to others. See PREVENTING COMPLICATIONS OR RECURRENCE.

MEDICATION

- Your doctor may prescribe anti-malaria drugs to kill the parasite.
- See Medications section for information regarding medicines your doctor may prescribe.

ACTIVITY

Your child should rest in bed until fever and chills subside and can then resume normal activities gradually as symptoms improve.

DIET & FLUIDS

No special diet. Give vitamin and mineral supplements until your child recovers.

OK FOR SCHOOL, PRESCHOOL, OR NURSERY?

Only when signs of infection have decreased, appetite returns, and alertness, strength, and feeling of well-being will allow.

CALL YOUR DOCTOR IF

- Your child has symptoms of malaria.
- Your child is weak for a prolonged time after an attack. This may indicate anemia.
- Symptoms of malaria recur after treatment.
- New, unexplained symptoms develop. Drugs used in treatment may produce side effects.

MEASLES
(Red Measles; Rubeola)

GENERAL INFORMATION

DESCRIPTION

Red measles is a serious virus illness that infects the respiratory tract and skin. This is one of the most contagious diseases known. The skin, eyes, and upper-respiratory tract are involved. Red measles affects all ages but is most common in children.

Appropriate health care includes:

- Home care after diagnosis.
- Physician's monitoring of general condition and medications.

SIGNS & SYMPTOMS

Measles symptoms usually occur in the following sequence:

- Temperature of 102F (38.9C) or higher.
- Fatigue.
- Loss of appetite.
- Sneezing and runny nose.
- Harsh, hacking cough.
- Red eyes and sensitivity to light.
- Koplik spots (tiny white spots) in the child's mouth and throat.
- Reddish rash on the child's forehead and around the ears that spreads to the body.

CAUSES

Measles is caused by a rubeola-virus infection that chiefly affects your child's skin and respiratory tract. The incubation period after exposure is 7 to 14 days.

RISK FACTORS

- Crowded or unsanitary living conditions.
- Population groups that are not immunized.
- Measles epidemics. The disease becomes more virulent as it spreads.

PREVENTING COMPLICATIONS OR RECURRENCE

- Immunize your child against measles. See Appendix 1 for the recommended schedule.
- If your child has not been immunized against measles and is exposed to it, a gamma globulin (antibodies) injection may prevent or reduce the severity of the disease.

? WHAT TO EXPECT

MEDICAL TESTS

- Your own observation of symptoms.
- Medical history and physical exam by a doctor.
- Blood counts by the laboratory (sometimes).

POSSIBLE COMPLICATIONS

- Pneumonia.
- Encephalitis or meningitis.

MEASLES (Red Measles; Rubeola)

PROBABLE OUTCOME

• A child who has been immunized against measles or has had the disease will probably never develop it.
• A child who has been passively immunized with gamma globulin is protected against measles for about 3 months.

TREATMENT

HOME CARE

• Urge your child not to read books or watch TV during the first days when the eyes are sensitive to light.
• Use a cool-mist humidifier to soothe the child's cough and to thin lung secretions so they can be coughed up more easily.
• Take morning and evening temperatures; keep a record. If the child's fever is 103F (39.4C) or higher, reduce it. See Appendix 17, How to Reduce Your Child's Fever.

MEDICATION

• Your doctor will not prescribe antibiotics for measles, which is a virus. However, if complications arise, such as pneumonia or a middle-ear infection, antibiotics may be necessary.
• Don't give aspirin to a child younger than 16. Use acetaminophen instead to relieve discomfort and reduce fever. Some research shows a link between the use of aspirin in children during a virus illness and the development of Reye's syndrome.

ACTIVITY

Encourage your child to rest—but don't force it—until the fever and rash disappear. Light activities are acceptable once the eyes are not painful. The child should not return to school until 7 to 10 days after the fever and rash disappear.

DIET & FLUIDS

No special diet. Your child should drink extra fluids, including water, tea, lemonade, cola, and fruit juice. Maintaining an adequate fluid intake is very important in keeping lung secretions thin and preventing lung complications.

OK FOR SCHOOL, PRESCHOOL, OR NURSERY?

Not until signs of infection have faded and when appetite has returned and alertness, strength, and feeling of well-being will allow.

CALL YOUR DOCTOR IF

• Your child has symptoms of measles.
• The following occurs during treatment: temperature above 103F (39.4C), accompanied by a sore throat; severe headache; earache; convulsion; excessive lethargy or drowsiness; breathing rate above 35 breaths-per-minute, or breathing difficulty; blue, gray or purple lips or nails; thick, discolored nasal discharge or sputum; cough that persists longer than 4 or 5 days.

MEASLES, GERMAN (Rubella)

GENERAL INFORMATION

DESCRIPTION

German measles is usually a mild, contagious virus illness. However, German measles is likely to cause serious birth defects to the unborn baby of a pregnant woman who develops the disease in the first 3 or 4 months of pregnancy. The skin and the lymph glands behind the ears and in the neck are involved.

Appropriate health care includes:

- Self-care.
- Physician's monitoring of general condition and medications.

SIGNS & SYMPTOMS

- Fever.
- Muscle aches and stiffness, especially in your child's neck.
- Fatigue.
- Headache.
- Reddish rash on the child's head and body after the 2nd or 3rd day. The rash lasts 1 or 2 days.
- Swollen lymph glands, especially behind the child's ears and at the back and sides of the neck.
- Joint pain (adolescents and adults).

CAUSES

RNA virus spread by person-to-person contact. Patients are contagious from 1 week before the rash appears until 1 week after it fades.

RISK FACTORS

Springtime weather when epidemics are common.

PREVENTING COMPLICATIONS OR RECURRENCE

- Your child should be immunized against German measles at approximately 15 months of age.
- Non-pregnant females of childbearing age should be immunized if they have not had German measles or been immunized. Pregnancy should be prevented for 3 months following immunization. (If you don't know whether or not you have had German measles, your doctor or local health department can determine it from a blood test.)
- A child should *not* be immunized if the child has an altered autoimmune system (as with cancer) or if the child currently takes cortisone or anti-cancer drugs or is receiving radiation therapy or has an illness with fever.
- Delay vaccinating a child whose mother is pregnant. The virus could pass to the mother and expose her.

MEASLES, GERMAN (Rubella)

? WHAT TO EXPECT

MEDICAL TESTS

Your own observation of symptoms; medical history and physical exam by a doctor; laboratory blood studies.

POSSIBLE COMPLICATIONS

Miscarriage or catastrophic birth defects; encephalitis; thrombocytopenia; agranulocytosis.

PROBABLE OUTCOME

Spontaneous recovery in 1 week in children (longer in adults). Symptoms are usually quite mild.

TREATMENT

HOME CARE

Contact any pregnant woman who has been exposed. Exposure includes contact with the infected child (or adult) 1 week prior to, during, or 1 week after the infection. This woman should consult her obstetrician immediately.

MEDICATION

For minor discomfort, use non-prescription drugs such as acetaminophen. Don't give aspirin to a child younger than 16. Some research shows a link between the use of aspirin in children during a virus illness and the development of Reye's syndrome (a type of encephalitis).

ACTIVITY

Your child should stay in bed until the fever disappears, then limit activities until the day after the rash disappears. The child can resume normal activity gradually as strength allows. Don't expose your child to others until 1 week after the rash disappears.

DIET & FLUIDS

No special diet.

OK FOR SCHOOL, PRESCHOOL, OR NURSERY?

Not until signs infection have decreased, appetite returns, and alertness, strength, and feeling of well-being will allow.

CALL YOUR DOCTOR IF

- Your child has symptoms of German measles.
- The following occurs during treatment:
  - — Fever of 103F (39.4C) or higher.
  - — Red eyes.
  - — Cough or shortness of breath.
  - — Severe headache, drowsiness, lethargy or convulsion.
- Unusual bleeding occurs 1 to 4 weeks after the illness (bleeding gums, nose or uterus, or scattered blood specks on the skin).

MENINGITIS, ASEPTIC
(Non-Bacterial Meningitis)

GENERAL INFORMATION

DESCRIPTION

Aseptic meningitis is inflammation of the meninges (thin membranes that cover the brain and spinal cord). This is contagious. The brain and spinal cord are involved.

Appropriate health care includes:
- Physician's monitoring of general condition and medications.
- Hospitalization, except in mild cases.
- Home care after hospitalization.

SIGNS & SYMPTOMS

- Fever.
- Headache.
- Irritability.
- Eyes that are sensitive to light.
- Stiff neck.
- Vomiting.
- Confusion, lethargy, and drowsiness.

CAUSES

- Viruses of several types, including the polio virus.
- Fungi, including yeasts.
- A reaction—probably an autoimmune response—following various viral illnesses, such as measles.

RISK FACTORS

- Recent measles, German measles, or various types of flu.
- Immunosuppressive treatment, such as for cancer or following an organ transplant.
- Poor nutrition.
- Recent illness that has lowered resistance.
- Meningitis epidemics. The disease becomes more virulent as it spreads from person to person.

PREVENTING COMPLICATIONS OR RECURRENCE

Keep your child's immunizations up to date against all viruses for which vaccines are available. See Appendix 1 for an immunization schedule.

WHAT TO EXPECT

MEDICAL TESTS

- Your own observation of symptoms.
- Medical history and physical exam by a doctor.
- Laboratory studies, such as blood-cell counts and examination of the cerebrospinal fluid.

POSSIBLE COMPLICATIONS

- Permanent brain damage (rare).
- Muscle impairment or paralysis (if caused by poliomyelitis).

PROBABLE OUTCOME

Most children recover fully from viral meningitis without specific therapy—unlike bacterial meningitis, in which antibiotics may be life-saving.

TREATMENT

HOME CARE

No special instructions except those listed under other headings.

MEDICATION

- If your child's aseptic meningitis is caused by a virus, there is no medication for it. The body defenses will usually cure it (although a polio virus may leave permanent damage).
- If your child's meningitis is caused by a fungus, your doctor may prescribe anti-fungal drugs, such as amphoterecin B.
- See Medications section for information regarding medicines your doctor may prescribe.

ACTIVITY

Your child should rest in bed in a darkened room and then resume normal activities as soon as symptoms improve.

DIET & FLUIDS

No special diet. Encourage drinking 6 to 8 glasses of fluid daily, even if your child doesn't feel like it.

OK FOR SCHOOL, PRESCHOOL, OR NURSERY?

When signs of infection have decreased, appetite returns, and alertness, strength, and feeling of well-being will allow.

CALL YOUR DOCTOR IF

- Your child has symptoms of aseptic meningitis.
- New, unexplained symptoms develop. Drugs used in treatment may produce side effects.

MENINGITIS, BACTERIAL (Spinal Meningitis)

GENERAL INFORMATION

DESCRIPTION

Bacterial meningitis is a bacterial infection or inflammation of the meninges (thin membranes that cover the brain and spinal cord). The central nervous system—including the brain, the coverings to the brain (meninges), and the spinal cord—and peripheral nerves are involved. Bacterial meningitis can affect all ages but is more severe in children under age 2.

Appropriate health care includes:

- Physician's monitoring of general condition and medications.
- Hospitalization.
- Self-care after hospitalization.

SIGNS & SYMPTOMS

- Fever, chills, and sweating (may be absent in acritically ill child).
- Headache.
- Irritability.
- Eyes sensitive to light; pupils may be different sizes.
- Stiff neck.
- Vomiting.
- Red or purple skin rash.
- Confusion, lethargy, drowsiness, or unconsciousness.
- Sore throat or other signs of respiratory illness may precede other symptoms.

CAUSES

Infection caused by bacteria, from the following sources:

- Infection in another body part, such as the lung, ear, or sinus, that spreads to the meninges.
- Head injury, such as a fractured skull, that allows infection to enter.

RISK FACTORS

- Infancy.
- Illness that has lowered resistance.
- Poor nutrition.
- Use of drugs that decrease the body's immune responses, such as anti-cancer drugs.

PREVENTING COMPLICATIONS OR RECURRENCE

- Consult your doctor for treatment of any infection in your child's body to prevent its spread.
- Urge your child to avoid contact with anyone who has meningitis. Those who have had close contact with a person with meningitis may need preventive antibiotic treatment even if they have no symptoms.

MENINGITIS, BACTERIAL
(Spinal Meningitis)

? WHAT TO EXPECT

MEDICAL TESTS

- Your own observation of symptoms.
- Medical history and physical exam by a doctor.
- Laboratory studies, such as blood-sugar tests and cultures of the throat, blood, nose, or other infection sites.
- Lumbar puncture (see Glossary).

POSSIBLE COMPLICATIONS

Death or permanent brain damage—including paralysis, hearing loss, speech difficulty, and intellectual impairment—if not treated quickly.

PROBABLE OUTCOME

Full recovery is likely in 2 to 3 weeks with treatment, if no complications arise.

TREATMENT

HOME CARE

Restrict your child's visitors until the doctor determines the disease is no longer contagious.

MEDICATION

- Your doctor may prescribe antibiotics, depending on what bacteria is causing the child's meningitis.
- See Medications section for information regarding medicines your doctor may prescribe.

ACTIVITY

While in the hospital, your child will need bed rest in a darkened room. After a 2- to 3-week recovery, the child should be as active as strength allows.

DIET & FLUIDS

Your child may be given intravenous nutrients in the hospital. At home, serve the child a normal, well-balanced diet. Vitamin and mineral supplements should not be necessary unless your child has a deficiency or cannot eat normally.

OK FOR SCHOOL, PRESCHOOL, OR NURSERY?

When signs of infection have decreased, appetite returns, and alertness, strength, and feeling of well-being will allow.

CALL YOUR DOCTOR IF

- Your child has symptoms of bacterial meningitis.
- Temperature rises to 101F (38.3C) or higher during treatment.
- New, unexplained symptoms develop. Drugs used in treatment may produce side effects.
- Your child has had contact with someone who has meningitis.

MOLLUSCUM CONTAGIOSUM

GENERAL INFORMATION

DESCRIPTION

Molluscum contagiosum is a contagious virus infection of the skin anywhere on the body. The virus usually occurs on the face in children. In older adolescents and adults, it usually occurs on the inner thighs, abdomen, and genitals.

Appropriate health care includes:

- Doctor's treatment to remove the papules with liquid nitrogen or currette.
- Self-care after removal.

SIGNS & SYMPTOMS

Papules (small, raised bumps on the child's skin) with the following characteristics:

- Bumps are firm, smooth, domed, and skin-colored or white. The overlying skin is transparent and thin.
- Bumps are usually 2mm to 3mm in diameter. A few may be as large as 10mm.
- Bumps cause eye irritation if they are on the child's eyelids.
- Bumps don't hurt or itch.

CAUSES

DNA virus of the pox group. This virus may be transmitted sexually. The incubation is 2 weeks to 6 months.

RISK FACTORS

- The child's previous allergies or a family history of allergy.
- Use of immunosuppressive drugs.

PREVENTING COMPLICATIONS OR RECURRENCE

To prevent spread to other parts of the body or to other people, urge your child not to scratch bumps.

WHAT TO EXPECT

MEDICAL TESTS

- Your own observation of symptoms.
- Medical history and physical exam by a doctor.

POSSIBLE COMPLICATIONS

Scarring or disfigurement.

PROBABLE OUTCOME

If untreated, a few of your child's papules may increase to 20 to 50 lesions in several weeks. They will disappear spontaneously in 10 to 24 months. However, they should be treated to prevent their spread to others.

TREATMENT

HOME CARE

- After treatment with liquid nitrogen, leave the child's blisters alone. The tops will come off spontaneously in 7 to 14 days.
- Keep the child's blisters dry. Cover with small adhesive bandages any that may be irritated by clothing.

MEDICATION

- Medicine usually is not necessary for this disorder. In some cases, your doctor may prescribe cantharidin (Cantherone) to apply topically to kill the virus.
- See Medications section for information regarding medicines your doctor may prescribe.

ACTIVITY

No restrictions, except to avoid sexual relations until bumps disappear.

DIET & FLUIDS

No special diet.

OK FOR SCHOOL, PRESCHOOL, OR NURSERY?

Yes.

CALL YOUR DOCTOR IF

- Your child has symptoms of molluscum contagiosum.
- The following occurs after treatment:
  - — Fever.
  - — Signs of infection (swelling, redness, pain, tenderness, or warmth) at the treatment site.

MONONUCLEOSIS, INFECTIOUS (Mono; "Kissing Disease")

GENERAL INFORMATION

DESCRIPTION

Infectious mononucleosis is an infectious viral disease that affects the respiratory system, liver, and lymphatic system. The lymph nodes, liver, spleen, throat, and bronchial tubes are involved. Infectious mononucleosis is most common in adolescents.

Appropriate health care includes:

- Self-care after diagnosis.
- Physician's monitoring of general condition and medications.
- Hospitalization (rare).

SIGNS & SYMPTOMS

- Fever.
- Sore throat (sometimes severe).
- Loss of appetite.
- Fatigue.
- Swollen lymph glands, usually in the child's neck, underarms, or groin.
- Enlarged spleen.
- Enlarged liver.
- Jaundice with yellow skin and eyes (sometimes).
- Headache.
- General aching.

CAUSES

A contagious virus (Epstein-Barr virus) transmitted from person to person by close contact, such as kissing, shared food, or coughing.

RISK FACTORS

- Stress.
- Illness that has lowered your child's resistance.
- Fatigue or overwork. The high incidence among college students and military recruits may result from inadequate rest and crowded living conditions.

PREVENTING COMPLICATIONS OR RECURRENCE

- Your child should avoid contact with persons having infectious mononucleosis.
- Vaccine (possibly). This is still in the experimental stages.

WHAT TO EXPECT

MEDICAL TESTS

Your own observation of symptoms; medical history and physical exam by a doctor; laboratory blood tests.

POSSIBLE COMPLICATIONS

- Meningitis or encephalitis (rare).
- Misdiagnosis as streptococcal sore throat, resulting in useless, unnecessary treatment with antibiotics.
- Ruptured spleen, resulting in surgery.

MONONUCLEOSIS, INFECTIOUS
(Mono; "Kissing Disease")

PROBABLE OUTCOME

Spontaneous recovery in 10 days to 6 months. The child's fatigue frequently persists for 3 to 6 weeks after other symptoms disappear.

TREATMENT

HOME CARE

- To relieve the sore throat, the child should gargle frequently with double-strength tea or warm salt water (1 teaspoon of salt to 8 oz. of water).
- Your child should not strain hard for bowel movements. This may injure an enlarged spleen.

MEDICATION

- For minor discomfort, use non-prescription drugs such as acetaminophen. Your child should not take aspirin because of its suspected association with Reye's syndrome.
- If symptoms are severe, your doctor may prescribe a short course of cortisone drugs. It is not safe to use cortisone drugs if your child has any of the following: a positive tuberculin skin test or history of tuberculosis, a viral eye infection, a chronic bacterial infection, diabetes, high blood pressure, diverticulitis, thrombophlebitis, or chronic kidney disease. It is also not safe to use cortisone drugs during pregnancy.

ACTIVITY

Instructions for your child:

- Rest in bed, especially when you have fever. Resume activity gradually. Rest when you are fatigued.
- Don't participate in contact sports until at least 1 month after complete recovery.

DIET & FLUIDS

No special diet. Your child may not feel like eating while ill. Maintaining an adequate fluid intake is important. Encourage the child to drink at least 8 glasses of water or juice a day—more during periods of high fever.

OK FOR SCHOOL, PRESCHOOL, OR NURSERY?

When signs of infection have decreased, appetite returns, and alertness, strength, and feeling of well-being will allow.

CALL YOUR DOCTOR IF

- Your child has symptoms of infectious mononucleosis.
- The following occurs during treatment:
  - — Fever over 102F (38.9C).
  - — Constipation, which may cause straining.
  - — Severe pain in the upper left abdomen that lasts for 5 minutes or more.
  - — Swallowing or breathing difficulty from severe throat inflammation.

MOTION SICKNESS

GENERAL INFORMATION

DESCRIPTION

Motion sickness is an unpleasant, temporary disturbance that occurs while traveling. It is characterized by dizziness and stomach upset. The semicircular canals in the inner ear are involved. These fluid-filled canals maintain balance.

Appropriate health care includes:

- Self-care.
- Physician's monitoring of general condition, and medications, and treatment, if your child has a chronic illness that may be worsened by vomiting.
- Psychotherapy or counseling, if your family's lifestyle requires travel and your child usually develops motion sickness.

SIGNS & SYMPTOMS

- Loss of appetite.
- Nausea and vomiting.
- Spinning sensation.
- Weakness and unsteadiness.

CAUSES

Travel by any means, especially airplane, boat, or car. Irregular motion causes fluid changes in the semicircular canals of your child's inner ear, which transmit signals to the brain's vomiting center.

RISK FACTORS

- Stress.
- Ear disorders.
- Smoky environment or poor ventilation.
- Excess alcohol consumption.

PREVENTING COMPLICATIONS OR RECURRENCE

Instructions for your child:

- Don't eat large meals or drink alcohol before and during travel.
- Sit in areas of the airplane or boat with the least motion.
- Recline in your seat, if possible.
- Breathe slowly and deeply.
- Avoid areas where others are smoking, if possible.
- On an airplane or bus, turn on the overhead air vent to improve air circulation.
- Take medication to prevent motion sickness ½ hour before you travel.

Some airlines have developed behavior-modification techniques for those who are afraid to fly or have motion sickness. Contact the airline or your travel agent for information.

WHAT TO EXPECT

MEDICAL TESTS

- Your own observation of symptoms.
- Medical history and physical exam by a doctor if motion sickness is recurrent and interferes with your child's life.

POSSIBLE COMPLICATIONS

- Dehydration from vomiting.
- Falls and injuries from unsteadiness.

PROBABLE OUTCOME

Spontaneous recovery when the trip is over.

TREATMENT

HOME CARE

Psychological factors contribute to motion sickness. Try to resolve your child's concerns about travel before leaving home. Maintain a positive attitude.

MEDICATION

- For minor discomfort, use non-prescription drugs, such as dimenhydrinate (Dramamine), before and during travel.
- Your doctor may prescribe scopolamine to control symptoms.
- See Medications section for information regarding medicines your doctor may prescribe.

ACTIVITY

To minimize symptoms during travel, urge your child to rest in a reclining position and gaze at a distant object.

DIET & FLUIDS

Your child should eat lightly or not at all before and during brief trips. For longer trips, encourage frequent sipping on beverages—not large drinks—to maintain fluid intake.

OK FOR SCHOOL, PRESCHOOL, OR NURSERY?

Yes.

CALL YOUR DOCTOR IF

You plan to travel and your child has had disabling motion sickness in the past.

MUMPS

GENERAL INFORMATION

DESCRIPTION

Mumps is a mild, contagious viral disease that causes painful swelling of the salivary glands. The parotid glands (salivary glands that lie between the ear and jaw) are involved. Other organs, including the testicles, ovaries, pancreas, breasts, brain, and meninges (membranes that cover the brain), sometimes become involved. Mumps is most common in children (2 to 12 years), but approximately 10% of adults are susceptible to mumps.

Appropriate health care includes:

- Home care after diagnosis.
- Doctor's examination to confirm the diagnosis and treat complications, if any occur.

SIGNS & SYMPTOMS

Mumps without complications:

- Inflammation, swelling, and pain of the parotid glands. The child's glands feel firm, and pain increases with chewing or swallowing.
- Fever.
- Headache.
- Sore throat.

Additional symptoms with complications:

- Painful, swollen testicles.
- Abdominal pain, if the ovaries or pancreas are involved.
- Severe headache, if the brain or meninges are involved.

CAUSES

Person-to-person transmission of the mumps virus. The virus can be transmitted anytime from 48 hours before symptoms begin to 6 days after symptoms appear. Virus incubation is 14 to 24 days after contact; the average is 18 days.

RISK FACTORS

Crowded living conditions.

PREVENTING COMPLICATIONS OR RECURRENCE

- Obtain mumps immunizations for your child at the appropriate age. For an immunization schedule, see Appendix 1.
- If your child has not had mumps or been vaccinated, and a close family member has mumps, your doctor may suggest an anti-mumps globulin. The infection *may* prevent the disease—it is not guaranteed—and it is expensive.

WHAT TO EXPECT

MEDICAL TESTS

- Your own observation of symptoms.
- Medical history and physical exam by a doctor.

POSSIBLE COMPLICATIONS

Infections of the child's brain or meninges (meningo-encephalitis), pancreas, ovaries, breasts, or testicles. Sterility may occur if both testicles become infected (rare).

PROBABLE OUTCOME

Spontaneous recovery in about 10 days if no complications occur. After having the disease, a person has lifetime immunity to mumps.

TREATMENT

HOME CARE

- It is not necessary to isolate the infected child from the family. By the time symptoms appear, the disease has usually already spread.
- Apply heat or ice—whichever feels better—intermittently to the swollen, painful glands (parotid or testicles). Use a hot-water bottle, hot towel, or ice pack.

MEDICATION

Once the disease begins, it must run its natural course. There is no safe, readily available medicine that can kill the virus or keep it from multiplying.

- For minor pain, use non-prescription drugs such as acetaminophen. Don't use aspirin. Aspirin, when taken by children with virus infections, increases the risk of developing Reye's syndrome.
- Your doctor may prescribe: stronger pain relievers; cortisone drugs, if testicles are involved.

ACTIVITY

Bed rest is not essential and does not reduce the possibility of complications. Allow as much activity as your child's strength and feeling of well-being allow. The child is no longer contagious when swelling disappears.

DIET & FLUIDS

No special diet, but your child should increase daily fluid intake to at least 6 to 8 glasses of liquid, including ginger ale, cola, tea, or water. Fruit juices or tart beverages may increase pain.

OK FOR SCHOOL, PRESCHOOL, OR NURSERY?

When signs of infection have decreased, appetite returns, and alertness, strength, and feeling of well-being will allow.

CALL YOUR DOCTOR IF

- Your child's fever (oral) rises above 101F (38.3C).
- The following occurs during the child's illness:
  - — Vomiting or abdominal pain.
  - — Severe headache that is not relieved by acetaminophen.
  - — Drowsiness or inability to stay awake.
  - — Swelling or pain in the testicle.
  - — Twitching of the face muscles.
  - — Convulsion.
  - — Discomfort or redness in the eyes.

MUSCLE CRAMPS

GENERAL INFORMATION

DESCRIPTION

Muscle cramps are painful involuntary contractions of muscles in swimmers and others caused by abnormalities of the nervous system or exercise-related changes in muscle-cell chemistry. Appropriate health care includes physical therapy, including warm soaks, applications of ice or heat, whirlpool, or gentle massage that may help with residual pain and soreness in a child's cramped muscles.

SIGNS & SYMPTOMS

Painful, involuntary contraction of muscles, usually in the child's leg. Swimming, more than other sports, causes leg cramps in athletes during exercise.

CAUSES

- Vigorous physical activity.
- Inadequate warm-up before engaging in strenuous physical activity.
- In swimmers, the cause of leg cramps is frequently unknown, and their presence does not suggest an underlying disorder.

RISK FACTORS

- Calcium deficiency.
- Nerve disorders, such as pressure on nerve roots near the child's spinal cord, or abnormalities of nerve fibers after they leave the spinal cord.
- Enzyme deficiency (temporary).
- Diabetes, alcoholism, chronic kidney disease, a variety of medications, Buerger's disease, all of which can cause damage to a child's peripheral nerves and thereby cause muscle cramps.

PREVENTING COMPLICATIONS OR RECURRENCE

Instructions for your child:

- Undertake a slow, thorough conditioning program prior to beginning vigorous physical activity, including swimming.
- Consult your doctor if you take any medicine and develop cramps. Discontinuing or modifying the dosage may prevent recurrent cramps.
- If you have an enzyme deficiency, there is no treatment except to reduce sports activities below the level that produces cramps.
- Don't smoke. Avoid polluted air while exercising. Both may decrease oxygen flow to muscles. Oxygen is needed in the muscles to avoid cramps.

? WHAT TO EXPECT

MEDICAL TESTS

- Your own observation of symptoms.
- Medical history and physical exam by a doctor.
- Blood studies (sometimes) to measure the child's enzyme levels.

POSSIBLE COMPLICATIONS

- Permanent muscle contractures (rare).
- Permanently weakened muscle groups (rare).
- Fear of recurrence, resulting in unwarranted abandonment of the child's exercise program.

PROBABLE OUTCOME

Can be controlled by treating any underlying medical disorder, using medication (carbamazepine), and undertaking a better conditioning program.

TREATMENT

HOME CARE

Instructions for your child:

- Stretch and rub the cramping muscles.
- Voluntarily contract the muscles that directly oppose those that are cramping. For example, if cramps affect the calf of the leg, force the front of the foot upward toward the knee and hold it until the cramp is diminished.

MEDICATION

Your doctor may prescribe the following medications:

- Carbamazepine for muscle cramps due to nerve damage.
- Aspirin or acetaminophen for pain following a muscle cramp.

ACTIVITY

Your child should decrease or discontinue vigorous physical activity until the muscle cramp relaxes.

DIET & FLUIDS

- If your child has frequent muscle cramps from any cause, provide foods high in potassium, such as dried apricots, whole-grain cereal (hot or cold), dried lentils, dried peaches, bananas, peanuts, citrus fruits, or fresh vegetables.
- Following a diet high in complex carbohydrates makes good nutritional sense to all those hoping to maintain or reach a good level of health and fitness. However, your child should not eat such a meal within 3 to 5 hours before competition, and should eat only lightly directly afterwards.
- Make sure you provide sufficient calcium in the child's diet through the use of dairy products or calcium supplements.

OK FOR SCHOOL, PRESCHOOL, OR NURSERY?

Yes, when condition and sense of well-being will allow.

CALL YOUR DOCTOR IF

- Your child has persistent or recurrent muscle cramps despite following the suggestions above.
- Your child develops new symptoms after starting any prescribed medicine. All effective medicines have potentially undesirable side effects. These can frequently be controlled by modifying the dosage.

MUSCLE, PULLED OR TORN

GENERAL INFORMATION

DESCRIPTION

Pulled or torn muscles are stretched or torn muscle fibers. Muscles attached to bones anywhere in the body are involved.

Appropriate health care includes:

- Self-care after diagnosis.
- Physician's monitoring of general condition and medications for severe injuries or if self-care is not successful.
- Rehabilitation and treatment by a physical therapist or athletic trainer.
- Completely torn muscles may require surgery.

SIGNS & SYMPTOMS

- Pain or tenderness in the injury area.
- Gradual stiffening or contraction of your child's injured muscle.
- Swelling, redness, or bruising at the injury site.

CAUSES

Injury caused by overuse or stress of a muscle group.

RISK FACTORS

- Poor nutrition, especially an electrolyte imbalance or vitamin deficiencies.
- Poor physical condition.
- Obesity.
- Fatigue or overwork.
- Lifting heavy weights improperly.
- Strenuous activity following excessive alcohol consumption.

PREVENTING COMPLICATIONS OR RECURRENCE

Your child should avoid vigorous exercise if unaccustomed to it. If your child is out of condition, urge the child to begin an exercise program to strengthen muscles gradually and prevent future injury. See Appendix 36.

WHAT TO EXPECT

MEDICAL TESTS

- Your own observation of symptoms.
- Medical history and physical exam by a doctor.
- X-rays of the painful area.

POSSIBLE COMPLICATIONS

Permanent weakness in the affected muscle.

PROBABLE OUTCOME

- Healing time for a pulled muscle depends on your child's age and general physical condition, on previous injuries, and on the severity of the present injury. Most partial tears or pulls heal with treatment within 1 month. Muscle function will be poor until the torn fibers heal.
- If the child's muscle is ruptured (torn in two), surgery may be necessary.

TREATMENT

HOME CARE

- Apply ice to the child's injured area during the first 24 hours. Place ice in a plastic bag and separate it from the skin with a thin towel. Let the child hold it against the muscle with the hand or an elastic bandage. Keep the ice pack on the area as long as your child can tolerate the cold.
- Wrap the injured area with a support bandage. Don't wrap it too tightly. If it swells *below* the bandage, loosen it. Elevate the injured part whenever possible.
- After 24 hours, apply heat in any form or continue ice packs, whichever feels better to the child. For heat, use a heating pad, heat lamp, whirlpool, ultrasound, hot baths, or hot compresses.

MEDICATION

- Your child may take non-prescription pain relievers such as aspirin. If the child's pain is severe or the affected area becomes badly swollen, your doctor may prescribe stronger pain relievers or muscle relaxants.
- See Medications section for information regarding medicines your doctor may prescribe.

ACTIVITY

- Urge your child not to use the pulled muscle as long as it is painful. However, the child should keep uninjured parts of the body active. Severe leg injuries may require crutches, and severe arm injuries may require slings.
- Physical therapy, with a graduated exercise program, may be necessary for your child to restore normal use and strength.

DIET & FLUIDS

Your child should eat a normal, well-balanced diet. Increase the child's protein intake by serving meat, poultry, fish, eggs, beans, and dairy products during healing.

OK FOR SCHOOL, PRESCHOOL, OR NURSERY?

Yes.

CALL YOUR DOCTOR IF

Your child has symptoms of a pulled or torn muscle, especially if any of the following occurs:

- Your child becomes unable to use the affected muscle.
- Your child's pain becomes intolerable.
- Swelling or bruising increase after 24 hours.
- You think medicine is causing symptoms.

MUSCLE WEAKNESS

GENERAL INFORMATION

DESCRIPTION

Muscle weakness refers to the profound muscle weakness that may follow hard or unaccustomed exercise. Appropriate health care must be individualized according to the underlying disorder.

SIGNS & SYMPTOMS

- Unaccustomed exercise.
- Symptoms that appear following a period of rest after the exercise, an hour or 2 later, or the next day. Frequently a child eats a high-carbohydrate meal after competition or vigorous physical exercise, followed by a night's sleep. The muscle weakness then appears the next day.
- Weakness that begins in the child's legs and progresses to the arms or other muscles in the body. Disabling fatigue accompanies the muscle weakness.

CAUSES

Decreased potassium levels in the circulating blood and muscle cells. The decreased potassium levels can be brought about by any of the following:

- An underlying inherited disorder called *periodic paralysis* that interferes with the child's muscle cellular metabolism.
- Excessive exercise in hot weather with loss of water, sodium, and potassium, leading to dehydration.
- Diuretic medications that cause sodium loss and excessive potassium loss through the child's kidneys. The sodium loss is desirable; the potassium loss is a significant undesirable side effect that may lead to major body disturbances. Customary doses of diuretics may require reduction during hot weather.

PREVENTING COMPLICATIONS OR RECURRENCE

Instructions for your child:

- Prevent potassium loss, increase fluid intake, and adjust exercise programs and medication dosages during hot weather.
- Avoid the combination of diuretic medications, alcohol, and heavy exercise during exceptionally hot weather. This combination can be lethal, causing strokes and life-threatening episodes of irregular heart rhythms.
- Increase potassium-rich foods in your diet.
- Take potassium supplements (with a doctor's prescription) prior to vigorous exercise if you have had an exercise-induced muscle weakness in the past.
- Modify your activity level to one below that which triggers attacks.

WHAT TO EXPECT

MEDICAL TESTS

- Your own observation of symptoms.
- Medical history and physical exam by a doctor.
- Blood studies (sometimes) to measure the child's potassium levels.
- Electromyography.

POSSIBLE COMPLICATIONS

- Permanently weakened muscle groups (rare).
- Fear of recurrence, resulting in unwarranted abandonment of the child's exercise program.

PROBABLE OUTCOME

Curable and preventable without long-lasting complications for your child by modifying the exercise program, taking potassium supplements, and avoiding dehydration.

TREATMENT

HOME CARE

- Your child should replace lost potassium with supplements or increase high-potassium foods in the diet.
- Your child should replace fluid loss with water instead of soft drinks.
- After vigorous exercise, the child should avoid a high-carbohydrate meal.

MEDICATION

Your doctor may prescribe potassium supplements for your child's muscle weakness.

ACTIVITY

If exercise-induced muscle weakness is a recurrent problem for your child, it may be necessary to cut back on the child's activity level permanently.

DIET & FLUIDS

- If your child has a potassium deficiency, provide foods high in potassium, such as dried apricots, whole-grain cereal (hot or cold), dried lentils, dried peaches, bananas, peanuts, citrus fruits, or fresh vegetables.
- Following a diet high in complex carbohydrates makes good nutritional sense to all those hoping to maintain or reach a good level of health and fitness. However, your child should not eat such a meal within 3 to 5 hours before competition, and should eat only lightly directly afterwards.

OK FOR SCHOOL, PRESCHOOL, OR NURSERY?

Yes, when condition and sense of well-being will allow.

CALL YOUR DOCTOR IF

- Your child has persistent or recurrent muscle weakness following exercise.
- Your child develops new symptoms after starting any prescribed medicine. All effective medicines have potentially undesirable side effects. These can frequently be controlled by modifying the dosage.

MUSCULAR DYSTROPHY

GENERAL INFORMATION

DESCRIPTION

Muscular dystrophy is a gradual deterioration of the body's muscles, leading to increasing difficulty in walking and moving. The muscular system—especially of the extremities, pelvis, and hips—is involved. Different types of muscular dystrophy exist, depending on the exact genes involved. They affect different areas of the body, such as the shoulders, hips, or face. Muscular dystrophy affects male children, usually between ages 5 and 12.

Appropriate health care includes:

- Home care.
- Physician's monitoring of general condition and medications.
- Psychotherapy or counseling for the child and the family to learn ways to cope with the child's disability and to adjust socially.
- Physical therapy.
- Nursing-home care, if the patient's needs exceed the resources available at home.

SIGNS & SYMPTOMS

- Early symptoms: weakness; ducklike gait; falling, with difficulty getting up; muscles that appear larger and stronger—but are weaker—than normal.
- Late symptoms: muscle deterioration severe enough to require confinement to a wheelchair by age 9 to 12; severe distortion of the child's body; recurrent respiratory infections.

CAUSES

Inherited. Muscular dystrophy is a genetic abnormality. It is carried by a female who does not have the disease; she passes it to male children. When a female carrier marries a male who does not carry the gene, half the male children will inherit the condition.

RISK FACTORS

Family history of muscular dystrophy.

PREVENTING COMPLICATIONS OR RECURRENCE

If you have a family history of muscular dystrophy:

- Obtain genetic counseling prior to starting a family.
- If you are pregnant, consider amniocentesis (see Glossary) to determine whether the fetus is male and whether the disorder is present.

WHAT TO EXPECT

MEDICAL TESTS

- Your own observation of symptoms.
- Medical history and physical exam by a doctor.
- Laboratory studies of muscle enzymes in the child's blood.
- Muscle biopsy (see Glossary).

POSSIBLE COMPLICATIONS

- Frequent fractures or injuries from falls.
- Spinal curvature caused by weakened muscles of the child's spine.
- Pneumonia caused by weakened chest muscles and a diminished cough response.
- Muscle shortening (contractures).
- Pressure sores.

PROBABLE OUTCOME

This condition is currently considered incurable. Children with this condition rarely reach adulthood. Scientific research into causes and treatment continues, so there is hope for better treatment and increased life expectancy for your child.

TREATMENT

HOME CARE

- Contact your local chapter of the Muscular Dystrophy Association for help.
- Your child should learn deep-breathing techniques. Your doctor can provide instructions.
- Your child should stay active in school as long as possible.

MEDICATION

No medicine can cure this condition. Your doctor may prescribe:

- Stool softeners to prevent constipation.
- Medications appropriate for complications.
- See Medications section for information regarding medicines your doctor may prescribe.

ACTIVITY

- Your child should be as physically and mentally active as possible. Many devices can help overcome handicaps caused by weakness. Your doctor will tell you if braces will help.
- If the child cannot voluntarily move muscle groups, family members or a visiting nurse should massage and passively exercise them to prevent contractures. Long periods of inactivity or bed rest should be avoided.

DIET & FLUIDS

No special diet. Overweight should be avoided, because it adds stress to weakened muscles.

OK FOR SCHOOL, PRESCHOOL, OR NURSERY?

Yes, so long as your child is able.

CALL YOUR DOCTOR IF

- You detect symptoms of muscular dystrophy in your child.
- Infection, especially of the lung, occurs after diagnosis. Symptoms include fever, cough, and chest pain.

MYASTHENIA GRAVIS

GENERAL INFORMATION

DESCRIPTION

Myasthenia gravis is a disorder of muscles, especially of the face and head, with increasing fatigue and weakness as muscles are used. Muscles, especially around the eyes, mouth and throat, and the extremities are involved.

Myasthenia gravis affects adolescents and young adults of both sexes but is more common in females.

Appropriate health care includes:

- Physician's monitoring of general condition and medications.
- Surgery to remove a thymus tumor, if present.

SIGNS & SYMPTOMS

- Drooping eyelids.
- Double vision.
- Loss of normal facial expression.
- Swallowing difficulty.
- Weakness of the child's arms and legs.
- Difficulty speaking clearly.
- Breathing difficulty.

Most flare-ups appear after a brief period of normal muscle function, and worsen as the muscle is used.

CAUSES

- Autoimmune disorder (probably).
- Tumor of the thymus (newborns only).

RISK FACTORS

- Medical history of other autoimmune diseases.
- Some cancers, especially thymus and lung cancer.
- Being an infant of a mother with myasthenia gravis. Newborns show symptoms in 2 to 3 weeks.

PREVENTING COMPLICATIONS OR RECURRENCE

Cannot be prevented at present.

OTHER

Pregnancy often results in temporary improvement.

WHAT TO EXPECT

MEDICAL TESTS

- Your own observation of symptoms.
- Medical history and physical exam by a doctor.
- Laboratory studies of antibodies in the child's blood and electrical muscle tests.
- X-rays of the child's chest.
- Therapeutic trial of anti-cholinesterase drugs.

POSSIBLE COMPLICATIONS

- Choking from swallowing difficulty.
- Respiratory paralysis.

PROBABLE OUTCOME

- This condition is currently considered incurable. However, the child's symptoms can be relieved or controlled. Worsening may be followed by improvement. Life expectancy is reduced, but your child can usually live many years with the disease.
- Scientific research into causes and treatment continues, so there is hope for increasingly effective treatment and cure.

TREATMENT

HOME CARE

Your child should maintain as normal a life as possible.

MEDICATION

Your doctor may prescribe:

- Anti-cholinesterase drugs to restore normal muscle function in the child. Excessive doses may cause weakness.
- Cortisone drugs at times when your child's symptoms worsen.
- See Medications section for information regarding medicines your doctor may prescribe.

ACTIVITY

No restrictions. Your child should remain as active as possible.

DIET & FLUIDS

No special diet.

OK FOR SCHOOL, PRESCHOOL, OR NURSERY?

Yes, when appetite has returned and alertness, strength, and feeling of well-being will allow.

CALL YOUR DOCTOR IF

- Your child has symptoms of myasthenia gravis.
- Your child develops swallowing or breathing difficulty. (You should have emergency medications—anti-cholinesterase drugs—available at all times to use if these symptoms develop.)

MYOCARDITIS

GENERAL INFORMATION

DESCRIPTION

Myocarditis is inflammation of the heart muscle (myocardium) that usually occurs as a complication of underlying illness, hypersensitive immune reactions, injury, or radiation therapy. All the chambers of the heart are involved.

Appropriate health care includes:

- Self-care after diagnosis.
- Physician's monitoring of general condition and medications.
- Hospitalization for the underlying disorder (frequently).

SIGNS & SYMPTOMS

- Fatigue.
- Shortness of breath.
- Irregular heartbeat.
- Fever.
- Other symptoms caused by the underlying disorder.

If myocarditis causes congestive heart failure, the following symptoms will also occur:

- Swollen feet and ankles.
- Distended neck veins.
- Rapid heartbeat, even when at rest.
- Breathing difficulty, even when the child is sleeping or at rest.

CAUSES

- Viral infections, such as measles, influenza, or adenovirus.
- Bacterial infections, such as tetanus, gonorrhea, typhoid fever, tuberculosis, or diphtheria.
- Surgery on the heart.
- Rheumatic fever.
- Parasite infections.

RISK FACTORS

- Excess alcohol consumption.
- Geographic location. Parasite infections are common in underdeveloped countries.

PREVENTING COMPLICATIONS OR RECURRENCE

- Urge your child not to drink more than 1 or 2 alcoholic drinks—if any—a day.
- Keep your child's immunizations current against diphtheria, tetanus, measles, German measles, and polio. See Appendix 1.

WHAT TO EXPECT

MEDICAL TESTS

- Your own observation of symptoms.
- Medical history and physical exam by a doctor.
- Laboratory blood studies.
- EKG (see Glossary).
- Other studies appropriate for the underlying disorder.

POSSIBLE COMPLICATIONS

Even with excellent treatment of the underlying disorder, a few children develop:

- Congestive heart failure.
- Permanent damage to the heart muscle or valves.
- A blood clot inside the heart muscle that can break away and lodge elsewhere in the body. This may be life-threatening.

PROBABLE OUTCOME

Usually curable with detection and treatment of the underlying cause.

TREATMENT

HOME CARE

Your child must have complete nursing care, including help with bathing and eating.

MEDICATION

Your doctor may prescribe:

- Antibiotics to fight infection, if your child's myocarditis is caused by a bacterial infection.
- Cortisone drugs to reduce inflammation.
- Appropriate medications, if the myocarditis develops into congestive heart failure. These include:
  - — Diuretics to reduce fluid retention.
  - — Digitalis to stimulate a stronger heartbeat.
  - — Anticoagulants to prevent clot formation.
- See Medications section for information regarding medicines your doctor may prescribe.

ACTIVITY

- Your child should rest in bed until symptoms disappear. Recovery time varies, depending on the underlying cause. Your child may read or watch TV.
- Your child should use a bedside commode for bowel movements while at complete bed rest. This causes less stress than a bedpan.
- After recovery, the child can resume normal activities gradually.

DIET & FLUIDS

Your child should eat a low-salt diet (see Appendix 29).

OK FOR SCHOOL, PRESCHOOL, OR NURSERY?

When signs of infection have decreased, appetite returns, and alertness, strength, and feeling of well-being will allow.

CALL YOUR DOCTOR IF

- Your child has symptoms of myocarditis.
- The following occurs during treatment:
  - — Recurrence of fever of chills.
  - — Increased shortness of breath.
- New, unexplained symptoms develop. Drugs used in treatment may produce side effects.

NAIL SPLITTING

GENERAL INFORMATION

DESCRIPTION

Nail splitting occurs in fingernails and toenails.
Appropriate health care includes:

- Self-care after diagnosis.
- Doctor's treatment for diagnosis, if splitting becomes severe.

SIGNS & SYMPTOMS

Painless splitting of the nail. Cracks may be parallel to the length of the finger, or flakes of nail may chip off the end.

CAUSES

- Scar formation from injury to the nail bed (sometimes).
- Family history of nail-splitting.
- Unknown (usually).

RISK FACTORS

Aging.

PREVENTING COMPLICATIONS OR RECURRENCE

Your child should protect fingernails from trauma, especially excessive irritation from soap and water.

WHAT TO EXPECT

MEDICAL TESTS

- Your own observation of symptoms.
- Medical history and physical exam by a doctor.

POSSIBLE COMPLICATIONS

None expected.

PROBABLE OUTCOME

Splitting may never disappear completely, but it may improve from time to time.

TREATMENT

HOME CARE

Instructions for your child:

- Apply multiple layers of clear fingernail polish so cracks, fissures, and flakes are cemented together. This can provide a splint or shield to protect nails. Nail polishes that contain nylon fibers will thicken and strengthen nails.
- Don't remove nail polish too often. Polish remover has a drying effect and may increase splitting. Instead, patch chips in the nail polish as they occur.
- Cement false fingernails over the split nail (older children and adolescents).
- Wear rubber gloves with cotton lining for household chores that involve water.
- Use a hand cream often. Massage it into the skin around the nails.

MEDICATION

- Medicine usually is not necessary for this disorder.
- See Medications section for information regarding medicines your doctor may prescribe.

ACTIVITY

No restrictions.

DIET & FLUIDS

No special diet. Many people say the condition improves if they drink large quantities of plain gelatin each day, but there is no evidence to support this theory.

OK FOR SCHOOL, PRESCHOOL, OR NURSERY?

Yes.

CALL YOUR DOCTOR IF

- Your child has severe nail splitting that has become a problem.
- Your child's self-care produces no improvement in 6 months.

NAILS, RINGWORM INFECTION OF (Onychomycosis; Tinea Unguium)

GENERAL INFORMATION

DESCRIPTION

Ringworm is a fungus infection of the toenails (usually) or fingernails (occasionally) in which nails become pliable, opaque, white, and thickened. This is contagious. Ringworm can affect both sexes, all ages, but is most common in older adolescents.

Appropriate health care includes:

- Self-care.
- Physician's monitoring of general condition and medications.
- Surgical removal of the nail.

SIGNS & SYMPTOMS

- Begins with a small separation between the end of the child's nail and the nail bed.
- Soft yellow material gradually builds up in the separation.
- The condition usually doesn't itch and is painless, unless the area is extensive and becomes infected.
- Eventually the child's entire nail is separated, resulting in a partially destroyed, misshapen, yellow nail.

CAUSES

Infection with the trichophyton fungus. Fingernail infection occurs only if your child's nail has been injured or if the nail is affected by another skin disease on the hand. Toenail infections can occur without injury.

RISK FACTORS

- Exposure to heat, wetness, and humidity, such as with cooking, dishwashing, and household chores.
- Hot, humid weather.

PREVENTING COMPLICATIONS OR RECURRENCE

- Encourage your child to keep feet cool, dry, and exposed to sunlight as much as possible.
- Urge your child to wear cotton or wool socks and to avoid footwear made from synthetic fibers.

WHAT TO EXPECT

MEDICAL TESTS

- Your own observation of symptoms.
- Medical history and physical exam by a doctor.
- Laboratory fungal cultures of the material under nails.

POSSIBLE COMPLICATIONS

Permanent nail loss or deformity.

NAILS, RINGWORM INFECTION OF (Onychomycosis; Tinea Unguium)

PROBABLE OUTCOME

Most fingernail infections are curable with 6 months of continuous treatment. Toenails require 12 to 24 months of treatment because of their slower growth rate. Most fingernail infections respond well to treatment, but toenail infections are more resistant to treatment. Recurrence is likely.

TREATMENT

HOME CARE

Instructions for your child:

- Dry feet and hands with extra care after bathing—even after the infection clears.
- Wear light footwear, such as sandals, to allow free air circulation. Don't wear socks or shoes made of synthetic materials. During acute phases, go barefoot as much as possible. Keep feet and hands cool, dry, and exposed to sunlight.
- For fingernail infections, wear cotton-lined latex or rubber gloves for dishwashing or other cleaning that requires immersion in water or chemicals.

MEDICATION

- Non-prescription anti-fungal ointments, creams, and powders are available, but they are ineffective in curing these infections. Your doctor may prescribe oral anti-fungal drugs, such as griseofulvin or ketoconazole, to cure the child's infection.
- See Medications section for information regarding medicines your doctor may prescribe.

ACTIVITY

No restrictions, but your child should avoid heat and excess sweating.

DIET & FLUIDS

No special diet.

OK FOR SCHOOL, PRESCHOOL, OR NURSERY?

Yes, unless school rules prohibit. Not readily contagious to others except with prolonged, intimate contact.

CALL YOUR DOCTOR IF

- Your child has a minor nail infection that becomes a problem.
- After 2 weeks of medication, your child's symptoms fail to improve.
- New, unexplained symptoms develop. Drugs used in treatment may produce side effects.

NARCOLEPSY

GENERAL INFORMATION

DESCRIPTION

Narcolepsy is a rare sleep disorder characterized by uncontrollable episodes of falling asleep at any place or time. After a 10 or 15 minute sleep attack, the person feels rested only briefly, then returns to an uncomfortable feeling of sleepiness. Attacks may occur while driving, talking, or working. The central nervous system is involved. This disorder begins in adolescence or young adulthood and continues throughout life.

Appropriate health care includes:

- Self-care after diagnosis.
- Doctor's treatment.

SIGNS & SYMPTOMS

Any of the following (10% of children and adults with narcolepsy have all the signs):

- Sleep attacks that may occur up to 10 times a day. These can occur during conversations or other activities. An attack leaves the child feeling refreshed, but another may occur again quickly.
- Vivid dreams, sounds, or hallucinations at the beginning of a sleep attack or upon awakening.
- Temporary paralysis (sudden loss of muscle strength) when falling asleep or just before complete awakening.
- Momentary paralysis not related to sleep when the child feels sudden emotion, such as anger, fear, or joy.
- Irresistible drowsiness during the day.

CAUSES

Unknown. Occasionally, it follows brain infection or head injury.

RISK FACTORS

Either of the following may trigger an attack:

- Monotonous activity.
- Prolonged laughter.

PREVENTING COMPLICATIONS OR RECURRENCE

Reduce the frequency of the child's attacks by avoiding risks listed above, if possible.

WHAT TO EXPECT

MEDICAL TESTS

- Your own observation of symptoms.
- Medical history and physical exam by a doctor.
- EEG (see Glossary).
- Studies in a sleep laboratory.

POSSIBLE COMPLICATIONS

Accidental injury during a sudden sleep attack.

PROBABLE OUTCOME

This disorder lasts throughout life, but it has no effect on your child's life expectancy. Medication can decrease the frequency of sleep attacks.

TREATMENT

HOME CARE

Your child should wear a Medic-Alert bracelet or pendant (see Glossary).

MEDICATION

- Your doctor may prescribe stimulants or antidepressants (but not both).
- See Medications section for information regarding medicines your doctor may prescribe.

ACTIVITY

Your child should not engage in any activity that carries the risk of injury from a sudden sleep attack. These include activities such as driving long distances, climbing ladders, or working around dangerous machinery.

DIET & FLUIDS

No special diet.

OK FOR SCHOOL, PRESCHOOL, OR NURSERY?

When appetite returns and alertness, strength, and feeling of well-being will allow.

CALL YOUR DOCTOR IF

- Your child has symptoms of narcolepsy.
- New, unexplained symptoms develop. Drugs used in treatment may produce side effects.

NASAL POLYPS

GENERAL INFORMATION

DESCRIPTION

Nasal polyps are non-malignant growths in the nasal cavities, usually in both sides of the nose. The nasal mucous membranes are involved. Nasal polyps occur in children but are most common in adults.

Appropriate health care includes:

- Self-care (only if surgery cannot be performed).
- Physician's monitoring of general condition and medications.
- Surgery to remove polyps under local anesthesia—a minor surgical procedure.

SIGNS & SYMPTOMS

- Obstruction of air through the nose (chronic "stuffy-nose" feeling).
- Impaired sense of smell.
- Feelings of fullness in the face.
- Nasal discharge.
- Facial pain (sometimes).
- Headaches (sometimes).

CAUSES

Chronic infection or allergy in the nose (allergic rhinitis) that causes the child's nasal mucous membranes to swell and produce excess fluid in the nasal cells.

RISK FACTORS

Sinusitis or chronic nasal infection.

PREVENTING COMPLICATIONS OR RECURRENCE

Obtain medical treatment for the child's underlying allergy. Consult your doctor about allergy testing and desensitizing procedures.

WHAT TO EXPECT

MEDICAL TESTS

- Your own observation of symptoms.
- Medical history and physical exam by a doctor.
- Laboratory skin tests to identify the child's allergies.

POSSIBLE COMPLICATIONS

- Repeated infections.
- Nosebleeds.

PROBABLE OUTCOME

Your child's symptoms can be controlled with treatment (usually surgery). Recurrence is common, even with surgical treatment.

TREATMENT

HOME CARE

If nosebleeds occur, see treatment described under Nosebleed (in Illnesses section).

MEDICATION

- For minor pain, use acetaminophen. Avoid giving your child aspirin, which may increase the tendency to bleed.
- Your doctor may prescribe cortisone drugs in nasal spray or oral form for a short while before surgery to shrink the child's polyps.
- See Medications section for information regarding medicines your doctor may prescribe.

ACTIVITY

Your child should resume normal activities gradually after surgery.

DIET & FLUIDS

No special diet.

OK FOR SCHOOL, PRESCHOOL, OR NURSERY?

Yes.

CALL YOUR DOCTOR IF

- Your child has symptoms of nasal polyps.
- The following occurs during treatment:
  — Nosebleeds that cannot be stopped.
  — Fever.
  — Pain that persists despite the use of acetaminophen.

NEPHROSIS
(Nephrotic Syndrome)

GENERAL INFORMATION

DESCRIPTION

Nephrosis is a form of chronic kidney disease that begins in childhood. Nephrosis is characterized by protein in the urine, swelling of the skin and organs, and low protein and high cholesterol in the blood. Early stages of the disease involve only the kidneys, but late or complicated stages involve all body cells. Nephrosis usually occurs in children between ages 1 and 6—especially ages 2 and 3. It affects more boys than girls. Appropriate health care includes: physician's monitoring of general condition and medications; self-care after diagnosis.

SIGNS & SYMPTOMS

- Fluid retention that appears first as puffy eyes and ankles, then as general puffiness of the child's skin, and eventually as a swollen abdomen.
- Reduced urine production, sometimes to 20% of normal.
- Loss of appetite.
- Weakness.
- General ill feeling.

CAUSES

Unknown. May be primary (of unknown cause) or may occur as a complication of other problems which affect kidney functions, such as diabetes, lupus erythematosus, glomerulonephritis, autoimmune disorders, serum sickness and other severe allergic disorders, a blood clot in the kidney, infections (especially of the skin), or congenital heart disease.

RISK FACTORS

Family history of nephrosis (primary form only). The following may reactivate a childhood case: pregnancy, exposure to chemical toxins, and congestive heart failure.

PREVENTING COMPLICATIONS OR RECURRENCE

Obtain prompt medical treatment for your child for any causes listed, especially skin and throat infections.

WHAT TO EXPECT

MEDICAL TESTS

Your own observation of symptoms; medical history and physical exam by a doctor; laboratory studies, such as urinalysis and blood studies of protein and cholesterol.

POSSIBLE COMPLICATIONS

- Kidney disease that resembles chronic glomerulonephritis.
- Kidney failure.
- Increased susceptibility to infections.

NEPHROSIS (Nephrotic Syndrome)

PROBABLE OUTCOME

• Nephrosis can't be cured or prevented. However, medication and diet can control swelling and reverse kidney abnormalities in many children.
• Although symptoms usually disappear in 2 weeks with treatment, medication is continued for 6 to 8 weeks. Nephrosis can be arrested with treatment, but relapses are common and the treatment must be repeated. If kidney failure develops, dialysis or a kidney transplant can prolong your child's life.

TREATMENT

HOME CARE

During the acute phase:
• Keep a record of the child's temperature each morning and evening.
• Collect all urine the child passes during each 24 hours and record every amount.
• Record all fluids the child consumes. Portions of the child's urine will be analyzed in the doctor's office.

MEDICATION

Your doctor may prescribe:
• Cortisone or immunosuppressive drugs to reduce kidney inflammation.
• Diuretics, including potassium-saving diuretics, to reduce fluid retention.
• Antibiotics to control infection.
• See Medications section for information regarding medicines your doctor may prescribe.

ACTIVITY

Keep your child in bed (except for trips to the bathroom) until the edema (fluid retention) improves. After the swelling decreases, the child may be as mildly active as strength allows.

DIET & FLUIDS

• Cook and serve the child's food without salt. Avoid serving prepared foods that contain salt. Include more protein than usual, such as fish, meat, eggs, and low-salt cheese.
• You may need to restrict your child's fluid intake. Ask your doctor.

OK FOR SCHOOL, PRESCHOOL, OR NURSERY?

When appetite has returned and alertness, strength and feeling of well-being will allow.

CALL YOUR DOCTOR IF

• Your child has symptoms of nephrosis.
• The following occurs during treatment: Severe headache; convulsion; extreme weakness; signs of infection, such as fever, sores on the skin, cough, or burning on urination; failure to pass 1 quart of urine in a 24-hour period; increased fluid retention; vomiting, diarrhea, or nausea.

NOSE FRACTURE

GENERAL INFORMATION

DESCRIPTION

A nose fracture is a fracture or damage to the bones and cartilage of the nose. This often happens when other facial bones are also fractured. The nose and adjacent structures are involved. Nose fracture is usually confined to older children (over age 8) and adults. Young children's noses have only cartilage.

Appropriate health care includes:

- Self-care after diagnosis of minor injuries.
- Physician's monitoring of general condition and medications.
- Emergency-room treatment for heavy bleeding.
- Surgery, if the nose is crooked or your child's breathing is impaired.

SIGNS & SYMPTOMS

- Pain in the nose.
- Nosebleed.
- Swollen, discolored nose.
- Inability to breathe through the nose.
- Crooked or misshapen nose (sometimes).

CAUSES

Injury to the child's nose.

RISK FACTORS

Previous nose injury.

PREVENTING COMPLICATIONS OR RECURRENCE

Your child should protect the nose from injury, whenever possible. Urge your child to wear protective headgear for contact sports or when riding motorcycles or bicycles and to wear auto seat belts.

WHAT TO EXPECT

MEDICAL TESTS

- Your own observation of symptoms.
- Medical history and physical exam by a doctor.
- Laboratory blood tests, if bleeding is heavy.
- X-ray of the nose.

POSSIBLE COMPLICATIONS

- Infection of the child's nose and sinuses.
- Shock from loss of blood (rare).
- Permanent breathing difficulty.
- Permanent change in the child's appearance.

PROBABLE OUTCOME

Minor fractures with no deformity usually heal in 4 weeks. Major fractures can be repaired with surgery. If surgery is necessary for your child, it should be done within 2 weeks or not until 6 months after the injury.

TREATMENT

HOME CARE

- Apply ice packs to the child's nose immediately after an injury to minimize swelling.
- If the child's nosebleed is heavy or cannot be stopped, obtain emergency medical treatment.

MEDICATION

- For minor discomfort, use non-prescription drugs such as acetaminophen.
- Your doctor may prescribe:
  — Stronger pain relievers, if needed.
  — Antibiotics, if infection develops.
- See Medications section for information regarding medicines your doctor may prescribe.

ACTIVITY

Your child should rest until bleeding stops.

DIET & FLUIDS

No special diet.

OK FOR SCHOOL, PRESCHOOL, OR NURSERY?

Yes, as soon as appetite has returned and alertness, strength, and feeling of well-being will allow.

CALL YOUR DOCTOR IF

- Your child has symptoms of a fractured nose, especially bleeding that is heavy or cannot be stopped.
- Your child has had a fractured nose and you think surgery is needed.

NOSE INJURY

GENERAL INFORMATION

DESCRIPTION

Nose injuries include fractures of the nasal bones, dislocations of nasal bones and cartilage, contusions of the nose, and nosebleed. Appropriate health care includes: self-care (see HOME CARE); doctor's treatment or emergency room treatment if self-care is unsuccessful; surgery (for severe bleeding only) to tie off the artery feeding the bleeding area; surgery, if the nose is crooked or breathing is impaired.

SIGNS & SYMPTOMS

- Pain or tenderness in the child's nose.
- A swollen, bruised nose.
- Inability to breathe through the nose.
- Crooked or misshapen nose (sometimes).
- Brisk bleeding or blood oozing from the nostril. If the child's nosebleed is close to the nostril, the blood is bright red. If the nosebleed is deeper in the nose, the blood may be bright or dark.
- Lightheadedness from blood loss.
- Rapid heartbeat, shortness of breath, and pallor (with significant blood loss only).

CAUSES

Direct blow to the child's nose.

RISK FACTORS

Contact sports, particularly boxing and wrestling; previous nose injury; blood disorders, including leukemia and hemophilia; use of certain drugs, such as anticoagulants, aspirin, or prolonged use of nosedrops; exposure to irritating chemicals; high altitude or dry climate.

PREVENTING COMPLICATIONS OR RECURRENCE

Your child should protect the nose from injury whenever possible. Urge your child to wear protective headgear for contact sports or when riding motorcycles or bicycles.

WHAT TO EXPECT

MEDICAL TESTS

Your own observation of symptoms; medical history and physical exam by a doctor; laboratory blood tests if bleeding is heavy; X-rays of the child's nose.

POSSIBLE COMPLICATIONS

Infection of the nose and sinuses; shock from loss of blood (rare); permanent breathing difficulty or change in the child's appearance.

PROBABLE OUTCOME

Minor fractures and contusions with no deformity usually heal in 4 weeks. Major fractures can be repaired with surgery—if surgery is necessary, it should be done within 2 weeks or not until 6 months after injury. Most bleeding can be controlled with home treatment—severe bleeding requires hospitalization.

TREATMENT

FIRST AID

- Apply ice packs to the child's nose immediately after injury to minimize swelling and decrease bleeding.
- If the child's nose is deformed or if the nosebleed is heavy or cannot be stopped, obtain emergency medical treatment. Gauze packing may be inserted to absorb blood, stop dripping, and exert pressure on ruptured blood vessels. Continued bleeding may require cauterization (see Glossary).

HOME CARE

- If surgery is required to set your child's broken nose or to insert a nasal pack, your surgeon will give you postoperative instructions.

Instructions for your child for a nosebleed from injury without fracture:

- Sit up with your head bent forward.
- Clamp your nose closed with your fingers for 5 uninterrupted minutes. During this time, breathe through your mouth.
- Don't talk, to avoid gagging.
- If bleeding stops and recurs, repeat—but pinch your nose firmly on both sides for 8 to 10 minutes. Holding your nose tightly closed allows the blood to clot and seal the damaged blood vessels.
- Apply cold compresses at the same time.
- Don't swallow blood. It may upset your stomach or make you gag, causing you to inhale blood.
- Don't blow your nose for 12 hours after the bleeding stops to avoid dislodging the blood clot.

MEDICATION

- For minor discomfort, use non-prescription drugs such as acetaminophen. Don't give the child aspirin, which can aggravate bleeding.
- Your doctor may prescribe stronger pain relievers, if needed; antibiotics if infection develops; drugs to treat any underlying serious disorder.

ACTIVITY

Your child can resume normal activities as soon as the bleeding stops or other symptoms improve.

DIET & FLUIDS

No special diet.

OK FOR SCHOOL, PRESCHOOL, OR NURSERY?

Yes, when condition and sense of well-being will allow.

CALL YOUR DOCTOR IF

- Your child has a nosebleed that won't stop with self-care described above.
- After the nosebleed, your child becomes nauseous or vomits.
- After the nose has been packed, your child's temperature rises to 101F (38.3C) or higher.

NOSEBLEED
(Epistaxis)

GENERAL INFORMATION

DESCRIPTION

Nosebleed is bleeding from the nose. The blood vessels (arteries and veins) in the nose are involved. In children, nosebleeds occur close to the nose opening. In adults, they usually occur deeper in the nose. Nosebleeds are twice as common in children as adults.

Appropriate health care includes:

- Self-care (see HOME CARE).
- Doctor's treatment or emergency-room treatment if self-care is unsuccessful.

Gauze packing may be inserted to absorb blood, stop dripping, and exert pressure on the ruptured blood vessels. Continued bleeding may require cauterization (see Glossary).

- Surgery (for severe bleeding only) to tie off the artery feeding the bleeding areas.

SIGNS & SYMPTOMS

- Blood oozing from your child's nostril. If the nosebleed is close to the nostril, the blood is bright red. If the nosebleed is deeper in the nose, the blood may be bright or dark.
- Lightheadedness from blood loss.
- Rapid heartbeat, shortness of breath, and pallor (with significant blood loss only).

CAUSES

- Injury to the nose or nasal polyps—even simple injury caused by picking the nose.
- Nasal or sinus infection.
- A foreign body in the nose.
- Scarlet fever.
- Malaria or typhoid fever.
- Dry mucous membranes in the nose from any cause.
- High blood pressure.
- Bleeding tendencies associated with aplastic anemia, leukemia, thrombocytopenia, or liver disease.

RISK FACTORS

Any disorder listed as a cause; Hodgkin's disease; scurvy; rheumatic fever; blood disorders, including leukemia and hemophilia; use of certain drugs such as anticoagulants, aspirin, or prolonged use of nose drops; exposure to irritating chemicals; high altitude or dry climate.

PREVENTING COMPLICATIONS OR RECURRENCE

- Urge your child to avoid injury to the nose if possible.
- Obtain medical treatment for the underlying cause of your child's nosebleed.
- Humidify the air in your home if you live in a dry climate or at a high altitude.

WHAT TO EXPECT

MEDICAL TESTS

- Your own observation of symptoms.
- Medical history and physical exam by a doctor.
- Laboratory blood studies.

NOSEBLEED (Epistaxis)

POSSIBLE COMPLICATIONS

Bleeding severe enough to require transfusion.

PROBABLE OUTCOME

Your child's symptoms can be controlled with treatment. Severe bleeding requires hospitalization and usually is caused by an underlying disorder, such as liver disease, blood disease, or hypertension. In these causes, the underlying disorder should be treated also.

TREATMENT

HOME CARE

Instructions for your child:

- Sit up with head bent forward.
- Clamp nose closed with fingers for 5 uninterrupted minutes. During this time, breathe through mouth.
- If bleeding stops and recurs, repeat—but pinch nose firmly on both sides for 8 to 10 minutes. Holding nose tightly closed allows the blood to clot and seal the damaged blood vessels.
- You may apply cold compresses at the same time.
- Don't blow nose for 12 hours after bleeding stops to avoid dislodging the blood clot.
- Don't swallow blood. It may upset the stomach or make you "gag," causing inhalation of blood.
- Don't talk (also to avoid gagging).

MEDICATION

Your doctor may prescribe drugs to treat any underlying serious disorder.

ACTIVITY

Your child can resume normal activities as soon as symptoms improve.

DIET & FLUIDS

No special diet.

OK FOR SCHOOL, PRESCHOOL, OR NURSERY?

Yes, when nosebleed has been halted for 24 hours.

CALL YOUR DOCTOR IF

- Your child has a nosebleed that won't stop with self-care described above.
- After the nosebleed, your child becomes nauseous or vomits.
- After the nose has been packed, your child's temperature rises to 101F (38.3C) or higher.

OBESITY

GENERAL INFORMATION

DESCRIPTION

Obesity exists when your child's weight is 20% or more above that considered normal for height. It may affect children of all ages and both sexes. Obese children are usually large at birth and gain weight rapidly. The tendency to be overweight is probably inherited. Most obese children are born with an excess of fat cells and an increased ability to store fats. Appropriate health care includes ruling out certain endocrine problems (hypopituitarism, Cushing's disease, hypothyroidism), treating any underlying health problems, and establishing life-long good eating habits. Patience, determination, high motivation, and a good sense of humor are constant requirements for successful treatment.

SIGNS & SYMPTOMS

Weight 20% or more than normal for your child's height. Most obese children have no symptoms except associated emotional problems and poor exercise tolerance.

CAUSES

- Inherited excess of body fat cells and eating more food than your child's body can use. The body cannot store carbohydrates or proteins, so excess calories are converted to fat and stored. One pound of fat represents about 3,500 excess calories, depending on individual metabolism.
- Copying poor eating patterns of parents.
- Decreased physical activity.
- Psychological factors, including stress, nervous tension, boredom, frustration, absence of friendships, depression, and poor self-esteem.

RISK FACTORS

Fat parents and siblings.

PREVENTING COMPLICATIONS OR RECURRENCE

Encourage your child to have an active lifestyle. Teach good physical conditioning. Serve your child foods low in fat, low in refined sugar, and low in salt.

WHAT TO EXPECT

MEDICAL TESTS

Observation of your child's symptoms; medical history and physical exam by a doctor; blood tests and X-rays to rule out endocrine problems.

POSSIBLE COMPLICATIONS

Diabetes, high blood pressure, heart disease, gallbladder disease, breathing problems, bloating, and stomach upsets, varicose veins, and severe psychological problems (same as those listed under "CAUSES").

PROBABLE OUTCOME

Your child's obesity can be controlled if basic causes are treated and motivation stays high for an entire lifetime.

TREATMENT

HOME CARE

Involve your child in outside social activities. Spare time fosters nibbling in everyone. Most snacking occurs between 3 and 6 p.m. Help your child find a part-time job when old enough, or occupy your child with music, drama, sports, Scouts, or other clubs.

MEDICATION

None offer any permanent help.

ACTIVITY

Daily exercise to the point of breathing hard can increase your child's rate of weight loss and sense of physical well-being. your child should participate in a gym program in school, or spend 10 minutes per day exercising at home. If possible, walk places instead of riding in a car. Use the stairs instead of elevators. Limit TV time to 2 hours or less per day. As your child loses weight, exercise will be less tiring. Encourage learning new sports that especially appeal to your child. Swimming, bicycling, skiing, and jogging are sports that burn the most calories.

DIET & FLUIDS

See Appendix 31, Obesity: Guidelines for Losing Weight.

OK FOR SCHOOL, PRESCHOOL, OR NURSERY?

Yes. Encourage full participation in any possible area of interest, particularly those requiring physical effort.

CALL YOUR DOCTOR IF

Obesity increases, despite self-help.

ORAL CANCER

GENERAL INFORMATION

DESCRIPTION

Oral cancer is a growth of malignant cells in the mouth or tongue. It is rare but dangerous. The lips, gums, palate, tongue, membranes inside the lip or cheek, and the floor of the mouth are involved. Oral cancer may affect adolescents or younger children if they smoke, chew tobacco, or dip snuff.

Appropriate health care includes:

- Self-care after diagnosis.
- Physician's monitoring of general condition and medications.
- Surgery to remove the cancerous area.
- Radiation therapy.
- Speech therapy, if surgery impairs the child's speech.

SIGNS & SYMPTOMS

A pale lump—usually painless—with a hard rim that appears in any part of the child's mouth or tongue. It has the following characteristics:

- It enlarges, ulcerates, and bleeds easily.
- It may make the child's tongue stiff and difficult to control, causing speaking and swallowing difficulty.

CAUSES

Unknown.

RISK FACTORS

- Use of tobacco in any form.
- Family history of oral cancer.

PREVENTING COMPLICATIONS OR RECURRENCE

Your child should not use tobacco.

WHAT TO EXPECT

MEDICAL TESTS

- Your own observation of symptoms.
- Medical history and physical exam by a doctor.
- Laboratory blood studies.
- Biopsy (see Glossary) of the lump.
- X-rays of the child's head.

POSSIBLE COMPLICATIONS

- Slow healing after surgery.
- Spread to lymph nodes in the child's neck, requiring radical head and neck surgery.
- Permanent disfigurement.
- Permanent speech impairment.

PROBABLE OUTCOME

Usually curable with early detection and treatment. The child's normal facial appearance can often be restored by plastic surgery.

TREATMENT

HOME CARE

After surgery, cleanse the child's mouth 3 to 4 times a day with a soothing salt-water solution (1 teaspoon salt to 8 oz. warm water).

MEDICATION

Your doctor may prescribe:

- Anti-cancer drugs.
- Pain relievers after surgery.
- Antibiotics, if infection coexists.
- See Medications section for information regarding medicines your doctor may prescribe.

ACTIVITY

Your child can resume normal activities gradually after surgery.

DIET & FLUIDS

No special diet after recovery. The child may require a liquid diet for several days after surgery.

OK FOR SCHOOL, PRESCHOOL, OR NURSERY?

Yes, when appetite has returned and alertness, strength, and feeling of well-being will allow.

CALL YOUR DOCTOR IF

- Your child has signs of a mouth or tongue tumor.
- The following occurs after surgery:
  - — Increasing pain.
  - — Fever.
  - — New lumps.
  - — Excessive bleeding.

OSGOOD-SCHLATTER DISEASE (Osteochondrosis)

GENERAL INFORMATION

DESCRIPTION

Osgood-Schlatter disease is a temporary condition of the leg at the knee, characterized by swelling, tenderness, and pain. The tibial tubercle, a prominence just below the knee cap attached to a large thigh muscle connecting the bone of the upper leg (femur) to the large bone in the lower leg (tibia), is involved. This disorder often affects both knees. Osgood-Schlatter disease is most likely to affect adolescents. It is uncommon after age 16.

Appropriate health care includes:

- Physician's monitoring of general condition and medications.
- Self-care after diagnosis.

SIGNS & SYMPTOMS

- A slightly swollen, warm and tender bump below the child's knee.
- Pain with activity, especially straightening the leg against force, as in stair-climbing, jumping, or weight-lifting.

CAUSES

Stress or injury of the tibial tubercle, which is still developing during adolescence. Repeated stress or injury interferes with development, causing inflammation.

RISK FACTORS

- Overzealous conditioning routines, such as running, jumping, or jogging.
- Being overweight.

PREVENTING COMPLICATIONS OR RECURRENCE

- Help an overweight child lose weight. A reducing diet appears in Appendix 31.
- Encourage your child to exercise moderately, avoiding extremes.

WHAT TO EXPECT

MEDICAL TESTS

- Your own observation of symptoms.
- Medical history and physical exam by a doctor.
- X-ray of the knee.

POSSIBLE COMPLICATIONS

- Bone infection.
- Recurrence of the condition in adulthood.

PROBABLE OUTCOME

Usually curable with treatment in 4 to 8 months.

OSGOOD-SCHLATTER DISEASE
(Osteochondrosis)

TREATMENT

HOME CARE

Use heat to relieve your child's pain. Warm compresses, heating pads, warm whirlpool baths, heat lamps, diathermy, or ultrasound are effective.

MEDICATION

- For minor discomfort, use non-prescription drugs such as aspirin.
- Your doctor may prescribe cortisone injections if other treatment fails.

Cortisone injections may weaken your child's tendons, so it is better to give the condition more time to heal than to use them.

- See Medications section for information regarding medicines your doctor may prescribe.

ACTIVITY

Resting the child's affected leg is the most important treatment. This is done with:

- Crutches.
- A leg cast or splint.
- An elastic knee brace that prevents the child's knee from bending fully.

The child should not participate in sports during treatment. This is temporary, and normal activity can be resumed when inflammation subsides.

DIET & FLUIDS

No special diet, unless the child is overweight. See Appendix 31 for a reducing diet.

OK FOR SCHOOL, PRESCHOOL, OR NURSERY?

Yes, when strength and feeling of well-being will allow.

CALL YOUR DOCTOR IF

- Your child has symptoms of Osgood-Schlatter disease.
- The following occurs during treatment:
  - — Symptoms don't improve in 4 weeks, despite treatment.
  - — Pain increases.
  - — Temperature rises to 101F (38.3C).

OSTEOMYELITIS

GENERAL INFORMATION

DESCRIPTION

Osteomyelitis is an infection of the bone and bone marrow. Any bone in the body can be involved. In a child, the femur (upper-leg bone), the tibia (lower-leg bone), or the humerus or radius (bones in the arm) are usually affected. In an adult, the pelvis or spine are usually affected. Osteomyelitis occurs in both sexes but is more common in males. It can affect all ages but is most common in rapidly growing children (5 to 14 years).

Appropriate health care includes:

- Physician's monitoring of general condition and medications.
- Hospitalization for surgery to drain abscesses or to remove pockets of infected bone, and to administer high doses of antibiotics—sometimes intravenously.
- Self-care after diagnosis and when hospitalization is no longer necessary.

SIGNS & SYMPTOMS

- Fever. Sometimes this is the only symptom.
- Pain, swelling, redness, warmth, and tenderness in the area over the infected bone, especially when moving a nearby joint. Nearby joints—especially the knee—may also be red, warm, and swollen.
- If a child is too young to talk, signs of pain include reluctance to move an arm or a leg, or refusing to walk, or limping, or screaming when the limb is touched or moved.
- Pus drainage through a skin abscess, without fever or severe pain (chronic osteomyelitis only).
- General ill feeling.

CAUSES

Usually staphylococcal infection, but many other bacteria may be responsible. The bacteria may spread to the child's bone through the bloodstream from the following sources: compound fracture or other injury; boil, carbuncle, or any break in the skin; middle-ear infection; pneumonia.

RISK FACTORS

- Illness that has lowered resistance.
- Rapid growth during childhood.

PREVENTING COMPLICATIONS OR RECURRENCE

Obtain prompt medical treatment for your child for any bacterial infection to prevent its spread to bone or other body parts.

WHAT TO EXPECT

MEDICAL TESTS

- Your own observation of symptoms; medical history and physical exam by a doctor; laboratory blood studies and blood cultures to identify the bacteria.
- X-rays of the bone. X-rays often don't show changes until 2 to 3 weeks after the infection begins.
- CAT or CT Scan (see Glossary).

POSSIBLE COMPLICATIONS

- Abscess that breaks through the child's skin and won't heal until the underlying bone heals.
- Permanent stiffness in a nearby joint (rare).
- Blood poisoning that makes amputation necessary (rare).

PROBABLE OUTCOME

Usually curable with prompt and aggressive treatment.

TREATMENT

HOME CARE

- Wear sterile gloves to change your child's dressings.
- Keep the involved limb level or slightly elevated and immobilized with pillows. Don't let it dangle.
- Keep unaffected parts of the child's body as active as possible to prevent pressure sores during required prolonged bed rest.

MEDICATION

Your doctor may prescribe:

- Large doses of antibiotics, usually intravenously. Antibiotics may be necessary—either orally or by injection—for 8 to 10 weeks.
- Pain relievers.
- Laxatives, if constipation develops during prolonged bed rest.

ACTIVITY

Your child should rest in bed until 2 to 3 weeks after symptoms disappear. Normal activities may be resumed gradually.

DIET & FLUIDS

No special diet. Urge your child to eat heartily. Give the child vitamin and mineral supplements.

OK FOR SCHOOL, PRESCHOOL, OR NURSERY?

When signs of infection have decreased, appetite returns, and alertness, strength, and feeling of well-being will allow.

CALL YOUR DOCTOR IF

- Your child has symptoms of osteomyelitis.
- The following occurs during treatment: An abscess forms over the infected bone, or drainage from an existing abscess increases; fever rises to 101F (38.3C) or higher; pain becomes intolerable.
- New, unexplained symptoms develop. Drugs used in treatment may produce side effects.

OTITIS, SEROUS
(Serous Otitis Media)

GENERAL INFORMATION

DESCRIPTION

Serous otitis media is a disorder of the middle ear resulting in accumulation of sterile fluid and temporary decrease or loss of hearing.

Appropriate health care includes:

- Doctor's treatment to surgically open the eardrum to remove fluid. Frequently it is necessary to insert a small plastic tube through the opening in the eardrum to prevent fluid reaccumulating.
- Self-care after diagnosis.
- Physician's monitoring of general condition and medications.

SIGNS & SYMPTOMS

- Decreased hearing on the affected side.
- The physician may visualize with an otoscope the following changes:
  - — Retraction of the child's eardrum.
  - — Bubbles of air in the fluid behind the eardrum.

CAUSES

- Infections or inflammation in the nose and throat.
- Allergies.
- Enlarged adenoids.
- Tumors.

RISK FACTORS

- Repeated upper respiratory infections.
- Bottle-feeding your baby in a lying down position.
- High altitude.
- Cold climate.
- Flying in a non-pressurized aircraft.

PREVENTING COMPLICATIONS OR RECURRENCE

Provide your child with early and complete treatment of all ear and throat infections.

WHAT TO EXPECT

MEDICAL TESTS

- Your own observation of symptoms.
- Medical history and physical exam by a doctor.

POSSIBLE COMPLICATIONS

- Permanent (partial or rarely) hearing loss.
- Delay of normal language development in a child.

PROBABLE OUTCOME

Usually completely curable with early, adequate treatment.

OTITIS, SEROUS
(Serous Otitis Media)

TREATMENT

HOME CARE

- If your doctor has inserted tubes into the child's eardrum, leave them alone. They will come out on their own when no longer needed.
- Apply heat to the area around the child's ear if there is pain.

MEDICATION

- Use non-prescription nasal sprays or drops to help open the eustachian tube and relieve pressure in the middle ear.
- Use non-prescription drugs, such as acetaminophen, to reduce pain and fever.
- Your doctor may prescribe antibiotics. Finish the medication. The infection may remain active for several days after the symptoms disappear.
- See Medications section for information regarding medicines your doctor may prescribe.

ACTIVITY

- Your child should reduce normal activity until the condition clears.
- Urge your child not to go swimming!
- Your child should avoid extreme atmospheric pressures as in mountain climbing or flying.

DIET & FLUIDS

No special diet.

OK FOR SCHOOL, PRESCHOOL, OR NURSERY?

When signs of infection have decreased, appetite returns, and alertness, strength, and feeling of well-being will allow.

CALL YOUR DOCTOR IF

- Your child has symptoms of serous otitis.
- The following occurs during treatment:
  - Fever above 102F (38.9C), despite treatment.
  - Severe headache.
  - Earache that persists longer than 2 days, despite treatment.
  - Swelling around the child's ear.
  - Convulsions.
  - Twitching of the child's face muscles.
  - Dizziness.

OTOSCLEROSIS

GENERAL INFORMATION

DESCRIPTION

Otosclerosis is the slow formation of abnormal spongy bone growth in the middle ear. The growth prevents one of the small bones in the middle ear from vibrating sound waves, leading to hearing loss. The middle-ear bones and the nerves in the ear that allow us to hear are involved. Otosclerosis usually affects both ears. Otosclerosis is twice as likely to affect females as males and occurs most commonly from ages 15 to 30.

Appropriate health care includes:

- Physician's monitoring of general condition and medications.
- Surgery to remove the stapes (a bone in the middle ear).

SIGNS & SYMPTOMS

- Slow, progressive hearing loss.
- Ringing in the ears.
- Hearing that is better in noisy environments than quiet ones.

CAUSES

Inherited. This is a dominant genetic trait.

RISK FACTORS

- Family history of hearing loss.
- Caucasian heritage. Otosclerosis affects to some degree about 10% of all white people.
- Pregnancy, which may trigger the onset.

PREVENTING COMPLICATIONS OR RECURRENCE

Cannot be prevented at present. Obtain genetic counseling before starting a family if you or your spouse have otosclerosis.

WHAT TO EXPECT

MEDICAL TESTS

- Your own observation of symptoms.
- Medical history and physical exam by a doctor.
- Laboratory studies such as audiogram and Rinne test (see Glossary).

POSSIBLE COMPLICATIONS

Total deafness in 10 to 15 years without treatment. The younger the patient, the more rapid the hearing loss.

PROBABLE OUTCOME

In most cases, your child's hearing can be at least partially restored with surgery.

TREATMENT

HOME CARE

Instructions for your child to prevent complications after surgery:

- Don't blow your nose for 1 week.
- Avoid unnecessary contact with persons who have a respiratory infection, such as a cold, flu, or bronchitis.
- Protect your ears against cold.
- Avoid activities that might cause dizziness, such as bending, lifting, or straining.
- Avoid loud noises and sudden pressure changes (flying or scuba diving) for 6 months or until healing is complete.

MEDICATION

- Your doctor may prescribe antibiotics after surgery.
- See Medications section for information regarding medicines your doctor may prescribe.

ACTIVITY

After surgery, your child can resume normal activities gradually.

DIET & FLUIDS

No special diet.

OK FOR SCHOOL, PRESCHOOL, OR NURSERY?

Yes.

CALL YOUR DOCTOR IF

- Your child has symptoms of otosclerosis.
- Signs of infection, such as fever, pain, or excessive dizziness, develop after treatment.

OVARIAN CANCER

GENERAL INFORMATION

DESCRIPTION

Ovarian cancer is a malignant growth in the ovary that is likely to spread to other body parts and threaten life. One or both ovaries are involved. It may spread to the lungs and bone. Ovarian cancer can affect females of all ages but is more common in adults than in children.

Appropriate health care includes:

- Physician's monitoring of general condition and medications.
- Surgery to remove the cancerous ovary and other affected areas, including the Fallopian tubes, the uterus, and the other ovary (sometimes).
- Radiation treatment.
- Psychotherapy or counseling to learn to accept and cope with cancer.

SIGNS & SYMPTOMS

Frequently no symptoms occur until the tumor becomes large. The earliest symptoms include:

- Vague discomfort in the lower abdomen.
- Gastrointestinal upsets.
- Irregular menstrual periods.

Later symptoms:

- Deep voice.
- Excessive hair growth.
- Unexplained weight loss.
- Anemia.
- An enlarged, hard, and sometimes tender mass in the lower abdomen.
- Pain with intercourse.

CAUSES

Unknown.

RISK FACTORS

Unknown.

PREVENTING COMPLICATIONS OR RECURRENCE

Your daughter should have yearly pelvic examinations, which offer the best chance of early detection and cure, starting in her late teens or when she become sexually active.

WHAT TO EXPECT

MEDICAL TESTS

- Your own observation of symptoms.
- Medical history and physical exam by a doctor.
- Laboratory blood studies.
- Sonogram (see Glossary) of the abdomen.
- X-rays of the abdomen.
- Surgical diagnostic procedures, such as culdoscopy and laparoscopy (see Glossary).

POSSIBLE COMPLICATIONS

Death from spread of cancer to other body parts.

PROBABLE OUTCOME

25% to 50% of women with ovarian cancer survive at least 5 years after treatment.

TREATMENT

HOME CARE

Follow your surgeon's instructions for home care following surgery.

MEDICATION

Your doctor may prescribe:

- Anti-cancer drugs.
- Pain relievers.
- Female hormones until menopause.
- See Medications section for information regarding medicines your doctor may prescribe.

ACTIVITY

No restrictions after recovery from surgery.

DIET & FLUIDS

Your daughter should eat a normal, well-balanced diet that is high in protein to promote repair of body tissues.

OK FOR SCHOOL, PRESCHOOL, OR NURSERY?

When appetite has returned and alertness, strength, and feeling of well-being will allow.

CALL YOUR DOCTOR IF

- Your daughter has symptoms of an ovarian tumor.
- The following occurs after surgery:
  - — Increased pain, swelling, redness, or drainage from the surgical wound.
  - — Pain or swelling in the leg.
  - — Signs of infection, such as fever, chills, headache, or muscle aches.

OVARIAN CYST

GENERAL INFORMATION

DESCRIPTION

An ovarian cyst is a closed cavity or sac containing liquid or semisolid material which develops in an ovary. Ovarian cysts are rarely cancerous. The ovaries, Fallopian tubes, peritoneum, and colon are involved. Ovarian cysts can affect females of all ages. Appropriate health care includes: physician's monitoring of general condition and medications; surgery to drain the cyst through a laparoscope (see Glossary) or surgery to remove the ovary.

SIGNS & SYMPTOMS

Some ovarian cysts produce no symptoms. Others produce any of the following:

- Swelling without pain in the lower abdomen.
- Stinging or burning on urination (if the cyst presses on the bladder).
- Difficulty emptying the bladder completely.
- Brownish vaginal discharge.
- Irregular menstruation or increased hairiness (if the cyst produces excess hormones).
- Precocious breast development and perhaps premature menstruation in young girls—even as young as 2-5 years.
- Painful sexual intercourse.

The following may occur if the cyst twists, bleeds, or breaks: severe abdominal pain; fever; vomiting.

CAUSES

Hormone disturbance. Ovarian cysts sometimes develop during pregnancy.

RISK FACTORS

Pregnancy; use of hormones.

PREVENTING COMPLICATIONS OR RECURRENCE

Cannot be prevented at present.

WHAT TO EXPECT

MEDICAL TESTS

- Your own observation of symptoms; medical history and physical exam—including a complete pelvic examination—by a doctor; X-ray of the abdomen.
- Special studies that may include:
  - — Ultrasonography: A non-invasive technique that translates sound waves into images displayed on a screen and photographed (see Glossary).
  - — CAT or CT Scan (computerized axial tomography): Non-invasive computerized X-ray images that show sections (or "slices") of an organ or region of the body clearly and precisely (see Glossary).
  - — MRI (magnetic resonance imaging): A non-invasive (non-X-ray) computerized test that uses radio frequency energy and a powerful magnetic field to produce images with excellent detail (see Glossary).
  - — Radionuclide Scan: A nuclear medicine procedure that uses radioactive isotopes injected into a patient. The isotope tracers are absorbed in various concentrations by targeted organs, which are then photographed (see Glossary).

POSSIBLE COMPLICATIONS

- Rupture of the cyst or twisting of the cyst's stalk. This requires emergency surgery.
- Urinary obstruction.
- Increased risk of ovarian cancer.

PROBABLE OUTCOME

Ovarian cysts are curable with surgery. Without surgery, they often recur.

TREATMENT

HOME CARE

Follow your surgeon's instructions for home care following surgery.

MEDICATION

- Medicine is usually not necessary for this disorder. For minor discomfort, use non-prescription drugs such as acetaminophen.
- See Medications section for information regarding medicines your doctor may prescribe.

ACTIVITY

No restrictions. If surgery is necessary, your daughter can resume activities gradually.

DIET & FLUIDS

No special diet.

OK FOR SCHOOL, PRESCHOOL, OR NURSERY?

Yes, after recuperating from surgery.

CALL YOUR DOCTOR IF

- Your daughter has symptoms of an ovarian cyst.
- Any of the following develops in your daughter after diagnosis:
  — Weight loss for no apparent reason.
  — Generally ill feeling.
  — Pain in the lower abdomen.
  — Severe abdominal pain, nausea, and fever that comes on suddenly. This may indicate rupture of a cyst.

OVARIAN TUMOR, BENIGN

GENERAL INFORMATION

DESCRIPTION

A benign ovarian tumor is a cystic (saclike) tumor on the ovary that contains fluid or semisolid material. These tumors are usually small, but in some cases they may grow large enough to make a young woman appear pregnant. Ovarian tumors are usually benign, but a few undergo malignant change. One or both ovaries are involved. Benign ovarian tumors may affect one or both ovaries in females between puberty and menopause.

Appropriate health care includes:

- Physician's monitoring of general condition and medications.
- Surgery to remove the tumor or diseased ovary (sometimes).

SIGNS & SYMPTOMS

- May not cause symptoms. If symptoms occur in your daughter, they may include:
  - Mild pelvic pain.
  - Pain in the lower back.
  - Abnormal menstruation, including changes in menstrual flow, length of periods, and intervals between periods.
  - Excessive hair growth, deep voice, and weight gain (sometimes).
  - Discomfort with sexual intercourse.
- If a large ovarian tumor twists or ruptures, the following will occur in the lower abdomen:
  - Severe pain.
  - Rigid muscles.
  - Swelling.

CAUSES

Unknown, but it is probably related to abnormalities of female hormone production and secretion.

RISK FACTORS

Unknown.

PREVENTING COMPLICATIONS OR RECURRENCE

No specific preventive measures.

WHAT TO EXPECT

MEDICAL TESTS

- Your own observation of symptoms.
- Medical history and physical exam by a doctor.
- Laboratory blood studies.
- Laparoscopy, a surgical diagnostic procedure. A small tube is inserted in the abdomen under local anesthesia. The tube allows the doctor to see the organs and biopsy or drain the tumor, if necessary.

POSSIBLE COMPLICATIONS

Emergency abdominal surgery caused by twisting, rupture, or bleeding of a tumor.

PROBABLE OUTCOME

• Most ovarian tumors require no treatment and disappear spontaneously within 2 months.

• Some tumors require surgery to diagnose accurately, ruling out malignancy, or to treat. If one ovary must be removed, normal conception and childbirth is possible as long as a normal ovary remains on the other side.

TREATMENT

HOME CARE

• Your daughter should have yearly medical checkups and pelvic exams after puberty to detect tumors early. Treatment may not be necessary, except to have regular pelvic examinations so the tumor's growth can be monitored.

MEDICATION

• Your doctor may prescribe female hormones or clomiphene for your daughter. These help shrink or destroy some tumors.

• See Medications section for information regarding medicines your doctor may prescribe.

ACTIVITY

No restrictions if surgery is not necessary.

DIET & FLUIDS

No special diet.

OK FOR SCHOOL, PRESCHOOL, OR NURSERY?

Yes, when condition and sense of well-being will allow.

CALL YOUR DOCTOR IF

• Your daughter has symptoms of an ovarian tumor, especially severe pain, rigidity, and abdominal distention.

• New, unexplained symptoms develop. Drugs used in treatment may produce side effects.

PARAPLEGIA or QUADRIPLEGIA

GENERAL INFORMATION

DESCRIPTION

Paraplegia is partial or complete paralysis of both legs. Quadriplegia is partial or complete paralysis of both arms *and* both legs. The spinal cord and all body parts below the spinal-cord damage are involved.

Appropriate health care includes:

- Physician's monitoring of general condition and medications.
- Surgery to limit further spinal-cord damage, or to remove bones or a tumor.
- Time in an extended-care facility or nursing home (sometimes).
- Occupational rehabilitation.
- Psychotherapy or counseling for depression or for sexual problems.

SIGNS & SYMPTOMS

The following vary, depending on the site and extent of your child's spinal-cord damage:

- Loss of movement and sensation in affected arms or legs.
- Loss of urinary and bowel control.
- Loss of normal blood pressure.
- Loss of body-temperature control.
- Constipation.
- Impaired sexual function.

CAUSES

Paraplegia is caused by spinal-cord damage in the back. Quadriplegia is caused by spinal-cord damage in the neck. Spinal-cord damage results from accidents, spinal-cord tumors, or birth defects.

RISK FACTORS

- Sports or other activities with a high risk of injury.
- Excess alcohol consumption or drug use, which increase the risk of accidents—especially vehicle accidents.

PREVENTING COMPLICATIONS OR RECURRENCE

Instructions for your child:

- Observe safety precautions and don't take risks.
- Don't dive into shallow swimming pools or into water of unknown depth.
- Don't drink alcohol or use mind-altering drugs and drive.
- Use seat belts in cars.
- Wear protective headgear during contact sports or while riding a bicycle or motorcycle.

WHAT TO EXPECT

MEDICAL TESTS

- Your own observation of symptoms.
- Medical history and physical exam by a doctor.
- Laboratory studies of blood and urine.
- Special studies that may include ultrasonography, CAT or CT scan, MRI, and radionuclide scan (see Glossary for all).

POSSIBLE COMPLICATIONS

Kidney infections, especially if a urinary catheter is needed; lung infections; fecal impaction; pressure sores; deep-vein blood clots; depression.

PROBABLE OUTCOME

Depends on the extent of your child's injury. A damaged spinal cord is limited in its ability to recover from injury. With rehabilitation, uninjured areas can take over some lost functions.

TREATMENT

HOME CARE

- If someone is in an accident and has neck pain or possible spinal-cord injury, *don't move the person unless absolutely necessary.* Immobilize the neck with splints or pillows to avoid movement and additional damage until Emergency Medical Services arrive.
- If your child has had a spinal-cord injury, family and friends need to offer emotional support. Encourage the child not to be afraid to ask for help.
- Put thigh-length elastic stockings on your child during convalescence—and knee-length stockings later—to reduce the chance of deep-vein blood clots.
- Let your child sleep on a waterbed or egg-crate foam mattress to reduce the chance of pressure sores.

MEDICATION

No medication can heal a damaged spinal cord. Your doctor may prescribe:

- Antibiotics to fight infection. Urinary-tract infections are most common.
- Stool softeners and laxatives to prevent constipation.

ACTIVITY

Encourage your child to stay as active as strength and condition allow. The body can be retrained to compensate for or restore some lost functions.

DIET & FLUIDS

- Serve the child a high-fiber diet to prevent constipation.
- If your child has a urinary catheter, urge the child to drink up to 16 glasses of water a day to prevent bladder stones and urinary-tract infections.

OK FOR SCHOOL, PRESCHOOL, OR NURSERY?

Yes, after special rehabilitation. Encourage your child to try to stay in life's mainstream.

CALL YOUR DOCTOR IF

- You observe signs of a neck or spine injury in your child.
- Signs of infection occur during treatment. These include fever, chills, cloudy urine, muscle aches, and headache.

ILLNESSES

PARONYCHIA

GENERAL INFORMATION

DESCRIPTION

Paronychia is inflammation of the tissue folds that surround the fingernails. The inflammation can be bacterial or fungal and is not contagious.

Appropriate health care includes:

- Self-care after diagnosis.
- Physician's monitoring of general condition and medications.

SIGNS & SYMPTOMS

Bacterial paronychia:

- Pain or tenderness, redness, warmth, and swelling in the affected finger.
- Drops of pus that can be squeezed out of swollen tissue.

Fungal paronychia:

- Redness and swelling around the fingernail.
- No pain, warmth, itching, or pus.

CAUSES

- Bacterial paronychia is preceded by injury, such as a torn hangnail. The infecting germ is usually staphylococcus.
- Fungal paronychia is caused by a fungus or yeast infection.

RISK FACTORS

- Injury around the fingernail.
- Exposure to constant wetness (washing dishes or other cleaning chores involving liquids).

PREVENTING COMPLICATIONS OR RECURRENCE

Instructions for your child:

- Protect hands from wetness.
- Leave hangnails alone.
- Avoid fingertip injury.

WHAT TO EXPECT

MEDICAL TESTS

- Your own observation of symptoms.
- Medical history and physical exam by a doctor.
- Laboratory studies, such as culture of the discharge, to identify the germ.

POSSIBLE COMPLICATIONS

If untreated, may permanently damage the child's fingernail and nail bed.

PROBABLE OUTCOME

- Bacterial paronychia is curable with treatment in 2 weeks.
- Fungal paronychia is chronic and may require 6 months to heal.
- Recurrence is common with both forms.

TREATMENT

HOME CARE

Instructions for your child:

- Wear heavy-duty vinyl gloves to prevent contact with irritating substances, such as water, soap, detergent, metal scrubbing pads, scouring pads, scouring powder, and other chemicals.
- Dry the insides of gloves after use. Discard a glove that develops a hole. A glove with a hole harms the hand more than not wearing a glove.
- Wear gloves when you peel or squeeze lemons, oranges, grapefruit, tomatoes, or potatoes.
- Wear leather or heavy-duty fabric gloves for housework or gardening.
- Use a dishwashing machine or ask someone else to wash dishes.
- Avoid contact with irritating chemicals, such as paint, paint thinner, turpentine, and polish for cars, floors, shoes, furniture, or metal.
- Use lukewarm water and very little mild soap to shower or bathe. All soaps are irritating. Expensive soaps offer no more protection against irritation than less-expensive ones.
- For bacterial paronychia, apply warm soaks.

MEDICATION

- For minor pain, use non-prescription drugs, such as aspirin or acetaminophen.
- Your doctor may prescribe antibiotics or anti-fungal medicine (depending on the type of infection).
- See Medications section for information regarding medicines your doctor may prescribe.

ACTIVITY

No restrictions.

DIET & FLUIDS

No special diet.

OK FOR SCHOOL, PRESCHOOL, OR NURSERY?

Yes. Not contagious.

CALL YOUR DOCTOR IF

- Your child has symptoms of paronchia.
- Fever develops.
- Your child's pain is not relieved by treatment.

PELVIC INFLAMMATORY DISEASE (PID)

GENERAL INFORMATION

DESCRIPTION

Pelvic inflammatory disease is infection of the female internal reproductive organs. This is contagious if it is caused by a sexually transmitted organism. The Fallopian tubes, cervix, uterus, ovaries, and urinary bladder are involved. Pelvic inflammatory disease can affect sexually active females after puberty. The peak incidence occurs in the late teens and early 20s.

Appropriate health care includes:

- Physician's monitoring of general condition and medications. Your daughter's sexual partner may also need examination and treatment.
- Self-care after diagnosis.
- Hospitalization (usually).
- Surgery to drain a pelvic abscess (sometimes).
- Psychotherapy or counseling, if infertility occurs.

SIGNS & SYMPTOMS

Early symptoms (up to 1 week):

- Pain in the lower pelvis on one or both sides, especially during menstrual periods. Menstrual flow may be heavy.
- Bad-smelling vaginal discharge.
- General ill feeling.
- Low fever (up to 101F or 38.3C).
- Frequent, painful urination.

Later symptoms (1 to 3 weeks later):

- Severe pain and tenderness in the lower abdomen.
- Temperature over 101F (38.3C).
- Increased bad-smelling vaginal discharge.

CAUSES

- Bacterial infection (chlamydia, gonorrhea, or mycoplasma) or a virus. This may be transmitted by an infected sexual partner.
- Childbirth.
- Abortion.
- Pelvic surgery.

RISK FACTORS

Many sexual partners; use of an intrauterine contraceptive device (IUD).

PREVENTING COMPLICATIONS OR RECURRENCE

Using rubber condoms helps to prevent sexually transmitted infections.

WHAT TO EXPECT

MEDICAL TESTS

- Your own observation of symptoms; medical history and physical exam by a doctor; laboratory blood studies and culture of the vaginal discharge; surgical diagnostic procedures, such as laparoscopy or culdocentesis (see Glossary).
- Special studies that may include ultrasonography, CAT or CT scan, MRI, and radionuclide scan (see Glossary for all).

POSSIBLE COMPLICATIONS

- Pelvic abscess and rupture. This can be life-threatening to your daughter.
- Adhesions (bands of scar tissue) inside the pelvis.
- Infertility.
- Blood poisoning.
- Thrombophlebitis (blood clots that break off and travel to the lungs).

PROBABLE OUTCOME

Usually curable with early treatment. Complications may be fatal to your daughter. The illness lasts from 1 to 6 weeks, depending on its severity.

TREATMENT

HOME CARE

Instructions for your daughter:

- Use heat to relieve pain:

— Place a heating pad or hot water bottle on your abdomen or back.

— Take frequent hot baths. This may reduce the bad odor of the vaginal discharge, as well as relax muscles and relieve discomfort. Sit in a tub of hot water for 10 to 15 minutes as often as needed.

- Use sanitary pads to absorb the discharge or menstrual flow.
- Don't douche during treatment.

MEDICATION

Your doctor may prescribe:

- Intravenous antibiotics to fight infection during hospitalization. Oral antibiotics may be necessary for about 1 month following hospitalization.
- Pain relievers.

ACTIVITY

Your daughter should avoid sexual intercourse until she is well. She should rest in bed until the fever subsides. She may have to sit and lie in different positions until she finds one that is comfortable. Allow 6 weeks for recovery.

DIET & FLUIDS

No special diet.

OK FOR SCHOOL, PRESCHOOL, OR NURSERY?

When signs of infection have decreased, appetite returns, and alertness, strength, and feeling of well-being will allow.

CALL YOUR DOCTOR IF

- Your daughter has symptoms of pelvic inflammatory disease.
- Symptoms recur after treatment.
- New, unexplained symptoms develop. Drugs used in treatment may produce side effects.

PERICARDITIS, ACUTE

GENERAL INFORMATION

DESCRIPTION

Acute pericarditis is inflammation of the pericardium (the thin membrane around the heart). This is not contagious or cancerous unless it is caused by the spread of cancer elsewhere. The pericardium, blood vessels, and sensory nerves are involved.

Appropriate health care includes:

- Physician's monitoring of general condition and medications.
- Surgery (sometimes) to remove fluid through a needle if fluid collects in the pericardium.
- Self-care after diagnosis.

SIGNS & SYMPTOMS

- Dull or sharp pain in the front of the chest, radiating to the neck and shoulder. The pain worsens with movement and eases when the child is sitting up or leaning forward.
- Rapid breathing.
- Cough.
- Fever and chills.
- Weakness.
- Anxiety.
- The most important signs are apparent only with medical examination: friction rub heard through a stethoscope, elevated white blood cell count, rapid sedimentation rate (see Glossary), and abnormal EKG (see Glossary).

CAUSES

Sometimes unknown. The most common known causes are:

- Viral infection.
- Rheumatic fever and other diseases of connective tissue, such as lupus erythematosus.
- Chronic kidney failure.
- Complication of a heart attack.
- Complication following heart surgery.
- Complication of a chest injury, including use of a cardiac catheter.
- Spread of cancer to the pericardium.

RISK FACTORS

- Recent illness, such as a heart attack, viral illness, or rheumatic fever.
- Medical history of tuberculosis.

PREVENTING COMPLICATIONS OR RECURRENCE

No specific preventive measures except medical treatment for your child for the disorders that cause pericarditis.

WHAT TO EXPECT

MEDICAL TESTS

- Your own observation of symptoms; medical history and physical exam by a doctor; EKG; chest X-ray.
- Thoracentesis (fluid removal with a needle). This procedure may be diagnostic or therapeutic.

POSSIBLE COMPLICATIONS

Fluid in the pericardium may cause pressure on your child's heart. This can be fatal unless fluid is removed quickly.

PROBABLE OUTCOME

Usually curable in 6 months unless the pericarditis is caused by cancer. After cure, there should be no functional disability in your child.

TREATMENT

HOME CARE

Apply a heating pad or warm compresses to the child's chest to relieve pain.

MEDICATION

- Your doctor may prescribe steroid drugs if your child's pericarditis is a complication of a heart attack, connective-tissue disease, or a metabolic disorder. No medication is needed if the pericarditis is caused by a virus.
- Use non-prescription drugs, such as acetaminophen, for minor pain.

ACTIVITY

Your child should rest in bed until the fever and pain subside. The child may read or watch TV and may resume normal activities gradually.

DIET & FLUIDS

No special diet.

OK FOR SCHOOL, PRESCHOOL, OR NURSERY?

When signs of infection have decreased, appetite returns, and alertness, strength, and feeling of well-being will allow.

CALL YOUR DOCTOR IF

- Your child has symptoms of pericarditis.
- The following occurs during treatment:
  - — Fever above 102F (38.9C).
  - — Shortness of breath and rapid heartbeat.
  - — Cough with blood.
  - — Unexplained weight loss.
  - — Pain not controlled by acetaminophen.
- New, unexplained symptoms develop. Steroids used in treatment may produce side effects, especially restlessness.

PERINEAL CONTUSION

GENERAL INFORMATION

DESCRIPTION

A perineum contusion results from a direct blow to the floor of the pelvis and associated structures including the genitals, causing bruising of the skin and underlying tissues. Contusions cause bleeding from ruptured small capillaries that allow blood to infiltrate muscles, tendons, nerves, or other soft tissue. The perineum, vaginal lips, mons pubis (pubic mound), vagina, anus, penis, scrotum, and testicles can be involved, as well as the skin, subcutaneous tissue, tendons, ligaments, blood vessels (both large vessels and capillaries), periosteum (the outside lining of bone), muscles, and connective tissue.

Appropriate health care includes:

- Doctor's care unless the injury is quite small.
- Self-care for minor contusions.

SIGNS & SYMPTOMS

- Swelling in the perineal area—either superficial or deep.
- Pain in the perineum.
- Feeling of firmness when pressure is exerted from outside.
- Tenderness.
- Discoloration under the skin, beginning with redness and progressing to characteristic "black and blue" discoloration.

CAUSES

- Direct blow to the perineum, usually by a blunt object or because of a fall.
- Damage to tiny blood vessels causing bleeding that infiltrates into the child's muscle and other surrounding tissue.

RISK FACTORS

Ice skating; gymnastics; cycling; horseback riding; medical history of any bleeding disorder, such as hemophilia; poor nutrition; inadequate protection of exposed areas during sports; obesity.

PREVENTING COMPLICATIONS OR RECURRENCE

Usually cannot be prevented.

WHAT TO EXPECT

MEDICAL TESTS

- Your own observation of symptoms.
- Medical history and physical exam by a doctor for all except minor injuries. The total extent of your child's injury may not be apparent for 48 to 72 hours.
- X-rays of the child's pelvis to assess total injury to perineal soft tissue and to rule out the possibility of underlying fracture.

POSSIBLE COMPLICATIONS

- Excessive bleeding leading to disability. Infiltrative type bleeding can (rarely) lead to calcification and impaired function of the child's injured muscle.
- Prolonged healing time if the child's usual activities are resumed too soon.
- Infection if the skin over the injury site was broken.
- Scarring and narrowing of the birth canal in females.

PROBABLE OUTCOME

Healing is usually complete in 1 to 4 weeks, depending on the extent of injury.

TREATMENT

FIRST AID

Use instructions for R.I.C.E., the first letters of *rest*, *ice*, *compression*, and *elevation* (if possible). See Appendix 39 for details.

HOME CARE

- Use an ice pack 3 or 4 times a day. Wrap ice chips or cubes in a plastic bag, and wrap the bag in a moist towel. Place it over the child's injured area for 20 minutes at a time.
- After 72 hours, apply heat instead of ice, if it feels better. Use heat lamps, hot soaks, hot showers, heating pads, or heat liniments or ointments.
- Provide the child with whirlpool treatments, if available.
- Protect the child's injured area with pads between treatments.

MEDICATION

- For minor discomfort, use non-prescription medicines such as acetaminophen or ibuprofen (available under many different brand names). Do not use aspirin for injuries involving bleeding.
- Your doctor may prescribe stronger medicine for pain, if needed.

ACTIVITY

Your child should begin activities slowly and stop exercise as soon as pain begins but may increase activity as healing progresses. Sexual activity should be delayed until healing is complete.

DIET & FLUIDS

Your child should eat a well-balanced diet that includes extra protein, such as meat, fish, poultry, cheese, milk, and eggs. Increasing fiber and fluid intake helps prevent constipation that may result from decreased activity.

OK FOR SCHOOL, PRESCHOOL, OR NURSERY?

Yes, when condition and sense of well-being will allow.

CALL YOUR DOCTOR IF

- The injured perineum doesn't improve within a day or two.
- Signs of infection (drainage from the skin, headache, muscle aches, dizziness, fever, or a general ill feeling) occur if the child's skin was broken.
- There is discomfort with sexual activity after healing.

PERITONITIS

GENERAL INFORMATION

DESCRIPTION

Peritonitis is a serious infection or inflammation of part or all of the peritoneum, the covering of the intestinal tract. The abdomen, including the intestines and peritoneum (a thin membrane that covers all the organs and walls of the abdomen), is involved.

Appropriate health care includes:

- Physician's monitoring of general condition and medications.
- Hospitalization.
- Surgery to repair the organ damage or the injury that allowed foreign material into your child's abdomen.
- Self-care after treatment.

SIGNS & SYMPTOMS

- Pain in one area or throughout the child's abdomen. Pain usually starts suddenly and becomes increasingly severe. Pain may be crampy at first, and then steady. The patient often prefers to lie quietly on the back because movement or pressure on the abdomen increases pain.
- Shoulder pain (sometimes).
- Chills and fever (often high).
- Dizziness and weakness.
- Rapid heartbeat.
- Low blood pressure.

CAUSES

Intense inflammation of the peritoneum lining that occurs when foreign material enters the abdominal cavity. Foreign material includes bacteria or gastrointestinal contents, such as digestive juices, blood, partly digested food, or feces. These materials can enter your child's abdomen after any of the following occurs:

- Rupture or perforation of any organ in the abdomen, such as an inflamed appendix, peptic ulcer, or infected diverticulum or gallbladder.
- Injury to the abdominal wall, such as from a knife or bullet wound.
- Pelvic inflammatory disease.
- Rupture of an ectopic pregnancy.

RISK FACTORS

- Delay in treatment of causes listed above.
- Recent abdominal surgery.

PREVENTING COMPLICATIONS OR RECURRENCE

Obtain prompt medical treatment for your child's underlying disorders.

WHAT TO EXPECT

MEDICAL TESTS

- Your own observation of symptoms.
- Medical history and physical exam by a doctor.
- Laboratory white blood cell count to detect inflammation, red blood cell count to detect bleeding, and measurement of fluid and electrolyte levels.
- Surgical diagnostic procedures, such as passing a small needle into the child's abdomen to obtain fluid, blood, or other material.
- Special studies that may include ultrasonography, CAT or CT scan, MRI, and radionuclide scan (see Glossary for all).

POSSIBLE COMPLICATIONS

Shock; blood poisoning (septicemia); intestinal obstruction caused by later adhesions (bands of scar tissue).

PROBABLE OUTCOME

Usually curable with early diagnosis and treatment. Treatment delay and complications can be fatal to your child.

TREATMENT

HOME CARE

Early diagnosis and treatment of the child's underlying disorder, such as appendicitis, ulcer, or ectopic pregnancy, are essential. If abdominal pain develops, don't waste valuable time with home treatments—especially laxative use. Laxatives may cause your child's inflamed abdominal organs to rupture.

MEDICATION

Your doctor may prescribe antibiotics to fight infection; pain relievers (sometimes) after diagnosis or surgery.

ACTIVITY

Your child should rest in bed after treatment until symptoms disappear. The child may read or watch TV. If surgery is necessary, normal activities may be resumed gradually after surgery.

DIET & FLUIDS

Your child should not eat or drink anything, so the intestinal tract can rest until the acute infection subsides. Intravenous nourishment and fluids will be given.

OK FOR SCHOOL, PRESCHOOL, OR NURSERY?

When signs of infection have decreased, appetite returns, and alertness, strength, and feeling of well-being will allow.

CALL YOUR DOCTOR IF

- Your child has symptoms of peritonitis. This is an emergency!
- The following occurs during treatment: constipation; signs of new infection, including fever, chills, muscle aches, dizziness, headache, and increasing abdominal pain.

PHARYNGITIS

GENERAL INFORMATION

DESCRIPTION

Pharyngitis is throat inflammation and infection from a variety of germs. The throat area, including the tonsils, is involved. Pharyngitis can affect both sexes, all ages, except during infancy.

Appropriate health care includes:

- Self-care after diagnosis.
- Physician's monitoring of general condition and medications.
- Hospitalization if the pharyngitis is caused by diphtheria or the hemophilus bacteria.

SIGNS & SYMPTOMS

- Sore throat.
- Swallowing difficulty.
- Tickle or "lump" in the child's throat.
- Fever.
- Swollen glands in the child's neck (sometimes).
- Throat may be red or covered with a grayish membrane (sometimes).
- Generalized aching.

CAUSES

Infection from bacteria, viruses, or fungi. Following are the most common germs.

- Bacteria—streptococci, diphtheria, gonococci, hemophilus, pneumococci, or staphylococci.
- Viruses—Epstein-Barr and many types of respiratory viruses.
- Fungi—monilia.

RISK FACTORS

- Illness that has lowered resistance.
- Fatigue or overwork.
- Diabetes mellitus.
- Immune deficiencies.
- Smoking.
- Excess alcohol consumption.
- Epidemics, during which all persons are at increased risk.

PREVENTING COMPLICATIONS OR RECURRENCE

- Urge your child to avoid contact with anyone with a sore throat.
- Keep your child's immunizations, including diphtheria, up to date. An immunization schedule appears in Appendix 1.

WHAT TO EXPECT

MEDICAL TESTS

- Your own observation of symptoms.
- Medical history and physical exam by a doctor.
- Laboratory throat culture and blood count.

POSSIBLE COMPLICATIONS

- Epiglottitis, leading to complete breathing obstruction.
- Pneumonia.
- Rheumatic fever, scarlet fever, or glomerulonephritis, if the child's pharyngitis is caused by strep bacteria and does not receive adequate antibiotic treatment.

PROBABLE OUTCOME

Spontaneous recovery for most cases of viral pharyngitis. Other cases are curable with antibiotic or anti-fungal drugs.

TREATMENT

HOME CARE

- Use gargles to relieve your child's throat pain. Prepare double-strength tea, hot or cold, or a salt-water solution (1 teaspoon salt in 8 ounces warm water). Use to gargle as often as your child wishes.
- Use a cool-mist humidifier to increase the air moisture around the child. This will relieve the dry, tight feeling in the child's throat.
- To reduce a high fever, or for fever in a child who has had a convulsion, see Appendix 17, How to Reduce Your Child's Fever.
- If the child's glands are large and tender, apply moist, warm soaks at least 4 times a day for 30 to 60 minutes. The compresses will be more effective if they are kept warm. Be careful not to burn the child's skin.

MEDICATION

- For minor discomfort, use non-prescription drugs such as acetaminophen. Don't give aspirin to a child for any viral illness. Studies link its use with the development of Reye's syndrome, a form of encephalitis.
- Your doctor may prescribe antibiotics or anti-fungal agents to fight bacterial or fungal infections.

ACTIVITY

Bed rest is necessary for your child until symptoms disappear. Reading or watching TV is acceptable.

DIET & FLUIDS

Extra fluids are necessary—at least 8 glasses of water daily, more for high fevers. If swallowing solid food is painful for your child, a liquid diet may be necessary.

OK FOR SCHOOL, PRESCHOOL, OR NURSERY?

When signs of infection have decreased, appetite returns, and alertness, strength, and feeling of well-being will allow.

CALL YOUR DOCTOR IF

- Your child has symptoms of pharyngitis.
- The following occurs during treatment: breathing or swallowing difficulty; fever (oral) over 102F (38.9C); severe headache; thick mucous drainage from the nose; cough that produces green, yellow, brown or bloody sputum; skin rash.

PICA

GENERAL INFORMATION

DESCRIPTION

Pica is eating bizarre substances that have no food value. The brain and gastrointestinal tract are involved. Pica can affect children between ages 1 and 6, and pregnant females. Pica does not apply to infants and children up to 18 months old who "put everything" in the mouth. That is normal.

Appropriate health care includes:

- Self-care after diagnosis.
- Physician's monitoring of general condition and medications.
- Psychotherapy or counseling.

SIGNS & SYMPTOMS

- Eating non-food substances, such as starch, clay, ice, plaster, paint, hair, or gravel.
- Abdominal pain (sometimes).

CAUSES

- Instinctive need to replace minerals absent in the diet. This is especially true of eating clay for iron content.
- Psychological factors that are not well-understood, related to substandard housing, low income, or emotional deprivation.

RISK FACTORS

- Family history of pica.
- Poor nutrition.
- Poverty.
- Mental retardation.

PREVENTING COMPLICATIONS OR RECURRENCE

- Remove substances from the reach of your child.
- Repaint homes in which lead-base paints have been used. Don't use older baby cribs painted with lead-base paint.
- Provide a well-balanced diet for yourself and your child.
- Provide a loving, supportive home environment for your child.

WHAT TO EXPECT

MEDICAL TESTS

- Your own observation of symptoms.
- Medical history and physical exam by a doctor.
- Laboratory blood studies to detect anemia and measure fluids and electrolytes.
- X-rays of the abdomen.

POSSIBLE COMPLICATIONS

- Lead poisoning from paint or plaster.
- Intestinal infections or parasites from soil.
- Anemia.
- Malnutrition.
- Intestinal obstruction.

PROBABLE OUTCOME

Pica during pregnancy usually ends with childbirth. Other forms can be controlled with treatment.

TREATMENT

HOME CARE

- Childproof your home by removing substances the child is eating.
- Examine your home environment and family interactions. If you feel they are not what they should be, seek ways to create a healthier atmosphere. Consult a counselor, if necessary.

MEDICATION

- Medicine usually is not necessary for this disorder.
- See Medications section for information regarding medicines your doctor may prescribe.

ACTIVITY

No restrictions.

DIET & FLUIDS

Provide a well-balanced diet for your child. Vitamin and mineral supplements may be necessary. If you need help planning meals, consult the home-extension service, a dietitian, or a visiting nurse.

OK FOR SCHOOL, PRESCHOOL, OR NURSERY?

Yes.

CALL YOUR DOCTOR IF

- Your child has symptoms of pica.
- You are pregnant and have symptoms of pica.
- Pica does not improve in 2 weeks, despite treatment.

PILONIDAL CYST

GENERAL INFORMATION

DESCRIPTION

A pilonidal cyst is a small, hair-containing skin sac at the base of the spine. The cyst looks like a small opening—sometimes no more than a dimple—with a few hairs protruding (sometimes). The skin and hair follicles are involved. It is prone to infection. Pilonidal cysts are uncommon in black people. Pilonidal cysts can affect both sexes but are more common in males. Cyst infections usually begin in young adulthood.

Appropriate health care includes:

- Self-care after diagnosis.
- Physician's monitoring of general condition and medications.
- Surgery to remove the cyst, if it repeatedly becomes infected.

SIGNS & SYMPTOMS

No symptoms when not infected. When infected, it causes:

- Pain, redness, tenderness, and swelling in the area.
- Fever and chills.
- Discharge of pus.

CAUSES

A pilonidal cyst is a minor abnormality that occurs during fetal development. Infection is usually caused by staphylococcal bacteria.

RISK FACTORS

- Heavy perspiration. Obesity increases perspiration.
- Tight clothing.

PREVENTING COMPLICATIONS OR RECURRENCE

- Urge your child to bathe or shower daily to keep the area clean. Hot tub baths seem more effective in preventing infection of the cyst.
- Encourage your child to wear light, loose-fitting clothing.
- Help your child avoid becoming overweight.

WHAT TO EXPECT

MEDICAL TESTS

- Your own observation of symptoms.
- Medical history and physical exam by a doctor.
- Laboratory culture of the discharge.

POSSIBLE COMPLICATIONS

Spread of infection (rare).

PROBABLE OUTCOME

Curable with antibiotic treatment.

TREATMENT

HOME CARE

If the cyst is infected, the child should take warm baths to relieve pain. Encourage your child to sit in a tub of warm water for 10 to 15 minutes as often as it feels good.

MEDICATION

- Your doctor may prescribe antibiotics to fight infection.
- See Medications section for information regarding medicines your doctor may prescribe.

ACTIVITY

No restrictions, unless the cyst becomes infected. Then, limit the child's activities until the infection is cured.

DIET & FLUIDS

Losing weight is beneficial if your child is overweight. A reducing diet appears in Appendix 31.

OK FOR SCHOOL, PRESCHOOL, OR NURSERY?

Yes, after surgery has healed and appetite has returned and alertness, strength, and feeling of well-being will allow.

CALL YOUR DOCTOR IF

- Your child has symptoms of a pilonidal cyst. It should be diagnosed.
- After diagnosis, your child's cyst shows signs of infection.

PINWORMS
(Enterobiasis; Seatworm; Threadworm; Oxyuriasis)

GENERAL INFORMATION

DESCRIPTION

Pinworms are intestinal parasites. Pinworm infestations are a common occurrence in children. They are more a nuisance than a major health problem. The cecum (the pouchlike beginning of the large intestine on the right side to which the appendix is attached), large intestine, anus, and skin around the anus are involved. Pinworms can affect both sexes, all ages, but is most common in children of elementary school age.

Appropriate health care includes:

- Home care after diagnosis.
- Physician's monitoring of general condition and medications.

SIGNS & SYMPTOMS

- Skin irritation and painful itching around your child's anus.
- Restless sleep.
- Vaginal discharge, itching, and discomfort if pinworms migrate into the vaginal opening.
- Poor appetite and stomach pain (sometimes).
- Paleness (sometimes).

CAUSES

- Infestation of the cecum by a very small worm (oxyuria) that measures only 10mm in its adult form.
- Pinworms travel from the cecum to the rectum to lay eggs around the anus and buttocks. The tiny eggs are picked up on the fingers by scratching.
- Eggs are transferred to others on toilet seats or by hand-to-hand or hand-to-mouth contact. They also drift in the air, where they are inhaled or swallowed.
- Eggs hatch in the small intestine. The larvae travel to the cecum, where they mature, mate and repeat the cycle.

RISK FACTORS

Groups of children, as in schools or large families; poor personal hygiene; dishwashing water that is not hot enough to kill eggs.

PREVENTING COMPLICATIONS OR RECURRENCE

- Teach your child to wash hands carefully after using the toilet and before meals.
- Keep the child's nails short and clean.
- Urge the child to wash the anus and genitals at least once a day, rinsing well, preferably under a shower.
- Have your child wear snug cotton underpants day and night, and change them daily.
- Encourage the child not to scratch the anus or put fingers near the nose or mouth.
- Use very hot water to wash dishes.

WHAT TO EXPECT

MEDICAL TESTS

Your own observation of symptoms; medical history and physical exam by a doctor; microscopic study of the worms or eggs.

POSSIBLE COMPLICATIONS

No serious complications expected.

PROBABLE OUTCOME

- Usually curable in one treatment—two treatments at the most. Treatment should include all family members at once. Recurrence is common.
- If worms reappear soon after treatment, they usually represent a new infection—not treatment failure.

TREATMENT

HOME CARE

The following should be done on the day the family is treated with medicine:

- Clean the house with extra care. Wash the sheets and clothing with extra bleach or ammonia, or boil them.
- Scrub washable toys. Sterilize metal toys and similar objects in a hot oven.
- Cut and clean your fingernails and your child's.
- Change towels.
- Scrub toilet bowls.
- Take extra-long showers.

About 2 weeks after treatment, your doctor will probably check your child to be sure all parasites have been destroyed.

MEDICATION

Your doctor may prescribe anti-worm medicine. Follow directions carefully. Give your child the medicine on an empty stomach. The medicine may cause nausea, vomiting, and diarrhea. It is not absorbed by the stomach or intestines, so the bowel movement following treatment will probably be the color of the medicine.

ACTIVITY

No restrictions.

DIET & FLUIDS

No special diet.

OK FOR SCHOOL, PRESCHOOL, OR NURSERY?

Yes.

CALL YOUR DOCTOR IF

- Your child has symptoms of pinworms.
- Pinworms reappear after treatment.
- You think medicine is causing side effects that don't disappear quickly.

PITUITARY GLAND, UNDERACTIVE (Hypopituitarism)

GENERAL INFORMATION

DESCRIPTION

Underactivity of the pituitary gland results in inadequate amounts of hormones produced by the pituitary. The anterior lobe of the pituitary produces the following hormones: a growth hormone; prolactin, which stimulates the breasts to produce milk; a thyroid-stimulating hormone; an adrenal-stimulating hormone; ovarian- or testicular-stimulating hormones. The posterior lobe of the pituitary gland produces two hormones: an anti-diuretic hormone, which affects the kidneys in regulating the concentration and quantity of urine, and oxytocin, which stimulates contractions of the uterus during childbirth and releases milk during breast-feeding.

Appropriate health care includes:

- Physician's monitoring of general condition and medications. This requires close supervision and continuing treatment.
- Surgery to remove underlying tumors or blood clots, if necessary.

SIGNS & SYMPTOMS

- Menstrual irregularities.
- Infertility.
- Low blood sugar and weakness.
- Retarded growth in children (evident after 6 months of age).
- Lack of secondary sexual features that develop in puberty, such as voice changes, breast development, and growth of pubic hair.
- Mental changes, including psychosis.
- Extreme lethargy.
- Persistent headaches.
- Impotence.

CAUSES

- Unknown (sometimes).
- Serious head injury with pressure (usually from bleeding) on the pituitary gland.
- Reduced blood supply to the pituitary gland in a mother following severe hemorrhage and shock during childbirth.
- Tumor of the pituitary gland.
- Infection in the child's brain.
- Aneurysm of blood vessels in the base of the child's brain.

RISK FACTORS

- Family history of pituitary disorders.
- Pregnancy.

PREVENTING COMPLICATIONS OR RECURRENCE

Obtain medical treatment for your child for the underlying injury, infection, or tumor, if possible.

PITUITARY GLAND, UNDERACTIVE (Hypopituitarism)

WHAT TO EXPECT

MEDICAL TESTS
- Your own observation of symptoms.
- Medical history and physical exam by a doctor.
- Laboratory blood studies of hormone levels and function.
- CAT scan (see Glossary) of the head.

POSSIBLE COMPLICATIONS
Hormonal failure and death without treatment.

PROBABLE OUTCOME
Usually curable with surgery or replacement therapy of pituitary, thyroid, adrenal, and sex hormones.

TREATMENT

HOME CARE
No specific instructions except those listed under other headings.

MEDICATION
Your doctor may prescribe:
- Hormones to replace those the child's pituitary is not producing.
- Pain relievers after your child's surgery.
- Antibiotics or anti-viral medications, if infection is causing the child's disorder.
- See Medications section for information regarding medicines your doctor may prescribe.

ACTIVITY
Your child should stay as active as the condition allows.

DIET & FLUIDS
No special diet.

OK FOR SCHOOL, PRESCHOOL, OR NURSERY?
Yes, when appetite has returned and alertness, strength, and feeling of well-being will allow.

CALL YOUR DOCTOR IF

- Your child has symptoms of an underactive pituitary gland.
- After surgery, your child develops signs of infections, such as fever, lethargy, and muscle aches.
- New, unexplained symptoms develop. Drugs used in treatment may produce side effects.

PITUITARY TUMOR

GENERAL INFORMATION

DESCRIPTION

A pituitary tumor is an abnormal growth in the pituitary gland. Pituitary tumors may be benign or malignant—but even malignant pituitary tumors rarely spread to other body parts. The pituitary gland (which is located at the base of the brain) and adjacent structures are involved. Because of changing functions due to a pituitary tumor, all parts of the endocrine system eventually become involved. Appropriate health care includes:

- Physician's monitoring of general condition and medications.
- Surgery to remove the tumor, cryohypophysectomy (freezing the tumor with liquid nitrogen), or surgery to implant tiny radioactive pellets in the tumor.
- Postoperative radiation therapy.
- Self-care after surgery and radiation.

SIGNS & SYMPTOMS

- Blurred vision, double vision, dizziness, or a drooping eyelid caused by tumor pressure on nerves to the eye.
- Headache in the forehead.
- Nausea and vomiting.
- Seizures.
- Runny nose.
- Excessive thirst.
- Menstrual changes.
- Unexplained weight gain.
- Retarded or excessive growth in your child.
- Low blood sugar.
- Low blood pressure.
- Symptoms of abnormalities in other endocrine glands. See Hyperparathyroidism, Cushing's Syndrome, and Ovarian Tumor (all in Illnesses section).

CAUSES

Unknown, but it may be caused by a dominant genetic trait.

RISK FACTORS

Unknown.

PREVENTING COMPLICATIONS OR RECURRENCE

No specific preventive measures.

WHAT TO EXPECT

MEDICAL TESTS

- Your own observation of symptoms.
- Medical history and physical exam by a doctor.
- Laboratory studies of cerebrospinal fluid and blood.
- X-rays of the skull.
- Special studies that may include ultrasonography, CAT or CT scan, MRI, and radionuclide scan (see Glossary for all).

POSSIBLE COMPLICATIONS

The following complications may diminish or be reversed after surgery:

- Blindness.
- Loss of sense of smell.
- Extreme hormone imbalance.

PROBABLE OUTCOME

Curable with surgery if your child's tumor has not spread from the pituitary gland. If it has, fatal complications usually develop.

TREATMENT

HOME CARE

No specific instructions except those listed under other headings.

MEDICATION

Your doctor may prescribe:

- Pain relievers.
- Hormone replacement medication for life. This may require frequent dosage adjustments.
- Anti-cancer drugs.
- See Medications section for information regarding medicines your doctor may prescribe.

ACTIVITY

Your child can resume normal activities gradually after surgery.

DIET & FLUIDS

No special diet.

OK FOR SCHOOL, PRESCHOOL, OR NURSERY?

When effects of surgery have healed and when appetite has returned and alertness, strength, and feeling of well-being will allow.

CALL YOUR DOCTOR IF

- Your child has symptoms of a pituitary tumor.
- The following occurs after surgery:
  - — Bleeding at the surgical site.
  - — Signs of general infections, such as fever, chills, muscle aches, and headache.
  - — Clear discharge from the child's nose.

PITYRIASIS ALBA

GENERAL INFORMATION

DESCRIPTION

Pityriasis alba is a benign disorder of the skin in which the child's skin temporarily loses pigmentation in patches. The skin of the cheeks and arms is involved. Pityriasis alba occurs most in children but may occur up to age 25. Appropriate health care includes:

- Self-care after diagnosis.
- Physician's monitoring of general condition and medications.

SIGNS & SYMPTOMS

Skin lesions with the following characteristics:

- The lesions are small white patches with vague borders. They sometimes have pinpoint-sized white papules (small, raised bumps).
- The patches are most apparent in summer because the lesions cannot tan, and tanning heightens the contrast between the areas.
- A child may have 1 to 12 patches at a time.
- The patches feel smooth.
- The patches may itch the child occasionally, but they are not painful.

CAUSES

Unknown. The tendency may be inherited.

RISK FACTORS

Family history of allergies of any kind.

PREVENTING COMPLICATIONS OR RECURRENCE

No specific preventive measures.

WHAT TO EXPECT

MEDICAL TESTS

- Your own observation of symptoms.
- Medical history and physical exam by a doctor.

POSSIBLE COMPLICATIONS

None expected.

PROBABLE OUTCOME

Your child's patches may come and go for years. Between ages 20 and 30 they disappear completely.

TREATMENT

HOME CARE

- Apply prescribed topical steroids to your child's patches only once or twice a day unless directed otherwise. Apply immediately after bathing for better spreading and penetration. For the child's face, use only low-potency steroid products without fluorine. Apply a thin layer; a heavy layer wastes medicine and is no more beneficial to the child than a thin layer. Rub in gently for several minutes until the cream disappears.
- Use sunscreen or protective clothing on your child to prevent sunburn in affected areas.

MEDICATION

- Your doctor may prescribe prescription or non-prescription topical steroid medicine to control your child's itching and to prevent papules.
- See Medications section for information regarding medicines your doctor may prescribe.

ACTIVITY

No restrictions.

DIET & FLUIDS

No special diet.

OK FOR SCHOOL, PRESCHOOL, OR NURSERY?

Yes.

CALL YOUR DOCTOR IF

- Your child has symptoms of pityriasis alba.
- New, unexplained symptoms develop. Drugs used in treatment may produce side effects.

PITYRIASIS ROSEA

GENERAL INFORMATION

DESCRIPTION

Pityriasis rosea is a non-contagious inflammatory skin disorder with a faint rash that lasts 3 to 4 weeks. The skin, especially of the chest and abdomen, is involved. Pityriasis rosea can affect both sexes, all ages, but is most common in adolescents and young adults.

Appropriate health care includes:

- Self-care after diagnosis.
- Physician's monitoring of general condition and medications.

SIGNS & SYMPTOMS

- A faint rash—often found in skin creases—of oval or round, pale-pink or brown areas. One larger patch (the "herald patch") may appear first.
- Mild fatigue.
- Itching, usually mild.
- Occasional slight fever and headache.

CAUSES

Unknown, but may be caused by a virus or autoimmune disorder.

RISK FACTORS

Fall and spring seasons.

PREVENTING COMPLICATIONS OR RECURRENCE

Cannot be prevented at present.

WHAT TO EXPECT

MEDICAL TESTS

- Your own observation of symptoms.
- Medical history and physical exam by a doctor to rule out other disorders.

POSSIBLE COMPLICATIONS

Secondary bacterial infection of the rash area.

PROBABLE OUTCOME

- Pityriasis rosea usually runs its natural course in 5 weeks to 4 months. No medication or treatment is available to shorten its course, but your child's itching and discomfort can be relieved.
- The skin eruptions won't leave scars on the child unless complicated by a secondary infection. New rash areas continue to break out for several weeks. Once over, one episode seems to confer lifelong immunity.
- Although pityriasis is probably caused by an infectious agent, it is not contagious. Even close family contacts are unlikely to develop the disease.

TREATMENT

HOME CARE

- Your child should bathe as usual with a mild soap. You don't need to sterilize the tub or shower after the child bathes.
- Your child should expose the skin to moderate amounts of sunlight. This may decrease the rash.

MEDICATION

For minor discomfort, use non-prescription drugs, such as:

- Calamine lotion to decrease your child's itching.
- Acetaminophen to reduce fever.
- See Medications section for information regarding medicines your doctor may prescribe.

ACTIVITY

Usually no restrictions. Your child should be as active as strength allows.

DIET & FLUIDS

No special diet.

OK FOR SCHOOL, PRESCHOOL, OR NURSERY?

When signs of infection have decreased, appetite returns, and alertness, strength, and feeling of well-being will allow.

CALL YOUR DOCTOR IF

- Your child has symptoms of pityriasis rosea.
- The following occurs during treatment:
  — Fever over 101F (38.3C).
  — Signs of infection (warmth, redness, tenderness, pain, and swelling) in the rash area.

PITYRIASIS VERSICOLOR
(Tinea Versicolor)

GENERAL INFORMATION

DESCRIPTION

Pityriasis versicolor is a yeast infection of the skin that changes the color of the skin it affects. The skin of the chest, back, shoulders, upper arms, trunk, or groin is involved. This infection rarely affects the face. Pityriasis versicolor seldom affects children prior to adolescence.

Appropriate health care includes:

- Physician's monitoring of general condition and medications.
- Self-care after diagnosis.

SIGNS & SYMPTOMS

Lesions on your child with the following characteristics:

- Lesions on exposed skin are white; on covered areas, they are brown or brownish red.
- Lesions are flat with clearly defined borders. They don't scale unless scraped.
- Lesions begin at 3 to 4mm in diameter and spread. They often join together to form large patches.

CAUSES

A developing stage of the yeast, pityrosborum orbiculare. High heat and high humidity favor the growth of this yeast. The infection is contagious, but how it spreads is unknown.

RISK FACTORS

Environmental exposure to heat and high humidity.

PREVENTING COMPLICATIONS OR RECURRENCE

No specific preventive measures.

WHAT TO EXPECT

MEDICAL TESTS

- Your own observation of symptoms.
- Medical history and physical exam by a doctor.
- Laboratory culture of scrapings for positive diagnosis.

POSSIBLE COMPLICATIONS

Unlimited recurrence without treatment.

PROBABLE OUTCOME

Untreated pityriasis versicolor persists indefinitely but seems to come and go at times. It frequently recurs, even with treatment. Following treatment, the white patches will remain on your child for months after the yeast infection has been cured.

PITYRIASIS VERSICOLOR
(Tinea Versicolor)

TREATMENT

HOME CARE

Instructions for your child:

- Apply prescribed medicine with cotton balls to affected parts once a day for 3 weeks. Rinse off in 30 minutes if you wish.
- Expose affected skin to air as much as possible.
- Repeat treatment prior to the tanning season each year.

MEDICATION

- Your doctor may prescribe selenium sulfide shampoo (Exgel and Selsun) or other anti-fungal medication to apply to affected areas.
- See Medications section for information regarding medicines your doctor may prescribe.

ACTIVITY

No restrictions.

DIET & FLUIDS

No special diet.

OK FOR SCHOOL, PRESCHOOL, OR NURSERY?

Yes.

CALL YOUR DOCTOR IF

- Your child has symptoms of pityriasis versicolor.
- Infection doesn't improve despite treatment.

PLEURISY

GENERAL INFORMATION

DESCRIPTION

Pleurisy is inflammation and irritation of the pleura, a thin two-layered membrane that encloses the lung and lines the inside of the chest. The pleura, blood vessels, sensory nerves, and the diaphragm are involved.

Appropriate health care includes:
- Self-care after diagnosis.
- Physician's monitoring of general condition and medications.

SIGNS & SYMPTOMS

- Sudden chest pain that worsens with breathing and coughing. The pain varies from vague discomfort that occurs only with deep breathing or coughing to intense, stabbing pain. The pain is usually over the area of the pleura, but it may also occur in the lower chest or abdomen.
- Fever.
- Discomfort on moving the affected side.
- Rapid, shallow breathing.

If fluid develops at the site of inflammation between the two membrane layers, the liquid is called pleural effusion. When this happens, the pleurisy pain usually subsides, but breathlessness worsens.

CAUSES

Complication of:
- Lung or chest infections, such as pneumonia or tuberculosis.
- Bronchiectasis.
- Collapse of part of the lung.
- Blood clot in the lung.
- Injury to the chest or rib fracture.
- Cancer in other parts of the body.
- Collagen vascular disease, such as systemic lupus erythematosus or rheumatoid arthritis.
- Congestive heart failure.
- Kidney disorders.
- Liver disorders.

RISK FACTORS

Obesity; smoking; use of immunosuppressive drugs.

PREVENTING COMPLICATIONS OR RECURRENCE

Obtain medical treatment for the child's underlying disorder.

WHAT TO EXPECT

MEDICAL TESTS

- Your own observation of symptoms.
- Medical history and physical exam by a doctor.
- Laboratory blood studies to detect infection or autoimmune disease.
- X-rays of the chest.

POSSIBLE COMPLICATIONS

- Pneumonia.
- Lung compression and impaired breathing from leakage of pleural effusion.
- Scarring and adhesions at the site of inflammation, restricting lung expansion.

PROBABLE OUTCOME

Successful treatment of your child's pleurisy depends on successful treatment of the disorder causing it. Often, symptoms without complications clear completely and spontaneously in 2 weeks.

TREATMENT

HOME CARE

- For your child's chest pain, wrap the entire chest loosely with 2 or 3 non-adhesive, 6-inch-wide elastic bandages.
- For your child's coughing, use a cool-mist humidifier to help loosen bronchial secretions so they can be coughed up easily.

MEDICATION

- Your doctor may prescribe antibiotics or pain relievers after diagnosis of the child's underlying disorder. You may give your child simple pain relievers, such as acetaminophen or aspirin, to relieve pain if no complicating disorders exist.
- See Medications section for information regarding medicines your doctor may prescribe.

ACTIVITY

Your child should reduce activity until the pain and fever disappear. Then the child can resume normal activities gradually.

DIET & FLUIDS

No special diet.

OK FOR SCHOOL, PRESCHOOL, OR NURSERY?

When signs of infection have decreased, appetite returns, and alertness, strength, and feeling of well-being will allow.

CALL YOUR DOCTOR IF

- Your child has symptoms of pleurisy.
- The following occurs during treatment:
  - — Temperature spikes (rises suddenly) to over 101F (38.3C).
  - — Increased pain.
  - — Increased breathlessness.
  - — Cough that is dry and non-productive.
  - — Blue or dark fingernails, toenails, or lips.
  - — Blood in the sputum.

PNEUMONIA, BACTERIAL

GENERAL INFORMATION

DESCRIPTION

Bacterial pneumonia is an infection and inflammation of the lungs with bacterial germs. This is not usually contagious. The lungs and bronchial tubes are involved. Pneumonia can affect both sexes, all ages, but is most severe in young children.

Appropriate health care includes:

- Self-care after diagnosis.
- Physician's monitoring of general condition and medications.
- Hospitalization (severe cases only).

SIGNS & SYMPTOMS

- High fever (over 102F or 38.9C) and chills.
- Shortness of breath.
- Cough with sputum that may contain blood or blood streaks.
- Rapid breathing.
- Chest pain that worsens with inhalations.
- Abdominal pain.
- Fatigue.
- Bluish lips and nails (rare).

CAUSES

Infection with bacteria, such as pneumococci, hemophilus, streptococci, or staphylococci.

RISK FACTORS

- Being a newborn or infant.
- Use of anti-cancer drugs.
- Smoking.
- Illness that has lowered your child's resistance, such as heart disease, recent surgery, cancer, tuberculosis, congestive heart failure, diabetes, alcoholism, or chronic lung disease.
- Poor general health from any cause.
- Crowded or unsanitary living conditions.

PREVENTING COMPLICATIONS OR RECURRENCE

- Obtain prompt medical treatment for your child's respiratory infections.
- Arrange for pneumococcal and influenza immunizations of a child at risk.

WHAT TO EXPECT

MEDICAL TESTS

- Your own observation of symptoms.
- Medical history and physical exam by a doctor.
- Laboratory studies, such as a sputum culture, blood culture, and blood count.
- X-rays of lungs.

POSSIBLE COMPLICATIONS

- Pleurisy.
- Pleural effusion (fluid between the membranes that cover the lung).
- Spread of infection to the brain or meninges (meningitis).

PROBABLE OUTCOME

Usually curable in 1 to 2 weeks with treatment, but may take longer for the very young (or the elderly).

TREATMENT

HOME CARE

- Use a cool-mist humidifier to increase air moisture around the child. Putting medicine in the humidifier probably will not help.
- Don't suppress the child's cough with medicine if the cough produces sputum or mucus. It is useful in ridding the body of lung secretions.
- Suppress the child's cough with medicine if it is dry, non-productive, and painful. Consult your doctor about a cough suppressant.
- Use a heating pad or hot compresses to relieve the child's chest pain.

MEDICATION

- Your doctor may prescribe antibiotics to fight your child's infection.
- Use non-prescription drugs, such as acetaminophen, to relieve minor discomfort.
- See Medications section for information regarding medicines your doctor may prescribe.

ACTIVITY

Your child should rest in bed until fever declines and pain and shortness of breath disappear. Your child may read or watch TV and, after treatment, may resume normal activity as soon as possible.

DIET & FLUIDS

No special diet. Urge your child to increase fluid intake; drinking at least 1 glass of water or other beverage every hour is beneficial. Extra fluid helps thin lung secretions so they are easier to cough up.

OK FOR SCHOOL, PRESCHOOL, OR NURSERY?

When signs of infection have decreased, appetite returns, and alertness, strength, and feeling of well-being will allow.

CALL YOUR DOCTOR IF

- Your child has symptoms of pneumonia.
- The following occurs during treatment: fever higher than 102F (38.9C); pain not relieved by heat or prescribed medication; increased shortness of breath; dark or bluish fingernails, skin, or toenails; blood in the sputum; nausea, vomiting, or diarrhea.
- New, unexplained symptoms develop. Drugs used in treatment may produce side effects.

PNEUMONIA, MYCOPLASMA (Primary Atypical Pneumonia; Eaton-Agent Pneumonia)

GENERAL INFORMATION

DESCRIPTION

Mycoplasma pneumonia is a contagious lung inflammation caused by mycoplasma germ. This germ can cause infection in other body parts. The respiratory system—including the nose, sinuses, pharynx, trachea, bronchial tubes, and lungs—is involved. Mycoplasma pneumonia can affect both sexes, all ages, but is most common in children (1 to 12 years).

Appropriate health care includes:

- Home care after diagnosis.
- Physician's monitoring of general condition and medications.
- Hospitalization of a seriously ill child.

SIGNS & SYMPTOMS

- Cough (with or without sputum).
- Fever.
- Labored breathing.
- Chest pain.
- Abdominal pain.
- Bluish skin (severe cases).

CAUSES

Preceding mycoplasma infection in the nose, throat, or bronchial tubes.

RISK FACTORS

- Stress.
- Illness that has lowered your child's resistance.
- Exposure to cold, harsh weather.
- Crowded or unsanitary living conditions.

PREVENTING COMPLICATIONS OR RECURRENCE

- Your child should avoid exposure to persons who are ill with respiratory infections.
- Your child should not get chilled or wet in cold weather.

WHAT TO EXPECT

MEDICAL TESTS

- Your own observation of symptoms.
- Medical history and physical exam by a doctor.
- Laboratory culture of sputum and blood studies.
- Chest and lung X-rays.

POSSIBLE COMPLICATIONS

Prolonged illness.

PROBABLE OUTCOME

This form of pneumonia is characteristically slow to heal. It is usually curable in 4 to 6 weeks with treatment. Your child's lungs should not have residual scars.

PNEUMONIA, MYCOPLASMA (Primary Atypical Pneumonia; Eaton-Agent Pneumonia)

TREATMENT

HOME CARE

- Use a cool-mist humidifier to increase air moisture around your child. Putting medicine in the humidifier probably will not help.
- Don't suppress the child's cough with medicine if it produces sputum or mucus. Coughing is useful in ridding the body of lung secretions.
- Suppress the child's cough with medicine it if it dry, non-productive, and painful. Consult your doctor about a cough suppressant.
- Use a heating pad on low heat or hot compresses to relieve the child's chest pain.
- Urge your child to catch sneezes and coughs with disposable tissue.

MEDICATION

Your doctor may prescribe:

- Antibiotics, such as erythromycin, to fight your child's infection.
- Cough medicine to make the cough more tolerable.
- Nose drops, sprays, or oral decongestants to reduce congestion in the child's upper-respiratory system.
- See Medications section for information regarding medicines your doctor may prescribe.

ACTIVITY

Bed rest is necessary for your child until fever subsides. Normal activities should be resumed gradually.

DIET & FLUIDS

No special diet. Your child should increase fluids to at least 1 glass of water or other beverage every hour. Extra fluid helps thin lung secretions so they can be coughed up more easily.

OK FOR SCHOOL, PRESCHOOL, OR NURSERY?

When signs of infection have decreased, appetite returns, and alertness, strength, and feeling of well-being will allow.

CALL YOUR DOCTOR IF

- Your child has symptoms of mycoplasma pneumonia.
- The following occurs during treatment:
  - — Fever higher than 102F (38.9C).
  - — Pain that is not relieved by heat or prescribed medication.
  - — Increased shortness of breath.
  - — Dark or bluish fingernails, skin, or toenails.
  - — Blood in the sputum.
  - — Nausea, vomiting, or diarrhea.
- New, unexplained symptoms develop. Drugs used in treatment may produce side effects.

PNEUMONIA, VIRAL

GENERAL INFORMATION

DESCRIPTION

Viral pneumonia is a lung infection caused by a virus. It is unlikely that others will develop pneumonia from exposure to a child with viral pneumonia. The lower respiratory tract (bronchial tubes, bronchioles, and lungs) and the upper respiratory tract (nose, throat, tonsils, sinuses, trachea, and larynx) are involved. Appropriate health care includes:

- Self-care after diagnosis.
- Physician's monitoring of general condition and medications.
- Hospitalization (rare).

SIGNS & SYMPTOMS

- Fever and chills.
- Muscle aches and fatigue.
- Cough, with or without sputum or "croup."
- Rapid, labored (sometimes) breathing.
- Chest pain.
- Sore throat.
- Loss of appetite.
- Enlarged lymph glands in the neck.
- Bluish nails.

CAUSES

Virus infections, including influenza, chickenpox (especially in adults), respiratory viruses, measles, and cytomegalovirus (especially in infants).

RISK FACTORS

- Infancy.
- Asthma.
- Cystic fibrosis.
- Inhalation of a foreign body into the lung.
- Smoking.
- Crowded or unsanitary living conditions.

PREVENTING COMPLICATIONS OR RECURRENCE

No specific preventive measures.

WHAT TO EXPECT

MEDICAL TESTS

- Your own observation of symptoms.
- Medical history and physical exam by a doctor.
- Laboratory blood studies.
- X-rays of the chest and lungs.

POSSIBLE COMPLICATIONS

- Secondary bacterial infections of the lungs.
- Post-infectious depression.

PROBABLE OUTCOME

Usually curable in 4 weeks.

TREATMENT

HOME CARE

- Use a cool-mist humidifier to increase air moisture around your child. Putting medicine in the vaporizer probably will not help.
- Use a heating pad on the child's chest to relieve chest pain.

MEDICATION

- If the cough produces sputum, it is ridding the child's lungs of secretions and should not be suppressed with medicine. If the cough is dry, non-productive and painful, you may suppress it with non-prescription cough medicine that contains dextromethorphan.
- For minor pain and fever, use non-prescription drugs, such as acetaminophen or decongestant nose drops, nasal sprays, or tablets. Avoid aspirin to decrease the possibility of Reye's syndrome.
- Your doctor may prescribe antibiotics to fight secondary bacterial infections.
- See Medications section for information regarding medicines your doctor may prescribe.

ACTIVITY

Bed rest is necessary for your child until fever, pain, and shortness of breath have been gone at least 48 hours. Then normal activity may be resumed slowly. Many children are fatigued and weak for up to 6 weeks after recovery, so don't expect a quick return to normal strength.

DIET & FLUIDS

No special diet, but do everything possible to encourage your child to maintain a normal intake of nutritious foods and drinks. Extra fluids help thin lung secretions so they are easier to cough up.

OK FOR SCHOOL, PRESCHOOL, OR NURSERY?

When signs of infection have decreased, appetite returns, and alertness, strength, and feeling of well-being will allow.

CALL YOUR DOCTOR IF

- Your child has symptoms of pneumonia.
- The following occurs during treatment:
  - — Temperature spikes (rises suddenly) to over 102F (38.9C).
  - — Intolerable pain, despite medication and heat treatment.
  - — Increasing shortness of breath.
  - — Increasing blueness of nails and skin.
  - — Blood in the sputum.
  - — Nausea, vomiting, or diarrhea.

PNEUMOTHORAX

GENERAL INFORMATION

DESCRIPTION

Pneumothorax is collapse of part or all of a lung caused by pressure from free air in the chest between the two layers of the pleura (thin membranes that cover the lung). The lung, pleura, blood vessels, and sensory nerves are involved. Pneumothorax can affect both sexes, all ages, but is most common in active young men.

Appropriate health care includes:

- Self-care after diagnosis.
- Physician's monitoring of general condition and medications.
- Hospitalization, if the extent of lung collapse is disabling.

SIGNS & SYMPTOMS

The following symptoms vary according to the degree of lung collapse and extent of underlying lung disease. Symptoms may be less acute if the child's pneumothorax develops slowly:

- Sharp chest pain. Pain may extend to a shoulder or across the chest or abdomen.
- Shortness of breath.
- Dry, hacking cough (occasionally).

CAUSES

Spontaneous pneumothorax:

- Rupture of a small air sac in the child's lung resulting from asthma, lung abscess or empyema, or physical exertion, such as diving, high-altitude flying, or stretching. Causes related to activity occur most often in healthy children (and young adults).

Pneumothorax due to trauma:

- Penetrating wounds to the chest, which permit outside air to rush into the pleural space and cause the lung to collapse.
- Complication of removing fluid from the lung (thoracentesis).

RISK FACTORS

- Chest injury.
- Chronic lung disease.
- Smoking.

PREVENTING COMPLICATIONS OR RECURRENCE

- Obtain medical treatment for your child's lung disorders, such as asthma or emphysema.
- Urge your child not to smoke.

WHAT TO EXPECT

MEDICAL TESTS

- Your own observation of symptoms.
- Medical history and physical exam by a doctor.
- X-rays of the chest and lungs to confirm the diagnosis.

POSSIBLE COMPLICATIONS

- Respiratory failure.
- Lung infection.

PROBABLE OUTCOME

- A small pneumothorax is inconsequential and heals itself. However, if the collapse is extensive and the child's lungs have been damaged by any previous lung trouble, it can lead to respiratory failure and critical illness.
- Treatment depends on the size of the pneumothorax and the condition of the child's lung. The disorder may heal itself, but hospitalization and treatment may be necessary to remove the air.

TREATMENT

HOME CARE

Instructions for your child:

- Don't smoke.
- Try not to cough.
- Avoid loud talking, laughing, or singing.
- You may be more comfortable if you rest in a sitting position.

MEDICATION

- Medication usually is not necessary. However, you may give your child non-prescription drugs, such as acetaminophen, for minor pain. For severe pain, your doctor may prescribe stronger pain relievers.
- See Medications section for information regarding medicines your doctor may prescribe.

ACTIVITY

Your child should stay as active as strength allows but should rest often. Normal activities may be resumed as soon as possible. Allow about 2 weeks for your child's recovery.

DIET & FLUIDS

No special diet.

OK FOR SCHOOL, PRESCHOOL, OR NURSERY?

When breathing and stamina return to normal and when signs of infection have decreased, appetite returns, and alertness, strength, and feeling of well-being will allow.

CALL YOUR DOCTOR IF

- Your child has symptoms of pneumothorax.
- The following occurs during treatment:
  - — Temperature rises to 101F (38.3C).
  - — Chest pain or shortness of breath increases.
  - — Painful, debilitating coughing or sputum production begins.

POLYARTERITIS (Polyarteritis Nodosa; Periarteritis Nodosa; Necrotizing Angiitis)

GENERAL INFORMATION

DESCRIPTION

Polyarteritis is a disorder of connective tissue that is one of several related diseases of collagen tissue. Collagen is a protein molecule that forms the major part of all connective tissue. Polyarteritis causes inflammation of small and medium arteries, decreasing the blood supply to tissues supplied by the affected blood vessels. It is not contagious. All body parts are involved. It is more common in males than females and affects all ages.

Appropriate health care includes:

- Self-care after diagnosis.
- Doctor's treatment.
- Surgery to remove part of the child's intestines, if they are involved.
- Hospitalization for intensive treatment (severe cases).

SIGNS & SYMPTOMS

Varies, depending on which organ is affected by the decreased blood supply. The most common include:

- Chest pain (heart involvement).
- Shortness of breath (lung involvement).
- Abdominal pain (intestinal and liver involvement).
- Blood in the child's urine (kidney involvement).
- Numbness and tingling of the child's hands and feet (nerve involvement).

The course may be acute, with fever, weight loss, and rapid deterioration. If the course is chronic, body tissues will waste away over several years.

CAUSES

This is considered a disease of autoimmunity or hypersensitivity, although the cause is uncertain. In many children, no predisposing factors can be found. Following are the most common preceding factors:

- Bacterial infections.
- Viral infections.
- Use of certain drugs, including sulfa drugs, penicillin, antithyroid drugs, gold, and thiazide diuretics.
- Vaccines.

RISK FACTORS

- Family history of collagen or hypersensitivity disease; smoking.

PREVENTING COMPLICATIONS OR RECURRENCE

No specific preventive measures.

WHAT TO EXPECT

MEDICAL TESTS

- Your own observation of symptoms.
- Medical history and physical exam by a doctor.
- Laboratory studies of the child's kidneys and blood, including sedimentation rate (see Glossary).

POLYARTERITIS (Polyarteritis Nodosa; Periarteritis Nodosa; Necrotizing Angiitis)

POSSIBLE COMPLICATIONS

Kidney failure and death, despite treatment.

PROBABLE OUTCOME

This condition is currently considered incurable. However, your child's symptoms can be relieved or controlled. Many patients live many years with the disease, and medical literature cites a few instances of unexplained recovery. Scientific research into causes and treatment continues, so there is hope for increasingly effective treatment and cure.

TREATMENT

HOME CARE

No specific instructions except those listed under other headings.

MEDICATION

- Your doctor may prescribe:

  —Cortisone drugs in high doses until acute symptoms diminish. Then symptoms may be controlled by a schedule of 1 cortisone dose every other day. Give these to the child only as long as necessary. Long-term use of cortisone produces serious adverse effects.

  —Drugs to treat disorders of organs involved with this serious disease, such as heart medications for heart involvement or antihypertensives for high blood pressure.

  —Immunosuppressive drugs—either alone or with steroids—if other drugs fail. These drugs pose additional risks to your child, including severe generalized septic bacterial infections.
- See Medications section for information regarding medicines your doctor may prescribe.

ACTIVITY

Your child can resume normal activities gradually as symptoms improve.

DIET & FLUIDS

Low-salt diet (see Appendix 29).

OK FOR SCHOOL, PRESCHOOL, OR NURSERY?

When appetite returns and alertness, strength, and feeling of well-being will allow.

CALL YOUR DOCTOR IF

- Your child has symptoms of polyarteritis.
- New, unexplained symptoms develop. Drugs used in treatment may produce side effects.

POLYMYOSITIS & DERMATOMYOSITIS

GENERAL INFORMATION

DESCRIPTION

The conditions refer to inflammation of connective tissue, with degenerative changes in the muscles (polymyositis) and the skin (dermatomyositis). This causes weakness and muscle wasting, especially in the arms and legs. This disease has many similarities to rheumatoid arthritis and lupus erythematosus. Body parts involved include the large muscles of the skeleton and the tiny muscles that control small arteries, the skin, and connective tissue. It is twice as common in females as males and can affect all ages.

Appropriate health care includes:

- Self-care after diagnosis.
- Doctor's treatment.
- Hospitalization during early, active phases.
- Surgery, if intestinal obstruction occurs.
- Time in an extended-care facility for physical therapy and rehabilitation.

SIGNS & SYMPTOMS

Sudden or slow onset of the following:

- Weakness in the child's pelvic-girdle and shoulder-girdle muscles.
- Skin rash that may itch on the child's face, shoulders, and arms and over the joints.
- Cold hands and feet.
- Frequent falls and difficulty in getting up.
- Speaking or swallowing difficulty.
- Infection with fever, muscle weakness, weight loss, and joint pain (sometimes) preceding other symptoms.

CAUSES

Probably a disease of hypersensitivity or autoimmunity, although the cause is uncertain. This disease has been associated with the use of certain drugs and preceding bacterial infections, viral infections, and vaccines.

RISK FACTORS

- Allergies.
- Use of sulfa drugs, penicillin, antithyroid drugs, gold, and thiazide diuretics.
- Family history of hypersensitivity diseases from illness or drugs, such as lupus.
- Cancer of the lung, colon, or breast.

PREVENTING COMPLICATIONS OR RECURRENCE

No specific preventive measures.

? WHAT TO EXPECT

MEDICAL TESTS

- Your own observation of symptoms.
- Medical history and physical exam by a doctor.
- Laboratory blood studies to measure antinuclear antibodies (ANA) and muscle enzymes.
- Surgical diagnostic procedures, such as biopsy of muscle and electromyography (see Glossary for both).

POSSIBLE COMPLICATIONS

- Muscle and body wasting.
- Congestive heart failure.
- High blood pressure.
- Intestinal obstruction.
- Kidney damage.

PROBABLE OUTCOME

The disease may begin suddenly or gradually. Most patients become wheelchair-bound or bedridden because of muscle weakness. Some of your child's symptoms can be controlled briefly with treatment, but the disease is often fatal in a short time. However, remissions or spontaneous recovery can occur—especially in children. Scientific research into causes and treatment continues, so there is hope for increasingly effective treatment and cure.

TREATMENT

HOME CARE

- The child may need a wheelchair and attendants to help with the daily routine.
- If confined to bed, the child should be moved frequently to prevent pressure sores.
- Passive exercise should be provided to prevent contractures (muscle shortening).
- Cool-water compresses may relieve the child's itching.

MEDICATION

- Your doctor may prescribe:
  —Cortisone drugs in high doses until acute symptoms diminish, then in lower doses.
  —Immunosuppressive drugs, if other treatment is not effective. These drugs impose additional risks to your child, including life-threatening septic bacterial infections.
- See Medications section for information regarding medicines your doctor may prescribe.

ACTIVITY

No restrictions, except those imposed by muscle weakness.

DIET & FLUIDS

No special diet.

OK FOR SCHOOL, PRESCHOOL, OR NURSERY?

When appetite returns and alertness, strength, and feeling of well-being will allow.

CALL YOUR DOCTOR IF

- Your child has symptoms or polymyositis and dermatomyositis.
- The following occurs during treatment:
  —Blood in the urine.
  —Shortness of breath.
  —Chest pain.
  —Bloody bowel movements.
  —Severe abdominal pain.
  —Fever.

PORPHYRIA

GENERAL INFORMATION

DESCRIPTION

Porphyria is a rare inherited disorder characterized by excessive formation and excretion of porphyrins (chemicals in all living things). The skin, liver, digestive system, and central nervous system—including the brain, the coverings of the brain (meninges), and the spinal cord—and peripheral nerves are involved. Porphyria can affect both sexes but is more common and severe in females.
Appropriate health care includes:

- Physician's monitoring of general condition and medications.
- Psychotherapy or counseling.
- Hospitalization during attacks for supportive care.

SIGNS & SYMPTOMS

- Increased sensitivity to light.
- Mental changes, including depression and mania.
- Skin changes, including itching and blistering.
- Dark urine that darkens more if left standing in a specimen jar.
- Abdominal pain and vomiting.
- Muscle cramps and weakness.
- Numbness and tingling in the feet and hands.

CAUSES

An inherited disturbance in the metabolism of porphyrins.

RISK FACTORS

- Family history of porphyria.
- Use of drugs, such as birth-control pills, alcohol, barbiturates. These don't cause the disease, but they may trigger attacks.
- Exposure to sunlight. This may trigger attacks.

PREVENTING COMPLICATIONS OR RECURRENCE

Cannot be prevented at present. To reduce the frequency and severity of attacks, urge your child to do the following:

- Avoid all drugs, including non-prescription medicines, until discussing it with your doctor.
- Avoid taking birth-control pills.
- Avoid bright sunlight.

OTHER

If you are a female and your disease is severe, pregnancy may not be advisable. Any person with a family history of porphyria should seek genetic counseling before starting a family.

WHAT TO EXPECT

MEDICAL TESTS

- Your own observation of symptoms.
- Medical history and physical exam by a doctor.
- Laboratory studies to measure porphyrins in the urine, blood, and stool.

POSSIBLE COMPLICATIONS

- A fatal porphyria crisis may occur during pregnancy. Special medical care is necessary in prenatal and postnatal stages.
- Misdiagnosis as a psychological or emotional problem may delay recognition and appropriate treatment.

PROBABLE OUTCOME

- This condition is currently considered incurable, but many patients live several years with the disorder. Symptoms can be relieved or controlled.
- Scientific research into causes and treatment continues, so there is hope for increasingly effective treatment and cure.

TREATMENT

HOME CARE

Your child should avoid bright sunlight. If your child must be in bright sun, using a hat and protective clothing is necessary.

MEDICATION

- Medicine usually is not necessary for this disorder, and some drugs may trigger attacks. Your child should not take any medicine without asking the doctor. Your doctor may prescribe tranquilizers to decrease anxiety.
- See Medications section for information regarding medicines your doctor may prescribe.

ACTIVITY

No restrictions.

DIET & FLUIDS

No special diet.

OK FOR SCHOOL, PRESCHOOL, OR NURSERY?

Between active episodes of the disease.

CALL YOUR DOCTOR IF

- Your child has symptoms of porphyria.
- Dark urine or other symptoms of an attack recur.

POTASSIUM IMBALANCE

GENERAL INFORMATION

DESCRIPTION

Potassium imbalance is above- or below-normal levels of potassium in the blood, which eventually affects all body fluids and body cells.

Appropriate health care includes:
- Self-care after diagnosis.
- Physician's monitoring of general condition and medications.
- Hospitalization (severe cases).

SIGNS & SYMPTOMS

For above-normal levels (hyperkalemia):
- Weakness and paralysis.
- Dangerously rapid, irregular heartbeat or slow heartbeat (sometimes).
- Nausea and diarrhea.

For below-normal levels (hypokalemia):
- Weakness and paralysis.
- Low blood pressure.
- Life-threatening rapid, irregular heartbeat. This is more severe than with hyperkalemia.

CAUSES

Hyperkalemia:
- Chronic kidney disease with kidney failure. Failing kidneys eliminate potassium too slowly, causing an excess in the child's body.
- Use of oral potassium supplements.
- Burns or crushing injuries. These may release potassium from the child's body tissues into body fluids.
- Addison's disease.

Hypokalemia:
- The use of diuretic drugs for hypertension or heart failure.
- Prolonged loss of body fluids from vomiting or diarrhea.
- Chronic kidney disease with kidney failure. At certain stages, this may cause the child's body to lose potassium.

RISK FACTORS

- Diabetes mellitus.
- Adrenal disease.
- Use of drugs, such as diuretics, potassium supplements, and digitalis. Low potassium levels—especially in persons who take digitalis—often lead to serious heartbeat disturbances.

PREVENTING COMPLICATIONS OR RECURRENCE

- If your child has a disorder or takes drugs that affect potassium levels (see CAUSES and RISK FACTORS), learn as much as you can about the condition, the drugs, and the ways to prevent a potassium imbalance.
- If your child takes digitalis and diuretics, frequent blood studies to monitor potassium levels are necessary.
- Obtain medical care for your child's prolonged vomiting or diarrhea.

OTHER

A normal medium to high blood level of potassium may help protect against coronary-artery disease.

WHAT TO EXPECT

MEDICAL TESTS

- Your own observation of symptoms, especially muscle weakness and heart-rhythm changes.
- Medical history and physical exam by a doctor.
- Laboratory blood and urine studies of potassium and other electrolytes.
- EKG (see Glossary).

POSSIBLE COMPLICATIONS

Cardiac arrest and death.

PROBABLE OUTCOME

Usually can be corrected with intravenous fluids and treatment of the child's underlying disorder.

TREATMENT

HOME CARE

If your child takes diuretics and digitalis, friends and family members should learn cardiopulmonary resuscitation (CPR). Learn to count a pulse at the wrist or neck.

MEDICATION

Your doctor may prescribe:

- Oral potassium supplements to raise low levels.
- Diuretics to increase urination and decrease high potassium levels.
- Intravenous fluids to correct a serious imbalance.
- Medications appropriate for the child's underlying disease.
- See Medications section for information regarding medicines your doctor may prescribe.

ACTIVITY

Your child can resume normal activities as soon as symptoms improve.

DIET & FLUIDS

Depends on the condition. Mild hypokalemia can be corrected by increasing your child's consumption of potassium-containing foods, such as orange juice and bananas.

OK FOR SCHOOL, PRESCHOOL, OR NURSERY?

Only after balance has been restored to normal and appetite has returned and alertness, strength, and feeling of well-being will allow.

CALL YOUR DOCTOR IF

Your child has symptoms of a potassium imbalance or is having problems with a disorder that affects potassium levels.

PREMATURE INFANTS

GENERAL INFORMATION

DESCRIPTION

Premature infants are babies born before 37 weeks of pregnancy. All the newborn's body systems are involved.

Appropriate health care includes:

- Physician's monitoring of general condition and medications.
- Hospitalization in a nursery for premature infants. This provides temperature-controlled bassinets, mechanical breathing machines, and continuous nursing care.

SIGNS & SYMPTOMS

- Birth weight of less than 5-1/2 pounds (2.5kg).
- Low body temperature.
- Breathing difficulty.
- Weak sucking and swallowing reflexes.
- Susceptibility to infection.
- Fluid and electrolyte imbalance (sometimes).
- Jaundice caused by poor elimination of bilirubin, a byproduct of the breakdown of red blood cells.

CAUSES

- Premature labor.
- Induced (artificially-started) labor or Cesarean section because of serious injury or illness in the mother.

RISK FACTORS

Poor nutrition; smoking; injury to the uterus; excess alcohol consumption; use of mind-altering drugs; inadequate prenatal care; damage to the cervix in previous deliveries; vaginal infections that spread to the uterus; urinary-tract infection; more than one fetus (twins or more); previous premature delivery; being an adolescent mother.

PREVENTING COMPLICATIONS OR RECURRENCE

- Obtain good prenatal care throughout pregnancy.
- Don't smoke, use mind-altering drugs, or drink alcohol during pregnancy.
- Eat a normal, well-balanced diet during pregnancy (see Appendix 32). Take prenatal vitamin and mineral supplements, if your doctor prescribes them.
- Don't use medications of any kind, including non-prescription drugs, without consulting your doctor.
- If you have a weak cervix, which is sometimes evident before pregnancy, ask your doctor about a minor operation to strengthen the cervix.
- Rest more and decrease activity in the 3rd trimester, especially if you have bloody spotting or other warning signs.

WHAT TO EXPECT

MEDICAL TESTS

- Medical history and physical exam by a doctor.
- Laboratory blood studies to detect anemia or infection in the infant and to determine the degree of jaundice.

POSSIBLE COMPLICATIONS

- Anemia.
- Serious infections, such as meningitis or colitis.
- Hyaline-membrane disease (see Glossary).
- Blindness, if excessive oxygen is necessary to maintain the infant's life.

PROBABLE OUTCOME

The infant's survival chances depend on its maturity. With good care, most premature infants "catch up" developmentally with other children and lead normal lives.

TREATMENT

HOME CARE

Premature infants require special care once they are mature enough to leave the hospital. Ask for assistance from a visiting-nurse service or your local health department.

MEDICATION

- Medicine usually is not necessary for prematurity, but your doctor may prescribe drugs for complications.
- See Medications section for information regarding medicines your doctor may prescribe.

ACTIVITY

No restrictions.

DIET & FLUIDS

Feeding by stomach tube may be necessary if your infant's sucking reflex is too weak. When normal feeding is possible, most premature infants tolerate mother's milk best. Return to the hospital as often as possible to feed the baby. Use a breast pump to express and store milk for feedings when you cannot be present. Hold the baby often. Bonding is important.

OK FOR SCHOOL, PRESCHOOL, OR NURSERY?

Only after your child has reached a degree of normal development. Your physician will be your guide.

CALL YOUR DOCTOR IF

After returning home, your baby has any of the following:

- Fever.
- Poor appetite or poor weight gain.
- Excessive crying that persists even when the child is picked up.

PREMENSTRUAL SYNDROME
(Premenstrual Tension; PMS)

GENERAL INFORMATION

DESCRIPTION

Premenstrual syndrome consists of symptoms that begin 7 to 14 days prior to a menstrual period and usually stop when menstruation begins. Body parts involved include the gastrointestinal system, the central nervous system—including the brain, the coverings of the brain (meninges), and the spinal cord—and peripheral nerves, as well as the skin, reproductive system, and breasts. Premenstrual syndrome affects about half of all females beyond puberty at some time—some very frequently.

Appropriate health care includes:

- Self-care.
- Physician's monitoring of general condition and medications (sometimes).

SIGNS & SYMPTOMS

- Nervousness and irritability.
- Dizziness or fainting.
- Emotional instability.
- Increased or decreased sex drive.
- Headaches.
- Tender, swollen breasts.
- Bloating, constipation, diarrhea, or other digestive disturbances.
- Fluid retention that causes puffiness in ankles, hands, and face.
- Higher incidence of minor infections such as colds.
- Acne outbreaks.
- Decreased urination.

CAUSES

- Fluctuations in the circulating level of hormones (especially estrogen and progesterone). These fluctuations cause retention of sodium in the bloodstream, resulting in edema in body tissues—including the brain.
- Increased levels of prostaglandin (a chemical) in the bloodstream.

RISK FACTORS

The older a woman is and the more children she has, the more likely she is to have PMS. Stress in younger women increases the likelihood of PMS.

PREVENTING COMPLICATIONS OR RECURRENCE

No specific preventive measures.

WHAT TO EXPECT

MEDICAL TESTS

- Your own observation of symptoms.
- Medical history and physical exam by a doctor.

POSSIBLE COMPLICATIONS

Emotional stress caused by symptoms severe enough to disrupt your daughter's life.

PREMENSTRUAL SYNDROME (Premenstrual Tension; PMS)

PROBABLE OUTCOME

Present treatments may or may not be effective. Medication can relieve some symptoms. However, many new treatments are in the experimental stage, offering hope for the future.

TREATMENT

HOME CARE

Reduce your daughter's stress whenever possible. See Appendix 19.

MEDICATION

Your doctor may prescribe:

- Tranquilizers or sedatives to relieve tension.
- Non-steroidal anti-inflammatory drugs to decrease prostaglandin levels.
- Diuretics to reduce fluid retention.
- See Medications section for information regarding medicines your doctor may prescribe.

ACTIVITY

No restrictions.

DIET & FLUIDS

- Your daughter should decrease salt intake during the premenstrual phase.
- Your doctor may prescribe vitamin B-6 (50mg to 100mg daily) and extra calcium (either in tablets or in milk or milk products). These supplements decrease symptoms in some females.

OK FOR SCHOOL, PRESCHOOL, OR NURSERY?

Yes. Try to keep activities normal.

CALL YOUR DOCTOR IF

- Your daughter has symptoms of PMS that interfere with normal activities or relationships, and self-care is not sufficient.
- Symptoms don't improve, despite treatment.
- New, unexplained symptoms develop. Drugs used in treatment may produce side effects.

ILLNESSES

PRICKLY HEAT
(Heat Rash; Miliaria Rubra; Sweat Retention)

GENERAL INFORMATION

DESCRIPTION

Prickly heat is a skin disorder characterized by a non-inflammatory, itchy rash caused by obstructed sweat-gland ducts. The skin, particularly in the diaper area, is involved. Prickly heat can affect both sexes, all ages, but is most common in infants.

Appropriate health care includes:

- Home care.
- Physician's monitoring of general condition and medications, if home care fails.

SIGNS & SYMPTOMS

Clusters of vesicles (small, fluid-filled skin blisters) or red rash without vesicles in areas of heavy perspiration.

CAUSES

Obstruction of sweat-gland ducts for unknown reasons.

RISK FACTORS

- Obesity.
- Stress.
- Hot, humid weather.
- Genetic factors, such as fair, sensitive skin.

PREVENTING COMPLICATIONS OR RECURRENCE

Your child should stay indoors in refrigerated air-conditioned buildings during hot, humid weather.

WHAT TO EXPECT

MEDICAL TESTS

- Your own observation of symptoms.
- Medical history and physical exam by a doctor (severe cases only).

POSSIBLE COMPLICATIONS

Secondary skin infection.

PROBABLE OUTCOME

Usually curable with treatment in 6 weeks to 6 months. Recurrence is common.

PRICKLY HEAT
(Heat Rash; Miliaria Rubra; Sweat Retention)

TREATMENT

HOME CARE

- Change diapers on infants as soon as they are wet.
- Expose the affected skin to air as much as possible.
- Apply lubricating ointment or cream to the child's skin 6 or 7 times a day.
- Use cool-water soaks to relieve the child's itching and hasten healing. Pat the skin dry, and dust with cornstarch after and between soaks.
- Your child should take frequent cool showers or tub baths.
- Your child should wear cotton socks and leather-soled footwear rather than shoes made of man-made materials.
- Don't use binding materials, such as adhesive tape, on your child.
- Your child should avoid sunburn after having had prickly heat. The body's inflammatory reaction to sunburn may trigger a new outbreak of prickly heat.
- Urge your older child not to wear tight pantyhose or girdles.

MEDICATION

- Your doctor may suggest non-prescription steroid cream to apply 2 or 3 times a day.
- See Medications section for information regarding medicines your doctor may prescribe.

ACTIVITY

Your child should decrease activity during hot, humid weather or until skin heals.

DIET & FLUIDS

No special diet.

OK FOR SCHOOL, PRESCHOOL, OR NURSERY?

Yes.

CALL YOUR DOCTOR IF

Your child's prickly heat doesn't improve in 10 days, despite home care.

PROCTITIS

GENERAL INFORMATION

DESCRIPTION

Proctitis is inflammation of the rectum and tissues around the anus. Proctitis affects adolescents and adults of both sexes.

Appropriate health care includes:

- Self-care after diagnosis.
- Physician's monitoring of general condition and medications.
- Surgery to remove any underlying tumor.

SIGNS & SYMPTOMS

- Rectal pain.
- Constant urge to have a bowel movement, often when little or no stool is present.
- Blood or mucus discharge from the child's rectum.
- Cramping pain in the left lower abdomen.

CAUSES

- Sexually transmitted infections of gonorrhea, syphilis, and herpes.
- Chronic constipation.
- Ulcerative colitis (early stages).
- Cancer of the rectum.
- Rectal injury.
- Aftereffects of radiation therapy for cancer of the cervix and uterus.
- Endocrine disorders.
- Bacterial infections, including food poisoning.
- Food allergies.

RISK FACTORS

- Being a homosexual male.
- Use of laxatives.

PREVENTING COMPLICATIONS OR RECURRENCE

Instructions for your child:

- To prevent constipation, establish a regular pattern for bowel movements. Eat a diet high in fiber and drink many fluids.
- Don't use laxatives regularly.
- Don't eat foods to which you are sensitive.
- Avoid anal intercourse.

WHAT TO EXPECT

MEDICAL TESTS

- Your own observation of symptoms.
- Medical history and physical exam by a doctor.
- Laboratory studies, such as blood counts; tests for gonorrhea, syphilis, and other sexually transmitted diseases; and stool cultures.
- Surgical diagnostic procedures such as proctoscopy (see Glossary).

POSSIBLE COMPLICATIONS

Anal scarring and stricture (permanent narrowing of the anus).

PROBABLE OUTCOME

The outcome of proctitis depends on the outcome of the underlying cause:

- Infections can usually be cured with antibiotics.
- Cancer is often curable with surgery.
- Food allergies can be minimized if the offending foods are avoided.
- Symptoms of other disorders in your child can be relieved or controlled with treatment.

TREATMENT

HOME CARE

Instructions for your child:

- Keep the anal area clean with frequent bathing.
- Take sitz baths often to relieve pain. Sit in a tub of hot water for 10 to 15 minutes as often as necessary.

MEDICATION

- Use non-prescription topical anesthetics to relieve your child's discomfort.
- Your doctor may prescribe:
  — Antibiotics for sexually transmitted infections.
  — Steroid suppositories to reduce inflammation from other causes.
- See Medications section for information regarding medicines your doctor may prescribe.

ACTIVITY

No restrictions.

DIET & FLUIDS

- Your child should eat a high-fiber diet and drink at least 8 glasses of water a day.
- Avoid serving foods to which the child is sensitive.

OK FOR SCHOOL, PRESCHOOL, OR NURSERY?

Yes, after treatment is complete.

CALL YOUR DOCTOR IF

- Your child has symptoms of proctitis, or symptoms recur after treatment.
- New, unexplained symptoms develop. Drugs used in treatment may produce side effects.

PRURITIS ANI

GENERAL INFORMATION

DESCRIPTION

Pruritis ani is itching around the anus and genitals. The anus, vulva (vaginal lips) in females, and scrotum in males are involved.

Appropriate health care includes:

- Self-care after diagnosis.
- Physician's monitoring of general condition and medications, if self-care is not successful.

SIGNS & SYMPTOMS

Itching, often intense and worse at night.

CAUSES

- Yeast infection.
- Pinworms.
- Scabies.
- Contact dermatitis caused by soaps, contraceptive foams or jellies, perfumed toilet paper, deodorant sprays, douches, or underwear made of synthetic fabric.
- Various skin disorders, including psoriasis or seborrheic dermatitis.
- Vaginal discharge or skin atrophy in females caused by low estrogen levels.
- Chronic diarrhea.
- Unknown (often).

RISK FACTORS

- Stress.
- Diabetes mellitus.
- Excessive sweating.

PREVENTING COMPLICATIONS OR RECURRENCE

- Encourage your child to keep the body clean with regular showers or baths.
- Teach your child to cleanse carefully after bowel movements with moistened tissue.
- Avoid contact with substances to which the child is sensitive (see CAUSES).

WHAT TO EXPECT

MEDICAL TESTS

- Your own observation of symptoms.
- Medical history and physical exam by a doctor.
- Laboratory studies, such as cultures for fungi, or microscopic examinations for pinworm eggs or scabies in skin burrows.

POSSIBLE COMPLICATIONS

- Skin damage, allowing secondary bacterial infection to develop.
- Skin thickening and chronic inflammation.
- Fatigue from chronic sleep disturbance.

PROBABLE OUTCOME

Your child's symptoms can be controlled with treatment, even if the cause cannot be determined.

TREATMENT

HOME CARE

Instructions for your child:

- Keep showers or baths brief to minimize dryness and soap irritation. Use plain, unscented soap—if any.
- Keep the rectal area clean, dry, and cool. Wear loose clothing and underclothing. Clean carefully after bowel movements, using moist tufts of cotton or plain soap and water.
- Don't use irritants listed as causes.
- Wear underwear with a cotton crotch or underwear made of cotton, rather than nylon or other synthetics.
- If you are menstruating, you may be more comfortable using tampons for menstrual periods, rather than sanitary napkins.

MEDICATION

- You may use non-prescription cortisone ointment or cream on your child. Apply 3 times a day, and rub in gently until it disappears.
- Your doctor may prescribe:
  - — More potent topical cortisone drugs.
  - — Zinc oxide.
- See Medications section for information regarding medicines your doctor may prescribe.

ACTIVITY

Your child should avoid activities that cause excessive perspiration.

DIET & FLUIDS

Your child should avoid spicy or highly seasoned foods. These irritate mucous membranes of the anus.

OK FOR SCHOOL, PRESCHOOL, OR NURSERY?

Yes.

CALL YOUR DOCTOR IF

- Your child has symptoms of pruritis ani that persist, despite self-care.
- Your child develops a fever.
- The irritated area seems infected.

PRURITUS VULVAE
(Female Genital Itching)

GENERAL INFORMATION

DESCRIPTION

Pruritus vulvae is an acute or chronic disorder of the skin around the vulva (the vaginal lips) and anus. This disorder is characterized by severe itching. It is not contagious. The vulva and skin surrounding the vulva and anus are involved. Females of all ages are affected.

Appropriate health care includes:

- Self-care after diagnosis has been established.
- Physician's monitoring of general condition and medications.

SIGNS & SYMPTOMS

- Intense itching, sensitivity, and irritation in the genital area. The skin may be dry and red. With secondary infection the skin may become moist and ooze.
- Thin, white vaginal discharge (sometimes).
- Discomfort during sexual intercourse.

CAUSES

- Skin disease, such as psoriasis or lichen planus.
- Systemic disease, such as diabetes.
- Atrophy and dryness caused by estrogen deficiency.
- Skin reaction to irritants, such as toilet tissue, sanitary pads, soap, douches, deodorants, powders, perfume, and fabric.
- Systemic allergies, including food allergies.
- Disorder of the vagina or rectum, such as vaginitis or hemorrhoids.

RISK FACTORS

- Stress.
- Days prior to menstruation.
- Hot, humid weather.
- Diabetes mellitus.
- Lack of urinary control.

PREVENTING COMPLICATIONS OR RECURRENCE

Instructions for your daughter:

- Wear cotton panties rather than nylon.
- Avoid contact with irritants listed above.
- Obtain medical treatment for underlying causes.

WHAT TO EXPECT

MEDICAL TESTS

- Your own observation of symptoms.
- Medical history and physical exam by a doctor.
- Diagnostic measures including cultures of involved skin to test for yeast or fungus infection.

POSSIBLE COMPLICATIONS

Secondary bacterial infection of the inflamed skin.

PRURITIS VULVAE
(Female Genital Itching)

PROBABLE OUTCOME

Home treatment usually provides relief in 4 to 7 days. If medical treatment becomes necessary, allow 2 weeks for recovery.

TREATMENT

HOME CARE

Instructions for your daughter:

- Follow suggestions under PREVENTING COMPLICATIONS OR RECURRENCE.
- Keep the area as dry and cool as possible. Wear loose clothing.
- Don't scratch the itchy area. Scratching will aggravate soreness and irritation.
- Wash the genital area with water and unscented soap only once a day.
- After urinating or having a bowel movement, clean the genital area gently with absorbent cotton or antiseptic wipes. Wipe from front to back (vagina to anus).
- During menstruation, use tampons rather than sanitary napkins until the disorder heals.
- Use a lubricant such as K-Y Lubricating Jelly or baby oil during intercourse.

MEDICATION

Your daughter may use low-potency, non-prescription steroid creams or ointments. If these are not effective, your doctor may prescribe:

- More potent steroid creams or lotions to reduce inflammation. These require 24 to 36 hours to provide relief.
- Ointments that contain hormones.
- Benzodiazepines or antihistamines at night to ensure rest.
- See Medications section for information regarding medicines your doctor may prescribo.

ACTIVITY

Your daughter should avoid overexertion, heat, and excessive sweating.

DIET & FLUIDS

No special diet, except for your daughter to avoid foods to which she may be allergic.

OK FOR SCHOOL, PRESCHOOL, OR NURSERY?

Yes.

CALL YOUR DOCTOR IF

- Your daughter has symptoms of pruritis vulvae.
- Symptoms don't improve in 2 weeks, despite treatment.
- Scratching leads to skin infection.
- New, unexplained symptoms develop. Drugs used in treatment may produce side effects.

ILLNESSES

PSEUDOMEMBRANOUS ENTEROCOLITIS

GENERAL INFORMATION

DESCRIPTION

Pseudomembranous enterocolitis is a rare, severe illness in the small and large intestines. It usually follows 5 to 7 days after extensive gastrointestinal surgery and antibiotic treatment in a person who was debilitated before surgery. It is characterized by inflammation and tissue death of the lining membrane and deeper layers of the intestine. The large and small intestines are involved. Pesudomembranous enterocolitis can affect both sexes, all ages, but is more common in adults than children.

Appropriate health care includes:

- Physician's monitoring of general condition and medications.
- Hospitalization for intravenous nutrition and intensive care.
- Self-care during convalescence after hospitalization.

SIGNS & SYMPTOMS

- Watery diarrhea (sometimes bloody) with abdominal cramps.
- Fever.
- High white blood cell count.
- Drop in blood pressure, sometimes to shock levels, with weak pulse and rapid heartbeat.
- Nausea and vomiting.
- Disorientation.

CAUSES

Infection from bacteria, usually the germ clostridium difficile, which manufactures a toxin that causes the symptoms, or from the staphylococcus germ. These germs normally inhabit your child's intestinal tract. They cause enterocolitis when other normal bacteria of the intestinal tract have been killed by heavy use of broad-spectrum antibiotics. This upsets the bacterial balance of the intestinal tract. The illness usually occurs as a complication of surgery.

RISK FACTORS

Recent surgery with a drop in blood pressure during surgery; kidney failure; obesity; poor nutrition; use of antibiotics, especially lincomycin, clindamycin, ampicillin, chloramphenicol, cephalosporins, penicillin, or sulfa drugs.

PREVENTING COMPLICATIONS OR RECURRENCE

No specific preventive measures.

? WHAT TO EXPECT

MEDICAL TESTS

- Your own observation of symptoms.
- Medical history and physical exam by a doctor.
- Biopsy (see Glossary) of the membrane lining of the large intestine through a colonoscope (see Glossary).

Note: A barium enema should *not* be administered to your child. It may cause intestinal perforation.

POSSIBLE COMPLICATIONS

The following occur only if the child's problem is not recognized and treated:

- Shock and severe dehydration.
- Peritonitis caused by perforation of the intestine.

PROBABLE OUTCOME

Your child's symptoms will usually disappear in 1 to 2 weeks after the offending antibiotic is discontinued. A substitute antibiotic is usually not prescribed; the body's defense mechanisms must take over for the withdrawn antibiotic. The worst cases are fatal.

TREATMENT

HOME CARE

The most important treatment is to discontinue use of the antibiotic causing the child's illness.

MEDICATION

- Your doctor may prescribe:
  — Cholestyramine, vancomycin, or metronidazole to prevent secondary, non-bacterial infections that occur when the balance of intestinal organisms is upset.
  — High doses of cortisone for a short time to decrease inflammation.
- Your child should not take anti-diarrheal drugs unless prescribed by the doctor. They may contribute to intestinal perforation.

ACTIVITY

Your child should rest in bed until all symptoms of the illness disappear. Flexing the legs often while in bed decreases the likelihood of deep-vein blood clots. The child can resume normal activities gradually.

DIET & FLUIDS

Intravenous nourishment will be necessary for your child at first, progressing to a liquid diet, to a soft diet, and finally to a normal diet.

OK FOR SCHOOL, PRESCHOOL, OR NURSERY?

When signs of infection have decreased, appetite returns, and alertness, strength, and feeling of well-being will allow.

CALL YOUR DOCTOR IF

- Your child has symptoms of pseudomembranous enterocolitis following intestinal surgery.
- Symptoms return after treatment.
- New, unexplained symptoms develop. Drugs used in treatment may produce side effects.

PSITTACOSIS
(Parrot Fever; Ornithosis)

GENERAL INFORMATION

DESCRIPTION

Psittacosis is an infectious form of pneumonia transmitted by birds. The lungs and other parts of the respiratory tract are involved.

Appropriate health care includes:

- Self-care after diagnosis.
- Physician's monitoring of general condition and medications.

SIGNS & SYMPTOMS

- Fever and chills.
- General ill feeling.
- Loss of appetite.
- Cough without sputum that progresses to cough with occasional discolored sputum.
- Shortness of breath.

CAUSES

- Infection by the germ chlamydia. Microscopic chlamydia organisms are not bacteria, viruses, or fungi. However, they can be destroyed with antibiotics.
- Psittacosis is found in psittacine birds (parrots, parakeets, lovebirds), poultry, pigeons, canaries, and some sea birds. Germs enter the human body by inhalation of air that contains the germ, or by a bite from an infected bird. Incubation is 1 to 3 weeks after exposure.

RISK FACTORS

Exposure to birds, especially in zoos, in pet shops, or on farms.

PREVENTING COMPLICATIONS OR RECURRENCE

- Your child should avoid dust from bird feathers and cage contents.
- Your child should not handle any sick bird. Imported psittacine birds must be treated for 45 days with feed that contains chlortetracycline. This eliminates the organisms from the birds' blood and feces.

WHAT TO EXPECT

MEDICAL TESTS

- Your own observation of symptoms.
- Medical history and physical exam by a doctor.
- Laboratory blood studies and sputum culture.
- X-rays of the lungs.

POSSIBLE COMPLICATIONS

Severe or fatal pneumonia.

PROBABLE OUTCOME

Usually curable in 7 to 14 days with early diagnosis and treatment. The child's fever may remain for 2 or 3 weeks before falling slowly, unless antibiotics are used.

PSITTACOSIS
(Parrot Fever; Ornithosis)

TREATMENT

HOME CARE

- Keep your child isolated to avoid transmitting the disease through cough droplets and sputum.
- Use a cool-mist humidifier to increase air moisture around the child and loosen lung secretions. Use pure water; don't put medication in the humidifier.
- Use a heating pad on the chest to relieve pain.
- The patient should not smoke.

MEDICATION

- Your doctor may prescribe tetracycline (an antibiotic) for at least 10 days to control the child's fever and other symptoms.
- Don't suppress the child's cough if it produces sputum. It is performing a useful function in ridding the lungs of mucus. If the cough is non-productive and painful, you may suppress it with prescribed medication.
- For minor pain, use non-prescription drugs such as aspirin or acetaminophen.
- See Medications section for information regarding medicines your doctor may prescribe.

ACTIVITY

Bed rest is necessary for your child until the fever, pain, and shortness of breath have been gone at least 48 hours. Then normal activities may be resumed gradually. Fatigue and weakness may persist for a long time, so don't expect a quick return to normal strength.

DIET & FLUIDS

No special diet. Your child should increase fluid intake to at least 1 glass of fluid every hour. This helps to thin lung secretions so they can be coughed up more easily.

OK FOR SCHOOL, PRESCHOOL, OR NURSERY?

When signs of infection have decreased, appetite returns, and alertness, strength, and feeling of well-being will allow.

CALL YOUR DOCTOR IF

- Your child has symptoms of psittacosis.
- The following occurs during treatment:
  - — Fever rises to 102F (38.9C) or higher.
  - — Pain is not relieved by heat or prescribed medication.
  - — Shortness of breath increases.
  - — Fingernails become dark or bluish.
  - — Blood appears in the sputum.
  - — Nausea, vomiting, or diarrhea occur.

PSORIASIS

GENERAL INFORMATION

DESCRIPTION

Psoriasis is a chronic scaly skin disorder characterized by frequent remissions and recurrences. The skin—especially of the scalp, elbows, knees, chest, back, arms, legs, toenails, fingernails, and the fold between the buttocks—is involved. Psoriasis begins in late childhood or young adulthood and continues throughout life. Appropriate health care includes:

- Self-care after diagnosis.
- Physician's monitoring of general condition and medications.
- Psychotherapy or counseling (sometimes) to help in adapting to the disorder.

SIGNS & SYMPTOMS

- Skin areas that are slightly raised, have red borders, and are covered with large white or silver-white scales. The areas crack and become painful.
- Itching (sometimes).
- Joint pain.

CAUSES

Unknown, but probably caused by autoimmune disorder.

RISK FACTORS

- Rheumatoid arthritis.
- Local injury.
- Infections (viral and bacterial) elsewhere in the body.
- Family history of psoriasis.
- Stress.
- Cold climates.
- Genetic factors. Persons with psoriasis have HLA antigens, and the incidence is highest among Caucasians.

PREVENTING COMPLICATIONS OR RECURRENCE

Cannot be prevented at present.

WHAT TO EXPECT

MEDICAL TESTS

- Your own observation of symptoms.
- Medical history and physical exam by a doctor.
- Laboratory blood tests.

POSSIBLE COMPLICATIONS

- Secondary bacterial infection in the affected areas.
- Generalized secondary bacterial infection—sometimes fatal—characterized by the eruption of many pustules, fever, and joint pain.

PROBABLE OUTCOME

Your child's symptoms can be controlled but not cured. The disease may have long periods of inactivity. In females, severity decreases during pregnancy.

TREATMENT

HOME CARE

Instructions for your child:

- Maintain good skin hygiene with daily baths or showers.
- Avoid skin injury, including harsh scrubbing, which can trigger new outbreaks.
- Avoid skin dryness to decrease the frequency of recurrences. To reduce scaling, use non-prescription waterless cleansers and hair preparations containing coal tar or cortisone.
- Expose skin to moderate amounts of sunlight as often as possible.
- Oatmeal baths may loosen scales. Use 1 cup of oatmeal to a tub of warm water.
- Move to a warm climate, if possible. Severity increases during cold weather.

MEDICATION

Your doctor may prescribe the following to decrease inflammation and scaling:

- Ointments containing coal tar.
- Topical cortisone drugs to use under plastic dressings.
- Ultraviolet light.
- Immunosuppressive drugs (severest cases).
- See Medications section for information regarding medicines your doctor may prescribe.

ACTIVITY

No restrictions.

DIET & FLUIDS

No special diet.

OK FOR SCHOOL, PRESCHOOL, OR NURSERY?

Yes. Encourage your child to stay in life's mainstream.

CALL YOUR DOCTOR IF

- Your child has symptoms of psoriasis, or symptoms recur after treatment.
- During an outbreak, pustules erupt on the skin, accompanied by fever, muscle aches, and fatigue.
- New, unexplained symptoms develop. Drugs used in treatment may produce side effects.

PTOSIS

GENERAL INFORMATION

DESCRIPTION

Ptosis (pronounced: tosis; the "p" is silent) is drooping of the upper eyelid, partially or completely covering the eye. The upper eyelid, the eye, and the motor and sensory nerves to the eye are involved.

Appropriate health care includes:

- Self-care after diagnosis.
- Physician's monitoring of general condition and medications. Some ophthalmologists recommend keeping the lid raised with a support that is part of eyeglasses.
- Surgery to strengthen the muscles of the eyelid (sometimes).

SIGNS & SYMPTOMS

Drooping of one or both eyelids, accompanied by poor blinking reflexes. The extent of droop may vary at different times of the day.

CAUSES

May be present at birth or may accompany other problems, including:

- Paralysis of nerve fibers to the eyelids.
- Myasthenia gravis.
- Muscular dystrophy.
- Diabetes.
- Brain tumor.
- Birth injury.
- Head or eyelid injury.
- Tumor in the upper lobe of a lung.

RISK FACTORS

Family history of ptosis.

PREVENTING COMPLICATIONS OR RECURRENCE

No specific preventive measures.

WHAT TO EXPECT

MEDICAL TESTS

- Your own observation of symptoms.
- Medical history and physical exam by a doctor.
- X-rays of various body regions to look for the underlying cause.

POSSIBLE COMPLICATIONS

- Permanent disfigurement.
- Irritation and infection in the child's eye caused by poor blinking reflexes and continuous contact between the eyelid and eye surface.
- Visual disturbance.

PROBABLE OUTCOME

Sometimes curable if the underlying cause can be corrected by surgery or medication.

TREATMENT

HOME CARE

- Keep the child's eye moist with non-prescription, artificial tears.
- Urge your child to wear safety goggles to protect the eye from injury when exposed to dust or flying debris.

MEDICATION

- Medicine usually is not necessary for ptosis, but it may be necessary for the underlying disorder.
- See Medications section for information regarding medicines your doctor may prescribe.

ACTIVITY

No restrictions.

DIET & FLUIDS

No special diet.

OK FOR SCHOOL, PRESCHOOL, OR NURSERY?

Yes. Try to maintain normal activities for your child's age.

CALL YOUR DOCTOR IF

- Your child has symptoms of ptosis.
- The ptosis worsens or the child's vision is affected.

PULMONARY-VALVE STENOSIS

GENERAL INFORMATION

DESCRIPTION

Pulmonary-valve stenosis is narrowing of the pulmonary valve. The pulmonary valve separates the right ventricle (major chamber) of the heart from the pulmonary artery (the large artery that goes from the heart to the lungs). When this valve becomes narrowed, heart function is impaired. Special parts of the right side of the heart are involved.

Appropriate health care includes:

- Self-care after diagnosis.
- Physician's monitoring of general condition and medications.
- Surgery (only if the defective valve must be repaired).

SIGNS & SYMPTOMS

Early stages:

- No symptoms.

Later stages:

- Chest pain.
- Dizziness.
- Faintness upon exertion.
- Congestive heart failure, with the following symptoms:
  - — Fatigue.
  - — Swelling in the lower parts of the child's body—the feet if standing or sitting and the back if lying down.
  - — Breathlessness with exertion—walking or climbing stairs.
  - — Later, breathlessness appears without exertion—sometimes even after going to sleep.
  - — Cough, sometimes with frothy or bloody sputum.
  - — Nausea and loss of appetite.

CAUSES

- Congenital (present at birth).
- Complication of rheumatic fever (rare).

RISK FACTORS

Prior streptococcal infection.

PREVENTING COMPLICATIONS OR RECURRENCE

- Obtain a throat culture and prompt medical treatment for strep infections to prevent rheumatic fever.
- If your child has had rheumatic fever, give the child prescribed antibiotics before any surgery, even dental procedures.

WHAT TO EXPECT

MEDICAL TESTS

- Your own observation of symptoms.
- Medical history and physical exam by a doctor.
- Laboratory studies such as EKG, cardiac catheterization, and echocardiography (see Glossary for all).
- X-rays of the heart and lungs.

POSSIBLE COMPLICATIONS

Congestive heart failure.

PROBABLE OUTCOME

Mild pulmonary-valve stenosis may cause your child little if any disability. Severe impairment is usually curable with surgery to stretch the defective pulmonary heart valve.

TREATMENT

HOME CARE

- Weigh your child daily and keep a record.
- Advise any doctor or dentist who treats your child that the child has a disease of the heart valves.

MEDICATION

- Your doctor may prescribe diuretics for your child to reduce the fluid retention of congestive heart failure.
- See Medications section for information regarding medicines your doctor may prescribe.

ACTIVITY

If surgery is not advised and your child's condition allows, normal activity should be continued. The child should avoid strenuous activity but should not be treated as an invalid—even if there is some disability. Walks and other light exercise may be possible.

DIET & FLUIDS

Low-salt diet (see Appendix 29).

OK FOR SCHOOL, PRESCHOOL, OR NURSERY?

When strength and feeling of well-being will allow.

CALL YOUR DOCTOR IF

- Your child has symptoms of pulmonary-valve stenosis.
- The following occurs during treatment:
  - — Unexplained weight gain of 3 to 4 pounds in 2 to 3 days, indicating fluid retention.
  - — Increased breathlessness.
  - — Wheezing at night.
  - — Fever.
  - — Rapid heartbeat.
  - — Cough.

PUNCTURE WOUNDS

GENERAL INFORMATION

DESCRIPTION

A puncture wound is produced by any object that penetrates the skin to the soft tissue, bones, or joints below. Puncture wounds are likely to be full of dirt and should cause immediate concern because of the danger of tetanus. Tetanus is an extremely serious infection, caused by a poison secreted by tetanus bacteria. These are found in soil, particularly soil contaminated by animal droppings. The toxin from the bacteria spreads through the bloodstream and sets off muscle spasms throughout the body that produce the characteristic locked jaw. Tetanus bacteria thrive on low concentrations of oxygen, exactly the condition that exists in a sealed-over puncture wound.

Appropriate health care includes:

- Self care for minor wounds if tetanus boosters are current (if in doubt—call your doctor).
- Physician's treatment for a serious wound to clean the wound and sometimes to explore it surgically to determine the extent of the damage.

SIGNS & SYMPTOMS

A hole in the child's skin with a puckered and discolored edge. The hole may appear smaller than the object that caused it, due to partial re-expansion of the damaged tissues.

CAUSES

Any foreign body that penetrates the child's skin and underlying tissue (cleats, javelin, splinters, glass).

RISK FACTORS

- Contact sports.
- Activities on rough terrain.
- Stepping on rusty nails.

PREVENTING COMPLICATIONS OR RECURRENCE

A baby should receive a series of tetanus inoculations before 1 year, a booster shot at 1-1/2 years, and another booster before entering school. To keep the immunization to tetanus effective, everyone—children and adults—should have a tetanus booster shot every 10 years. Record the dates of the shots and take them with you whenever your child needs emergency treatment. In general, if your child has had the basic 4 tetanus immunizations or a booster injection within the past 5 years, it may not be necessary to have another booster after a puncture wound.

? WHAT TO EXPECT

MEDICAL TESTS

- Your own observation of symptoms.
- Medical history and physical exam by a doctor.
- Culture of the wound.
- X-rays of underlying tissue to rule out fractures and joint damage.

POSSIBLE COMPLICATIONS

- Fluid collection under a closed penetrating wound.
- Wound infection.

PROBABLE OUTCOME

With treatment, a child's puncture wound usually heals without complications.

TREATMENT

FIRST AID

- Remove any foreign material (splinter, glass, or others) if you can.
- Clean the area of the child's wound with warm water and soap.

HOME CARE

- Extensive or deep penetrating wounds may need to be enlarged and explored surgically under antiseptic conditions.
- If bleeding occurs, control it by applying firm pressure to the child's wound with a cloth.
- Use warm immersion soaks to relieve the child's pain and swelling. Use plain warm water or warm water with Epsom salt or table salt (4 tablespoons to 1 quart of water).
- Your child should rest the injured part until it heals and should wear a snug elastic bandage over the injured area, if possible. This will decrease fluid collection under the child's wound and minimize further bleeding.
- Get a tetanus booster shot for your child, if needed.
- Keep the injured part elevated when possible; for example, prop an injured foot on a footstool while the child is sitting, or on a pillow while sleeping.

MEDICATION

- For minor discomfort, use non-prescription drugs such as acetaminophen.
- Your doctor may prescribe antibiotics to fight infection or a tetanus booster, if needed.

ACTIVITY

Your child can resume normal activity slowly after clearance by your doctor.

DIET & FLUIDS

For a serious puncture wound, your child should eat a well-balanced diet that includes extra protein, such as meat, fish, poultry, cheese, milk, and eggs.

OK FOR SCHOOL, PRESCHOOL, OR NURSERY?

Yes, if there are no signs of infection.

CALL YOUR DOCTOR IF

- Your child receives a puncture wound and has not had a tetanus booster in 10 years.
- Signs of a wound infection (fever, headache, or increasing pain, redness, and fluid with pus at the puncture site) develop.

PURPURA, ALLERGIC (Anaphylactoid Purpura; Henoch-Schönlein Purpura)

GENERAL INFORMATION

DESCRIPTION

Allergic purpura is an allergic disorder. The joints (usually knees, ankles, hips, wrists, and elbows), the skin of the legs, thighs, and abdomen, the gastrointestinal tract, and the kidneys are involved. Allergic purpura can affect both sexes, all ages, but is more common in boys (2 to 8 years).

Appropriate health care includes:

- Home care after diagnosis.
- Physician's monitoring of general condition and medications.
- Hospitalization (for complications).

SIGNS & SYMPTOMS

- Sore throat about 2 weeks prior to other symptoms.
- Itching skin rash that seems to be just beneath the skin surface. The rash usually consists of large hives with small bruises or blood spots in the centers. The rash is most often on the legs, thighs, and lower abdomen, but it may be scattered over your child's body.
- Joint inflammation at the knees, ankles, hips, wrists, or elbows.
- Cramping abdominal pain and vomiting.
- Protein and blood in the urine.
- Low fever.

CAUSES

Purpura is probably an allergic reaction in the inflamed small blood vessels throughout the body. The allergic trigger is not known, but attacks often follow an upper-respiratory infection or the use of some drugs, especially sulfa drugs.

RISK FACTORS

- Recent illness, especially a bacterial sore throat.
- Use of sulfa drugs.

PREVENTING COMPLICATIONS OR RECURRENCE

- Don't allow your child to be exposed to respiratory infections, if possible.
- Obtain prompt medical treatment of any bacterial throat infection.
- Avoid the use of any drug that has triggered allergic purpura in your child. Consult the doctor before giving any medication to a child.

WHAT TO EXPECT

MEDICAL TESTS

- Your own observation of symptoms.
- Medical history and physical exam by a doctor.
- Laboratory blood studies and a urinalysis.

POSSIBLE COMPLICATIONS

- Kidney failure, resulting from kidney inflammation and damage.
- Permanent joint deformity.

PURPURA, ALLERGIC (Anaphylactoid Purpura; Henoch-Schönlein Purpura)

PROBABLE OUTCOME

- Allergic purpura usually lasts 1 to 3 weeks. Some children only have a few spots and fever. Others require hospitalization for severe abdominal pain and kidney inflammation.
- Most children with allergic purpura recovery completely. In some, however, allergic purpura recurs or persists for years.

TREATMENT

HOME CARE

Use warm soaks to relieve your child's joint pain.

MEDICATION

- Your doctor may prescribe cortisone drugs or immunosuppressive drugs, such as cyclophosphamide, for your child to suppress inflammation. Effectiveness of treatment varies.
- See Medications section for information regarding medicines your doctor may prescribe.

ACTIVITY

If your child has fever or pain, encourage bed rest. The child may sit up for meals and walk to the bathroom. When fever and pain are gone, the child may gradually resume normal activities as strength and well-being allow.

DIET & FLUIDS

Your child should eat a normal, well-balanced diet. Vitamin and mineral supplements should not be necessary unless the child shows evidence of deficiency.

OK FOR SCHOOL, PRESCHOOL, OR NURSERY?

When appetite has returned and alertness, strength, and feeling of well-being will allow.

CALL YOUR DOCTOR IF

- Your child has symptoms of allergic purpura.
- The following symptoms occur during treatment:
  - — Unrelenting abdominal pain.
  - — Blood in the stool.
  - — Black, tarry bowel movements.
  - — New bleeding under the skin.
  - — Blood in the urine.

PYLORIC STENOSIS, CONGENITAL (Hypertrophic Pyloric Stenosis)

GENERAL INFORMATION

DESCRIPTION

Congenital pyloric stenosis is a condition of infancy in which encircling muscles at the end of the stomach enlarge and cause obstruction. The pylorus (a muscular tube that carries food from the stomach to the small intestine) is involved. Congenital pyloric stenosis can affect both sexes but is more common in firstborn males. The condition usually begins between 2 and 5 weeks of age, but it can occur as late as 4 months.

Appropriate health care includes:

- Physician's monitoring of general condition and medications.
- Surgery to cut the thickened muscle (pyloromyotomy).
- Hospitalization for about 3 days after surgery.

SIGNS & SYMPTOMS

- Recurrent vomiting after feedings that becomes increasingly forceful.
- Muscular mass in the upper abdomen (sometimes).
- No pain or fever. The infant seems happy but hungry after vomiting.
- Constipation.
- Gradual weight loss and dehydration.

CAUSES

The muscular band that encircles the pylorus thickens and eventually closes off the outlet from the baby's stomach.

RISK FACTORS

Family history of pyloric stenosis.

PREVENTING COMPLICATIONS OR RECURRENCE

Cannot be prevented at present.

WHAT TO EXPECT

MEDICAL TESTS

- Your own observation of symptoms.
- Medical history and physical exam by a doctor.
- Laboratory blood counts and studies of fluids and electrolytes.
- X-rays of the stomach (sometimes).

POSSIBLE COMPLICATIONS

Weight loss, dehydration, shock, and death without treatment.

PROBABLE OUTCOME

Curable with surgery. The child usually recovers quickly.

PYLORIC STENOSIS, CONGENITAL (Hypertrophic Pyloric Stenosis)

TREATMENT

HOME CARE

After surgery:

- A firm ridge will appear at the incision site. This is a healthy sign and requires no treatment.
- Wash the incision site gently several times a day.
- If the baby seems uncomfortable, apply warm compresses to the incision site.

MEDICATION

- Intravenous fluids and electrolytes until the baby is ready for surgery.

Medication is usually not necessary after surgery.

- See Medications section for information regarding medicines your doctor may prescribe.

ACTIVITY

No restrictions.

DIET & FLUIDS

The baby may tolerate small feedings of half-strength formula while awaiting surgery—check with your doctor. If not, formula will be given by stomach tube.

OK FOR SCHOOL, PRESCHOOL, OR NURSERY?

When strength and feeling of well-being will allow.

CALL YOUR DOCTOR IF

- Your baby vomits repeatedly.
- The following occurs after surgery:
  - — Pain, swelling, redness, bleeding, or drainage at the surgical site.
  - — Temperature spike (sudden rise) to 101F (38.3C).

ILLNESSES

RABIES
(Hydrophobia)

GENERAL INFORMATION

DESCRIPTION

Rabies is a serious virus infection of the central nervous system, transmitted by the bite of an infected animal. Body parts involved include the central nervous system—including the brain, the coverings of the brain (meninges), and the spinal cord—and peripheral nerves as well as body parts bitten by the rabid animal. Appropriate health care includes: physician's monitoring of general condition and medications; surgery to clean and repair the bite wound (sometimes); hospitalization, if symptoms develop.

SIGNS & SYMPTOMS

- Symptoms may appear 3 to 7 weeks after the bite. Early symptoms are: restlessness and irritability; fatigue; slight fever; cough; sore throat; increased saliva and tears.
- 2 to 10 days later: violent spasms of throat muscles that make swallowing impossible; hyperactivity and violent behavior; confusion; high fever; irregular heartbeat; irregular breathing.

CAUSES

- A virus in the saliva of infected animals passes to humans through broken skin or a mucous membrane. The virus travels slowly from the bite area to the brain.
- Animals that are commonly infected include dogs (especially wild dogs), bats, skunks, foxes, coyotes, and raccoons. Other animals can also be infected, so consult your local health department after *any* animal bite.

RISK FACTORS

- Multiple bites or bites on the child's face, head, neck, or upper body.
- Outdoor activities that expose your child to wild animals, especially cave exploration and hunting (in which animals are handled).

PREVENTING COMPLICATIONS OR RECURRENCE

- Vaccinate your dog or cat against rabies, report stray animals in the neighborhood and teach your child to avoid them, and anyone whose work involves animals should have a rabies immunization.
- Keep your child's tetanus immunizations up-to-date. See Appendix 1 for an immunization schedule.

WHAT TO EXPECT

MEDICAL TESTS

- Your own observation of the animal's behavior. Try to determine if the animal was provoked. Unprovoked attacking animals are more likely to be infected.
- Medical history and physical exam by a doctor.
- Laboratory blood tests, and fluid and electrolyte measurements.
- Pathological exam of the animal's tissue.

POSSIBLE COMPLICATIONS

Dehydration and shock; coma; paralysis; death.

RABIES (Hydrophobia)

PROBABLE OUTCOME

Rabies can be prevented with early treatment for your child following an animal bite. Once symptoms begin, survival is unlikely. The mortality rate is 80%.

TREATMENT

HOME CARE

- Wash the bite area for 10 minutes with soap and water to remove all saliva.
- Cover the child's wound with a clean bandage.
- Call your doctor or local emergency room for advice.
- Call your local animal-control center to catch the animal, if possible.
- If the animal is killed, remove the head and refrigerate or freeze it until it can be examined by pathologists.
- Don't panic. The incubation period allows time for diagnosis and treatment of your child.

MEDICATION

Painful injections in the abdomen are no longer necessary.

Your doctor may prescribe one of the following:

- Injections of rabies-immune globulin.
- Injections of human-diploid-cell-strain vaccine, if the animal is proven rabid.
- Tetanus booster.

ACTIVITY

No restrictions unless symptoms begin. If they do, bed rest in a hospital is necessary for your child.

DIET & FLUIDS

No special diet during outpatient treatment before symptoms begin. Intravenous fluids and nutrients are necessary during the child's hospitalization.

OK FOR SCHOOL, PRESCHOOL, OR NURSERY?

Not until signs of infection have decreased, appetite returns, and alertness, strength, and feeling of well-being will allow.

CALL YOUR DOCTOR IF

Your child is bitten by an animal.

RADIATION SICKNESS

GENERAL INFORMATION

DESCRIPTION

Radiation sickness consists of the side effects that accompany radiation treatment for cancer or the aftereffects of accidental exposure to radiation. Body parts involved depend on the location of treatment or exposure. See SIGNS & SYMPTOMS below.

Appropriate health care includes: physician's monitoring of general condition and medications; psychotherapy or counseling to reduce the stress of radiation treatment; hospitalization for radiation treatment or complications.

SIGNS & SYMPTOMS

The following vary widely, and are often temporary, depending on the radiation dosage and the area radiated: nausea, vomiting, and diarrhea; headache; fatigue and shortness of breath; rapid heartbeat; yeast infection in the mouth; dry mouth and loss of taste; swallowing difficulty; worsening of tooth or gum disease; hair loss; dry cough; heart inflammation with chest pain; burning, inflammation, or scarring of skin; permanent skin darkening; bleeding spots anywhere under the skin; anemia.

CAUSES

Radiation damage to the immune system and to healthy tissues.

RISK FACTORS

For radiation treatment: poor nutrition and illness that has lowered resistance.

PREVENTING COMPLICATIONS OR RECURRENCE

Your child should have a thorough dental checkup to detect tooth or gum disease before head or neck radiation treatment. Your child should eat well before radiation treatment to be in optimal nutritional condition. Anyone who works around radiation should learn and observe safety regulations.

WHAT TO EXPECT

MEDICAL TESTS

Laboratory blood studies of hemoglobin, platelet counts, and white blood cell counts, and X-rays of treated areas.

POSSIBLE COMPLICATIONS

Susceptibility to infections due to decreased resistance; sterility or birth defects; increased susceptibility to cancer—especially bone-marrow cancer or leukemia. With radiation treatment, other complications depend on the area involved. Your doctor will explain possible complications for your child. Modern radiation equipment makes serious complications unlikely.

PROBABLE OUTCOME

With radiation treatment, most side effects or complications disappear gradually afterward. With radiation accidents not severe enough to cause immediate death, side effects may not appear for years.

TREATMENT

HOME CARE

If you are undergoing radiation treatments:

• Use effective birth-control measures to prevent pregnancy until your doctor determines it is safe to have children.

If your child is undergoing radiation treatments:

• Encourage your child to join a support group of people with similar experiences.

• During radiation treatment, keep your doctor informed of how your child is feeling. Treatments can sometimes be interrupted until the child feels better.

• If the radiation treatments result in hair loss, get the child a wig to wear until hair growth resumes.

MEDICATION

Your doctor may prescribe:

• Anti-nausea drugs.

• Pain relievers.

• Blood transfusions for anemia.

• Antibiotics to fight infections.

ACTIVITY

Your child should be as active as strength allows, but the child should rest often.

DIET & FLUIDS

Your child should eat a balanced diet. The child may temporarily need a liquid diet or food prepared in a blender if there is a problem with swallowing. Intravenous feeding or use of a small stomach tube is also possible until your child can resume normal eating. A dietitian can help.

OK FOR SCHOOL, PRESCHOOL, OR NURSERY?

When appetite has returned and alertness, strength, and feeling of well-being will allow.

CALL YOUR DOCTOR IF

• Your child is accidentally exposed to radiation.

• Your child feels very ill during radiation treatment, especially if there are unexpected symptoms.

• Your child develops signs of infection, such as fever and chills, muscle aches, headache, and dizziness, during or after exposure or treatment.

• New, unexplained symptoms develop. Drugs used in treatment may produce side effects.

RAPE CRISIS SYNDROME

GENERAL INFORMATION

DESCRIPTION

Rape crisis syndrome consists of the physical and emotional aftereffects of rape (forced sexual entry into the body). The genitals, rectum, mouth, and brain are involved. Rape crisis syndrome can affect both sexes, all ages, but is more common in females. Appropriate health care includes: doctor's treatment *always*—regardless of whether there are physical injuries; surgery to repair any wounds; hospitalization (rare); psychotherapy or counseling to learn to cope with fear, sexual trauma, and unrealistic feelings of guilt or worthlessness.

SIGNS & SYMPTOMS

- Cuts, bruises or other injuries, including vaginal and rectal tears.
- Effects of exposure to the elements, if the attack occurred outdoors or in a remote place.
- Fear, anger, crying, or unusual behavior such as hysterical laughter.
- Unwarranted self-blame and guilt.
- Depression and withdrawal, even from family and friends.
- No outward signs (sometimes).

CAUSES

Rape is not a sexual act for pleasure. It is a show of power—often an act of violence—and an attempt to degrade or humiliate the victim. Some rapists have been victims of sexual abuse. Many know their victims—at least casually—and their attacks may be planned, not impulsive.

RISK FACTORS

Economically depressed areas; excess alcohol consumption or drug abuse by the potential rapist.

PREVENTING COMPLICATIONS OR RECURRENCE

At home:

- Keep doors and windows locked.
- Install security devices.

Instructions for your child away from home:

- Avoid dark, quiet, or isolated places. Stay within sight of others.
- Never hitchhike.
- Always lock your car.
- Check the back seat of your car before getting in.
- Take a self-defense course.
- Carry a rape siren or whistle. Most authorities don't recommend that you carry a weapon. It might be taken away by the rapist and used on you.
- If you are threatened with rape, remain calm. Panic may worsen the situation.
- Sometimes a rapist can be stopped by unexpected behavior, such as asking for help with a task or mentioning that you have a disease such as herpes or AIDS—you can lie to a rapist. Try to speak in a calm, matter-of-fact manner.

WHAT TO EXPECT

MEDICAL TESTS

- Your own observation of your child's appearance and demeanor. Some rape victims are too traumatized to talk about what happened.
- Medical history and physical exam by a doctor.
- Laboratory studies, such as: cultures and blood tests for gonorrhea or other venereal disease; detailed examination of the child's body for evidence from the rapist, such as hair, sperm, or bits of clothing; X-rays, if fractures are suspected.

POSSIBLE COMPLICATIONS

Prolonged psychological trauma; pregnancy; venereal disease.

PROBABLE OUTCOME

Your child's complete physical and psychological recovery is often possible with professional treatment.

TREATMENT

HOME CARE

Instructions for your child who has been raped:

- Report the rape to police or a rape crisis center. If you don't, the rapist will probably attack others.
- Call your doctor or go to the nearest emergency room. Many cities have rape-crisis teams to help you through the stress of the medical examination.
- Don't bathe, douche, or change clothes before being examined.
- Talk over your feelings with trusted friends and family. Suppressing your feelings increases distress.

MEDICATION

Your doctor may prescribe:

- Antibiotics, if venereal infection is suspected or diagnosed.
- Hormones to prevent pregnancy ("day-after pill").
- Sedatives or tranquilizers for a short time to reduce anxiety.

ACTIVITY

Your child should resume normal life as quickly as possible.

DIET & FLUIDS

No special diet.

OK FOR SCHOOL, PRESCHOOL, OR NURSERY?

When crisis has passed and appetite has returned and alertness, strength, and feeling of well-being will allow.

CALL YOUR DOCTOR IF

You know or suspect your child has been raped.

RAYNAUD'S DISEASE

GENERAL INFORMATION

DESCRIPTION

Raynaud's disease is a primary disorder of the circulatory system that affects blood circulation to the fingers and occasionally the toes. This is different from Raynaud's phenomenon, which is a circulatory-system disorder that occurs as a complication of other diseases. The small arteries to the hands and feet are involved. Both sexes can be affected but it is most common in females after age 12.

Appropriate health care includes:

- Self-care after diagnosis.
- Doctor's treatment.
- Biofeedback training (see Glossary).
- Surgery to sever sympathetic nerves to the involved extremities. Surgery usually relieves symptoms for 1 to 2 years before they recur.

SIGNS & SYMPTOMS

Early symptoms:

- Fingers that turn pale when exposed to cold or stress. Paleness is followed by a bluish tinge, then redness. Pain, numbness and tingling accompany the color changes. Warmth relieves these symptoms.

Late symptoms:

- Chronic infections around the child's fingernails and toenails.
- Ulcers on fingertips caused by inadequate blood circulation in fingers.

Symptoms develop gradually over a period of years. With Raynaud's phenomenon, symptoms may begin suddenly.

CAUSES

Spasms of arteries that supply blood to the fingers and toes caused by extreme sensitivity to cold. The sensitivity may be due to poor function of the child's autoimmune system.

RISK FACTORS

Stress; smoking, which impairs circulation to the extremities; cold, wet weather.

PREVENTING COMPLICATIONS OR RECURRENCE

Your child should not start smoking. Tobacco triggers the problem. This disease is rare among non-smokers.

OTHER

There are many similarities between Raynaud's disease and Raynaud's phenomenon. Diagnosis between the two may require years of observation.

WHAT TO EXPECT

MEDICAL TESTS

- Your own observation of symptoms.
- Medical history and physical exam by a doctor.
- Laboratory blood studies.
- X-rays of the child's hands and feet.

POSSIBLE COMPLICATIONS

- Permanent weakness and numbness in the child's toes and fingers.
- Gangrene and amputation (worst cases only).

PROBABLE OUTCOME

This condition is currently considered incurable. The disease worsens gradually over many years. However, your child's symptoms can be relieved or controlled. Most children cope well with Raynaud's disease and live a normal life span if complications don't arise. Scientific research into causes and treatment continues, so there is hope for increasingly effective treatment and cure.

TREATMENT

HOME CARE

Instructions for your child:

- Stop smoking. Symptoms will improve if you do.
- Avoid exposure to cold in any form. Wear mittens and gloves outdoors and when handling ice or frozen foods.
- Wear comfortable, roomy shoes and wool socks.
- Avoid stressful situations. See Appendix 19.
- Move to a warm climate, if possible.

MEDICATION

- Your doctor may prescribe:
  —Vasodilator drugs to dilate the small arteries and improve circulation.
  —Sedatives to reduce the child's stress.
- See Medications section for information regarding medicines your doctor may prescribe.

ACTIVITY

No restrictions, except for your child to keep warm and to avoid chilling while participating in active sports.

DIET & FLUIDS

- No special diet.
- Because alcohol dilates blood vessels and may temporarily improve circulation slightly, your child may have an occasional alcoholic drink if your doctor suggests this.

OK FOR SCHOOL, PRESCHOOL, OR NURSERY?

When appetite returns and alertness, strength, and feeling of well-being will allow.

CALL YOUR DOCTOR IF

- Your child has symptoms of Raynaud's disease.
- Discomfort worsens, despite treatment.
- Ulcers that do not heal appear on the child's fingers or toes.

RAYNAUD'S PHENOMENON

GENERAL INFORMATION

DESCRIPTION

Raynaud's phenomenon is a circulatory-system disorder affecting fingers and toes that is a complication of an underlying disease or emotional disturbance. This is different from Raynaud's disease, which is a primary disease. Symptoms arise suddenly with Raynaud's phenomenon. With Raynaud's disease, they appear slowly over several years. The small arteries to the hands and feet are involved. It affects both sexes and all ages, but is most common in young women.

Appropriate health care includes:

- Self-care after diagnosis.
- Doctor's treatment.
- Surgery to sever sympathetic nerves to the child's affected extremities.

Surgery sometimes relieves symptoms for 1 or 2 years before they recur.

SIGNS & SYMPTOMS

Early symptoms:

- Fingers that turn pale when exposed to cold or stress. Paleness is followed by a bluish tinge and then redness. Numbness and tingling accompany the color changes, and the child's symptoms are relieved by warmth.

Late symptoms:

- Ulcers on the child's fingertips caused by lack of normal blood flow to the fingers.
- Chronic infections under and around the child's fingernails and toenails.

CAUSES

Spasms of arteries that supply blood to the child's fingers and toes. Spasms may be caused by:

- Scleroderma, lupus erythematosus, or other connective-tissue disorders.
- Buerger's disease.
- Cor pulmonale.
- Certain medications, including ergot preparations, antihypertensives, alpha- and beta-adrenergic blockers, and calcium-channel blockers.

RISK FACTORS

- Stress.
- Smoking.
- Cold, wet weather.
- Activities that involve working with heavy equipment that vibrates forcefully, such as a chain saw or pneumatic drill.

PREVENTING COMPLICATIONS OR RECURRENCE

Instructions for your child:

- Don't smoke.
- Avoid exposure to the cold.
- Obtain medical treatment for diseases listed as causes.
- Avoid exposure to cigarette smoke from other people.

OTHER

Because of the similarities between Raynaud's disease and Raynaud's phenomenon, an accurate diagnosis between the two may require years of observation.

WHAT TO EXPECT

MEDICAL TESTS

- Your own observation of symptoms.
- Medical history and physical exam by a doctor.
- Laboratory blood studies.
- X-rays of the child's hands and feet.

POSSIBLE COMPLICATIONS

- Permanent weakness and numbness in the child's toes and fingers caused by blockage of the blood supply.
- Gangrene that necessitates amputation, caused by loss of blood supply (worst cases only).

PROBABLE OUTCOME

Curable if the underlying cause can be cured.

TREATMENT

HOME CARE

Instructions for your child:

- Don't smoke.
- Avoid exposure to cold in any form. Wear mittens and gloves outdoors and when handling ice or frozen food.
- Wear comfortable, roomy shoes and wool socks. Don't go barefoot outdoors.
- Avoid stressful situations whenever possible. See Appendix 19.
- Move to a warm climate, if possible.

MEDICATION

Your doctor may prescribe:

- Vasodilator drugs to dilate small arteries and improve the child's circulation.
- Sedatives to relieve the child's tension and anxiety.

ACTIVITY

No restrictions, except for your child to keep warm and to avoid chilling, which may happen following any active recreational sport.

DIET & FLUIDS

No special diet. Alcohol dilates blood vessels and may temporarily improve circulation slightly. An occasional alcoholic beverage may be helpful to your child if the doctor suggests this.

OK FOR SCHOOL, PRESCHOOL, OR NURSERY?

When appetite returns and alertness, strength, and feeling of well-being will allow.

CALL YOUR DOCTOR IF

- Your child has symptoms of Raynaud's phenomenon.
- Discomfort worsens, despite treatment.
- Ulcers appear on the child's fingers or toes and do not heal.

REITER'S SYNDROME

GENERAL INFORMATION

DESCRIPTION

Reiter's syndrome is an inflammatory disease characterized by a complex of symptoms resembling those of arthritis, urethritis, conjunctivitis, and psoriasis. This is probably a sexually transmitted disease. The joints, eyes (including white eye covering), urethra and head of the penis, and skin are involved. Reiter's syndrome affects adolescent and young adult males.

Appropriate health care includes:

- Physician's monitoring of general condition and medications, diagnosis, and supervision of treatment.
- Self-care after diagnosis.

SIGNS & SYMPTOMS

- Inflammation of the urethra and discharge within 7 to 14 days after sexual intercourse.
- Frequent urinary urgency.
- Small ulcers inside the mouth, on the tongue, and on the penis tip.
- Low fever.
- Red eyes.
- Painful joints, especially toes, legs, hips, and back.
- Aching in the pelvis.
- Skin lesions similar to psoriasis on the soles and palms and around the fingernails and toenails.

CAUSES

Unknown. The predisposition is inherited, and the disease usually follows sexual contact. It probably represents an unusual response to a sexually transmitted infection.

RISK FACTORS

- Recent gastrointestinal illness with diarrhea.
- Previous sexually transmitted infections.
- Family history of Reiter's syndrome.
- Genetic factors. Most persons with this disease carry antigen HLA-B27.

PREVENTING COMPLICATIONS OR RECURRENCE

Advise your son to use rubber condoms for sexual intercourse.

WHAT TO EXPECT

MEDICAL TESTS

- Your own observation of symptoms.
- Medical history and physical exam by a doctor.
- Laboratory blood studies and culture of the urethral discharge.

POSSIBLE COMPLICATIONS

Osteoporosis.

PROBABLE OUTCOME

Your son's arthritis symptoms may continue up to 4 months; others disappear sooner. Most patients recover in 2 to 16 weeks with no residual signs of the disease, but some have recurrent flare-ups and remissions.

TREATMENT

HOME CARE

To relieve foot pain, your son should wear cushion pads and arch supports in his shoes.

MEDICATION

Your doctor may prescribe:

- Non-steroidal anti-inflammatory drugs.
- Antibiotics, such as tetracyclines, for urethritis.
- See Medications section for information regarding medicines your doctor may prescribe.

ACTIVITY

- Your son should stay as active as the condition allows, but it is important to avoid sexual excitement and activity during the illness.
- Your son should exercise the affected joints according to instructions from your doctor or physical therapist. Don't immobilize affected joints.

DIET & FLUIDS

No special diet.

OK FOR SCHOOL, PRESCHOOL, OR NURSERY?

When signs of infection have decreased, appetite returns, and alertness, strength, and feeling of well-being will allow.

CALL YOUR DOCTOR IF

- Your child has symptoms of Reiter's syndrome.
- Symptoms recur after recovery.
- New, unexplained symptoms develop. Drugs used in treatment may produce side effects.

RETINAL DETACHMENT

GENERAL INFORMATION

DESCRIPTION

Retinal detachment is a separation or tear of the retina (the light-sensitive tissue at the back of the eye) from the remainder of the eye. It requires immediate treatment! It affects all ages and both sexes but is more common in males than females. Appropriate health care includes:

- Doctor's (ophthalmologist's) treatment. This is an emergency!
- Surgery to reattach the retina using special lasers or cryotherapy (see Glossary), or by changing the shape of the eye (sometimes).

SIGNS & SYMPTOMS

The following usually affect one eye, but sometimes both of the child's eyes are affected:

- Light flashes in the field of vision.
- Floating spots in the field of vision.
- Blurred vision.
- Wavy visual images (sometimes).
- Gradual loss of vision. This may not be noticed because it is so gradual.
- No pain.

CAUSES

- Extreme nearsightedness (myopia).
- Complications of eye surgery.
- Eye injury.
- Inherited tendency (possibly).

RISK FACTORS

- Age.
- Diabetes mellitus.
- Vascular disease.
- Previous retinal detachment.
- Family history of retinal detachment.

PREVENTING COMPLICATIONS OR RECURRENCE

Instructions for your child:

- Wear protective eye shields when participating in sports.
- If you have diabetes mellitus or vascular disease, obtain medical treatment to control the disorder. See an opthalmologist at least once a year.

WHAT TO EXPECT

MEDICAL TESTS

- Your own observation of symptoms.
- Medical history and physical exam by a doctor.

POSSIBLE COMPLICATIONS

- Without treatment: Partial or complete blindness in the affected eye.
- With delayed treatment: Detachment that extends to the macula (the area of most detailed vision). This causes permanent loss of detailed (central) vision.

PROBABLE OUTCOME

Often treatable with early surgical treatment using laser-beam surgery.

TREATMENT

HOME CARE

The following instructions for your child apply after surgery:

- Both eyes will be patched for a time. Your family and friends can help overcome this stress by providing companionship and assistance.
- Use dark glasses after the patches are removed.
- Don't rub your eyes.
- Don't bend over.
- Avoid straining, such as from constipation, heavy lifting, or harsh coughing. This may increase pressure in the eyes.

MEDICATION

- Your doctor may prescribe:
  —Mydriatic eye drops to dilate the pupil. Dilation reduces eye activity during healing. If your child cannot instill the drops, someone should be available to help at the appropriate times.
  —Sedatives or tranquilizers to reduce anxiety during the child's convalescence.
- See Medications section for information regarding medicines your doctor may prescribe.

ACTIVITY

After surgery, your child should lie on the back in bed with the head elevated. Moving the legs frequently helps prevent blood clots from forming in deep veins. Your child can resume normal activities when your ophthalmologist considers it safe.

DIET & FLUIDS

No special diet.

OK FOR SCHOOL, PRESCHOOL, OR NURSERY?

Wait for clearance from your doctor.

CALL YOUR DOCTOR IF

- Your child has flashes or floating spots in the field of vision.
- Any sign of infection (bleeding, redness, pain, swelling, or fever) occurs after surgery.
- Your child's vision worsens after full recovery from surgery.

REYE'S SYNDROME

GENERAL INFORMATION

DESCRIPTION

Reye's syndrome is a disease that involves the brain and other major organs, including the liver, kidneys, and heart. Reye's syndrome affects children from infancy through adolescence.

Appropriate health care includes:

- Physician's monitoring of general condition and medications.
- Hospitalization for intensive care to monitor pressure on the brain.
- Home care during convalescence.

SIGNS & SYMPTOMS

- Confusion.
- Lethargy.
- Personality changes.
- Seizures.
- Weakness and paralysis in an arm or leg.
- Double vision.
- Speech impairment.
- Hearing loss.
- Drowsiness that progresses to coma.

CAUSES

Unknown. Reye's syndrome usually follows a virus infection. Some studies link it to the use of aspirin during a viral illness, especially chickenpox and influenza.

RISK FACTORS

- Recent illness, such as chickenpox, influenza, or other respiratory illness.
- Use of aspirin.
- Genetic factors. This is more common in Caucasians than in blacks.

PREVENTING COMPLICATIONS OR RECURRENCE

Don't give a child aspirin for any illness with fever until the doctor has diagnosed it. If the illness is diagnosed as viral, *don't use aspirin.*

WHAT TO EXPECT

MEDICAL TESTS

- Your own observation of symptoms.
- Medical history and physical exam by a doctor.
- Laboratory studies, such as blood studies of liver function and an analysis of cerebrospinal fluid.

POSSIBLE COMPLICATIONS

Permanent brain damage, coma, or death caused by pressure on the brain.

PROBABLE OUTCOME

With treatment, 80% of patients survive. Most children recover completely, but some have varying degrees of brain damage.

TREATMENT

HOME CARE

No specific instructions except those listed under other headings.

MEDICATION

Your doctor may prescribe:
- Intravenous fluids.
- Anticoagulant drugs to prevent blood-clot formation during prolonged bed rest.
- Drugs, such as dexamethasone, to reduce cerebral swelling.
- Antibiotics to fight secondary bacterial infections, if they develop.
- See Medications section for information regarding medicines your doctor may prescribe.

ACTIVITY

Bed rest is necessary for your child until the acute stage is over. Reading or watching TV is acceptable. Normal activities may then be resumed gradually.

DIET & FLUIDS

No special diet.

OK FOR SCHOOL, PRESCHOOL, OR NURSERY?

When signs of infection have decreased, appetite returns, and alertness, strength, and feeling of well-being will allow.

CALL YOUR DOCTOR IF

- Your child has symptoms of Reye's syndrome. Call at the first sign of confusion, lethargy, or other mental changes!
- After hospitalization, any symptoms of Reye's syndrome recur or the child develops fever of 100F (37.8C) or higher.
- New, unexplained symptoms develop. Drugs used in treatment may produce side effects.

RHEUMATIC FEVER

GENERAL INFORMATION

DESCRIPTION

Rheumatic fever is an inflammatory complication of Group A streptococcal infections. It affects many parts of the body, especially the joints, heart, and heart valves, and sometimes the skin and brain. Strep infections are contagious, but rheumatic fever is not. Rheumatic fever affects children between ages 4 and 18. Appropriate health care includes: physician's monitoring of general condition and medications; home care after diagnosis (mild cases); hospitalization (severe cases).

SIGNS & SYMPTOMS

- Joint inflammation, characterized by pain, redness, swelling, and warmth. The child's wrists, elbows, knees, or ankles are most often affected. Joint inflammation usually subsides in 10 to 14 days, but without treatment, other joints may become inflamed.
- Fever.
- Loss of appetite.
- General ill feeling.
- Mild skin rash on the chest, back, and abdomen.
- Small, painless bumps just under the skin in body areas such as the elbows or knees.
- Fatigue.
- Paleness.

If the heart is involved:

- Shortness of breath.
- Fluid retention that causes swelling of the legs and back.
- Rapid heartbeat, especially when lying down.

CAUSES

Rheumatic fever is caused by a preceding strep infection, usually in the throat, that occurs 1 to 6 weeks prior to the onset of the child's symptoms. It is probably an autoimmune disorder in which antibodies produced to attack the strep bacteria also attack tissues of the joints or heart.

RISK FACTORS

Poor nutrition; family history of rheumatic fever; crowded or unsanitary living conditions; untreated streptococcal infections.

PREVENTING COMPLICATIONS OR RECURRENCE

- Request a throat culture for strep for your child from your doctor's office for any throat infection.
- Obtain prompt antibiotic treatment for your child for any strep infection, including those of the skin. Strep infections must be treated with antibiotics, usually penicillin, for *a minimum of 10 days orally or by long-lasting injection.*

WHAT TO EXPECT

MEDICAL TESTS

- Your own observation of symptoms.
- Medical history and physical exam by a doctor.
- Laboratory studies, such as blood studies, a throat culture, and EKG (see Glossary).
- X-rays of the chest and heart.

POSSIBLE COMPLICATIONS

Permanently damaged heart valves, leading to congestive heart failure.

PROBABLE OUTCOME

Usually curable with treatment. In some cases, rheumatic fever may damage the child's heart valves. A damaged valve can be replaced with surgery. In rare cases, rheumatic fever is fatal—even with treatment.

TREATMENT

HOME CARE

- Take your child's temperature and count the pulse; keep a record for your doctor.
- Use a cool-mist humidifier if the child has a sore throat or cough.

MEDICATION

Your doctor may prescribe:

- Steroids (anti-inflammatory drugs) or aspirin to reduce inflammation.
- Diuretics to reduce fluid retention.
- Antibiotics to fight any remaining strep bacteria. Once rheumatic fever reaches the inactive stage, your child may continue taking low-dose antibiotics indefinitely to prevent recurrence.

ACTIVITY

Your child should stay in bed until laboratory studies show the disease has subsided. Bed rest for 2 to 5 weeks is usually required, but some cases require months. Provide a bedpan or bedside commode so the child won't have to get up to use the bathroom.

DIET & FLUIDS

Serve your child a liquid or soft diet in the early stages, progressing to a normal diet high in protein, calories, and vitamins.

OK FOR SCHOOL, PRESCHOOL, OR NURSERY?

When signs of infection have decreased, appetite returns, and alertness, strength, and feeling of well-being will allow.

CALL YOUR DOCTOR IF

- Your child has symptoms of rheumatic fever.
- The following symptoms occur during treatment: swelling of the legs or back; shortness of breath; vomiting or diarrhea; cough; severe abdominal pain; fever of 101F (38.3C) or higher.

RIB FRACTURE

GENERAL INFORMATION

DESCRIPTION

A rib fracture is a complete or incomplete fracture of any of the 12 ribs on either side. Most rib fractures are accompanied by sprain or rupture of muscles, tendons, or ligaments between the ribs (intercostal structures). Rib fractures are relatively common injuries in athletes, particularly those who compete in contact sports. Appropriate health care includes:

- Doctor care and X-rays to confirm the diagnosis.
- Application of a wide elastic binder to decrease movement of chest muscles and reduce pain with breathing.
- Hospitalization if symptoms of lung, spleen, or liver injury appear.

SIGNS & SYMPTOMS

- Severe pain at the fracture site.
- Tenderness to the touch.
- A feeling that the "wind has been knocked out" of the child (sometimes).
- Abdominal pain if the fractured ribs are below the diaphragm (the 11th and 12th ribs).
- Severe chest pain when the child coughs, sneezes, or breathes deeply.
- A feeling of small air pockets under the skin of the chest or neck if the child's lung has been injured and has leaked air.
- Swelling and bruising over the fracture site.

CAUSES

- Direct blow to the child's chest from a blunt object, such as a steering wheel.
- Compression of the chest, such as being crushed in a sports pileup.

RISK FACTORS

Contact sports, especially football, hockey, boxing, wrestling, or rugby; history of bone or joint disease; poor nutrition, especially calcium deficiency; reckless driving.

PREVENTING COMPLICATIONS OR RECURRENCE

Use seat belts and shoulder restraints in your automobile.

WHAT TO EXPECT

MEDICAL TESTS

Your own observation of symptoms; medical history and physical exam by a doctor; repeated X-rays of the child's ribs and vertebral column. (Early X-rays may not show fractures if they are not dislocated, but repeat X-rays taken 4 or more days later usually reveal them.) The early treatment for an uncomplicated rib fracture is the same as for bruised ribs, so a delay in diagnosis does not hinder treatment.

POSSIBLE COMPLICATIONS

Rupture of the child's lung with bleeding or escape of air into the chest wall or under the skin in the neck; injury to the liver if the right 11th or 12th ribs are fractured and have jagged edges; injury or rupture of the spleen if the 11th and 12th ribs on the left are fractured and have jagged edges; prolonged pain and slow healing.

PROBABLE OUTCOME

If this is a child's first-time chest injury and there are no complications of internal injury. Healing is usually complete in 4 to 6 weeks.

TREATMENT

FIRST AID

If injury to the lung, liver, or spleen is suspected, transport the child to the nearest emergency facility.

HOME CARE

- Use the chest binder as long as needed to ease the child's pain and provide support—usually 4 to 6 weeks.
- Use an ice pack 3 or 4 times a day. Place chips in a plastic bag. Wrap the bag in a moist towel and place over the injured area. Use for 20 minutes at a time.
- After 2 or 3 days, if heat is more soothing to the child than ice, use heat lamps, hot soaks, hot showers, or heating pads.

MEDICATION

- For minor discomfort, use aspirin, acetaminophen, or ibuprofen; topical liniments and ointments.
- Your doctor may prescribe stronger pain relievers.
- Injection of long-acting local anesthesia into the fracture site to reduce the child's pain and allow normal breathing (sometimes).

ACTIVITY

Your child can resume normal activities gradually after clearance from the doctor.

DIET & FLUIDS

No restrictions.

OK FOR SCHOOL, PRESCHOOL, OR NURSERY?

Yes, when condition and sense of well-being will allow.

CALL YOUR DOCTOR IF

- Your child has symptoms of a fractured rib.
- Any of the following occur after diagnosis: shortness of breath; uncontrollable chest pain; sudden or severe abdominal pain; nausea or vomiting; swelling of the abdomen.
- New, unexplained symptoms develop. Drugs used in treatment may produce side effects.

RINGWORM

GENERAL INFORMATION

DESCRIPTION

Ringworm is a fungus (tinea) infection of the skin. This is transmitted by person-to-person contact or by contact with infected surfaces, such as towels, shoes, or shower stalls. The scalp (tinea capitis), skin (tinea corporis), groin skin (tinea cruris), nails (tinea unguium), feet (tinea pedis), and skin with beard (tinea barbae) are involved. Ringworm can affect both sexes but is more common in males.

Appropriate health care includes:

- Self-care after diagnosis.
- Physician's monitoring of general condition and medications.

SIGNS & SYMPTOMS

Lesions that itch (sometimes) and have the following characteristics:

- On the scalp, lesions cause patchy hair loss and scaling scalp.
- On the body skin, lesions are red, circular, flat, and scaling, and have well-defined borders.
- On the bearded area of the face, lesions cause an itchy, scaling rash.
- On the feet: see Athlete's Foot in the Illnesses section.
- On the nails: see Paronychia and Nails, Ringworm Infection of, in the Illnesses section.

CAUSES

Fungus infection with one or more of 5 different fungi.

RISK FACTORS

- Diabetes mellitus.
- Exposure to darkness, moisture, and warmth.
- Crowded or unsanitary living conditions.

PREVENTING COMPLICATIONS OR RECURRENCE

The fungi are so prevalent that total prevention is impossible. To minimize risk your child should:

- Avoid continuous exposure to overheated humid environments.
- Avoid contact with pets that have skin problems.

? WHAT TO EXPECT

MEDICAL TESTS

- Your own observation of symptoms.
- Medical history and physical exam by a doctor.
- Microscopic exam of skin scrapings in potassium hydroxide solution.
- Laboratory culture of skin scrapings.
- Examination with ultraviolet light (Wood's lamp) for ringworm on the scalp.

POSSIBLE COMPLICATIONS

Secondary bacterial infection of ringworm lesions.

PROBABLE OUTCOME

Usually curable in 6 weeks with treatment, but recurrence is common. Ringworm becomes chronic in 20% of cases.

TREATMENT

HOME CARE

For ringworm on the child's body:

• Boil or chemically sterilize all clothing, towels, or bed linens that have touched the lesions.

• Keep the child's skin dry. Moist areas favor fungus growth.

• The child should wear cotton underwear, which should be changed more than once a day. Don't let the child wear tight clothes.

• If the area is red, swollen, and weeping, use compresses made of 1 teaspoon salt to 1 pint water. Apply 4 times a day for 2 to 3 days before starting the local anti-fungal medication.

For ringworm of the child's scalp:

• Shampoo the hair every day.

• Have the hair cut short, but don't shave the child's scalp. Place large sheets of paper under and around the hair and chair to catch all the clippings. Place a cloth drape around the child's shoulders, chest, and back. The child should not wear street clothes for a haircut but instead should wear something that can be sterilized, such as pajamas, a housecoat, or a smock. Repeat this procedure every 2 weeks, or whenever the hair grows back.

MEDICATION

• Your doctor may prescribe oral or topical anti-fungal drugs.

• See Medications section for information regarding medicines your doctor may prescribe.

ACTIVITY

No restrictions.

DIET & FLUIDS

No special diet.

OK FOR SCHOOL, PRESCHOOL, OR NURSERY?

Yes, if the school allows.

CALL YOUR DOCTOR IF

• Your child has symptoms of ringworm.

• Ringworm lesions become redder, painful, and ooze pus.

• Symptoms don't improve in 3 or 4 weeks, despite treatment.

• New, unexplained symptoms develop. Drugs used in treatment may produce side effects.

ROCKY MOUNTAIN SPOTTED FEVER (Tick Fever; Tick Typhus; Spotted Fever)

GENERAL INFORMATION

DESCRIPTION

Rocky Mountain spotted fever is an acute illness with fever caused by a germ transmitted by infected ticks. This is not contagious from person to person. The skin, the central nervous system—including the brain, the coverings of the brain (meninges), and the spinal cord—and peripheral nerves, as well as the gastrointestinal tract and muscles are involved.

Appropriate health care includes:

- Physician's monitoring of general condition and medications. This may be a medical emergency.
- Home care during convalescence.

SIGNS & SYMPTOMS

The following occur 2 to 5 days after a tick bite:

- Fever up to 105F (40.6C) with chills.
- Red skin rash that begins on hands and feet and spreads to ankles, wrists, legs, trunk, and abdomen.
- Headache.
- Muscle aches and weakness; stiff back.
- Nausea and vomiting.
- Mental confusion; coma.

CAUSES

Rickettsia germs that live inside ticks. People are infected through tick bites, usually in the spring or summer. Rickettsia also infect rodents, squirrels, and chipmunks. The disease occurs in all states of the U.S., especially on the Eastern seaboard from Georgia to Maryland, and in heavy brush areas, such as Long Island.

RISK FACTORS

Outdoor activities in tick-infested areas.

PREVENTING COMPLICATIONS OR RECURRENCE

- Urge your child to wear protective clothing in tick-infested areas, and to use insect repellant.
- During outdoor activity, carefully inspect the child's body frequently to remove ticks. Don't crush them during removal—the whole tick must be removed. Hold a lighted cigarette near the tick, or apply gasoline, kerosene, or oil to the tick's body. Pull it off with tweezers.

ROCKY MOUNTAIN SPOTTED FEVER
(Tick Fever; Tick Typhus; Spotted Fever)

? WHAT TO EXPECT

MEDICAL TESTS

- Your own observation of symptoms.
- Medical history and physical exam by a doctor.
- Laboratory studies, such as blood counts and serological tests (see Glossary).

POSSIBLE COMPLICATIONS

Rocky Mountain spotted fever is often fatal if untreated.

PROBABLE OUTCOME

Curable if antibiotic treatment is begun in the early stages.

TREATMENT

HOME CARE

No specific instructions except those listed under other headings.

MEDICATION

- Your doctor may prescribe antibiotics, such as tetracycline or chloramphenicol.
- See Medications section for information regarding medicines your doctor may prescribe.

ACTIVITY

Your child should rest in bed until the fever and other symptoms disappear. Reading or watching TV are acceptable activities.

DIET & FLUIDS

No special diet.

OK FOR SCHOOL, PRESCHOOL, OR NURSERY?

When appetite has returned and alertness, strength, and feeling of well-being will allow.

CALL YOUR DOCTOR IF

- Your child has symptoms of Rocky Mountain spotted fever.
- New, unexplained symptoms develop. Drugs used in treatment may produce side effects.

ILLNESSES

ROSEOLA INFANTUM
(Exanthem Subitum; Pseudorubella)

GENERAL INFORMATION

DESCRIPTION

Roseola infantum is a common, contagious childhood disease characterized by a high fever and skin rash. The skin and central nervous system—including the brain, the coverings of the brain (meninges), and the spinal cord—and peripheral nerves are involved. Roseola infantum affects infants and young children (1 to 3 years).

Appropriate health care includes:

- Home care after diagnosis.
- Physician's monitoring of general condition and medications.

SIGNS & SYMPTOMS

- Fever of 103F (39.4C) to 105F (40.6C) for 3 to 4 days.
- Irritability.
- Drowsiness.
- Flat, reddish skin rash after 3 or 4 days of high fever. When the rash appears, fever and other symptoms disappear.

CAUSES

Unknown. Because roseola has many features of viral illness, it is commonly believed to be caused by a virus—but the organism has not been identified. Incubation is 5 to 15 days.

RISK FACTORS

- Spring and autumn seasons.
- Exposure to others in public places.

PREVENTING COMPLICATIONS OR RECURRENCE

Your child should avoid exposure to others with roseola, if possible.

WHAT TO EXPECT

MEDICAL TESTS

- Your own observation of symptoms.
- Medical history and physical exam by a doctor.
- Laboratory studies, such as urinalysis and blood counts, to rule out other reasons for your child's high fever, such as middle-ear infection, meningitis, pneumonia, or urinary-tract infection.

POSSIBLE COMPLICATIONS

- Convulsions caused by high fever.
- Dehydration.

PROBABLE OUTCOME

Spontaneous recovery in 1 week.

ROSEOLA INFANTUM (Exanthem Subitum; Pseudorubella)

TREATMENT

HOME CARE

Try to reduce your child's fever if it reaches 102F (38.9C) or higher. See How to Reduce Your Child's Fever, Appendix 17.

MEDICATION

- For minor discomfort and to reduce fever, use non-prescription drugs such as acetaminophen.
- See Medications section for information regarding medicines your doctor may prescribe.

ACTIVITY

Your child should rest in bed until the fever disappears.

DIET & FLUIDS

Your child should eat a normal, well-balanced diet. Continue baby-vitamin supplements if the child is accustomed to taking them.

OK FOR SCHOOL, PRESCHOOL, OR NURSERY?

When signs of infection have decreased, appetite returns, and alertness, strength, and feeling of well-being will allow.

CALL YOUR DOCTOR IF

- Fever exceeds 103F (38.4C) rectally.
- Twitching or other signs of a convulsion begin.
- The child refuses liquids.
- The child cries loudly and persistently, and does not stop when picked up.
- The child is listless and has a stiff neck.

ROUNDWORMS (Ascariasis)

GENERAL INFORMATION

DESCRIPTION

Roundworms are intestinal parasites shaped like earthworms that can be seen easily without a microscope. Roundworms thrive in the gastrointestinal tract. They are contagious. The gastrointestinal tract and lungs (sometimes) are involved.

Appropriate health care includes:

- Home care after diagnosis.
- Physician's monitoring of general condition and medications.

SIGNS & SYMPTOMS

- Irritability.
- Restlessness at night.
- Erratic or poor appetite.
- Frequent fatigue.
- Weight loss or lack of weight gain.
- Colicky abdominal discomfort.
- Diarrhea (sometimes).
- Cough and wheezing (rare).

CAUSES

A parasite called ascaris whose eggs enter the human body through contaminated water or food or soil-contaminated hands.

RISK FACTORS

Crowded or unsanitary living conditions.

PREVENTING COMPLICATIONS OR RECURRENCE

- Teach your child to wash hands frequently—*always* before eating.
- Urge your child to keep fingers away from the mouth.
- Have pets treated for worms. Your child should avoid strange animals.

OTHER

Worms may sometimes be seen in bowel movements or in the child's bed. Rarely, one may be vomited.

WHAT TO EXPECT

MEDICAL TESTS

- Your own observation of symptoms.
- Medical history and physical exam by a doctor.
- Laboratory studies to identify the worm.

POSSIBLE COMPLICATIONS

If untreated:

- Anemia or malnutrition. May cause failure to thrive and abnormal physical and mental development in your child.
- Intestinal obstruction (rare).

ROUNDWORMS (Ascariasis)

PROBABLE OUTCOME

Usually curable in 1 week with treatment.

TREATMENT

HOME CARE

- Your child should wash hands carefully after using the toilet or before meals. It is important to keep fingers away from the mouth and to keep nails short and clean.
- Your child should wash the anus and genitals with warm soap and water at least twice a day, rinsing well, preferably under a shower. Tub baths are not advisable.
- If possible, boil all soiled linen, nightclothes, underwear, towels, and washcloths that have been used by anyone with roundworms. Fabrics that cannot be boiled can be soaked in an ammonia solution (1 cup of household ammonia to 5 gallons of cold water).
- After treatment, scrub all toilet seats, bathroom floors, and fixtures. Vacuum rugs, table tops, curtains, sofas, and chairs carefully. Sterilize metal toys or similar objects in a hot oven.

MEDICATION

Your doctor may prescribe drugs to kill the child's roundworms, such as:

- Pyrantel pamoate or piperazine.
- Mebendazole. This medication may cause fetal abnormalities. A pregnant woman should not use mebendazole.
- See Medications section for information regarding medicines your doctor may prescribe.

ACTIVITY

Your child may resume normal activities as soon as symptoms improve.

DIET & FLUIDS

No special diet.

OK FOR SCHOOL, PRESCHOOL, OR NURSERY?

When signs of infection have decreased, appetite returns, and alertness, strength, and feeling of well-being will allow.

CALL YOUR DOCTOR IF

- Your child has symptoms of roundworms.
- Roundworms reappear after treatment.
- New, unexplained symptoms develop. Drugs used in treatment may produce side effects.

ST. VITUS' DANCE
(Sydenham's Chorea; Rheumatic Chorea)

GENERAL INFORMATION

DESCRIPTION

St. Vitus' dance is a temporary disorder of the parts of the brain that control movement and coordination. St. Vitus' dance is not contagious. The central nervous system—including the brain, the coverings of the brain (meninges), and the spinal cord—and peripheral nerves are involved. St. Vitus' dance can affect children of both sexes but is more common in girls.

Appropriate health care includes:

- Home care after diagnosis.
- Physician's monitoring of general condition and medications.
- Psychotherapy or counseling for the patient and family. Parents and teachers should understand that the unusual movements are temporary, and the condition is not contagious.

SIGNS & SYMPTOMS

- Uncontrollable, purposeless and non-repetitive movements that are wandering or jerky. The eyes are not involved.
- Facial grimacing that disappears during sleep.

Symptoms are similar to those of cerebral palsy, except these last for a limited time, while cerebral palsy lasts a lifetime.

CAUSES

A delayed (up to 6 months) complication of inadequately treated Group A streptococcal infections, usually of the throat or skin. St. Vitus' dance is more likely to occur in summer and early autumn.

RISK FACTORS

Prior strep infection.

PREVENTING COMPLICATIONS OR RECURRENCE

- Obtain prompt antibiotic treatment for strep infections of the throat, tonsils, or skin. Your child should take medication at least 10 days.
- A child who has had St. Vitus' dance should take daily antibiotics (usually penicillin or erythromycin) until adulthood to prevent strep infections.

OTHER

Use of phenothiazine drugs and other tranquilizers may produce symptoms identical to those of St. Vitus' dance, leading to misdiagnosis. If your child has these symptoms and takes these drugs, consult your doctor.

? WHAT TO EXPECT

MEDICAL TESTS

- Your own observation of symptoms. Sometimes the symptoms are so mild that you may think only that the child seems unusually clumsy.
- Medical history and physical exam by a doctor.
- Laboratory throat culture and tests of spinal fluid (to rule out other causes of symptoms).
- EEG (see Glossary).

ST. VITUS' DANCE
(Sydenham's Chorea; Rheumatic Chorea)

POSSIBLE COMPLICATIONS

- Injury from involuntary movements.
- Psychosocial problems.

PROBABLE OUTCOME

Spontaneous recovery in 3 to 6 months without lasting effects on personality, intelligence, emotions, or muscle control.

TREATMENT

HOME CARE

- Keep your child away from dangerous implements, such as knives. Use plastic tableware with dull edges to prevent mouth injury.
- Help the child dress and eat, if necessary.
- Provide the child with love, support, and reassurance.

MEDICATION

Your doctor may prescribe:

- Mild sedatives, tranquilizers, or muscle relaxants to control abnormal, unintentional movements and help prevent self-injury.
- Cortisone drugs to control the child's movements if the above drugs fail.
- Penicillin or other antibiotics until adulthood to prevent strep infections.
- See Medications section for information regarding medicines your doctor may prescribe.

ACTIVITY

Your child should resume normal activities as soon as possible. Try to educate teachers and classmates so the child can return to school—even before all involuntary movements cease. Avoid bed rest.

DIET & FLUIDS

No special diet.

OK FOR SCHOOL, PRESCHOOL, OR NURSERY?

When appetite has returned and alertness, strength, and feeling of well-being will allow.

CALL YOUR DOCTOR IF

- Your child has symptoms of St. Vitus' dance.
- Injury occurs from uncontrolled movements.

SALMONELLA INFECTIONS

GENERAL INFORMATION

DESCRIPTION

A salmonella infection is a general infection caused by one of the 12,000 or more germs in the salmonella family. The gastrointestinal tract and lymphatic system are involved. Appropriate health care includes: self-care; physician's monitoring of general condition and medications, if symptoms continue longer than 48 hours or for complications; hospitalization (rare).

SIGNS & SYMPTOMS

- Diarrhea, often accompanied by abdominal cramps. In mild cases, diarrhea may be only 2 or 3 loose bowel movements a day. In severe cases, it may be watery diarrhea as often as every 10 or 15 minutes.
- Vomiting; fever; blood in the stool (sometimes).

A relatively mild salmonella infection may be mistaken for simple gastroenteritis.

CAUSES

- Infection with salmonella bacteria after eating meat that contains the bacteria. Salmonella bacteria survive freezing, but thorough cooking kills them. Pet turtles can also carry salmonella bacteria.
- Salmonella epidemics often occur when many people eat the same contaminated food at a picnic, social gathering, or restaurant. The infection can be transmitted from person to person.

RISK FACTORS

Recent gastrointestinal illness; crowded or unsanitary living conditions.

PREVENTING COMPLICATIONS OR RECURRENCE

- Follow these recommendations for your child and yourself in any area with a substandard water supply:
  — Drink purified water, boil water, or add 2 to 4 drops of 4% to 6% chlorine bleach to each quart of water 30 minutes before use.
  — If in a hotel, draw hot water from the faucet, let it cool and use it as drinking water.
  — Don't use ice.
  — Don't eat raw fruits and vegetables unless you can peel them.

Other instructions for your family:

- Drink only pasteurized milk.
- Wash your hands after bowel movements and before handling food.
- Isolate anyone in the family who has the infection.
- Ask your doctor about preventive antibiotics before traveling in countries with unsanitary water and food supplies.

WHAT TO EXPECT

MEDICAL TESTS

- Your own observation of symptoms.
- Medical history and physical exam by a doctor.
- Laboratory stool studies.

POSSIBLE COMPLICATIONS

- Dehydration from excessive diarrhea and vomiting. Severe dehydration can be fatal, especially in infants.
- Infection of other organs, such as the kidneys, gallbladder, spleen, and lungs, from salmonella bacteria in the bloodstream (rare).

PROBABLE OUTCOME

Most salmonella infections are mild and curable with treatment in 24 to 48 hours. Children with severe infections require hospitalization and isolation. The infection may last 2 to 3 weeks.

TREATMENT

HOME CARE

- Isolate the ill child, if possible.
- Use a heating pad or hot-water bottle to relieve your child's abdominal cramps.
- If diarrhea is severe, use a bedside commode.

MEDICATION

Medicine is usually not necessary for mild cases. Anti-diarrhea medications may retard the child's recovery. For severe cases, your doctor may prescribe anti-diarrhea medication, antibiotics to fight infection, and intravenous fluids for severe dehydration.

ACTIVITY

Your child should stay in bed, except for trips to the bathroom, until at least 3 days after diarrhea, fever, and other symptoms disappear. Then the child can resume normal activities gradually. Flexing the legs regularly in bed helps prevent the formation of blood clots.

DIET & FLUIDS

Offer your child only clear liquids until diarrhea stops. Then serve the child a high-calorie, well-balanced diet. Vitamin and mineral supplements may be helpful after prolonged illness.

OK FOR SCHOOL, PRESCHOOL, OR NURSERY?

When signs of infection have decreased, appetite returns, and alertness, strength, and feeling of well-being will allow.

CALL YOUR DOCTOR IF

- Your infant has symptoms of a salmonella infection and shows signs of dehydration, such as dry, wrinkled skin, decreased urination, or dark urine.
- Your child has symptoms of a salmonella infection that persist longer than 48 hours.
- The following occurs during the illness: fever of 102F (38.9C) or higher; jaundice; cough with blood; worsening diarrhea.

SCABIES

GENERAL INFORMATION

DESCRIPTION

Scabies is a disease of the skin caused by a mite (the "itch" mite) with a characteristic pattern of distribution. Scabies is contagious from person to person (by shared clothing or bed linen) and from one site to another in the same person. The skin of the finger webs and the folds under the arms, breasts, elbows, genitals, and buttocks are involved.

Appropriate health care includes:

- Self-care after diagnosis.
- Physician's monitoring of general condition and medications.

SIGNS & SYMPTOMS

- Small, itchy blisters in several parts of your child's body. The blisters break easily when scratched.
- Broken blisters leave scratch marks and thickened skin, crisscrossed by grooves and scaling.

CAUSES

A mite that burrows into deep skin layers, where the female mite deposits eggs. Eggs mature into adult mites in 3 weeks. Mites are 0.1mm in diameter and can be seen only under a microscope. Scratching collects mites and eggs under the fingernails, so they spread to other parts of the child's body.

RISK FACTORS

Crowded or unsanitary living conditions.

PREVENTING COMPLICATIONS OR RECURRENCE

- Your child should avoid contact with persons or linen and clothing that may have been infected with scabies.
- Your child should maintain personal cleanliness by doing the following:
  - — Bathing daily, or at least 2 to 3 times a week.
  - — Washing hands before eating.
  - — Laundering clothes often.

WHAT TO EXPECT

MEDICAL TESTS

- Your own observation of symptoms.
- Medical history and physical exam by a doctor. The diagnosis is confirmed by discovering the mite, lifting it from its burrow, and identifying it under a microscope.

POSSIBLE COMPLICATIONS

Secondary bacterial infection of mite-infested areas of inflammation.

PROBABLE OUTCOME

- Itching usually disappears quickly, and evidence of your child's disease is gone in 1 to 2 weeks with treatment.
- In 20% of cases, re-treatment is necessary in 20 days. If your child's skin irritation persists longer than this, oral antihistamines or topical steroids may be necessary to break the itch-scratch cycle.
- Scabies may last for years if left untreated. This accounts for the term "seven-year itch."

TREATMENT

HOME CARE

- Bathe the child thoroughly before applying the prescribed medicine.
- Apply from the neck down, and cover the child's entire body.
- Wait 15 minutes before letting the child get dressed.
- Carefully wash all clothes and toys used prior to or during treatment. You don't need to clean furniture or floors with special care.
- Leave medicine on the child's skin for 2 hours before bathing.
- Keep the child's fingernails short.
- You may need to repeat the treatment in 1 week. Ask your doctor.

MEDICATION

- Your doctor may prescribe a pediculicide, such as gamma benzene hexachloride or crotamiton cream.
- Infants and pregnant females may need a pediculicide that is less toxic, such as a 6% solution of sulfur.
- See Medications section for information regarding medicines your doctor may prescribe.

ACTIVITY

No restrictions.

DIET & FLUIDS

No special diet.

OK FOR SCHOOL, PRESCHOOL, OR NURSERY?

Yes, after treatment.

CALL YOUR DOCTOR IF

- Your child has symptoms of scabies.
- After treatment, the lesions show signs of infection (redness, pus, swelling, or pain).
- New, unexplained symptoms develop. Drugs used in treatment may produce side effects.

SCARLET FEVER

GENERAL INFORMATION

DESCRIPTION

Scarlet fever is a childhood disorder characterized by a bright red rash. Scarlet fever is preceded by a streptococcal throat infection. Both are very contagious. The throat, tonsils, and skin are involved. Scarlet fever can affect children and adolescents, especially between ages 2 and 10.

Appropriate health care includes:

- Home care after diagnosis.
- Physician's monitoring of general condition and medications.

SIGNS & SYMPTOMS

Symptoms may vary. Following is the usual course of the disease:

- Day 1—Fever as high as 104F (40C), a red sore throat, swollen tonsils (tonsils may have a whitish coating), enlarged lymph glands in the neck, a cough, and vomiting.
- Day 2—Bright red rash on the child's face, except around the mouth.
- Day 3—Reddened tongue and rash in body creases, spreading to the neck, chest and back, then to the entire body. The rash resembles a sunburn with bumps.
- Day 6—Faded rash and skin that begins peeling, continuing for 10 to 14 days.

CAUSES

Strep infection caused by a specific type of strep germ that manufactures a scarlet-fever toxin (poison). Not all strep infections cause scarlet fever, because not everyone is susceptible to the rash-producing toxin. In one family, one child may contract scarlet fever, another may have a strep throat only, and a third may carry the germ and transmit it to others without being sick.

RISK FACTORS

Family history of recurrent strep infections, recent impetigo, crowded or unsanitary living conditions, and exposure to others in public places.

PREVENTING COMPLICATIONS OR RECURRENCE

Cannot be prevented completely, because some healthy children are carriers of the strep germ without being ill. However, partial preventive measures include:

- Antibiotic treatment for at least 10 days for any strep infection.
- Avoidance of persons with sore throats.

WHAT TO EXPECT

MEDICAL TESTS

Your own observation of symptoms; medical history and physical exam by a doctor; laboratory throat culture.

POSSIBLE COMPLICATIONS

Without treatment: rheumatic fever; impaired hearing; glomerulonephritis; meningitis; pneumonia; encephalitis.

PROBABLE OUTCOME

Usually curable in 10 days or more with treatment. Scarlet fever is not as prevalent as it once was, and it is rarely fatal. With antibiotic treatment, the severity and likelihood of complications decrease.

TREATMENT

HOME CARE

- Prepare a soothing tea gargle for a child old enough to gargle. Double the usual strength of tea. This may be gargled warm or cold as often as it feels soothing to your child.
- Use a cool-mist humidifier to relieve the dry, tight feeling in the child's throat.
- Use moist, warm soaks to relieve tender, enlarged glands in the child's neck.
- Isolate the ill child from other people, including family members.

MEDICATION

Your doctor may prescribe penicillin to shorten the course of scarlet fever and prevent complications. If your child is allergic to penicillin, other antibiotics, such as erythromycin, are also effective.

ACTIVITY

Bed rest is necessary until all signs of illness have disappeared. Your child may read or watch TV.

DIET & FLUIDS

No special diet.

OK FOR SCHOOL, PRESCHOOL, OR NURSERY?

When signs of infection have decreased, appetite returns, and alertness, strength, and feeling of well-being will allow.

CALL YOUR DOCTOR IF

- Your child has symptoms of strep throat or scarlet fever.
- The following occurs during treatment:
  —Temperature becomes normal for 2 days, then rises over 101F (38.3C).
  —New symptoms begin such as nausea; vomiting; earache; cough; headache; thick, colored, nasal drainage; chest pain; or labored breathing.

SCHIZOPHRENIA

GENERAL INFORMATION

DESCRIPTION

"Schizo" means "split," and "phrenia" refers to the mind. So schizophrenia refers to a disorder characterized by disorganization of mind processes. It occurs in about 1 in 10,000 children, 5 times more commonly in boys than girls. Appropriate health care includes:
Psychiatric consultation and continued treatment if deemed necessary.

SIGNS & SYMPTOMS

- Your child is more concerned with inner thoughts and emotions than with the external world.
- The child feels conflicting thoughts and feelings simultaneously.
- The child has difficulty in keeping the mind and speech on one topic.
- There is severe limitation of emotions, with inappropriate expression.
- There are disorders of thought, language, and learning.
- There are disorders of perception.
- There are disorders of emotions and social relations.
- There is poor muscle tone and coordination.
- Hallucinations and delusions with some or all of the above equal an *active psychosis.*

CAUSES

Unknown. Probably genetic.

RISK FACTORS

- History of schizophrenia in the family.
- Environmental stress that may trigger episodes of active psychosis.

PREVENTING COMPLICATIONS OR RECURRENCE

None known.

WHAT TO EXPECT

MEDICAL TESTS

Evaluation by a university-affiliated developmental evaluation clinic after age 4 or 5. An accurate diagnosis may require a long period of time.

POSSIBLE COMPLICATIONS

Life-time disability.

PROBABLE OUTCOME

Continuing problems of varying degree throughout the child's life, with interspersed periods of near-normal functioning and active psychosis.

TREATMENT

HOME CARE

- Accept a competent diagnosis of your child's condition.
- Discourage the child's concentration on one endless activity.
- Forbid the child to disrupt the activities of others.
- Challenge and contradict the child's illusions.
- Discourage loud talking.
- Arrange for your child to have public school education for handicapped children. Federal law mandates its provision.
- Work constantly toward the goal of preparing the child to function as well as possible as an adult in society.

MEDICATION

None except during severe active psychosis or for severe insomnia.

ACTIVITY

Your child should live as normal a life as possible.

DIET & FLUIDS

No restrictions.

OK FOR SCHOOL, PRESCHOOL, OR NURSERY?

Under special arrangements.

CALL YOUR DOCTOR IF

- Your child has signs or symptoms of schizophrenia.
- A diagnosis of schizophrenia has been established and hallucinations, delusions, or paranoid feelings develop.

SCLERITIS

GENERAL INFORMATION

DESCRIPTION

Slceritis is deep, localized inflammation of the sclera, the outermost white layer of tissue covering the eyeball. Scleritis is not contagious. The sclera, which includes the conjunctiva and cornea, is involved. Scleritis may affect one or both eyes. Appropriate health care includes:

- Self-care after diagnosis.
- Doctor's treatment.
- Surgery to close a perforation, if perforation occurs as a complication.

SIGNS & SYMPTOMS

- Eye pain (usually dull).
- Purple-red, inflamed areas in one or more areas of the white of the child's eye.
- Partial vision loss (sometimes).

CAUSES

Unknown, but scleritis frequently occurs with rheumatoid arthritis, Crohn's disease, and other connective-tissue disorders. It is probably an autoimmune disorder.

RISK FACTORS

- Rheumatoid arthritis.
- Crohn's disease (regional ileitis).
- Chronic gastrointestinal disorder.

PREVENTING COMPLICATIONS OR RECURRENCE

No specific preventive measures.

WHAT TO EXPECT

MEDICAL TESTS

- Your own observation of symptoms.
- Medical history and physical exam by a doctor.

POSSIBLE COMPLICATIONS

Rupture of the scleral tissue, perforating the eyeball and causing loss of the eye. The child's eye can sometimes be saved with surgery after perforation.

PROBABLE OUTCOME

Usually curable with treatment. If partial vision loss occurs, it is usually permanent.

TREATMENT

HOME CARE

Use warm-water soaks to relieve the child's pain.

MEDICATION

- Your doctor may prescribe immunosuppressive drugs, oral cortisone drugs, or cortisone eye drops to reduce inflammation.
- For minor pain, use non-prescription drugs, such as acetaminophen.
- See Medications section for information regarding medicines your doctor may prescribe.

ACTIVITY

Your child should reduce normal activity until inflammation subsides.

DIET & FLUIDS

No special diet.

OK FOR SCHOOL, PRESCHOOL, OR NURSERY?

When appetite returns and alertness, strength, and feeling of well-being will allow.

CALL YOUR DOCTOR IF

- Your child has symptoms of scleritis.
- The following occurs during treatment:
  —Symptoms don't improve in 48 hours.
  —Temperature rises to 100F (37.8C) or higher.
  —Pain becomes worse.
  —Vision is affected.

SCOLIOSIS
(Curvature of the Spine)

GENERAL INFORMATION

DESCRIPTION

Scoliosis is a painless, progressive bending and twisting of the upper spinal column, which eventually distorts the chest and back. The spinal vertebrae (bones) are involved. Scoliosis can affect adolescents between ages 12 and 15. It is more common in girls than boys.

Appropriate health care includes:

- Physician's monitoring of general condition and medications.
- Exercises to strengthen back muscles.
- Orthopedic back brace.
- Surgery to correct the deformity (severe cases only).

SIGNS & SYMPTOMS

- Early stages: No obvious symptoms or signs, but your child's scoliosis can be detected by your doctor or school nurse with a simple screening test.
- Later states: Visible curving of the child's upper body. The spine becomes S-shaped and the shoulders become uneven.

CAUSES

Usually unknown. Scoliosis is sometimes a result of:

- Diseases of the central nervous system, such as polio or muscular dystrophy.
- Congenital defects of the spine.

RISK FACTORS

Family history of scoliosis.

PREVENTING COMPLICATIONS OR RECURRENCE

Cannot be prevented at present.

WHAT TO EXPECT

MEDICAL TESTS

- Your own observation of symptoms.
- Medical history and physical exam by a doctor.

POSSIBLE COMPLICATIONS

- Severe distortion of the child's spine and ribs.
- Breathing difficulty.
- Lung infection.
- Muscle spasms and pain in the back and legs.
- Arthritis of the spine.
- Congestive heart failure.

SCOLIOSIS
(Curvature of the Spine)

PROBABLE OUTCOME

When diagnosed early, scoliosis can usually be corrected completely. Your child may have to wear a back brace daily for as long as several years.

TREATMENT

HOME CARE

A teenager may be embarrassed to wear a brace. Be sure your teenager understands that the brace is temporary. Explain the eventual consequences of not wearing the brace. Insist on keeping doctor appointments for follow-up evaluation.

MEDICATION

- Medicine usually is not necessary for this disorder. For minor discomfort from muscle imbalance or complications, use non-prescription drugs, such as aspirin or acetaminophen.
- See Medications section for information regarding medicines your doctor may prescribe.

ACTIVITY

Consult your doctor. Special exercises may be part of your child's therapy. If a brace is necessary, your child's participation in sports will be restricted.

DIET & FLUIDS

No special diet.

OK FOR SCHOOL, PRESCHOOL, OR NURSERY?

Yes. Your child should maintain as normal physical activities as possible.

CALL YOUR DOCTOR IF

You suspect your child is developing scoliosis.

SEBACEOUS CYST
(Epidermoid Cyst; Wen)

GENERAL INFORMATION

DESCRIPTION

A sebaceous cyst is a dome-shaped cyst filled with semisolid material (keratin, the same material that forms skin, hair, and nails). The name *sebaceous cyst* is in error, because a real sebaceous cyst would be filled with material called sebum and manufactured in hair follicles. The skin of the trunk, face, neck, and scalp is involved. Sebaceous cysts can affect both sexes, all ages, but are most common in adolescents.

Appropriate health care includes:

- Self-care.
- Physician's monitoring of general condition and medications.
- Surgery to remove the cyst (sometimes).
  — A small cyst can be removed through a simple incision, but rupture of the cyst—and corresponding incomplete removal—frequently results in recurrence.
  — A large cyst does better if incised and drained in an initial procedure, with removal of the complete cyst at another time.

SIGNS & SYMPTOMS

A cyst with the following characteristics:

- The cyst has sloped shoulders or a dome-shaped, nodular appearance and a smooth surface.
- The cyst is whitish or skin-colored.
- Cysts range from 1cm to 4cm in diameter.
- If the cyst becomes injured or infected, it may become bright red and painful.

CAUSES

Sebaceous cysts are caused by plugged ducts in malformed hair follicles. They may enlarge from hormonal stimulation or injury.

RISK FACTORS

- Skin injury.
- Hormonal stimulation at puberty.

PREVENTING COMPLICATIONS OR RECURRENCE

Cannot be prevented at present.

WHAT TO EXPECT

MEDICAL TESTS

- Your own observation of symptoms.
- Medical history and physical exam by a doctor.

POSSIBLE COMPLICATIONS

- Infection of a cyst.
- Injury to a cyst, causing rupture or inflammation.

SEBACEOUS CYST
(Epidermoid Cyst; Wen)

PROBABLE OUTCOME

- Cysts that cause no symptoms to your child require no medical treatment. Those that are unsightly or are repeatedly injured can be removed.
- Infected cysts may require incision, drainage, and packing with gauze.

TREATMENT

HOME CARE

Before surgery, apply warm compresses to your child's cyst to reduce inflammation and size.

MEDICATION

- Medicine usually is not necessary for this disorder. If your child's cyst becomes infected, your doctor may prescribe antibiotics.
- See Medications section for information regarding medicines your doctor may prescribe.

ACTIVITY

Your child can resume normal activities as soon as symptoms improve.

DIET & FLUIDS

No special diet.

OK FOR SCHOOL, PRESCHOOL, OR NURSERY?

Yes.

CALL YOUR DOCTOR IF

- After removal, signs of infection (pain, redness, warmth, and increased tenderness) occur at the surgical site.
- Fever of 101F (38.3C) or higher develops.
- The treated area does not appear to be healing well within 1 week.
- Your child is taking antibiotics, and new, unexplained symptoms develop. Antibiotics may produce side effects.

SERUM SICKNESS

GENERAL INFORMATION

DESCRIPTION

Serum sickness is an allergic reaction usually appearing 7 to 12 days (sometimes much sooner) after giving or taking a foreign serum (such as antivenom following snakebites or horse serum antitoxins) or any of a number of drugs.

Appropriate health care includes:

- Self-care after diagnosis.
- Physician's monitoring of general condition and medications.

SIGNS & SYMPTOMS

- Hives.
- Skin rash.
- Joint pains, including the jaw.
- Swollen lymph glands.
- Enlarged spleen.
- Peripheral neuritis.

CAUSES

Allergic reaction to a foreign substance in the body.

RISK FACTORS

Positive skin test of the foreign serum.

PREVENTING COMPLICATIONS OR RECURRENCE

To avoid the need for tetanus antitoxin (a horse serum used to protect against tetanus), make sure your children (and the entire family) have had basic immunizations with tetanus toxoid, and boosters as required. This way, your child will never need tetanus antitoxin.

WHAT TO EXPECT

MEDICAL TESTS

- Your own observation of symptoms.
- Medical history and physical exam by a doctor.

POSSIBLE COMPLICATIONS

Precipitous drop in the child's blood pressure.

PROBABLE OUTCOME

Complete cure within 1 to 2 weeks.

TREATMENT

HOME CARE

Bed rest if the child's joints are painful.

MEDICATION

- Your physician may prescribe antihistamines, salicylates, or corticosteroids.
- See Medications section for information regarding medicines your doctor may prescribe.

ACTIVITY

Your child can resume normal activity as soon as the condition and sense of well-being will allow.

DIET & FLUIDS

No restriction.

OK FOR SCHOOL, PRESCHOOL, OR NURSERY?

When appetite has returned and alertness, strength, and feeling of well-being will allow.

CALL YOUR DOCTOR IF

- Your child has symptoms of serum sickness.
- New, unexplained symptoms develop. Drugs used in treatment may produce side effects.

SHIN SPLINTS

GENERAL INFORMATION

DESCRIPTION

Shin splints is a catchall phrase for pain in the lower leg brought on by exercise or athletic activity. The discomfort is due to inflammation of one or several body tissues. Pain worsens with exercise using the legs. The muscles (causing myositis), tendons (causing tendinitis), or the bone covering (causing periostitis) may be involved. Appropriate health care sometimes includes physical therapy.

SIGNS & SYMPTOMS

- Anterior shin splints: pain in front of the lower leg. The pain radiates down the front and outer side of the child's leg.
- Posterior shin splints: pain along the back and inner side of the child's lower leg and ankle.

CAUSES

Inflammation of muscles, tendons, and covering of the bone (periosteum), usually due to an imbalance of the calf muscles (which pull the forefoot down) and the shin muscles (which pull the forefoot up).

RISK FACTORS

Shin splints are most common with marathon running, walking, or jogging, particularly on rough terrain.

PREVENTING COMPLICATIONS OR RECURRENCE

Instructions for your child:

- Avoid hard and uneven surfaces—use soft surfaces such as dirt or grass for jogging, running, and walking.
- Warm up adequately before exercise or competition. Keep shins warm during exercise.
- Wear well-fitting shoes with good arch support during physical activities.

WHAT TO EXPECT

MEDICAL TESTS

Your own observation of symptoms; medical history and physical exam by a doctor; X-rays of the child's lower leg, knee, and ankle.

POSSIBLE COMPLICATIONS

- Mistaken diagnosis. Similar symptoms can be caused by stress fractures or increased pressure caused by constricted tissue covering muscles or nerves.
- Prolonged healing time if activity is resumed too soon.
- Proneness to recurrence.
- Inflammation and arthritic changes in nearby joints (such as the ankle, knee, hip, back) caused by a changed gait and posture due to lower-leg pain.

PROBABLE OUTCOME

Complete cure requires rest and slow rehabilitation. Total time may range from 2 weeks to 2 months. Tough competition should be delayed until the child can exercise regularly for 4 to 6 weeks without pain.

TREATMENT

HOME CARE

- The child should stop exercising until there is no pain. If there is pain with walking, the child should not try to run.
- Use frequent ice massage. Fill a large Styrofoam cup with water and freeze. Tear a small amount of foam from the top so ice protrudes. Massage firmly over the injured area in a circle about the size of a softball. Do this for 15 minutes at a time, 3 or 4 times a day, and before workouts or competition.
- Apply heat instead of ice, if it feels better to the child. Use heat lamps, hot soaks, hot showers, heating pads, or heat liniments or ointments.
- Provde the child with whirlpool treatments, if available.
- Massage gently and often to provide comfort to the child and decrease swelling. Apply lubricating oil to the skin over the painful area during massage.
- For anterior shin splints, raise the heel of the child's shoe with 1/8 inch of adhesive felt.
- For posterior shin splints, the child should wear an extra pair of socks and run with the body erect, not leaning forward. The child should try not to land directly on the toes.

MEDICATIONS

For minor discomfort, use non-prescription drugs such as aspirin or ibuprofen. Your doctor may prescribe other non-steroidal anti-inflammatory medicines.

ACTIVITY

Instructions after treatment, when the child is ready to resume normal activity:

- Cut back on your training schedule in proportion to the time it took for the pain to stop.
- Ice your legs 6 to 10 minutes before warmup and after running.
- Wear long socks to keep your legs warm.
- Run only every other day during first few weeks after treatment.
- For anterior shin splints, shave your legs and use criss-cross adhesive taping over the front half of your lower leg, with or without an elbow brace.

DIET & FLUIDS

Your child should eat a well-balanced diet that includes extra protein, such as meat, fish, poultry, cheese, milk, and eggs. Increasing fiber and fluid intake helps prevent constipation that may result from decreased activity.

OK FOR SCHOOL, PRESCHOOL, OR NURSERY?

Yes, when condition and sense of well-being will allow.

CALL YOUR DOCTOR IF

Your child has symptoms of shin splints that persist despite treatment.

SHINGLES
(Herpes Zoster; Zona; Acute Posterior Ganglionitis)

GENERAL INFORMATION

DESCRIPTION

Shingles is a viral infection of the central nervous system. Shingles is contagious to persons who have not had chickenpox. The sensory nerves of the skin on one side of the body only are involved. Shingles can affect both sexes, all ages, but is more common in adults than children.

Appropriate health care includes:

- Self-care after diagnosis.
- Physician's monitoring of general condition and medications.

SIGNS & SYMPTOMS

- Mild chills and fever.
- General ill feeling.
- Mild nausea, abdominal cramps, or diarrhea.
- Painful red blisters anywhere on your child's body. Blisters appear 4 to 5 days after early symptoms begin. The blisters appear on a broad streak of reddened skin along sensory-nerve routes to a particular area of skin. They occur most often on the child's chest, and spread only on one side of the body.
- Chest pain, face pain, or burning pain in the skin of the abdomen, depending on the affected area.

CAUSES

Shingles is caused by the varicella-zoster virus, the same virus that causes chickenpox. It may lie dormant in the spinal cord until triggered by risk factors.

RISK FACTORS

- Stress.
- Hodgkin's disease.
- Illness that has lowered your child's resistance.
- Use of immunosuppressive or anti-cancer drugs.

PREVENTING COMPLICATIONS OR RECURRENCE

Cannot be prevented at present.

WHAT TO EXPECT

MEDICAL TESTS

- Your own observation of symptoms.
- Medical history and physical exam by a doctor.

POSSIBLE COMPLICATIONS

- Secondary infection in the shingles blisters.
- Chronic pain (especially in the elderly) that persists for months or years in the sensory nerves where the blisters have been.

PROBABLE OUTCOME

Most children recover spontaneously without lasting complications, except for mild scarring. One attack usually provides immunity against shingles, but a few persons have had more than one attack.

SHINGLES
(Herpes Zoster; Zona; Acute Posterior Ganglionitis)

TREATMENT

HOME CARE

Instructions for your child:

- Avoid chilling drafts.
- When bathing, wash blisters gently.
- Don't bandage the sores.
- Apply heat or moist compresses if this decreases the pain.

MEDICATION

- For minor discomfort, use non-prescription drugs such as acetaminophen.
- Your doctor may prescribe:
  - Pain relievers.
  - Tranquilizers for a short time.
  - Cortisone drugs to relieve pain in severe cases.
  - Anti-viral drugs. These may be useful, but they are still experimental.
- See Medications section for information regarding medicines your doctor may prescribe.

ACTIVITY

No restrictions.

DIET & FLUIDS

No special diet.

OK FOR SCHOOL, PRESCHOOL, OR NURSERY?

When appetite has returned and alertness, strength, and feeling of well-being will allow.

CALL YOUR DOCTOR IF

- Your child has symptoms of shingles.
- Pain is intolerable, despite treatment.
- New, unexplained symptoms develop. Drugs used in treatment may produce side effects.

SHOCK

GENERAL INFORMATION

DESCRIPTION

Shock is low blood pressure that is extensive enough so the body cannot maintain normal functions. Shock does not include a person's reaction to emotional trauma. The heart, blood vessels, blood, and body electrolytes are involved.

Appropriate health care includes:

- Physician's monitoring of general condition and medications.
- Surgery to stop hemorrhaging.
- Hospitalization for inatravenous fluids and medications to raise blood pressure and treat the underlying cause.

SIGNS & SYMPTOMS

- Cold hands and feet.
- Fast, weak pulse.
- Disorientation or confusion.
- Anxiety with feelings of impending doom.
- Skin that is pale, moist, and sweaty.
- Shortness of breath and rapid breathing.
- Lack of urination.
- Low blood pressure. This may be so low that it cannot be measured by the usual means.

CAUSES

- Sudden loss of blood from injury or disorders, such as a bleeding peptic ulcer, a ruptured aneurysm or a ruptured ectopic pregnancy.
- Fluid loss, such as occurs with severe burns, fluid and electrolyte imbalance, or peritonitis.
- Impaired heart-pumping function from a heart attack, heart-rhythm irregularities, pericarditis, or a pulmonary embolism.
- Blood poisoning, which causes blood vessels to greatly expand, such as occurs with toxic shock syndrome or major infections.
- Some endocrine diseases, such as Addison's disease or diabetes mellitus.

RISK FACTORS

- Recent serious injury.
- Recent surgery.
- Infection.
- Childbirth.
- Anemia.
- Cancer.
- Use of drugs that cause anaphylactic (allergic) shock as an adverse reaction, such as penicillin, local anesthetics, and many others.

PREVENTING COMPLICATIONS OR RECURRENCE

Your child should avoid causes and risk factors when possible.

WHAT TO EXPECT

MEDICAL TESTS

- Medical history and physical exam by a doctor.
- Laboratory blood studies to measure the amount of blood in circulation and to measure the child's fluids and electrolytes.

POSSIBLE COMPLICATIONS

- Cardiac arrest.
- Permanent brain damage.

PROBABLE OUTCOME

Usually curable with early diagnosis and treatment. Without treatment, shock can be fatal to your child.

TREATMENT

HOME CARE

If you observe signs of shock in your child, do the following until medical help arrives:

- Stop external bleeding by applying pressure.
- Keep the victim lying down with legs elevated. Cover the child for warmth.
- Make sure the victim's airway is open to allow breathing. If your child's breathing stops, give mouth-to-mouth resuscitation. If breathing *and* pulse stop, give cardiopulmonary resuscitation.

MEDICATION

Depends on the underlying disorder:

- If shock is from blood or fluid loss, treatment includes blood transfusion or intravenous fluids.
- If blood pressure is at a life-threatening low level, hypertensive drugs to raise blood pressure may be given to your child.
- If infection is present, antibiotics will be used.

ACTIVITY

Your child should rest in bed until completely recovered. Moving the legs actively while in bed decreases the likelihood of deep-vein blood clots.

DIET & FLUIDS

No special diet.

OK FOR SCHOOL, PRESCHOOL, OR NURSERY?

When appetite has returned and alertness, strength, and feeling of well-being will allow.

CALL YOUR DOCTOR IF

Your child has symptoms of shock or you observe them in someone else. Call immediately. This is a life-threatening emergency!

SHOULDER BURSITIS, SUBACROMIAL (Subdeltoid Bursitis)

GENERAL INFORMATION

DESCRIPTION

Subacromial shoulder bursitis refers to inflammation of the subdeltoid bursa, one of the important bursas of the shoulder. Bursitis develops slowly and may vary in degree from mild irritation to an abscess formation that causes excruciating pain. Appropriate health care includes: doctor's diagnosis and treatment; surgery (sometimes) in worse cases, particularly for a frozen shoulder.

SIGNS & SYMPTOMS

Pain in the shoulder area; tenderness; swelling; redness (sometimes) over the affected bursa; fever if infection is present; limitation of motion in the shoulder.

CAUSES

Injury to the shoulder; acute or chronic infection; arthritis; gout; unknown (frequently).

RISK FACTORS

Participation in competitive athletics, particularly contact sports such as football, especially if protective equipment is inadequate; previous history of bursitis in any joint; previous shoulder injury involving the "rotator cuff" (see Glossary); exposure to cold weather; poor conditioning and inadequate warmup.

PREVENTING COMPLICATIONS OR RECURRENCE

Instructions for your child:
Use protective gear for contact sports; warm up adequately before athletic practice or competition; wear warm clothing in cold weather; to prevent recurrence, continue to wear extra protection over the shoulder until healing is complete.

WHAT TO EXPECT

MEDICAL TESTS

Your own observation of symptoms; medical history and physical exam by a doctor; X-rays of the child's shoulder.

POSSIBLE COMPLICATIONS

Frozen shoulder, with temporary or permanent limitation of the shoulder's normal mobility; prolonged healing time if the child resumes activity too soon; proneness to repeated flare-ups; an unstable or arthritic shoulder following repeated episodes of bursitis; spontaneous rupture of bursa if severe infection is present.

PROBABLE OUTCOME

Mild, subdeltoid bursitis is a common—but not a serious—problem. Symptoms usually subside in 7 to 14 days with treatment. Chronic bursitis in any bursa of the shoulder can cause recurrent flare-ups.

SHOULDER BURSITIS, SUBACROMIAL
(Subdeltoid Bursitis)

TREATMENT

HOME CARE

- Use frequent ice massage. Fill a large Styrofoam cup with water and freeze. Tear a small amount of foam from the top so ice protrudes. Massage firmly over the injured area in a circle about the size of a softball. Do this for 15 minutes at a time, 3 or 4 times a day, and before workouts or competition.
- Apply heat instead of ice, if it feels better to the child. Use heat lamps, hot soaks, hot showers, heating pads, or heat liniments or ointments. Sometimes heat makes pain worse. If so, discontinue and use ice only.
- Use a sling to support the child's shoulder joint, if needed.
- Elevate the shoulder above the level of the child's heart to reduce swelling and prevent accumulation of fluid. Use pillows for propping.
- Gentle massage will frequently provide comfort and decrease swelling.
- Urge your child to do the rehabilitation exercises prescribed by your doctor.

MEDICATION

Your doctor may prescribe:

- Non-steroidal anti-inflammatory drugs.
- Prescription pain relievers for severe pain. Use non-prescription aspirin, acetaminophen, or ibuprofen (available under many trade names) for mild pain.
- Injections into the inflamed bursa of a long-lasting local anesthetic mixed with a corticosteroid drug, such as triamcinolone.

ACTIVITY

Instructions for your child:

Rest the inflamed area as much as possible. If you must resume normal activity immediately, wear a sling until the pain becomes more bearable. To prevent a frozen shoulder, begin normal, slow joint movement as soon as possible.

DIET & FLUIDS

Your child should eat a well-balanced diet that includes extra protein, such as meat, fish, poultry, cheese, milk, and eggs. Increasing fiber and fluid intake helps prevent constipation that may result from decreased activity. Your doctor may suggest vitamin and mineral supplements to promote healing.

OK FOR SCHOOL, PRESCHOOL, OR NURSERY?

Yes, when condition and sense of well-being will allow.

CALL YOUR DOCTOR IF

- Your child has symptoms of shoulder bursitis; pain increases despite treatment; pain, swelling, tenderness, drainage, or bleeding increases in the surgical area; your child develops signs of infection (headache, muscle aches, dizziness, or a general ill feeling and fever).
- New, unexplained symptoms develop. Drugs used in treatment may produce side effects.

SHOULDER DISLOCATION

GENERAL INFORMATION

DESCRIPTION

Shoulder dislocation is the displacement of the humerus (upper-arm bone) from its socket in the shoulder joint. Injury to nerves in the axilla (armpit) is quite common. Appropriate health care includes: doctor's treatment, including manipulation of the joint to reposition the bones; surgery (sometimes) to restore the joint to its normal position—acute or recurring dislocations may require surgical reconstruction or replacement of the joint; self-care during rehabilitation.

SIGNS & SYMPTOMS

Excruciating pain at the time of injury; loss of function of the dislocated shoulder joint and severe pain when attempting to move it; visible deformity if the child's dislocated bones lock in the dislocated position—if they spontaneously reposition themselves, no deformity will be visible, but the damage will be the same; tenderness over the dislocation; swelling and bruising at the injury site; numbness or paralysis in the child's arm from pressure, pinching, or cutting of blood vessels or nerves.

CAUSES

Direct upward blow to the shoulder or backward force on an extended arm; powerful muscle twisting or a violent muscle contraction—some children can willfully produce a recurrent dislocation.

RISK FACTORS

Contact sports; any activity that involves forceful throwing, lifting, hitting, or twisting; previous shoulder dislocation or sprain; repeated shoulder injury of any sort; arthritis of any type; poor muscle conditioning.

PREVENTING COMPLICATIONS OR RECURRENCE

Your child should build overall strength and muscle tone with an appropriate long-term conditioning program.

? WHAT TO EXPECT

MEDICAL TESTS

X-rays of the child's shoulder joint and adjacent bones.

POSSIBLE COMPLICATIONS

Temporary or permanent damage to nearby nerves or major blood vessels, causing numbness, coldness, and paleness; excessive internal bleeding; shock or loss of consciousness; recurrent dislocations, particularly if the child's previous dislocation is not healed completely.

PROBABLE OUTCOME

Immobilization with a cast or sling for 2 to 8 weeks. Complete healing of injured ligaments requires a minimum of 6 weeks. If customary treatment does not prevent a recurrence, then the child should modify athletic activities until surgery can be done to cure the problem. Surgery should be followed by rehabilitation to prevent reinjury.

TREATMENT

FIRST AID

Keep the child warm with blankets to decrease the possibility of shock. Cut away clothing if possible, but don't move the injured area to remove clothing. Untrained persons should not attempt to reposition a dislocated shoulder. Immobilize the child's neck, dislocated shoulder, and elbow with padded splints or a sling. Follow instructions for R.I.C.E., the first letters of *rest*, *ice*, *compression*, and *elevation*. (See Appendix 39 for details.) The doctor will manipulate the child's dislocated bones to return them to their normal position. Manipulation should be done within 6 hours, if possible.

HOME CARE

- Use an ice pack 3 or 4 times a day. Wrap ice chips or cubes in a plastic bag, and wrap the bag in a moist towel. Place it over the injured area for 20 minutes at a time.
- Exercise all the child's muscle groups not immobilized in a cast or sling.
- Massage gently and often to provide comfort to the child and decrease swelling.

MEDICATION

Your doctor may prescribe general anesthesia or muscle relaxants to make joint manipulation possible; acetaminophen to relieve moderate pain; narcotic pain relievers for severe pain; antibiotics to fight infection if surgery is necessary.

ACTIVITY

Your child can resume normal activities gradually after treatment.

DIET & FLUIDS

No restrictions after surgery.

OK FOR SCHOOL, PRESCHOOL, OR NURSERY?

Yes, when condition and sense of well-being will allow.

CALL YOUR DOCTOR IF

- Your child has difficulty moving the shoulder after dislocation.
- Your child's arm becomes numb, pale, or cold after a dislocation. This is an emergency!
- Any of the following occur after surgery: increased pain, swelling, or drainage in the surgical area; signs of infection (headache, muscle aches, dizziness, or a general ill feeling and fever); constipation.
- New, unexplained symptoms develop. Drugs used in treatment may produce side effects.
- Dislocations occur repeatedly that you can "pop" back into normal position.

ILLNESSES

SHOULDER, FROZEN (Adhesive Capsulitis)

GENERAL INFORMATION

DESCRIPTION

Frozen shoulder means pain and stiffness in the shoulder joint that progresses to inability to use the shoulder. In this case, "frozen" does not relate to freezing temperatures. The shoulder tendons, bursa, joint capsules, muscles, blood vessels and nerves are involved. It affects all ages but is most common in athletic adolescents.

Appropriate health care includes:

- Self-care after diagnosis.
- Doctor's treatment, including manipulation of the child's shoulder to break up adhesions. This is done in a hospital or outpatient surgical facility under general anesthesia.
- Physical therapy and exercises.

SIGNS & SYMPTOMS

Early stages:

- Pain in the shoulder, often slight, that progresses to severe pain that interferes with the child's sleep and normal activities. Pain worsens with shoulder movement.
- Stiffness in the child's shoulder that prevents normal movement. Reduced movement increases stiffness.

Later stages:

- Pain in the child's arm or neck.
- Inability to move the shoulder.
- Intolerable shoulder pain.

CAUSES

Minor shoulder injury or inflammation, such as bursitis or tendinitis, that worsens from lack of use. Adhesions (constricting bands of tissue) form with disuse in 7 to 10 days. Adhesions increase disuse. After 3 weeks of disuse, adhesions grow so severe that the joint cannot move.

RISK FACTORS

- Neglect of your child's minor injuries, including bursitis or tendinitis.
- Poor nutrition, especially lack of adequate protein.
- Poor physical conditioning and occasional athletic activity.

PREVENTING COMPLICATIONS OR RECURRENCE

Obtain medical treatment for your child's bursitis and tendinitis, including exercises to prevent formation of adhesions.

WHAT TO EXPECT

MEDICAL TESTS

- Your own observation of symptoms.
- Medical history and physical exam by a doctor.
- X-rays of the child's shoulder.

POSSIBLE COMPLICATIONS

Permanent shoulder disability and pain without treatment or with delayed treatment.

PROBABLE OUTCOME

Usually curable with treatment and rehabilitation.

TREATMENT

HOME CARE

After treatment and rehabilitation begin, your doctor will prescribe ice treatment and exercises for your child.

MEDICATION

- Your doctor may prescribe:
  —Pain relievers.
  —Non-steroidal anti-inflammatory drugs.
  —Injections of cortisone and local anesthesia into the child's joints to reduce pain and inflammation.
- For minor pain, use non-prescription drugs such as aspirin.
- See Medications section for information regarding medicines your doctor may prescribe.

ACTIVITY

Your child can resume normal activities as soon as symptoms improve.

DIET & FLUIDS

No special diet. Vitamins and mineral supplements don't help unless your child can't eat a normal, well-balanced diet.

OK FOR SCHOOL, PRESCHOOL, OR NURSERY?

When appetite returns and alertness, strength, and feeling of well-being will allow.

CALL YOUR DOCTOR IF

- Your child has symptoms of a frozen shoulder.
- Your child has persistent shoulder pain, indicating possible bursitis or tendinitis.
- New, unexplained symptoms develop. Drugs used in treatment may produce side effects.

SICKLE-CELL ANEMIA

GENERAL INFORMATION

DESCRIPTION

Sickle-cell anemia is an inherited blood disorder that causes anemia, episodes of severe pain, low resistance to infection and chronic poor health. It is not cancerous. The bone marrow, lymph glands, spleen, liver, and thymus are involved. Symptoms of sickle-cell anemia usually begin around 6 months of age and last a lifetime.

Appropriate health care includes:

- Physician's monitoring of general condition and medications. If your child has the condition, seek special treatment from a pediatrician with special knowledge of this condition.
- Psychotherapy or counseling may be helpful in adapting to this condition, especially for children.
- Hospitalization at times of severe attacks.

SIGNS & SYMPTOMS

- Anemia with shortness of breath, rapid heartbeat, fatigue, and jaundice.
- Episodes of pain in joints, chest, abdomen, and back.
- Frequent infections, especially pneumonia.
- Nerve impairment.
- Delayed growth and development.
- Skin ulcers, especially on the legs.

CAUSES

This disease is hereditary. Persons with the gene may pass it on to their children. Red blood cells change from round to sickle shapes; this causes blockage in the capillaries. Low oxygen in the tissues is partly responsible for the changed shape. The change occurs in attacks that cause pain and disability. The disease occurs mostly in black people.

RISK FACTORS

Family history of sickle-cell anemia. The following may aggravate symptoms:

- Ascending to high altitude, as in driving up a mountain or flying.
- Pregnancy.
- Surgery.
- Injury.

PREVENTING COMPLICATIONS OR RECURRENCE

If you have a family history of sickle-cell anemia, ask your doctor to test you. If the condition is present, obtain genetic counseling before starting a family. A less serious condition, sickle-cell trait, may be present. It will not cause the disease, but genetic counseling is still desirable.

WHAT TO EXPECT

MEDICAL TESTS

- Your own observation of symptoms.
- Medical history and physical exam by a doctor.
- Laboratory blood studies. Simple screening tests are also available. They may be done at birth if there is a family history of sickle-cell anemia.
- X-rays of bones and lungs.

POSSIBLE COMPLICATIONS

- Infections of the lungs and bones.
- Kidney failure.
- Eye disease.
- Stroke.

PROBABLE OUTCOME

Sickle-cell anemia is incurable and your child's life expectancy is reduced. A few patients reach adulthood. Most patients die prematurely of infection or stroke.

TREATMENT

HOME CARE

- During an attack, keep your child warm. Apply warm compresses to painful areas.
- Maintain your child's immunization schedule, including a pneumonia vaccine.
- Don't let your child fly, even in pressurized planes, without oxygen. Check with your airline.
- Urge your child to wear a Medic-Alert bracelet or pendant (see Glossary).

MEDICATION

No medications are yet available to control this condition. For severe attacks, intravenous fluids, blood transfusions, and pain relievers are helpful.

ACTIVITY

Your child should avoid strenuous exercise and exposure to cold temperatures. Bedrest is necessary during acute attacks.

DIET & FLUIDS

Your child should drink at least 8 glasses of water a day—more if there is a fever. This helps keep blood cells from collecting and blocking capillaries.

OK FOR SCHOOL, PRESCHOOL, OR NURSERY?

Yes. OK between attacks or injury.

CALL YOUR DOCTOR IF

- Your child has signs and symptoms of sickle-cell anemia.
- You want to know if you have the sickle-cell gene.
- Your child has the disease, and symptoms recur after a period of remission or your child develops fever or other signs of infection.

SINUS INFECTION (Sinusitis)

GENERAL INFORMATION

DESCRIPTION

Sinusitis is an inflammation of the sinuses adjacent to the nose. Germs that cause sinusitis are contagious. Any one or all of the eight sinuses in the skull close to the nasal passages are involved. Appropriate health care includes: self-care; physician's monitoring of general condition and medications; surgery to drain blocked sinuses (rare).

SIGNS & SYMPTOMS

Early stages:

- Nasal congestion with green-yellow (sometimes blood-tinged) discharge.
- Feeling of pressure inside the head.
- Eye pain.
- Headache that is worse in the morning or when bending forward.
- Cheek pain that may resemble a toothache.
- Post-nasal drip.
- Cough (sometimes) that is usually non-productive.
- Disturbed sleep (sometimes).
- Fever (sometimes).

Late stages:

- Complete blockage of the sinus openings, blocking the discharge and increasing pain.

CAUSES

- Infection (usually initiated by a cold or other upper-respiratory infection). The infection may be complicated by a bacterial invasion of organisms that normally inhabit your child's nose and throat.
- Irritation of the nasal passages from allergies, smoking, harsh sneezes with the mouth closed, chilling, swimming (especially jumping into the water without holding the nose) and fatigue.

RISK FACTORS

- Illness that has lowered resistance.
- Smoking.
- Exposure to cold, damp weather outdoors and dry heat indoors.
- Exposure to others in public places.
- Excessive nose-blowing during an upper-respiratory infection.

PREVENTING COMPLICATIONS OR RECURRENCE

- Keep the humidity level at 45% to 50% in heated buildings during the winter.
- Encourage your child not to stifle sneezes.

WHAT TO EXPECT

MEDICAL TESTS

- Your own observation of symptoms.
- Medical history and physical exam by a doctor.
- X-rays of the sinuses.

SINUS INFECTION (Sinusitis)

POSSIBLE COMPLICATIONS

Meningitis or brain abscess (rare).

PROBABLE OUTCOME

Usually curable with intense treatment. Recurrence is common.

TREATMENT

HOME CARE

- Use a cool-mist humidifier around your child to help thin secretions so they will drain more easily.
- For an infant or young child who cannot blow the nose, use a nasal aspirator to suction each nostril gently before applying nose drops. Suction again 10 minutes after using nose drops.
- Apply heat to relieve pain in the child's sinuses and nose. Use an electric heating pad or warm compresses.
- Don't allow other persons to use your child's nose drops. They will be contaminated by the infection. Discard them after treatment.
- Don't give your child nose drops after the prescribed time. They can interfere with normal nasal and sinus function and become addictive, causing a rebound phenomenon (see Glossary).

MEDICATION

- Your doctor may prescribe:
  — Nasal sprays, nose drops, or decongestant medicine to reduce congestion.
  — Antibiotics to fight infection.
- For minor pain, use non-prescription drugs such as acetaminophen.
- See Medications section for information regarding medicines your doctor may prescribe.

ACTIVITY

Your child can resume normal activities gradually.

DIET & FLUIDS

No special diet, but the child should drink extra fluids to help thin secretions.

OK FOR SCHOOL, PRESCHOOL, OR NURSERY?

When appetite has returned and alertness, strength, and feeling of well-being will allow.

CALL YOUR DOCTOR IF

- Your child has symptoms of sinusitis.
- The following occurs during treatment:
  — Fever of 101F (38.3C) or higher.
  — Bleeding from the nose.
  — Severe headache.
  — Swelling of the face (forehead, eyes, side of the nose, or cheek).
  — Blurred vision.

SKIN ABRASION

GENERAL INFORMATION

DESCRIPTION

A skin abrasion refers to scraped skin or mucous membrane. An abrasion is usually a minor injury, but it can be serious if it covers a large area or if foreign materials become imbedded in it. The most common sites are usually over bone or other firm tissue.

Appropriate health care includes:

- Self-care for minor, non-infected wounds.
- Doctor's care for extensive contaminated abrasions.

SIGNS & SYMPTOMS

- Skin that looks scraped or irritated.
- Bleeding at the abrasion site.
- Immediate pain that lasts a short time.
- Crusting over of the abraded area in 3 to 5 days.

CAUSES

- Falling on a hard, rough, or jagged surface.
- Rough fabric, seams in clothing, ill-fitting shoes, or other parts of athletic equipment such as helmets and shoulder pads that constantly irritate the child's skin.

RISK FACTORS

- Athletic activity on rough terrain, such as bicycling, or playing football or baseball (sliding).
- Skin that is not properly covered or protected, especially when the child is playing on rough terrain.

PREVENTING COMPLICATIONS OR RECURRENCE

Instructions for your child:

- Wear protective clothing, including long sleeves, high socks, knee and elbow pads, and special clothing designed for your sport.
- Wear good-quality, well-fitting footgear to help avoid falls and to prevent foot abrasion.
- Choose athletic clothing wisely to avoid irritating fabric and poorly placed seams. A combination of cotton and synthetic may be the most comfortable. Seams on the inside of the thigh of shorts can be particularly irritating, and should be checked for roughness before purchase.
- Avoid poor-quality playing fields.

WHAT TO EXPECT

MEDICAL TESTS

- Your own observation of symptoms.
- Medical history and physical exam by a doctor.
- X-rays of underlying tissue (sometimes) to rule out other injuries.

POSSIBLE COMPLICATIONS

- Infection.
- "Tattooing," if imbedded dark-colored foreign material is not carefully removed.
- Scarring, if deeper layers of skin are affected (rare).

PROBABLE OUTCOME

The child's wound will heal in 3 to 10 days, depending on its location.

TREATMENT

FIRST AID

- For a scrape, wash the abraded area with plain soap and warm water as soon as possible. Scrub the child with a soft brush if possible. Soap acts as a solvent for imbedded dirt.
- For an irritation, protect the area against further abrasion. Use gauze or moleskin.

HOME CARE

- If foreign material is imbedded too deeply or the wound is too painful to the child to cleanse thoroughly, seek medical help.
- Cleanse lightly each day. If crusting or oozing occurs, soak in warm water with a little dishwashing or laundry detergent.
- Between soakings, apply non-prescription antibiotic ointment.
- Cover lightly with a bandage during the day, but leave the wound open to air at night.
- If infection occurs, use warm soaks more frequently. Keep the injured area elevated above the level of the child's heart, when possible.

MEDICATION

- Your doctor may decide to administer a tetanus booster to the child.
- Apply non-prescription antibiotic ointment to prevent infection.
- Spray with tincture of benzoin to reduce the child's pain, if necessary.
- Don't use strong antiseptics such as iodine, Merthiolate, mercurochrome, or alcohol. They will further irritate the child's skin.
- For minor discomfort, use aspirin, acetaminophen, or ibuprofen.
- Your doctor may prescribe antibiotics if the abrasion becomes infected.

ACTIVITY

Your child can resume normal activities as healing progresses but should not overuse the abraded area until it heals. Protect it against repeat injury.

DIET & FLUIDS

No special diet.

OK FOR SCHOOL, PRESCHOOL, OR NURSERY?

Yes, when condition and sense of well-being will allow.

CALL YOUR DOCTOR IF

- You cannot clean all the debris from your child's abrasion.
- Signs of infection begin (fever, headache, or tenderness, increased oozing, redness, swelling, and pain at the injury site).
- New, unexplained symptoms develop. Drugs used in treatment may produce side effects.

ILLNESSES

SKIN CANCER, MALIGNANT MELANOMA

GENERAL INFORMATION

DESCRIPTION

A malignant melanoma is a skin cancer that spreads to other areas of the body, primarily the lymph nodes, liver, lungs, and central nervous system. Most melanomas begin in a mole or other pre-existing skin lesion. Excessive exposure to sun is a major factor in causing malignant melanoma. It usually affects the skin of the head, neck, legs, or back, but rarely occurs in the eye, mouth, vagina, or anus. Melanomas are more likely to occur in adults, but some affect children. The incidence of melanomas has increased since 1970.

Appropriate health care includes:

- Surgery to remove suspicious skin lesions or to remove nearby lymph glands if the child's tumor has spread.
- Hospitalization for radiation treatment and chemotherapy, if the child's tumor has spread.

SIGNS & SYMPTOMS

A flat or slightly raised skin lesion that can be black, brown, blue, red, white, or a mixture of all colors. Its borders are often irregular and may bleed.

CAUSES

Uncontrolled growth of cells that give skin its brownish color (melanocytes). When the cells grow down into deep skin layers, they invade the child's blood vessels and lymph vessels and are spread to other body areas.

RISK FACTORS

The following factors increase the likelihood of developing a melanoma:

- Moles on the child's skin.
- Excessive sun exposure.
- Pregnancy.
- Genetic factors. This is most common in light-complexioned, blond people, and is rare in black people.
- Radiation treatment or excessive exposure to ultraviolet light, as with sun lamps.

PREVENTING COMPLICATIONS OR RECURRENCE

Instructions for a child in a high-risk group:

- Protect yourself from excessive sun exposure. Wear broad-rimmed hats and protective clothing. Use maximum protection sun-block preparations on exposed skin.
- Examine your skin, including genitals and soles of the feet, regularly for changes in pigmented areas. Ask a family member to examine your back. See your doctor about any skin area (especially brown or black) that becomes multi-colored, develops irregular edges or surfaces, bleeds, or changes in any way.

SKIN CANCER, MALIGNANT MELANOMA

WHAT TO EXPECT

MEDICAL TESTS

- Your own observation of symptoms.
- Medical history and physical exam by a doctor.
- Biopsy of suspicious lesions. The melanoma's depth must be established to determine appropriate treatment.

POSSIBLE COMPLICATIONS

Fatal spread to the child's lungs, liver, brain, or other internal organs.

PROBABLE OUTCOME

Varies greatly. Early melanomas that have not grown downward are curable with surgical removal. Once a child's tumor has spread to distant organs, this condition is currently considered incurable. However, symptoms can be relieved or controlled. Scientific research into causes and treatment continues, so there is hope for increasingly effective treatment and cure.

TREATMENT

HOME CARE

No specific instructions except those listed under other headings.

MEDICATION

- Your doctor may prescribe anti-cancer drugs.
- See Medications section for information regarding medicines your doctor may prescribe.

ACTIVITY

No restrictions.

DIET & FLUIDS

No special diet.

OK FOR SCHOOL, PRESCHOOL, OR NURSERY?

Yes, when condition and sense of well-being will allow.

CALL YOUR DOCTOR IF

- Your child has a skin lesion with any characteristics of a malignant melanoma.
- During treatment, changes occur in another skin area on the child.
- New, unexplained symptoms develop. Drugs used in treatment may produce side effects.

SKIN LESIONS, BENIGN

GENERAL INFORMATION

DESCRIPTION

Benign skin lesions are non-cancerous growths or areas of pigment or color change on the skin. The skin in any region of the body is involved.

Appropriate health care includes:

- Self-care after diagnosis.
- Physician's monitoring of general condition and medications.
- Surgery to remove lesions that enlarge, bleed, change color, are slow to heal, or are unsightly.
- Radiation treatment following removal of keloids to prevent their recurrence.

SIGNS & SYMPTOMS

Benign skin lesions fall into the following categories:

- Tags—Soft, flesh-colored buds, often on stalks, found on the neck, armpits, or groin.
- Moles—Flat or raised lesions with clearly defined borders. Moles may be black, blue, red, yellow, or brown.
- Cherry spots—Pinhead-sized, bright-red lesions on the chest or back.
- Strawberry marks—Bright-red raised areas in infants that grow until they are removed.
- Keloids—Thick, pale, irregular growths that begin at the site of a scar and gradually increase in size.
- Dermatofibromas—Rounded nodules, usually brownish and usually on the legs.
- Freckles—Flat, brownish spots of pinhead-size or larger.

CAUSES

Unknown, but most children have a few benign skin lesions.

RISK FACTORS

- Family history of benign skin lesions.
- Pregnancy or use of oral contraceptives (brownish, frecklelike patches only).

PREVENTING COMPLICATIONS OR RECURRENCE

To decrease freckles, your child should avoid excessive sun exposure. Other forms cannot be prevented.

WHAT TO EXPECT

MEDICAL TESTS

- Your own observation of symptoms.
- Medical history and physical exam by a doctor.
- Skin biopsy (see Glossary).

POSSIBLE COMPLICATIONS

- Malignant change in moles.
- Bleeding in strawberry marks.

PROBABLE OUTCOME

Treatment is usually unnecessary because most skin lesions are harmless. Suspicious or unsightly lesions can be removed surgically. If the affected area is large or in a prominent place, plastic surgery may be necessary for your child after removal of a skin lesion.

TREATMENT

HOME CARE

- Examine your child's skin lesions regularly—especially those that are constantly rubbed or irritated by clothing—for signs of growth, color change, pain, infection, or bleeding.
- If a lesion is removed, cover the area with a clean dressing and protect against injury. Ointments are rarely needed.

MEDICATION

- Medicine usually is not necessary for this disorder. Makeup may be helpful in covering unsightly blemishes.
- See Medications section for information regarding medicines your doctor may prescribe.

ACTIVITY

No restrictions.

DIET & FLUIDS

No special diet.

OK FOR SCHOOL, PRESCHOOL, OR NURSERY?

Yes.

CALL YOUR DOCTOR IF

Your child has a skin lesion that enlarges, bleeds, changes color, is painful, or doesn't heal.

SLEEP APNEA IN INFANTS

GENERAL INFORMATION

DESCRIPTION

Sleep apnea in infants is unexplained lapses in breathing during sleep, leading to lack of oxygen to the brain and heart with life-threatening heartbeat irregularity. This can cause sudden infant death syndrome (SIDS), a mysterious tragedy that kills apparently healthy infants. The central nervous system—including the brain, the coverings of the brain (meninges), and the spinal cord—and peripheral nerves are involved. Sleep apnea can affect infants of both sexes.

Appropriate health care includes:

- Home care that includes monitoring equipment and close, constant observation.
- Doctor's supervision.

SIGNS & SYMPTOMS

Episodes when the infant's breathing stops and skin color changes. Episodes may last several minutes. Breathing usually resumes spontaneously. Unless death occurs, these episodes are apparent only with careful observation by hospital nurses or parents during the first weeks after birth.

CAUSES

Unknown.

RISK FACTORS

- Prematurity or low birth weight.
- Being a young mother (under 20 years old). Older mothers (over age 35) do *not* have a higher incidence of infants with sleep apnea, as has been theorized.
- Belonging to lower socioeconomic groups.

PREVENTING COMPLICATIONS OR RECURRENCE

Special equipment (a respiration monitor) is used continuously to monitor breathing in infants that experience sleep apnea or in those suspected of being at risk for SIDS.

WHAT TO EXPECT

MEDICAL TESTS

None, except the observations of breathing lapses by persons caring for the infant.

POSSIBLE COMPLICATIONS

Sudden infant death syndrome. When this occurs, infants die in their sleep without signs of struggle or injury. Autopsies show no apparent cause of death. There are approximately 6,000 to 7,000 such deaths each year in the U.S. Autopsies must be performed on all SIDS victims.

PROBABLE OUTCOME

As long as SIDS can be averted, infants with sleep apnea grow and develop normally. Most children are considered out of danger and can be taken off the monitor between 6 months and 1 year of age.

TREATMENT

HOME CARE

- If your baby suffers from sleep apnea, obtain and use a respiration monitor. The manufacturer and your doctor or nurse will demonstrate and provide full instructions.
- If your baby has a monitor, obtain detailed cardiopulmonary resuscitation training (CPR). In many cases, CPR can revive an infant who has stopped breathing, and the child experiences no serious aftereffects.

MEDICATION

- No medication is currently available to prevent sleep apnea in infants.
- See Medications section for information regarding medicines your doctor may prescribe.

ACTIVITY

No restrictions.

DIET & FLUIDS

No special diet. Bottle-feeding has *no* association with SIDS, as was once theorized.

OK FOR SCHOOL, PRESCHOOL, OR NURSERY?

After monitoring is no longer needed and appetite has returned and alertness, strength, and feeling of well-being will allow.

CALL YOUR DOCTOR IF

Your baby has lapses in breathing (apnea). Call immediately!

SMALL-INTESTINE TUMOR

GENERAL INFORMATION

DESCRIPTION

A small-intestine tumor is an abnormal new growth in the small intestine. Only 10% of small-intestine tumors are cancerous. The various segments of the small intestine are involved. Small-intestine tumors can affect both sexes, all ages, but is less common in children than adults.

Appropriate health care includes:

- Physician's monitoring of general condition and medications.
- Surgery to remove the tumor (sometimes).
- Radiation treatment (sometimes).
- Self-care after surgery or during treatment.

SIGNS & SYMPTOMS

- No symptoms (sometimes).
- Tiredness.
- Paleness.
- Blood in stools or black, tarry stools.
- Unexplained weight loss.

CAUSES

Unknown.

RISK FACTORS

- Regional ileitis (Crohn's disease).
- Celiac disease.

PREVENTING COMPLICATIONS OR RECURRENCE

No specific preventive measures.

WHAT TO EXPECT

MEDICAL TESTS

- Your own observation of symptoms.
- Medical history and physical exam by a doctor.
- Laboratory blood studies for anemia.
- X-rays of the intestinal tract (upper and lower GI series).

POSSIBLE COMPLICATIONS

Intestinal obstruction. Symptoms include a distended abdomen, severe colicky pain, nausea, vomiting, and fever.

PROBABLE OUTCOME

Most tumors are removed surgically, regardless of whether they are malignant. With surgery or other treatment, the disorder is curable and a normal life span is expected for your child.

TREATMENT

HOME CARE

No specific instructions except those under other headings.

MEDICATION

Your doctor may prescribe:
- Anti-cancer drugs.
- Cortisone drugs to reduce bowel inflammation that may cause obstruction.
- See Medications section for information regarding medicines your doctor may prescribe.

ACTIVITY

No restrictions. Your child can resume normal activities as soon as possible after surgery.

DIET & FLUIDS

Your doctor may prescribe a special diet for the child following surgery or during treatment with radiation or anti-cancer drugs.

OK FOR SCHOOL, PRESCHOOL, OR NURSERY?

After recovery from treatment, including surgery, if needed.

CALL YOUR DOCTOR IF

- Your child has symptoms of a tumor of the small intestine.
- Your child has symptoms of intestinal obstruction (see POSSIBLE COMPLICATIONS).
- New, unexplained symptoms develop. Drugs used in treatment may produce side effects.

SNAKEBITE

GENERAL INFORMATION

DESCRIPTION

Snakebite is a bite from a poisonous snake. Bites on the extremities are the most common, but bites on the head and trunk are the most dangerous. Exposed skin, blood, and the lymphatic system are involved.

Appropriate health care includes:

- Immediate self-care.
- Doctor's treatment as soon as possible.
- Surgery (sometimes) to remove injured or gangrenous tissue 2 to 3 days after the bite.

SIGNS & SYMPTOMS

Early symptoms:

- Severe pain and swelling around the bite.

Late symptoms:

- Fever.
- Skin discoloration that resembles bruising around the bite.
- Bleeding spots under the skin all over the body.
- Numbness and tingling around the mouth and in the hands and feet.
- Excessive sweating.
- Low blood pressure and shock.
- Breathing difficulty.
- Blurred vision.
- Headache.
- Seizures.
- Coma.

Signs:

- Multiple fang marks and small cuts, if the bite is from a coral snake. Symptoms may not appear for 3 to 4 hours.
- Deep single or double fang marks, if the bite is from another snake. Symptoms begin quickly.

CAUSES

Bite from a poisonous snake, including rattlesnake, copperhead, water moccasin, or coral snake.

RISK FACTORS

Outdoor activities during warm months in areas where poisonous snakes live.

PREVENTING COMPLICATIONS OR RECURRENCE

Your child should wear protective shoes, boots, and clothing for hiking, camping, fishing, and hunting. Prevent complications by carrying a snakebite kit and instructions.

WHAT TO EXPECT

MEDICAL TESTS

Your own observation of symptoms; medical history and physical exam by a doctor; laboratory blood studies.

POSSIBLE COMPLICATIONS

- Gangrene, requiring amputation of the affected part.
- DIC (disseminated intravascular coagulation).
- Severe immunological response, if your child has had a previous venomous snakebite.

PROBABLE OUTCOME

Usually curable with rapid medical care. Severe bites involving a large amount of poisonous venom may be fatal to your child—even with treatment. After one snakebite, succeeding snakebites may produce more severe reactions.

TREATMENT

HOME CARE

- Don't panic! Venom will spread more quickly through the body if your child runs or becomes excited.
- Before giving the child first aid, identify the snake.
- Don't pack the affected part in ice.
- If the child's bite is from a coral snake, elevate and immobilize the bitten part and go to the nearest emergency facility.
- If the bite is from another poisonous snake:
  — Put a *light* tourniquet (constricting band of any sort) 3 or 4 inches above the bite, toward the body. Don't use a tourniquet if 30 minutes or more have passed since the bite.
  — Wash the bite with soap and water.
  — Immobilize the bitten area.
  — Go to the nearest emergency facility.

MEDICATION

Your doctor may prescribe:

- Antivenin to neutralize snake poison.
- Tetanus booster injection.
- Antibiotics to prevent infection.
- Pain relievers. (Narcotics cannot be used for coral-snake bites. They may cause shock.)

ACTIVITY

Your child can resume normal activities as soon as symptoms improve.

DIET & FLUIDS

No special diet.

OK FOR SCHOOL, PRESCHOOL, OR NURSERY?

When appetite has returned and alertness, strength, and feeling of well-being will allow.

CALL YOUR DOCTOR IF

Your child or someone you are with receives a snakebite.

SODIUM IMBALANCE

GENERAL INFORMATION

DESCRIPTION

Sodium imbalance is above- or below-normal levels of sodium in the blood. All body cells are involved.

Appropriate health care includes:

- Self-care after diagnosis and treatment.
- Physician's monitoring of general condition and medications.
- Hospitalization (frequently, particularly for the very young who require regulation of dehydration by receiving intravenous fluids).

SIGNS & SYMPTOMS

- Confusion.
- Restlessness and anxiety.
- Weakness.
- Muscle cramps (usually in the legs).
- Changes in pulse rate and blood pressure.
- Tissue swelling (edema).
- Stupor or coma.

Sodium imbalance in your child may be part of a disease with other symptoms that predominate, such as fever, vomiting, diarrhea, or excessive sweating.

CAUSES

Hyponatremia (below-normal sodium):

- Prolonged loss of body fluids from vomiting or diarrhea.
- Addison's disease.
- Congestive heart failure.
- Prolonged, excessive drinking of water. (This is usually a psychiatric condition.)
- Some cancers of the adrenal glands.
- Infections with high fever.

Hypernatremia (above-normal sodium):

- Inability to drink water, as with stroke or gastrointestinal diseases.
- Use of cortisone drugs.
- Excessive intake of salty food or liquid, as in near-drowning in salt water.

RISK FACTORS

- Diabetes mellitus.
- Congestive heart failure.
- Use of diuretics.
- Kidney diseases. Healthy kidneys can usually control sodium levels.

PREVENTING COMPLICATIONS OR RECURRENCE

Because sodium disturbance is the result of underlying disease, obtain early medical treatment for your child to prevent a sodium imbalance.

WHAT TO EXPECT

MEDICAL TESTS

- Your own observation of symptoms.
- Medical history and physical exam by a doctor.
- Laboratory blood and urine studies of sodium and other electrolytes.

POSSIBLE COMPLICATIONS

Shock and death.

PROBABLE OUTCOME

Usually can be corrected with intravenous fluids and treatment of the child's underlying disorder.

TREATMENT

HOME CARE

If your child has a disorder or takes drugs that affect sodium balance, learn as much as possible about the drugs, your child's condition, and ways to prevent a sodium imbalance.

MEDICATION

Your doctor may prescribe:

- Intravenous sodium if your child's sodium levels are low.
- Diuretics to decrease high sodium levels.
- Medications to correct underlying disorders.
- See Medications section for information regarding medicines your doctor may prescribe.

ACTIVITY

Your child can resume normal activities after recovery.

DIET & FLUIDS

No special diet for low sodium levels. Most children with high sodium levels benefit from a low-salt diet (see Appendix 29). Low-salt diets contain enough sodium to prevent hyponatremia. However, sodium levels are not influenced by diet alone.

OK FOR SCHOOL, PRESCHOOL, OR NURSERY?

When appetite has returned and alertness, strength, and feeling of well-being will allow.

CALL YOUR DOCTOR IF

- Your child has symptoms of a sodium imbalance.
- Your child is having problems with a disorder that affects sodium levels.

SORES, PRESSURE
(Bed Sores; Decubitus Ulcers)

GENERAL INFORMATION

DESCRIPTION

Pressure sores are skin ulcerations, usually in an area of pressure over a bony prominence. Pressure sores are not contagious or cancerous. The skin over pressure points in the lower back, buttocks, elbows, knees, shoulders, heels, ankles, and other areas with bony prominences is involved.

Appropriate health care includes:
- Home care.
- Doctor's treatment.
- Surgery to remove dead tissue (sometimes).

SIGNS & SYMPTOMS

Spots of skin that are red and shiny. Spots progress to blisters, then ulcers, leading to a breakdown of tissue under the ulcer. Ulcers are usually painless.

CAUSES

Constant pressure on the child's skin, especially over bony areas. Pressure reduces the blood supply, causing death in the tissue layers. Pressure sores usually develop in children who cannot move because of chronic illness or disability that confines them to bed.

RISK FACTORS
- Poor circulation.
- Decreased or absent sensation.
- Malnutrition.
- Obesity.
- Illness or accident requiring prolonged bed confinement, especially with unsanitary living conditions and wrinkled or wet bed linen.

PREVENTING COMPLICATIONS OR RECURRENCE

Provide good nursing care for the disabled child, including the following:
- Frequent changes of the child's position in bed.
- Protective, soft padding, such as gel flotation pads or sheepskin, over the child's bony areas.
- A water mattress, egg-crate rubber mattress, or alternating-pressure mattress.
- Dry, clean, smooth bed linen.
- Frequent inspection of skin areas at risk.

WHAT TO EXPECT

MEDICAL TESTS
- Your own observation of symptoms.
- Medical history and physical exam by a doctor.

POSSIBLE COMPLICATIONS
- Local or general infection.
- Infection of bone (osteomyelitis) adjacent to the ulcer.

SORES, PRESSURE
(Bed Sores; Decubitus Ulcers)

PROBABLE OUTCOME

Usually curable with treatment. Sores may heal very slowly. Healing time varies with the site and size of the ulcer and the child's general health.

TREATMENT

HOME CARE

- Provide good nursing care for the child (see PREVENTING COMPLICATIONS).
- Provide warm whirlpool treatments, if a pressure sore is on the child's arm, hand, foot, or leg.
- Apply lotions or ointment if prescribed for the child by your doctor. Apply a thin layer of the cream, ointment, or lotion 3 or 4 times daily. A heavy layer wastes medicine and is no more beneficial than a thin layer. Rub in gently for several minutes until it disappears.

MEDICATION

- Your doctor may prescribe:
  —Antibiotics to fight infection.
  —Ointments, dressings and drying agents, such as zinc oxide, granulated sugar, povidone-iodine packs or 3% hydrogen peroxide.
- Avoid harsh soaps, tincture of benzoin or hexachlorophene.
- See Medications section for information regarding medicines your doctor may prescribe.

ACTIVITY

Your child can resume normal activities as soon as symptoms improve.

DIET & FLUIDS

Your child should eat a normal, well-balanced diet that includes extra protein. Vitamin and mineral supplements may be necessary.

OK FOR SCHOOL, PRESCHOOL, OR NURSERY?

When appetite returns and alertness, strength, and feeling of well-being will allow.

CALL YOUR DOCTOR IF

- Your child has symptoms of pressure sores or you observe them in someone else.
- The following occurs during treatment:
  —Skin inflammation or breakdown.
  —Signs of infection, such as: pain, redness, tenderness, swelling or increased warmth of the affected area.
  —Fever.

SPINAL-CORD TUMOR

GENERAL INFORMATION

DESCRIPTION

A spinal-cord tumor is an abnormal growth that compresses the spinal cord or its nerve roots. The growth may be benign or malignant—but a non-malignant tumor may be as disabling as a malignant tumor unless treated appropriately. The spinal cord and the nerves below the level of the spinal-cord tumor are involved. Spinal-cord tumors can affect both sexes, all ages, but are most common in adults.

Appropriate health includes:

- Self-care after diagnosis and treatment.
- Physician's monitoring of general condition and medications.
- Surgery to remove tumors and surrounding bone that compress the spinal cord.
- Radiation therapy following surgery.
- Physical therapy.

SIGNS & SYMPTOMS

- Progressive weakness, numbness, and wasting of muscles whose nerve supply comes from the affected area of the spinal cord.
- Difficult urination or bowel movements; incontinence.
- Chronic back pain.

CAUSES

- Tumors originating in the spinal cord (primary tumors) are rare—especially in childhood or old age—and their cause is unknown.
- A spinal-cord tumor usually results from cancer that has spread from another part of the body, such as lung, breast, intestinal tract, prostate, kidney, thyroid, or lymphatic system.

RISK FACTORS

Cancer in any of the body parts listed above.

PREVENTING COMPLICATIONS OR RECURRENCE

- Because spinal-cord tumors frequently result from the spread of cancer, be alert to early symptoms of cancer in other organs.
- Encourage your child to eat a high-fiber diet to reduce the likelihood of intestinal cancer.
- Be alert to enlargement of the child's thyroid gland.
- Encourage your adolescent daughter to practice breast self-exam.
- Urge your child not to smoke.

WHAT TO EXPECT

MEDICAL TESTS

- Your own observation of symptoms.
- Medical history and physical exam by a doctor.
- Laboratory studies of blood and spinal fluid.
- X-rays of the spine.

POSSIBLE COMPLICATIONS

Total paralysis caused by a blockage of blood vessels that nourish spinal-cord cells.

PROBABLE OUTCOME

- The success of your child's treatment depends on the type, size, and location of the growth.
- Surgery to remove bone surrounding the spinal cord can relieve pressure on spinal nerves and nerve pathways. This operation generally relieves your child's pain and other symptoms immediately but may impair motor functions. Physical therapy and rehabilitation may restore lost function.
- If the tumor originated on the exterior of the spinal cord and has not spread, surgery restores a normal life expectancy.

TREATMENT

HOME CARE

No specific instructions except those listed under other headings.

MEDICATION

Your doctor may prescribe:

- Pain relievers.
- Cortisone drugs to decrease swelling around the tumor and reduce pressure on the spinal cord.
- Anti-cancer drugs, if your child's tumor is malignant.
- See Medications section for information regarding medicines your doctor may prescribe.

ACTIVITY

Your child should stay as active as strength allows. Work and exercise should be done in moderation. The child should rest when tired.

DIET & FLUIDS

The child should eat a normal, well-balanced diet. Vitamin and mineral supplements should not be necessary unless your child shows evidence of deficiency or cannot eat normally.

OK FOR SCHOOL, PRESCHOOL, OR NURSERY?

After surgery has healed and appetite has returned and alertness, strength, and feeling of well-being will allow.

CALL YOUR DOCTOR IF

Your child has any symptoms of a spinal-cord tumor.

SPLEEN RUPTURE

GENERAL INFORMATION

DESCRIPTION

Bleeding of a ruptured spleen can be fatal. The spleen is vulnerable to injury, particularly if it is enlarged due to any underlying disorder (infectious mononucleosis is the most common). Spleen injuries are infrequent in athletes but, when they do occur, they can be disastrous. Appropriate health care usually involves surgery.

SIGNS & SYMPTOMS

- Recent injury to the child's abdomen or flank.
- Rib fracture on the left side.
- Vomiting.
- Abdominal pain and tenderness.
- Pain in the child's left shoulder or the left side of the neck.
- Rapid heart rate.
- Low blood pressure.
- Other signs of shock: pale, moist and sweaty skin; anxiety with feelings of impending doom; shortness of breath and rapid breathing; disorientation and confusion.

CAUSES

Direct injury to the child's left upper abdomen or left side of the chest.

RISK FACTORS

Contact sports; bleeding disorders such as hemophilia; infectious mononucleosis or any other illness that causes spleen enlargement in the child.

PREVENTING COMPLICATIONS OR RECURRENCE

Your child should avoid causes and risk factors when possible and should not return to athletic activities until a spleen enlarged by disease has returned to normal.

WHAT TO EXPECT

MEDICAL TESTS

- Before surgery: blood and urine studies; X-rays of the abdomen and chest.
- After surgery: examination of all removed tissue; additional blood studies.

POSSIBLE COMPLICATIONS

- At the time of the child's injury: rapid deterioration due to internal bleeding, possibly leading to death.
- Following surgery: excessive bleeding; infection; incisional hernia; lung collapse; inflammation of the pancreas; deep-vein blood clots; pneumonia.

PROBABLE OUTCOME

Expect the child to heal completely if no complications occur. Allow about 4 weeks for recovery from surgery.

TREATMENT

FIRST AID

Cover the child with a blanket to combat shock, and go to the nearest emergency facility. Do not give the child any water, food, or pain relievers.

HOME CARE

If surgery is required, your surgeon will supply postoperative instructions.

MEDICATION

- Do not give pain relievers at the time of injury. They may mask symptoms.
- After the child's surgery, your doctor may prescribe:
  - — Pain relievers. Don't give the child prescription pain medication longer than 4 to 7 days. Use only as much as your child needs.
  - — Antibiotics to fight infection.
  - — Pneumonia vaccinations.
  - — Stool softeners to prevent constipation.
  - — Non-prescription drugs such as acetaminophen for minor pain.

ACTIVITY

- The child should return to school, work, play, and normal activity as soon as possible. This reduces postoperative depression, which is common.
- The child should avoid vigorous exercise for 6 weeks after surgery.
- The child can resume driving 4 weeks after returning home.

DIET & FLUIDS

- No food or water for the child before surgery.
- The child should drink a clear liquid diet until the gastrointestinal tract functions again. Then serve the child a well-balanced diet that includes extra protein, such as meat, fish, poultry, cheese, milk, and eggs. Increase the child's fiber and fluid intake to prevent constipation that may result from decreased activity.

REHABILITATION

Your child's rehabilitation exercises must be individualized. Follow your doctor's or surgeon's directions.

OK FOR SCHOOL, PRESCHOOL, OR NURSERY?

Yes, when condition and sense of well-being will allow.

CALL YOUR DOCTOR IF

- Your child receives any abdominal injury and the symptoms last longer than a few minutes, worsen, or recur within hours or days. This may be an emergency!
- Any of the following occur after surgery: your child develops signs of infection (headache, muscle aches, dizziness, or a general ill feeling and fever); pain, swelling, redness, drainage, or bleeding increase in the surgical area.
- New, unexplained symptoms develop. Drugs used in treatment may produce side effects.

SPRAINS & STRAINS

GENERAL INFORMATION

DESCRIPTION

Sprains and strains are injuries to ligaments that hold joints together and in position. A strain is a stretched ligament. A sprain is a stretched and torn ligament. Sprains occur most often in ankles, knees, or fingers, although any joint can be sprained. Sprained joints can function—but only with pain. Any ligament (tendon) attached to any joint can be involved. The most commonly injured joint is the ankle, followed by the knee, wrist, and back.

Appropriate health care includes:

- Self-care if the injury is not severe.
- Physician's monitoring of general condition and medications, if the joint cannot move or bear weight normally.
- Cast for a severely sprained joint.
- Surgery to repair badly torn ligaments.
- Physical therapy to regain strength and normal use of the joint.

SIGNS & SYMPTOMS

- Pain or tenderness in the area of injury; severity varies with the extent of your child's injury.
- Swelling of the affected joint.
- Redness or bruising in the area of the child's injury, either immediately or several hours after injury.
- Loss of normal mobility in the injured joint.

CAUSES

Overuse or stress of a ligament or membrane around a joint. A sprain usually occurs when the body weight is placed abnormally on ligaments, causing them to stretch and tear. The ankle is injured most often because of its anatomical weakness, its exposed position, and the stress it sustains in athletic and recreational activities.

RISK FACTORS

Obesity.

PREVENTING COMPLICATIONS OR RECURRENCE

Your child should avoid injury:

- Wrap the child's weak joints with support bandages before strenuous activity.
- Strengthen the child's weak joints with rehabilitative exercises to prevent a recurrence. Consult your doctor or a physical therapist for exercises.
- Accident-proof your home.

WHAT TO EXPECT

MEDICAL TESTS

- Your own observation of symptoms.
- Medical history and physical exam by a doctor.
- X-rays of the injured area.

POSSIBLE COMPLICATIONS

Permanent weakness if your child's sprain is severe or if a joint is sprained repeatedly.

PROBABLE OUTCOME

Strains usually heal in 1 to 2 weeks. Sprains generally heal in 2 weeks without complications.

TREATMENT

HOME CARE

- Apply ice to the child's injured joint during the first 24 hours. Place ice in a plastic bag and separate it from the child's skin with a thin towel. Hold it against the joint with your hand or an elastic bandage. Keep the ice pack on the joint up to 2 hours at a time—either constantly or intermittently—depending on your child's ability to tolerate the cold. Continue the ice treatment at 2-hour intervals for 24 hours.
- After 24 hours, some doctors recommend continued ice treatment. Others recommend heat.
- To use heat, soak the child's joint in hot water or apply heat for 15 minutes every 2 hours or whenever possible. Don't apply heat during the first 24 hours. It may increase bleeding and swelling and prolong healing time.
- Whenever possible, elevate the child's joint so fluid can drain and diminish swelling.
- A cast may be necessary for severe sprains or following surgery. See Care of Casts, Appendix 41. Following cast removal, your child will wear support bandages for a while.
- Your child will have to learn how to use crutches, if needed.

MEDICATION

- Use non-prescription pain relievers such as aspirin. If the child's sprain is severe, your doctor may prescribe a stronger pain reliever.
- See Medications section for information regarding medicines your doctor may prescribe.

ACTIVITY

Allow the child's joint to rest 1 or 2 days. Then the child can begin exercising the joint gently, without putting weight on it.

DIET & FLUIDS

No special diet.

OK FOR SCHOOL, PRESCHOOL, OR NURSERY?

Yes, when mobility has returned with or without crutches.

CALL YOUR DOCTOR IF

- Your child has a sprained joint that won't bear weight or move normally.
- Pain becomes intolerable.
- Swelling or bruising increases, despite treatment.

STRABISMUS
(Crossed Eyes)

GENERAL INFORMATION

DESCRIPTION

Strabismus is a lack of coordinated muscle movement or focusing ability between the eyes, causing the eyes to point in different directions. One or both eyes may turn inward (crossed eyes) or outward ("walleye"). The eyes, the brain area that controls vision, and the muscles attached to the eyeball are involved. Strabismus can affect both sexes, all ages, but it usually begins during early childhood, frequently before age 5.

Appropriate health care includes:

- Home care after diagnosis.
- Doctor's (opthalmologist's) treatment.
- Surgery to correct the condition of the eye muscles (sometimes).
- Tedious but necessary muscle re-training exercises by a qualified specialist.

SIGNS & SYMPTOMS

- Uncoordinated eye movements. This is sometimes evident only when the child is looking in certain directions.
- Double vision (sometimes).
- Vision in one eye only, with loss of depth perception.

CAUSES

Your child's eye movement is controlled by brain signals to four muscles around each eye. Loss of coordinated movement results from:

- Muscle imbalance between the eyes.
- Lack of equal focusing ability in the eyes. The brain cannot tolerate differing focused images, so it ignores signals from one field of vision. The weaker eye eventually becomes useless from disuse, and a "lazy" or wandering eye results.
- Brain damage or head injury.

RISK FACTORS

Family history of strabismus.

PREVENTING COMPLICATIONS OR RECURRENCE

No specific preventive measures.

WHAT TO EXPECT

MEDICAL TESTS

- Your own observation of symptoms. Note particularly if your young child covers one eye—this may indicate the eyes are not focusing together.
- Medical history and physical exam by a doctor, including tests of your child's visual acuity, a retina examination, a total neurological exam, and muscle tests.

POSSIBLE COMPLICATIONS

- Loss of normal vision in one eye.
- Psychological distress from an unattractive facial appearance.

STRABISMUS
(Crossed Eyes)

PROBABLE OUTCOME

- With early diagnosis, your child's strabismus can be corrected with glasses, an eye patch, eye exercises, or surgery. Without prompt treatment, vision loss in one eye may become permanent.
- Many children adapt well to single-eye vision and eventually learn to drive a car or fly an airplane.
- If vision is lost in one eye, your child should take extra precautions against injury in the other eye. The child should wear goggles for sports and other activities, such as carpentry, that carry the risk of injury.

TREATMENT

HOME CARE

Your doctor may recommend:

- Glasses or an eye patch over the child's stronger eye to correct focusing imbalance. These force the weak eye to work.
- Eye-muscle exercises.

MEDICATION

- Medicine usually is not necessary for this disorder.
- See Medications section for information regarding medicines your doctor may prescribe.

ACTIVITY

No restrictions. Protect your child against falls or injury while adjusting to an eye patch.

DIET & FLUIDS

No special diet.

OK FOR SCHOOL, PRESCHOOL, OR NURSERY?

Yes. Try to make the environment the same as for a child without strabismus.

CALL YOUR DOCTOR IF

Your child has symptoms of strabismus.

STREP THROAT
(Streptococcal Sore Throat)

GENERAL INFORMATION

DESCRIPTION

Strep throat is infection and inflammation of the pharynx by streptococcal bacteria. Strep throat is contagious. One out of 4 family members usually catches it within 2 to 7 days after exposure. The throat, tonsils, and frequently the nose and trachea are involved.

Appropriate health care includes self-care after diagnosis; physician's monitoring of general condition and medications.

SIGNS & SYMPTOMS

- Fever.
- Throat pain that is worse when swallowing.
- Very young children may complain of stomach pain rather than throat pain.
- Loss of appetite.
- Headache.
- General ill feeling.
- Ear pain when swallowing (sometimes).
- Swollen glands in the neck.
- Bright-red tonsils that may have specks of pus.

CAUSES

Streptococcal bacteria.

RISK FACTORS

- Recent strep infection in the household.
- Smoking.
- Fatigue.
- Cold, wet weather.
- Crowded living conditions.

PREVENTING COMPLICATIONS OR RECURRENCE

Your child should avoid contact with infected people.

WHAT TO EXPECT

MEDICAL TESTS

- Your own observation of symptoms.
- Medical history and physical exam by a doctor.
- Laboratory studies, such as a throat culture and blood count. A throat culture is the only way to diagnose a strep-throat infection in your child. This is an inexpensive, quick, painless procedure in a doctor's office.

POSSIBLE COMPLICATIONS

- Dehydration (if your child's throat is too sore to swallow liquid).
- The following complications can be prevented with at least 10 days of treatment with penicillin or other effective antibiotics:
  - — Abscess next to the tonsil.
  - — Rheumatic fever.
  - — Glomerulonephritis.

STREP THROAT
(Streptococcal Sore Throat)

PROBABLE OUTCOME

Usually curable in 10 to 12 days with antibiotic treatment.

TREATMENT

HOME CARE

- For children old enough to gargle, prepare a soothing tea gargle. Double the usual strength of tea, and let the child gargle warm or cold as often as it feels good.
- Use a cool-mist humidifier to provide moisture. This relieves the dry, tight feeling in the child's throat.
- Use warm soaks (see Glossary) to relieve pain in the child's swollen glands.

MEDICATION

- Your doctor may prescribe penicillin or another antibiotic for the child to take orally or by injection.
- See Medications section for information regarding medicines your doctor may prescribe.

ACTIVITY

- Your child should rest in bed until fever drops below 100F (37.8C), reading or watching TV.
- After treatment, your child can resume normal activity as symptoms improve. Children may return to school 5 days after beginning antibiotics, if symptoms have improved.

DIET & FLUIDS

A liquid diet may be necessary while the child's throat is sore. Your child should drink as many fluids as possible, including milk shakes, soups, tea, carbonated drinks, and iced coffee. Any type and amount of solid food is acceptable as long as it can be swallowed without too much pain.

OK FOR SCHOOL, PRESCHOOL, OR NURSERY?

When signs of infection have decreased, appetite returns, and alertness, strength, and feeling of well-being will allow.

CALL YOUR DOCTOR IF

- Your child has symptoms of a strep throat.
- The following occurs during treatment:
  - — Temperature is normal for 1 or 2 days, then rises to 101F (38.3C).
  - — New symptoms appear, such as nausea, vomiting, earache, cough, swollen glands, skin rash, severe headache, nasal drainage, chest pain, or shortness of breath.
  - — Convulsions occur.
  - — Joints become red or painful.
  - — Cough begins that produces green, yellow-brown, or bloody sputum.

STY
(Hordeolum)

GENERAL INFORMATION

DESCRIPTION

A sty is a small abscess of hair-follicle glands in the eyelid. The eyelid, eyelashes, and conjunctiva (white of the eye) are involved.

Appropriate health care includes:

- Self-care.
- Physician's monitoring of general condition and medications.
- Surgery to drain the abscess (sometimes).

SIGNS & SYMPTOMS

- Redness, swelling, warmth, tenderness, or pain on the edge of the top or bottom eyelid. The head of the sty is usually on the outside, but it may be on the underside of the lid.
- Increased tear production.
- Sensitivity to bright light.
- A gritty feeling in the child's eye.

CAUSES

Bacterial infection (usually staphylococcal). The infection may be limited to the child's eyelid or may have spread from somewhere else in the body. A sty may result from general poor health or may occasionally indicate a need for glasses.

RISK FACTORS

- Stress.
- Illness that has lowered resistance.
- Eye irritation from smoking.
- Exposure to chemical or environmental irritants.
- Crowded or unsanitary living conditions.
- Poor nutrition.

PREVENTING COMPLICATIONS OR RECURRENCE

- Your child should wash hands frequently, and dry with clean towels.
- Urge your child to avoid environments with excessive dust or other irritating substances.
- Encourage your child to eat a normal, well-balanced diet.

WHAT TO EXPECT

MEDICAL TESTS

- Your own observation of symptoms.
- Medical history and physical exam by a doctor.
- Laboratory culture of the discharge from the child's sty.

POSSIBLE COMPLICATIONS

Spread of infection to other glands in the eyelid.

PROBABLE OUTCOME

Usually curable within 1 week after the sty discharges its pus. Sties frequently recur in children, even with treatment.

TREATMENT

HOME CARE

Use warm-water soaks to relieve the child's pain and inflammation and hasten healing. Apply soaks for 20 minutes, then let the child rest at least 1 hour. Repeat as often as needed.

MEDICATION

Your doctor may prescribe:

• Antibiotic eye drops to prevent the spread of infection to other parts of the child's eye. Oral antibiotics or antibiotic injections are usually not needed.

• Topical antibiotic ointments or creams, such as erythromycin or bacitracin. Apply a thin layer of medication to the edge of the child's eyelid 3 or 4 times daily. A heavy layer wastes medicine and is no more beneficial to your child than a thin layer.

• See Medications section for information regarding medicines your doctor may prescribe.

ACTIVITY

No restrictions.

DIET & FLUIDS

No special diet.

OK FOR SCHOOL, PRESCHOOL, OR NURSERY?

Yes. Not contagious directly to others if your child keeps hands clean and away from eyes.

CALL YOUR DOCTOR IF

• A ripened sty does not drain spontaneously or after gentle removal of the affected eyelash.
• Pain occurs in the child's eye.
• Vision changes.

SUBARACHNOID HEMORRHAGE

GENERAL INFORMATION

DESCRIPTION

A subarachnoid hemorrhage is sudden bleeding into the subarachnoid space (the area between 2 of the membranes that cover the brain). The space is normally filled with cerebrospinal fluid. The brain, meninges (membranes that cover the brain), blood vessels to the brain, and cranial nerves are involved.
Appropriate health care includes:
- Physician's monitoring of general condition and medications. This is an emergency!
- Surgery to stop bleeding and remove collected blood.
- Long-term rehabilitation.
- Self-care after treatment.

SIGNS & SYMPTOMS

- Acute, severe headache, often followed by unconsciousness.
- Drowsiness, dizziness, convulsions, or coma.
- Eye pain with extreme sensitivity to light.
- Vomiting.
- Rapid heartbeat and breathing.
- Stiff neck with pain on movement.
- Fever.
- Numbness, weakness, or inability to move an arm or leg.

CAUSES

- Head injury (the most common cause).
- Hardening of the arteries.
- Infection in any part of the central nervous system.
- Rupture of an aneurysm (weakened part of an artery) that has been present since birth. Rupture is often preceded by high blood pressure or hardening of the arteries.
- Bleeding disorder, such as sickle-cell anemia, leukemia, or any that is a side effect of prescription drugs.

RISK FACTORS

- High blood pressure.
- Family history of bleeding disorders.
- Family history of subarachnoid hemorrhage. Cerebral aneurysms run in families.

PREVENTING COMPLICATIONS OR RECURRENCE

- Avoiding head injury is important. Your child should use seat belts in cars and protective head gear in contact sports.
- Have your child's blood pressure checked regularly. If it is high, consult your doctor for treatment to reduce it.

? WHAT TO EXPECT

MEDICAL TESTS

- Your own observation of symptoms.
- Medical history and physical exam by a doctor.
- Laboratory studies of blood and cerebrospinal fluid.
- X-rays of the skull.
- Special studies that may include ultrasonography, CAT or CT scan, MRI, and radionuclide scan (see Glossary for all).

POSSIBLE COMPLICATIONS

Death or permanent disability if treatment does not begin soon enough.

PROBABLE OUTCOME

- If surgery is possible, recovery chances for your child are good. Partial paralysis, weakness or numbness, and speech and visual difficulties may remain in some cases.
- The damaged area of the brain cannot be restored. However, undamaged areas of the child's brain often can be taught the lost functions. This usually requires rehabilitation, including physical therapy or speech therapy. Determination and a positive attitude greatly affect the success of the rehabilitation process for your child.

TREATMENT

HOME CARE

At home, consider installing hand bars at the tub and toilet, and ramps at each entry to the house.

MEDICATION

Your doctor may prescribe cortisone drugs to reduce the child's brain swelling and pressure.

ACTIVITY

- If your child has lost some motor functions, occupational and physical therapists will help the child use the affected limbs to regain basic skills, such as eating, dressing, and toilet functions.
- After recovery, your child can resume as many former activities as strength and sense of well-being allow. Allow 6 to 12 months for recovery.

DIET & FLUIDS

No special diet. Vitamin and mineral supplements should not be necessary unless your child cannot eat normally.

OK FOR SCHOOL, PRESCHOOL, OR NURSERY?

When appetite has returned and alertness, strength, and feeling of well-being will allow.

CALL YOUR DOCTOR IF

- Your child has any symptoms of a subarachnoid hemorrhage. This is an emergency!
- Symptoms recur after surgery.

SUBCONJUNCTIVAL HEMORRHAGE

GENERAL INFORMATION

DESCRIPTION

A subconjunctival hemorrhage is a sudden appearance of blood in the white area of the eye. Although the bleeding may appear frightening, it is not painful or serious. The conjunctiva (white of the eye) is involved.

Appropriate health care includes:

- Self-care after diagnosis.
- Physician's monitoring of general condition and medications, but only if there has been injury or a change in the child's vision.

SIGNS & SYMPTOMS

A small, painless collection of bright red blood over the white of the eye. Swelling may occur in the affected area of the conjunctiva. The blood changes color gradually to brown or green before disappearing. The condition doesn't interfere with your child's vision.

CAUSES

Usually spontaneous bleeding with no known cause. It may follow coughing, sneezing, or vomiting.

RISK FACTORS

- Use of mind-altering drugs.
- Use of anticoagulant drugs.

PREVENTING COMPLICATIONS OR RECURRENCE

No specific preventive measures.

WHAT TO EXPECT

MEDICAL TESTS

- Your own observation of symptoms.
- Medical history and physical exam by a doctor (sometimes).

POSSIBLE COMPLICATIONS

None expected.

PROBABLE OUTCOME

The blood should be absorbed in 2 or 3 weeks. It is very unlikely that any scarring will occur.

TREATMENT

HOME CARE

- Use cold compresses on your child's eye for several days to prevent additional bleeding. Fold a clean cloth in several layers, dip it in ice water, and wring it out a little. Apply it to the child's eye for 10 minutes every hour.
- Use warm compresses on your child's eye when signs of bleeding have stopped for 2 days. This will hasten blood absorption. Dip the compress in warm water instead of cold water. Apply to the child's eye for 10 minutes 3 times a day.

MEDICATION

- Medicine is usually not necessary for this disorder.
- See Medications section for information regarding medicines your doctor may prescribe.

ACTIVITY

No restrictions.

DIET & FLUIDS

No special diet.

OK FOR SCHOOL, PRESCHOOL, OR NURSERY?

Yes. Activity not likely to worsen the child's condition, nor cause recurrence.

CALL YOUR DOCTOR IF

Your child has symptoms of a subconjunctival hemorrhage, especially if there is eye pain or vision changes.

SUBDURAL HEMORRHAGE & HEMATOMA

GENERAL INFORMATION

DESCRIPTION

Subdural hemorrhage and hematoma is bleeding (hemorrhage) that causes blood to collect and clot (hematoma) beneath the outermost of 3 membranes that cover the brain (meninges). There are 2 types of subdural hematomas. An acute subdural hematoma occurs soon after a severe head injury. A chronic subdural hematoma is a complication that may develop weeks after a head injury. The injury may have been so minor that the child does not remember it. The brain, meninges, (membranes that cover the brain), and blood vessels to the brain are involved.

Appropriate health care includes:

- Physician's monitoring of general condition and medications.
- Surgical exploration and removal of the clot.

SIGNS & SYMPTOMS

- Recurrent headaches that worsen each day.
- Fluctuating drowsiness, dizziness, mental changes, or confusion.
- Weakness or numbness on one side of the child's body.
- Vision disturbances.
- Vomiting without nausea.
- Pupils of different size (sometimes).

CAUSES

Head injury.

RISK FACTORS

Injuries occur more often after:

- Excess alcohol consumption.
- Use of mind-altering drugs.

PREVENTING COMPLICATIONS OR RECURRENCE

Your child should avoid head injury in the following ways:

- Use seat belts in cars.
- Wear protective head gear during contact sports, or while riding a bicycle or motorcycle.
- Don't drink alcohol or use mind-altering drugs and drive.

WHAT TO EXPECT

MEDICAL TESTS

- Your own observation of symptoms.
- Medical history and physical exam by a doctor.
- Laboratory studies of blood and cerebrospinal fluid.
- Hospital diagnostic tests, including arteriography (see Glossary).
- Special studies that may include ultrasonography, CAT or CT scan, MRI, and radionuclide scan (see Glossary for all).

POSSIBLE COMPLICATIONS

Death or permanent brain damage, including partial or complete paralysis, behavioral and personality changes, and speech problems.

SUBDURAL HEMORRHAGE & HEMATOMA

PROBABLE OUTCOME

The degree of your child's recovery depends upon general health, age, severity of the injury, rapidity of the treatment, and extensiveness of the bleeding or clot. After the clot is removed, brain tissue that has been compressed usually expands slowly to fill its original space. The outlook is good under the best circumstances.

TREATMENT

HOME CARE

There is no self-treatment for your child. These suggestions apply to care at home following surgery.

MEDICATION

- Your doctor may prescribe cortisone drugs to reduce swelling inside the child's skull.
- See Medications section for information regarding medicines your doctor may prescribe.

ACTIVITY

- Your child should stay as active as strength allows, working and exercising moderately and resting when tired.
- If your child's speech or muscle control has been damaged, there may be a need for physical therapy or speech therapy.

DIET & FLUIDS

Your child should eat a normal, well-balanced diet. Vitamin and mineral supplements should not be necessary unless your child cannot eat normally.

OK FOR SCHOOL, PRESCHOOL, OR NURSERY?

When signs of infection have decreased, appetite returns, and alertness, strength, and feeling of well-being will allow. May take *months* following surgery.

CALL YOUR DOCTOR IF

- Your child has had a head injury—even if it seems minor—and symptoms of subdural hemorrhage develop. This is an emergency!
- The following occurs during or after treatment:
  - — Temperature rises to 101F (38.3C) or higher.
  - — The surgical wound becomes red, swollen, or tender.
  - — Headache worsens.

ILLNESSES

SUN POISONING

GENERAL INFORMATION

DESCRIPTION

Sun poisoning is a reaction to overexposure to the sun. The skin in areas most exposed to sunlight is involved.

Appropriate health care includes:

- Self-care after diagnosis.
- Physician's monitoring of general condition and medications (sometimes).

SIGNS & SYMPTOMS

- Red skin rash, sometimes with small blisters, in areas exposed to sunlight.
- Fever.
- Fatigue or dizziness.

CAUSES

Sun poisoning is most likely to occur during hot seasons when ultraviolet light is strongest. It is triggered by exposure to the sun, usually in conjunction with sunburn. It is especially likely in children who take medications that cause photosensitivity (increased sensitivity to ultraviolet light). The most common drugs include tetracycline antibiotics, thiazide diuretics, sulfa drugs, and oral contraceptives. Some cosmetics, including lipstick, perfume, and soaps, can also cause a photosensitive reaction in your child.

RISK FACTORS

- Underlying infection.
- Previous episodes of sun poisoning.
- Metabolic disorders, such as diabetes mellitus or thyroid disease.
- Use of immunosuppressive drugs or any drugs listed under CAUSES.

PREVENTING COMPLICATIONS OR RECURRENCE

Your child should stay out of the sun when possible if there is a history of sun poisoning.

WHAT TO EXPECT

MEDICAL TESTS

- Your own observation of symptoms.
- Medical history and physical exam by a doctor.

POSSIBLE COMPLICATIONS

Recurrence of the child's rash and other symptoms when exposed to the sun—even for short periods—especially in spring and summer.

PROBABLE OUTCOME

Symptoms can be controlled with treatment if the child stays out of the sun. Allow up to 1 week for recovery.

TREATMENT

HOME CARE

• Your child should stay out of the sun during the hours of strongest ultraviolet light (10 a.m. to 2 p.m.).

• If your child must go out in the sun, wearing protective clothing and the most protective sun-screen preparation available is beneficial.

MEDICATION

Your doctor may prescribe:

• Beta-carotene to reduce discomfort.

• Chloroquine prior to sun exposure to prevent a recurrence of symptoms.

• See Medications section for information regarding medicines your doctor may prescribe.

ACTIVITY

No restrictions, except for the child to avoid prolonged sun exposure.

DIET & FLUIDS

No special diet. Your child should drink extra fluids to prevent dehydration.

OK FOR SCHOOL, PRESCHOOL, OR NURSERY?

Yes. When fever has returned to normal and appetite has returned and alertness, strength, and feeling of well-being will allow.

CALL YOUR DOCTOR IF

• Your child has symptoms of sun poisoning.

• New, unexplained symptoms develop. Drugs used in treatment may produce side effects.

SUNBURN

GENERAL INFORMATION

DESCRIPTION

Sunburn is inflammation of the skin that follows overexposure to the sun, sun lamps, or occupational light sources. Exposed skin on any part of the body is involved.

Appropriate health care includes:

• Self-care for minor sunburn.

• Doctor's treatment, but usually only necessary for severe sunburn.

SIGNS & SYMPTOMS

• Red, swollen, painful, and sometimes blistered skin.

• Chills and fever.

• Nausea and vomiting (severe burns).

• Delirium (severe, extensive burns).

• Tanning or peeling of the child's skin after recovery, depending on severity of the burn.

CAUSES

Excess exposure to ultraviolet (UV) light. This is not screened out by thin clouds on overcast days, but it is partially screened by smoke and smog. A great deal of ultraviolet light reflects from snow, water, sand, and sidewalks.

RISK FACTORS

• Genetic factors, especially fair skin, blue eyes, and red or blonde hair.

• Exposure to industrial light sources, such as welding arcs.

• Use of drugs, including sulfa, tetracyclines, amoxicillon, or oral contraceptives.

PREVENTING COMPLICATIONS OR RECURRENCE

Instructions for your child to avoid sunburn:

• Avoid the sun from noon to 3 p.m.

• Use a sun-block preparation for outdoor activity. Products with a sun-protective value of 20 or more protect almost totally. Those with lower values offer partial protection and allow minimal tanning. Some of these resist water and perspiration, but reapply them after swimming or after prolonged exposure. Baby oil, mineral oil, or cocoa butter offer no protection from the sun.

• For maximum protection, use a physical-barrier agent such as zinc-oxide ointment. Reapply after swimming and at frequent intervals during exposure. Barrier agents are especially helpful on skin areas that are most susceptible to burns, such as the nose, ears, backs of the legs, and back of the neck.

• If you rarely burn, use a sun-screen product that permits tanning and provides minimal protection.

• Wear muted colors such as tan. Avoid brilliant colors and whites, which reflect the sun into your face.

• If you insist on tanning, limit your sun exposure on the first day to 5 to 10 minutes on each side. Add 5 minutes per side each day.

WHAT TO EXPECT

MEDICAL TESTS
- Your own observation of symptoms.
- Medical history and physical exam by a doctor.

POSSIBLE COMPLICATIONS
- Skin changes leading to skin cancer, including life-threatening malignant melanoma.
- Keratoses, pre-malignant skin lesions.
- Premature wrinkling and loss of skin elasticity.
- Temporary delirium in worst cases.

PROBABLE OUTCOME
Spontaneous recovery in 3 days to 3 weeks, depending on the severity of the child's sunburn.

TREATMENT

HOME CARE
- To reduce heat and pain, dip gauze or towels in cool water and lay these on the child's burned areas.
- After skin swelling subsides, apply cold cream or baby lotion.
- For badly blistered skin, apply a light coating of petroleum jelly. This prevents anything from sticking to the child's blisters.

MEDICATION
- Use non-prescription drugs, such as aspirin or acetaminophen, to relieve pain and reduce fever. Non-prescription burn remedies that contain local anesthetics, such as benzocaine or lidocaine, may be useful, but they produce allergic reactions in some children.
- Your doctor may prescribe pain relievers or cortisone drugs for your child to use briefly.

ACTIVITY
Your child should rest in any comfortable position until fever and discomfort diminish. Covering the child with an upside-down "cradle" or tent of cardboard or other material helps to keep bed linens off the burned skin.

DIET & FLUIDS
No special diet. Your child should increase fluid intake.

OK FOR SCHOOL, PRESCHOOL, OR NURSERY?
When appetite has returned and alertness, strength, and feeling of well-being will allow.

CALL YOUR DOCTOR IF

The following occurs after sunburn:
- Oral temperature spikes (rises suddenly) to 101F (38.C).
- Vomiting or diarrhea.
- Delirium.
- Pain and fever that persist longer than 48 hours.

SURGICAL-WOUND INFECTION

GENERAL INFORMATION

DESCRIPTION

A surgical-wound infection is from bacterial contamination during or after a surgical procedure. Infections occur following surgery in 1.5% to 30% of cases, depending on the type of procedure. Any body part with a recent surgical incision can be involved.

Appropriate health care includes:

- Physician's monitoring of general condition and medications.
- Surgery to incise and drain a wound abscess.
- Self-care during convalescence.

SIGNS & SYMPTOMS

The following usually begin within 5 to 10 days after your child's surgery, but in some cases, they may begin months later:

- Fever.
- Pain and redness around the surgical wound.
- Edema (collection of fluid) around the incision, making the sutures tighter.

CAUSES

- Infection with bacteria, including streptococcal, staphylococcal, or other germs. These sometimes cause infection in spite of elaborate precautions against them and scrupulous surgical technique. They occur most often in children (and adults) who must have emergency surgery on the gastrointestinal tract, such as for perforation of an ulcer or intestinal bleeding.
- Infection from any material left in the surgical area, including instruments or gauze.

RISK FACTORS

- Poor nutrition.
- Any chronic illness, especially diabetes mellitus.
- Gastrointestinal surgery.
- Use of immunosuppressive drugs.

PREVENTING COMPLICATIONS OR RECURRENCE

Skillful surgical techniques and presurgical procedures that include the following:

- Use of certain antibiotics, such as neomycin, before gastrointestinal surgery, to sterilize the child's intestinal tract.
- Meticulous cleansing of the child's skin before surgery.
- Use of as few sutures as possible.

WHAT TO EXPECT

MEDICAL TESTS

- Your own observation of symptoms.
- Medical history and physical exam by a doctor.
- Laboratory culture of pus from the infection site.

POSSIBLE COMPLICATIONS

- Peritonitis.
- Blood poisoning.
- Interference with normal incision healing after surgery, sometimes necessitating further surgery and repairs.

PROBABLE OUTCOME

Usually curable in most patients with drainage of pus and antibiotic treatment. Allow about 2 weeks for your child's surgical-wound infection to heal.

TREATMENT

HOME CARE

- Relieve pain with heat. Use a heat lamp or apply a heating pad or warm compress 3 or 4 times a day for 30 to 40 minutes.
- Change dressings frequently if the wound oozes.

MEDICATION

Your doctor may prescribe:

- Antibiotics to fight infection.
- Vitamin and mineral supplements to hasten healing.
- Pain relievers. Use non-prescription drugs, such as acetaminophen, to relieve minor pain.
- See Medications section for information regarding medicines your doctor may prescribe.

ACTIVITY

Your child should rest in bed until all signs of infection disappear. The child may read or watch TV.

DIET & FLUIDS

Your surgeon will prescribe a diet for your child.

OK FOR SCHOOL, PRESCHOOL, OR NURSERY?

When signs of infection have decreased, appetite returns, and alertness, strength, and feeling of well-being will allow.

CALL YOUR DOCTOR IF

- Your child has symptoms of a surgical-wound infection.
- Your child develops a high fever and a general ill feeling, or infection seems to worsen after treatment.
- New, unexplained symptoms develop. Drugs used in treatment may produce side effects.

SYPHILIS

GENERAL INFORMATION

DESCRIPTION

Syphilis is a contagious, sexually transmitted disease that causes widespread tissue destruction. Syphilis is known as the "great mimic," because its symptoms resemble those of many other diseases. The genitals, skin, and central nervous system—including the brain, the coverings of the brain (meninges), and the spinal cord—and peripheral nerves are involved. Syphilis can affect newborns (0 to 2 weeks) born to mothers with syphilis (congenital form), and it can affect persons of all ages and both sexes who have sexual contact (contagious form).

Appropriate health care includes:

- Physician's monitoring of general condition, medications, and treatment.

SIGNS & SYMPTOMS

First stage (contagious; appears 3 to 6 days after contact):

- A painless red sore (chancre) on the genitals, mouth, or rectum. The sore affects the penis in males and the vagina or cervix in females.

Second stage (contagious; begins 6 or more weeks after the chancre appears):

- Fever (sometimes).
- Enlarged lymph glands in the neck, armpit, or groin.
- Headache.
- Rash on skin and mucous membranes of the penis, vagina, or mouth. The rash has small red scaly bumps.

Third stage (non-contagious; may appear years after the first and second stages):

- Mental deterioration.
- Sexual impotence.
- Loss of balance.
- Loss of feeling, or shooting pains in the legs.
- Heart disease.

CAUSES

The infecting germ for both forms is treponema pallidum.

- The congenital form is spread to the fetus through the bloodstream.
- The contagious form is spread by intimate sexual contact with someone who has syphilis in the first or second stages.

RISK FACTORS

Having many sexual partners.

PREVENTING COMPLICATIONS OR RECURRENCE

- Obtain a blood serum test for syphilis early in your pregnancy. If infected, consult your doctor immediately for treatment.
- Use rubber condoms during intercourse.
- Avoid any sexual contact if you suspect a partner is infectious.

WHAT TO EXPECT

MEDICAL TESTS

- Your own observation of symptoms.
- Medical history and physical exam by a doctor.
- Laboratory studies, such as a blood serum test for syphilis, a microscopic exam of discharge from the chancre, and a study of spinal fluid. Tests are repeated after treatment.

POSSIBLE COMPLICATIONS

Widespread tissue destruction and death without treatment.

PROBABLE OUTCOME

Usually curable in 3 months with treatment. In spite of treatment, syphilis returns within 1 year in 10% of patients. If this happens, re-treatment is necessary.

TREATMENT

HOME CARE

Instructions for anyone with syphilis:

- Ensure that all your sexual partners obtain treatment. The public health department will work with you to notify contacts confidentially and help them obtain treatment.
- After treatment, have blood studies done each month for 6 months to check for recurrence. Then repeat blood studies every 3 months for 2 years.

MEDICATION

Your doctor will probably prescribe penicillin unless the patient is allergic to it. If penicillin cannot be used, other antibiotics can be equally as effective.

ACTIVITY

Anyone with syphilis should avoid sexual intercourse for at least 2 months after treatment begins. Then use rubber condoms during sexual intercourse.

DIET & FLUIDS

No special diet.

OK FOR SCHOOL, PRESCHOOL, OR NURSERY?

After full course of treatment and when signs of infection have decreased, appetite returns, and alertness, strength, and feeling of well-being will allow.

CALL YOUR DOCTOR IF

- Your or your child has symptoms of syphilis.
- The following occurs during or after treatment: fever over 101F (38.3C); skin rash; sore throat; swelling in any joint, such as the ankle or knee.
- New, unexplained symptoms develop. Drugs used in treatment may produce side effects.
- You or your child once had syphilis and have not had a medical checkup in the past year.
- You or your child have had sexual contact with someone who has syphilis.

TAPEWORM
(Taenia Saginata)

GENERAL INFORMATION

DESCRIPTION

Tapeworm is an infestation of the intestinal tract by the tapeworm, a parasite. This is not contagious from person to person.
Appropriate health care includes:
Physician's monitoring of general condition and medications.

SIGNS & SYMPTOMS

Most children with this problem have no symptoms. However, some experience the following:
- Pain in the upper abdomen.
- Diarrhea.
- Unexplained weight loss.
- Symptoms of anemia (weakness, fatigue, and shortness of breath).
- Bowel movements containing worm eggs and worm body parts.

CAUSES

An intestinal parasite called taenia saginata. Your child can become infected by eating improperly cooked or raw beef muscle infected with the parasite.

RISK FACTORS

Travel to Africa, the Middle East, Eastern Europe, Mexico, and South America. This is uncommon in the U.S. except in California and New England.

PREVENTING COMPLICATIONS OR RECURRENCE

- Cook beef long enough for all parts to reach at least 133F (56.1C), and hold it at that temperature at least 5 minutes.
- Buy only meat that has been inspected.

WHAT TO EXPECT

MEDICAL TESTS

- Your own observation of symptoms.
- Medical history and physical exam by a doctor.
- Laboratory stool studies to identify the worm.

POSSIBLE COMPLICATIONS

Anemia.

PROBABLE OUTCOME

Usually curable in 1 day with treatment.

TREATMENT

HOME CARE

- Teach your child to wash hands before eating.
- Have all family members examined by a doctor for possible infection.

MEDICATION

- Your doctor may prescribe an anti-helminthic drug, such as niclosamide or paromomycin, to kill the parasite. Either drug cures a child with a single dose.
- See Medications section for information regarding medicines your doctor may prescribe.

ACTIVITY

No restrictions.

DIET & FLUIDS

No special diet.

OK FOR SCHOOL, PRESCHOOL, OR NURSERY?

When appetite has returned and alertness, strength, and feeling of well-being will allow.

CALL YOUR DOCTOR IF

- Your child has symptoms of a tapeworm.
- New, unexplained symptoms develop. Drugs used in treatment may produce side effects.

TAY-SACHS DISEASE

GENERAL INFORMATION

DESCRIPTION

Tay-Sachs disease is a rare, inherited disorder of the central nervous system in infants and young children. It causes progressive impairment and early death. Fewer than 100 children are born with the disease each year in the U.S. The central nervous system—including the brain, the coverings of the brain (meninges), and the spinal cord—and peripheral nerves are involved.

Appropriate health care includes:

- Physician's monitoring of general condition and medications.
- Time in an extended-care facility for basic care if parents are unable to provide it for the child at home.
- Psychotherapy or counseling for parents and siblings to learn to cope with the distress produced by this condition.

SIGNS & SYMPTOMS

The child seems normal at birth. Between 3 and 6 months, the following symptoms begin to appear:

- Loss of alertness and retarded mental development.
- Loss of muscle strength, such as difficulty sitting up or turning over.
- Deafness.
- Blindness.
- Severe constipation caused by an impaired nerve supply to the colon.
- Seizures.

CAUSES

An inherited disease resulting from a recessive gene that causes an enzyme deficiency. If both parents have the gene, they have a 25% chance of having a child with Tay-Sachs disease. If only one parent is a carrier, the children will not have the disease.

RISK FACTORS

Genetic factors. Most parents who carry the recessive gene are of Eastern European Jewish origin (Ashkenazi).

PREVENTING COMPLICATIONS OR RECURRENCE

- Obtain genetic screening for children in families with Tay-Sachs.
- Obtain genetic counseling if you or your spouse have a family history of Tay-Sachs or are of Ashkenazi background.
- If you are expecting a child and have a family history of Tay-Sachs, consider amniocentesis (see Glossary) to detect if the fetus has the disease.

WHAT TO EXPECT

MEDICAL TESTS
- Your own observation of symptoms.
- Medical history and physical exam by a doctor.
- Laboratory blood tests to detect the hexosaminidase A enzyme deficiency.

POSSIBLE COMPLICATIONS
- Pneumonia.
- Pressure sores.

PROBABLE OUTCOME
Death usually occurs before age 5.

TREATMENT

HOME CARE
Seek out support groups for families of Tay-Sachs victims.

MEDICATION
Your doctor may prescribe:
- Anti-convulsants to control the child's seizures.
- Stool softeners and laxatives to relieve constipation.
- Other medicines to control complicating disorders as they arise.
- See Medications section for information regarding medicines your doctor may prescribe.

ACTIVITY
In the early stages, encourage your child to be as active as possible. Increasing mental, nervous and muscular deficiencies will eventually confine the child to bed much of the time.

DIET & FLUIDS
Provide adequate fluids and a normal, high-fiber diet to minimize the child's constipation. Feeding by tube usually becomes necessary as the disease progresses.

OK FOR SCHOOL, PRESCHOOL, OR NURSERY?
Not likely.

CALL YOUR DOCTOR IF
- You are concerned about your infant's mental and physical development.
- You think you or any member of your family carries the abnormal gene. A genetic counselor can advise you on how to prevent having children with this disease.

TEAR DUCT, INFECTION OR BLOCKAGE OF (Dacryocystitis or Dacryostenosis)

GENERAL INFORMATION

DESCRIPTION

A blockage or infection of the tear duct, sac, or gland is called dacryocystitis. The germs that cause the infection can be spread to other people. Scarring or blockage of the tear duct—usually from an inherited abnormality or prior infection—is called dacryostenosis. The eye and the tear (nasolacrimal) gland, sac, or duct are involved. Blockage or infection of the tear duct or sac occurs in all ages, but it is most common in children. Inherited blockage of the tear duct usually appears in infants at 3 to 12 weeks. Blockage caused by infection can occur at any age following an infection.

Appropriate health care includes:

- Home care after diagnosis.
- Physician's monitoring of general condition and medications.
- Surgery to dilate and probe the tear-duct canal. In infants, this usually requires a brief general anesthesia in an out-patient surgical facility. In adolescents and adults, it is often done in the doctor's office with local anesthesia. After dilation, the tear-duct system is irrigated with a saline solution. Complete obstruction may require a surgical opening from your child's eye into the nasal passage.

SIGNS & SYMPTOMS

The following symptoms may apply to either blockage or infection:

- Persistent tearing of one or both of your child's eyes.
- Drainage of mucus and pus instead of water from the tear duct. The drainage may flow spontaneously or with pressure on the area.
- Pain below the child's eye.
- Redness and swelling of the tear duct.
- Redness of the white of the eye surrounding the tear duct.

CAUSES

Obstruction of your child's tear duct resulting from the following:

- Inherited abnormality.
- Bacterial infection of the duct.
- Sinus or nasal infection, especially chronic nasal infection.
- Nasal polyps.
- Eye injury.
- Eye infection, including severe pinkeye (conjunctivitis).
- Fracture of the nose or facial bones.

RISK FACTORS

- Being a newborn or an infant, especially with a family history of blocked tear ducts.
- Recent infection, such as those listed above.

PREVENTING COMPLICATIONS OR RECURRENCE

Obtain prompt medical treatment for your child's eye, nose, or sinus infections.

TEAR DUCT, INFECTION OR BLOCKAGE OF (Dacryocystitis or Dacryostenosis)

? WHAT TO EXPECT

MEDICAL TESTS

- Your own observation of symptoms.
- Medical history and physical exam by a doctor.

POSSIBLE COMPLICATIONS

- Without treatment, an obstruction may cause chronic infection.
- Without treatment, infection may spread to the child's cornea and other parts of the eye or permanently scar the tear duct.

PROBABLE OUTCOME

- Infection is usually curable with antibiotics.
- Obstruction is usually curable with dilation of the duct or surgery. Allow 3 weeks for your child's recovery.

TREATMENT

HOME CARE

- For obstruction (if surgery is not necessary): Massage the child's tear duct twice a day with fingertips to milk the contents.
- For infection: Relieve your child's pain by applying warm soaks.

MEDICATION

- Your doctor may prescribe oral or topical antibiotics for your child's infection.
- See Medications section for information regarding medicines your doctor may prescribe.

ACTIVITY

Your child should reduce activity during treatment for the infection. Avoiding swimming and contact sports is necessary.

DIET & FLUIDS

No special diet.

OK FOR SCHOOL, PRESCHOOL, OR NURSERY?

When signs of infection have decreased, appetite returns, and alertness, strength, and feeling of well-being will allow.

CALL YOUR DOCTOR IF

- Your child has symptoms of a tear-duct infection or blockage.
- Your child has a temperature of 101F (38.3C) or more.
- Your child's symptoms don't improve, despite treatment.
- Your child's vision is affected.

TEETHING
(Cutting Teeth; Tooth Eruption)

GENERAL INFORMATION

DESCRIPTION

Teething is the sequential appearance of baby teeth and adult teeth. New teeth erupt continually from age 6 months to 3 years. Between ages 6 and 12, children lose baby teeth, which are replaced with adult teeth. The mouth, teeth, and gums are involved. Cutting teeth often causes discomfort to babies and children.

Appropriate health care includes:

- Home care for teething discomfort.
- Dentist's treatment (complications only).

SIGNS & SYMPTOMS

- Excess saliva production and drooling.
- Pain. (This symptom cannot be proved, but it probably does occur.)
- Blood or blood blisters at the site of tooth eruption (rarely). This usually requires no treatment.

Signs & Symptoms *not* related to teething:

- Fever.
- Infection.
- Personality or sleep disturbance. These problems are most likely occurring concurrently; there is no cause-and-effect relationship.

CAUSES

Normal physiological development.

RISK FACTORS

Teething problems are not related to any known risk factor.

PREVENTING COMPLICATIONS OR RECURRENCE

Teething problems cannot be prevented, but your child's symptoms can be relieved.

OTHER

The sequence of normal tooth eruption in children is:

- First teeth (lower front teeth) at about 6 months, sooner in girls than boys.
- First adult teeth at about age 6.
- Bicuspids (side teeth) between ages 10 and 12.
- Permanent molars at about age 12.

WHAT TO EXPECT

MEDICAL TESTS

Your own observation of teething symptoms.

POSSIBLE COMPLICATIONS

- If not cared for properly, baby teeth may decay and need filling.
- Teething may be misdiagnosed as a fever-causing illness.

TEETHING
(Cutting Teeth; Tooth Eruption)

PROBABLE OUTCOME

Your child's teething discomfort can be partially relieved.

TREATMENT

HOME CARE

- Rub the child's gums with your finger; this is very comforting.
- Freeze a coarse washcloth and allow the child to chew it.
- Offer the child a teething biscuit or teething ring (you may chill it).
- Don't use any *imported,* fluid-filled teething rings—even if they are less expensive. The liquid inside may be contaminated.
- Clean new teeth with a cotton swab and water if you notice any collection of tartar. Otherwise, wait until the child is 2 or 3 years old before brushing teeth regularly. By this age, children want to imitate parents by brushing teeth.
- Begin regular dental visits at age 2 or 3.
- At age 5, explain to the child that losing baby teeth is normal. This prevents the child from becoming concerned when tooth loss begins.

MEDICATION

- Medicine usually is not necessary for teething discomfort. Don't use tooth powder, ointment, or cream to relieve your child's discomfort.
- See Medications section for information regarding medicines your doctor may prescribe.

ACTIVITY

No restrictions.

DIET & FLUIDS

Children may find biting apples and other firm foods uncomfortable when teeth are loose. Try to maintain a full, well-balanced diet for your child.

OK FOR SCHOOL, PRESCHOOL, OR NURSERY?

Yes.

CALL YOUR DOCTOR IF

- Your child's temperature rises above normal.
- Signs of infection, such as pain, pus, excessive swelling, or very red gums, occur at the site of the erupting tooth.

TELOGEN EFFLUVIUM

GENERAL INFORMATION

DESCRIPTION

Telogen effluvium is generalized hair loss in which numerous scattered hair follicles simultaneously change from the growing phase to the resting stage of the hair-growth cycle. Children with telogen effluvium rarely progress to significant baldness, and it is not contagious. The hair and scalp are involved. Telogen effluvium can affect both sexes and all ages but is most common in young females (age 8 through adolescence).

Appropriate health care includes:

Self-care.

SIGNS & SYMPTOMS

- Hair loss of 4 to 5 times the normal rate. Normal hair loss is approximately 400 hairs a day, mostly during washing or brushing.
- No itching or pain.

CAUSES

- Hormonal changes, such as those that occur during adolescence, following childbirth, or after discontinuing use of oral contraceptives.
- Severe psychological or physical stress—including that of serious illness, such as high fever, serious infection, injury, or loss of a loved one.

RISK FACTORS

- Stress.
- Pregnancy.

PREVENTING COMPLICATIONS OR RECURRENCE

No specific preventive measures.

WHAT TO EXPECT

MEDICAL TESTS

- Your own observation of symptoms.
- Medical history and physical exam by a doctor (severe, prolonged cases only).

POSSIBLE COMPLICATIONS

None expected.

PROBABLE OUTCOME

Spontaneous recovery in 6 to 12 months.

TREATMENT

HOME CARE

Instructions for your child:

- Continue to wash and brush your hair as usual.
- Confront and define areas of conflict in your family and school life and in your leisure-time activities. If you cannot resolve conflicts, ask for help from family, friends, or competent counselors.
- Aim for a balance of work, study, recreation, reflection, and rest.
- Concentrate on feeling positive. A good attitude toward yourself and others is a powerful asset.

MEDICATION

- Medicine usually is not necessary for this disorder.
- See Medications section for information regarding medicines your doctor may prescribe.

ACTIVITY

No restrictions. Your child should engage in a regular exercise program at least 3 times a week to reduce stress and maintain good overall fitness.

DIET & FLUIDS

No special diet or supplements. Your child should eat a normal, well-balanced diet to provide the nutrients necessary for healthy hair growth.

OK FOR SCHOOL, PRESCHOOL, OR NURSERY?

Yes.

CALL YOUR DOCTOR IF

- Your child's hair loss doesn't improve in 4 months.
- Signs of infection (pain, redness, tenderness, swelling) begin at the site of hair loss.

TEMPORO-MANDIBULAR JOINT SYNDROME (TMJ) (Myofascial Pain-Dysfunction Syndrome; MPD)

GENERAL INFORMATION

DESCRIPTION

Temporo-mandibular joint syndrome means pain and inflammation in the temporo-mandibular joint (the joint on either side of the jaw that opens and closes the mouth) and adjoining muscles. The temporo-mandibular joint, facial muscles, and sensory nerves are involved. TMJ affects both sexes of older children, adolescents, and adults.

Appropriate health care includes:

- Self-care after diagnosis.
- Doctor's or dentist's treatment. Your dentist may manufacture, fit and install a night-guard prosthesis to prevent tooth-grinding while the child is asleep. A night-guard prosthesis consists of removable splints that fit over the tops of the child's teeth to eliminate incorrect biting pressure.
- Psychotherapy or counseling, including biofeedback training, to help the child learn new ways to cope with stress.

SIGNS & SYMPTOMS

- Dull, aching pain on one side of the child's jaw (below the ear) that radiates to the temples, back of the head and along the jaw line.
- Tenderness of the muscles used to chew.
- "Clicking" or "popping" sounds when opening the mouth.
- Inability to open the jaw completely.

CAUSES

Grinding teeth and contracting jaw muscles in an unconscious attempt by the child to:

- Relieve muscle tension caused by stress.
- Correct a faulty alignment ("bite") between the upper and lower jaws.

RISK FACTORS

- Stress.
- Osteoarthritis.

PREVENTING COMPLICATIONS OR RECURRENCE

Your child should not grind the teeth and should learn techniques for relaxing muscles and relieving tension, such as biofeedback, meditation, and exercise.

WHAT TO EXPECT

MEDICAL TESTS

- Your own observation of symptoms.
- Medical history and physical exam by a doctor or dentist.
- X-rays of the child's temporo-mandibular joint.

POSSIBLE COMPLICATIONS

Without treatment, bone in the child's temporo-mandibular joint may erode and deteriorate.

TEMPORO-MANDIBULAR JOINT SYNDROME (TMJ) (Myofascial Pain-Dysfunction Syndrome; MPD)

PROBABLE OUTCOME

With treatment, the child's symptoms can be controlled, and behavior that produces symptoms can be modified. A jaw misalignment can also be corrected.

TREATMENT

HOME CARE

- No specific instructions except those listed under other headings.
- Ice and/or heat may be of slight benefit in relieving the child's discomfort, but will not cure.

MEDICATION

- Your doctor may prescribe:
  —Tranquilizers or muscle relaxants for a short time.
  —Non-steroidal anti-inflammatory drugs.
- For minor pain, use non-prescription drugs, such as aspirin or acetaminophen.
- See Medications section for information regarding medicines your doctor may prescribe.

ACTIVITY

No restrictions.

DIET & FLUIDS

Your child should eat a soft diet until symptoms subside.

OK FOR SCHOOL, PRESCHOOL, OR NURSERY?

When appetite returns and alertness, strength, and feeling of well-being will allow.

CALL YOUR DOCTOR IF

- Your child has symptoms of temporo-mandibular joint syndrome.
- New, unexplained symptoms develop. Drugs used in treatment may produce side effects.

TENDINITIS

GENERAL INFORMATION

DESCRIPTION

Tendinitis is painful inflammation of a tendon. Tendon fibers merge into muscle fibers. A typical skeletal muscle has a tendon on each end that attaches to bone. The force of a muscle contraction is transmitted through the tendon to produce movement. Tendons, bones, and joints are involved. Tendinitis can affect children but is more common in adolescents and adults.

Appropriate health care includes:

- Self-care for mild cases.
- Physician's monitoring of general condition and medications, it self-care is not successful.

SIGNS & SYMPTOMS

- Restricted movement, tenderness and swelling around your child's inflamed tendon. Common sites are the shoulder, elbow, Achilles' tendon, or hamstring muscle.
- Weakness in the tendon caused by calcium deposits that often accompany tendinitis.

CAUSES

- Injury, usually from strenuous athletic activity.
- Musculo-skeletal disorders, including congenital defects and rheumatism.
- Poor posture.

RISK FACTORS

- Overuse of certain tendons and joints from participation in active, competitive sports.
- Incorrect movement and strain during activity. For example, repeatedly holding and swinging a tennis racket incorrectly may cause tendinitis at the elbow (tennis elbow).

PREVENTING COMPLICATIONS OR RECURRENCE

Instructions for your child:

- Precondition your body and build up strength gradually for a sport before beginning it on a regular, competitive basis.
- Warm up before each workout.
- Learn the proper techniques for any sport you intend to play regularly.

WHAT TO EXPECT

MEDICAL TESTS

- Your own observation of symptoms.
- Medical history and physical exam by a doctor.
- X-rays of the involved area.

POSSIBLE COMPLICATIONS

Large deposits of calcium in the inflamed tendon, leading to permanent impairment ("frozen joint").

PROBABLE OUTCOME

Usually curable with treatment and rest of the tendon. Allow 6 weeks for your child to heal.

TREATMENT

HOME CARE

Treatment varies with the cause, severity and duration of the condition. Your child should do the following:

- With severe pain, stiffness, and tenderness, relax completely with the injured area resting in a splint or on a pillow until the pain becomes more bearable.
- Apply ice packs to the affected area during the acute stage or after receiving injections.
- When pain diminishes, wear a sling or use crutches until pain becomes bearable.
- After the acute phase, apply heat. Take hot showers, apply hot compresses, use a heat lamp or heating pad, or rub in deep-heating ointment.
- If you have a shoulder injury, perform shoulder exercises that your doctor or physical therapist will give you. If done conscientiously, these exercises help prevent stiffness and increase strength.

MEDICATION

Your doctor may prescribe:

- Anti-inflammatory drugs.
- Pain relievers.
- Injections of local anesthetics.
- Injections of cortisone into painful and calcified tendons. This reduces the child's pain and inflammation and allows movement, preventing a frozen joint.
- See Medications section for information regarding medicines your doctor may prescribe.

ACTIVITY

Your child can resume normal activities as soon as symptoms improve.

DIET & FLUIDS

No special diet.

OK FOR SCHOOL, PRESCHOOL, OR NURSERY?

Yes.

CALL YOUR DOCTOR IF

- Your child has symptoms of tendinitis.
- Pain and swelling increases, despite treatment.
- New, unexplained symptoms develop. Drugs used in treatment may produce side effects.

TESTES, UNDESCENDED (Cryptorchidism)

GENERAL INFORMATION

DESCRIPTION

Undescended testes is a disorder present at birth in which one or both testicles have not descended from the pelvis into their normal position in the scrotum. The condition exists in 3% of full-term newborn males and 30% of premature newborn males. Most undescended testes descend spontaneously without treatment by age 1. One or both testes (the testicles), the scrotum, and the spermatic cord are involved.

Appropriate health care includes:

- Physician's monitoring of general condition and medications.
- Surgery to move the testes into the scrotum.

SIGNS & SYMPTOMS

- The boy's scrotum appears undeveloped on one or both sides.
- The testicle can't be felt in its normal position in the scrotum.

CAUSES

Unknown, but probably related to a hormone deficiency in the mother or fetus.

RISK FACTORS

Unknown.

PREVENTING COMPLICATIONS OR RECURRENCE

No specific preventive measures.

WHAT TO EXPECT

MEDICAL TESTS

- Your own observation of symptoms.
- Medical history and physical exam by a doctor.
- Laboratory blood studies of gonadotrophin (hormone) levels. Normal levels indicate normally functioning testes that are undescended. Abnormal levels indicate a congenital absence of testes.

POSSIBLE COMPLICATIONS

- Increased likelihood of testicular cancer.
- Sterility, if your son's testes are not repositioned before puberty.
- Psychological problems associated with an altered male self-image, if your son's problem is not corrected.
- Lack of normal sexual development, if the boy's testes are not present.

PROBABLE OUTCOME

Usually curable if treated before puberty with surgery or hormones.

TREATMENT

HOME CARE

Surgery is the only treatment for those boys who don't respond to hormone treatment. Surgery ideally should be performed at about age 5 and *must* be performed prior to puberty to preserve reproductive function.

MEDICATION

- Your doctor may prescribe human chorionic gonadotrophins by injection. These are usually given 3 times a week for 4 to 6 weeks. This treatment causes your son's testes to descend normally in about 25% of cases.
- See Medications section for information regarding medicines your doctor may prescribe.

ACTIVITY

No restrictions.

DIET & FLUIDS

No special diet.

OK FOR SCHOOL, PRESCHOOL, OR NURSERY?

Yes, during and after treatment or after recovery from surgery.

CALL YOUR DOCTOR IF

Your son has undescended testes. Call as soon as you identify this abnormality.

TESTICLE, CANCER OF (Testicular Cancer)

GENERAL INFORMATION

DESCRIPTION

Cancer of the testicle is uncontrolled growth of malignant cells in the testicle. There are several types of testicular cancer, some more dangerous than others. This is the most common form of cancer in young men. The testicles (usually one only) are involved. It affects older adolescent and young adult males.

Appropriate health care includes:

- Doctor's treatment.
- Surgery to remove the cancerous testicle.
- Radiation therapy or chemotherapy for some types of tumors.
- Hospitalization for treatment.

SIGNS & SYMPTOMS

- A firm swelling in one testicle discovered by accident or by self-examination.
- No pain (usually).

CAUSES

Unknown.

RISK FACTORS

Undescended testicle(s) in infancy—even if the testicle was surgically moved into the scrotum.

PREVENTING COMPLICATIONS OR RECURRENCE

Your son should examine his testicles routinely at least once a month.

WHAT TO EXPECT

MEDICAL TESTS

- Your own observation of symptoms. Testicular self-examination is the most important diagnostic measure.
- Medical history and physical exam by a doctor.
- Laboratory and radioactive studies of hormone levels.
- Biopsy (see Glossary).
- X-rays of your son's chest or kidneys to determine if the cancer has spread.

POSSIBLE COMPLICATIONS

Without treatment, some tumors may spread to other parts of your son's body.

PROBABLE OUTCOME

- Most types of testicular tumors are curable with surgery and other treatment. A few types are extremely malignant and have a high death rate unless discovered and treated early.
- Removal of one testicle does not interfere with normal sexual function or the ability to have normal children.

TREATMENT

HOME CARE
No special instructions except those listed under other headings.

MEDICATION
- Your doctor may prescribe anticancer drugs for your son for some types of tumors.
- See Medications section for information regarding medicines your doctor may prescribe.

ACTIVITY
- Your son should resume normal activities as soon as possible. Radiation and chemotherapy may cause temporary fatigue requiring extra rest.
- Your sexually active son can resume sexual relations when he is able. Contraception may be necessary for 12 to 18 months because some forms of treatment cause temporary genetic damage to sperm in the remaining testicle.

DIET & FLUIDS
No special diet.

OK FOR SCHOOL, PRESCHOOL, OR NURSERY?
When appetite returns and alertness, strength, and feeling of well-being will allow.

CALL YOUR DOCTOR IF
- Your son has a firm swelling or mass in the scrotum.
- New, unexplained symptoms develop. Drugs used in treatment may produce side effects.

TESTICLE TORSION

GENERAL INFORMATION

DESCRIPTION

Testicle torsion is twisting of the spermatic cord of the testicle, damaging the testicle—sometimes irreversibly. Testicle torsion usually occurs on one side only. Prompt treatment is necessary to salvage the affected testicle. The testicle, the spermatic cord, and the blood supply to each are involved. Testicle torsion can affect males of all ages but is most common in adolescents (12 to 20 years).

Appropriate health care includes:

- Physician's monitoring of general condition and medications.
- Surgery to untangle the twisted spermatic cord and to attach the affected testicle to the inside scrotal wall, which prevents recurrence. The surgeon will probably operate on the boy's unaffected testicle also to prevent torsion.

SIGNS & SYMPTOMS

- Sudden pain in one testicle.
- Swelling, redness, and tenderness of the scrotum.
- Nausea and vomiting.
- Sweating.
- Rapid heartbeat, if pain is severe.

CAUSES

Usually unknown. It is occasionally present at birth, or it may rarely be caused by an injury or the sudden forceful contraction of muscles attached to the testicle and spermatic cord.

RISK FACTORS

Unknown.

PREVENTING COMPLICATIONS OR RECURRENCE

Your son should wear an athletic supporter or cup when participating in contact sports to prevent genital injury.

WHAT TO EXPECT

MEDICAL TESTS

- Your own observation of symptoms.
- Medical history and physical exam by a doctor.

POSSIBLE COMPLICATIONS

Death of cells in the testicle caused by a diminished or blocked blood supply. This strangulation requires removal of the boy's affected testicle and spermatic cord.

PROBABLE OUTCOME

- Sometimes the torsion will correct itself, symptoms will disappear and no treatment will be needed for your son. However, the testicle is usually injured beyond repair unless surgery is done within 3 to 4 hours after symptoms begin.
- If one of your son's testicles must be removed, the remaining healthy testicle should provide enough hormones for normal male maturation, sex life, and reproduction.

TREATMENT

HOME CARE

• After surgery, use ice packs to relieve the boy's pain and swelling. Wrap the ice in plastic. Apply it to the affected side, separating the ice from the boy's skin with a cloth towel. Apply ice 5 to 10 minutes at a time. Repeat as often as necessary.

• Your son will need to return to your doctor for suture removal in about 7 days.

MEDICATION

• After surgery, your doctor may prescribe pain relievers.

• See Medications section for information regarding medicines your doctor may prescribe.

ACTIVITY

Your son can resume normal activities gradually after surgery.

DIET & FLUIDS

No special diet.

OK FOR SCHOOL, PRESCHOOL, OR NURSERY?

After surgery, when appetite has returned and alertness, strength, and feeling of well-being will allow.

CALL YOUR DOCTOR IF

• Your son has symptoms of testicular torsion. This is an emergency!

• Signs of infection begin after surgery. These include fever, chills, muscle aches, headache, dizziness, and a general ill feeling.

• Excessive bleeding occurs at the surgical site.

TETANUS
(Lockjaw)

GENERAL INFORMATION

DESCRIPTION

Tetanus is an infection in a wound or injury that causes severe muscle spasms. Tetanus is not contagious from person to person. The injured tissue and muscles throughout the body, especially the jaw, neck, back, and abdomen are involved.

Appropriate health care includes:

- Physician's monitoring of general condition and medications.
- Surgery to remove infected tissue.
- Hospitalization in a quiet, dark room. Your child's treatment may include the use of breathing tubes, a respirator, and 24-hour nursing care.

SIGNS & SYMPTOMS

- Muscle pain, irritability, and frequent, severe spasms.
- Severe swallowing difficulty.
- Fever.
- Difficulty using chest muscles to breathe.

CAUSES

Bacteria (clostridium tetani) that are present almost everywhere—especially in soil, manure, or dust. They can enter your child's body through a puncture caused by a nail or other object. Toxins produced by the bacteria travel to nerves that control muscle contraction, producing muscle spasms and seizures.

RISK FACTORS

- Diabetes mellitus.
- Lack of up-to-date tetanus immunizations.
- Warm, humid weather.
- Crowded or unsanitary living conditions, especially for newborn infants born to non-immunized mothers.
- Use of street drugs administered with unclean needles and syringes.

PREVENTING COMPLICATIONS OR RECURRENCE

Obtain tetanus immunizations for your child. These consist of 3 immunization shots, with a booster shot every 10 years. An additional booster shot may be necessary for your child at the time of injury. Private doctors or local health departments may provide immunizations at little or no cost.

WHAT TO EXPECT

MEDICAL TESTS

- Your own observation of symptoms.
- Medical history and physical exam by a doctor.

POSSIBLE COMPLICATIONS

- Pneumonia.
- Pressure sores.
- Irregular heartbeat.
- Respiratory paralysis and death.

PROBABLE OUTCOME

The death rate from tetanus is 50%. With early diagnosis and treatment, however, full recovery is likely. Allow 4 weeks for your child's recovery.

TREATMENT

HOME CARE

Provide your child with reassurance and psychological support. Despite the seriousness of tetanus, patients are usually conscious.

MEDICATION

Your doctor may prescribe:

- Antitoxins to neutralize the nerve toxin.
- Muscle relaxants to control spasms.
- Sedatives to relieve anxiety.
- See Medications section for information regarding medicines your doctor may prescribe.

ACTIVITY

During hospitalization, bed rest is necessary for your child with as little disturbance as possible. During recovery, the child's activities should be resumed gradually.

DIET & FLUIDS

During hospitalization, intravenous fluids will be necessary for the child because of swallowing difficulty.

OK FOR SCHOOL, PRESCHOOL, OR NURSERY?

When signs of infection have decreased, appetite returns, and alertness, strength, and feeling of well-being will allow.

CALL YOUR DOCTOR IF

- Your child has symptoms of tetanus or you observe them in someone else. Call immediately. This is an emergency!
- Your child or someone in your family needs basic or booster tetanus immunizations.
- Your child has a puncture wound or injury that breaks the skin, and there has not been an immunization or booster in 5 years.

THALASSEMIA
(Mediterranean Anemia; Hereditary Leptocytosis)

GENERAL INFORMATION

DESCRIPTION

Thalassemia is an inherited form of anemia in which red blood cells contain less hemoglobin than normal.

Appropriate health care includes:

- Self-care.
- Physician's monitoring of general condition and medications.
- Hospitalization for repeated transfusions as needed.

SIGNS & SYMPTOMS

- Fatigue.
- Paleness.
- Breathlessness.
- Irregular heartbeat, especially with exertion.
- Bloody or dark urine.
- Jaundice (yellow skin and eyes).
- Leg ulcers.
- Enlarged spleen.

CAUSES

- Destruction of abnormal blood cells in your child's spleen and other sites.
- Inadequate manufacture of normal amounts of hemoglobin-A.

RISK FACTORS

- Poor nutrition, especially a diet likely to produce other anemias.
- Obesity.
- Family history of thalassemia.
- Genetic factors, including absence of the gene necessary to manufacture hemoglobin-A. The disorder first appeared in persons of Mediterranean heritage; it also affects people from the Middle East and Far East.

PREVENTING COMPLICATIONS OR RECURRENCE

Cannot be prevented at present, especially if the mother *and* father have thalassemia or the thalassemia genetic trait. If you have a family history of thalassemia, obtain genetic counseling before having children.

WHAT TO EXPECT

MEDICAL TESTS

- Your own observation of symptoms.
- Medical history and physical exam by a doctor.
- Laboratory blood tests and bone-marrow examinations.

POSSIBLE COMPLICATIONS

- Many years of thalassemia produce gallstones.
- Repeated transfusions increase your child's risk of transfusion reaction or kidney damage.

THALASSEMIA (Mediterranean Anemia; Hereditary Leptocytosis)

PROBABLE OUTCOME

This condition is currently considered incurable. However, your child's symptoms can be relieved or controlled. It usually causes death by early adulthood or middle age, depending on the severity of the symptoms. Scientific research into causes and treatment continues, so there is hope for increasingly effective treatment and cure.

TREATMENT

HOME CARE

The only treatment for thalassemia is periodic hospitalization for blood transfusions when the child's symptoms become disabling.

MEDICATION

- Medicine usually is not necessary for this disorder. For minor pain, use non-prescription drugs such as acetaminophen.
- See Medications section for information regarding medicines your doctor may prescribe.

ACTIVITY

After treatment, your child can resume normal activity as soon as possible.

DIET & FLUIDS

No special diet. Don't give the child iron supplements; they make symptoms worse.

OK FOR SCHOOL, PRESCHOOL, OR NURSERY?

Yes.

CALL YOUR DOCTOR IF

Your child has symptoms of anemia (fatigue, paleness, irregular heartbeat, breathlessness).

THIGH INJURY, HAMSTRING

GENERAL INFORMATION

DESCRIPTION

A hamstring thigh injury is an injury to a hamstring tendon. The hamstrings connect the muscles of the thigh to the back and side of the knee. These tendons can be felt behind the knee on either side. They feel like tough rope. Hamstring tendons, muscles and bone comprise units that stabilize the knee and allow its motion. The injury, usually a strain, occurs at the weakest part of a unit. Severe strains require surgical repair. Acute strains are caused by direct injury or overstress. Chronic strains are caused by overuse. Appropriate health care includes: doctor's care; application of tape, plaster splints, or a cast (sometimes) if a muscle ruptures or the muscle-tendon-bone attachment loosens; self-care during rehabilitation; physical therapy (moderate and severe injury); surgery (severe injury).

SIGNS & SYMPTOMS

Pain when moving or stretching the child's leg; muscle spasm of the injured muscles; swelling over the injury; weakened leg (moderate or severe strain); crepitation ("crackling") feeling and sound when the injured area is pressed with fingers; calcification of the child's hamstring tendon or muscles (visible with X-rays); inflammation of the sheath covering the hamstring tendon.

CAUSES

Prolonged overuse of muscle-tendon units in the child's leg; a single violent injury or force applied to the muscle-tendon unit in the leg.

RISK FACTORS

Contact sports; running, jumping, and quick-start sports; medical history of any bleeding disorder; obesity; poor nutrition; previous pelvic or knee injury; poor muscle conditioning.

PREVENTING COMPLICATIONS OR RECURRENCE

Your child should build strength with a long-term conditioning program, warming up adequately before participating in sports. The child should use proper protective equipment, such as knee pads and thigh pads, during contact sports.

WHAT TO EXPECT

MEDICAL TESTS

X-rays of the child's pelvis, femur, and knee to rule out fracture.

POSSIBLE COMPLICATIONS

Prolonged healing time if activity is resumed too soon; proneness to repeated injury; an unstable or arthritic knee following repeated injury; inflammation at the attachment to bone (periostitis); prolonged disability (sometimes).

PROBABLE OUTCOME

If this is a first-time injury, proper care and sufficient healing time before the child resumes activity should prevent permanent disability. Torn ligaments and tendons require as long to heal as fractured bones. Average healing times are: mild strain— 2 to 10 days; moderate strain—10 days to 6 weeks; severe strain—6 to 10 weeks. If this is a repeat injury, complications listed above are more likely to occur.

TREATMENT

FIRST AID

Use instructions for R.I.C.E., the first letters of *rest*, *ice*, *compression*, and *elevation*. See Appendix 39 for details.

HOME CARE

Continue using an ice pack 3 or 4 times a day. Place ice chips or cubes in a plastic bag. Wrap the bag in a moist towel, and place it over the injured area. Use for 20 minutes at a time. Provide the child with whirlpool treatments, if available. Wrap the injured leg with an elasticized bandage between ice or heat treatments. Massage gently and often to provide comfort to the child and decrease swelling.

MEDICATION

- For minor discomfort, use non-prescription medicines such as aspirin, acetaminophen, or ibuprofen; topical liniments and ointments.
- Your doctor may prescribe stronger medicine for pain, if needed; injection of a long-acting local anesthetic to reduce pain; injection of a corticosteroid, such as triamcinolone, to reduce inflammation.

ACTIVITY

For a moderate or severe injury, the child should use crutches for at least 72 hours, then resume normal activities gradually.

DIET & FLUIDS

During recovery, serve the child a well-balanced diet.

OK FOR SCHOOL, PRESCHOOL, OR NURSERY?

Yes, when condition and sense of well-being will allow.

CALL YOUR DOCTOR IF

- Your child has symptoms of a hamstring injury, or a mild injury.
- Pain or swelling worsens despite treatment.
- Any of the following occurs with a cast or splints: pain, numbness, or coldness below the injury; dusky, blue, or gray toenails.

THROMBOCYTOPENIA

GENERAL INFORMATION

DESCRIPTION

Thrombocytopenia is reduction of platelets in the blood, which reduces blood clotting and increases the risk of bleeding. This blood condition simultaneously affects all body parts.

Appropriate health care includes:

- Physician's monitoring of general condition and medications.
- Hospitalization to transfuse platelets.
- Self-care after diagnosis.

SIGNS & SYMPTOMS

- Abnormal bleeding in the mouth.
- A rash of pinpoint-size dots that doesn't fade when the child's skin is pressed.
- Unexplained bruising.
- Spontaneous nosebleeds.
- Blood in the urine.
- Unexplained vaginal bleeding.
- Black, tarry stools.
- Signs of anemia: weakness, fatigue, paleness (if bleeding is prolonged).

CAUSES

Frequently unknown. The following often precede the disorder:

- Allergies.
- Virus infections.
- Use of drugs, such as non-steroidal anti-inflammatory drugs including ibuprofen, aspirin, indomethacin, and phenylbutazone; tricyclic antidepressants; antihistamines; and phenothiazines.
- Collagen disorders, such as lupus erythematosus.
- Blood transfusions and surgery.
- Blood poisoning.
- Liver disease.
- Radiation treatment for cancer.
- Enlarged spleen from any cause.
- Uremia.
- Scurvy.
- Pernicious anemia.
- Leukemia.

RISK FACTORS

- Family history of a bleeding disorder.
- Use of any drug.
- Poor nutrition.

PREVENTING COMPLICATIONS OR RECURRENCE

- Your child should avoid any drug that has lowered the platelet count in the past.
- The child should take only drugs that are necessary.
- Encourage the child to eat a well-balanced diet.

WHAT TO EXPECT

MEDICAL TESTS

- Your own observation of symptoms.
- Medical history and physical exam by a doctor.
- Laboratory blood studies.

POSSIBLE COMPLICATIONS

The child's spleen may enlarge and require surgical removal.

PROBABLE OUTCOME

Usually curable in 2 to 3 weeks if the cause can be treated.

TREATMENT

HOME CARE

- To stop bleeding at any accessible site, apply cold compresses or ice packs and pressure until bleeding stops.
- Inform your doctor or dentist that your child has thrombocytopenia.
- Avoid surgery for your child, including dental surgery, unless it is essential.
- Avoid injections. If your child must have a shot, apply pressure continuously to the injection site for 5 minutes.
- Your child should avoid injury whenever possible.

MEDICATION

- Your child should stop taking all drugs, including non-prescription drugs (especially aspirin) and vitamins.
- Your doctor may prescribe cortisone drugs to reduce the child's autoimmune response.
- See Medications section for information regarding medicines your doctor may prescribe.

ACTIVITY

- Do not get pregnant while thrombocytopenia is active.
- Your child with this condition should not engage in contact sports.
- The child should avoid overexertion or dehydration.
- If an activity involves a risk of injury, urge your child not to participate until cured.

DIET & FLUIDS

No special diet.

OK FOR SCHOOL, PRESCHOOL, OR NURSERY?

When appetite has returned and alertness, strength, and feeling of well-being will allow.

CALL YOUR DOCTOR IF

- Your child has symptoms of thrombocytopenia.
- The following occurs during treatment: bleeding that can't be stopped; enlargement of the child's abdomen; black, tarry stools or vomit that looks like coffee grounds; a rash (described under SIGNS & SYMPTOMS)—especially if fever is present.
- New, unexplained symptoms develop. Drugs used in treatment may produce side effects.

THROMBOPHLEBITIS, SUPERFICIAL (Phlebitis; Phlebothrombosis)

GENERAL INFORMATION

DESCRIPTION

Superficial thrombophlebitis is inflammation and small blood clots in a superficial vein, usually caused by infection or injury. This type of inflammation seldom causes clots to break loose and flow in the bloodstream, as does deep-vein thrombosis. Superficial veins, usually in the legs, are involved. Superficial thrombophlebitis can affect both sexes, all ages, but is most common in adult females.

Appropriate health care includes:

- Physician's monitoring of general condition and medications, which sometimes includes sclerosing injections into tiny veins.
- Self-care after diagnosis.

SIGNS & SYMPTOMS

- Hardness of a superficial vein (feels like a cord).
- Redness, tenderness, and pain in the affected area.
- Fever (sometimes).

CAUSES

Increased fibrin and clotting of red blood cells in a vein due to:

- Injury to the vein's membrane lining from injections. This allows bacteria to enter.
- Spread of malignant blood cancer.
- Pooling of blood following surgery or prolonged bed rest.

RISK FACTORS

- Illness with prolonged bed confinement.
- Smoking.
- Use of birth-control pills. The combination of birth-control pills and smoking greatly increases the risk.

PREVENTING COMPLICATIONS OR RECURRENCE

Instructions for your child:

- Don't smoke if you take birth-control pills.
- If confined to bed for any reason, move your legs as much as possible to prevent pooling of blood in the veins.
- Don't use any drug intravenously, if you can avoid it.

WHAT TO EXPECT

MEDICAL TESTS

- Your own observation of symptoms.
- Medical history and physical exam by a doctor.
- Laboratory blood studies, if the cause is not immediately apparent.

POSSIBLE COMPLICATIONS

Embolism, in which part of the clot breaks off and travels through the child's bloodstream, lodging in the lung or elsewhere (extremely rare).

THROMBOPHLEBITIS, SUPERFICIAL (Phlebitis; Phlebothrombosis)

PROBABLE OUTCOME

Usually curable in 2 weeks.

TREATMENT

HOME CARE

Instructions for your child:

• Stop smoking and stop taking birth-control pills. If you continue both, the next episode of vein clots may be a dangerous, deep-vein clot.

• Wear elastic stockings or wrapped elastic bandages to hasten the blood flow through the veins, relieving discomfort and helping prevent further clot formation. Don't wear garters or knee-high hosiery.

• To relieve pain, use wrapped soaks.

MEDICATION

Your doctor may prescribe:

• Non-steroidal anti-inflammatory drugs to decrease the child's inflammation and pain.

• Antibiotics, if bacterial infection is suspected (rare).

• See Medications section for information regarding medicines your doctor may prescribe.

ACTIVITY

Bed rest with the affected limb elevated may be helpful for 1 or 2 days. Encourage your child to move the feet, ankles, and legs often. When the inflammation begins to subside, the child can resume normal activity slowly. The child should rest often, being careful not to sit or stand for prolonged periods, nor to cross legs.

DIET & FLUIDS

No special diet.

OK FOR SCHOOL, PRESCHOOL, OR NURSERY?

When appetite has returned and alertness, strength, and feeling of well-being will allow.

CALL YOUR DOCTOR IF

• Your child has symptoms of superficial thrombophlebitis.

• The following occurs during treatment:
  — Fever of 102F (38.9C) or higher.
  — Intolerable pain.
  — Coughing blood.
  — Shortness of breath.
  — Chest pain.

• New, unexplained symptoms develop. Drugs used in treatment may produce side effects.

ILLNESSES

THROMBOSIS, DEEP-VEIN

GENERAL INFORMATION

DESCRIPTION

Deep-vein thrombosis is a blood clot that forms inside a vein. It may partially or completely block the blood flow, or break off and travel to the lung. This is different from clots in superficial veins, where clots rarely break off. Usually the lower legs (calves) or lower abdomen are involved, but occasionally this condition affects other veins in the body.

Appropriate health care includes:

- Physician's monitoring of general condition and medications.
- Hospitalization for anticoagulant injections (usually with heparin).
- Self-care after hospitalization.

SIGNS & SYMPTOMS

- Swelling and pain in the area drained by the vein, usually the ankle, calf, or thigh. Swelling in the leg includes everything below the clot, extending to the child's toes.
- Tenderness and redness of the affected parts.
- Soreness or pain when walking. The soreness does not disappear when your child rests.
- Pain when raising the leg and flexing the foot (sometimes).
- Fever (sometimes).
- Increased heartbeat (sometimes).

CAUSES

Pooling of blood in the child's vein, which triggers blood-clotting mechanisms. The pooling may occur after prolonged bed rest following surgery, or from debilitating illness, such as a severe injury, or serious infections, stroke, or bone fractures.

RISK FACTORS

- Obesity.
- Smoking.
- Use of estrogen in oral contraceptives. This is especially hazardous if estrogen use is combined with smoking.

PREVENTING COMPLICATIONS OR RECURRENCE

- Your child should avoid prolonged bed rest during illnesses. The child should start moving the lower limbs as soon as possible after any surgical procedure or during any bed-confining illness.
- On long auto or airplane trips, encourage the child to exercise the legs at least every 1 or 2 hours.
- Urge the child to stop smoking, especially if taking estrogen for any purpose.

WHAT TO EXPECT

MEDICAL TESTS

- Your own observation of symptoms.
- Medical history and physical exam by a doctor.
- Laboratory studies, such as ultrasound, radioactive fibrinogen, and prothrombin time (see Glossary for all).
- X-rays of veins after dye is injected into a foot vein.

POSSIBLE COMPLICATIONS

Pulmonary embolism, in which the clot breaks away and travels to your child's lung. The lung's blood supply is blocked, causing affected lung tissue to die.

PROBABLE OUTCOME

Usually curable with anti-coagulant treatment, if pulmonary embolism can be avoided.

TREATMENT

HOME CARE

The following suggestions apply to your child after hospitalization or if the condition can be treated safely at home:

- Wear fitted elastic stockings or wrapped elastic bandages, but don't wear garters or knee-high hosiery.
- Don't cross your legs or ankles while sitting, lying in bed, or traveling.
- Elevate the feet higher than the hips when sitting for long periods.
- Elevate the foot of the bed.

MEDICATION

After your child's hospitalization, your doctor may prescribe oral anti-coagulant drugs, such as coumarin. To minimize the danger of pulmonary embolism, blood tests to monitor the anticoagulant levels are mandatory. Oral anticoagulants may be necessary up to 6 months.

ACTIVITY

Your child should rest in bed until all signs of inflammation have disappeared. While resting, the child should make it a habit to move the leg muscles, bend the ankles, and wiggle the toes.

DIET & FLUIDS

No special diet.

OK FOR SCHOOL, PRESCHOOL, OR NURSERY?

When appetite has returned and alertness, strength, and feeling of well-being will allow.

CALL YOUR DOCTOR IF

- Your child has symptoms of deep-vein thrombosis.
- The following occurs during treatment: unexpected bleeding anywhere; chest pain; coughing up blood; shortness of breath; continued or increased swelling and pain, despite treatment.

THRUSH
(Oral Thrush)

GENERAL INFORMATION

DESCRIPTION

Thrush is a common fungus infection of the mouth. The mouth, gums, tongue, soft palate, cheeks, and lips are involved. Thrush can affect newborns and infants, but it may also affect older children and adults.

Appropriate health care includes:

- Self-care.
- Physician's monitoring of general condition and medications, if self-care is not successful.

SIGNS & SYMPTOMS

Patches appear in the child's mouth with the following characteristics:

- Patches are white to creamy yellow and slightly raised. They are similar to milk curds, but they don't wipe off.
- Patches are not painful to the child unless they are rubbed off. Then they leave small, painful ulcers.
- The child's mouth is dry.

CAUSES

A fungus called candida albicans, which may develop under the following circumstances:

- Treatment with antibiotics. This may upset the natural balance of organisms in the child's mouth and allow thrush to develop.
- Birth. Newborns may acquire the infection during passage through the birth canal—especially if the mother has a vaginal yeast infection. Thrush appears within hours or up to 7 days after birth.

RISK FACTORS

- Poor nutrition.
- Illness that has lowered resistance.
- Diabetes.
- Use of immunosuppressive drugs.

PREVENTING COMPLICATIONS OR RECURRENCE

If your child has had thrush and must take antibiotics, urge the child to drink buttermilk or eat yogurt during treatment to replenish helpful bacteria in the digestive tract.

WHAT TO EXPECT

MEDICAL TESTS

- Your own observation of symptoms.
- Medical history and physical exam by a doctor.

POSSIBLE COMPLICATIONS

Can spread to the child's vagina, skin, larynx, gastrointestinal tract, or respiratory system.

THRUSH (Oral Thrush)

PROBABLE OUTCOME

Treatment usually clears this infection in 3 days. It is not dangerous or serious, but it has a tendency to recur.

TREATMENT

HOME CARE

- To avoid transmitting thrush to others, boil your child's eating utensils or use disposable items. Boil anything that touches the child's mouth or saliva.
- Your child should rinse the mouth with a salt solution (1/2 teaspoon salt to 8 ounces water) 3 times a day or more after eating.
- If an infant has the infection, boil bottle nipples separately for 20 minutes before the final sterilization.

MEDICATION

- Gently swab patches of thrush in the child's mouth with antiseptic mouthwash or non-prescription 1% gentian-violet solution.
- If these simple medicines don't cure your child's infection, your doctor may prescribe an anti-fungal drug, nystatin, to apply to the patches.
- See Medications section for information regarding medicines your doctor may prescribe.

ACTIVITY

No restrictions.

DIET & FLUIDS

No changes in infants. Older children and adults should maintain an adequate fluid intake with milk, liquid gelatin, ice cream, custard, water, tea, or other beverages and foods that are easy to swallow. Let the child use a straw for drinking if the patches are painful.

OK FOR SCHOOL, PRESCHOOL, OR NURSERY?

When signs of infection have decreased, appetite returns, and alertness, strength, and feeling of well-being will allow.

CALL YOUR DOCTOR IF

- Signs of dehydration (sunken eyes, poor elasticity of the skin, and lethargy) appear in your child.
- An infant fails to gain weight, or an unexplained weight loss occurs in an older child.
- Fever develops.
- Lesions on the child's skin or vagina appear.
- Signs of secondary bacterial infection (pain, redness, tenderness, swelling, sometimes fever) appear in the child's mouth.

THUMB-SUCKING

GENERAL INFORMATION

DESCRIPTION

Thumb-sucking refers to placing the finger or thumb on the roof of the mouth behind the teeth and sucking with lips and teeth closed. Thumb-sucking is a behavior—not a disorder. The mouth, teeth, tongue, pharynx, finger, or thumb are involved. Thumb-sucking can affect children of both sexes up to age 12 but is most common in young children.

Appropriate health care includes:

- Home care.
- Doctor's or dentist's treatment.
- Psychotherapy or counseling (prolonged or excessive thumb-sucking only).

SIGNS & SYMPTOMS

Protruding front teeth. Thumb-sucking may put enough pressure on front teeth to move them forward eventually.

CAUSES

Some psychiatrists believe thumb-sucking provides a mother substitute and is caused by a child's need to cling to the mother. Others believe it is an instinctive behavior that becomes habitual.

RISK FACTORS

Lack of love and attention during infancy and childhood.

PREVENTING COMPLICATIONS OR RECURRENCE

- Provide a loving and secure environment for your child.
- Provide other comfort mechanisms early in infancy, such as orthodontic pacifiers designed to minimize tooth misalignment.

OTHER

Thumb-sucking does not cause serious damage until the permanent teeth begin cutting through gums at age 6 or 7. Most children have outgrown the habit by this age. If not, parents should work with the child to change the habit for the sake of appearance and dental health.

? WHAT TO EXPECT

MEDICAL TESTS

- Your own observation of symptoms.
- Medical history and physical exam by a doctor.

POSSIBLE COMPLICATIONS

Unsightly facial appearance without treatment.

PROBABLE OUTCOME

If your child develops protruding front teeth, they should improve in 6 months to 2 years with dental treatment.

TREATMENT

HOME CARE

For a child over 6 or 7 who sucks the fingers or thumb:

• Give your child extra attention. Observe if conflicts or anxiety-producing situations provoke sucking. Help the child explore other solutions to stress.

• If the child decides to try to stop sucking, help set goals. Give rewards for *any* progress toward the goal. Reward is not a bribe, but something earned through effort.

MEDICATION

• Medicine usually is not necessary for this disorder.

• See Medications section for information regarding medicines your doctor may prescribe.

ACTIVITY

No restrictions.

DIET & FLUIDS

No special diet.

OK FOR SCHOOL, PRESCHOOL, OR NURSERY?

Yes.

CALL YOUR DOCTOR IF

• Your child wishes to stop and behavior-modification efforts (rewards for progress) have not solved the problem. The dentist may fit a training device in the child's mouth to prevent the thumb from touching the roof of the mouth.

• The child becomes intolerant of the training device or it loosens.

• The sucking behavior does not diminish in 6 months, despite treatment. Referral for psychological counseling may be necessary at this point.

THYROID TUMOR

GENERAL INFORMATION

DESCRIPTION

A thyroid tumor is a benign or malignant thyroid nodule. Benign tumors are unlikely to spread to other body parts. These growths may be cystic or solid (thyroid adenoma). Malignant thyroid nodules can spread and threaten your child's life. Early symptoms of both types are the same. The thyroid gland in the front of the neck is involved. Thyroid tumors can affect both sexes, but benign nodules are more common in females than males. Thyroid tumors can affect all ages, but malignant nodules are more likely in children between ages 4 and 7.

Appropriate health care includes:

- Home care after diagnosis.
- Physician's monitoring of general condition and medications.
- Surgery to aspirate a cystic tumor or to remove a solid tumor and the affected lobe of the thyroid.
- Radioactive iodine treatment (see Glossary).
- Speech therapy, if your child's voice is affected after surgery.

SIGNS & SYMPTOMS

- Swelling or lump in the child's thyroid gland.
- Pain and tenderness in the child's thyroid gland.
- Swallowing difficulty.
- Hoarseness.
- Breathing difficulty (rare).
- Symptoms of hypothyroidism or hyperthyroidism.

CAUSES

Unknown.

RISK FACTORS

- Radiation treatment during childhood—even in small doses—to the head, neck, and upper chest.
- Family history of thyroid tumors.

PREVENTING COMPLICATIONS OR RECURRENCE

Avoid having the child receive radiation treatments to the neck for acne, tonsillitis, enlarged thymus gland, or other minor conditions.

WHAT TO EXPECT

MEDICAL TESTS

- Your own observation of symptoms.
- Medical history and physical exam by a doctor.
- Laboratory tests, such as radioactive-iodine uptake studies, CAT or CT scan (see Glossary for both) and blood studies of thyroid function.
- Biopsy (see Glossary).

POSSIBLE COMPLICATIONS

- Spread of a malignant tumor to adjacent parts, requiring radical surgery to remove lymph nodes and muscles of one side of the child's neck.
- Hypothyroidism or hypoparathyroidism, caused by inadvertent injury to the child's thyroid or parathyroid glands during surgery.
- Permanent hoarseness and loss of voice following surgery for some thyroid cancers.

PROBABLE OUTCOME

Usually curable with surgery or a combination of surgery and radioactive-iodine treatment.

TREATMENT

HOME CARE

- If your child no longer has a voice, special equipment is available from the telephone company and other agencies to assist with speech.
- After thyroid surgery, when the child rises from a lying to a sitting position, put a pillow under the head and support it with your hands to prevent neck-muscle strain.

MEDICATION

Your doctor may prescribe:

- Anti-thyroid medications *or* replacement thyroid hormone.
- Radioactive iodine to treat cancer.
- Pain relievers.
- See Medications section for information regarding medicines your doctor may prescribe.

ACTIVITY

Your child can resume normal activities as soon as symptoms improve after surgery.

DIET & FLUIDS

No special diet.

OK FOR SCHOOL, PRESCHOOL, OR NURSERY?

After recovery from surgery.

CALL YOUR DOCTOR IF

- Your child has symptoms of thyroid nodules or thyroid enlargement.
- The following occurs after surgery:
  - — Symptoms of hypothyroidism (fatigue, puffy face, rapid weight gain, and coarse hair).
  - — Bleeding, pain, or swelling at the surgical site.
  - — Fever.
  - — Twitching muscles.
  - — Breathing difficulty.
- New, unexplained symptoms develop. Drugs used in treatment may produce side effects.

TOENAIL, INGROWN

GENERAL INFORMATION

DESCRIPTION

Ingrown toenail is a condition in which the sharp edge of a nail grows into the flesh of a toe, usually the great (big) toe. Ingrown toenail can affect both sexes, all ages, but is most common in adolescents and adults.

Appropriate health care includes:

- Self-care.
- Physician's monitoring of general condition and medications.
- Surgery to remove the nail.

SIGNS & SYMPTOMS

Pain, tenderness, redness, swelling, and heat in your child's toe where the sharp nail edge pierces the surrounding fold of tissue. Once tissue surrounding the nail becomes inflamed, infection usually develops in the injured area.

CAUSES

An ingrown toenail is likely to accompany one of the following conditions:

- Your child's nail formation is more curved than normal.
- The child's toenail is clipped back too far, allowing tissue to grow up over it.
- Shoes fit poorly, forcing the toe of the shoe against the nail and surrounding tissue.
- The child participates in activities that require sudden stops ("toe jamming").

RISK FACTORS

Any of the circumstances listed as causes.

PREVENTING COMPLICATIONS OR RECURRENCE

- Your child should wear roomy, well-fitting shoes.
- Cut the child's toenails carefully. Children with diabetes mellitus or peripheral vascular disease should be especially careful in trimming toenails. Foot injury is dangerous with these disorders because of impaired blood circulation to the feet.

WHAT TO EXPECT

MEDICAL TESTS

- Your own observation of symptoms.
- Medical history and physical exam by a doctor.

POSSIBLE COMPLICATIONS

Chronic infection that cannot be cured without surgery.

PROBABLE OUTCOME

Curable with treatment. Oral antibiotics usually relieve symptoms of infection within 1 week. Then part or all of the child's toenail is removed surgically and the nail bed is scraped so the problem will not recur. The child's nail should grow back, but it probably won't look the same.

TREATMENT

HOME CARE

The following home treatment is appropriate either before or after surgery:

- Use immersion soaks.
- Lift the nail corners free of surrounding inflamed tissue by wedging a small piece of cotton under the child's nail around the edges. Protect the inflamed tissue from further injury.

MEDICATION

- Your doctor may prescribe antibiotics to fight infection.
- See Medications section for information regarding medicines your doctor may prescribe.

ACTIVITY

Your child can resume normal activities as soon as symptoms improve. The child may need to wear a shoe with the toe cut out until the toe heals.

DIET & FLUIDS

No special diet.

OK FOR SCHOOL, PRESCHOOL, OR NURSERY?

After surgery, when appetite has returned and alertness, strength, and feeling of well-being will allow.

CALL YOUR DOCTOR IF

- Your child has symptoms of an ingrown toenail.
- The following occurs during treatment or after surgery:
  - — Fever.
  - — Increased pain.
  - — Signs of infection (pain, redness, tenderness, swelling, or heat) in the toe.

TONGUE INFLAMMATION (Glossitis)

GENERAL INFORMATION

DESCRIPTION

Glossitis is an acute or chronic inflammation of the tongue from a variety of causes. This is sometimes contagious, but is not cancerous. Adjacent parts of the mouth are frequently inflamed as well as the tongue.

SIGNS & SYMPTOMS

Any of the following:

- Bright red, swollen tongue.
- Ulcers on the tongue.
- Hairy-looking tongue.
- A tongue with red tip and edges.

CAUSES

- Infections, including herpes.
- Burns.
- Injury from jagged teeth, mouth-breathing, or repeated biting during convulsive seizures.
- Excessive consumption of alcohol, tobacco, hot food, or spices.
- Poor dental health.
- Allergy to toothpaste, mouthwash (especially mouthwash containing peroxide), candy, dye, or material used in dental work.
- Lack of B-vitamins, resulting in pellagra, B-12 deficiency anemia, or iron-deficiency anemia.
- Adverse reaction to antibiotic drugs.

RISK FACTORS

- Poor nutrition, especially vitamin deficiencies.
- Smoking.
- Chemical or environmental exposure to irritating or corrosive chemicals.

PREVENTING COMPLICATIONS OR RECURRENCE

- Have the child practice good oral hygiene. Brush teeth and tongue at least twice a day, and floss teeth daily. Get regular dental checkups.
- Keep the child away from tobacco smoke.
- Prevent tongue injury by having the child wear protective headgear for contact sports or cycling.

WHAT TO EXPECT

MEDICAL TESTS

- Your own observation of symptoms.
- Medical history and physical exam by a doctor.

POSSIBLE COMPLICATIONS

Tongue inflammation can become chronic and spread to other parts of the body if not adequately treated.

TONGUE INFLAMMATION
(Glossitis)

PROBABLE OUTCOME

Usually curable in 2 weeks with home care and medical treatment.

TREATMENT

HOME CARE

- Observe if there is an association between eating specific foods and tongue inflammation. Irritating foods may include chocolate, citrus, acid foods (vinegar, pickles), salted nuts, or potato chips.
- Rinse the child's mouth 3 or more times a day with a salt solution (1/2 teaspoon salt to 8 oz. water).
- If tongue inflammation is caused by a rough tooth or braces, consult your dentist. Inflammation won't heal until the cause is eliminated.

MEDICATION

- For minor pain, use non-prescription drugs, such as anesthetic mouthwashes or acetaminophen.
- For infection and pain, your doctor may prescribe antibiotics or topical anesthetics.
- See Medications section for information regarding medicines your doctor may prescribe.

ACTIVITY

No restrictions.

DIET & FLUIDS

No special diet, except to avoid foods that aggravate inflammation. Have the child drink as many fluids and eat as well-balanced a diet as possible while healing. To minimize pain, let him sip liquids through straws. Foods that cause the least pain are milk, liquid gelatin, yogurt, ice cream and custard.

OK FOR SCHOOL, PRESCHOOL, OR NURSERY?

When appetite and activity at home return to normal. Approximately 4 days.

CALL YOUR DOCTOR IF

- Fever develops.
- Symptoms don't improve in 3 days despite treatment.
- Pain is unbearable and isn't relieved by treatment.
- Skin rash appears.
- Weight loss occurs.

TONSILLITIS (Pharyngitis)

GENERAL INFORMATION

DESCRIPTION

Tonsillitis is inflammation of the tonsils (clumps of lymphoid tissue at the back of the throat). Tonsils are small at birth, enlarge during childhood, and become smaller at puberty. When not infected, tonsils help prevent infection in the sinuses, mouth, and throat from spreading to other body parts. Tonsillitis is contagious.

SIGNS & SYMPTOMS

- Throat pain, either mild or severe.
- Swallowing difficulty.
- Chills and fever as high as 104F (40C) or more.
- Swollen lymph glands on either side of the jaw.
- Headache.
- Ear pain.
- Cough (sometimes).
- Vomiting (sometimes).

CAUSES

Viral or bacterial infection of the tonsils.

RISK FACTORS

- Crowded or unsanitary living conditions.
- Exposure to others in public places.

PREVENTING COMPLICATIONS OR RECURRENCE

Avoid exposure to people with upper-respiratory infections.

WHAT TO EXPECT

MEDICAL TESTS

- Your own observation of symptoms.
- Medical history and physical exam by a doctor.
- Surgery to remove the tonsils (occasionally).

POSSIBLE COMPLICATIONS

- Abscess of the tonsils and nearby throat area, requiring surgery to drain.
- Chronic tonsillitis, with a recurrent sore throat and greatly enlarged tonsils, caused by repeated attacks.
- Rheumatic fever, if the bacterial infection is streptococcal and it is not treated with antibiotics.

PROBABLE OUTCOME

Usually spontaneous recovery. Symptoms generally begin to improve in 2 to 3 days, but treatment may last longer. If attacks of tonsillitis are so severe and frequent that they affect one's general health or interfere with schooling, hearing, or breathing, your doctor may recommend surgery to remove the tonsils. A tonsillectomy involves small risk to a child, but the risk increases with age.

TREATMENT

HOME CARE

- Use a cool-mist humidifier to relieve throat irritation and cough.
- Prepare a soothing tea or other gargle. Double the usual strength of tea. This may be gargled warm or cold as often as is soothing.

MEDICATION

- If the tonsillitis is caused by a streptococcal infection, your doctor will prescribe penicillin or other antibiotics for at least 10 days.
- To relieve pain, you may use acetaminophen.
- See Medications section for information regarding medicines your doctor may prescribe.

ACTIVITY

- Keep the patient away from others until fever, pain, and other symptoms disappear.
- Bed rest, except to use the bathroom, is necessary until fever subsides. Normal activity may be resumed when temperature has been normal for 2 or 3 days.

DIET & FLUIDS

Increase all fluid intake. While the throat is very sore, use liquid nourishment, such as milkshakes, soups, and high-protein fluids (diet or instant-breakfast milk drinks).

OK FOR SCHOOL, PRESCHOOL, OR NURSERY?

When appetite and activity at home return to normal. Approximately 2 weeks.

CALL YOUR DOCTOR IF

- Your child has symptoms of tonsillitis. If tonsils cover the opening of the throat (hold down the tongue with a spoon and look with a flashlight), call your doctor immediately.
- Symptoms worsen or the following occurs during treatment:
  - — Temperature is normal for 1 to 2 days, then rises above 101F (38.3C) orally or 102F (38.9C) rectally.
  - — New symptoms begin, such as nausea, vomiting, skin rash, thick nasal drainage, chest pain, or shortness of breath.
  - — Your child has a convulsion.
  - — Joints become red and painful.
  - — Cough produces a discolored (green, yellow, brown, or bloody) sputum.

TOOTH ABSCESS
(Periapical Abscess; Periodontal Abscess)

GENERAL INFORMATION

DESCRIPTION

Tooth abscess is an abscess around a tooth root, which is imbedded in the bone of the upper or lower jaw. The gums and jawbone are involved.

Appropriate health care includes:

• Tooth abscesses can be drained in one of 3 ways: If the tooth has poor bone and gum support, the tooth can be extracted, allowing the abscess to drain through the socket and heal.

• A hole can be drilled through the top of the child's tooth, and a tiny metal or plastic wick inserted into the narrow nerve canal through the center of the tooth. This allows the abscess to drain.

• An incision can be made in the child's gum at the site of infection, which dramatically relieves pain and pressure. Your dentist may place a small rubber wick in the incision for a few days. When the infection improves, the dentist can perform root-canal therapy on your child.

SIGNS & SYMPTOMS

• Persistent toothache or throbbing, extreme pain upon biting or chewing.

• Swelling and tenderness in the child's neck glands and on the side of the face.

• Earache.

• Fever.

• General ill feeling.

• Foul taste and bad breath (if the abscess opens spontaneously).

CAUSES

• Tartar beneath the gum.

• Deep decay which has entered the tooth nerve. The infection spreads down the nerve and into surrounding bone and gum tissue, but does not affect the child's adjacent teeth.

RISK FACTORS

Poor nutrition; improper diet; inadequate fluoride in drinking water.

PREVENTING COMPLICATIONS OR RECURRENCE

• Your child should follow these instructions to prevent decay with good brushing and flossing:

— Use a soft-bristle toothbrush to remove plaque from the teeth's front and back surfaces, especially at the gum line.

— Learn to use dental floss correctly. Ask your dentist or hygienist to demonstrate the technique.

• Use fluoride mouthwash, toothpaste, tablets, or liquid supplements if your dentist recommends them.

• Reduce sugar consumption. Tooth decay increases as sugar consumption increases.

TOOTH ABSCESS
(Periapical Abscess; Periodontal Abscess)

? WHAT TO EXPECT

MEDICAL TESTS

Your own observation of symptoms; medical history and physical exam by a dentist; X-rays of the mouth.

POSSIBLE COMPLICATIONS

- Rupture into the sinus of an abscess in the upper jaw.
- Loss of the tooth.
- Spread of infection through the bloodstream to other body parts.

PROBABLE OUTCOME

Usually curable with oral surgery.

TREATMENT

HOME CARE

Instructions for your child:

- Rinse your mouth with warm water to draw infection from the abscess. Repeat each hour or as often as it feels good.
- Don't chew on the affected side of your mouth for at least 2 days.
- If a tube has been used to drain the abscess, keep the small hole free of obstruction. Carefully remove impacted food.
- If a drain has been placed in gum tissue, return to your dentist in several days to have it removed.

MEDICATION

- For minor pain, use non-prescription drugs such as acetaminophen.
- Your doctor or dentist may prescribe:
  - — Antibiotics to control infection.
  - — Pain relievers.

ACTIVITY

Your child can resume normal activities as soon as possible.

DIET & FLUIDS

A liquid diet may be necessary for 1 or 2 days until pain subsides.

OK FOR SCHOOL, PRESCHOOL, OR NURSERY?

When appetite has returned and alertness, strength, and feeling of well-being will allow.

CALL YOUR DOCTOR IF

- Your child has symptoms of a tooth abscess.
- The following occurs during treatment:
  - — Fever spikes to 101F (38.3C) or higher.
  - — Pain becomes intolerable.
- New, unexplained symptoms develop. Drugs used in treatment may produce side effects.

TOOTH DECAY (Caries; Dental Decay; Cavities)

GENERAL INFORMATION

DESCRIPTION

Tooth decay is disintegration of tooth enamel, allowing injury to the dentin (layer below the enamel) and eventual involvement of the pulp (the layer below the dentin), which contains nerves and blood vessels. Tooth decay and the common cold are the most common human disorders. Dental caries can involve any tooth or possibly all teeth.

Appropriate health care includes:

- Self-care.
- Dentist's treatment to remove all decay in your child's tooth and replace it with a restorative material (filling). The filling prevents further decay.

SIGNS & SYMPTOMS

- Tooth sensitivity to heat and cold.
- Tooth discomfort after eating sugar.
- Darkening on or between your child's teeth (cavity) when the decay has progressed enough to be seen. The most common tooth-cavity sites are the gum line, biting surfaces, and surfaces between adjacent teeth.
- Unpleasant taste in the child's mouth and bad breath because of stagnant food and bacteria trapped in the cavity.
- Persistent tooth pain (in the final stages of decay when the pulp becomes inflamed).

CAUSES

- Cavities are caused by acid destruction of tooth material. Acid is produced by bacteria in the child's mouth. The bacteria feed on food debris—usually sugar—and produce the acid that dissolves tooth material.
- The combination of sugars from food debris, bacteria, and chemicals in the child's saliva form a substance called plaque. Plaque becomes a localized site of acid production, which forms continuously at the neck of each tooth. This plaque must be thoroughly cleaned away at the gum line daily or it fosters tooth decay.

RISK FACTORS

- Poor nutrition and improper diet.
- Poor dental hygiene.

PREVENTING COMPLICATIONS OR RECURRENCE

- Your child should brush and floss teeth regularly.
- Consult your dentist about your child using fluoride mouthwash, liquid or tablets, or having fluoride treatments once or twice a year.
- Drinking fluoridated water or taking fluoride supplements during pregnancy has not proven to protect the unborn child's teeth.

TOOTH DECAY (Caries; Dental Decay; Cavities)

? WHAT TO EXPECT

MEDICAL TESTS

- Your own observation of symptoms.
- Examination by a dentist. The decayed area feels soft when the dentist probes it with a sharp instrument.
- X-rays of the child's teeth and mouth.

POSSIBLE COMPLICATIONS

- Abscess around a decayed tooth.
- Death of the tooth, caused by destruction of the tooth pulp that contains the tooth's nerve and blood supply.

PROBABLE OUTCOME

Usually curable with dental treatment.

TREATMENT

HOME CARE

No specific instructions except those listed under other headings.

MEDICATION

- For minor pain, use non-prescription drugs such as acetaminophen.
- Your dentist may prescribe stronger pain relievers or fluoride supplements.
- See Medications section for information regarding medicines your doctor may prescribe.

ACTIVITY

No restrictions.

DIET & FLUIDS

For 48 hours after your dentist fills the child's decayed tooth, urge the child not to put pressure on the tooth, as by eating apples, hard candy, or raw vegetables, or by chewing on ice. The child should avoid very hot or cold foods. The tooth remains sensitive for 48 hours to 10 days after a cavity has been filled.

OK FOR SCHOOL, PRESCHOOL, OR NURSERY?

Yes.

CALL YOUR DOCTOR IF

- Your child has symptoms of tooth decay.
- The following occurs after treatment:
  — Fever.
  — Increased pain that is not relieved by non-prescription medication.
  — Discomfort with hot or cold food that persists longer than 2 weeks after the filling procedure.
  — Brown spots on the tops of any other teeth.

TOOTH-GRINDING (Bruxism)

GENERAL INFORMATION

DESCRIPTION

Bruxism is the habit of grinding teeth. Tooth-grinding is often done while your child is asleep, but grinding or tapping teeth during the day is also common. Continual tooth-grinding may erode gums and supporting bones in the mouth. The teeth, gums, and tempero-mandibular joints are affected.

Appropriate health care includes:

- Self-care after diagnosis.
- Dentist's care. Your dentist may manufacture, fit, and install a night-guard prosthesis to prevent tooth-grinding while your child is asleep. A night-guard prosthesis consists of removable splints which fit over the tops of the child's teeth to eliminate incorrect biting pressure.
- Biofeedback training or counseling for the child to learn ways to cope more effectively with stress.

SIGNS & SYMPTOMS

- Frequent contraction of muscles on the side of the face.
- Annoying tooth-grinding noises at night. These may be loud enough to awaken others.
- Damaged teeth, supporting gums, and bone (apparent in a dental exam).
- Headaches.

CAUSES

- Anxiety.
- Unconscious attempts to correct a faulty "bite" (contact between the upper and lower teeth when the child's jaws are closed).

RISK FACTORS

Stress or anxiety.

PREVENTING COMPLICATIONS OR RECURRENCE

Help your child avoid stressful situations. See Appendix 19.

WHAT TO EXPECT

MEDICAL TESTS

- Your own observation of symptoms.
- Medical history and physical exam by a dentist.
- X-rays of the mouth.

POSSIBLE COMPLICATIONS

Without treatment, your child's teeth, bones, and gums may erode from the pressure of grinding.

PROBABLE OUTCOME

Usually curable in 6 months without treatment.

TREATMENT

HOME CARE

No specific instructions except those listed under other headings.

MEDICATION

- Medicine usually is not necessary for this disorder.
- See Medications section for information regarding medicines your doctor may prescribe.

ACTIVITY

No restrictions.

DIET & FLUIDS

No special diet.

OK FOR SCHOOL, PRESCHOOL, OR NURSERY?

Yes.

CALL YOUR DOCTOR IF

- Your child grinds the teeth at night.
- Your child develops pain around the ears, dizziness, or ringing in the ears.
- Your child develops pain or clicking in the jaw.
- Your child loses or breaks the night-guard prosthesis.

TOOTH INJURY & LOSS
(Tooth Avulsion)

GENERAL INFORMATION

DESCRIPTION

Tooth avulsion is damage to a tooth severe enough to separate it completely from the gum and bone without fracture. Children whose front teeth have short, slender roots are most likely to lose teeth through injury. The teeth, the bones that hold teeth, and the gums and soft tissue surrounding the tooth, including nerves, blood vessels and covering to bone (periosteum) are involved.

Appropriate health care includes:

Dentist's or oral surgeon's evaluation and replantation of an avulsed tooth, with blood studies after surgery to evaluate blood loss and infection.

The dentist or oral surgeon will:

- Cleanse the socket.
- Remove the nerve from the child's tooth and fill the root canal with a plasticlike material before the tooth is replaced.
- Replace the child's tooth in its socket.
- Anchor the tooth to neighboring teeth with wire or plastic. The child's tooth must be held in place for 6 to 8 weeks.

SIGNS & SYMPTOMS

- A missing tooth.
- Pain and bleeding from the tooth site.
- Swelling of the child's gums soon after injury.

CAUSES

Direct blow to the child's tooth and gum.

RISK FACTORS

Contact sports, especially football and boxing; poor nutrition, especially calcium deficiency; poor dental hygiene or gum disease.

PREVENTING COMPLICATIONS OR RECURRENCE

Your child should wear a helmet, strong face guard, and mouthpiece whenever possible during contact sports.

WHAT TO EXPECT

MEDICAL TESTS

Your own observation of symptoms; medical history and physical exam by your dentist or oral surgeon; X-rays of the child's mouth and jaw to detect additional injuries.

POSSIBLE COMPLICATIONS

Permanent tooth loss if the replantation fails; excessive bleeding; infection.

PROBABLE OUTCOME

Allow about 4 weeks for recovery from surgery if complications don't occur. After it heals, the child's tooth often appears normal. If it darkens, a plastic or porcelain dental veneer can be applied to make it cosmetically acceptable.

TOOTH INJURY & LOSS
(Tooth Avulsion)

TREATMENT

FIRST AID

- Find and wash the missing tooth or teeth.
- Replace the child's tooth in its socket as soon as possible.
- If you cannot replace the tooth in its socket, wash it and keep it wet in a wet cloth until you reach a dentist or doctor. Put a moist cloth in the empty socket and have the child bite on it.
- Go to the child's dentist or to the emergency room immediately. *Hurry!* The longer the tooth stays out of the mouth, the less the chance of saving it.

HOME CARE

Instructions for your child after replantation:

- Don't rinse your mouth, spit, smoke, or suck on straws for 24 hours after tooth replantation.
- After 24 hours, brush your other teeth often with a soft toothbrush. A clean mouth heals faster. Don't brush the injured tooth until you have clearance from your dentist.
- Beginning 24 hours after surgery, rinse your mouth every 1 to 2 hours with a solution of 1/2 teaspoon salt in 8 oz. of lukewarm water.
- Don't bite down on the affected tooth until healing is complete.

MEDICATION

- Use non-prescription drugs such as acetaminophen for minor pain.
- Your doctor may prescribe:
  - — Pain relievers. Don't give the child prescription pain medication longer than 4 to 7 days. Use only as much as the child needs.
  - — Antibiotics to fight infection.
  - — Mouthwashes.

ACTIVITY

Your child should avoid vigorous physical exercise for 4 to 6 weeks following surgery and should wear a face mask when resuming sports activity.

DIET & FLUIDS

Adequate food and fluid intake following surgery will promote more rapid healing. If your child can't avoid putting pressure on the tooth by eating a normal diet, use a liquid high-protein diet for 2 to 3 days. The child should avoid all alcoholic beverages during healing.

OK FOR SCHOOL, PRESCHOOL, OR NURSERY?

Yes, when condition and sense of well-being will allow.

CALL YOUR DOCTOR IF

- Your child has a tooth knocked out.
- Any of the following occur after surgery: increased mouth pain, swelling, redness, drainage, or bleeding; signs of infection (headache, muscle aches, dizziness, or a general ill feeling and fever).

TORTICOLLIS (Wryneck)

GENERAL INFORMATION

DESCRIPTION

Torticollis is shortened neck muscles or chronic neck-muscle spasm that causes the head to turn and bend. The central nervous system—including the brain, the coverings of the brain (meninges), and the spinal cord—and peripheral nerves and the muscular system are involved. Torticollis can affect both sexes but is more common in females of all ages.

Appropriate health care includes:

- Self-care after diagnosis.
- Physician's monitoring of general condition and medications.
- Psychotherapy or counseling if the cause is stress-related.
- Surgery to lengthen neck muscles if the cause is congenital.
- Physical therapy (sometimes), including gentle massage.

SIGNS & SYMPTOMS

The following may be permanent or intermittent:

- Head that turns sideways and bends down.
- Neck-muscle spasm that is sometimes painful.

CAUSES

For constant torticollis:

- Birth defect.
- Injury to neck muscles or vertebrae at birth or later.
- Neck-muscle inflammation.

For intermittent torticollis:

- Stress and psychological conflict.

RISK FACTORS

- Sleeping in an awkward position.
- Emotional disturbances, such as neurosis or hyponchondriasis.

PREVENTING COMPLICATIONS OR RECURRENCE

Stress-related forms can be prevented in your child with stress-reduction techniques, including biofeedback.

WHAT TO EXPECT

MEDICAL TESTS

- Your own observation of symptoms.
- Medical history and physical exam by a doctor.
- Laboratory blood tests for infection and inflammation.
- X-rays of the spinal column in your child's neck.

POSSIBLE COMPLICATIONS

Without treatment, the congenital form becomes permanent, causing an unattractive, abnormal appearance of the child's head and neck.

PROBABLE OUTCOME

- Congenital torticollis can usually be corrected with muscle-stretching exercises or surgery.
- Other forms will improve or heal with treatment. Healing time varies. Some cases require treatment for several years.

TREATMENT

HOME CARE

If your infant has signs of torticollis:

- Ask your doctor or physical therapist for muscle-stretching exercises to do with the child twice a day.
- Place attention-getting objects in the crib opposite the side that the head turns.

For non-congenital forms of torticollis:

- Your doctor may recommend that your child wear a neck brace.
- Relieve pain from neck spasms with heat. The child should take hot showers or use hot compresses, deep-heating ointments, or heat lamps.

MEDICATION

- If the child's condition is caused by injury or inflammation, your doctor may prescribe muscle relaxants and pain relievers.
- See Medications section for information regarding medicines your doctor may prescribe.

ACTIVITY

Normal activities may be resumed as soon as symptoms improve.

DIET & FLUIDS

No special diet.

OK FOR SCHOOL, PRESCHOOL, OR NURSERY?

Yes.

CALL YOUR DOCTOR IF

- Your infant has symptoms of torticollis.
- Your child has neck pain or spasms that persist longer than 1 week.

TOXIC SHOCK SYNDROME (TSS)

GENERAL INFORMATION

DESCRIPTION

Toxic shock syndrome is a form of blood poisoning caused by poisons (toxins) released by staphylococcal bacteria. It must be treated immediately! The reproductive system and respiratory system are involved. TSS affects all ages and both sexes but is most common in females after puberty.

Appropriate health care includes:

- Doctor's treatment. This is an emergency!
- Immediate hospitalization for intravenous fluids to administer antibiotics and correct fluid and electrolyte loss and dehydration.

SIGNS & SYMPTOMS

- Sudden, high fever in a previously healthy child.
- Vomiting and watery diarrhea.
- A rash that resembles sunburn.
- Low blood pressure.
- Thirst.
- Rapid pulse.
- A feeling of impending doom.
- Mental changes, such as confusion.
- Extreme fatigue and weakness.
- Headache.
- Sore throat.

CAUSES

Some strains of staphylococcal bacteria produce toxins that enter the bloodstream, causing sudden symptoms. Most serious cases have come from staphylococci in the vagina of women using tampons. Toxic shock syndrome can also arise from wounds or infections in the throat, skin, lungs, or bone.

RISK FACTORS

- Continuous use of tampons during menstrual periods.
- Any infection.

PREVENTING COMPLICATIONS OR RECURRENCE

Instructions for your daughter:

- Change tampons frequently, and alternate them at night with sanitary napkins.
- Don't use superabsorbent tampons. Use those made of cotton.
- Don't use tampons if you have a skin infection, especially near the genitals.
- Wash your hands thoroughly before inserting tampons. Staphylococci are commonly found on hands.

TOXIC SHOCK SYNDROME (TSS)

WHAT TO EXPECT

MEDICAL TESTS

- Your own observation of symptoms.
- Medical history and physical exam by a doctor.
- Laboratory studies, such as blood counts, blood cultures, and cultures from the vagina or other areas of infection.

POSSIBLE COMPLICATIONS

- Severe shock.
- Kidney failure.
- Congestive heart failure.

PROBABLE OUTCOME

Most patients recover with early diagnosis and prompt hospital treatment, but some cases are fatal. Skin of the palms and soles often peels during recovery.

TREATMENT

HOME CARE

No specific instructions except those listed under other headings.

MEDICATION

- Your doctor may prescribe:
  —Antibiotics, usually intravenous, for your child's infection.
  —Intravenous fluids and electrolytes.
- See Medications section for information regarding medicines your doctor may prescribe.

ACTIVITY

Your child can resume normal activities as soon as symptoms improve.

DIET & FLUIDS

No special diet after recovery. Intravenous nourishment is usually necessary during hospitalization.

OK FOR SCHOOL, PRESCHOOL, OR NURSERY?

When appetite returns and alertness, strength, and feeling of well-being will allow.

CALL YOUR DOCTOR IF

- Your child has symptoms of toxic shock syndrome. Call immediately! Shock develops rapidly.
- New, unexplained symptoms develop. Drugs used in treatment may produce side effects.

ILLNESSES

TOXOCARA
(Toxocariasis, Visceral Larva Migrans)

GENERAL INFORMATION

DESCRIPTION

Toxocara is a disorder resulting from invasion of larvae of worms normally found in the intestines of dogs and cats. These same larvae cause a skin disease (larva migrans or creeping eruption) if they invade no deeper than the skin. If they invade deeper tissues of humans they may affect many organs, including the eye, liver, lungs, and heart, and the central nervous system. Toxocara may affect older children and adults, but it normally affects young children aged 2 to 4. The incubation period inside the human body varies from weeks to months after ingesting the larvae. This disease is not contagious from one infected child to another.

Appropriate health care includes:

- Self-care after diagnosis.
- Physician's monitoring of general condition and medications.

SIGNS & SYMPTOMS

- Loss of appetite.
- Fever.
- Cough or wheezing.
- Abdominal pain.
- Enlarged liver.
- Skin rash.
- Enlarged spleen.
- Eye lesions and vision problems.

CAUSES

The embryonated eggs of *Toxocara canis* and *cati,* parasites found in soil contaminated by the feces of dogs and cats.

RISK FACTORS

- Playing in children's sandboxes.
- Owning a dog or cat.

PREVENTING COMPLICATIONS OR RECURRENCE

- Your child should avoid areas likely to be contaminated by dog and cat feces.
- Deworm pet dogs and cats regularly.
- Cover your child's sandbox when not in use.
- Your child should always wash hands after playing with animals.

WHAT TO EXPECT

MEDICAL TESTS

- Your own observation of symptoms.
- Medical history and physical exam by a doctor.
- Skin test, blood test for eosinophiles, liver biopsy, and fluorescent antibody tests.

POSSIBLE COMPLICATIONS

Serious complications if the child's liver, heart, or eye are involved.

TOXOCARA
(Toxocariasis, Visceral Larva Migrans)

PROBABLE OUTCOME

Complete cure. Self-limited (6 to 18 months) for mild cases. Appropriate treatment results in a quicker cure.

TREATMENT

HOME CARE

- Employ preventive measures to keep your child from getting re-infected.
- Give your child the prescribed medication as directed.

MEDICATION

- Your physician may prescribe a special anti-parasite drug such as thiabendazole.
- See Medications section for information regarding medicines your doctor may prescribe.

ACTIVITY

- If actively infected, your child should keep away from all animals and potentially contaminated areas for a minimum of 6 months.
- Otherwise, no restrictions.

DIET & FLUIDS

No restrictions.

OK FOR SCHOOL, PRESCHOOL, OR NURSERY?

Yes, when condition and sense of well-being will allow.

CALL YOUR DOCTOR IF

- Your child has symptoms of toxocara.
- New, unexplained symptoms develop. Drugs used in treatment may produce side effects.

TRENCH MOUTH (Necrotizing Ulcerative Gingivitis; Vincent's Disease; Fusospirochetosis)

GENERAL INFORMATION

DESCRIPTION

Trench mouth is an infection of tissue between the teeth. This is not contagious or cancerous. The gums are involved. If untreated, trench mouth can spread to the lymph glands in the neck, or to the tonsils, vocal cords, bronchial tubes, rectum, or vagina.

Appropriate health care includes:

- Self-care after diagnosis.
- Physician's monitoring of general condition and medications.
- Scaling of teeth by a dentist to remove plaque.
- Frequent dental checkups—up to once a month—after treatment.

SIGNS & SYMPTOMS

- Painful gums.
- Gums that bleed when pressed.
- Excess salivation.
- Bad breath.
- Ulcers covered with gray membrane on the child's gums.
- Swallowing difficulty.
- Speaking difficulty.

CAUSES

- Spirochetes, a fusiform bacteria.
- Tartar, plaque, or food debris between the child's teeth.

RISK FACTORS

Poor nutrition; illness that has lowered resistance; smoking; stress.

PREVENTING COMPLICATIONS OR RECURRENCE

Instructions for your child:

- Maintain good oral hygiene.
  — To brush teeth: Scrub clear, sticky plaque off teeth daily with a soft toothbrush. Place the brush at the gum line and gently rotate, pointing bristles toward the gum. Brush one section of teeth at a time. Then brush the tongue. A soft brush is less likely to damage teeth and gums than a hard brush.
  — To floss: Use waxed or unwaxed dental floss according to instructions on the package label or your dentist's instructions.
- Eat a well-balanced diet.
- Don't smoke.

WHAT TO EXPECT

MEDICAL TESTS

- Your own observation of symptoms.
- Medical history and physical exam by a doctor.
- Laboratory culture to identify the infecting germs.

TRENCH MOUTH (Necrotizing Ulcerative Gingivitis; Vincent's Disease; Fusospirochetosis)

POSSIBLE COMPLICATIONS

Surgery may be necessary to trim your child's rough, infected gums.

PROBABLE OUTCOME

Usually curable in 2 weeks with treatment.

TREATMENT

HOME CARE

Instructions for your child:

- Rinse your mouth every 2 hours, alternating the following rinses:
  - — Mixture of 1 teaspoon salt in large glass of very warm water.
  - — Mixture of equal parts 2% hydrogen peroxide and warm water.
- Avoid any gum irritation until gums heal completely.
- Don't smoke.

MEDICATION

- Your doctor may prescribe penicillin or another antibiotic for your child to fight the infection.
- Use non-prescription drugs, such as acetaminophen, for minor pain.
- See Medications section for information regarding medicines your doctor may prescribe.

ACTIVITY

Your child should rest at home for the first 2 days of treatment. Then the child can resume normal activities.

DIET & FLUIDS

- A liquid diet may be necessary for 2 or 3 days because of gum tenderness. When the pain subsides, your child should eat many fresh fruits and vegetables. Don't serve the child spicy or hot (temperature) food.
- Your child should drink juices and 4 to 6 glasses of water each day, but not carbonated beverages or alcohol.

OK FOR SCHOOL, PRESCHOOL, OR NURSERY?

When signs of infection have decreased, appetite returns, and alertness, strength, and feeling of well-being will allow.

CALL YOUR DOCTOR IF

- Your child has symptoms of trench mouth.
- The following occurs during treatment:
  - — Fever of 101F (38.3C) or higher.
  - — Swelling of the neck or face.
  - — Swallowing difficulty.
  - — Inability to eat.

TRICHINOSIS

GENERAL INFORMATION

DESCRIPTION

Trichinosis is an infection caused by larvae of parasites that live in the intestines of pigs and bears. Body parts involved include the gastrointestinal tract (where larvae enter), the lymphatic system and bloodstream (through which they are transported), and the large muscles of the body, especially the diaphragm large muscle used in breathing that separates the chest from the abdomen, arms, and legs (in which larvae become embedded).

Appropriate health care includes:
- Self-care after diagnosis.
- Physician's monitoring of general condition and medications.
- Hospitalization (worst cases).

SIGNS & SYMPTOMS

Early stages (usually begin in 7 to 10 days):
- Loss of appetite, nausea, vomiting, diarrhea, and abdominal cramps.

Later stages:
- Puffy eyelids and face.
- Muscle pain.
- Itching, burning skin.
- Sweating.
- High fever (102F to 104F or 38.9C to 40C).

Late stages:
- Symptoms subside, but some muscle tissues remain permanently infected with microscopic cysts. In rare cases these may cause your child heart and central nervous system disorders.

CAUSES

Infection with a parasite, trichina spiralis, which is transmitted to children when they eat infected animals. Thorough cooking kills the parasite and makes infected meat safe to eat. The parasites pass from animal to animal in contaminated food—usually raw garbage.

RISK FACTORS

- Eating improperly cooked or raw pork or bear meat.
- Use of immunosuppressive drugs.

PREVENTING COMPLICATIONS OR RECURRENCE

Your child should not eat raw or undercooked pork (including sausage) or bear meat.

WHAT TO EXPECT

MEDICAL TESTS

- Your own observation of symptoms.
- Medical history and physical exam by a doctor.
- Laboratory blood studies.
- Muscle biopsy.

POSSIBLE COMPLICATIONS

Overwhelming infection, which can lead to:

- Congestive heart failure.
- Respiratory failure.
- Permanent damage to the child's central nervous system.

PROBABLE OUTCOME

Usually curable in most children with anti-parasite drugs and, in severe cases, expert supportive care. Some deaths have been reported. Allow up to 6 months for your child's recovery.

TREATMENT

HOME CARE

Reduce the child's fever if it goes over 103F (39.4C). See Appendix 17, How to Reduce Your Child's Fever.

MEDICATION

- Your doctor may prescribe anti-helminthic drugs (usually thiabendazole) to kill the parasites.
- You may give the child non-prescription drugs, such as acetaminophen, to reduce fever and discomfort.
- See Medications section for information regarding medicines your doctor may prescribe.

ACTIVITY

Your child should rest in bed until the symptoms subside. While the child is confined to bed, moving the legs frequently reduces the likelihood of deep-vein blood clots. Normal activities may be resumed gradually.

DIET & FLUIDS

Your child should eat a special high-protein diet to help rebuild damaged muscle tissue. The diet will be prescribed by your doctor and explained by a dietitian. Usually the child can progress to an unrestricted, well-balanced diet within 6 months.

OK FOR SCHOOL, PRESCHOOL, OR NURSERY?

When signs of infection have decreased, appetite returns, and alertness, strength, and feeling of well-being will allow.

CALL YOUR DOCTOR IF

- Your child has symptoms of trichinosis.
- The following occurs during treatment:
  - — Fever spikes (rises suddenly) to over 104F (40C).
  - — Irregular heartbeat.
  - — Shortness of breath.
  - — Puffy ankles.
  - — Clumsy finger or thumb movement.
- New, unexplained symptoms develop. Drugs used in treatment may produce side effects, especially nausea, vomiting, skin rash, or fever.

ILLNESSES

TUBERCULOSIS (TB)

GENERAL INFORMATION

DESCRIPTION

Tuberculosis is an acute or chronic contagious bacterial infection. The lungs are primarily involved, but the disease may spread to other organs. Childhood tuberculosis is usually confined to the middle of the lungs, but it may spread to cause meningitis.

Appropriate health care includes:

- Self-care after diagnosis.
- Physician's monitoring of general condition and medications.

SIGNS & SYMPTOMS

- Early stages: no symptoms (often); symptoms that resemble those of influenza.
- Second stages: low fever; weight loss; chronic fatigue; heavy sweating, especially at night.
- Later stages: cough with sputum that becomes progressively bloody, yellow, thick, or gray; chest pain; shortness of breath; reddish or cloudy urine (sometimes).

CAUSES

Infection by the germ mycobacterium tuberculosis. The germ is transmitted in the air from one person to another. Cattle are also susceptible and can transmit TB through non-pasteurized milk.

RISK FACTORS

Infancy; chronic illness that has lowered your child's resistance; use of cortisone or immunosuppressive drugs may reactivate inactive TB in your child; crowded or unsanitary living conditions.

PREVENTING COMPLICATIONS OR RECURRENCE

- Vaccination with BCG, a strain of the tuberculosis bacteria. This may prevent infection, or it may shorten and diminish the severity of the infection.
- Preventive treatment for several months with isonicotinic acid if your child's tuberculin skin test is positive.

OTHER

Health authorities recommend vaccination and preventive treatment for the following groups:

- Persons who have positive reactions to TB tests, but show no symptoms of disease—especially children under age 5.
- Children with negative reactions to TB tests in areas where 20% or more of classmates have positive reactions.
- Persons traveling to countries where TB is prevalent.
- Persons who must take immuno-suppressive or cortisone drugs for a long time.
- Post-gastrectomy patients whose X-rays show evidence of inactive TB.
- Persons with silicosis.

WHAT TO EXPECT

MEDICAL TESTS

Your own observation of symptoms; medical history and physical exam by a doctor; tuberculin skin test; laboratory cultures of your child's sputum and urine; X-rays of the child's chest; pulmonary function studies. This disease must be reported to the health department. All family members and close associates need tuberculin skin tests and treatment if needed.

POSSIBLE COMPLICATIONS

Lung abscess; bronchiectasis; COPD (see Glossary); spread of infection to other organs (brain, bone, spine, and kidneys); respiratory failure.

PROBABLE OUTCOME

Usually curable with treatment. Without treatment, it can be fatal to your child.

TREATMENT

HOME CARE

- It may not be necessary to isolate or hospitalize a child with TB. The disease is usually spread before diagnosis. Patients are probably not infectious after 10 days to 2 weeks of treatment.
- Occasionally you will need to collect a 24-hour sputum specimen from your child for laboratory analysis to see if the TB is still active.

MEDICATION

Your doctor may prescribe anti-tubercular drugs, including INH (isonicotinic acid hydrizide), ethambutol, para-aminosalicylic acid, or rifampin.

ACTIVITY

Your child should rest in bed until symptoms disappear and tests show TB germs are gone. You may need to restrict the child's activities for 6 months.

DIET & FLUIDS

No special diet.

OK FOR SCHOOL, PRESCHOOL, OR NURSERY?

When all signs, symptoms, and laboratory studies verify complete healing. Various health departments have varying policies or laws to obey. Check with them before sending your child back.

CALL YOUR DOCTOR IF

- Your child has symptoms of tuberculosis.
- Symptoms persist or worsen, despite treatment.
- New, unexplained symptoms develop. Drugs used in treatment may produce side effects.

TYPHOID FEVER

GENERAL INFORMATION

DESCRIPTION

Typhoid fever is a bacterial infection of the gastrointestinal tract. Body parts involved include the gastrointestinal tract, the skin and the central nervous system—including the brain, the coverings of the brain (meninges), and the spinal cord—and peripheral nerves. Typhoid fever can affect both sexes, all ages, but infants can have especially severe cases.

Appropriate health care includes:

- Physician's monitoring of general condition and medications.
- Self-care during the convalescent stage.
- Hospitalization for severe cases.

SIGNS & SYMPTOMS

- Diarrhea. In mild cases, this may be only 2 or 3 loose bowel movements a day. In severe cases, it may be watery diarrhea as often as every 10 or 15 minutes.
- Vomiting.
- Fever.
- Headache.
- Muscle aches.
- Skin rash on the child's abdomen.
- Abdominal cramps (sometimes).
- Blood in the child's stool (sometimes).

A relatively mild attack may be mistaken for simple gastroenteritis.

CAUSES

- Infection with the salmonella typhi bacteria. The bacteria is found in infected animals and transmitted to children (or adults) in contaminated meat or milk. Thorough cooking kills the germ.
- The infection can also be transmitted by ill persons or non-ill carriers who handle food without careful hand-washing after bowel movements.

RISK FACTORS

- Illness that has lowered your child's resistance.
- Crowded or unsanitary living conditions.

PREVENTING COMPLICATIONS OR RECURRENCE

- Your child should follow these recommendations in any area with a substandard water supply:
  - — Drink purified water, boil water, or add 2 to 4 drops of 4% to 6% chlorine bleach to each quart of water 30 minutes before use.
  - — If in a hotel, draw hot water from the faucet, let it cool and use it as drinking water.
  - — Don't use ice.
  - — Don't eat raw fruits and vegetables unless you can peel them.
- Drink only pasteurized milk.
- Wash your hands after bowel movements and before handling food.
- Obtain a vaccination if exposed to typhoid.

WHAT TO EXPECT

MEDICAL TESTS

Your own observation of symptoms; medical history and physical exam by a doctor; laboratory studies, such as stool studies and a blood culture; X-rays of the child's gastrointestinal tract; sigmoidoscopy (see Glossary).

POSSIBLE COMPLICATIONS

Dehydration; perforation of the child's intestines; gastrointestinal hemorrhage or abscess; deep-vein blood clot; pneumonia; bone infection; congestive heart failure.

PROBABLE OUTCOME

Usually curable in 2 to 3 weeks with treatment. Without treatment, it can be fatal to your child.

TREATMENT

HOME CARE

- Isolate ill children and have them use bedside commodes or a separate bathroom; use a heating pad or hot-water bottle to relieve the child's abdominal cramps.
- Wash hands carefully and often while treating the child; turn the child frequently in bed.
- Apply lukewarm wet towels to the child's groin and underarms to reduce fever. *Don't* use aspirin or acetaminophen; both irritate the gastrointestinal tract.

MEDICATION

Your doctor may prescribe antibiotics, such as ampicillin or sulfa drugs.

ACTIVITY

Bed rest is necessary for your child until all symptoms have been gone at least 3 days. The child's legs should be flexed often in bed to prevent formation of deep-vein blood clots.

DIET & FLUIDS

A clear-liquid diet is necessary during the diarrhea phase. Later, a high-calorie, well-balanced diet is necessary. In addition, vitamin and mineral supplements may be helpful to your child.

OK FOR SCHOOL, PRESCHOOL, OR NURSERY?

When signs of infection have decreased, appetite returns, and alertness, strength, and feeling of well-being will allow.

CALL YOUR DOCTOR IF

- Your child has symptoms of typhoid fever.
- The following occurs during treatment: fever of 102F (38.9C) or higher; sore throat; severe cough or coughing up blood; shortness of breath; severe abdominal pain or swelling; rectal bleeding; pain in the child's calf or leg; headache, earache, or swollen joints.

ULCER, PEPTIC, IN THE DUODENUM, STOMACH, OR ESOPHAGUS

GENERAL INFORMATION

DESCRIPTION

A peptic ulcer (or "sore") in the duodenum causes symptoms similar to those of a stomach ulcer. An ulcer is not contagious or cancerous. The duodenum (the first 12 inches of small intestine beyond the stomach) is involved. Peptic ulcers are more common in males. Similar ulcerations with the same causes can occur in the lower end of the esophagus and in the stomach. Stomach or gastric ulcers are rare in children but affect both sexes of young adults. Appropriate health care includes self-care after diagnosis; physician's monitoring of general condition and medications; hospitalization (for complications). Stomach ulcers may require surgery to remove part of the stomach or cut nerves that stimulate acid production, if conservative treatment fails.

SIGNS & SYMPTOMS

- Pain with the following characteristics: a burning, boring, or gnawing feeling lasting 30 minutes to 3 hours, often interpreted as heartburn, indigestion, or hunger; pain in the upper abdomen, or occasionally below the breastbone; pain immediately after eating, or even hours later, frequently awakening a child at night; pain that comes and goes; weeks of intermittent pain alternating with short pain-free periods; pain relieved by drinking milk, eating, resting, or taking antacids.
- Appetite and weight loss; recurrent vomiting; blood in the stool.
- Anemia; sometimes no pain.

CAUSES

Unknown. An ulcer can develop wherever stomach acid comes in contact with the gastrointestinal lining. Ulcers seem to run in families. An ulcer is most likely to develop in an anxious, tense, or worried child with many emotional conflicts and an overactive stomach that manufactures too much hydrochloric acid. Children with ulcers often have irregular living habits.

RISK FACTORS

Family history of ulcers; stress and anxiety; fatigue and overwork; improper diet, irregular mealtimes, and skipped meals; smoking; excess alcohol consumption; use of drugs, including caffeine, which irritate the stomach.

PREVENTING COMPLICATIONS OR RECURRENCE

Your child should avoid as many risk factors as possible.

WHAT TO EXPECT

MEDICAL TESTS

Your own observation of symptoms; medical history and physical exam by a doctor; analysis of gastric acid; gastroscopy to determine the ulcer size and location and cell types in gastric scrapings; X-rays of stomach, esophagus, and duodenum.

ULCER, PEPTIC, IN THE DUODENUM, STOMACH, OR ESOPHAGUS

POSSIBLE COMPLICATIONS

Perforation (erosion of the ulcer through the intestinal wall) or dangerous bleeding; unrelenting pain, failure to heal, and scarring; extensive peptic-ulcer disease, with increased likelihood of stomach cancer.

PROBABLE OUTCOME

Usually curable with lifestyle changes and medical treatment for your child. For perforation or hemorrhaging, surgery is mandatory. It usually produces a complete cure.

TREATMENT

HOME CARE

- Urge your child not to smoke.
- Check the stool daily for bleeding. If the stool is black, remove it from the toilet and take it to your doctor's office for analysis.
- Review your child's lifestyle and goals in life, and try to identify ways to decrease or eliminate disabling frustrations.
- Children who live the healthiest lives eat 3 or 4 regular meals daily, exercise regularly, sleep 7 or 8 hours each night, do not smoke at all nor drink alcohol, and keep an optimistic outlook.

MEDICATION

Your doctor may prescribe antacids to help neutralize excess stomach acid; H-2 blockers to reduce stomach acid. Don't give your child aspirin or other non-steroidal anti-inflammatory drugs, as they may cause bleeding.

ACTIVITY

Your child can resume normal activities as soon as symptoms improve. Bed rest may be necessary for a week or two.

DIET & FLUIDS

Drastic changes in the child's diet are no longer considered necessary. Your child should eat small frequent meals for at least 2 weeks, should not drink alcohol, and should avoid caffeine and any food that makes symptoms worse.

OK FOR SCHOOL, PRESCHOOL, OR NURSERY?

When appetite has returned and alertness, strength, and feeling of well-being will allow.

CALL YOUR DOCTOR IF

- Your child has symptoms of an ulcer; vomiting begins that is bloody or looks like coffee grounds; stool is bloody, black, or tarry-looking; diarrhea begins which may be caused by antacids; pain is severe, despite treatment; your child is unusually weak or pale; any sign of internal bleeding occurs—this is an emergency! *Call for help immediately.*
- New, unexplained symptoms develop during treatment. Drugs used may produce side-effects or adverse reactions.

UMBILICAL CORD INFECTIONS

GENERAL INFORMATION

DESCRIPTION

An umbilical cord infection is an infection of the stump of the umbilical cord—the tubular structure that once connected the baby to the mother through the placenta.

Appropriate health care includes:

- Home care unless simple measures fail to clear the infection.
- Physician's monitoring of general condition and medications if infection is severe.
- Hospitalization may rarely be needed.

SIGNS & SYMPTOMS

- The umbilical stump remaining too long—the normal stump withers and drops off within 10 days of birth.
- The umbilical stump exhibiting one or all of the following symptoms of infection:
  - — Weeping and oozing of yellow fluid with a bad odor, sometimes pus.
  - — Crusting in the navel area.
  - — Redness and swelling around the umbilical stump.

CAUSES

- Too infrequent diaper changes.
- Bacterial infection.

RISK FACTORS

- Prematurity.
- Unclean surroundings for the infant.

PREVENTING COMPLICATIONS OR RECURRENCE

Clean the infant's navel area and umbilical stump at every diaper change, because it probably becomes wet with urine.

WHAT TO EXPECT

MEDICAL TESTS

- Your own observation of symptoms.
- Medical history and physical exam by a doctor.

POSSIBLE COMPLICATIONS

Systemic infection reaching the infant's blood stream from the infected umbilical stump.

PROBABLE OUTCOME

Complete cure with appropriate and timely care.

TREATMENT

HOME CARE

- Clean the stump and the surrounding area thoroughly at every diaper change with a moist cloth or a piece of cotton soaked in alcohol.
- Allow the stump to fall off naturally—don't twist or pull it in an attempt to hasten its dropping off.

MEDICATION

- Antibiotics (sometimes).
- See Medications section for information regarding medicines your doctor may prescribe.

ACTIVITY

No restrictions.

DIET & FLUIDS

No special instructions.

OK FOR SCHOOL, PRESCHOOL, OR NURSERY?

Yes.

CALL YOUR DOCTOR IF

- Your infant has symptoms of an umbilical cord stump infection.
- Symptoms don't improve within two days of beginning treatment.

URETHRITIS

GENERAL INFORMATION

DESCRIPTION

Urethritis is inflammation or infection of the urethra (the tube through which urine travels from the bladder to the outside), frequently accompanied by bladder infection or inflammation (cystitis). The female urethra is much shorter than the male's. The urethra, bladder (sometimes), and prostate (sometimes) are involved. Urethritis can affect all ages, both sexes, but is 10 times more common in females.

Appropriate health care includes:

- Self-care after diagnosis.
- Physician's monitoring of general condition and medications.

SIGNS & SYMPTOMS

- Painful or burning urination with cloudy, yellow-green mucus discharge from the urethra.
- Frequent urge to urinate, even when there is not much urine in the child's bladder.

CAUSES

Bacterial infection. *In females,* the infection is associated with:

- Bacteria that enter the urethra from the skin around the genitals and anal area.
- Bruising during sexual intercourse.

In males, infection is associated with:

- Non-specific urethritis, which may be caused by sexual contact or irritation of the urethra.
- Infections that reach the urethra through the bloodstream from the prostate gland or through the penis.

In both sexes: The infection may be associated with gonorrhea, which is spread by contact with an infected sexual partner.

RISK FACTORS

- Use of a urinary catheter.
- Use of drugs to which bacteria causing infection have become resistant.
- Previous kidney stones, prostatitis, epididymitis, or genital injury.
- Multiple sexual partners.

PREVENTING COMPLICATIONS OR RECURRENCE

- For causes related only to females: After bowel movements, wipe from front to back and wash with soap and water; take showers rather than tub baths.
- For both sexes: Drink 8 glasses of water every day.

WHAT TO EXPECT

MEDICAL TESTS

Your own observation of symptoms; medical history and physical exam by a doctor; urinalysis and urine culture; cystoscopy (sometimes—see Glossary); for chronic urethritis, some doctors dilate the child's urethra with blunt surgical instruments.

POSSIBLE COMPLICATIONS

- Chronic urethritis and cystitis, if treatment is inadequate.
- Spread of infection to your child's ureters and kidneys.

PROBABLE OUTCOME

Urethritis is usually a "low grade" infection, seldom producing serious, long-term illness. Recurrence is common.

TREATMENT

HOME CARE

- To relieve pain, encourage your child to take sitz baths by sitting in a tub of hot water for 15 minutes at least twice a day.
- Males should not irritate the urethra by pulling the penis skin down to open it and see if the discharge is still present. The penis may be inspected but should not be squeezed.
- Your child should keep the area around the genitals clean with unscented plain soap.

MEDICATION

Your doctor may prescribe antibiotics to fight your child's infection. Be sure the child finishes the prescribed dose, even if symptoms subside sooner.

ACTIVITY

No restrictions, except to avoid any sexual activity until free of symptoms for 2 weeks.

DIET & FLUIDS

Instructions for your child:

- Drink 8 glasses of water every day.
- Drink cranberry juice to acidify urine. Some drugs are more effective with acid urine.
- Avoid caffeine and alcohol during treatment.

OK FOR SCHOOL, PRESCHOOL, OR NURSERY?

When signs of infection have decreased, appetite returns, and alertness, strength, and feeling of well-being will allow.

CALL YOUR DOCTOR IF

- Your child has symptoms of urethritis.
- The following occurs during treatment:
  - — Oral temperature of 101F (38.3C) or higher.
  - — Bleeding from the urethra, or blood in the child's urine.
  - — No improvement in 1 week, despite treatment.
- New, unexplained symptoms develop. Drugs used in treatment may produce side effects.

UTERINE BLEEDING, ABNORMAL

GENERAL INFORMATION

DESCRIPTION

Abnormal uterine bleeding refers to unexpected, menstrual-like bleeding. The vulva (vaginal lips), vagina, cervix (lower third of the uterus), and endometrium (inner uterine lining) are involved. It affects females of all ages.

Appropriate health care includes:

- Doctor's treatment.
- Surgery (hysterectomy) to remove the uterus (sometimes).
- Psychotherapy or counseling to reduce your daughter's anxiety about the bleeding.

SIGNS & SYMPTOMS

- Vaginal bleeding, which may be a light-brown discharge or heavy, red bleeding (with or without clots). Mucus may accompany the bleeding. Bleeding episodes vary in length—there is no expected range.
- Pelvic pain.

CAUSES

- Cancer of the reproductive system.
- Irritation, infection, or thinning of the membranes lining the vulva.
- Injury or trauma to the vagina, associated with reduced estrogen levels.
- Polyps or benign tumors of the cervix.
- Polyps on the inner uterine lining, myomas (see Glossary), or fibroid tumors of the uterus.
- Hormone therapy that stimulates the endometrium (uterine lining), causing sloughing similar to normal menstruation. Estrogens (female hormones) taken irregularly are a common cause of this.
- Disorders of the blood cells, lymphatic system, or bone marrow.
- High blood pressure.
- Congestive heart failure.
- Liver disorders.
- Anticoagulant or aspirin-containing drugs.

RISK FACTORS

Recent vaginal infection.

PREVENTING COMPLICATIONS OR RECURRENCE

No specific preventive measures.

WHAT TO EXPECT

MEDICAL TESTS

- Your own observation of symptoms.
- Medical history and physical exam by a doctor.
- Laboratory studies, such as a Pap smear (see Glossary), blood studies and pregnancy test.
- Surgical diagnostic procedures, such as dilatation and curettage (D & C) and colposcopy (see Glossary).
- Biopsy (see Glossary) of suspicious areas.

POSSIBLE COMPLICATIONS

- Anemia.
- If cancer is the cause, it may spread to other body parts and cause death.

PROBABLE OUTCOME

Depends on the underlying cause and treatment chosen. Hysterectomy cures bleeding immediately. Hormone treatment may require up to 6 months.

TREATMENT

HOME CARE

Instructions for your daughter:

- Use heat to relieve pain. Place a heating pad or hot-water bottle on the abdomen or back.
- Take frequent hot baths to relax muscles and relieve discomfort. Sit in a tub of hot water for 10 to 15 minutes as often as necessary.
- Use sanitary pads instead of tampons.

MEDICATION

- Your doctor may prescribe:
  —Hormones.
  —Medication to treat your daughter's underlying disorder, such as antihypertensives for high blood pressure.
- See Medications section for information regarding medicines your doctor may prescribe.

ACTIVITY

- Your daughter can resume her normal activities as soon as symptoms improve.
- Your sexually active daughter can resume sexual relations as soon as possible after diagnosis and treatment.

DIET & FLUIDS

No special diet.

OK FOR SCHOOL, PRESCHOOL, OR NURSERY?

When appetite returns and alertness, strength, and feeling of well-being will allow.

CALL YOUR DOCTOR IF

- Your daughter has bleeding that persists for 1 week, despite treatment.
- Your daughter's bleeding becomes excessive (saturates a pad more frequently than once each hour).
- Your daughter develops signs of infection: fever, a general feeling of ill health, headache, dizziness, and muscle aches.
- New, unexplained symptoms develop. Drugs used in treatment may produce side effects.

VAGINA, FOREIGN BODY IN

GENERAL INFORMATION

DESCRIPTION

A foreign body in the vagina refers to any kind of foreign material introduced into the vagina that remains there. These can include safety pins, sticks, and other materials in very young girls or retained tampons in girls who have begun menstruating.

Appropriate health care includes:

Doctor's care for diagnosis and treatment. Foreign bodies occasionally must be removed with the child under anesthesia.

SIGNS & SYMPTOMS

- Unpleasant-smelling or blood-stained vaginal discharge.
- Soreness or tenderness around the vagina.

CAUSES

Accidental or intentional introduction of a foreign body into the vagina.

RISK FACTORS

- Mental retardation.
- Unusually inquisitive children.
- An older child or adult molesting your daughter.

PREVENTING COMPLICATIONS OR RECURRENCE

Discourage your child from using any instruments when playing "nurse and doctor."

WHAT TO EXPECT

MEDICAL TESTS

- Your own observation of symptoms.
- Medical history and physical exam by a doctor.
- Self-care after diagnosis.
- Physician's monitoring of general condition and medications.
- X-rays of the pelvis to identify and locate the foreign body.

POSSIBLE COMPLICATIONS

- Bacterial infection of the genital area.
- Pelvic inflammatory disease.

PROBABLE OUTCOME

Complete cure with timely treatment.

TREATMENT

HOME CARE

- Don't attempt to remove the foreign body from your daughter yourself unless it has been in only a short while and is unlikely to cause injury if you try.
- After removal, give your daughter warm, soapy baths twice a day until all symptoms clear.
- Have your daughter wear absorbent cotton panties—not nylon or any man-made fiber.
- Don't make too much fuss about the incident if you think your daughter did it to herself. A little girl is naturally curious about her vagina and she will investigate it with her fingers or perhaps objects.
- If you suspect that an older child or an adult has molested your daughter, pursue the matter with health care or social workers or with the police.

MEDICATION

- Antibiotics prescribed by your physician if needed to treat any secondary infection.
- See Medications section for information regarding medicines your doctor may prescribe.

ACTIVITY

No restrictions after the foreign body has been removed.

DIET & FLUIDS

No restrictions.

OK FOR SCHOOL, PRESCHOOL, OR NURSERY?

Yes.

CALL YOUR DOCTOR IF

- Your daughter has symptoms of a foreign body in the vagina.
- New, unexplained symptoms develop. Drugs used in treatment may produce side effects.

VAGINA OR VULVA, CANCER OF

GENERAL INFORMATION

DESCRIPTION

This cancer refers to the uncontrolled growth of malignant cells in the vagina or on the vulva (vaginal lips). It affects females of all ages. One type (rhabdomyosarcoma) occurs in children.

Appropriate health care includes:

- Doctor's treatment.
- Surgery (usually) to remove the vaginal lips.
- Radiation treatment (sometimes). External radiation shrinks the primary tumor. Internal radiation (implants) affects cancer that has spread to adjoining tissues. Implants of radium or cesium are used for 48 to 72 hours.
- Self-care after diagnosis, radiation treatment, or surgery.

SIGNS & SYMPTOMS

- Itching.
- Abnormal vaginal bleeding.
- Discomfort or bleeding with intercourse.
- Small or large, firm, ulcerated, painless lesion of the vulva. Cancers on the vulva have thick, raised edges and bleed easily.
- Uncomfortable urination, if cancer spreads to your daughter's bladder.
- Rectal bleeding, if it spreads to the rectum.

CAUSES

Unknown.

RISK FACTORS

- Family history of cancer of the reproductive organs.
- Infants born to mothers who take estrogen during pregnancy.

PREVENTING COMPLICATIONS OR RECURRENCE

- No specific preventive measures. Your daughter should have a yearly pelvic exam beginning at about age 16 to detect the disease during early stages, when treatment is most effective.
- Your daughter should become familiar with the appearance of her genitals. (She should use a mirror and examine them once a month.)

WHAT TO EXPECT

MEDICAL TESTS

- Your own observation of symptoms.
- Medical history and physical exam by a doctor.
- Laboratory studies, such as a Pap smear and culposcopy (see Glossary for both).
- Surgical diagnostic procedures such as dilatation and curettage (D & C, see Glossary).

POSSIBLE COMPLICATIONS

Fatal spread to other body parts. Common sites of spread are the lymph nodes in the groin, the wall of the pelvis, the bladder, rectum, bone, lungs, or liver.

VAGINA OR VULVA, CANCER OF

PROBABLE OUTCOME

This condition is currently considered incurable, but early detection and treatment offer a good chance for normal life expectancy. Your daughter's symptoms can be relieved or controlled during treatment. Scientific research into causes and treatment continues, so there is hope for increasingly effective treatment and cure.

TREATMENT

HOME CARE

No specific instructions except those listed under other headings.

MEDICATION

- Your doctor may prescribe:
  - —Pain relievers.
  - —Antibiotics, if your daughter develops a urinary-tract infection that results from the use of a bladder catheter during radiation treatment.
  - —Stool softeners beginning a week after treatment.
- See Medications section for information regarding medicines your doctor may prescribe.

ACTIVITY

A catheter will remain in your daughter's bladder for about 2 weeks following surgery or during radiation treatment. Instructions for your daughter:

- If you have radiation implants, lie on your back while the radiation source is in place. Move your arms and legs often to prevent formation of deep-vein blood clots.
- After radiation treatment—internal or external—resume your normal activities in about 5 days.
- After surgery, resume your normal activities gradually, allowing 6 weeks for full recovery.
- Resume sexual relations when healing is complete in 8 to 10 weeks.

DIET & FLUIDS

No special diet after treatment.

OK FOR SCHOOL, PRESCHOOL, OR NURSERY?

When appetite returns and alertness, strength, and feeling of well-being will allow.

CALL YOUR DOCTOR IF

- Your child has symptoms of cancer of the vagina or vulva.
- The following occurs at the treatment site after surgery or radiation treatment:
  - —Signs of infection, such as increasing pain, fever and swelling.
  - —Excessive bleeding.

ILLNESSES

VAGINISMUS

GENERAL INFORMATION

DESCRIPTION

Vaginismus is spasm of the muscles around the opening to the vagina. The muscles surrounding the vagina and the muscles of the lower vagina are involved. Vaginismus affects females of all ages.

Appropriate health care includes:

- Self-care after diagnosis.
- Doctor's treatment. Your doctor or nurse will probably teach your daughter how to dilate the vaginal opening gently and gradually with rubber or glass dilators. Office treatments will probably be necessary 3 times a week, and your daughter should practice at home at least twice a day.
- Psychotherapy or counseling, if medical treatment is unsuccessful.

SIGNS & SYMPTOMS

Involuntary contraction of the muscles around the vagina and rectum. The vagina closes so tightly that the penis cannot penetrate for sexual intercourse.

CAUSES

- An unconscious desire to prevent penile penetration because of emotional or psychological factors. These may include fear, anxiety, hostility, anger, or a distaste for sex.
- An insensitive sexual partner, insufficient or unskillful foreplay, or inadequate vaginal lubrication prior to attempted penetration.
- Physical disorders (rare), such as infections, allergic reactions, or a rigid, non-perforated hymen.

RISK FACTORS

- First sexual experiences.
- Previous sexual trauma.
- Stress.

PREVENTING COMPLICATIONS OR RECURRENCE

Pelvic examination by a doctor and counseling prior to your daughter beginning sexual activity.

WHAT TO EXPECT

MEDICAL TESTS

- Your own observation of symptoms.
- Medical history and physical exam by a doctor.

POSSIBLE COMPLICATIONS

- Psychological trauma caused by guilt, anxiety, loss of self-esteem, and feelings of inadequacy, or interpersonal problems resulting from the disorder.
- Painful intercourse for sexual partner.

PROBABLE OUTCOME

Usually curable if the underlying cause can be cured or a coping method can be developed for your daughter through medical treatment and psychological counseling.

TREATMENT

HOME CARE

Instructions for your sexually active daughter:

- Learn dilation techniques and practice twice daily at home.
- Prior to dilation exercises or attempted intercourse, sit in a tub of hot water for 10 to 15 minutes. Baths often relax muscles and relieve discomfort. Repeat baths as often as is helpful.
- Before attempting intercourse, you and your partner should use a lubricant, such as K-Y Lubricating Jelly or baby oil.

MEDICATION

- Medicine is usually not necessary for vaginismus, but your doctor may prescribe mild sedatives or tranquilizers for your daughter for short periods of time.
- See Medications section for information regarding medicines your doctor may prescribe.

ACTIVITY

No restrictions.

DIET & FLUIDS

No special diet.

OK FOR SCHOOL, PRESCHOOL, OR NURSERY?

When appetite returns and alertness, strength, and feeling of well-being will allow.

CALL YOUR DOCTOR IF

- Your daughter has symptoms of vaginismus.
- Symptoms don't improve after 3 weeks, despite treatment.
- Symptoms recur after treatment.

VAGINITIS, GARDNERELLA OR NON-SPECIFIC

GENERAL INFORMATION

DESCRIPTION

Vaginitis means infection or inflammation of the vagina. Non-specific vaginitis implies that any of several infecting germs, including gardnerella, escherichia coli, mycoplasma, streptococci, staphylococci, and viruses, have caused the infection. These infections are contagious. The vagina, urethra, bladder, and skin around the genitals are involved. Non-specific vaginitis can affect females of all ages, including children and adolescents.

Appropriate health care includes:

- Self-care after diagnosis.
- Physician's monitoring of general condition and medications.

SIGNS & SYMPTOMS

Severity of the following symptoms varies between females and from time to time in the same female:

- Vaginal discharge that has an unpleasant odor.
- Genital itching.
- Vaginal discomfort.
- Change in vaginal color from pale pink to red.

CAUSES

- The germs normally present in the vagina can multiply and cause infection when the pH and hormone balance of the vagina and surrounding tissue are disturbed.
- The E. coli bacteria that normally inhabit the rectum can cause infection if spread to the vagina.

RISK FACTORS

- Diabetes mellitus.
- Illness that has lowered resistance.
- General poor health.
- Hot weather, non-ventilating clothing—especially underwear—or any other condition that increases genital moisture, warmth, and darkness. These foster the growth of germs.

PREVENTING COMPLICATIONS OR RECURRENCE

Instructions for your daughter:

- Keep the genital area clean. Use plain unscented soap.
- Take showers rather than tub baths.
- Wear cotton panties or pantyhose with a cotton crotch. Avoid panties made from non-ventilating materials, such as nylon.
- Don't sit around in wet clothing—especially a wet bathing suit.
- After urination or bowel movements, cleanse by wiping or washing from front to back (vagina to anus).
- Lose weight if you are obese.
- Avoid frequent douches or vaginal sprays.
- If you have diabetes, adhere strictly to your treatment program.

VAGINITIS, GARDNERELLA OR NON-SPECIFIC

? WHAT TO EXPECT

MEDICAL TESTS

- Your own observation of symptoms.
- Medical history and physical exam (including pelvic exam) by a doctor.
- Laboratory studies, such as a Pap smear (see Glossary) and culture of the vaginal discharge.

POSSIBLE COMPLICATIONS

Secondary bacterial infection of the vagina.

PROBABLE OUTCOME

Usually curable in 2 weeks with treatment. If there are sexual partners involved, they may need treatment also.

TREATMENT

HOME CARE

Instructions for your daughter:

- Follow the first 4 instructions under PREVENTING COMPLICATIONS OR RECURRENCE.
- Don't douche unless your doctor recommends it.
- If urinating causes burning:
  - — Urinate through a tubular device, such as a toilet-paper roll or plastic cup with the end cut out.
  - — Urinate while bathing.

MEDICATION

Your doctor may prescribe:

- Antibiotics or anti-parasitic drugs for gardnerella vaginitis.
- Soothing vaginal creams or lotions for non-specific forms of vaginitis.
- Using a thin sanitary pad will protect clothing from creams or suppositories.

Keep the creams and suppositories in the refrigerator. After treatment, you may want to keep a refill of the medication so you can begin treatment for your daughter quickly if the infection recurs. Follow the prescription directions carefully.

ACTIVITY

Your daughter should avoid overexertion, heat, and excessive sweating.

DIET & FLUIDS

No special diet.

OK FOR SCHOOL, PRESCHOOL, OR NURSERY?

Yes.

CALL YOUR DOCTOR IF

- Your daughter has symptoms of vaginitis.
- Symptoms persist longer than 1 weeks or worsen, despite treatment.
- Unusual vaginal bleeding or swelling develops.

VAGINITIS IN FEMALE ATHLETES

GENERAL INFORMATION

DESCRIPTION

Vaginitis is irritation, infection, or inflammation of the vagina. This condition is slightly more common in female athletes than in the female population at large. Appropriate health care includes visiting the doctor for the application of special medication to the vagina.

SIGNS & SYMPTOMS

- Vaginal discharge, with or without an unpleasant odor.
- Swollen, red, tender vaginal lips (labia) and surrounding skin.
- Burning on urination, if urine touches inflamed tissue.
- Change in vaginal color from pale-pink to red.
- Genital itching and pain.
- Discomfort during sexual intercourse.

CAUSES

- For irritation: friction of clothing, especially tight clothing, that rubs against the skin or mucous membranes in the vaginal area. This occurs often in girls involved in sports such as cycling, gymnastics, or horseback riding.
- For infection: germs multiplying and causing infection when the vagina's hormone and pH balance is disturbed. These germs may be yeast, fungi, parasites, or bacteria.

RISK FACTORS

Factors that may disturb the vagina's pH balance include pregnancy; diabetes mellitus; use of oral contraceptives; high intake of simple carbohydrates; non-ventilating clothing or underwear made from man-made fibers, which increases darkness, moisture, and warmth in the vaginal area; hot weather; immunosuppression from drugs or disease, including antibiotic treatment.

PREVENTING COMPLICATIONS OR RECURRENCE

Instructions for your daughter:

- Take showers rather than tub baths.
- Shower and dry off carefully after any vigorous physical activity.
- Wear cotton panties or pantyhose with a cotton crotch. Avoid panties made from non-ventilating materials.
- Don't sit around in wet clothing—especially a wet bathing suit.
- When you take antibiotics, ask your doctor about eating yogurt, sour cream, or buttermilk containing active cultures, or taking acidophilus tablets.
- After urination or bowel movements, cleanse by wiping or washing from front to back (vagina to anus), never back to front.
- Lose weight if you are obese.
- If you have diabetes, adhere strictly to your treatment program.
- Avoid frequent douches.

VAGINITIS IN FEMALE ATHLETES

WHAT TO EXPECT

MEDICAL TESTS

Your own observation of symptoms; medical history and physical exam (including pelvic exam) by a doctor; laboratory studies, such as a Pap smear, and culture and microscopic exam of the vaginal discharge.

POSSIBLE COMPLICATIONS

Spread of infection from the vagina or skin surrounding the genitals to other female organs (cervix, uterus, Fallopian tubes, ovaries).

PROBABLE OUTCOME

- Vaginal irritation usually disappears once the irritant is removed.
- Vaginal infection is usually curable with 2 weeks of medication. Recurrence is common.

TREATMENT

HOME CARE

Instructions for your daughter:

- Follow the instructions under PREVENTING COMPLICATIONS AND RECURRENCE.
- Don't douche unless your doctor recommends it.
- If urination burns, urinate through a tubular device, such as a toilet-paper roll or plastic cup with the end cut out, or urinate while bathing.

MEDICATION

Your doctor may prescribe:

- Antibiotics, hormones, or topical cortisone cream or ointment.
- Anti-fungal drugs, either in oral form (rare) or in vaginal creams or suppositories (usually). Keep creams or suppositories in the refrigerator.

ACTIVITY

- For irritation, your daughter should modify her athletic activity if causes and risk factors have been eliminated and intolerable irritation persists.
- For infection, your daughter should avoid overexertion, heat, and excessive sweating during treatment. She should delay sexual activity until symptoms cease.

DIET & FLUIDS

Your daughter should increase consumption of yogurt, acidophilus milk, buttermilk, or sour cream.

OK FOR SCHOOL, PRESCHOOL, OR NURSERY?

Yes, when condition and sense of well-being will allow.

CALL YOUR DOCTOR IF

- Your daughter has symptoms of vaginitis.
- Symptoms worsen or persist longer than a week despite treatment.
- Unusual vaginal bleeding or swelling develops.

VAGINITIS, MONILIAL
(Vaginal Yeast Infection; Vaginal Candidiasis)

GENERAL INFORMATION

DESCRIPTION

Monilial vaginitis is an infection or inflammation of the vagina caused by a yeastlike fungus (monilia or candida albicans). The vagina and adjacent skin are involved. Monilial vaginitis causes at least 50% of the infections found in the vagina. Monilial vaginitis can affect females of all ages, especially after puberty. Appropriate health care includes: self-care after diagnosis; physician's monitoring of general condition and medications.

SIGNS & SYMPTOMS

Severity of the following symptoms varies between females and from time to time in the same female:

- White, "curdy" vaginal discharge, (resembles lumps of cottage cheese). The odor may be unpleasant but not foul.
- Swollen, red, tender, itching vaginal lips (labia) and surrounding skin.
- Burning on urination.
- Change in vaginal color from pale pink to red.

CAUSES

Monilia (or candida) live in a healthy vagina, rectum, and mouth. When your daughter's vaginal hormone and pH balance is disturbed, the organisms multiply and cause infections. Monilial vaginitis tends to appear before a menstrual period and improves as soon as the period begins. Factors that may disturb the vagina's balance include: pregnancy; diabetes mellitus; antibiotic treatment; oral contraceptives; high carbohydrate intake; hot weather or non-ventilating clothing, which increase moisture, warmth, and darkness, fostering fungal growth; immunosuppression from drugs or disease.

RISK FACTORS

Factors listed under CAUSES.

PREVENTING COMPLICATIONS OR RECURRENCE

Instructions for your daughter:

- Keep the genital area clean. Use plain unscented soap.
- Take showers rather than tub baths.
- Wear cotton panties or pantyhose with a cotton crotch. Avoid panties made from non-ventilating materials.
- Don't sit around in wet clothing—especially a wet bathing suit.
- Avoid frequent douches and vaginal sprays.
- Ask your doctor about eating yogurt, sour cream, or buttermilk, or taking acidophilus tablets when you take antibiotics.
- After urination or bowel movements, cleanse by wiping or washing from front to back (vagina to anus).
- Lose weight if you are obese.
- If you have diabetes, adhere strictly to your treatment program.

VAGINITIS, MONILIAL
(Vaginal Yeast Infection; Vaginal Candidiasis)

WHAT TO EXPECT

MEDICAL TESTS

- Your own observation of symptoms.
- Medical history and physical exam (including pelvic exam) by a doctor.
- Laboratory studies, such as a Pap smear (see Glossary), and culture and microscopic exam of the vaginal discharge.

POSSIBLE COMPLICATIONS

Secondary bacterial infections of the vagina and other pelvic organs.

PROBABLE OUTCOME

Usually curable with 2 weeks of treatment. Recurrence is common.

TREATMENT

HOME CARE

Instructions for your daughter:

- Follow the first 4 instructions under PREVENTING COMPLICATIONS OR RECURRENCE.
- Don't douche unless your doctor recommends it.
- If urinating causes burning:
  - — Urinate through a tubular device, such as a toilet-paper roll or a plastic cup with the end cut out.
  - — Urinate while bathing.

MEDICATION

- Your doctor may prescribe anti-fungal drugs, either in oral form (rare) or in vaginal creams or suppositories (usually). Keep the creams or suppositories in the refrigerator.
- After treatment, you may want to keep a refill of the medication so you can begin treatment for your daughter quickly if the infection recurs. Follow the prescription carefully.

ACTIVITY

Your daughter should avoid overexertion, heat, and excessive sweating.

DIET & FLUIDS

Your daughter should increase consumption of yogurt, buttermilk, or sour cream.

OK FOR SCHOOL, PRESCHOOL, OR NURSERY?

Yes.

CALL YOUR DOCTOR IF

- Your daughter has symptoms of monilial vaginitis.
- Despite treatment, symptoms worsen or persist longer than 1 week.
- Unusual vaginal bleeding or swelling develops.
- After treatment, symptoms recur.

VAGINITIS, TRICHOMONAL (Trichomoniasis)

GENERAL INFORMATION

DESCRIPTION

Trichomonal vaginitis is infection or inflammation of the vagina caused by a parasite that lives in the lower genitourinary tract of males and females. This is very contagious between sexual partners. The vagina, urethra, and bladder in females are involved, as are the prostate gland and urethra in males.

Trichomonal vaginitis can affect males and females of all ages but is most likely in adolescent and adult females.

Appropriate health care includes:

- Self-care after diagnosis.
- Physician's monitoring of general condition and medications. Both sexual partners require simultaneous treatment.

SIGNS & SYMPTOMS

- Foul-smelling, frothy vaginal discharge that is most noticeable several days after a menstrual period.
- Vaginal itching and pain.
- Redness of the vaginal lips (labia) and vagina.
- Painful urination, if urine touches inflamed tissue.

The severity of discomfort varies greatly from female to female and from time to time in the same female. Infected males may have no symptoms.

CAUSES

Infection from a tiny parasite, trichomonas vaginalis. The parasite passes from person to person during sexual intercourse. It may live in its host for years without producing symptoms. Then, perhaps from altered resistance, it will suddenly multiply rapidly and cause distressing symptoms. Since it thrives in both the male and female, both sexual partners must receive treatment.

RISK FACTORS

Frequent changes of sexual partners.

PREVENTING COMPLICATIONS OR RECURRENCE

Using rubber condoms during sexual intercourse helps.

WHAT TO EXPECT

MEDICAL TESTS

- Your own observation of symptoms.
- Medical history and physical exam (including pelvic exam) by a doctor.
- Microscopic exam of the vaginal discharge or prostate secretions.

POSSIBLE COMPLICATIONS

Secondary bacterial infections.

PROBABLE OUTCOME

Usually curable with treatment.

VAGINITIS, TRICHOMONAL (Trichomoniasis)

TREATMENT

HOME CARE

Instructions for your child:

- Don't douche unless recommended by your doctor.
- Wear cotton panties or pantyhose with a cotton crotch. Avoid panties made from non-ventilating materials, such as nylon.
- Take showers rather than tub baths.
- If urinating causes burning:
  - — Urinate through a tubular device, such as a toilet-paper roll or plastic cup with the end cut out.
  - — Urinate while bathing.
- Don't sit around in wet clothing—especially a wet bathing suit.
- Don't wear tight garments, such as jeans.

MEDICATION

- Your doctor may prescribe metronidazole for your child as well as any sexual partner or partners. Urge your child to follow directions carefully, especially *not to drink alcohol or use vinegar when taking metronidazole.* Alcohol or vinegar and metronidazone interact to cause a violent reaction with nausea, vomiting, sweating, weakness, and other symptoms.
- See Medications section for information regarding medicines your doctor may prescribe.

ACTIVITY

Your child should avoid overexertion, heat, and excessive sweating. Sexual relations should be delayed until your child is well. Allow about 10 days for recovery.

DIET & FLUIDS

No special diet.

OK FOR SCHOOL, PRESCHOOL, OR NURSERY?

Yes.

CALL YOUR DOCTOR IF

- Your child has symptoms of trichomonal vaginitis.
- Symptoms persist longer than 1 week or worsen despite treatment.
- Unusual vaginal bleeding or swelling develops.
- After treatment, symptoms recur.

ILLNESSES

VALLEY FEVER (San Joaquin Valley Fever; Coccidioidomycosis; "Cocci")

GENERAL INFORMATION

DESCRIPTION

Valley fever is an infection caused by a fungus whose spores are found in soil. Valley fever is not contagious from person to person. The upper respiratory tract (including the nose, throat, sinuses, and trachea) and the lymph glands are involved. Appropriate health care includes: self-care after diagnosis; physician's monitoring of general condition and medications; hospitalization (severe cases only).

SIGNS & SYMPTOMS

The infection is usually so mild that it produces no symptoms. In a few cases your child's symptoms may be quite severe. They include cough; sore throat; chills and fever; headache; muscle aches; shortness of breath; skin rash; general ill feeling; depression; sweating at night; weight loss; stiff neck (sometimes).

CAUSES

Infection by the fungus, coccidioides immitis, which thrives in soil—especially soil that lines rodent burrows. Susceptible persons become infected when they breathe the dust from such soil and the fungi lodge in the lungs. Incubation is 1 to 4 weeks after exposure.

RISK FACTORS

- Geographic location. The disease is most common in California's San Joaquin Valley, scattered regions in southern and central Arizona, and southwest Texas.
- Occupational or environmental exposure to dust, such as from construction or archeological sites.
- Illness that has lowered your child's resistance, especially uremia, diabetes mellitus, chronic lung disease, tuberculosis, Hodgkin's disease, leukemia, or severe burns.

PREVENTING COMPLICATIONS OR RECURRENCE

Cannot be prevented at present.

WHAT TO EXPECT

MEDICAL TESTS

- Your own observation of symptoms.
- Medical history and physical exam by a doctor.
- Laboratory skin tests and blood studies.
- If your family has moved from an area where the disease is common, ask your doctor about the valley fever skin test.

VALLEY FEVER (San Joaquin Valley Fever; Coccidioidomycosis; "Cocci")

POSSIBLE COMPLICATIONS

Spread of infection throughout the child's body and severe illness, especially in the brain or membranes that cover the brain.

PROBABLE OUTCOME

- Spontaneous recovery in 3 to 6 weeks. Most children continue to feel ill for 3 to 6 weeks after signs of infection disappear.
- Anti-fungal drugs are reserved for persons with severe, widespread infection, in which case they are life-saving.

TREATMENT

HOME CARE

- Use a cool-mist humidifier, without medicine added, to increase moisture and help relieve your child's cough and sore throat.
- Keep a daily weight chart for the child.

MEDICATION

- Medicine is usually not necessary. For severe infection, hospitalization may be necessary for treatment with intravenous anti-fungal drugs, such as amphotericin B or ketoconazole. Both drugs are potent and have potential severe adverse reactions.
- See Medications section for information regarding medicines your doctor may prescribe.

ACTIVITY

Your child should stay as active as strength allows, resting often.

DIET & FLUIDS

No special diet.

OK FOR SCHOOL, PRESCHOOL, OR NURSERY?

When signs of infection have decreased, appetite returns, and alertness, strength, and feeling of well-being will allow.

CALL YOUR DOCTOR IF

- Your child has symptoms of valley fever.
- The following occurs during treatment:
  - — Continued weight loss.
  - — Fever of 101F (38.3C) orally.
  - — Diarrhea that cannot be controlled.
  - — Stiff neck with severe headache.

VITAMIN B DEFICIENCIES

GENERAL INFORMATION

DESCRIPTION

Vitamin B deficiencies are diseases caused by inadequate or absent B vitamins: B-1 (thiamine), B-2 (riboflavin), niacin, B-6 (pyridoxine), and B-12 (cyanocobalamin). Vitamins are organic chemicals that occur in many natural foods. They are necessary for normal body function. B vitamins are water soluble, and excess amounts cannot be stored by the body. Body parts involved include the central nervous system—including the brain, the coverings of the brain (meninges), and the spinal cord—and peripheral nerves, as well as the heart, skin, eyes, and blood.

Appropriate health care includes:

- Self-care after diagnosis.
- Physician's monitoring of general condition and medications.
- Hospitalization for severe malnutrition.

SIGNS & SYMPTOMS

One or several of the following deficiencies may exist in your child at the same time:

- B-1 deficiency (beriberi).
  Tingling or loss of sensation in the legs; weakness; congestive heart failure; mental changes, including poor memory or psychosis; lack of urinary control; abdominal pain.
- B-2 deficiency.
  Cracked lips; pallor; sore tongue.
- Niacin deficiency (pellagra).
  Fatigue and weakness; poor appetite; inflamed skin that may blister, weep, and split; sore, burning mouth and tongue; indigestion, nausea, vomiting, and diarrhea; mental changes, including confusion and psychosis.
- B-6 deficiency.
  Dermatitis; sore mouth and tongue; abdominal pain, vomiting, and diarrhea; convulsions.
- B-12 deficiency.
  Pernicious anemia (uncommon in children).

CAUSES

- Malnutrition, including malnutrition incurred from fad diets or malnutrition present in infants born to malnourished mothers.
- Gastrointestinal diseases with poor absorption.
- Stomach surgery (B-12 deficiency only).
- Use of some medications, such as isoniazid or oral contraceptives, which inactivate vitamin B-6.
- Alcoholism.

RISK FACTORS

Improper diet; prolonged illness; pregnancy; smoking (maybe). Smoking decreases absorption of vitamin C and may affect other vitamins.

PREVENTING COMPLICATIONS OR RECURRENCE

- Your family should eat a well-balanced, nutritious diet.
- Your child may need to take multiple-vitamin supplements if the diet is deficient.

WHAT TO EXPECT

MEDICAL TESTS

- Your own observation of symptoms.
- Medical history and physical exam by a doctor.
- Laboratory blood studies of vitamin levels.

POSSIBLE COMPLICATIONS

Permanent brain or nerve damage; severe heart disease.

PROBABLE OUTCOME

Prompt recovery if your child's vitamin B deficiency is treated with proper nutrition and oral supplements in the early stages. Without treatment, severe malnutrition can cause permanent disability or death.

TREATMENT

HOME CARE

No specific instructions except those listed under other headings.

MEDICATION

Your doctor may prescribe vitamin supplements, depending on the type of deficiency. The child should not take more than the prescribed amount. Excessive doses of vitamin B-6 can *cause* the same symptoms produced by deficiency.

ACTIVITY

No restrictions.

DIET & FLUIDS

No special diet. Prepare well-balanced meals for your child. Don't overcook food or expose it to the air for prolonged periods—these destroy vitamins. Use fresh fruits, vegetables, and meats rather than processed foods, if possible.

OK FOR SCHOOL, PRESCHOOL, OR NURSERY?

Yes.

CALL YOUR DOCTOR IF

Your child has symptoms of vitamin B deficiency.

VITAMIN C DEFICIENCY (Scurvy)

GENERAL INFORMATION

DESCRIPTION

Vitamin C deficiency is an illness caused by inadequate intake of vitamin C. Vitamin C is essential for the body to manufacture collagen, the connective tissue that helps form healthy bones, teeth, and capillaries, and promotes wound healing. The bones, teeth, gums, and capillaries are involved.

Appropriate health care includes:

- Self-care after diagnosis.
- Physician's monitoring of general condition and medications.

SIGNS & SYMPTOMS

Infants and children:

- Tender, swollen legs. The child prefers to lie with legs partly bent, and cries if moved.
- Bleeding and bruising under the skin.
- Anemia.
- Tender ribs (sometimes)
- Bleeding gums (if teeth are present).
- Fever.

Adolescents and adults:

- Swollen, bleeding gums.
- Loss of teeth.
- Rough skin.
- Bleeding or bruising under your child's skin or into joints.
- Weakness and fatigue.
- Mental changes, including hallucinations and bizarre behavior.

Both children and adults:

- Increased susceptibility to infection.

CAUSES

Diet that is lacking in adequate vitamin C.

RISK FACTORS

- Improper diet, including following fad diets that don't include fruits and vegetables.
- Loss of vitamin C from foods by overcooking or improper or prolonged storage.
- Maintaining an infant on formula without vitamin supplements.
- Hyperthyroidism.
- Pregnancy.

PREVENTING COMPLICATIONS OR RECURRENCE

Your child should eat a diet rich in vitamin C-containing foods. These include citrus fruits, tomatoes, and green vegetables, such as green peppers, broccoli, and cabbage. Your child can drink 4 to 6 ounces of orange juice a day for the minimum daily requirement of vitamin C.

VITAMIN C DEFICIENCY (Scurvy)

WHAT TO EXPECT

MEDICAL TESTS

- Your own observation of symptoms.
- Medical history and physical exam by a doctor.
- Laboratory blood studies, such as blood counts for anemia, tests for blood levels of vitamin C, and bleeding and clotting tests.
- X-rays of bones.

POSSIBLE COMPLICATIONS

Fractures or dislocations, especially in children with tenderness (soreness) upon pressing the legs or ribs.

PROBABLE OUTCOME

Curable with vitamin C (ascorbic acid) supplements and a balanced diet that contains foods high in vitamin C. All symptoms and effects, except tooth loss, are reversible. Without treatment, vitamin C deficiency can be fatal.

TREATMENT

HOME CARE

No specific instructions except those listed under other headings.

MEDICATION

- Your doctor will prescribe vitamin C tablets. Your child should not take more than the prescribed amount. Excessive doses of vitamin C can contribute to kidney-stone formation. If massive doses are suddenly decreased, scurvy can result.
- See Medications section for information regarding medicines your doctor may prescribe.

ACTIVITY

Handle infants and children carefully to avoid bone or joint injury until the deficiency is corrected.

DIET & FLUIDS

- Your family should eat a well-balanced diet that includes foods rich in vitamin C (see PREVENTING COMPLICATIONS).
- Take prenatal vitamin supplements if you are pregnant.
- Provide your infant with vitamin supplements or vitamin-fortified formula.

OK FOR SCHOOL, PRESCHOOL, OR NURSERY?

Yes.

CALL YOUR DOCTOR IF

- Your child has symptoms of vitamin C deficiency.
- Symptoms don't improve in 3 weeks despite treatment.

VITAMIN D DEFICIENCY

GENERAL INFORMATION

DESCRIPTION

Vitamin D deficiency is an insufficient intake or absorption of vitamin D, coupled with too little exposure to sunlight. This deficiency causes rickets in children and osteomalacia (softening of the bone) in adults. The total body is involved, but bones are more affected than other tissues. Vitamin D deficiency can affect both sexes, all ages, but is most common in infants and young children up to age 10. Appropriate health care includes: self-care after diagnosis; physician's monitoring of general condition and medications.

SIGNS & SYMPTOMS

In infants:

- Restlessness.
- Poor sleep habits.
- Profuse sweating.
- Delayed sitting, crawling, or walking.
- Delayed closing of the fontanels ("soft spots" on the infant's head).
- Poor muscular development, causing a pot belly.
- Bowed legs, "knock knees," and "pigeon breast" after weight-bearing activities begin (standing and walking).

In older children and adults:

- No symptoms until late stages (sometimes).
- Bone pain.
- Muscle weakness.
- Shortening of the vertebral column and flattening of pelvic bones.

CAUSES

- Insufficient dietary intake of vitamin D.
- Poor absorption of vitamin D, causing poor absorption of calcium and phosphorous necessary for healthy bone. Vitamin D absorption is affected by chronic diseases, such as pancreatitis, celiac disease, cystic fibrosis, colitis, bile-duct disorders, liver disorders, and kidney disease, or surgery on the stomach or small bowel.
- Inadequate exposure to sunlight. This is especially likely if your child is confined to bed or home.
- Poor function of the parathyroid glands (sometimes).

RISK FACTORS

Genetic factors, such as black skin, which decrease the absorption of sunlight; use of anti-convulsant drugs; exposure to polluted air (smog reduces sunlight penetration); improper diet as a result of poverty, food faddism, bulimia, or anorexia nervosa; pregnancy, in which the body needs additional vitamin D.

PREVENTING COMPLICATIONS OR RECURRENCE

Provide vitamin D supplements for yourself and your family—including breast-fed babies—unless you are sure your diet supplies a satisfactory amount; encourage your child to exercise outdoors in sunlight; urge your child not to follow fad diets, which may be deficient in many nutrients, including vitamin D.

? WHAT TO EXPECT

MEDICAL TESTS

Your own observation of symptoms; medical history and physical exam by a doctor; laboratory blood studies of calcium, phosphorous, and alkaline levels.

POSSIBLE COMPLICATIONS

- Spontaneous fractures in your child's softened bones.
- Difficult or impossible vaginal childbirth in females with flattened pelvic bones. Delivery by Cesarean section is usually necessary.

PROBABLE OUTCOME

Usually curable with an adequate diet, vitamin D supplements, and treatment for any underlying disease. Bone malformation cannot be reversed.

TREATMENT

HOME CARE

Your child should sleep on a firm mattress.

MEDICATION

- Your doctor may prescribe vitamin D tablets or injections.
- See Medications section for information regarding medicines your doctor may prescribe.

ACTIVITY

Instructions for your child:

- Exercise whenever possible, especially in sunlight. Weight-bearing exercise, such as walking or running, is especially beneficial.
- Avoid excessive bed rest.
- Stoop—don't bend—to lift heavy objects.

DIET & FLUIDS

Increase your family's intake of foods rich in vitamin D—even if they take vitamin D supplements. Dietary sources include fortified milk, liver, eggs, margarine, green vegetables, cauliflower, tomatoes, and cheese.

OK FOR SCHOOL, PRESCHOOL, OR NURSERY?

Yes.

CALL YOUR DOCTOR IF

- Your child has symptoms of vitamin D deficiency.
- Your child's symptoms don't improve in a month, despite treatment.
- Pain or suspected fracture occurs following an injury—even minor injury.

VITAMIN E DEFICIENCY

GENERAL INFORMATION

DESCRIPTION

Vitamin E deficiency is the effect of inadequate intake of vitamin E. Vitamin E is present in many foods, so deficiency is rare in otherwise healthy children.

Vitamin E promotes normal growth and development. It also enhances the enzyme action necessary for body cells to use oxygen efficiently. The blood and body cells are involved.

Appropriate health care includes:

- Self-care after diagnosis.
- Physician's monitoring of general condition and medications.

SIGNS & SYMPTOMS

- Muscle weakness or cramps in your child.
- Swelling of the ankles, abdomen, and face in an infant.
- Anemia in a premature infant.

CAUSES

- Malnutrition.
- Malabsorption.

RISK FACTORS

Poor nutrition.

PREVENTING COMPLICATIONS OR RECURRENCE

- Determine if your infant's formula has adequate vitamin E.
- Provide your family with a well-balanced diet.
- Give your family vitamin supplements if their diet is inadequate.

OTHER

No evidence exists that vitamin E has any effect on human sexual reproduction or activity.

WHAT TO EXPECT

MEDICAL TESTS

- Your own observation of symptoms.
- Medical history and physical exam by a doctor.
- Laboratory studies to measure blood level of vitamin E.

POSSIBLE COMPLICATIONS

Chronic anemia, resulting in fatigue and underachievement.

PROBABLE OUTCOME

Curable with proper diet and vitamin E supplements.

TREATMENT

HOME CARE

No specific instructions except those listed under other headings.

MEDICATION

- Your doctor may prescribe vitamin E supplements.
- See Medications section for information regarding medicines your doctor may prescribe.

ACTIVITY

No restrictions.

DIET & FLUIDS

Your family should eat a well-balanced diet and avoid fad reducing diets. Good sources of vitamin E include salad and cooking oil, margarine, peanuts, beef, eggs, and green vegetables.

OK FOR SCHOOL, PRESCHOOL, OR NURSERY?

Yes.

CALL YOUR DOCTOR IF

Your child has symptoms of vitamin E deficiency.

VITAMIN K DEFICIENCY

GENERAL INFORMATION

DESCRIPTION

Vitamin K deficiency is inadequate or absent vitamin K, a fat-soluble vitamin necessary for proper blood clotting. Some vitamin K is produced in the gastrointestinal tract. The liver and blood are involved. Vitamin K deficiency can affect both sexes, all ages. A newborn infant lacks vitamin K until its body begins to produce it.

Appropriate health care includes:
- Self-care after diagnosis.
- Physician's monitoring of general condition and medications.

SIGNS & SYMPTOMS

- Unusual bleeding, such as from the child's gums, nose, or gastrointestinal tract.
- Unexplained bruising.

CAUSES

- Excessive amounts of anticoagulant drugs, such as warfarin or dicumarol.
- Prolonged use of antibiotics. Vitamin K is produced by intestinal bacteria that are destroyed by antibiotics.
- Gallbladder disease.
- Malabsoprtion disorders, such as celiac disease, pellagra, Crohn's disease, ulcerative colitis, or cystic fibrosis.

RISK FACTORS

Poor nutrition, especially an unbalanced diet with inadequate amounts of vitamin K.

PREVENTING COMPLICATIONS OR RECURRENCE

Injections of vitamin K are given to newborn infants, and to children (or adults) with gallbladder disease or malabsorption disorders, to prevent deficiency. For most children, a well-balanced diet should provide all the vitamin K necessary.

WHAT TO EXPECT

MEDICAL TESTS

- Your own observation of symptoms.
- Medical history and physical exam by a doctor.
- Laboratory studies of blood clotting.

POSSIBLE COMPLICATIONS

Severe or fatal hemorrhage.

PROBABLE OUTCOME

Curable with vitamin K supplements by mouth or injection.

TREATMENT

HOME CARE

If your child takes anticoagulants, give only the prescribed amount. Have the child take frequent blood tests to monitor prothrombin time (see Glossary) and prevent unexpected bleeding.

MEDICATION

- Your doctor will prescribe vitamin K orally or by injection.
- See Medications section for information regarding medicines your doctor may prescribe.

ACTIVITY

No restrictions.

DIET & FLUIDS

Your family should eat a well-balanced diet that includes foods high in vitamin K, such as green leafy vegetables, cauliflower, tomatoes, cheese, egg yolks, and liver.

OK FOR SCHOOL, PRESCHOOL, OR NURSERY?

Yes.

CALL YOUR DOCTOR IF

Your child has unexplained bleeding or bruising, especially if the child takes anticoagulants, or has gallbladder disease or a malabsorptive disorder.

VITILIGO

GENERAL INFORMATION

DESCRIPTION

Vitiligo is loss of skin pigmentation in patches. This can affect children of any race or ethnic group. The skin on the back of the hands, face, and armpits is involved. Vitiligo can affect both sexes from late childhood (9 to 12 years) to mid-adulthood.

Appropriate health care includes:

- Self-care.
- Physician's monitoring of general condition and medications.

SIGNS & SYMPTOMS

Macules (small areas of different skin color) or patches on your child, with the following characteristics:

- They are flat and white and can't be felt with the fingers.
- They spread to form very large, irregularly-shaped areas without pigmentation.
- They are usually on both sides of the child's body in approximately the same place.
- Their size varies from 2mm or 3mm to several centimeters in diameter.
- They don't hurt or itch the child.

CAUSES

Probably autoimmune disease. The pigment-producing cells (melanocytes) don't function normally, allowing destruction of pigment. Once the child's pigment has been destroyed, melanocytes can't produce more pigment.

RISK FACTORS

- Family history of vitiligo.
- Thyroid or adrenal disease.
- Diabetes mellitus.

PREVENTING COMPLICATIONS OR RECURRENCE

Cannot be prevented at present.

WHAT TO EXPECT

MEDICAL TESTS

- Your own observation of symptoms.
- Medical history and physical exam by a doctor.

POSSIBLE COMPLICATIONS

The disorder may never disappear completely, causing permanent disfigurement of the child.

PROBABLE OUTCOME

- Treatment is prolonged and often unsatisfactory. Complete and permanent repigmentation is rarely possible. Treatment consists of using an oral medication called psoralens. When discontinued, most of the pigmentation your child has regained is usually lost.
- It is impossible to predict how much improvement will occur in your child with treatment. Children and young adults and those who obtain treatment early usually respond best. Allow 1 year to evaluate results.

TREATMENT

HOME CARE

- If your child chooses not to use oral medication (of if it is unsuccessful), the lesions can be covered with waterproof, opaque makeup such as Lydia O'Leary's Cover Mark.
- If your child doesn't use cosmetic makeup, sunscreen should be applied to protect areas without pigment from sun damage.

MEDICATION

- Your doctor may prescribe psoralens, which stimulates pigmentation from healthy pigment cells bordering damaged cells. Results may be disappointing and adverse effects are frequent.
- See Medications section for information regarding medicines your doctor may prescribe.

ACTIVITY

No restrictions.

DIET & FLUIDS

No special diet.

OK FOR SCHOOL, PRESCHOOL, OR NURSERY?

Yes.

CALL YOUR DOCTOR IF

- Your child has symptoms of vitiligo.
- New, unexplained symptoms develop. Drugs used in treatment may produce side effects.

VULVOVAGINITIS BEFORE PUBERTY

GENERAL INFORMATION

DESCRIPTION

Vulvovaginitis before puberty is an infection or inflammation of the vagina or vulva before a young girl reaches puberty. The vagina, cervix, vulva (vaginal lips), and skin around the genitals are involved. Vulvovaginitis before puberty can affect female infants and children.

Appropriate health care includes:

- Physician's monitoring of general condition, medications, and treatment, including removal of any foreign object in the vagina.
- Home care after diagnosis.

SIGNS & SYMPTOMS

- Redness, pain, and itching around your daughter's genital area.
- Vaginal discharge, which may or may not smell bad.
- Pain with urination.
- Bleeding from the affected area (sometimes).

CAUSES

- Infections caused by bacteria, parasites (including pinworms), yeastlike fungi, or viruses. See Vaginitis (several charts in Illnesses section).
- Allergies to synthetic fabrics, soap, or other items in contact with your daughter's genitals.
- Scratches, abrasions, or genital injury from insertion of foreign bodies in the vagina by the child or a playmate.
- Genital injury from sexual abuse.

RISK FACTORS

- Diabetes mellitus.
- Infrequent bathing or unsanitary living conditions.

PREVENTING COMPLICATIONS OR RECURRENCE

- Teach your daughter to wipe after bowel movements from the vagina toward the anus.
- Don't let your daughter sit around in wet clothing—especially a wet bathing suit.
- Don't provide your daughter with colored or perfumed toilet tissue, scented soap, or bubble baths.
- Buy your daughter cotton panties or nylon panties with a cotton crotch—not panties made of non-ventilating materials.
- If antibiotics are prescribed for any reason, your daughter should eat more yogurt and sour cream. This helps prevent vaginal yeast infections.
- Teach your daughter to resist and report any attempted sexual contact by an older person.

VULVOVAGINITIS BEFORE PUBERTY

? WHAT TO EXPECT

MEDICAL TESTS

- Your own observation of symptoms.
- Medical history and physical exam by a doctor.
- Laboratory culture and microscopic exam of the discharge.

POSSIBLE COMPLICATIONS

Psychological trauma if your daughter's condition is caused by sexual abuse.

PROBABLE OUTCOME

Usually curable in 10 days with treatment.

TREATMENT

HOME CARE

- Follow suggestions under PREVENTING COMPLICATIONS OR RECURRENCE.
- Remove the source of any irritation or allergy, such as soap.
- Don't try to remove a foreign object from your daughter's vagina. This may be painful or cause her further injury. Take your child to the doctor for removal.
- If urinating causes burning, your daughter may urinate while bathing or urinate through a toilet-paper roll or plastic cup with the end cut out. This prevents urine from stinging inflamed skin.

MEDICATION

Your doctor may prescribe:

- Medication appropriate for the infection, including antibiotics, anti-fungal or anti-parasitic drugs.
- Topical ointments to relieve your daughter's pain and itching.
- See Medications section for information regarding medicines your doctor may prescribe.

ACTIVITY

No restrictions.

DIET & FLUIDS

No special diet.

OK FOR SCHOOL, PRESCHOOL, OR NURSERY?

Yes.

CALL YOUR DOCTOR IF

- Your daughter has symptoms of vulvovaginitis.
- You suspect your daughter has been sexually abused.
- Symptoms don't improve in 7 to 10 days, or symptoms worsen despite treatment.
- Unusual vaginal bleeding or swelling develops.

WARTS
(Verruca Vulgaris)

GENERAL INFORMATION

DESCRIPTION

Warts are benign tumors caused by a virus in the outer skin layer. Warts are not cancerous. They are contagious from person to person and from one area to another on the same person. The skin anywhere on the body is involved, but warts are most likely to appear on the fingers, hands, and arms. Warts are most common in children and young adults between ages 1 and 30, but they may occur at any age.

Appropriate health care includes:

- Home care after diagnosis and treatment.
- Physician's monitoring of general condition and medications.
- Cryotherapy (freezing cells to destroy them). This is an office procedure that doesn't require anesthesia or cause bleeding. Freezing stings or hurts slightly during application, and your child's pain may increase a bit after thawing. Destroying the wart usually requires 3 to 5 weekly treatments.
- Electrosurgery (using heat to destroy cells). This treatment can usually be completed in a single office visit, but healing takes longer and secondary bacterial infections and scarring are more common.

SIGNS & SYMPTOMS

A small, raised bump on the child's skin with the following characteristics:

- Warts begin very small (1mm to 3mm) and grow larger.
- Warts have a rough surface and clearly defined borders.
- They are usually the same color as the child's skin but sometimes are darker.
- Warts often appear on your child in clusters around a "mother wart."
- Small black dots or bleeding points appear just below the wart's surface.
- Warts are painless and don't itch your child.

CAUSES

- Invasion of the outer skin layer (epidermis) by the papilloma virus. The virus stimulates some cells to grow more rapidly than normal.
- Warts are very common in children. By adulthood, 90% of all people have antibodies to the virus, indicating a history of at least one wart infection.

RISK FACTORS

Unknown.

PREVENTING COMPLICATIONS OR RECURRENCE

To keep from spreading warts, urge your child not to scratch them. Warts spread readily to small cuts and scratches.

WHAT TO EXPECT

MEDICAL TESTS

- Your own observation of symptoms.
- Medical history and physical exam by a doctor.

POSSIBLE COMPLICATIONS

- Spread to other body parts.
- Secondary infection of a wart.

PROBABLE OUTCOME

Within a month, 20% of warts disappear spontaneously in children. Without treatment, it may take 2 or 3 years for the remainder to disappear in most children.

TREATMENT

HOME CARE

- If your child has electrosurgery, keep the treatment site clean with soap and water. Cover with an adhesive bandage, if you wish.
- If your child has cryotherapy, a blister (sometimes with blood) will develop at the treatment site. The roof of the blister will come off without further treatment in 10 to 14 days. There should be little or no scarring. Your child can wash and use make-up or cosmetics as usual. If clothing irritates the blister, cover with a small adhesive bandage.

MEDICATION

- Your doctor may prescribe chemicals, such as mild salicylic acid, to destroy your child's warts. If so, apply twice a day for 4 to 6 weeks.
- See Medications section for information regarding medicines your doctor may prescribe.

ACTIVITY

No restrictions.

DIET & FLUIDS

No special diet.

OK FOR SCHOOL, PRESCHOOL, OR NURSERY?

Yes.

CALL YOUR DOCTOR IF

- Your child has warts and you want them removed.
- After removal by cryosurgery or electrocautery, signs of infection appear at the treatment site.
- After treatment, your child's temperature rises over 101F (38.3C).
- Warts don't disappear completely after treatment.
- Other warts appear after treatment.

WARTS, FLAT

GENERAL INFORMATION

DESCRIPTION

Flat warts are benign small tumors of the skin caused by a virus. This type of wart is not passed by sexual activity, but it is contagious. The skin along scratch marks or other areas of injury is involved. In children, flat warts occur most often on the face or injured surfaces of the arms and legs. In young adult males, they usually occur on areas of the face that are shaved. In young adult females, they are common on the legs or other areas that are shaved.

Appropriate health care includes:

- Self-care to apply topical medications.
- Doctor's treatment to remove warts with chemicals, cryotherapy, or curettage (see Glossary), with or without electrosurgery (see Glossary).

SIGNS & SYMPTOMS

Flat warts have the following characteristics:

- They are flat-topped, square-shouldered, solid elevations barely raised above the child's skin surface.
- They appear along scratch marks or other areas of skin injury and accumulate in lines or clusters.
- They don't hurt or itch the child.

CAUSES

Flat warts are caused by the contagious papilloma virus. The virus is shed from the child's fingers and spaces beneath the fingernails.

RISK FACTORS

Use of immunosuppressive drugs.

PREVENTING COMPLICATIONS OR RECURRENCE

No specific preventive measures except to protect your child's skin from injury and to wash hands frequently.

WHAT TO EXPECT

MEDICAL TESTS

- Your own observation of symptoms.
- Medical history and physical exam by a doctor.

POSSIBLE COMPLICATIONS

None expected.

PROBABLE OUTCOME

In children, flat warts spread rapidly, reach a plateau period and disappear soon after. In adults, flat warts are stubborn and may last for years without treatment.

TREATMENT

HOME CARE

Remove the source of trauma, if possible:

- Males with flat warts on the face should shave with an electric shaver or grow a beard.
- Females with flat warts on areas that are shaved should use other methods to remove hair, such as depilatory cream or wax.

MEDICATION

Your doctor may prescribe:

- Retinoic acid (Retin-A) or benzoyl peroxide. Either should be applied once or twice a day for 4 to 6 weeks. Apply a small amount to each of your child's warts with the tip of a toothpick.
- Duofilm (16% salicylic acid). Follow directions on the medication label.
- See Medications section for information regarding medicines your doctor may prescribe.

ACTIVITY

No restrictions.

DIET & FLUIDS

No special diet.

OK FOR SCHOOL, PRESCHOOL, OR NURSERY?

Yes.

CALL YOUR DOCTOR IF

- Your child has symptoms of flat warts.
- Warts continue to spread despite treatment.
- Signs of infection (redness, pain, or fever) develop in a treated area.

WARTS, PLANTAR

GENERAL INFORMATION

DESCRIPTION

Plantar warts appear on the soles of the feet. The skin of the plantar surface (bottom) of the foot is involved.

Appropriate health care includes:

- Self-care after diagnosis.
- Physician's monitoring of general condition and medications. Your doctor will probably treat your child by paring away the overlying calloused skin and applying chemical cauterants, such as trichloracetic acid, 20% salicylic acid, or 20% formalin.

SIGNS & SYMPTOMS

- A pinhead-sized bump that grows to 2mm or 3mm. Accidental scraping off the top reveals small black dots, pinpoint bleeding, and an underlying translucent core.
- Pain when your child walks. The wart compresses underlying tender tissue.

CAUSES

Infection with the human papilloma virus, which passes from person to person by direct contact. The virus invades your child's skin, making infected cells reproduce faster than normal cells.

RISK FACTORS

Unknown.

PREVENTING COMPLICATIONS OR RECURRENCE

Instructions for your child:

- Don't touch warts on other people.
- Don't wear another person's shoes.
- Wear footwear in public locker rooms or showers.

WHAT TO EXPECT

MEDICAL TESTS

- Your own observation of symptoms.
- Medical history and physical exam by a doctor.

POSSIBLE COMPLICATIONS

None expected.

PROBABLE OUTCOME

Usually curable in 6 to 10 weeks with treatment, but some cases are resistant to treatment. Recurrence is common.

TREATMENT

HOME CARE

Insert pads or cushions in your child's shoes to make walking more comfortable.

MEDICATION

- For minor discomfort, use non-prescription drugs such as acetaminophen.
- Your doctor may prescribe a chemically treated plaster to apply to your child's foot. Follow instructions carefully.
- See Medications section for information regarding medicines your doctor may prescribe.

ACTIVITY

No restrictions. Because walking aggravates the wart, your child should find the most comfortable way to walk without putting weight on the wart, such as walking on the heels.

DIET & FLUIDS

No special diet.

OK FOR SCHOOL, PRESCHOOL, OR NURSERY?

Yes.

CALL YOUR DOCTOR IF

- Your child has a plantar wart.
- The treated area becomes infected, with redness, heat, increased pain, and tenderness.

WARTS, VENEREAL (Condylomata Acuminata; Genital Warts; Moist Warts)

GENERAL INFORMATION

DESCRIPTION

Venereal warts appear in the genital area. These are more contagious than other warts. The urethra, genitals, and rectum are involved. Venereal warts can affect sexually active adolescents and adults.

Appropriate health care includes:

- Self-care after diagnosis.
- Physician's monitoring of general condition, medications, and treatment, which may include application of liquid nitrogen to warts.

SIGNS & SYMPTOMS

Venereal warts have the following characteristics:

- They appear on moist surfaces, especially the penis, the entrance to the vagina, and the entrance to the rectum.
- They are thin, flexible, solid elevations of the skin, growing in stalks or clusters. They are taller than they are wide.
- Each wart measures 1mm to 2mm in diameter, but clusters may be quite large.
- They don't hurt or itch.

CAUSES

Venereal warts are caused by a subtype of the same virus that causes other warts, but they are more contagious. They spread easily on the skin of the infected person and pass easily to other people. They are usually transmitted sexually, often as a result of poor hygiene. They have an incubation period of 1 to 6 months.

RISK FACTORS

- Poor nutrition.
- Other venereal disease.
- Crowded or unsanitary living conditions.

PREVENTING COMPLICATIONS OR RECURRENCE

Instructions for your child to prevent spread of warts to other parts of the body or to other persons:

- Don't scratch warts.
- Avoid sexual activity until warts heal completely.
- Use rubber condoms during sexual intercourse.

WHAT TO EXPECT

MEDICAL TESTS

- Your own observation of symptoms.
- Medical history and physical exam by a doctor.

POSSIBLE COMPLICATIONS

Medication used to treat venereal warts (podophyllin) may damage an unborn child. Systemic toxicity (poisoning) to the fetus has occurred after intravaginal application. Don't use podophyllin if you are pregnant.

WARTS, VENEREAL (Condylomata Acuminata; Genital Warts; Moist Warts)

PROBABLE OUTCOME

These small warts usually cause your child no symptoms. If untreated, they probably will disappear eventually. However, because the virus may be associated with a genital malignancy, obtain medical treatment for your child.

TREATMENT

HOME CARE

These warts are generally treated with chemicals: podophyllin, trichloracetic acid, or liquid nitrogen. After the application of any of these, your child should wait 4 hours; then the child should wash the treated area carefully.

MEDICATION

- If your doctor prescribes podophyllin, a topical medication, it should be applied carefully to your child to avoid damaging surrounding healthy tissue. Use petroleum jelly on surrounding tissue first. Don't apply to large areas at one time. This may cause irritation or absorption of the drug. Keep podophyllin out of the child's eyes.
- See Medications section for information regarding medicines your doctor may prescribe.

ACTIVITY

No restrictions, except to avoid sexual relations until warts are completely gone.

DIET & FLUIDS

No special diet.

OK FOR SCHOOL, PRESCHOOL, OR NURSERY?

Yes.

CALL YOUR DOCTOR IF

- Your child has symptoms of venereal warts.
- The following occurs after treatment.
  - — The treated area becomes infected (red, swollen, painful, or tender).
  - — Temperature rises to 101F (38.3C) or above.
  - — Your child feels generally ill.

ILLNESSES

WHIPLASH
(Acceleration-Deceleration Cervical Injury)

GENERAL INFORMATION

DESCRIPTION

Whiplash is an injury to the neck caused when it is whipped backward forcefully—usually in an accident. The muscles, tendons, disks, and nerves in the neck are involved.

Appropriate health care includes:

- Self-care after diagnosis.
- Physician's monitoring of general condition and medications.
- Diathermy or ultrasound treatments (see Glossary).
- Surgery to remove an injured spinal disk (rare).

SIGNS & SYMPTOMS

- Pain or stiffness in the front and back of your child's neck—either immediately following or up to 24 hours after injury.
- Dizziness.
- Headache.
- Nausea and vomiting (sometimes).

CAUSES

Injury, usually from contact sports or motor-vehicle accidents.

RISK FACTORS

- Osteoarthritis of the spine.
- Situations your child might be in that make accidents more likely, such as:
  - — Driving in rainy, icy or snowy weather.
  - — "Tail-gaiting" or other poor driving habits.
  - — Driving after excess alcohol consumption or use of mind-altering drugs.

PREVENTING COMPLICATIONS OR RECURRENCE

Driving instructions for your child:

- Use the padded headrests in your auto. These have decreased the frequency and severity of auto whiplash injuries.
- Drive carefully and defensively.
- Don't drink or use mind-altering drugs and drive.

WHAT TO EXPECT

MEDICAL TESTS

- Your own observation of symptoms.
- Medical history and physical exam by a doctor.
- X-rays of the neck.
- Myelograms (see Glossary).

POSSIBLE COMPLICATIONS

Temporary numbness and weakness in your child's arms, if nerve roots are injured. This may persist until recovery.

PROBABLE OUTCOME

Usually curable in 1 week to 3 months with treatment.

WHIPLASH
(Acceleration-Deceleration Cervical Injury)

TREATMENT

HOME CARE

Instructions for your child:

- Apply ice packs to the injured area for 10 to 20 minutes each hour during the first 24 hours.
- After 24 hours, use ice packs or heat to relieve pain. Heat may include hot showers twice a day, in which the water beats on your neck and shoulders for 10 to 20 minutes. Between showers, apply hot soaks to the neck, or use a heat lamp several times a day for 10 to 15 minutes.
- Try to improve your posture. Pull in your chin and abdomen when sitting or standing. Sit in a firm chair and force your buttocks to touch the chair's back.
- If the symptoms are severe, buy and wear a soft padded fabric collar (Thomas collar) until the pain subsides.
- Sleep without a pillow. Instead roll a small towel to 2 inches in diameter, or use a cervical pillow or a Thomas collar. Poor sleeping positions delay healing.
- If you have nerve-root pressure, with numbness and weakness in the hand or arm, buy or rent a cervical-traction apparatus. This can be hung over a doorway. Ask your doctor for specific instructions.

MEDICATION

- Your doctor may prescribe pain relievers or muscle relaxants (sometimes).
- Use non-prescription drugs, such as aspirin or acetaminophon, for your child's minor pain.
- See Medications section for information regarding medicines your doctor may prescribe.

ACTIVITY

Depends on the severity of symptoms. During the acute or severe stage, your child should rest as much as possible. As symptoms improve, the child can resume normal activity gradually.

DIET & FLUIDS

No special diet.

OK FOR SCHOOL, PRESCHOOL, OR NURSERY?

Yes.

CALL YOUR DOCTOR IF

- Your child has a painful neck injury.
- Pain, numbness, tingling, or weakness develop in the child's arm or face.
- New, unexplained symptoms develop. Drugs used in treatment may produce side effects.

WHOOPING COUGH (Pertussis)

GENERAL INFORMATION

DESCRIPTION

Whooping cough is a serious contagious bacterial infection of the bronchial tubes and lungs. Immunization throughout the world has greatly decreased the incidence of whooping cough. The bronchial tubes, larynx, and lungs are involved. Whooping cough can affect all ages but is most common in children. Appropriate health care includes:

- Physician's monitoring of general condition and medications.
- Hospitalization with intensive care for severely ill infants. Older children can usually be treated at home.

SIGNS & SYMPTOMS

Early stages:

- Runny nose.
- Dry cough that progresses to a cough with thick sputum.
- Slight fever.

Late stages:

- Severe, continual coughing bouts that last up to a minute. The child's face turns red or blue from lack of oxygen while coughing. At the end of each coughing effort, the child gasps for breath with a "whooping" sound.
- Vomiting and diarrhea.
- Fever.

CAUSES

Infection with bordetella pertussis bacteria. The disease is transmitted by direct contact with a contagious person, or by indirect contact, such as breathing air containing infected droplets or handling linen or other contaminated articles. The incubation period is 5 to 7 days.

RISK FACTORS

- Non-immunized populations.
- Epidemics in late winter or early spring. The bacteria become more virulent as they spread.
- Crowded or unsanitary living conditions.

PREVENTING COMPLICATIONS OR RECURRENCE

Obtain immunizations against whooping cough for your child. Immunizations normally begin at 2 months. See Appendix 1 for an immunization schedule.

WHAT TO EXPECT

MEDICAL TESTS

Your own observation of symptoms; medical history and physical exam by a doctor; laboratory studies, such as culture of the sputum and fluorescent antibody studies (see Glossary); X-rays of the chest.

POSSIBLE COMPLICATIONS

Nosebleeds; retinal detachment; seizures and encephalitis; pneumonia; apnea (slowed or stopped breathing); middle-ear infection; ruptured blood vessels in the child's brain; death in its most severe form.

PROBABLE OUTCOME

Usually curable in about 6 weeks with treatment. The usual course of illness is 2 weeks with an ordinary cough, bouts of the characteristic "whooping" cough, and 2 weeks for convalescence. Some persistent cough may continue for months.

TREATMENT

HOME CARE

- Isolate your child until the fever disappears. Necessary visitors should wear masks.
- During a coughing bout in a baby, raise the foot of the crib. Place the baby face down with the head turned to one side to help drain the lungs. Older children usually prefer to sit up and lean forward during coughing bouts.
- Use a cool-mist humidifier to soothe the child's cough and help loosen bronchial and lung secretions.

MEDICATION

- Don't give your child cough medicine unless your doctor prescribes it.
- Your doctor may prescribe antibiotics for complications, such as middle-ear infection or pneumonia.

ACTIVITY

Keep the child in bed until the fever disappears. Normal activity should be resumed slowly, as the child's strength returns.

DIET & FLUIDS

- Encourage the child to drink extra fluids, such as fruit juice, tea, carbonated drinks, and bouillon.
- No special diet. Small, frequent meals may decrease vomiting.

OK FOR SCHOOL, PRESCHOOL, OR NURSERY?

When signs of infection have decreased, appetite returns, and alertness, strength, and feeling of well-being will allow.

CALL YOUR DOCTOR IF

- Your child has signs of whooping cough, especially blueness of the face with coughing bouts.
- Fever rises to 103F (39.4C).
- Vomiting persists more than 1 or 2 days.

WILM'S TUMOR
(Congenital Nephroblastoma)

GENERAL INFORMATION

DESCRIPTION

Wilm's tumor is a malignant mixed tumor (one that contains several cell types) of the kidney that occurs primarily in children. Only one kidney is involved in 90% of these tumors. Wilm's tumor affects children under age 7, with a peak incidence between ages 3 and 4. Appropriate health care includes: physician's monitoring of general condition, medications, and treatment; surgery to remove the child's affected kidney and adjacent tissue, if the cancer has spread; hospitalization for radiation treatment and anti-cancer drugs.

SIGNS & SYMPTOMS

Enlarged abdomen (a large, firm, smooth tumor can be felt easily within the child's abdominal wall); high blood pressure; blood in the urine; abdominal pain (sometimes); repeated vomiting; fever; weight loss.

CAUSES

Unknown. It is probably congenital but dormant until it becomes active at some point before age 7.

RISK FACTORS

Genetic factors. It is most likely in children with other congenital abnormalities.

PREVENTING COMPLICATIONS OR RECURRENCE

Cannot be prevented at present.

WHAT TO EXPECT

MEDICAL TESTS

- Your own observation of symptoms.
- Medical history and physical exam by a doctor.
- Laboratory studies, such as 24-hour urine studies.
- X-rays of the child's abdomen, kidneys, and chest.
- Special studies that may include:
  - — Ultrasonography: A non-invasive technique that translates sound waves into images displayed on a screen and photographed (see Glossary).
  - — CAT or CT Scan (computerized axial tomography): Non-invasive computerized X-ray images that show sections (or "slices") of an organ or region of the body clearly and precisely (see Glossary).
  - — MRI (magnetic resonance imaging): A non-invasive (non-X-ray) computerized test that uses radio frequency energy and a powerful magnetic field to produce images with excellent detail (see Glossary).
  - — Radionuclide Scan: A nuclear medicine procedure that uses radioactive isotopes injected into a patient. The isotope tracers are absorbed in various concentrations by targeted organs, which are then photographed (see Glossary).

WILM'S TUMOR (Congenital Nephroblastoma)

POSSIBLE COMPLICATIONS

- Kidney failure.
- Tumor spread to the lungs, bones, liver, or brain if untreated.
- Adverse reactions, including hair loss, from radiation treatment and anti-cancer drugs.

PROBABLE OUTCOME

With appropriate treatment, the outlook is better than for most malignant tumors in children. In most cases, Wilm's tumor is curable with surgery, radiation treatment, and anti-cancer drugs. If the tumor is detected before it spreads, the 5-year survival rate is 90%.

TREATMENT

HOME CARE

Follow surgeon's instructions for postoperative care.

MEDICATION

Your doctor may prescribe:

- Anti-cancer drugs.
- Anti-nausea drugs.
- Pain relievers.
- Antibiotics, if infection occurs during anti-cancer drug treatment.
- Stool softeners to prevent constipation following surgery.
- See Medications section for information regarding medicines your doctor may prescribe.

ACTIVITY

No restrictions. The child may be as active as strength allows.

DIET & FLUIDS

No special diet.

OK FOR SCHOOL, PRESCHOOL, OR NURSERY?

After successful surgery and recuperation.

CALL YOUR DOCTOR IF

- Your child has symptoms of Wilm's tumor.
- The following occurs during treatment:
  - — Vomiting, abdominal pain, or constipation.
  - — Shortness of breath.
  - — Swelling in the child's feet or ankles.
- New, unexplained symptoms develop. Drugs used in treatment may produce side effects.

ILLNESSES

WINTER ITCH
(Xerotic Eczema)

GENERAL INFORMATION

DESCRIPTION

Winter itch refers to severely chapped skin that becomes cracked, fissured, and inflamed. The disorder is most common in winter. It is not contagious. The skin anywhere on the body can be involved, but it occurs most commonly on the legs. Appropriate health care includes:
- Self-care after diagnosis.
- Physician's monitoring of general condition and medications.

SIGNS & SYMPTOMS

Lesions on your child, with the following characteristics:
- The lesions are round plaques (flat-topped patches), 2cm to 5cm in diameter. The plaques are sometimes piled like flat discs on top of each other. They usually have very definite borders.
- The plaques itch, burn, and sting.
- Redness is most pronounced within the cracks and fissures which crisscross the plaque surface.
- The plaques usually don't weep or become crusty.

CAUSES

Insufficient oil on the skin's surface, which allows evaporation of water through the child's skin. Skin cells shrink so much that islands of cells begin to separate, causing cracks and fissures. Oil in the skin decreases with aging, excessive bathing, and excessive rubbing of the skin.

RISK FACTORS

An environment with low humidity, especially in homes heated with hot-air fans in the winter.

PREVENTING COMPLICATIONS OR RECURRENCE

Instructions for your child to reduce water loss from the skin:
- Bathe less frequently and use cool water.
- Use soap sparingly.
- Pat dry skin rather than rubbing it.
- Apply skin lubricants to dry skin before chapped areas become inflamed.
- Use humidifiers in rooms with very dry air.

WHAT TO EXPECT

MEDICAL TESTS
- Your own observation of symptoms.
- Medical history and physical exam by a doctor.

POSSIBLE COMPLICATIONS

Secondary bacterial infection in the affected area.

PROBABLE OUTCOME

Usually curable with treatment, but recurrence is common unless environmental conditions around your child can be controlled.

TREATMENT

HOME CARE

- See instructions under PREVENTING COMPLICATIONS OR RECURRENCE.
- To apply lubricants: Use hand cream 4 to 8 times per day on the child's hands and twice daily on the trunk and extremities. When possible, the child should apply cream immediately after bathing—while the skin is wet—to trap additional moisture before evaporation occurs. Bath oils probably don't help.

MEDICATION

- For minor discomfort, use non-prescription skin lubricants, such as petroleum jelly, mineral oil, or cold cream.
- For serious discomfort, your doctor may prescribe topical cortisone creams or lotions.
- See Medications section for information regarding medicines your doctor may prescribe.

ACTIVITY

No restrictions.

DIET & FLUIDS

No special diet.

OK FOR SCHOOL, PRESCHOOL, OR NURSERY?

Yes. This problem is not contagious.

CALL YOUR DOCTOR IF

- Your child has severely chapped skin, and self-care does not relieve symptoms in 1 week.
- Chapped skin becomes inflamed.

ZINC DEFICIENCY

GENERAL INFORMATION

DESCRIPTION

Zinc deficiency refers to inadequate amounts of zinc in body cells. This deficiency affects the function of the testes, liver, and muscles and the structure of bones, teeth, hair, and skin. Zinc is a vital part of many enzymes that facilitate chemical reactions necessary for normal body function—including the immune function and skin healing. All body cells are involved. Zinc deficiency can affect both sexes, all ages, but is most common in children during periods of rapid growth (10 to 18 years).

Appropriate health care includes:

- Home care after diagnosis.
- Physician's monitoring of general condition and medications.

SIGNS & SYMPTOMS

Two or more of the following:

- Poor appetite.
- Sensations of unpleasant tastes and odors, and decreased sense of taste and smell.
- Darkening of skin all over the body.
- Sparse hair growth.
- Deformed nails.

CAUSES

- Excessive consumption of substances that bind zinc and prevent its absorption from the child's gastrointestinal tract. These include calcium, vitamin D, and phytate enzyme (found in unleavened bread).
- Surgical removal of any part of the child's gastrointestinal tract, especially the stomach.
- Parasite infection in the child's gastrointestinal tract.

RISK FACTORS

- Use of cortisone drugs, which increase zinc excretion.
- Alcoholism. Alcohol increases the excretion of zinc.

PREVENTING COMPLICATIONS OR RECURRENCE

Instructions for your child:

- Children and adolescents should not drink or eat more than the recommended amounts of milk, other dairy products, or unleavened bread. Keep calcium intake at 1500mg or less daily.
- Don't take large doses of vitamin D supplements.
- Take zinc supplements if you have had gastrointestinal surgery.
- Don't drink more than 1 or 2 alcoholic drinks—if any—a day.

WHAT TO EXPECT

MEDICAL TESTS

- Your own observation of symptoms.
- Medical history and physical exam by a doctor.
- Laboratory blood studies of zinc levels.

POSSIBLE COMPLICATIONS

- Iron-deficiency anemia. Zinc is necessary for iron absorption.
- Poor wound healing.
- Liver and spleen enlargement.
- Excess zinc replacement or overdose may interfere with the manufacture of necessary enzymes in your child's body.

PROBABLE OUTCOME

Usually curable in 2 months with zinc supplements and removal or treatment of the underlying causes.

TREATMENT

HOME CARE

No specific instructions except those listed under other headings.

MEDICATION

- Your doctor may prescribe zinc supplements. Your child should take them with milk or meals to prevent stomach upset.
- See Medications section for information regarding medicines your doctor may prescribe.

ACTIVITY

No restrictions.

DIET & FLUIDS

Your child should eat foods high in zinc, such as red meat.

OK FOR SCHOOL, PRESCHOOL, OR NURSERY?

Yes.

CALL YOUR DOCTOR IF

Your child has symptoms of zinc deficiency.

Medications

ACETAMINOPHEN

BRAND & GENERIC NAMES

See complete list of brand and generic names in the Brand & Generic Name Directory.

BASIC INFORMATION

Habit forming? No
Prescription needed? No
Available as generic? Yes
Drug class: Analgesic, fever-reducer

USES

Treatment of mild to moderate pain and fever. Acetaminophen does not relieve redness, stiffness or swelling of joints or tissue inflammation. Use aspirin or other drugs for inflammation.

DOSAGE & USAGE INFORMATION

How to take:
- Tablet or capsule—Swallow with liquid.
- Effervescent granules—Dissolve granules in 4 oz. of cool water. Drink all the water.
- Elixir—Swallow with liquid.
- Suppositories—Remove wrapper and moisten suppository with water. Gently insert larger end into rectum. Push well into rectum with finger.

When to take:
As needed, no more often than every 3 hours.

If you forget a dose:
Take as soon as you remember. Wait 3 hours for next dose.

Continued next column

OVERDOSE

SYMPTOMS:
Stomach upset, irritability, sweating, anorexia, convulsions, coma. (See Acetaminophen Poisoning in Illness Section.)
WHAT TO DO:
- **Call your doctor or poison-control center for advice if you suspect overdose, even if not sure. Symptoms may not appear until damage has occurred.**
- **See emergency information at the back of this book.**

What drug does:
May affect hypothalamus—part of brain that helps regulate body heat and receives body's pain messages.

Time lapse before drug works:
15 to 30 minutes. May last 4 hours.

Don't take with:
Any other medicines, even over-the-counter drugs such as cough and cold medicines, nose drops, diet pills, laxatives or caffeine, without consulting your doctor.

POSSIBLE ADVERSE REACTIONS OR SIDE EFFECTS

Life-threatening:
None expected.

Common:

Lightheadedness.	Continue. Call doctor when convenient.

Infrequent:

Trembling.	Continue. Call doctor when convenient.

Rare:

• Extreme fatigue; rash, itch, hives; sore throat and fever after taking regularly a few days; unexplained bleeding or bruising; blood in urine; painful or frequent urination; jaundice; anemia.	Discontinue. Call doctor right away.
• Decreased volume of urine output.	Continue. Call doctor when convenient.

WARNINGS & PRECAUTIONS

Don't take if:
- You are allergic to acetaminophen.
- Your symptoms don't improve after 2 days use. Call your doctor.

Before you start, consult your doctor:
If you have kidney disease or liver damage.

Pregnancy:
No proven harm to unborn child. Avoid if possible.

Infants & children:
Use only under medical supervision.

Prolonged use:
May affect blood system and cause anemia. Limit use to 5 days for children 12 and under, and 10 days for adults.

Skin & sunlight:
No age-related problems expected.

Driving or hazardous activities:
Avoid if you feel drowsy. Otherwise, no restrictions.

Discontinuing:
Discontinue in 2 days if symptoms don't improve.

Others:
No age-related problems expected.

POSSIBLE INTERACTION WITH OTHER DRUGS

GENERIC NAME OR DRUG CLASS	COMBINED EFFECT
Anticoagulants (oral, see Drugs Glossary)	May increase anticoagulant effect. If combined frequently, prothrombin time should be monitored.
Phenobarbital	Quicker elimination of and decreased effect of acetaminophen.
Zidovudine (AZT)	Increased toxic effect of zidovudine.

POSSIBLE INTERACTION WITH OTHER SUBSTANCES

INTERACTS WITH	COMBINED EFFECT
Alcohol:	Drowsiness, long-term use may cause toxic effect in liver.
Beverages:	None expected.
Cocaine (or crack):	None expected. However, cocaine may slow body's recovery. Avoid.
Foods:	None expected.
Marijuana:	Increased pain relief. However, marijuana may slow body's recovery. Avoid.
Tobacco:	None expected.

ACYCLOVIR (ORAL & TOPICAL)

BRAND NAMES

Zovirax **Zovirax Ointment**

BASIC INFORMATION

Habit forming? No
Prescription needed? Yes
Available as generic? No
Drug class: Antiviral

USES

- Treatment of severe herpes infections of genitals occurring for first time in special cases.
- Treatment of severe herpes infections on mucous membrane of mouth and lips in special cases.
- Used (although not yet approved by FDA) for shingles (herpes zoster) and chickenpox (varicella) in special cases.

DOSAGE & USAGE INFORMATION

How to take:
- Capsule—Swallow with liquid.
- Ointment—Apply to skin and mucous membranes every 3 hours (6 times a day) for 7 days. Use rubber glove when applying. Apply 1/2-inch strip to each sore or blister. Wash before using.

When to use:
As directed on label.

If you forget a dose:
Take as soon as you remember up to 2 hours late. If more than 2 hours, wait for next scheduled dose (don't double this dose).

What drug does:
Inhibits reproduction of virus in cells without killing normal cells.

Time lapse before drug works:
2 hours.

Continued next column

OVERDOSE

SYMPTOMS:
Hallucinations, seizures, kidney shutdown.
WHAT TO DO:
- **Dial 0 (operator) or 911 (emergency) for an ambulance or medical help. Then give first aid immediately.**
- **See emergency information at the back of this book.**

Don't take with:
Any other medicines, even over-the-counter drugs such as cough and cold medicines, nose drops, diet pills, laxatives or caffeine, without consulting your doctor.

POSSIBLE ADVERSE REACTIONS OR SIDE EFFECTS

SYMPTOMS	WHAT TO DO
Life-threatening: None expected.	
Common: Rash, hives, itch, mild pain, burning or stinging of skin, lightheadedness, headache.	Continue. Call doctor when convenient.
Infrequent: Confusion, hallucinations, trembling.	Discontinue. Call doctor right away.
Rare: Abdominal pain, decreased appetite, nausea, vomiting, breathing difficulty, blood in urine, decreased urine volume.	Discontinue. Call doctor right away.

WARNINGS & PRECAUTIONS

Don't take if:
You are allergic to acyclovir.

Before you start, consult your doctor:
- If pregnant or plan pregnancy.
- If breast-feeding.
- If you have kidney disease.
- If you have any nerve disorder.

Pregnancy:
Risk to unborn child outweighs drug benefits. Don't use.

Infants & children:
Use only under special medical supervision by experienced clinician.

Prolonged use:
Don't use longer than prescribed time.

Skin & sunlight:
No age-related problems expected.

Driving or hazardous activities:
No age-related problems expected.

Discontinuing:
May be unnecessary to finish medicine. Follow doctor's instructions.

Others:
- Females: Get Pap smear every 6 months because women with herpes infections are more likely to develop cancer of cervix. Avoid sexual activity until all blisters or sores heal. Don't get medicine in eyes.
- Protect medicine from freezing.
- Check with doctor if no improvement in 1 week.

POSSIBLE INTERACTION WITH OTHER DRUGS

GENERIC NAME OR DRUG CLASS	COMBINED EFFECT
Interferon	Neurological abnormalities. Avoid.
Methotrexate	Neurological abnormalities. Avoid.
Other medications that can cause toxic effects on kidneys: **Amikacin** **Amphotericin B** **Capreomycin** **Colistimethate** **Colistin** **Gentamycin** **Kanamycin** **Neomycin** **Netilmicin** **Polymixin B** **Probenecid** **Streptomycin** **Tobramycin** **Vancomycin**	Possible increased kidney toxicity.

POSSIBLE INTERACTION WITH OTHER SUBSTANCES

INTERACTS WITH	COMBINED EFFECT
Alcohol:	Increased chance of brain and nervous system adverse reaction. Avoid.
Beverages:	None expected.
Cocaine (or crack):	Increased chance of brain and nervous system adverse reaction. Avoid.
Foods:	None expected.
Marijuana:	Increased chance of brain and nervous system adverse reaction. Avoid.
Tobacco:	None expected.

ADRENOCORTICOIDS (TOPICAL)

BRAND & GENERIC NAMES

Some of these brand names are available as oral medicine. Look under specific generic name for each brand. See complete list of brand and generic names in the Brand & Generic Name Directory.

BASIC INFORMATION

Habit forming? No
Prescription needed? For some
Available as generic? Yes
Drug class: Adrenocorticoid (topical)

USES

Relieves redness, swelling, itching, skin discomfort of hemorrhoids, insect bites, poison ivy, oak, sumac, soaps, cosmetics and jewelry.

DOSAGE & USAGE INFORMATION

How to use:
• Cream, lotion, ointment, gel—Apply small amount to skin and rub in gently.
• Topical aerosol—Follow directions on container. Don't breathe vapors.

When to use:
When needed or as directed. Don't use more often than directions allow.
If you forget an application:
Use as soon as you remember.

What drug does:
Reduces inflammation by affecting enzymes that produce inflammation.

Time lapse before drug works:
15 to 20 minutes.

Don't use with:
Any other medicines, even over-the-counter drugs such as cough and cold medicines, nose drops, diet pills, laxatives or caffeine, without consulting your doctor.

OVERDOSE

SYMPTOMS:
None expected.
WHAT TO DO:
If child swallows or inhales the drug, call doctor, poison-control center or hospital emergency room for instructions.

POSSIBLE ADVERSE REACTIONS OR SIDE EFFECTS

SYMPTOMS	WHAT TO DO
Life-threatening: None expected.	
Common: None expected.	
Infrequent: Infection on skin with pain, redness, blisters, pus; skin irritation with burning, itching, blistering or peeling; acne-like skin eruptions.	Continue. Call doctor when convenient.
Rare: None expected.	

WARNINGS & PRECAUTIONS

Don't take if:
You are allergic to any topical adrenocorticoid (cortisone) preparation.

Before you start, consult your doctor:
- If you plan pregnancy within medication period.
- If you have diabetes.
- If you have infection at treatment site.
- If you have stomach ulcer.
- If you have tuberculosis.

Pregnancy:
Risk to unborn child outweighs drug benefits. Don't use.

Infants & children:
Use only under medical supervision. Too much for too long can be absorbed into bloodstream through skin and retard growth. For infants in diapers, avoid plastic pants or tight diapers.

Prolonged use:
- Increases chance of absorption into bloodstream to cause side effects of oral cortisone drugs.
- May thin skin where used.

Skin & sunlight:
No age-related problems expected.

Driving or hazardous activities:
No age-related problems expected.

Discontinuing:
May be unnecessary to finish medicine. Follow doctor's instructions.

Others:
- Don't use a plastic dressing to cover skin with topical steroids underneath for longer than 2 weeks.
- Aerosol spray—Store in cool place. Don't use near heat or open flame or while smoking. Don't puncture, break or burn container.

POSSIBLE INTERACTION WITH OTHER DRUGS

GENERIC NAME OR DRUG CLASS	COMBINED EFFECT
Antibiotics, topical (see Drugs Glossary)	Decreased antibiotic effects.
Antifungals, topical (see Drugs Glossary)	Decreased antifungal effect.

POSSIBLE INTERACTION WITH OTHER SUBSTANCES

INTERACTS WITH	COMBINED EFFECT
Alcohol:	None expected.
Beverages:	None expected.
Cocaine (or crack):	None expected.
Foods:	None expected.
Marijuana:	None expected.
Tobacco:	None expected.

MEDICATIONS

ALLOPURINOL

BRAND NAMES

Alloprin
Aluline
Apo-Allopurinol
Caplenal
Lopurin
Novopurol
Purinol
Roucol
Zurinol
Zyloprim
Zyloric

BASIC INFORMATION

Habit forming? No
Prescription needed? Yes
Available as generic? Yes
Drug class: Anti-gout

USES

- Treatment for chronic gout.
- Prevention of kidney stones caused by uric acid.

DOSAGE & USAGE INFORMATION

How to take:
Tablet—Swallow with liquid or food to lessen stomach irritation.

When to take:
At the same times each day.

If you forget a dose:
- 1 dose per day—Take as soon as you remember up to 6 hours late. If more than 6 hours, wait for next scheduled dose (don't double this dose).
- More than 1 dose per day—Take as soon as you remember up to 3 hours late. If more than 3 hours, wait for next scheduled dose (don't double this dose).

What drug does:
Slows formation of uric acid by inhibiting enzyme (xanthine oxidase) activity.

Continued next column

OVERDOSE

SYMPTOMS:
None expected.
WHAT TO DO:
Overdose unlikely to threaten life. If child takes much larger amount than prescribed, call doctor, poison-control center or hospital emergency room for instructions.

Time lapse before drug works:
Reduces blood uric acid in 1 to 3 weeks. May require 6 months to prevent acute gout attacks.

Don't take with:
Any other medicines, even over-the-counter drugs such as cough and cold medicines, nose drops, diet pills, laxatives or caffeine, without consulting your doctor.

POSSIBLE ADVERSE REACTIONS OR SIDE EFFECTS

SYMPTOMS	WHAT TO DO
Life-threatening:	
None expected.	
Common:	
Rash, hives, itch.	Discontinue. Call doctor right away.
Infrequent:	
• Jaundice.	Discontinue. Call doctor right away.
• Drowsiness, diarrhea, stomach pain, nausea, vomiting, headache.	Continue. Call doctor when convenient.
Rare:	
• Sore throat, fever, unusual bleeding or bruising.	Discontinue. Call doctor right away.
• Numbness, tingling, pain in hands or feet.	Continue. Call doctor when convenient.

WARNINGS & PRECAUTIONS

Don't take if:
You are allergic to allopurinol.

Before you start, consult your doctor:
If you have had liver or kidney problems.

Pregnancy:
Studies inconclusive on harm to unborn child. Animal studies show fetal abnormalities. Decide with your doctor whether drug benefits justify risk to unborn child.

Infants & children
Don't give to infants or young children unless prescribed and monitored by your physician.

Prolonged use:
No age-related problems expected.

Skin & sunlight:
No age-related problems expected.

Driving or hazardous activities:
Avoid if you feel drowsy. Use may disqualify you for piloting aircraft.

Discontinuing:
Don't discontinue without doctor's advice until you complete prescribed dose, even though symptoms diminish or disappear.

Others:
Acute gout attacks may increase during first weeks of use. If so, consult doctor about additional medicine.

POSSIBLE INTERACTION WITH OTHER DRUGS

GENERIC NAME OR DRUG CLASS	COMBINED EFFECT
Ampicillin	Likely skin rash.
Anticoagulants, oral (see Drugs Glossary)	May increase anticoagulant effect.
Antidiabetics, oral (see Drugs Glossary)	Increased uric-acid elimination.
Azathioprine	Increased azathioprine effect.
Chlorpropamide	May increase chlorpropamide effect.
Chlorthalidone	Decreased allopurinol effect.
Cyclophosphamide	Increased cyclophosphamide toxicity.
Diuretics, thiazide (see Drugs Glossary)	Decreased allopurinol effect.
Ethacrynic acid	Decreased allopurinol effect.
Furosemide	Decreased allopurinol effect.
Indapamide	Decreased allopurinol effect.
Iron supplements (see Drugs Glossary)	Excessive accumulation of iron in tissues.
Mercaptopurine	Increased mercaptopurine effect.
Metolazone	Decreased allopurinol effect.
Probenecid	Increased allopurinol effect.
Theophylline	May increase theophylline effect.

POSSIBLE INTERACTION WITH OTHER SUBSTANCES

INTERACTS WITH	COMBINED EFFECT
Alcohol:	None expected, but may impair management of gout.
Beverages: Caffeine drinks.	Decreased allopurinol effect.
Cocaine (or crack):	Decreased allopurinol effect. Avoid.
Foods:	None expected. Low-purine diet recommended (see Glossary).
Marijuana:	Occasional use—None expected. Daily use—Possible increase in uric-acid level.
Tobacco:	None expected.

MEDICATIONS

AMILORIDE & HYDROCHLOROTHIAZIDE

BRAND NAMES

Moduret **Moduretic**

BASIC INFORMATION

Habit forming? No
Prescription needed? Yes
Available as generic? Yes
Drug class: Diuretic (thiazide), antihypertensive

USES

• Controls, but doesn't cure, high blood pressure.
• Reduces fluid retention (edema), decreasing likelihood of congestive heart failure.

DOSAGE & USAGE INFORMATION

How to take:
Tablet—Swallow with liquid. If you can't swallow whole, crumble tablet and take with liquid or food.

When to take:
At the same time each day, no later than 6 p.m.

If you forget a dose:
Take as soon as you remember up to 2 hours late. If more than 2 hours, wait for next scheduled dose (don't double this dose).

What drug does:
• Forces sodium and water excretion, conserves potassium, reducing body fluid.
• Relaxes muscle cells of small arteries.
• Reduced body fluid and relaxed arteries lower blood pressure.

Time lapse before drug works:
2-6 hours. May require several weeks to lower blood pressure.

Continued next column

OVERDOSE

SYMPTOMS:
Cramps, weakness, drowsiness, weak pulse, coma, rapid, irregular heartbeat.
WHAT TO DO:
• **Dial 0 (operator) or 911 (emergency) for an ambulance or medical help. Then give first aid immediately.**
• **See emergency information at the back of this book.**

Don't take with:
Any other medicines, even over-the-counter drugs such as cough and cold medicines, nose drops, diet pills, laxatives or caffeine, without consulting your doctor.

POSSIBLE ADVERSE REACTIONS OR SIDE EFFECTS

SYMPTOMS	WHAT TO DO
Life-threatening:	
None expected.	
Common:	
• Increased thirst, irregular heartbeat, cramps in muscles, numbness and tingling in hands and feet, thready pulse, shortness of breath.	Discontinue. Call doctor right away.
• Tiredness, weakness, dry mouth, diarrhea, headache, appetite loss, nausea.	Continue. Call doctor when convenient.
Infrequent:	
Mood changes, constipation, decreased sex function, dizziness, lightheadedness.	Continue. Call doctor when convenient.
Rare:	
Jaundice; unusual bleeding or bruising; abdominal pain with nausea and vomiting; sore throat, fever, sores in mouth; hives, skin rash; joint pain.	Discontinue. Seek emergency treatment.

WARNINGS & PRECAUTIONS

Don't take if:
You are allergic to amiloride or any thiazide diuretic drug.

Before you start, consult your doctor:
• If you are allergic to any sulfa drug.
• If you have gout, diabetes, heart disease.
• If you have liver, pancreas or kidney disorder.

Pregnancy:
Risk to unborn child outweighs drug benefits. Don't use.

Infants & children:
Don't give to infants or young children unless prescribed and monitored by your physician.

Prolonged use:
You may need medicine to treat high blood pressure for the rest of your life.

Skin & sunlight:
May cause rash or intensify sunburn in areas exposed to sun or sunlamp. Avoid overexposure.

Driving or hazardous activities:
Don't drive or pilot aircraft until you learn how medicine affects you. Don't work around dangerous machinery. Don't climb ladders or work in high places. Danger increases if you drink alcohol or take medicine affecting alertness and reflexes, such as antihistamines, tranquilizers, sedatives, pain medicine, narcotics and mind-altering drugs.

Discontinuing:
Don't discontinue without medical advice.

Others:
• Hot weather and fever may cause dehydration and drop in blood pressure. Dose may require temporary adjustment. Weigh daily and report any unexpected weight decreases to your doctor.
• May cause rise in uric acid, leading to gout.
• May cause blood-sugar rise in diabetics.
• Get periodic check-ups and potassium-level laboratory tests.

POSSIBLE INTERACTION WITH OTHER DRUGS

GENERIC NAME OR DRUG CLASS	COMBINED EFFECT
Allopurinol	Decreased allopurinol effect.
Antidepressants, tricyclic (TCA, see Drugs Glossary)	Dangerous drop in blood pressure. Avoid combination unless under medical supervision.
Antihypertensives (other, see Drugs Glossary)	Increased effect of both drugs.
Barbiturates (see Drugs Glossary)	Increased hydrochlorothiazide effect.
Beta-adrenergic blockers (see Drugs Glossary)	Increased antihypertensive effect. Dosages of both drugs may require adjustments.
Blood-bank blood	Increased potassium levels.
Cortisone drugs (see Drugs Glossary)	Excessive potassium loss that causes dangerous heart rhythms.
Digitalis preparations (see Drugs Glossary)	Excessive potassium loss that causes dangerous heart rhythms.
Diuretics (thiazide, see Drugs Glossary	Increased diuretic effect.
Diuretics (other, see Drugs Glossary)	Increased effect of both drugs.
Indapamide	Increased diuretic effect.
Lithium	Possible lithium toxicity.
MAO inhibitors (see Drugs Glossary)	Increased hydrochlorothiazide effect.
Nitrates (see Drugs Glossary)	Excessive blood-pressure drop.
Oxprenolol	Increased antihypertensive effect. Dosages may require adjustment.
Probenecid	Decreased probenecid effect.
Sodium bicarbonate	Decreased potassium levels.

POSSIBLE INTERACTION WITH OTHER SUBSTANCES

INTERACTS WITH	COMBINED EFFECT
Alcohol:	Dangerous blood-pressure drop.
Beverages: Low-salt milk.	Possible excess potassium levels. Low-salt milk has extra potassium.
Cocaine (or crack):	None expected.
Foods: Salt substitutes.	Possible excess potassium levels.
Marijuana:	May increase blood pressure.
Tobacco:	None expected.

AMOXICILLIN

BRAND NAMES

Amoxil
Apo-Amoxi
Augmentin
Clavulin
Larotid
Moxilean
Novamoxin
Penamox
Polymox
Robamox
Sumox
Trimox
Utimox
Wymox

BASIC INFORMATION

Habit forming? No
Prescription needed? Yes
Available as generic? Yes
Drug class: Antibiotic (penicillins)

USES

Treatment of bacterial infections that are susceptible to amoxicillin.

DOSAGE & USAGE INFORMATION

How to take:
• Tablet or capsule—Swallow with liquid on an empty stomach 1 hour before or 2 hours after eating.
• Chewable tablets—Chew well before swallowing.
• Liquid—Take with cold beverage. Liquid form is perishable and effective for only 7 days at room temperature. Effective for 14 days if stored in refrigerator. Don't freeze.

When to take:
Follow instructions on prescription label or side of package. Doses should be evenly spaced. For example, 4 times a day means before meals and at bedtime.

If you forget a dose:
Take as soon as you remember. Continue regular schedule.

Continued next column

OVERDOSE

SYMPTOMS:
Severe diarrhea, nausea or vomiting.
WHAT TO DO:
Overdose unlikely to threaten life. If child takes much larger amount than prescribed, call doctor, poison-control center or hospital emergency room for instructions.

What drug does:
Destroys susceptible bacteria. Does not kill viruses.

Time lapse before drug works:
May be several days before medicine affects infection.

Don't take with:
Any other medicines, even over-the-counter drugs such as cough and cold medicines, nose drops, diet pills, laxatives or caffeine, without consulting your doctor.

POSSIBLE ADVERSE REACTIONS OR SIDE EFFECTS

SYMPTOMS	WHAT TO DO
Life-threatening:	
Hives, rash, intense itching, faintness soon after a dose (anaphylaxis); difficulty breathing.	Seek emergency treatment immediately.
Common:	
Dark or discolored tongue.	Continue. Tell doctor at next visit.
Infrequent:	
Mild nausea, vomiting, diarrhea.	Continue. Call doctor when convenient.
Rare:	
Unexplained bleeding, weakness, sore throat.	Discontinue. Call doctor right away.

WARNINGS & PRECAUTIONS

Don't take if:
You are allergic to amoxicillin, cephalosporin antibiotics, other penicillins. Life-threatening: reaction may occur.

Before you start, consult your doctor:
If you are allergic to any substance or drug.

Pregnancy:
Studies inconclusive on harm to unborn child. Animal studies show fetal abnormalities. Decide with your doctor whether drug benefits justify risk to unborn child.

Infants & children:
No age-related problems expected.

Prolonged use:
You may become more susceptible to infections caused by germs not responsive to amoxicillin.

Skin & sunlight:
No age-related problems expected.

Driving or hazardous activities:
Usually not dangerous. Most hazardous reactions likely to occur a few minutes after taking amoxicillin.

Discontinuing:
Don't discontinue without doctor's advice until you complete prescribed dose, even though symptoms diminish or disappear.

Others:
No age-related problems expected.

POSSIBLE INTERACTION WITH OTHER DRUGS

GENERIC NAME OR DRUG CLASS	COMBINED EFFECT
Beta-adrenergic blockers (see Drugs Glossary)	Increased chance of anaphylaxis (see emergency information on inside front cover).
Chloramphenicol	Decreased effect of both drugs.
Erythromycins	Decreased effect of both drugs.
Loperamide	Decreased amoxicillin effect.
Paromomycin	Decreased effect of both drugs.
Tetracyclines (see Drugs Glossary)	Decreased effect of both drugs.
Troleandomycin	Decreased effect of both drugs.

POSSIBLE INTERACTION WITH OTHER SUBSTANCES

INTERACTS WITH	COMBINED EFFECT
Alcohol:	Occasional stomach irritation.
Beverages:	None expected.
Cocaine (or crack):	No proven problems.
Foods:	None expected.
Marijuana:	No proven problems.
Tobacco:	None expected.

AMPHETAMINE

BRAND NAMES

Amphaplex 10 & 20	**Biphetamine**
Benzedrine	**Declobese**
Bexedrine	**Obetrol 10 & 20**

BASIC INFORMATION

Habit forming? Yes
Prescription needed? Yes
Available as generic? Yes
Drug class: Central nervous system stimulant (amphetamine)

USES

- Prevents narcolepsy (attacks of uncontrollable sleepiness).
- Controls hyperactivity in children.

DOSAGE & USAGE INFORMATION

How to take:
Tablet—Swallow with liquid.

When to take:
- At the same times each day.
- Short-acting form—Don't take later than 6 hours before bedtime.
- Long-acting form—Take on awakening.

If you forget a dose:
- Short-acting form—Take up to 2 hours late. If more than 2 hours, wait for next dose (don't double this dose).
- Long-acting form—Take as soon as you remember. Wait 20 hours for next dose.

What drug does:
- Narcolepsy—Apparently affects brain centers to decrease fatigue or sleepiness and increase alertness and motor activity.
- Hyperactive children—Calms children, opposite to effect on narcoleptic adults.

Continued next column

OVERDOSE

SYMPTOMS:
Rapid heartbeat, hyperactivity, high fever, hallucinations, suicidal or homicidal feelings, convulsions, coma.
WHAT TO DO:
- **Dial 0 (operator) or 911 (emergency) for an ambulance or medical help. Then give first aid immediately.**
- **See emergency information at the back of this book.**

Time lapse before drug works:
15 to 30 minutes.

Don't take with:
Any other medicines, even over-the-counter drugs such as cough and cold medicines, nose drops, diet pills, laxatives or caffeine, without consulting your doctor.

POSSIBLE ADVERSE REACTIONS OR SIDE EFFECTS

SYMPTOMS	WHAT TO DO
Life-threatening: None expected.	
Common:	
• Irritability, nervousness, insomnia.	Continue. Call doctor when convenient.
• Dry mouth.	Continue. Tell doctor at next visit.
Infrequent:	
• Dizziness; reduced alertness; blurred vision; fast, pounding heartbeat; unusual sweating.	Discontinue. Call doctor right away.
• Headache.	Continue. Call doctor when convenient.
• Diarrhea or constipation, appetite loss, stomach pain, nausea, vomiting, weight loss, diminished sex drive, impotence.	Continue. Tell doctor at next visit.
Rare:	
• Rash, hives; chest pain or irregular heartbeat; uncontrollable movements of head, neck, arms, legs.	Discontinue. Call doctor right away.
• Mood changes, swollen breasts.	Continue. Call doctor when convenient.

WARNINGS & PRECAUTIONS

Don't take if:
- You are allergic to any amphetamine.
- You will have surgery within 2 months, including dental surgery, requiring general or spinal anesthesia.

Before you start, consult your doctor:
- If you plan to become pregnant within medication period.
- If you have glaucoma.
- If you have heart or blood-vessel disease, or high blood pressure.
- If you have overactive thyroid, anxiety or tension.
- If you have a severe mental illness (especially children).

Pregnancy:
Risk to unborn child outweighs drug benefits. Don't use.

Infants & children:
Not recommended for children under 12.

Prolonged use:
Habit forming.

Skin & sunlight:
No age-related problems expected.

Driving or hazardous activities:
Don't drive or pilot aircraft until you learn how medicine affects you. Don't work around dangerous machinery. Don't climb ladders or work in high places. Danger increases if you drink alcohol or take medicine affecting alertness and reflexes.

Discontinuing:
May be unnecessary to finish medicine. Follow doctor's instructions.

Others:
- This is a dangerous drug and must be closely supervised. Don't use for appetite control or depression. Potential for damage and abuse.
- During withdrawal phase, may cause prolonged sleep of several days.

POSSIBLE INTERACTION WITH OTHER DRUGS

GENERIC NAME OR DRUG CLASS	COMBINED EFFECT
Acetazolamide	Increased amphetamine effect.
Anesthesias (general, see Drugs Glossary)	Irregular heartbeat.
Antidepressants, tricyclic (TCA, see Drugs Glossary)	Decreased amphetamine effect.
Antihypertensives (see Drugs Glossary)	Decreased antihypertensive effect.
Carbonic anhydrase inhibitors (see Drugs Glossary)	Increased amphetamine effect.
Guanethidine	Decreased guanethidine effect.
Haloperidol	Decreased amphetamine effect.
MAO inhibitors (see Drugs Glossary)	May severely increase blood pressure.
Phenothiazines (see Drugs Glossary)	Decreased amphetamine effect.
Sodium bicarbonate	Increased amphetamine effect.

POSSIBLE INTERACTION WITH OTHER SUBSTANCES

INTERACTS WITH	COMBINED EFFECT
Alcohol:	Decreased amphetamine effect. Avoid.
Beverages: Caffeine drinks.	Overstimulation. Avoid.
Cocaine (or crack):	Dangerous stimulation of nervous system. Avoid.
Foods:	None expected.
Marijuana:	Frequent use—Severely impaired mental function.
Tobacco:	None expected.

MEDICATIONS

ANGIOTENSIN-CONVERTING ENZYME (ACE) INHIBITORS

BRAND NAMES

Captopril
Capoten
EnalaVasotec

BASIC INFORMATION

Habit forming? No
Prescription needed? Yes
Available as generic? No
Drug class: Antihypertensive, ACE inhibitor (see Drugs Glossary)

USES

Treatment for high blood pressure and congestive heart failure.

DOSAGE & USAGE INFORMATION

How to take:
Tablet—Swallow with liquid. Instructions to take on empty stomach mean 1 hour before or 2 hours after eating.

When to take:
At the same times each day, usually 2-3 times daily. Take first dose at bedtime and lie down immediately.

If you forget a dose:
Take as soon as you remember up to 2 hours late. If more than 2 hours, wait for next scheduled dose (don't double this dose).

What drug does:
- Reduces resistance in arteries.
- Strengthens heartbeat.

Time lapse before drug works:
60 to 90 minutes.

Don't take with:
Any other medicines, even over-the-counter drugs such as cough and cold medicines, nose drops, diet pills, laxatives or caffeine, without consulting your doctor.

OVERDOSE

SYMPTOMS:
Low blood pressure.
WHAT TO DO:
- **Dial 0 (operator) or 911 (emergency) for an ambulance or medical help. Then give first aid immediately.**
- **See emergency information at the back of this book.**

POSSIBLE ADVERSE REACTIONS OR SIDE EFFECTS

SYMPTOMS	WHAT TO DO
Life-threatening:	
Hives, rash, intense itching, faintness soon after a dose (anaphylaxis); difficulty breathing.	Seek emergency treatment immediately.
Common:	
Rash, loss of taste.	Discontinue. Call doctor right away.
Infrequent:	
• Swelling of mouth, face, hands or feet.	Discontinue. Seek emergency treatment.
• Dizziness, fainting, chest pain, fast or irregular heartbeat, coughing.	Discontinue. Call doctor right away.
Rare:	
• Sore throat, cloudy urine, fever, chills.	Discontinue. Call doctor right away.
• Nausea, vomiting, indigestion, abdominal pain.	Continue. Call doctor when convenient.

WARNINGS & PRECAUTIONS

Don't take if:
- You are allergic to any ACE inhibitor.
- You have any autoimmune disease, including AIDS or lupus.
- You are receiving blood from a blood bank.
- You take drugs for cancer.
- You will have surgery within 2 months, including dental surgery, requiring general or spinal anesthesia.

Before you start, consult your doctor:
- If you have had a stroke.
- If you have angina or heart or blood-vessel disease.
- If you have high level of potassium in blood.
- If you have kidney disease.
- If you are on severe salt-restricted diet.
- If you have lupus.

Pregnancy:
Risk to unborn child outweighs drug benefits. Don't use.

Infants & children
Don't give to infants or young children unless prescribed and monitored by your physician.

Prolonged use:
May decrease white cells in blood or cause protein loss in urine. Request periodic laboratory blood counts and urine tests.

Skin & sunlight:
No age-related problems expected.

Driving or hazardous activities:
Avoid if you become dizzy or faint. Otherwise, no problems expected.

Discontinuing:
Don't discontinue without consulting doctor. Dose may require gradual reduction if you have taken drug for a long time. Doses of other drugs may also require adjustment.

Others:
- Stop taking diuretics or increase salt intake 1 week before starting captopril.
- Avoid exercising in hot weather.

POSSIBLE INTERACTION WITH OTHER DRUGS

GENERIC NAME OR DRUG CLASS	COMBINED EFFECT
Amiloride	Possible excessive potassium in blood.
Antihypertensives (other, see Drugs Glossary)	Increased antihypertensive effect. Dosage of each may require adjustment.
Beta-adrenergic blockers (see Drugs Glossary)	Increased antihypertensive effect. Dosage of each may require adjustment.
Chloramphenicol	Possible blood disorders.
Diuretics (see Drugs Glossary)	Possible severe blood-pressure drop with first dose.
Enalapril	Possible excessive blood-pressure drop.
Guanfacine	Increased effect of both drugs.
Nitrates	Possible excessive blood-pressure drop.
Non-steroidal anti-inflammatory adrugs (NSAIDs, see Drugs Glossary)	Decreased ACE inhibitor effect.
Pentoxifylline	Increased antihypertensive effect.
Potassium supplements (see Drugs Glossary)	Possible increased potassium in blood.
Spironolactone	Possible excessive potassium in blood.
Triamterene	Possible excessive potassium in blood.

POSSIBLE INTERACTION WITH OTHER SUBSTANCES

INTERACTS WITH	COMBINED EFFECT
Alcohol:	Possible excessive blood-pressure drop.
Beverages: Low-salt milk.	Possible excessive potassium in blood.
Cocaine (or crack):	Increased dizziness and chest pain.
Foods: Salt substitutes.	Possible excessive potassium.
Marijuana:	Increased dizziness.
Tobacco:	May decrease ACE inhibitor effect.

ANTICOAGULANTS, ORAL

BRAND & GENERIC NAMES

ANISINDIONE
Anthrombin-K
Coumadin
Danilone
DICUMAROL
Dufalone
Hedulin
Liquamar
Marcumar
Marevan
Melitoxin
Miradon
Panwarfin
PHENINDIONE
PHENPROCOUMON
Sofarin
WARFARIN POTASSIUM
WARFARIN SODIUM
Warfilone
Warnerin

BASIC INFORMATION

Habit forming? No
Prescription needed? Yes
Available as generic? Yes
Drug class: Anticoagulant

USES

Reduces blood clots. Used for abnormal clotting inside blood vessels.

DOSAGE & USAGE INFORMATION

How to take:
Tablet—Swallow with liquid. If you can't swallow whole, crumble tablet and take with liquid or food.

When to take:
At the same time each day.

If you forget a dose:
Take as soon as you remember up to 12 hours late. If more than 12 hours, wait for next scheduled dose (don't double this dose). Inform your doctor of any missed doses.

What drug does:
Blocks action of vitamin K necessary for blood clotting.

Continued next column

OVERDOSE

SYMPTOMS:
Bloody vomit and bloody or black stools, red urine.
WHAT TO DO:
- **Dial 0 (operator) or 911 (emergency) for an ambulance or medical help. Then give first aid immediately.**
- **See emergency information at the back of this book.**

Time lapse before drug works:
36 to 48 hours.

Don't take with:
Any other medicines, even over-the-counter drugs such as cough and cold medicines, nose drops, diet pills, laxatives or caffeine, without consulting your doctor.

POSSIBLE ADVERSE REACTIONS OR SIDE EFFECTS

SYMPTOMS	WHAT TO DO
Life-threatening: None expected.	
Common: Bloating, gas.	Continue. Tell doctor at next visit.
Infrequent:	
• Black stools or bloody vomit, coughing up blood.	Discontinue. Seek emergency treatment.
• Rash, hives, itch, blurred vision, sore throat, easy bruising, bleeding, cloudy or red urine, back pain, jaundice, fever, chills, fatigue, weakness.	Discontinue. Call doctor right away.
• Diarrhea, cramps, nausea, vomiting, swollen feet or legs, hair loss.	Continue. Call doctor when convenient.
Rare:	
• Necrosis of skin	Discontinue. Seek emergency treatment
• Dizziness, headache, mouth sores.	Discontinue. Call doctor right away.

WARNINGS & PRECAUTIONS

Don't take if:
- You have been allergic to any oral anticoagulant.
- You have a bleeding disorder.
- You have an active peptic ulcer.
- You have ulcerative colitis.

Before you start, consult your doctor:
- If you take any other drugs, including nonprescription drugs.
- If you have high blood pressure.
- If you have heavy or prolonged menstrual periods.
- If you have diabetes.
- If you have a bladder catheter.
- If you have serious liver or kidney disease.
- If you will have surgery within 2 months, including dental surgery, requiring general or spinal anesthesia.

Pregnancy:
Risk to unborn child outweighs drug benefits. Don't use.

Infants & children:
Use only under doctor's supervision.

Prolonged use:
No age-related problems expected.

Skin & sunlight:
No age-related problems expected.

Driving or hazardous activities:
- Avoid hazardous activities that could cause injury.
- Don't drive if you feel dizzy or have blurred vision.

Discontinuing:
Don't discontinue without consulting doctor. Dose may require gradual reduction if you have taken drug for a long time. Doses of other drugs may also require adjustment.

Others:
Carry identification to state you take anticoagulants.

POSSIBLE INTERACTION WITH OTHER DRUGS

GENERIC NAME OR DRUG CLASS	COMBINED EFFECT
Acetaminophen	Increased effect of anticoagulant.
Allopurinol	Increased effect of anticoagulant.
Amiodarone	Increased effect of anticoagulant.
Androgens	Increased effect of anticoagulant.
Antacids (large doses, see Drugs Glossary)	Decreased effect of anticoagulant.
Antibiotics (see Drugs Glossary)	Increased effect of anticoagulant.
Anticonvulsants (hydantoin, see Drugs Glossary)	Increased effect of both drugs.
Antidepressants, tricyclic (TCA, see Drugs Glossary)	Increased effect of anticoagulant.
Antidiabetics (oral, see Drugs Glossary)	Increased effect of anticoagulant.
Antihistamines (see Drugs Glossary)	Unpredictable increased or decreased effect of anticoagulant.
Aspirin	Possible spontaneous bleeding.
Barbiturates (see Drugs Glossary)	Decreased effect of anticoagulant.
Benzodiazepines (see Drugs Glossary)	Unpredictable increased or decreased anticoagulant effect.

See Additional Drug Interactions Section

POSSIBLE INTERACTION WITH OTHER SUBSTANCES

INTERACTS WITH	COMBINED EFFECT
Alcohol:	Can increase or decrease effect of anticoagulant. Use with caution.
Beverages:	None expected.
Cocaine (or crack):	None expected.
Foods: High in vitamin K such as fish, liver, spinach, cabbage.	May decrease anticoagulant effect.
Marijuana:	None expected.
Tobacco:	None expected.

ANTICONVULSANTS, HYDANTOIN

BRAND & GENERIC NAMES

See complete list of brand and generic names in the Brand & Generic Name Directory.

BASIC INFORMATION

Habit forming? No
Prescription needed? Yes
Available as generic? Yes
Drug class: Anticonvulsant (hydantoin)

USES

- Prevents epileptic seizures.
- Stabilizes irregular heartbeat.

DOSAGE & USAGE INFORMATION

How to take:
- Capsule—Swallow with liquid.
- Chewable tablets—Chew carefully before swallowing.
- Suspension—Shake well before taking with liquid.

When to take:
At the same time each day.

If you forget a dose:
- If drug taken 1 time per day—Take as soon as you remember up to 12 hours late. If more than 12 hours, wait for next scheduled dose (don't double this dose).
- If taken several times per day—Take as soon as possible, then return to regular schedule.

Continued next column

OVERDOSE

SYMPTOMS:
Jerky eye movements; stagger; slurred speech; imbalance; drowsiness; blood-pressure drop; slow, shallow breathing; coma.
WHAT TO DO:
- **Dial 0 (operator) or 911 (emergency) for an ambulance or medical help. Then give first aid immediately.**
- **See emergency information at the back of this book.**

What drug does:
Promotes sodium loss from nerve fibers. This lessens excitability and inhibits spread of nerve impulses.

Time lapse before drug works:
7 to 10 days continual use.

Don't take with:
Any other medicines, even over-the-counter drugs such as cough and cold medicines, nose drops, diet pills, laxatives or caffeine, without consulting your doctor.

POSSIBLE ADVERSE REACTIONS OR SIDE EFFECTS

SYMPTOMS	WHAT TO DO
Life-threatening: None expected.	
Common: Enlarged, tender, receding gums with increased likelihood of bleeding; nausea; vomiting; constipation; mild dizziness; sleeplessness.	Continue. Call doctor when convenient.
Infrequent: • Hallucinations, confusion, slurred speech, stagger, rash, change in vision.	Discontinue. Call doctor right away.
• Headache, diarrhea, drowsiness, muscle twitching.	Continue. Call doctor when convenient.
• Increased body and facial hair.	Continue. Tell doctor at next visit.
Rare: Sore throat, fever, stomach pain, unusual bleeding or bruising, swollen lymph glands, jaundice.	Discontinue. Call doctor right away.

WARNINGS & PRECAUTIONS

Don't take if:
You are allergic to any hydantoin anticonvulsant.

Before you start, consult your doctor:
• If you have had impaired liver function or disease.
• If you will have surgery within 2 months, including dental surgery, requiring general or spinal anesthesia.

Pregnancy:
Risk to unborn child outweighs drug benefits. Don't use.

Infants & children:
Use only under medical supervision.

Prolonged use:
• Weakened bones.
• Lymph gland enlargement.
• Possible liver damage.
• Numbness and tingling of hands and feet.
• Continual back-and-forth eye movements.
• Bleeding, swollen or tender gums.

Skin & sunlight:
May cause rash or intensify sunburn in areas exposed to sun or sunlamp.

Driving or hazardous activities:
Don't drive or pilot aircraft until you learn how medicine affects you. Don't work around dangerous machinery. Don't climb ladders or work in high places. Danger increases if you drink alcohol or take medicine affecting alertness and reflexes.

Discontinuing:
Don't discontinue without consulting doctor. Dose may require gradual reduction if you have taken drug for a long time. Doses of other drugs may also require adjustment.

Others:
No age-related problems expected.

POSSIBLE INTERACTION WITH OTHER DRUGS

GENERIC NAME OR DRUG CLASS	COMBINED EFFECT
Anticoagulants (see Drugs Glossary)	Increased effect of anticoagulant.
Antidepressants, tricyclic (TCA, see Drugs Glossary)	Decreased hydantoin anticonvulsant effect. Dose may require adjustment.
Barbiturates (see Drugs Glossary)	Changed seizure pattern.
Carbamazepine	Possible increased hydantoin anticonvulsant metabolism.
Carbonic anhydrase inhibitors (see Drugs Glossary)	Increased chance of bone disease.
Chloramphenicol	Increased hydantoin anticonvulsant effect.
Cimetidine	Increased hydantoin anticonvulsant toxicity.
Contraceptives (oral, see Drugs Glossary)	Increased seizures. Menstrual irregularities.
Cortisone drugs (see Drugs Glossary)	Decreased cortisone effect.
Cyclosporine	May decrease cyclosporine effect.
Digitalis preparations (see Drugs Glossary)	Decreased digitalis effect.
Disopyramide	Decreased disopyramide effect.
Disulfiram	Increased hydantoin anticonvulsant effect.
Encainide	Increased effect of toxicity on heart muscle.
Estrogens (see Drugs Glossary)	Increased estrogen effect.

See Additional Drug Interactions Section

POSSIBLE INTERACTION WITH OTHER SUBSTANCES

INTERACTS WITH	COMBINED EFFECT
Alcohol:	Possible decreased anticonvulsant effect. Use with caution.
Beverages:	None expected.
Cocaine (or crack):	Possible seizures.
Foods:	None expected.
Marijuana:	Drowsiness, unsteadiness, decreased anticonvulsant effect.
Tobacco:	None expected.

ANTIDIABETICS, ORAL

BRAND & GENERIC NAMES

See complete list of brand and generic names in the Brand & Generic Name Directory.

BASIC INFORMATION

Habit forming? No
Prescription needed? Yes
Available as generic? No
Drug class: Antidiabetic (oral), sulfonurea

USES

Treatment for diabetes in adults and children who can't control blood sugar by diet, weight loss and exercise.

DOSAGE & USAGE INFORMATION

How to take:
Tablet—Swallow with liquid or food to lessen stomach irritation. If you can't swallow whole, crumble tablet and take with liquid or food.

When to take:
At the same times each day.

If you forget a dose:
Take as soon as you remember up to 2 hours late. If more than 2 hours, wait for next scheduled dose (don't double this dose).

What drug does:
Stimulates pancreas to produce more insulin. Insulin in blood forces cells to use sugar in blood.

Continued next column

Time lapse before drug works:
3 to 4 hours. May require 2 weeks for maximum benefit.

Don't take with:
Any other medicines, even over-the-counter drugs such as cough and cold medicines, nose drops, diet pills, laxatives or caffeine, without consulting your doctor.

OVERDOSE

SYMPTOMS:
Excessive hunger, nausea, anxiety, cool skin, cold sweats, drowsiness, rapid heartbeat, weakness, unconsciousness, coma.
WHAT TO DO:
- **Dial 0 (operator) or 911 (emergency) for an ambulance or medical help. Then give first aid immediately.**
- **See emergency information at the back of this book.**

POSSIBLE ADVERSE REACTIONS OR SIDE EFFECTS

SYMPTOMS	WHAT TO DO
Life-threatening: None expected.	
Common:	
• Dizziness.	Discontinue. Call doctor right away.
• Diarrhea, appetite loss, nausea, stomach pain, heartburn.	Continue. Call doctor when convenient.
Infrequent:	
Low blood sugar (hunger, anxiety, cold sweats, rapid pulse), drowsiness, nervousness, headache, weakness, rapid heartbeat.	Discontinue. Seek emergency treatment.
Rare:	
• Itching or rash, sore throat, fever, ringing in ears, unusual bleeding or bruising, fatigue, jaundice, joint pain, numbness or tingling in hands or feet.	Discontinue. Call doctor right away.
• Excess urination at night.	Continue. Call doctor when convenient.

WARNINGS & PRECAUTIONS

Don't take if:
- You are allergic to any sulfonurea.
- You have impaired kidney or liver function.

Before you start, consult your doctor
- If you have a severe infection.
- If you have thyroid disease.
- If you take insulin.
- If you have heart disease.

Pregnancy:
No proven harm to unborn child. Avoid if possible.

Infants & children:
Don't give to infants or young children unless prescribed and monitored by your physician.

Prolonged use:
None expected.

Skin & sunlight:
May cause rash or intensify sunburn in areas exposed to sun or sunlamp.

Driving or hazardous activities:
No age-related problems expected unless you develop hypoglycemia (low blood sugar). If so, avoid driving or hazardous activity.

Discontinuing:
Don't discontinue without consulting doctor. Dose may require gradual reduction if you have taken drug for a long time. Doses of other drugs may also require adjustment.

Others:
Don't exceed recommended dose. Hypoglycemia (low blood sugar) may occur, even with proper dose schedule. You must balance medicine, diet and exercise.

POSSIBLE INTERACTION WITH OTHER DRUGS

GENERIC NAME OR DRUG CLASS	COMBINED EFFECT
Androgens (see Drugs Glossary)	Increased antidiabetic effect.
Anticoagulants (oral, see Drugs Glossary)	Unpredictable prothrombin times.
Anticonvulsants (hydantoin, see Drugs Glossary)	Decreased antidiabetic effect.
Aspirin	Increased antidiabetic effect.
Beta-adrenergic blockers (see Drugs Glossary)	Increased antidiabetic effect. Possible increased difficulty in regulating blood-sugar levels.
Chloramphenicol	Increased antidiabetic effect.
Clofibrate	Increased antidiabetic effect.
Contraceptives (oral, see Drugs Glossary)	Decreased antidiabetic effect.
Cortisone drugs	Decreased antidiabetic effect.
Diuretics (thiazide, see Drugs Glossary)	Decreased antidiabetic effect.
Epinephrine	Decreased antidiabetic effect.
Estrogens	Increased antidiabetic effect.
Guanethidine	Unpredictable antidiabetic effect.
Labetolol	Increased antidiabetic effect, may mask hypoglycemia.
Non-steroidal anti-inflammatory drugs (NSAIDs, see Drugs Glossary)	Increased antidiabetic effect.

POSSIBLE INTERACTION WITH OTHER SUBSTANCES

INTERACTS WITH	COMBINED EFFECT
Alcohol:	Disulfiram reaction (see Drugs Glossary). Avoid.
Beverages:	None expected.
Cocaine (or crack):	No proven problems.
Foods:	None expected.
Marijuana:	Decreased antidiabetic effect. Avoid.
Tobacco:	None expected.

ANTIHISTAMINES

BRAND & GENERIC NAMES

See complete list of brand and generic names in the Brand & Generic Name Directory.

BASIC INFORMATION

Habit forming? No
Prescription needed? Yes
Available as generic? No
Drug class: Antihistamine

USES

Reduces allergic symptoms such as hay fever, hives, rash or itching.
Induces sleep.

DOSAGE & USAGE INFORMATION

How to take:
Tablet—Swallow with liquid or food to lessen stomach irritation.

When to take:
Varies with form. Follow label directions.

If you forget a dose:
Take as soon as you remember up to 2 hours late. If more than 2 hours, wait for next scheduled dose (don't double this dose).

What drug does:
Blocks action of histamine after an allergic response triggers histamine release in sensitive cells.

Continued next column

OVERDOSE

SYMPTOMS:
Convulsions, red face, hallucinations, coma.
WHAT TO DO:
- **Dial 0 (operator) or 911 (emergency) for an ambulance or medical help. Then give first aid immediately.**
- **If the child is unconscious and not breathing, give mouth-to-mouth breathing. If there is no heartbeat, use cardiac massage and mouth-to-mouth breathing (CPR). Don't try to make the child vomit. If you can't get help quickly, take the child to nearest emergency facility.**
- **See emergency information at the back of this book.**

Time lapse before drug works:
30 minutes.

Don't take with:
Any other medicines, even over-the-counter drugs such as cough and cold medicines, nose drops, diet pills, laxatives or caffeine, without consulting your doctor.

POSSIBLE ADVERSE REACTIONS OR SIDE EFFECTS

SYMPTOMS	WHAT TO DO
Life-threatening: None expected.	
Common: Drowsiness; dizziness; dry mouth, nose, throat; nausea.	Continue. Tell doctor at next visit.
Infrequent: • Changes in vision.	Discontinue. Call doctor right away.
• Less tolerance for contact lenses, difficult urination.	Continue. Call doctor when convenient.
• Appetite loss, gastric discomfort.	Continue. Tell doctor at next visit.
Rare: Nightmares, agitation, irritability, sore throat, fever, rapid or slow heartbeat, unusual bleeding or bruising, fatigue, weakness, decreased libido, impotence.	Discontinue. Call doctor right away.

WARNINGS & PRECAUTIONS

Don't take if:
You are allergic to any antihistamine.

Before you start, consult your doctor:
- If you have glaucoma.
- If you have enlarged prostate.
- If you have asthma.
- If you have kidney disease.
- If you have peptic ulcer.
- If you will have surgery within 2 months, including dental surgery, requiring general or spinal anesthesia.

Pregnancy:
Unknown effect on unborn child. Avoid if possible.

Infants & children:
Not recommended for premature or newborn infants. Otherwise, no problems expected.

Prolonged use:
Avoid. May damage bone-marrow and nerve cells.

Skin & sunlight:
May cause rash or intensify sunburn in areas exposed to sun or sunlamp.

Driving or hazardous activities:
Don't drive or pilot aircraft until you learn how medicine affects you. Don't work around dangerous machinery. Don't climb ladders or work in high places. Danger increases if you drink alcohol or take medicine affecting alertness and reflexes, such as antihistamines, tranquilizers, sedatives, pain medicine, narcotics and mind-altering drugs.

Discontinuing:
No age-related problems expected.

Others:
May mask symptoms of hearing damage from aspirin, other salicylates, cisplatin, paromomycin, vancomycin or anticonvulsants. Consult doctor if you use these.

POSSIBLE INTERACTION WITH OTHER DRUGS

GENERIC NAME OR DRUG CLASS	COMBINED EFFECT
Anticholinergics (see Drugs Glossary)	Increased anticholinergic effect.
Anticoagulants (oral, see Drugs Glossary)	Possible decreased anticoagulant effect.
Antidepressants (see Drugs Glossary)	Excess sedation. Avoid.
Antihistamines (other, see Drugs Glossary)	Excess sedation. Avoid.
Dronabinol	Increased effects of both drugs. Avoid.
Hypnotics (see Drugs Glossary)	Excess sedation. Avoid.
MAO inhibitors (see Drugs Glossary)	Increased antihistamine effect.
Mind-altering drugs	Excess sedation. Avoid.
Molindone	Increased antihistamine effect.
Narcotics (see Drugs Glossary)	Excess sedation. Avoid.
Sedatives (see Drugs Glossary)	Excess sedation. Avoid.
Sleep inducers (see Drugs Glossary)	Excess sedation. Avoid.
Tranquilizers (see Drugs Glossary)	Excess sedation. Avoid.

POSSIBLE INTERACTION WITH OTHER SUBSTANCES

INTERACTS WITH	COMBINED EFFECT
Alcohol:	Excess sedation. Avoid.
Beverages: Caffeine drinks.	Less azatadine sedation.
Cocaine (or crack):	Decreased antihistamine effect. Avoid.
Foods:	None expected.
Marijuana:	Excess sedation. Avoid.
Tobacco:	None expected.

ANTI-INFLAMMATORY ANALGESICS, NON-STEROIDAL (NSAIDS)

BRAND & GENERIC NAMES

See complete list of brand and generic names in the Brand & Generic Name Directory.

BASIC INFORMATION

Habit forming? No
Prescription needed? No
Available as generic? Yes
Drug class: Anti-inflammatory (non-steroidal)

USES

- Treatment for joint pain, stiffness, inflammation and swelling of arthritis and gout.
- Pain reliever.
- Treatment for dysmenorrhea (painful or difficult menstruation).
- Treats juvenile rheumatoid arthritis.

DOSAGE & USAGE INFORMATION

How to take:
Tablet or capsule—Swallow with liquid or food to lessen stomach irritation. If you can't swallow whole, crumble tablet and take with liquid or food.

When to take:
At the same times each day.

If you forget a dose:
Take as soon as you remember up to 2 hours late. If more than 2 hours, wait for next scheduled dose (don't double this dose).

What drug does:
Reduces tissue concentration of prostaglandins (hormones which produce inflammation and pain).

Continued next column

OVERDOSE

SYMPTOMS:
Confusion, agitation, incoherence, convulsions, possible hemorrhage from stomach or intestine, coma.
WHAT TO DO:
- **Dial 0 (operator) or 911 (emergency) for an ambulance or medical help. Then give first aid immediately.**
- **See emergency information at the back of this book.**

Time lapse before drug works:
Begins in 4 to 24 hours. May require 3 weeks regular use for maximum benefit.

Don't take with:
Any other medicines, even over-the-counter drugs such as cough and cold medicines, nose drops, diet pills, laxatives or caffeine, without consulting your doctor.

POSSIBLE ADVERSE REACTIONS OR SIDE EFFECTS

SYMPTOMS	WHAT TO DO
Life-threatening:	
Hives, rash, intense itching, faintness soon after a dose (anaphylaxis in aspirin-sensitive persons).	Seek emergency treatment immediately.
Common:	
• Dizziness, nausea, pain.	Continue. Call doctor when convenient.
• Headache.	Continue. Tell doctor at next visit.
Infrequent:	
Depression; drowsiness; ringing in ears; swollen feet, legs; constipation or diarrhea; vomiting.	Continue. Call doctor when convenient.
Rare:	
• Convulsions; confusion; rash, hives or itch; blurred vision; black, bloody, tarry stool; difficult breathing; tightness in chest; rapid heartbeat; unusual bleeding or bruising; blood in urine; jaundice; psychosis; frequent, painful urination; severe abdominal pain.	Discontinue. Call doctor right away.
• Frequent, painful, or difficult urination; fatigue; weakness; menstrual irregularities; swollen breasts in males; impotence.	Continue. Call doctor when convenient.

ANTI-INFLAMMATORY ANALGESICS, NON-STEROIDAL (NSAIDS)

WARNINGS & PRECAUTIONS

Don't take if:
- You are allergic to aspirin or any non-steroid, anti-inflammatory drug.
- You have gastritis, peptic ulcer, enteritis, ileitis, ulcerative colitis, asthma, heart failure, high blood pressure or bleeding problems.
- Patient is younger than 15.

Before you start, consult your doctor:
- If you have epilepsy.
- If you have Parkinson's disease.
- If you have been mentally ill.
- If you have had kidney disease or impaired kidney function.

Pregnancy:
Studies inconclusive on harm to unborn child. Decide with your doctor whether drug benefits justify risk to unborn child.

Infants & children:
Not recommended for anyone younger than 15. Use only under medical supervision.

Prolonged use:
- Eye damage.
- Reduced hearing.
- Sore throat, fever.
- Weight gain.

Skin & sunlight:
Possible increased sensitivity to sunlight.

Driving or hazardous activities:
Don't drive or pilot aircraft until you learn how medicine affects you. Don't work around dangerous machinery. Don't climb ladders or work in high places. Danger increases if you drink alcohol or take medicine affecting alertness and reflexes, such as antihistamines, tranquilizers, sedatives, pain medicine, narcotics and mind-altering drugs.

Discontinuing:
Don't discontinue without consulting doctor. Dose may require gradual reduction if you have taken drug for a long time. Doses of other drugs may also require adjustment.

Others:
No age-related problems expected.

POSSIBLE INTERACTION WITH OTHER DRUGS

GENERIC NAME OR DRUG CLASS	COMBINED EFFECT
ACE inhibitors: captopril, enalapril, lisinopril (see Drugs Glossary)	May decrease ACE inhibitor effect.
Anticoagulants (oral, see Drugs Glossary)	Increased risk of bleeding.
Aspirin	Increased risk of stomach ulcer.
Beta-adrenergic blockers (see Drugs Glossary)	Decreased antihypertensive effect.
Cortisone drugs	Increased risk of stomach ulcer.
Diuretics (see Drugs Glossary)	May decrease diuretic effect.
Lithium	Possible increase in effect and toxicity.
Methotrexate	May increase toxicity.
Minoxidil	Decreased minoxidil effect.
Oxyphenbutazone	Possible stomach ulcer.
Phenylbutazone	Possible stomach ulcer.
Probenecid	Increased NSAID effect.
Thyroid hormones	Rapid heartbeat, blood-pressure rise.

POSSIBLE INTERACTION WITH OTHER SUBSTANCES

INTERACTS WITH	COMBINED EFFECT
Alcohol:	Possible stomach ulcer or bleeding.
Beverages:	None expected.
Cocaine (or crack):	None expected.
Foods:	None expected.
Marijuana:	Increased pain relief from NSAIDs.
Tobacco:	None expected.

MEDICATIONS

APPETITE SUPPRESSANTS

BRAND & GENERIC NAMES

See complete list of brand and generic names in the Brand & Generic Name Directory.

BASIC INFORMATION

Habit forming? Yes
Prescription needed? Yes
Available as generic? Yes
Drug class: Appetite suppressant

USES

Suppresses appetite.

DOSAGE & USAGE INFORMATION

How to take:
- Tablet or capsule—Swallow with liquid. You may chew or crush tablet.
- Extended-release tablets or capsules—Swallow each dose whole with liquid; do not crush.
- Elixir—Swallow with liquid.

When to take:
- Long-acting forms—10 to 14 hours before bedtime.
- Short-acting forms—1 hour before meals. Last dose no later than 4 to 6 hours before bedtime.

If you forget a dose:
- Long-acting form—Take as soon as you remember up to 2 hours late. • If more than 2 hours, wait for next scheduled dose (don't double this dose).
- Short-acting form—Wait for next scheduled dose. Don't double this dose.

Continued next column

OVERDOSE

SYMPTOMS:
Irritability, overactivity, trembling, insomnia, mood changes, fever, rapid heartbeat, confusion, disorientation, hallucinations, convulsions, coma.
WHAT TO DO:
- **Dial 0 (operator) or 911 (emergency) for an ambulance or medical help. Then give first aid immediately.**
- **See emergency information at the back of this book.**

What drug does:
Apparently stimulates brain's appetite-control center.

Time lapse before drug works:
Begins in 1 hour. Short-acting form lasts 4 hours. Long-acting form lasts 14 hours.

Don't take with:
Any other medicines, even over-the-counter drugs such as cough and cold medicines, nose drops, diet pills, laxatives or caffeine, without consulting your doctor.

POSSIBLE ADVERSE REACTIONS OR SIDE EFFECTS

SYMPTOMS	WHAT TO DO
Life-threatening: None expected.	
Common: Irritability, nervousness, insomnia, false sense of well-being.	Continue. Call doctor when convenient.
Infrequent: • Irregular or pounding heartbeat, urgent or difficult urination.	Discontinue. Call doctor right away.
• Blurred vision, unpleasant taste or dry mouth, constipation or diarrhea, nausea, vomiting, cramps, changes in sex drive, increased sweating.	Continue. Call doctor when convenient.
Rare: • Mood changes, rash or hives, breathing difficulty.	Discontinue. Call doctor right away.
• Hair loss.	Continue. Call doctor when convenient.

WARNINGS & PRECAUTIONS

Don't take if:
- You are allergic to any sympathomimetic or phenylpropanolamine.
- You have glaucoma.
- You have taken MAO inhibitors within 2 weeks.
- You plan to become pregnant within medication period.
- You have a history of drug abuse.
- You have irregular or rapid heartbeat.

Before you start, consult your doctor:
- If you have high blood pressure or heart disease.
- If you have an overactive thyroid, nervous tension or "anxiety."
- If you have epilepsy.
- If you will have surgery within 2 months, including dental surgery, requiring general or spinal anesthesia.

Pregnancy:
Safety not established. Avoid.

Infants & children
Don't give to children younger than 12.

Prolonged use:
Loses effectiveness. Avoid.

Skin & sunlight:
No age-related problems expected.

Driving or hazardous activities:
Don't drive or pilot aircraft until you learn how medicine affects you. Don't work around dangerous machinery. Don't climb ladders or work in high places. Danger increases if you drink alcohol or take medicine affecting alertness and reflexes, such as antihistamines, tranquilizers, sedatives, pain medicine, narcotics and mind-altering drugs.

Discontinuing:
Dose may require gradual reduction if you have taken drug for a long time. Doses of other drugs may also require adjustment.

Others:
Don't increase dose.

POSSIBLE INTERACTION WITH OTHER DRUGS

GENERIC NAME OR DRUG CLASS	COMBINED EFFECT
Antihypertensives (see Drugs Glossary)	Decreased antihyper-tensive effect.
Appetite suppressants (other, see Drugs Glossary)	Dangerous overstimulation.
Caffeine	Increased nervous stimulant effect of appetite suppressants.
Guanethidine	Decreased guanethidine effect.
Hydralazine	Decreased hydralazine effect.
MAO inhibitors (see Drugs Glossary)	Dangerous blood-pressure rise.
Methyldopa	Decreased methyldopa effect.
Molindone	Decreased suppressant effect.
Phenothiazines (see Drugs Glossary)	Decreased appetite suppressant effect.
Rauwolfia alkaloids (see Drugs Glossary)	Decreased effect of rauwolfia alkaloids.
Sodium bicarbonate	Increased action of amphetamines.

POSSIBLE INTERACTION WITH OTHER SUBSTANCES

INTERACTS WITH	COMBINED EFFECT
Alcohol: Beer, chianti wines, vermouth.	Dangerous blood-pressure rise.
Beverages: Caffeine drinks.	Excessive stimulation.
Drinks containing tyramine (see Drugs Glossary).	Blood-pressure rise.
Cocaine (or crack):	Excessive stimulation.
Foods: Foods containing tyramine (see Drugs Glossary).	Blood-pressure rise.
Marijuana:	Frequent use—Irregular heartbeat.
Tobacco:	Increased heartbeat rate.

MEDICATIONS

ASPIRIN

BRAND & GENERIC NAMES

See complete list of brand and generic names in the Brand & Generic Name Directory.

BASIC INFORMATION

Habit forming? No
Prescription needed? No
Available as generic? Yes
Drug class: Analgesic, anti-inflammatory (salicylate)

USES

- Reduces pain, fever, inflammation.
- Relieves swelling, stiffness, joint pain of arthritis or rheumatism.
- Antiplatelet effect.

DOSAGE & USAGE INFORMATION

How to take:
- Tablet or capsule—Swallow with liquid.
- Extended-release tablets or capsules—Swallow each dose whole.
- Effervescent tablets—Dissolve in water.
- Chewing gum tablets—Chew completely. Don't swallow whole.
- Suppositories—Remove wrapper and moisten suppository with water. Gently insert into rectum, large end first.

When to take:
Pain, fever, inflammation—As needed, no more often than every 4 hours.

If you forget a dose:
- Pain, fever—Take as soon as you remember. Wait 4 hours for next dose.
- Arthritis—Take as soon as you remember up to 2 hours late. Return to regular schedule.

Continued next column

OVERDOSE

SYMPTOMS:
Ringing in ears; nausea; vomiting; dizziness; fever; deep, rapid breathing; hallucinations; convulsions; coma.
WHAT TO DO:
- **Dial 0 (operator) or 911 (emergency) for an ambulance or medical help. Then give first aid immediately.**
- **See emergency information at the back of this book.**

What drug does:
- Affects hypothalamus, the part of the brain which regulates temperature by dilating small blood vessels in skin.
- Prevents clumping of platelets (small blood cells) so blood vessels remain open.
- Decreases prostaglandin effect.
- Suppresses body's pain messages.

Time lapse before drug works:
30 minutes for pain, fever, arthritis.

Don't take with:
Any other medicines, even over-the-counter drugs such as cough and cold medicines, nose drops, diet pills, laxatives or caffeine, without consulting your doctor.

POSSIBLE ADVERSE REACTIONS OR SIDE EFFECTS

SYMPTOMS	WHAT TO DO
Life-threatening:	
Black or bloody vomit; blood in urine; difficulty breathing; hives, rash, intense itching, faintness soon after a dose (anaphylaxis).	Seek emergency treatment immediately.
Common:	
• Nausea, vomiting.	Discontinue. Seek emergency treatment.
• Heartburn, indigestion.	Continue. Call doctor when convenient.
• Ringing in ears.	Continue. Tell doctor at next visit.
Infrequent:	
None expected.	
Rare:	
• Black stools, unexplained fever.	Discontinue. Seek emergency treatment.
• Rash, hives, itch, diminished vision, shortness of breath, wheezing, jaundice, mental confusion.	Discontinue. Call doctor right away.
• Drowsiness.	Continue. Call doctor when convenient.

WARNINGS & PRECAUTIONS

Don't take if:
• You need to restrict sodium in your diet. Buffered effervescent tablets and sodium salicylate are high in sodium.
• You are sensitive to aspirin or aspirin has a strong vinegar-like odor, which means it has decomposed.
• You have a peptic ulcer of the stomach or duodenum or a bleeding disorder.

Before you start, consult your doctor:
• If you have had stomach or duodenal ulcers.
• If you have had gout.
• If you have asthma or nasal polyps.

Pregnancy:
Risk to unborn child outweighs drug benefits. Don't use.

Infants & children:
• Overdose frequent and severe. Keep bottles out of children's reach.
• Consult doctor before giving to persons under age 18 who have fever and discomfort of viral illness, especially chickenpox and influenza. Probably increases risk of Reye's syndrome.

Prolonged use:
Kidney damage. Periodic kidney-function test recommended.

Skin & sunlight:
Aspirin combined with sunscreen may decrease sunburn.

Driving or hazardous activities:
No restrictions unless you feel drowsy.

Discontinuing:
For chronic illness—Don't discontinue without doctor's advice until you complete prescribed dose, even though symptoms diminish or disappear.

Others:
• Aspirin can complicate surgery, pregnancy, labor and delivery, and illness.
• For arthritis—Don't change dose without consulting doctor.
• Urine tests for blood sugar may be inaccurate.

POSSIBLE INTERACTION WITH OTHER DRUGS

GENERIC NAME OR DRUG CLASS	COMBINED EFFECT
Acebutolol	Decreased antihypertensive effect of acebutolol.
ACE inhibitors: captopril, enalapril, lisinopril (see Drugs Glossary)	Decreased ACE inhibitor effect.
Allopurinol	Decreased allopurinol effect.
Antacids (see Drugs Glossary)	Decreased aspirin effect.
Anticoagulants (see Drugs Glossary)	Increased anticoagulant effect. Abnormal bleeding.
Antidiabetics (oral, see Drugs Glossary)	Low blood sugar.
Aspirin (other)	Likely aspirin toxicity.
Bumetanide	Possible aspirin toxicity.
Cortisone drugs (see Drugs Glossary)	Increased cortisone effect. Risk of ulcers and stomach bleeding.
Ethacrynic acid	Possible aspirin toxicity.

See Additional Drug Interactions Section

POSSIBLE INTERACTION WITH OTHER SUBSTANCES

INTERACTS WITH	COMBINED EFFECT
Alcohol:	Possible stomach irritation and bleeding. Avoid.
Beverages:	None expected.
Cocaine (or crack):	None expected.
Foods:	None expected.
Marijuana:	Possible increased pain relief, but marijuana may slow body's recovery. Avoid.
Tobacco:	None expected.

BARBITURATES

BRAND & GENERIC NAMES

See complete list of brand and generic names in the Brand & Generic Name Directory.

BASIC INFORMATION

Habit forming? Yes
Prescription needed? Yes
Available as generic? Yes
Drug class: Sedative, hypnotic (barbiturate), anticonvulsant

USES

- Relieves insomnia (higher bedtime dose).
- Prevents convulsions or seizures, such as epilepsy.

DOSAGE & USAGE INFORMATION

How to take:
Tablet, liquid or capsule—Swallow with liquid or food to lessen stomach irritation. If you can't swallow whole, crumble tablet or open capsule and take with liquid or food.

When to take:
At the same times each day.

If you forget a dose:
Take as soon as you remember up to 2 hours late. If more than 2 hours, wait for next scheduled dose (don't double this dose).

What drug does:
May partially block nerve impulses at nerve-cell connections.

Time lapse before drug works:
60 minutes.

Don't take with:
Any other medicines, even over-the-counter drugs such as cough and cold medicines, nose drops, diet pills, laxatives or caffeine, without consulting your doctor.

OVERDOSE

SYMPTOMS:
Deep sleep, weak pulse, coma.
WHAT TO DO:
- **Dial 0 (operator) or 911 (emergency) for an ambulance or medical help. Then give first aid immediately.**
- **See emergency information at the back of this book.**

POSSIBLE ADVERSE REACTIONS OR SIDE EFFECTS

SYMPTOMS	WHAT TO DO
Life-threatening:	
Hives, rash, intense itching, faintness soon after a dose (anaphylaxis).	Seek emergency treatment immediately.
Common:	
Dizziness, drowsiness, "hangover" effect.	Continue. Call doctor when convenient.
Infrequent:	
• Rash or hives, face or lip swelling, swollen eyelids, sore throat, fever.	Discontinue. Call doctor right away.
• Depression, confusion, slurred speech, diarrhea, nausea, vomiting, joint or muscle pain.	Continue. Call doctor when convenient.
Rare:	
• Agitation, slow heartbeat, difficult breathing, jaundice.	Discontinue. Call doctor right away.
• Unexplained bleeding or bruising.	Continue. Call doctor when convenient.

WARNINGS & PRECAUTIONS

Don't take if:
- You are allergic to any barbiturate.
- You have porphyria.

Before you start, consult your doctor:
- If you have epilepsy.
- If you have kidney or liver damage.
- If you have asthma.
- If you have anemia.
- If you have chronic pain.
- If you will have surgery within 2 months, including dental surgery, requiring general or spinal anesthesia.

Pregnancy:
Risk to unborn child outweighs drug benefits. Don't use.

Infants & children:
Use only under doctor's supervision.

Prolonged use:
- May cause addiction, anemia, chronic intoxication.
- May lower body temperature, making exposure to cold temperatures hazardous.

Skin & sunlight:
May cause rash or intensify sunburn in areas exposed to sun or sunlamp.

Driving or hazardous activities:
Don't drive or pilot aircraft until you learn how medicine affects you. Don't work around dangerous machinery. Don't climb ladders or work in high places. Danger increases if you drink alcohol or take medicine affecting alertness and reflexes.

Discontinuing:
May be unnecessary to finish medicine. Follow doctor's instructions. If you develop withdrawal symptoms of hallucinations, agitation or sleeplessness after discontinuing, call doctor right away.

Others:
Great potential for abuse.

POSSIBLE INTERACTION WITH OTHER DRUGS

GENERIC NAME OR DRUG CLASS	COMBINED EFFECT
Anticoagulants (oral, see Drugs Glossary)	Decreased anticoagulant effect.
Anticonvulsants	Changed seizure
(see Drugs Glossary)	patterns.
Antidepressants, tricyclics (TCA, see Drugs Glossary)	Decreased antidepressant effect. Possible dangerous oversedation.
Antidiabetics (oral, see Drugs Glossary)	Increased barbiturate effect.
Antihistamines (see Drugs Glossary)	Dangerous sedation. Avoid.
Aspirin	Decreased aspirin effect.
Beta-adrenergic blockers (see Drugs Glossary)	Decreased effect of beta-adrenergic blocker.
Contraceptives (oral, see Drugs Glossary)	Decreased contraceptive effect.
Cortisone drugs (see Drugs Glossary)	Decreased cortisone effect.
Cyclosporine	Decreased effect of cyclosporine.
Digitoxin	Decreased digitoxin effect.
Disulfiram	Possible increased barbiturate effect.
Doxycycline	Decreased doxycycline effect.
Dronabinol	Increased effects of both drugs. Avoid.
Estrogens (see Drugs Glossary)	Decreased estrogen effect.
Griseofulvin	Decreased griseofulvin effect.
Indapamide	Increased indapamide effect.
Leucovorin (large doses)	May counteract anti-convulsant effect of barbiturate anticonvulsants.
Loxapine	Decreased anticonvulsant effect of all barbiturate anticonvulsants.
MAO inhibitors (see Drugs Glossary)	Increased barbiturate effect.
Metronidazole	Possible decreased metronidazole effect.
Mind-altering drugs (see Drugs Glossary)	Dangerous sedation. Avoid.

See Additional Drug Interactions Section

POSSIBLE INTERACTION WITH OTHER SUBSTANCES

INTERACTS WITH	COMBINED EFFECT
Alcohol:	Possible fatal oversedation. Avoid.
Beverages:	None expected.
Cocaine (or crack):	Decreased barbiturate effect.
Foods:	None expected.
Marijuana:	Excessive sedation. Avoid.
Tobacco:	None expected.

BECLOMETHASONE

BRAND NAMES

Beclovent
Beclovent Rotacaps
Beconase Inhaler
Becotide
Propaderm
Vancenase Inhaler
Vanceril

BASIC INFORMATION

Habit forming? No
Prescription needed? Yes
Available as generic? No
Drug class: Cortisone drug (adrenal corticosteroid, see Drugs Glossary), antiasthmatic

USES

Prevents attacks of bronchial asthma and allergic hay fever. Does not stop an active asthma attack.

DOSAGE & USAGE INFORMATION

How to take:
- Aerosol—Follow package instructions. Don't inhale more than 4 times twice a day. Rinse mouth after use to prevent hoarseness, throat irritation and mouth infection. Wait at least 1 minute between inhalations.
- Use other inhaled asthma drugs before beclomethasone.

When to take:
Regularly at the same times each day.

If you forget a dose:
Take as soon as you remember up to 2 hours late. If more than 2 hours, wait for next scheduled dose (don't double this dose).

What drug does:
Reduces inflammation in bronchial tubes.

Continued next column

OVERDOSE

SYMPTOMS:
Fluid retention, flushed face, nervousness, stomach irritation.
WHAT TO DO:
Overdose unlikely to threaten life. If the child inhales much larger amount than prescribed, call doctor, poison-control center or hospital emergency room for instructions.

Time lapse before drug works:
1 to 4 weeks.

Don't take with:
Any other medicines, even over-the-counter drugs such as cough and cold medicines, nose drops, diet pills, laxatives or caffeine, without consulting your doctor.

POSSIBLE ADVERSE REACTIONS OR SIDE EFFECTS

SYMPTOMS	WHAT TO DO
Life-threatening: None expected.	
Common: Fungus infection with white patches in mouth, dryness, sore throat.	Continue. Call doctor when convenient.
Infrequent: • Rash.	Discontinue. Call doctor right away.
• Lung inflammation, spasm of bronchial tubes.	Continue. Call doctor when convenient.
Rare: None expected.	

WARNINGS & PRECAUTIONS

Don't take if:
- You are allergic to beclomethasone.
- You have had tuberculosis or a systemic fungal infection.
- You are having an asthma attack.

Before you start, consult your doctor:
- If you take other cortisone drugs.
- If you have an infection.

Pregnancy:
Risk to unborn child outweighs drug benefits. Don't use.

Infants & children:
Use only under medical supervision.

Prolonged use:
No age-related problems expected.

Skin & sunlight:
No age-related problems expected.

Driving or hazardous activities:
No age-related problems expected.

Discontinuing:
Don't discontinue without doctor's advice until you complete prescribed dose, even though symptoms diminish or disappear.

Others:
- Unrelated illness or injury may require cortisone drugs by mouth or injection. Notify your doctor.
- Consult doctor as soon as possible if your asthma returns while using beclamethasone as a preventive.
- Drug can reactivate tuberculosis or lung fungal infection. If you have ever had a positive skin test for tuberculosis, consult your doctor before taking.
- Consult doctor frequently if changing from oral cortisone drug to beclomethasone inhaler.

POSSIBLE INTERACTION WITH OTHER DRUGS

GENERIC NAME OR DRUG CLASS	COMBINED EFFECT
Albuterol	Increased beclomethasone effect.
Antiasthmatics (other, see Drugs Glossary)	Increased antiasthmatic effect.
Bitolerol	Increased beclomethasone effect.
Ephedrine	Increased beclomethasone effect.
Epinephrine	Increased beclomethasone effect.
Indapamide	Possible excessive potassium loss, causing dangerous heartbeat irregularity.
Isoetharine	Increased beclomethasone effect.
Isoproterenol	Increased beclomethasone effect.
Metaproterenol	Increased beclomethasone effect.
Potassium supplements (see Drugs Glossary)	Decreased potassium effect.
Terbutaline	Increased beclomethasone effect.
Theophylline	Increased beclomethasone effect.

POSSIBLE INTERACTION WITH OTHER SUBSTANCES

INTERACTS WITH	COMBINED EFFECT
Alcohol:	None expected.
Beverages:	None expected.
Cocaine (or crack):	None expected.
Foods:	None expected.
Marijuana:	Decreased beclomethasone effect.
Tobacco:	Decreased beclomethasone effect.

BELLADONNA ALKALOIDS & BARBITURATES

BRAND & GENERIC NAMES

See complete list of brand and generic names in the Brand & Generic Name Directory.

BASIC INFORMATION

Habit forming? Yes
Prescription needed? Yes
Available as generic? Some yes, some no
Drug class: Antispasmodic, anticholinergic, sedative (see Drugs Glossary)

USES

• Reduces spasms of digestive system, bladder and urethra.
• Reduces anxiety or nervous tension (low dose).
• Relieves insomnia (higher bedtime dose).

DOSAGE & USAGE INFORMATION

How to take:
• Tablet, liquid or capsule—Swallow with liquid or food to lessen stomach irritation. If you can't swallow whole, crumble tablet or open capsule and take with liquid or food.
• Extended-release tablets or capsules—Swallow each dose whole.
• Chewable tablets—Chew well before swallowing.
• Drops—Dilute dose in beverage before swallowing.

When to take:
At the same times each day.

If you forget a dose:
Take as soon as you remember up to 2 hours late. If more than 2 hours, wait for next scheduled dose (don't double this dose).

Continued next column

OVERDOSE

SYMPTOMS:
Blurred vision, confusion, convulsions, irregular heartbeat, hallucinations, coma.
WHAT TO DO:
• **Dial 0 (operator) or 911 (emergency) for an ambulance or medical help. Then give first aid immediately.**
• **See emergency information at the back of this book.**

What drug does:
• May partially block nerve impulses at nerve-cell connections.
• Blocks nerve impulses at parasympathetic nerve endings, preventing muscle contractions and gland secretions of organs involved.

Time lapse before drug works:
15 to 30 minutes.

Don't take with:
Any other medicines, even over-the-counter drugs such as cough and cold medicines, nose drops, diet pills, laxatives or caffeine, without consulting your doctor.

POSSIBLE ADVERSE REACTIONS OR SIDE EFFECTS

SYMPTOMS	WHAT TO DO
Life-threatening:	
Unusual excitement, restlessness, fast heartbeat, breathing difficulty.	Seek emergency treatment immediately.
Common:	
• Dry mouth, throat, nose; drowsiness; constipation; dizziness; nausea; vomiting; "hangover" effect; depression; confusion.	Discontinue. Call doctor right away.
• Reduced sweating, slurred speech, agitation.	Continue. Call doctor when convenient.
Infrequent:	
Difficult urination; difficult swallowing; rash or hives; face, lip or eyelid swelling; joint or muscle pain.	Discontinue. Call doctor right away.
Rare:	
Jaundice; unusual bruising or bleeding; hives, skin rash; pain in eyes; blurred vision; sore throat, fever, mouth sores; unexplained bleeding or bruising.	Discontinue. Call doctor right away.

WARNINGS & PRECAUTIONS

Don't take if:
- You are allergic to any barbiturate or any anticholinergic.
- You have porphyria, trouble with stomach bloating, difficulty emptying your bladder completely, narrow-angle glaucoma, severe ulcerative colitis.

Before you start, consult your doctor:
- If you have open-angle glaucoma, angina, chronic bronchitis or asthma, hiatal hernia, liver disease, enlarged prostate, myasthenia gravis, peptic ulcer, epilepsy, kidney or liver damage, anemia, chronic pain.
- If you will have surgery within 2 months, including dental surgery, requiring general or spinal anesthesia.

Pregnancy:
Risk to unborn child outweighs drug benefits. Don't use.

Infants & children:
Use only under doctor's supervision.

Prolonged use:
- May cause addiction, anemia, chronic intoxication.
- May lower body temperature, making exposure to cold temperatures hazardous.

Skin & sunlight:
May cause rash or intensify sunburn in areas exposed to sun or sunlamp.

Driving or hazardous activities:
Don't drive or pilot aircraft until you learn how medicine affects you. Don't work around dangerous machinery. Don't climb ladders or work in high places. Danger increases if you drink alcohol or take medicine affecting alertness and reflexes.

Discontinuing:
May be unnecessary to finish medicine. Follow doctor's instructions. If you develop withdrawal symptoms of hallucinations, agitation or sleeplessness after discontinuing, call doctor right away.

Others:
Great potential for abuse.

POSSIBLE INTERACTION WITH OTHER DRUGS

GENERIC NAME OR DRUG CLASS	COMBINED EFFECT
Acetaminophen	Possible decreased barbiturate effect.
Amantadine	Increased belladonna effect.
Anticoagulants (oral, see Drugs Glossary)	Decreased anticoagulant effect.
Anticholinergics (other, see Drugs Glossary)	Increased belladonna effect.
Anticonvulsants (see Drugs Glossary)	Changed seizure patterns.
Antidepressants, tricyclics (TCA, see Drugs Glossary)	Possible dangerous oversedation. Avoid.
Antidiabetics (oral, see Drugs Glossary)	Increased barbiturate effect.
Antihistamines (see Drugs Glossary)	Dangerous sedation. Avoid.
Aspirin	Decreased aspirin effect.
Beta-adrenergic blockers (see Drugs Glossary)	Decreased effects of beta-adrenergic blocker.
Contraceptives (oral, see Glossary)	Decreased contraceptive effect.

See Additional Drug Interactions Section.

POSSIBLE INTERACTION WITH OTHER SUBSTANCES

INTERACTS WITH	COMBINED EFFECT
Alcohol:	Possible fatal oversedation. Avoid.
Beverages:	None expected.
Cocaine (or crack):	Excessively rapid heartbeat. Avoid.
Foods:	None expected.
Marijuana:	Drowsiness and dry mouth. Avoid.
Tobacco:	Decreased effectiveness of acid reduction in stomach.

BENZODIAZEPINES

BRAND & GENERIC NAMES

See complete list of brand and generic names in the Brand & Generic Name Directory.

BASIC INFORMATION

Habit forming? Yes
Prescription needed? Yes
Available as generic? Yes
Drug class: Tranquilizer (benzodiazepine)

USES

- Treatment for nervousness or tension.
- Treatment for muscle spasm.
- Treatment for convulsive disorders.

DOSAGE & USAGE INFORMATION

How to take:
Tablet, extended-release capsule or liquid—Swallow with liquid. If you can't swallow whole, crumble tablet or open capsule and take with liquid or food.

When to take:
At the same time each day, according to instructions on prescription label.

If you forget a dose:
Take as soon as you remember up to 2 hours late. If more than 2 hours, wait for next scheduled dose (don't double this dose).

Continued next column

OVERDOSE

SYMPTOMS:
Drowsiness, weakness, tremor, stupor, coma.
WHAT TO DO:
- **Dial 0 (operator) or 911 (emergency) for an ambulance or medical help. Then give first aid immediately.**
- **If the child is unconscious and not breathing, give mouth-to-mouth breathing. If there is no heartbeat, use cardiac massage and mouth-to-mouth breathing (CPR). Don't try to make the child vomit. If you can't get help quickly, take the child to nearest emergency facility.**
- **See emergency information at the back of this book.**

What drug does:
Affects limbic system of brain—part that controls emotions.

Time lapse before drug works:
2 hours. May take 6 weeks for full benefit.

Don't take with:
Any other medicines, even over-the-counter drugs such as cough and cold medicines, nose drops, diet pills, laxatives or caffeine, without consulting your doctor.

POSSIBLE ADVERSE REACTIONS OR SIDE EFFECTS

SYMPTOMS	WHAT TO DO
Life-threatening:	
None expected.	
Common:	
Clumsiness, drowsiness, dizziness.	Continue. Call doctor when convenient.
Infrequent:	
• Hallucinations, confusion, depression, irritability, rash, itch, vision changes.	Discontinue. Call doctor right away.
• Constipation or diarrhea, nausea, vomiting, difficult urination, vivid dreams.	Continue. Call doctor when convenient.
Rare:	
• Slow heartbeat, breathing difficulty.	Discontinue. Seek emergency treatment.
• Mouth, throat ulcers; jaundice.	Discontinue. Call doctor right away.
• Decreased libido.	Continue. Call doctor when convenient.

WARNINGS & PRECAUTIONS

Don't take if:
- You are allergic to any benzodiazepine.
- You have myasthenia gravis.
- You are active or recovering alcoholic.
- Patient is younger than 6 months.

Before you start, consult your doctor:
- If you have liver, kidney or lung disease.
- If you have diabetes, epilepsy or porphyria.

Pregnancy:
Risk to unborn child outweighs drug benefits. Don't use.

Infants & children:
Use only under medical supervision for children older than 6 months.

Prolonged use:
May impair liver function.

Skin & sunlight:
No age-related problems expected.

Driving or hazardous activities:
Don't drive or pilot aircraft until you learn how medicine affects you. Don't work around dangerous machinery. Don't climb ladders or work in high places. Danger increases if you drink alcohol or take medicine affecting alertness and reflexes.

Discontinuing:
Don't discontinue without consulting doctor. Dose may require gradual reduction if you have taken drug for a long time. Doses of other drugs may also require adjustment.

Others:
- Hot weather, heavy exercise and profuse sweat may reduce excretion and cause overdose.
- Blood sugar may rise in diabetics, requiring insulin adjustment.

POSSIBLE INTERACTION WITH OTHER DRUGS

GENERIC NAME OR DRUG CLASS	COMBINED EFFECT
Anticonvulsants (see Drugs Glossary)	Change in seizure frequency or severity.
Antidepressants (see Drugs Glossary)	Increased sedative effect of both drugs.
Antihistamines (see Drugs Glossary)	Increased sedative effect of both drugs.
Antihypertensives (see Drugs Glossary)	Excessively low blood pressure.
Contraceptives (oral, see Drugs Glossary)	Increased benzodiazepine effect.
Disulfiram	Increased benzodiazepine effect.
Dronabinol	Increased effects of both drugs. Avoid.
Erythromycin	Increased benzodiazepine effect.
Ketoconazole	Increased benzodiazepine effect.
Levodopa	Possible decreased levodopa effect.
MAO inhibitors (see Drugs Glossary)	Convulsions, deep sedation, rage.
Molindone	Increased tranquilizer effect.
Narcotics	Increased sedative effect of both drugs.
Probenecid	Increased benzodiazepine effect.
Sedatives (see Drugs Glossary)	Increased sedative effect of both drugs.
Sleep inducers (see Drugs Glossary)	Increased sedative effect of both drugs.
Tranquilizers (see Drugs Glossary)	Increased sedative effect of both drugs.

POSSIBLE INTERACTION WITH OTHER SUBSTANCES

INTERACTS WITH	COMBINED EFFECT
Alcohol:	Heavy sedation. Avoid.
Beverages:	None expected.
Cocaine (or crack):	Decreased benzodiazepine effect.
Foods:	None expected.
Marijuana:	Heavy sedation. Avoid.
Tobacco:	Decreased benzodiazepine effect.

BENZTROPINE

BRAND NAMES

Apo-Benztropine
PMS-Benztropine
Bensylagentin

BASIC INFORMATION

Habit forming? No
Prescription needed? Yes
Available as generic? Yes
Drug class: Antidyskinetic, antiparkinsonism

USES

• Treatment of Parkinson's disease.
• Treatment of adverse effects of phenothiazines.

DOSAGE & USAGE INFORMATION

How to take:
Tablets—Take with food to lessen stomach irritation.

When to take:
At the same times each day.

If you forget a dose:
Take as soon as you remember up to 2 hours late. If more than 2 hours, wait for next scheduled dose (don't double this dose).

What drug does:
Improves muscle control and reduces stiffness.

Time lapse before drug works:
1 to 2 hours.

Continued next column

OVERDOSE

SYMPTOMS:
Agitation, dilated pupils, hallucinations, dry mouth, rapid heartbeat, sleepiness.
WHAT TO DO:
• Dial 0 (operator) or 911 (emergency) for an ambulance or medical help. Then give first aid immediately.
• If the child is unconscious and not breathing, give mouth-to-mouth breathing. If there is no heartbeat, use cardiac massage and mouth-to-mouth breathing (CPR). Don't try to make the child vomit. If you can't get help quickly, take the child to nearest emergency facility.
• See emergency information at the back of this book.

Don't take with:
Any other medicines, even over-the-counter drugs such as cough and cold medicines, nose drops, diet pills, laxatives or caffeine, without consulting your doctor.

POSSIBLE ADVERSE REACTIONS OR SIDE EFFECTS

Life-threatening:
None expected.

Common:

• Blurred vision, light sensitivity, constipation, nausea, vomiting.	Continue. Call doctor when convenient.
• Difficult or painful urination, dry mouth.	Continue. Tell doctor at next visit.

Infrequent:
None expected.

Rare:

• Rash, pain in eyes.	Discontinue. Call doctor right away.
• Confusion, dizziness, sore mouth or tongue, muscle cramps, numbness or weakness in hands or feet.	Continue. Call doctor when convenient.

WARNINGS & PRECAUTIONS

Don't take if:
You are allergic to any antidyskinetic.

Before you start, consult your doctor:
- If you have had glaucoma.
- If you have had high blood pressure or heart disease.
- If you have had impaired liver function.
- If you have had prostate trouble.
- If you have had myasthenia gravis.
- If you have had kidney disease, urination difficulty or ulcers.

Pregnancy:
Studies inconclusive on harm to unborn child. Animal studies show fetal abnormalities. Decide with your doctor whether drug benefits justify risk to unborn child.

Infants & children:
Not recommended for children 3 and younger. Use for older children only under doctor's supervision.

Prolonged use:
Possible glaucoma.

Skin & sunlight:
No age-related problems expected.

Driving or hazardous activities:
Don't drive or pilot aircraft until you learn how medicine affects you. Don't work around dangerous machinery. Don't climb ladders or work in high places. Danger increases if you drink alcohol or take medicine affecting alertness and reflexes, such as antihistamines, tranquilizers, sedatives, pain medicine, narcotics and mind-altering drugs.

Discontinuing:
Don't discontinue without consulting doctor. Dose may require gradual reduction if you have taken drug for a long time. Doses of other drugs may also require adjustment.

Others:
- Internal eye pressure should be measured regularly.
- Avoid becoming overheated.

POSSIBLE INTERACTION WITH OTHER DRUGS

GENERIC NAME OR DRUG CLASS	COMBINED EFFECT
Amantadine	Increased amantadine effect.
Antidepressants, tricyclic (TCA, see Drugs Glossary)	Increased benztropine effect. May cause glaucoma.
Antihistamines (see Drugs Glossary)	Increased benztropine effect.
Digoxin	May increase digoxin effect.
Levodopa	May decrease or increase levodopa effect. Improved results in treating Parkinson's disease.
Meperidine	Increased benztropine effect.
MAO inhibitors (see Drugs Glossary)	Increased benztropine effect.
Narcotics (see Drugs Glossary)	Increased benztropine effect.
Orphenadrine	Increased benztropine effect.
Phenothiazines (see Drugs Glossary)	Behavior changes.
Primidone	Excessive sedation.
Procainamide	Increased procainamide effect.
Quinidine	Increased benztropine effect.
Tranquilizers (see Drugs Glossary)	Excessive sedation.

POSSIBLE INTERACTION WITH OTHER SUBSTANCES

INTERACTS WITH	COMBINED EFFECT
Alcohol:	None expected.
Beverages:	None expected.
Cocaine (or crack):	Decreased benztropine effect. Avoid.
Foods:	None expected.
Marijuana:	None expected.
Tobacco:	None expected.

BETA-ADRENERGIC BLOCKING AGENTS

BRAND & GENERIC NAMES

See complete list of brand and generic names in the Brand & Generic Name Directory.

BASIC INFORMATION

Habit forming? No
Prescription needed? Yes
Available as generic? Yes
Drug class: Beta-adrenergic blocker

USES

- Reduces angina attacks.
- Stabilizes irregular heartbeat.
- Lowers blood pressure.
- Reduces frequency of migraine headaches. (Does not relieve headache pain.)
- Other uses prescribed by your doctor.

DOSAGE & USAGE INFORMATION

How to take:
Tablet, liquid or extended-release capsule—Swallow with liquid. If you can't swallow whole, crumble tablet or open capsule and take with liquid or food. Don't crush capsule.

When to take:
With meals or immediately after.

If you forget a dose:
Take as soon as you remember. Return to regular schedule, but allow 3 hours between doses.

Continued next column

What drug does:
- Blocks certain actions of sympathetic nervous system.
- Lowers heart's oxygen requirements.
- Slows nerve impulses through heart.
- Reduces blood vessel contraction in heart, scalp and other body parts.

Time lapse before drug works:
1 to 4 hours.

Don't take with:
Any other medicines, even over-the-counter drugs such as cough and cold medicines, nose drops, diet pills, laxatives or caffeine, without consulting your doctor.

OVERDOSE

SYMPTOMS:
Weakness, slow or weak pulse, blood-pressure drop, fainting, difficulty breathing, convulsions, cold and sweaty skin.
WHAT TO DO:
- **Dial 0 (operator) or 911 (emergency) for an ambulance or medical help. Then give first aid immediately.**
- **See emergency information at the back of this book.**

POSSIBLE ADVERSE REACTIONS OR SIDE EFFECTS

SYMPTOMS	WHAT TO DO
Life-threatening:	
Congestive heart failure.	Discontinue. Seek emergency treatment.
Common:	
• Pulse slower than 50 beats per minute.	Discontinue. Call doctor right away.
• Drowsiness, fatigue, numbness or tingling of fingers or toes, dizziness, diarrhea, nausea, weakness.	Continue. Call doctor when convenient.
• Cold hands or feet; dry mouth, eyes and skin.	Continue. Tell doctor at next visit.
Infrequent:	
• Hallucinations, nightmares, insomnia, headache, difficult breathing, joint pain, anxiety.	Discontinue. Call doctor right away.
• Confusion, reduced alertness, depression, impotence.	Continue. Call doctor when convenient.
• Constipation.	Continue. Tell doctor at next visit.
Rare:	
• Rash, sore throat, fever.	Discontinue. Call doctor right away.
• Unusual bleeding and bruising; dry, burning eyes; impotence.	Continue. Call doctor when convenient.

WARNINGS & PRECAUTIONS

Don't take if:
- You are allergic to any beta-adrenergic blocker.
- You have asthma.
- You have hay fever symptoms.
- You have taken MAO inhibitors in past 2 weeks.

Before you start, consult your doctor:
- If you have heart disease or poor circulation to the extremities.
- If you have hay fever, asthma, chronic bronchitis, emphysema.
- If you have overactive thyroid function.
- If you have impaired liver or kidney function.
- If you will have surgery within 2 months, including dental surgery, requiring general or spinal anesthesia.
- If you have diabetes or hypoglycemia.

Pregnancy:
Risk to unborn child outweighs drug benefits. Don't use.

Infants & children
Don't give to infants or young children unless prescribed and monitored by your physician.

Prolonged use:
Weakens heart muscle contractions.

Skin & sunlight:
No age-related problems expected.

Driving or hazardous activities:
Don't drive or pilot aircraft until you learn how medicine affects you. Don't work around dangerous machinery. Don't climb ladders or work in high places. Danger increases if you drink alcohol or take medicine affecting alertness and reflexes.

Discontinuing:
Don't discontinue without consulting doctor. Dose may require gradual reduction if you have taken drug for a long time. Doses of other drugs may also require adjustment.

Others:
May mask hypoglycemia.

POSSIBLE INTERACTION WITH OTHER DRUGS

GENERIC NAME OR DRUG CLASS	COMBINED EFFECT
ACE inhibitors: captopril, enalapril, lisinopril (see Drugs Glossary)	Increased antihypertensive effects of both drugs. Dosages may require adjustment.
Antidiabetics (see Drugs Glossary)	Increased antidiabetic effect.
Antihistamines (see Drugs Glossary)	Decreased antihistamine effect.
Antihypertensives (see Drugs Glossary)	Increased antihypertensive effect.
Barbiturates (see Drugs Glossary)	Increased barbiturate effect. Dangerous sedation.
Beta-agonists (see Drugs Glossary)	Decreased beta-agonist effect.
Betaxolol eyedrops	Possible increased beta-adrenergic blocker effect.
Digitalis preparations (see Drugs Glossary)	Can either increase or decrease heart rate. Improves irregular heartbeat.
Encainide	Increased effect of toxicity on heart muscle.

See Additional Drug Interactions Section

POSSIBLE INTERACTION WITH OTHER SUBSTANCES

INTERACTS WITH	COMBINED EFFECT
Alcohol:	Excessive blood-pressure drop. Avoid.
Beverages:	None expected.
Cocaine (or crack):	Irregular heartbeat. Avoid.
Foods:	None expected.
Marijuana:	Daily use—Impaired circulation to hands and feet.
Tobacco:	Possible irregular heartbeat.

BETA-ADRENERGIC BLOCKING AGENTS & THIAZIDE DIURETICS

BRAND & GENERIC NAMES

ATENOLOL & CHLORTHALIDONE
Co-Betaloc
Corzide
Inderide
Inderide LA
Lopressor HCT
METOPROLOL & HYDROCHLOROTHIAZIDE
NADOLOL & BENDROFLUMETHIAZIDE
Normozide
PINDOLOL & HYDROCHLOROTHIAZIDE
PROPRANOLOL & HYDROCHLOROTHIAZIDE
Tenoretic
Timolide
TIMOLOL & HYDROCHLOROTHIAZIDE
Trandate HCT
Viskazide

BASIC INFORMATION

Habit forming? No
Prescription needed? Yes
Available as generic? Yes
Drug class: Beta-adrenergic blocker, thiazide diuretic

USES

- Controls, but doesn't cure, high blood pressure.
- Reduces fluid retention (edema).
- Reduces angina attacks.
- Stabilizes irregular heartbeat.
- Lowers blood pressure.
- Reduces frequency of migraine headaches. (Does not relieve headache pain.)
- Other uses prescribed by your doctor.

DOSAGE & USAGE INFORMATION

How to take:
Extended-release capsules—Swallow with liquid. If you can't swallow whole, crumble tablet and take with liquid or food.

Continued next column

OVERDOSE

SYMPTOMS:
Irregular heartbeat (usually too slow), confusion, fainting, convulsions, coma.
WHAT TO DO:
- **Dial 0 (operator) or 911 (emergency) for an ambulance or medical help. Then give first aid immediately.**
- **See emergency information at the back of this book.**

When to take:
At the same time each day.

If you forget a dose:
Take as soon as you remember up to 4 hours late. If more than 4 hours, wait for next scheduled dose (don't double this dose).

What drug does:
- Forces sodium and water excretion, reducing body fluid.
- Relaxes muscle cells of small arteries.
- Reduced body fluid and relaxed arteries lower blood pressure.
- Blocks some of the actions of sympathetic nervous system.
- Lowers heart's oxygen requirements.
- Slows nerve impulses through heart.
- Reduces blood vessel contraction in heart, scalp and other body parts.

Time lapse before drug works:
- 1 to 4 hours for beta-blocker effect.
- May require several weeks to lower blood pressure.

Don't take with:
Any other medicines, even over-the-counter drugs such as cough and cold medicines, nose drops, diet pills, laxatives or caffeine, without consulting your doctor.

POSSIBLE ADVERSE REACTIONS OR SIDE EFFECTS

SYMPTOMS	WHAT TO DO
Life-threatening:	
Wheezing, chest pain, irregular heartbeat.	Seek emergency treatment immediately.
Common:	
• Dry mouth, weak pulse, vomiting, muscle cramps, increased thirst, mood changes.	Discontinue. Call doctor right away.
• Weakness, tiredness, dizziness, mental depression, diminished sex drive, constipation, nightmares, insomnia.	Continue. Call doctor when convenient.
Infrequent:	
Cold feet and hands, chest pain, breathing difficulty, anxiety, nervousness, headache, appetite loss, abdominal pain, numbness and tingling in fingers and toes.	Discontinue. Call doctor right away.

Rare:	
• Hives, skin rash; joint pain; jaundice; fever, sore throat, mouth ulcers.	Discontinue. Call doctor right away.
• Impotence.	Continue. Call doctor when convenient.

WARNINGS & PRECAUTIONS

Don't take if:
• You are allergic to any beta-adrenergic blocker or any thiazide diuretic drug.
• You have asthma or hay fever symptoms.
• You have taken MAO inhibitors in past two weeks.

Before you start, consult your doctor:
• If you have heart disease or poor circulation to the extremities.
• If you have hay fever, asthma, chronic bronchitis, emphysema, overactive thyroid function, impaired liver or kidney function, gout, diabetes, hypoglycemia, pancreas disorder, systemic lupus erythematosus.
• If you are allergic to any sulfa drug or tartrazine dye.
• If you will have surgery within 2 months, including dental surgery, requiring general or spinal anesthesia.

Pregnancy:
Risk to unborn child outweighs drug benefits. Don't use.

Infants & children
Don't give to infants or young children unless prescribed and monitored by your physician.

Prolonged use:
• Weakens heart muscle contractions.
• You may need medicine to treat high blood pressure for the rest of your life.

Skin & sunlight:
May cause rash or intensify sunburn in areas exposed to sun or sunlamp.

Driving or hazardous activities:
Don't drive or pilot aircraft until you learn how medicine affects you. Don't work around dangerous machinery. Don't climb ladders or work in high places. Danger increases if you drink alcohol or take medicine affecting alertness and reflexes, such as antihistamines, tranquilizers, sedatives, pain medicine, narcotics and mind-altering drugs.

Discontinuing:
Don't discontinue without consulting doctor. Dose may require gradual reduction if you have taken drug for a long time. Doses of other drugs may also require adjustment.

Others:
• May mask hypoglycemia symptoms.
• Hot weather and fever may cause dehydration and drop in blood pressure. Dose may require temporary adjustment. Weigh daily and report any unexpected weight decreases to your doctor.
• May cause rise in uric acid, leading to gout.
• May cause blood-sugar rise in diabetics.

POSSIBLE INTERACTION WITH OTHER DRUGS

GENERIC NAME OR DRUG CLASS	COMBINED EFFECT
Allopurinol	Decreased allopurinol effect.
Antidepressants, tricyclic (TCA, see Drugs Glossary)	Dangerous drop in blood pressure. Avoid combination unless under medical supervision.
Antidiabetics (see Drugs Glossary)	Increased antidiabetic effect.
Antihistamines (see Drugs Glossary)	Decreased antihistamine effect.

See Additional Drug Interactions Section

POSSIBLE INTERACTION WITH OTHER SUBSTANCES

INTERACTS WITH	COMBINED EFFECT
Alcohol	Dangerous blood-pressure drop. Avoid.
Beverages:	None expected.
Cocaine (or crack):	Irregular heartbeat. Avoid.
Foods:	
Licorice.	Excessive potassium loss that causes dangerous heart rhythms.
Marijuana:	May increase blood pressure.
Tobacco:	May increase blood pressure and make heart work harder. Avoid.

MEDICATIONS

BUTALBITAL & ASPIRIN (Also contains caffeine)

BRAND & GENERIC NAMES

Axotal	Fiorgen PF
B-A-C	Fiorinal
Buff-A-Comp	Isollyl (Improved)
Butalbital A-C	Lanorinal
BUTALBITAL, ASPIRIN & CAFFEINE	Marnal
Butal Compound	Protension
	Tenstan

BASIC INFORMATION

Habit forming? Yes
Prescription needed? Yes
Available as generic? Yes
Drug class: Analgesic, anti-inflammatory, sedative

USES

- Reduces anxiety or nervous tension (low dose).
- Reduces pain, fever, inflammation.

DOSAGE & USAGE INFORMATION

How to take:
- Tablet or capsule—Swallow with liquid or food to lessen stomach irritation. If you can't swallow whole, crumble tablet or open capsule and take with liquid or food.
- Suppositories—Remove wrapper and moisten suppository with water. Gently insert into rectum, large end first.

When to take:
At the same times each day. No more often than every 4 hours.

Continued next column

If you forget a dose:
Take as soon as you remember up to 2 hours late. If more than 2 hours, wait for next scheduled dose (don't double this dose).

What drug does:
- May partially block nerve impulses at nerve-cell connections.
- Affects hypothalamus, the part of the brain which regulates temperature by dilating small blood vessels in skin.
- Prevents clumping of platelets (small blood cells) so blood vessels remain open.
- Decreases prostaglandin effect.
- Suppresses body's pain messages.

Time lapse before drug works:
30 minutes.

Don't take with:
Any other medicines, even over-the-counter drugs such as cough and cold medicines, nose drops, diet pills, laxatives or caffeine, without consulting your doctor.

OVERDOSE

SYMPTOMS:
Deep sleep, weak pulse, ringing in ears, nausea, vomiting, dizziness, fever, deep and rapid breathing, hallucinations, convulsions, coma.
WHAT TO DO:
- **Dial 0 (operator) or 911 (emergency) for an ambulance or medical help. Then give first aid immediately.**
- **See emergency information at the back of this book.**

POSSIBLE ADVERSE REACTIONS OR SIDE EFFECTS

SYMPTOMS	WHAT TO DO
Life-threatening:	
Hives, rash, intense itching, faintness soon after a dose (anaphylaxis); wheezing; tightness in chest; black or bloody vomit; black stools; shortness of breath.	Seek emergency treatment immediately.
Common:	
Dizziness, drowsiness, heartburn.	Continue. Call doctor when convenient.
Infrequent:	
Jaundice; vomiting blood; easy bruising; skin rash, hives; confusion; depression; sore throat, fever, mouth sores; hearing loss; slurred speech; decreased vision.	Discontinue. Call doctor right away.
Rare:	
• Diminished vision, blood in urine, unexplained fever.	Discontinue. Call doctor right away.
• Insomnia, nightmares, constipation, headache, jaundice, nervousness.	Continue. Call doctor when convenient.

BUTALBITAL & ASPIRIN (Also contains caffeine)

WARNINGS & PRECAUTIONS

Don't take if:
• You are allergic to any barbiturate or aspirin.
• You have a peptic ulcer of stomach or duodenum, bleeding disorder, porphyria.

Before you start, consult your doctor:
• If you have had stomach or duodenal ulcers.
• If you have asthma, nasal polyps, epilepsy, kidney or liver damage, anemia, chronic pain.
• If you will have surgery within 2 months, including dental surgery, requiring general or spinal anesthesia.

Pregnancy:
Risk to unborn child outweighs drug benefits. Don't use.

Infants & children:
• Overdose frequent and severe. Keep bottles out of children's reach.
• Use only under doctor's supervision.

Prolonged use:
• Kidney damage. Periodic kidney-function test recommended.
• May cause addiction, anemia, chronic intoxication.
• May lower body temperature, making exposure to cold temperatures hazardous.

Skin & sunlight:
May cause rash or intensify sunburn in areas exposed to sun or sunlamp.

Driving or hazardous activities:
Don't drive or pilot aircraft until you learn how medicine affects you. Don't work around dangerous machinery. Don't climb ladders or work in high places. Danger increases if you drink alcohol or take medicine affecting alertness and reflexes, such as antihistamines, tranquilizers, sedatives, pain medicine, narcotics and mind-altering drugs.

Discontinuing:
May be unnecessary to finish medicine. Follow doctor's instructions. If you develop withdrawal symptoms of hallucinations, agitation or sleeplessness after discontinuing, call doctor right away.

Others:
• Aspirin can complicate surgery, pregnancy, labor and delivery, and illness.
• For arthritis—Don't change dose without consulting doctor.
• Urine tests for blood sugar may be inaccurate.
• Great potential for abuse.

POSSIBLE INTERACTION WITH OTHER DRUGS

GENERIC NAME OR DRUG CLASS	COMBINED EFFECT
Allopurinol	Decreased allopurinol effect.
Antacids (see Drugs Glossary)	Decreased aspirin effect.
Anticoagulants (oral, see Drugs Glossary)	Increased anticoagulant effect. Abnormal bleeding.
Anticonvulsants (see Drugs Glossary)	Changed seizure patterns.
Antidepressants (see Drugs Glossary)	Decreased antidepressant effect. Possible dangerous oversedation.
Antidiabetics (oral, see Drugs Glossary)	Increased butalbital effect. Low blood sugar.
Antihistamines (see Drugs Glossary)	Dangerous sedation. Avoid.
Aspirin (other)	Likely aspirin toxicity.

See Additional Drug Interactions Section

POSSIBLE INTERACTION WITH OTHER SUBSTANCES

INTERACTS WITH	COMBINED EFFECT
Alcohol:	Possible stomach irritation and bleeding, possible fatal oversedation. Avoid.
Beverages:	None expected.
Cocaine (or crack):	Decreased butalbital effect.
Foods:	None expected.
Marijuana:	Possible increased pain relief, but marijuana may slow body's recovery. Avoid.
Tobacco:	None expected.

CALCIUM CHANNEL BLOCKING AGENTS

BRAND & GENERIC NAMES

Adalat	**Isoptin**
Calan	**Isoptin SR**
Calan SR	**NIFEDIPINE**
Cardizem	**Procardia**
DILTIAZEM	**VERAPAMIL**

BASIC INFORMATION

Habit forming? No
Prescription needed? Yes
Available as generic? No
Drug class: Calcium-channel blocker, antiarrhythmic, antianginal

USES

- Prevents angina attacks.
- Treats Reynaud's disease.
- Treats high blood pressure.
- Treats spasm of the esophagus.

DOSAGE & USAGE INFORMATION

How to take:
Capsule or extended-release tablet—Swallow with liquid.

When to take:
At the same times each day 1 hour before or 2 hours after eating.

Continued next column

If you forget a dose:
Take as soon as you remember up to 2 hours late. If more than 2 hours, wait for next scheduled dose (don't double this dose).

What drug does:
- Reduces work that heart must perform.
- Reduces normal artery pressure.
- Increases oxygen to heart muscle.

Time lapse before drug works:
1 to 2 hours.

Don't take with:
Any other medicines, even over-the-counter drugs such as cough and cold medicines, nose drops, diet pills, laxatives or caffeine, without consulting your doctor.

OVERDOSE

SYMPTOMS:
Unusually fast or unusually slow heartbeat, loss of consciousness, cardiac arrest.
WHAT TO DO:
- **Dial 0 (operator) or 911 (emergency) for an ambulance or medical help. Then give first aid immediately.**
- **If the child is unconscious and not breathing, give mouth-to-mouth breathing. If there is no heartbeat, use cardiac massage and mouth-to-mouth breathing (CPR). Don't try to make the child vomit. If you can't get help quickly, take the child to nearest emergency facility.**
- **See emergency information at the back of this book.**

POSSIBLE ADVERSE REACTIONS OR SIDE EFFECTS

SYMPTOMS	WHAT TO DO
Life-threatening: None expected.	
Common: Tiredness, flushing, swelling of feet, ankles and abdomen.	Continue. Tell doctor at next visit.
Infrequent: • Unusually fast or unusually slow heart-beat, wheezing, cough, shortness of breath.	Discontinue. Call doctor right away.
• Dizziness; numbness or tingling in hands or feet; swelling of ankles, feet, legs; difficult urination.	Continue. Call doctor when convenient.
• Nausea, constipation.	Continue. Tell doctor at next visit.
Rare: • Transient blindness, increased angina.	Discontinue. Seek emergency treatment.
• Fainting, chest pain, fever, rash, jaundice, depression, psychosis.	Discontinue. Call doctor right away.
• Arthritis, hair loss. vivid dreams.	Continue. Call doctor when convenient.
• Headache.	Continue. Tell doctor at next visit.

WARNINGS & PRECAUTIONS

Don't take if:
• You are allergic to calcium channel blockers.
• You have very low blood pressure.

Before you start, consult your doctor:
• If you have kidney or liver disease.
• If you have high blood pressure.
• If you have heart disease other than coronary-artery disease.

Pregnancy:
No proven harm to unborn child. Avoid if possible.

Infants & children:
Don't give to infants or young children unless prescribed and monitored by your physician.

Prolonged use:
No age-related problems expected.

Skin & sunlight:
Increased sensitivity to sunlight.

Driving or hazardous activities:
Avoid if you feel dizzy. Otherwise, no problems expected.

Discontinuing:
Don't discontinue without doctor's advice until you complete prescribed dose, even though symptoms diminish or disappear.

Others:
• Learn to check your own pulse rate. If it drops to 50 beats per minute or lower, don't take calcium channel blockers until you consult your doctor.
• Drug may lower blood-sugar level if daily dose is more than 60 mg.

POSSIBLE INTERACTION WITH OTHER DRUGS

GENERIC NAME OR DRUG CLASS	COMBINED EFFECT
ACE inhibitors: captopril, enalapril, lisinopril (see Drugs Glossary)	Possible excessive potassium in blood. Dosages may need adjustment.
Antiarrhythmics (see Drugs Glossary)	Possible increased effect and toxicity of each drug.
Anticoagulants (oral, see Drugs Glossary)	Possible increased anticoagulant effect.
Anticonvulsants (hydantoin, see Drugs Glossary)	Increased anticonvulsant effect.
Antihypertensives (see Drugs Glossary)	Dangerous blood-pressure drop. Dosage may need adjustment.
Beta-adrenergic blockers (see Drugs Glossary)	Possible irregular heartbeat. May worsen congestive heart failure.
Calcium (large doses)	Possible decreased calcium channel blocker effect.
Carbamazepine	May increase carbamazepine effect and toxicity.
Cimetidine	Possible increased calcium channel blocker effect and toxicity.

See Additional Drug Interactions Section

POSSIBLE INTERACTION WITH OTHER SUBSTANCES

INTERACTS WITH	COMBINED EFFECT
Alcohol:	Dangerously low blood pressure. Avoid.
Beverages:	None expected.
Cocaine (or crack):	Possible irregular heartbeat. Avoid.
Foods:	None expected.
Marijuana:	Possible irregular heartbeat. Avoid.
Tobacco:	Possible rapid heartbeat. Avoid.

MEDICATIONS

CAPTOPRIL & HYDROCHLOROTHIAZIDE

BRAND NAMES

Capozide

BASIC INFORMATION

Habit forming? No
Prescription needed? Yes
Available as generic? No
Drug class: Antihypertensive, diuretic (thiazide), ACE inhibitor (see Drugs Glossary)

USES

- Treatment for high blood pressure and congestive heart failure.
- Reduces fluid retention.

DOSAGE & USAGE INFORMATION

How to take:
Tablet—Swallow with liquid. Instructions to take on empty stomach mean 1 hour before or 2 hours after eating.

When to take:
At the same times each day, usually 2 to 3 times daily. Take first dose at bedtime and lie down immediately.

If you forget a dose:
Take as soon as you remember up to 2 hours late. If more than 2 hours, wait for next scheduled dose (don't double this dose).

What drug does:
- Forces sodium and water excretion, reducing body fluid.
- Relaxes muscle cells of small arteries.
- Reduced body fluid and relaxed arteries lower blood pressure.
- Reduces resistance in arteries.
- Strengthens heartbeat.

Continued next column

OVERDOSE

SYMPTOMS:
Cramps, weakness, drowsiness, weak pulse, low blood pressure.
WHAT TO DO:
- **Dial 0 (operator) or 911 (emergency) for an ambulance or medical help. Then give first aid immediately.**
- **See emergency information at the back of this book.**

Time lapse before drug works:
4 to 6 hours. May require several weeks to lower blood pressure.

Don't take with:
Any other medicines, even over-the-counter drugs such as cough and cold medicines, nose drops, diet pills, laxatives or caffeine, without consulting your doctor.

POSSIBLE ADVERSE REACTIONS OR SIDE EFFECTS

SYMPTOMS	WHAT TO DO
Life-threatening:	
Irregular heartbeat (fast or uneven); hives, rash, intense itching, faintness soon after a dose (anaphylaxis).	Discontinue. Seek emergency treatment.
Common:	
• Dry mouth, thirst, tiredness, weakness, muscle cramps, vomiting, chest pain, skin rash, coughing.	Discontinue. Call doctor right away.
• Taste loss, dizziness.	Continue. Call doctor when convenient.
Infrequent:	
• Face, mouth, hands swell.	Discontinue. Call doctor right away.
• Nausea, diarrhea.	Continue. Call doctor when convenient.
Rare:	
None expected.	

WARNINGS & PRECAUTIONS

Don't take if:
- You are allergic to captopril, or any thiazide diuretic drug.
- You have any autoimmune disease, including AIDS or lupus.
- You are receiving blood from a blood bank.
- You take drugs for cancer.
- If you will have surgery within 2 months, including dental surgery, requiring general or spinal anesthesia.

Before you start, consult your doctor:
- If you have had a stroke.
- If you have angina, heart or blood-vessel disease, a high level of potassium in blood, lupus, gout, liver, pancreas or kidney disorder.
- If you are on severe salt-restricted diet.
- If you are allergic to any sulfa drug.

Pregnancy:
Risk to unborn child outweighs drug benefits. Don't use.

Infants & children
Don't give to infants or young children unless prescribed and monitored by your physician.

Prolonged use:
May decrease white cells in blood or cause protein loss in urine. Request periodic laboratory blood counts and urine tests.

Skin & sunlight:
May cause rash or intensify sunburn in areas exposed to sun or sunlamp.

Driving or hazardous activities:
Don't drive or pilot aircraft until you learn how medicine affects you. Don't work around dangerous machinery. Don't climb ladders or work in high places. Danger increases if you drink alcohol or take medicine affecting alertness and reflexes, such as antihistamines, tranquilizers, sedatives, pain medicine, narcotics and mind-altering drugs.

Discontinuing:
Don't discontinue without consulting doctor. Dose may require gradual reduction if you have taken drug for a long time. Doses of other drugs may also require adjustment.

Others:
- Hot weather and fever may cause dehydration and drop in blood pressure. Dose may require temporary adjustment. Weigh daily and report any unexpected weight decreases to your doctor.
- May cause rise in uric acid, leading to gout.
- May cause blood-sugar rise in diabetics.

POSSIBLE INTERACTION WITH OTHER DRUGS

GENERIC NAME OR DRUG CLASS	COMBINED EFFECT
Allopurinol	Decreased allopurinol effect.
Amiloride	Possible excessive potassium in blood.
Antidepressants, tricyclic (TCA, see Drugs Glossary)	Dangerous drop in blood pressure. Avoid combination unless under medical supervision.
Antihypertensives (other, see Drugs Glossary)	Increased antihypertensive effect. Dosage of each may require adjustment.
Barbiturates (see Drugs Glossary)	Increased hydrochlorothiazide effect.
Beta-adrenergic blockers (see Drugs Glossary)	Increased antihypertensive effect. Dosage of each may require adjustments.
Chloramphenicol	Possible blood disorders.
Cholestyramine	Decreased hydrochlorothiazide effect.
Cortisone drugs (see Drugs Glossary)	Excessive potassium loss that causes dangerous heart rhythms.
Digitalis preparations (see Drugs Glossary)	Excessive potassium loss that causes dangerous heart rhythms.
Diuretics (see Drugs Glossary)	Decreased blood pressure.
Lithium	Increased effect of lithium.
MAO inhibitors (see Drugs Glossary)	Increased hydrochlorothiazide effect.
Nitrates (see Drugs Glossary)	Excessive blood-pressure drop.

See Additional Drug Interactions Section

POSSIBLE INTERACTION WITH OTHER SUBSTANCES

INTERACTS WITH	COMBINED EFFECT
Alcohol:	Dangerous blood-pressure drop. Avoid.
Beverages: Low-salt milk.	Possible excessive potassium in blood.
Cocaine (or crack):	Increased dizziness, chest pain.
Foods: Salt substitutes.	Possible excessive potassium.
Marijuana:	Increased dizziness, may increase blood pressure.
Tobacco:	May decrease captopril effect.

CARBAMAZEPINE

BRAND NAMES

Apo-Carbamazepine
Epitol
Mazepine
Tegretol

BASIC INFORMATION

Habit forming? No
Prescription needed? Yes
Available as generic? Yes
Drug class: Analgesic, anticonvulsant

USES

• Decreased frequency, severity and duration of attacks of tic douloureaux (see Drugs Glossary).
• Prevents seizures.

DOSAGE & USAGE INFORMATION

How to take:
Regular or chewable tablet—Swallow with liquid or food to lessen stomach irritation.

When to take:
At the same times each day.

If you forget a dose:
Take as soon as you remember up to 2 hours late. If more than 2 hours, wait for next scheduled dose (don't double this dose).

Continued next column

OVERDOSE

SYMPTOMS:
Involuntary movements, irregular bleeding, decreased urination, decreased blood pressure, dilated pupils, flushed skin, stupor, coma.
WHAT TO DO:
• Dial 0 (operator) or 911 (emergency) for an ambulance or medical help. Then give first aid immediately.
• If the child is unconscious and not breathing, give mouth-to-mouth breathing. If there is no heartbeat, use cardiac massage and mouth-to-mouth breathing (CPR). Don't try to make the child vomit. If you can't get help quickly, take the child to nearest emergency facility.
• See emergency information at the back of this book.

What drug does:
• Reduces transmission of pain messages at certain nerve terminals.
• Reduces excitability of nerve fibers in brain, thus inhibiting repetitive spread of nerve impulses.

Time lapse before drug works:
• Tic douloureaux—24 to 72 hours.
• Seizures—1 to 2 weeks.

Don't take with:
Any other medicines, even over-the-counter drugs such as cough and cold medicines, nose drops, diet pills, laxatives or caffeine, without consulting your doctor.

POSSIBLE ADVERSE REACTIONS OR SIDE EFFECTS

SYMPTOMS	WHAT TO DO
Life-threatening: None expected.	
Common: Blurred vision.	Continue. Call doctor when convenient.
Infrequent: • Confusion, slurred speech, fainting, depression, headache, hallucinations, hives, rash, mouth sores, sore throat, fever, unusual bleeding or bruising, unusual fatigue, jaundice.	Discontinue. Call doctor right away.
• Diarrhea, nausea, vomiting, constipation, dry mouth.	Continue. Call doctor when convenient.
Rare: • Back-and-forth eye movements; breathing difficulty; irregular, pounding or slow heartbeat; chest pain; uncontrollable body jerks; numbness, weakness or tingling in hands and feet; tender, bluish legs or feet; less urine; swollen lymph glands.	Discontinue. Call doctor right away.
• Frequent urination. muscle pains, joint aches.	Continue. Call doctor when convenient.

WARNINGS & PRECAUTIONS

Don't take if:
- You are allergic to carbamazepine.
- You have had liver or bone-marrow disease.
- You have taken MAO inhibitors in the past 2 weeks.

Before you start, consult your doctor:
- If you have high blood pressure, thrombophlebitis or heart disease.
- If you have glaucoma.
- If you have emotional or mental problems.
- If you have liver or kidney disease.
- If you drink more than 2 alcoholic drinks per day.

Pregnancy:
Studies inconclusive on harm to unborn child. Animal studies show fetal abnormalities. Decide with your doctor whether drug benefits justify risk to unborn child.

Infants & children
Don't give to infants or young children unless prescribed and monitored by your physician.

Prolonged use:
- Jaundice and liver damage.
- Hair loss.
- Ringing in ears.
- Lower sex drive.

Skin & sunlight:
May cause rash or intensify sunburn in areas exposed to sun or sunlamp.

Driving or hazardous activities:
Don't drive or pilot aircraft until you learn how medicine affects you. Don't work around dangerous machinery. Don't climb ladders or work in high places. Danger increases if you drink alcohol or take medicine affecting alertness and reflexes.

Discontinuing:
Don't discontinue without doctor's advice until you complete prescribed dose, even though symptoms diminish or disappear.

Others:
- Use only if less-hazardous drugs are not effective. Stay under medical supervision.
- Periodic blood tests are needed.

POSSIBLE INTERACTION WITH OTHER DRUGS

GENERIC NAME OR DRUG CLASS	COMBINED EFFECT
Anticoagulants (oral, see Drugs Glossary)	Decreased anticoagulant effect.
Anticonvulsants (hydantoin, see Drugs Glossary)	Decreased effect of both drugs.
Antidepressants, tricyclic (TCA, see Drugs Glossary)	Confusion. Possible psychosis.
Cimetidine	Increased carbamazepine effect.
Contraceptives (oral, see Drugs Glossary)	Reduced contraceptive protection. Use another birth-control method.
Digitalis preparations (see Drugs Glossary)	Excess slowing of heart.
Doxycycline	Decreased doxycycline effect.
Erythromycin	Increased carbamazepine effect.
Ethinamate	Dangerous increased effects of ethinamate. Avoid combining.
Fluoxetine	Increased depressant effects of both drugs.

See Additional Drug Interactions Section

POSSIBLE INTERACTION WITH OTHER SUBSTANCES

INTERACTS WITH	COMBINED EFFECT
Alcohol:	Increased sedative effect of alcohol. Avoid.
Beverages:	None expected.
Cocaine (or crack):	Increased adverse effects of carbamazepine. Avoid.
Foods:	None expected.
Marijuana:	Increased adverse effects of carbamazepine. Avoid.
Tobacco:	None expected.

MEDICATIONS

CEPHALOSPORINS

BRAND & GENERIC NAMES

See complete list of brand and generic names in the Brand & Generic Name Directory.

BASIC INFORMATION

Habit forming? No
Prescription needed? Yes
Available as generic? Yes
Drug class: Antibiotic (cephalosporin)

USES

Treatment of bacterial infections. Will not cure viral infections such as cold and flu.

DOSAGE & USAGE INFORMATION

How to take:
- Capsule—Swallow with liquid. If you can't swallow whole, open capsule and take with liquid or food.
- Liquid—Use measuring spoon.

When to take:
At same times each day, 1 hour before or 2 hours after eating.
Take until gone or as directed.

If you forget a dose:
Take as soon as you remember or double next dose. Return to regular schedule.

What drug does:
Kills susceptible bacteria.

Time lapse before drug works:
May require several days to affect infection.

Don't take with:
Any other medicines, even over-the-counter drugs such as cough and cold medicines, nose drops, diet pills, laxatives or caffeine, without consulting your doctor.

OVERDOSE

SYMPTOMS:
Abdominal cramps, nausea, vomiting, severe diarrhea with mucus or blood in stool.
WHAT TO DO:
Overdose unlikely to threaten life. If child takes much larger amount than prescribed, call doctor, poison-control center or hospital emergency room for instructions.

POSSIBLE ADVERSE REACTIONS OR SIDE EFFECTS

SYMPTOMS	WHAT TO DO
Life-threatening:	
Hives, rash, intense itching, faintness soon after a dose (anaphylaxis); difficulty breathing.	Seek emergency treatment immediately.
Common:	
Rash, redness, itching.	Discontinue. Call doctor right away.
Infrequent:	
Rectal itching.	Continue. Call doctor when convenient.
Rare:	
Mild nausea, vomiting, cramps, severe diarrhea with mucus or blood in stool, unusual weakness, tiredness, weight loss, fever, oral or vaginal candidiasis.	Discontinue. Call doctor right away.

WARNINGS & PRECAUTIONS

Don't take if:
You are allergic to any cephalosporin antibiotic.

Before you start, consult your doctor:
- If you are allergic to any penicillin antibiotic.
- If you have a kidney disorder.
- If you have colitis or enteritis.

Pregnancy:
No proven harm to unborn child. Avoid if possible.

Infants & children:
No special warnings.

Prolonged use:
Kills beneficial bacteria that protect body against other germs. Unchecked germs may cause secondary infections.

Skin & sunlight:
No age-related problems expected.

Driving or hazardous activities:
No age-related problems expected.

Discontinuing:
Don't discontinue without doctor's advice until you complete prescribed dose, even though symptoms diminish or disappear.

Others:
No age-related problems expected.

POSSIBLE INTERACTION WITH OTHER DRUGS

GENERIC NAME OR DRUG CLASS	COMBINED EFFECT
Anticoagulants (see Drugs Glossary)	Increased anticoagulant effect.
Erythromycin	Decreased antibiotic effect of cephalosporin.
Chloramphenicol	Decreased antibiotic effect of cephalosporin.
Clindamycin	Decreased antibiotic effect of cephalosporin.
Probenecid	Increased cephalosporin effect.
Tetracycline	Decreased antibiotic effect of cephalexin.

POSSIBLE INTERACTION WITH OTHER SUBSTANCES

INTERACTS WITH	COMBINED EFFECT
Alcohol:	Increased kidney toxicity.
Beverages:	None expected.
Cocaine (or crack):	None expected, but cocaine may slow body's recovery. Avoid.
Foods:	Slow absorption. Take with liquid 1 hour before or 2 hours after eating.
Marijuana:	None expected, but marijuana may slow body's recovery. Avoid.
Tobacco:	None expected.

CHLORZOXAZONE

BRAND NAMES

Algisin	Paraflex
Chlorzone Forte	Parafon Forte DSC

BASIC INFORMATION

Habit forming? Possibly
Prescription needed? Yes
Available as generic? Yes
Drug class: Muscle relaxant (skeletal)

USES

Adjunctive treatment to rest, analgesics and physical therapy for muscle spasm.

DOSAGE & USAGE INFORMATION

How to take:
Tablet—Swallow with liquid.

When to take:
As needed, no more often than every 4 hours.

If you forget a dose:
Take as soon as you remember. Wait 4 hours for next dose.

What drug does:
Blocks body's pain messages to brain. Also causes sedation.

Time lapse before drug works:
60 minutes.

Don't take with:
Any other medicines, even over-the-counter drugs such as cough and cold medicines, nose drops, diet pills, laxatives or caffeine, without consulting your doctor.

OVERDOSE

SYMPTOMS:
Nausea, vomiting, diarrhea, headache, severe weakness, breathing difficulty, sensation of paralysis.
WHAT TO DO:
Overdose unlikely to threaten life. Depending on severity of symptoms and amount taken, call doctor, poison-control center or hospital emergency room for instructions.

POSSIBLE ADVERSE REACTIONS OR SIDE EFFECTS

SYMPTOMS	WHAT TO DO
Life-threatening:	
Hives, rash, intense itching, faintness soon after a dose (anaphylaxis); extreme weakness, transient paralysis, temporary loss of vision.	Seek emergency treatment immediately.
Common:	
• Drowsiness, dizziness.	Continue. Call doctor when convenient.
• Orange or red-purple urine.	No action necessary.
Infrequent:	
Agitation, constipation or diarrhea, nausea, cramps, vomiting, headache, depression.	Discontinue. Call doctor right away.
Rare:	
• Bloody or tarry, black stool.	Discontinue. Seek emergency treatment.
• Rash or itch, sore throat, fever, jaundice, tiredness, weakness, bleeding in skin, hiccups.	Discontinue. Call doctor right away.

WARNINGS & PRECAUTIONS

Don't take if:
You are allergic to any skeletal-muscle relaxant.

Before you start, consult your doctor:
• If you have had liver disease.
• If you plan pregnancy within medication period.
• If you are allergic to tartrazine dye.

Pregnancy:
Safety not proven. Avoid if possible.

Infants & children
Don't give to infants or young children unless prescribed and monitored by your physician.

Prolonged use:
No age-related problems expected.

Skin & sunlight:
No age-related problems expected.

Driving or hazardous activities:
Don't drive or pilot aircraft until you learn how medicine affects you. Don't work around dangerous machinery. Don't climb ladders or work in high places. Danger increases if you drink alcohol or take medicine affecting alertness and reflexes, such as antihistamines, tranquilizers, sedatives, pain medicine, narcotics and mind-altering drugs.

Discontinuing:
Don't discontinue without doctor's advice until you complete prescribed dose, even though symptoms diminish or disappear.

Others:
Periodic liver-function tests recommended If you use this drug for a long time.

POSSIBLE INTERACTION WITH OTHER DRUGS

GENERIC NAME OR DRUG CLASS	COMBINED EFFECT
Antidepressants (see Drugs Glossary)	Increased sedation.
Antihistamines (see Drugs Glossary)	Increased sedation.
Dronabinol	Increased effect of dronabinol on central nervous system. Avoid combination.
Ethinamate	Dangerous increased effects of ethinamate. Avoid combining.
Fluoxetine	Increased depressant effects of both drugs.
Guanfacine	May increase depressant effects of either drug.
Leucovorin	High alcohol content of leucovorin may cause adverse effects.
MAO inhibitors (see Drugs Glossary)	Increased effect of both drugs.
Methyprylon	Increased sedative effect, perhaps to dangerous level. Avoid.
Mind-altering drugs	Increased sedation.
Muscle relaxants (others, see Drugs Glossary)	Increased sedation.
Narcotics (see Drugs Glossary)	Increased sedation.
Sedatives (see Drugs Glossary)	Increased sedation.
Sleep inducers (see Drugs Glossary)	Increased sedation
Tranquilizers (see Drugs Glossary)	Increased sedation.

POSSIBLE INTERACTION WITH OTHER SUBSTANCES

INTERACTS WITH	COMBINED EFFECT
Alcohol:	Increased sedation.
Beverages:	None expected.
Cocaine (or crack):	Lack of coordination.
Foods:	None expected.
Marijuana:	Lack of coordination, drowsiness, fainting.
Tobacco:	None expected

CIMETIDINE

BRAND NAMES

Apo-Cimetidine
Novo-Cimetine
Peptol
Tagamet

BASIC INFORMATION

Habit forming? No
Prescription needed? Yes
Available as generic? No
Drug class: Histamine H-2 antagonist

USES

Treatment for duodenal ulcers and other conditions in which stomach produces excess hydrochloric acid.

DOSAGE & USAGE INFORMATION

How to take:
Tablet or liquid—Swallow with liquid.

When to take:
• 1 dose per day—Take at bedtime.
• 2 or more doses per day—Take at the same times each day.

If you forget a dose:
Take as soon as you remember up to 2 hours late. If more than 2 hours, wait for next scheduled dose (don't double this dose).

What drug does:
Blocks histamine release so stomach secretes less acid.

Time lapse before drug works:
Begins in 30 minutes. May require several days to relieve pain.

Don't take with:
Any other medicines, even over-the-counter drugs such as cough and cold medicines, nose drops, diet pills, laxatives or caffeine, without consulting your doctor.

OVERDOSE

SYMPTOMS:
Confusion, slurred speech, breathing difficulty, rapid heartbeat, delirium.
WHAT TO DO:
Overdose unlikely to threaten life. If child takes much larger amount than prescribed, call doctor, poison-control center or hospital emergency room for instructions.

POSSIBLE ADVERSE REACTIONS OR SIDE EFFECTS

SYMPTOMS	WHAT TO DO
Life-threatening: None expected.	
Common: None expected.	
Infrequent:	
• Diarrhea, jaundice.	Discontinue. Call doctor right away.
• Dizziness or headache, diarrhea, decreased sperm production.	Continue. Call doctor when convenient.
• Diminished sex drive, breast swelling and soreness in males, unusual milk flow in females, hair loss.	Continue. Tell doctor at next visit.
Rare: Confusion; rash, hives; sore throat, fever; slow, fast or irregular heartbeat; unusual bleeding or bruising; muscle cramps or pain; fatigue; weakness; peripheral neuritis; chronic kidney disease.	Discontinue. Call doctor right away.

WARNINGS & PRECAUTIONS

Don't take if:
You are allergic to cimetidine or other histamine H-2 antagonist.

Before you start, consult your doctor:
• If you plan to become pregnant during medication period.
• If you take aspirin. Aspirin may irritate stomach.

Pregnancy:
No proven harm to unborn child. Avoid if possible.

Infants & children
Don't give to infants or young children unless prescribed and monitored by your physician.

Prolonged use:
Possible liver damage.

Skin & sunlight:
No age-related problems expected.

Driving or hazardous activities:
Don't drive or pilot aircraft until you learn how medicine affects you. Don't work around dangerous machinery. Don't climb ladders or work in high places. Danger increases if you drink alcohol or take medicine affecting alertness and reflexes, such as antihistamines, tranquilizers, sedatives, pain medicine, narcotics and mind-altering drugs.

Discontinuing:
Don't discontinue without consulting doctor. Dose may require gradual reduction if you have taken drug for a long time. Doses of other drugs may also require adjustment.

Others:
Patients on kidney dialysis—Take at end of dialysis treatment.

POSSIBLE INTERACTION WITH OTHER DRUGS

GENERIC NAME OR DRUG CLASS	COMBINED EFFECT
Alprazolam	Increased effect and toxicity of alprazolam.
Antacids (see Drugs Glossary)	Decreased cimetidine absorption.
Anticoagulants (oral, see Drugs Glossary)	Increased anticoagulant effect.
Anticholinergics (see Drugs Glossary)	Increased cimetidine effect.
Carbamazepine	Increased effect and toxicity of carbamazepine.
Carmustine (BCNU)	Severe impairment of red-blood-cell production; some interference with white-blood-cell formation.
Chlordiazepoxide	Increased effect and toxicity of chlordiazepoxide.
Diazepam	Increased effect and toxicity of diazepam.
Digitalis preparations (see Drugs Glossary)	Increased digitalis effect.
Encainide	Increased effect of cimetidine.
Flurazepam	Increased effect and toxicity of flurazepam.
Glipizide	Increased effect and toxicity of glipizide.
Ketoconazole	Decreased ketoconazole absorption.
Labetolol	Increased anti-hypertensive effects.
Methadone	Increased effect and toxicity of methadone.
Metoclopramide	Decreased cimetidine absorption.
Metoprolol	Increased effect and toxicity of metoprolol.
Metronidazole	Increased effect and toxicity of metronidazole.

See Additional Drug Interactions Section

POSSIBLE INTERACTION WITH OTHER SUBSTANCES

INTERACTS WITH	COMBINED EFFECT
Alcohol:	No interactions expected, but alcohol may slow body's recovery. Avoid.
Beverages: Milk.	Enhanced effectiveness. Small amounts useful for taking medication.
Caffeine drinks.	May increase acid secretion and delay healing.
Cocaine (or crack):	Decreased cimetidine effect.
Foods:	Enhanced effectiveness. Protein-rich foods should be eaten in moderation to minimize secretion of stomach acid.
Marijuana:	Increased chance of low sperm count. Marijuana may slow body's recovery. Avoid.
Tobacco:	Reverses cimetidine effect. Tobacco may slow body's recovery. Avoid.

MEDICATIONS

CLONIDINE

BRAND NAMES

Catapres
Catapres-TTS
Combipres
Dixarit

BASIC INFORMATION

Habit forming? No
Prescription needed? Yes
Available as generic? Yes
Drug class: Antihypertensive

USES

- Treatment of high blood pressure.
- Prevention of vascular headaches.
- Treatment of dysmenorrhea and menopausal "hot flashes."
- Treatment of narcotic withdrawal syndrome.
- Treatment of congestive heart failure.

DOSAGE & USAGE INFORMATION

How to take:
- Tablet—Swallow with liquid.
- Patches that attach to skin—Apply to clean, dry, hairless skin on arm or trunk.

When to take:
Daily dose at bedtime.

If you forget a dose:
Bedtime dose—If you forget your once-a-day dose, take it as soon as you remember. *Don't* double dose.

Continued next column

OVERDOSE

SYMPTOMS:
Vomiting, fainting, slow heartbeat, coma, diminished reflexes.
WHAT TO DO:
- **Dial 0 (operator) or 911 (emergency) for an ambulance or medical help. Then give first aid immediately.**
- **If the child is unconscious and not breathing, give mouth-to-mouth breathing. If there is no heartbeat, use cardiac massage and mouth-to-mouth breathing (CPR). Don't try to make the child vomit. If you can't get help quickly, take the child to nearest emergency facility.**
- **See emergency information at the back of this book.**

What drug does:
Relaxes and allows expansion of blood vessel walls.

Time lapse before drug works:
1 to 3 hours.

Don't take with:
Any other medicines, even over-the-counter drugs such as cough and cold medicines, nose drops, diet pills, laxatives or caffeine, without consulting your doctor.

POSSIBLE ADVERSE REACTIONS OR SIDE EFFECTS

SYMPTOMS	WHAT TO DO
Life-threatening:	
None expected.	
Common:	
• Dizziness, drowsiness, weight gain, lightheadedness upon rising from sitting or lying, swollen breasts.	Continue. Call doctor when convenient.
• Dry mouth.	Continue. Tell doctor at next visit.
Infrequent:	
• Abnormal heart rhythm.	Discontinue. Call doctor right away.
• Headache; painful glands in neck; nightmares; nausea; vomiting; cold fingers and toes; dry, burning eyes.	Continue. Call doctor when convenient.
• Insomnia, constipation, appetite loss, diminished sex drive.	Continue. Tell doctor at next visit.
Rare:	
• Rash, itch.	Discontinue. Call doctor right away.
• Depression.	Continue. Call doctor when convenient.

WARNINGS & PRECAUTIONS

Don't take if:
- You are allergic to any alpha-adrenergic blocker.
- You are under age 12.

Before you start, consult your doctor:
- If you will have surgery within 2 months, including dental surgery, requiring general or spinal anesthesia.
- If you have heart disease or chronic kidney disease.
- If you have a peripheral circulation disorder (intermittent claudication, Buerger's disease).
- If you have history of depression.

Pregnancy:
Studies inconclusive on harm to unborn child. Animal studies show fetal abnormalities. Decide with your doctor whether drug benefits justify risk to unborn child.

Infants & children:
Use only under careful medical supervision after age 12. Avoid before age 12.

Prolonged use:
- Don't discontinue without consulting doctor. Dose may require gradual reduction if you have taken drug for a long time. Doses of other drugs may also require adjustment.
- Continued use may cause fluid retention, requiring addition of diuretic to treatment program.
- Request yearly eye examinations.

Skin & sunlight:
No age-related problems expected.

Driving or hazardous activities:
Don't drive or pilot aircraft until you learn how medicine affects you. Don't work around dangerous machinery. Don't climb ladders or work in high places. Danger increases if you drink alcohol or take medicine affecting alertness and reflexes.

Discontinuing:
Don't discontinue abruptly. May cause rebound high blood pressure, anxiety, chest pain, insomnia, headache, nausea, irregular heartbeat, flushed face, sweating.

Others:
No age-related problems expected.

POSSIBLE INTERACTION WITH OTHER DRUGS

GENERIC NAME OR DRUG CLASS	COMBINED EFFECT
ACE inhibitors: captopril, enalapril, lisinopril (see Drugs Glossary)	Possible excessive potassium in blood.
Antidepressants, tricyclic (TCA, Drugs see Glossary)	Decreased clonidine effect.
Antihypertensives (other, see Drugs Glossary)	Excessive blood-pressure drop.
Appetite suppressants (see Drugs Glossary)	Decreased clonidine effect.
Beta-adrenergic blockers (see Drugs Glossary)	Possible precipitous change in blood pressure.
Diuretics (see Drugs Glossary)	Excessive blood-pressure drop.
Ethinamate	Dangerous increased effects of ethinamate. Avoid combining.
Fenfluramine	Possible increased clonidine effect.
Fluoxetine	Increased depressant effects of both drugs.

See Additional Drug Interactions Section

POSSIBLE INTERACTION WITH OTHER SUBSTANCES

INTERACTS WITH	COMBINED EFFECT
Alcohol:	Increased sensitivity to sedative effect of alcohol and very low blood pressure. Avoid.
Beverages: Caffeine-containing drinks.	Decreased clonidine effect.
Cocaine (or crack):	Blood pressure rise. Avoid.
Foods:	None expected.
Marijuana:	Weakness on standing.
Tobacco:	None expected.

DICYCLOMINE

BRAND & GENERIC NAMES

See complete list of brand and generic names in the Brand & Generic Name Directory.

BASIC INFORMATION

Habit forming? No
Prescription needed?
Low strength: No
High strength: Yes
Available as generic? Yes
Drug class: Antispasmodic, anticholinergic

USES

Reduces spasms of digestive system, bladder and urethra.

DOSAGE & USAGE INFORMATION

How to take:
Tablet, syrup or capsule—Swallow with liquid or food to lessen stomach irritation.

When to take:
30 minutes before meals (unless directed otherwise by doctor).

If you forget a dose:
Take as soon as you remember up to 2 hours late. If more than 2 hours, wait for next scheduled dose (don't double this dose).

What drug does:
Blocks nerve impulses at parasympathetic nerve endings, preventing muscle contractions and gland secretions of organs involved.

Time lapse before drug works:
15 to 30 minutes.

Continued next column

OVERDOSE

SYMPTOMS:
Dilated pupils, blurred vision, rapid pulse and breathing, dizziness, fever, hallucinations, confusion, slurred speech, agitation, flushed face, convulsions, coma.
WHAT TO DO:
- **Dial 0 (operator) or 911 (emergency) for an ambulance or medical help. Then give first aid immediately.**
- **See emergency information at the back of this book.**

Don't take with:
Any other medicines, even over-the-counter drugs such as cough and cold medicines, nose drops, diet pills, laxatives or caffeine, without consulting your doctor.

POSSIBLE ADVERSE REACTIONS OR SIDE EFFECTS

SYMPTOMS	WHAT TO DO
Life-threatening:	
Hives, rash, intense itching, faintness soon after a dose (anaphylaxis).	Seek emergency treatment immediately.
Common:	
• Confusion, delirium, rapid heartbeat.	Discontinue. Call doctor right away.
• Nausea, vomiting, decreased sweating.	Continue. Call doctor when convenient.
• Constipation, loss of taste.	Continue. Tell doctor at next visit.
• Dry ears, nose, throat.	No action necessary.
Infrequent:	
Headache, difficult urination.	Continue. Call doctor when convenient.
Rare:	
Rash or hives, pain, blurred vision.	Discontinue. Call doctor right away.

WARNINGS & PRECAUTIONS

Don't take if:
- You are allergic to any anticholinergic.
- You have trouble with stomach bloating.
- You have difficulty emptying your bladder completely.
- You have narrow-angle glaucoma.
- You have severe ulcerative colitis.

Before you start, consult your doctor:
- If you have open-angle glaucoma.
- If you have angina, chronic bronchitis or asthma.
- If you have hiatal hernia, liver disease, enlarged prostate, myasthenia gravis, peptic ulcer.
- If you will have surgery within 2 months, including dental surgery, requiring general or spinal anesthesia.

Pregnancy:
Studies inconclusive on harm to unborn child. Animal studies show fetal abnormalities. Decide with your doctor whether drug benefits justify risk to unborn child.

Infants & children:
Use only under medical supervision.

Prolonged use:
Chronic constipation, possible fecal impaction. Consult doctor immediately.

Skin & sunlight:
No age-related problems expected.

Driving or hazardous activities:
Use disqualifies you for piloting aircraft. Otherwise, no problems expected.

Discontinuing:
May be unnecessary to finish medicine. Follow doctor's instructions.

Others:
No age-related problems expected.

POSSIBLE INTERACTION WITH OTHER DRUGS

GENERIC NAME OR DRUG CLASS	COMBINED EFFECT
Amantadine	Increased dicyclomine effect.
Antacids	Decreased dicyclomine absorption effect.
Anticholinergics (other, see Drugs Glossary)	Increased dicyclomine effect.
Antidepressants, tricyclic (TCA, see Drugs Glossary)	Increased dicyclomine effect. Increased sedation.
Antihistamines (see Drugs Glossary)	Increased dicyclomine effect.
Buclizine	Increased dicyclomine effect.
Cortisone drugs	Increased internal-eye pressure.
Digitalis	Possible decreased absorption of digitalis.
Haloperidol	Increased internal-eye pressure.
MAO inhibitors (see Drugs Glossary)	Increased dicyclomine effect.
Meperidine	Increased dicyclomine effect.
Methylphenidate	Increased dicyclomine effect.
Nitrates	Increased internal-eye pressure.
Orphenadrine	Increased dicyclomine effect.
Phenothiazines	Increased dicyclomine effect.
Pilocarpine	Loss of pilocarpine effect in glaucoma treatment.
Potassium supplements	Possible intestinal ulcers with oral potassium tablets.
Quinidine	Increased dicyclomine effect.
Vitamin C	Decreased dicyclomine effect. Avoid large doses of vitamin C.

POSSIBLE INTERACTION WITH OTHER SUBSTANCES

INTERACTS WITH	COMBINED EFFECT
Alcohol:	None expected.
Beverages:	None expected.
Cocaine (or crack):	Excessively rapid heartbeat. Avoid.
Foods:	None expected.
Marijuana:	Drowsiness and dry mouth.
Tobacco:	None expected.

DIGITALIS PREPARATIONS

BRAND & GENERIC NAMES

Crystodigin	Gitaligen
Crystogin	GITALIN
Digifortis	Lanoxicaps
Digiglusin	Lanoxin
DIGITALIS	Natigozine
DIGITOXIN	Novodigoxin
DIGOXIN	Purodigin

BASIC INFORMATION

Habit forming? No
Prescription needed? Yes
Available as generic? Yes
Drug class: Digitalis preparations

USES

- Strengthens weak heart-muscle contractions to prevent congestive heart failure.
- Corrects irregular heartbeat.

DOSAGE & USAGE INFORMATION

How to take:
- Tablet or capsule—Swallow with liquid. If you can't swallow whole, crumble tablet or open capsule and take with liquid or food.
- Liquid—Dilute dose in beverage before swallowing.

When to take:
At the same time each day.

If you forget a dose:
Take as soon as you remember up to 12 hours late. If more than 12 hours, wait for next scheduled dose (don't double this dose).

What drug does:
- Strengthens heart-muscle contraction.
- Delays nerve impulses to heart.

Continued next column

OVERDOSE

SYMPTOMS:
Nausea, vomiting, diarrhea, vision disturbances, halos around lights, fatigue, irregular heartbeat, confusion, hallucinations, convulsions.
WHAT TO DO:
- **Dial 0 (operator) or 911 (emergency) for an ambulance or medical help. Then give first aid immediately.**
- **See emergency information at the back of this book.**

Time lapse before drug works:
May require regular use for a week or more.

Don't take with:
Any other medicines, even over-the-counter drugs such as cough and cold medicines, nose drops, diet pills, laxatives or caffeine, without consulting your doctor.

POSSIBLE ADVERSE REACTIONS OR SIDE EFFECTS

SYMPTOMS	WHAT TO DO
Life-threatening:	
None expected.	
Common:	
Appetite loss, diarrhea.	Continue. Call doctor when convenient.
Infrequent:	
Drowsiness, lethargy, disorientation.	Discontinue. Call doctor right away.
Rare:	
• Rash, hives, cardiac arrhythmias, depression, hallucinations, psychosis.	Discontinue. Call doctor right away.
• Double or yellow-green vision; enlarged, sensitive male breasts; tiredness; weakness.	Continue. Call doctor when convenient.

WARNINGS & PRECAUTIONS

Don't take if:
- You are allergic to any digitalis preparation.
- Your heartbeat is slower than 50 beats per minute.

Before you start, consult your doctor:
- If you have taken another digitalis preparation in past 2 weeks.
- If you have taken a diuretic within 2 weeks.
- If you have liver or kidney disease.
- If you have a thyroid disorder.
- If you will have surgery within 2 months, including dental surgery, requiring general or spinal anesthesia.

Pregnancy:
Studies inconclusive on harm to unborn child. Consult your doctor.

Infants & children:
Use only under medical supervision.

Prolonged use:
No age-related problems expected.

Skin & sunlight:
No age-related problems expected.

Driving or hazardous activities:
Possible vision disturbances. Otherwise, no problems expected.

Discontinuing:
Don't stop without doctor's advice.

Others:
Some digitalis products contain tartrazine dye. Avoid, especially if you are allergic to aspirin.

POSSIBLE INTERACTION WITH OTHER DRUGS

GENERIC NAME OR DRUG CLASS	COMBINED EFFECT
Amiodarone	Increased digitalis effect.
Amphotericin B	Decreased potassium. Increased toxicity of amphotericin B.
Antacids	Decreased digitalis effect.
Anticonvulsants (hydantoin, see Drugs Glossary)	Increased digitalis effect at first, then decreased.
Anticholinergics (see Drugs Glossary)	Possible increased digitalis effect.
Beta-adrenergic blockers (see Drugs Glossary)	Increased digitalis effect.
Beta-agonists (see Drugs Glossary)	Increased risk of heartbeat irregularity.
Calcium supplements	Decreased digitalis effects.
Cholestyramine	Decreased digitalis effect.
Colestipol	Decreased digitalis effect.
Cortisone drugs	Digitalis toxicity.
Disopyramide	Possible decreased digitalis effect.
Diuretics (see Drugs Glossary)	Possible digitalis toxicity. Excessive potassium loss that may cause irregular heartbeat.
Ephedrine	Disturbed heart rhythm. Avoid.
Epinephrine	Disturbed heart rhythm. Avoid.
Erythromycin	May increase digitalis absorption.
Flecainide	May increase digitalis blood level.
Fluoxetine	May cause confusion, agitation, convulsions and high blood pressure. Avoid combining.
Hydroxychloroquine	Possible increased digitalis toxicity.
Laxatives	Decreased digitalis effect.
Metoclopramide	Decreased digitalis absorption.
Oxyphenbutazone	Decreased digitalis effect.
Phenobarbital	Decreased digitalis effect.
Phenylbutazone	Decreased digitalis effect.
Potassium supplements	Overdosage of either drug may cause severe heartbeat irregularity.
PTU/Metronidazole	Decreased digitalis effect.

See Additional Drug Interactions Section

POSSIBLE INTERACTION WITH OTHER SUBSTANCES

INTERACTS WITH	COMBINED EFFECT
Alcohol:	None expected.
Beverages: Caffeine drinks.	Irregular heartbeat. Avoid.
Cocaine (or crack):	Irregular heartbeat. Avoid.
Foods:	None expected.
Marijuana:	Decreased digitalis effect.
Tobacco:	Irregular heartbeat. Avoid.

DIPHENIDOL

BRAND NAMES

Vontrol

BASIC INFORMATION

Habit forming? No
Prescription needed? Yes
Available as generic? No
Drug class: Antiemetic, antivertigo

USES

• Prevents motion sickness.
• Controls nausea and vomiting (do not use during pregnancy).

DOSAGE & USAGE INFORMATION

How to take:
Tablet—Swallow with liquid or food to lessen stomach irritation. If you can't swallow whole, crumble tablet and chew or take with liquid or food.

When to take:
30 to 60 minutes before traveling.

If you forget a dose:
Take as soon as you remember. Wait 4 hours for next dose.

What drug does:
Reduces sensitivity of nerve endings in inner ear, blocking messages to brain's vomiting center.

Time lapse before drug works:
30 to 60 minutes.

Don't take with:
Any other medicines, even over-the-counter drugs such as cough and cold medicines, nose drops, diet pills, laxatives or caffeine, without consulting your doctor.

OVERDOSE

SYMPTOMS:
Drowsiness, confusion, incoordination, weak pulse, shallow breathing, stupor, coma.
WHAT TO DO:
• Dial 0 (operator) or 911 (emergency) for an ambulance or medical help. Then give first aid immediately.
• See emergency information at the back of this book.

POSSIBLE ADVERSE REACTIONS OR SIDE EFFECTS

SYMPTOMS	WHAT TO DO
Life-threatening: None expected.	
Common: Drowsiness.	Continue. Tell doctor at next visit.
Infrequent:	
• Headache, diarrhea or constipation, fast heartbeat.	Continue. Call doctor when convenient.
• Dry mouth, nose, throat.	Continue. Tell doctor at next visit.
Rare:	
• Hallucinations, confusion.	Discontinue. Seek emergency treatment.
• Rash or hives, depression, jaundice.	Discontinue. Call doctor right away.
• Restlessness; excitement; insomnia; blurred vision; urgent, painful or difficult urination.	Continue. Call doctor when convenient.
• Appetite loss, nausea.	Continue. Tell doctor at next visit.

WARNINGS & PRECAUTIONS

Don't take if:
- You have severe kidney disease.
- You are allergic to diphenidol or meclizine.

Before you start, consult your doctor:
- If you have prostate enlargement.
- If you have glaucoma.
- If you have heart disease.
- If you have intestinal obstruction or ulcers in the gastrointestinal tract.
- If you have kidney disease.
- If you have low blood pressure.
- If you will have surgery within 2 months, including dental surgery, requiring general or spinal anesthesia.

Pregnancy:
Animal studies show fetal abnormalities. Decide with your doctor whether drug benefits justify risk to unborn child.

Infants & children:
No age-related problems expected.

Prolonged use:
No age-related problems expected.

Skin & sunlight:
No age-related problems expected.

Driving or hazardous activities:
Don't fly aircraft. Don't drive until you learn how medicine affects you. Don't work around dangerous machinery. Don't climb ladders or work in high places. Danger increases if you drink alcohol or take medicine affecting alertness and reflexes, such as antihistamines, tranquilizers, sedatives, pain medicine, narcotics and mind-altering drugs.

Discontinuing:
No age-related problems expected.

Others:
No age-related problems expected.

POSSIBLE INTERACTION WITH OTHER DRUGS

GENERIC NAME OR DRUG CLASS	COMBINED EFFECT
Anticonvulsants (see Drugs Glossary)	Increased effect of both drugs.
Antidepressants, tricyclic (TCA, see Drugs Glossary)	Increased sedative effect of both drugs.
Antihistamines (see Drugs Glossary)	Increased sedative effect of both drugs.
Atropine	Increased chance of toxic effect of atropine and atropine-like medicines.
Narcotics	Increased sedative effect of both drugs.
Sedatives	Increased sedative effect of both drugs.
Tranquilizers	Increased sedative effect of both drugs.

POSSIBLE INTERACTION WITH OTHER SUBSTANCES

INTERACTS WITH	COMBINED EFFECT
Alcohol:	Increased sedation. Avoid.
Beverages: Caffeine.	May decrease drowsiness.
Cocaine (or crack):	Increased chance of toxic effects of cocaine. Avoid.
Foods:	None expected.
Marijuana:	Increased drowsiness, dry mouth.
Tobacco:	None expected.

MEDICATIONS

DIPHENOXYLATE & ATROPINE

BRAND NAMES

Colonil	Lomotil
Diphenatol	Lonox
Enoxa	Lo-Trol
Latropine	Low-Quel
Lofene	Nor-Mil
Lomanate	SK-Diphenoxylate

BASIC INFORMATION

Habit forming? Yes
Prescription needed? Yes
Available as generic? Yes
Drug class: Antidiarrheal

USES

Relieves diarrhea and intestinal cramps.

DOSAGE & USAGE INFORMATION

How to take:
• Tablet—Swallow with liquid or food to lessen stomach irritation.
• Drops or liquid—Follow label instructions and use marked dropper.

When to take:
No more often than directed on label.

If you forget a dose:
Take as soon as you remember up to 2 hours late. If more than 2 hours, wait for next scheduled dose (don't double this dose).

Continued next column

OVERDOSE

SYMPTOMS:
Excitement, constricted pupils, shallow breathing, coma.
WHAT TO DO:
• Dial 0 (operator) or 911 (emergency) for an ambulance or medical help. Then give first aid immediately.
• If the child is unconscious and not breathing, give mouth-to-mouth breathing. If there is no heartbeat, use cardiac massage and mouth-to-mouth breathing (CPR). Don't try to make the child vomit. If you can't get help quickly, take the child to nearest emergency facility.
• See emergency information at the back of this book.

What drug does:
Blocks digestive tract's nerve supply, which reduces propelling movements.

Time lapse before drug works:
May require 12 to 24 hours of regular doses to control diarrhea, but cramps usually improve in 30 to 90 minutes.

Don't take with:
Any other medicines, even over-the-counter drugs such as cough and cold medicines, nose drops, diet pills, laxatives or caffeine, without consulting your doctor.

POSSIBLE ADVERSE REACTIONS OR SIDE EFFECTS

SYMPTOMS	WHAT TO DO
Life-threatening:	
Hives, rash, intense itching, faintness soon after a dose (anaphylaxis).	Seek emergency treatment immediately.
Common:	
None expected.	
Infrequent:	
• Dry mouth, swollen gums, rapid heartbeat.	Discontinue. Call doctor right away.
• Dizziness, depression, drowsiness, rash or itch, blurred vision, decreased urination.	Continue. Call doctor when convenient.
Rare:	
Restlessness, flush, fever, headache, stomach pain, nausea, vomiting, bloating, constipation, numbness of hands or feet.	Discontinue. Call doctor right away.

WARNINGS & PRECAUTIONS

Don't take if:
- You are allergic to diphenoxylate and atropine or any narcotic or anticholinergic.
- You have jaundice.
- You have infectious diarrhea or antibiotic-associated diarrhea.
- Patient is younger than 2.

Before you start, consult your doctor:
- If you have had liver problems.
- If you have ulcerative colitis.
- If you plan to become pregnant within medication period.
- If you have any medical disorder.
- If you take any medication, including non-prescription drugs.

Pregnancy:
No proven harm to unborn child. Avoid because of many side effects.

Infants & children:
Don't give to infants or toddlers. Use only under doctor's supervision for children older than 2.

Prolonged use:
Habit forming.

Skin & sunlight:
No age-related problems expected.

Driving or hazardous activities:
Don't drive or pilot aircraft until you learn how medicine affects you. Don't work around dangerous machinery. Don't climb ladders or work in high places. Danger increases if you drink alcohol or take medicine affecting alertness and reflexes.

Discontinuing:
- May be unnecessary to finish medicine. Follow doctor's instructions.
- After discontinuing, consult doctor if you experience muscle cramps, nausea, vomiting, trembling, stomach cramps or unusual sweating.

Others:
If diarrhea lasts longer than 4 days, discontinue and call doctor.

POSSIBLE INTERACTION WITH OTHER DRUGS

GENERIC NAME OR DRUG CLASS	COMBINED EFFECT
Barbiturates	Increased effect of both drugs.
Ethinamate	Dangerous increased effects of ethinamate. Avoid combining.
Fluoxetine	Increased depressant effects of both drugs.
Guanfacine	May increase depressant effects of either drug.
Leucovorin	High alcohol content of leucovorin may cause adverse effects.
MAO inhibitors (see Drugs Glossary)	May increase blood pressure excessively.
Methyprylon	Increased sedative effect, perhaps to dangerous level. Avoid.
Sedatives	Increased effect of both drugs.
Tranquilizers	Increased effect of both drugs.

POSSIBLE INTERACTION WITH OTHER SUBSTANCES

INTERACTS WITH	COMBINED EFFECT
Alcohol:	Depressed brain function. Avoid.
Beverages:	None expected.
Cocaine (or crack):	Decreased effect of diphenoxylate and atropine.
Foods:	None expected.
Marijuana:	None expected.
Tobacco:	None expected.

DIPYRIDAMOLE

BRAND NAMES

Apo-Dipyridamole
Persantine
Pyridamole
SK-Dipyridamole

BASIC INFORMATION

Habit forming? No
Prescription needed?
U.S.: Yes
Canada: No
Available as generic? Yes
Drug class: Coronary vasodilator

USES

- May reduce frequency and intensity of angina attacks.
- Prevents blood clots after heart surgery.

DOSAGE & USAGE INFORMATION

How to take:
Tablet—Swallow with liquid. If you can't swallow whole, crumble tablet and take with liquid.

When to take:
1 hour before meals.

If you forget a dose:
Take as soon as you remember up to 2 hours late. If more than 2 hours, wait for next scheduled dose (don't double this dose).

Continued next column

OVERDOSE

SYMPTOMS:
Decreased blood pressure; weak, rapid pulse; cold, clammy skin; collapse.
WHAT TO DO:
- **Dial 0 (operator) or 911 (emergency) for an ambulance or medical help. Then give first aid immediately.**
- **If the child is unconscious and not breathing, give mouth-to-mouth breathing. If there is no heartbeat, use cardiac massage and mouth-to-mouth breathing (CPR). Don't try to make the child vomit. If you can't get help quickly, take the child to nearest emergency facility.**
- **See emergency information at the back of this book.**

What drug does:
- Probably dilates blood vessels to increase oxygen to heart.
- Prevents platelet clumping, which causes blood clots.

Time lapse before drug works:
3 months of continual use.

Don't take with:
Any other medicines, even over-the-counter drugs such as cough and cold medicines, nose drops, diet pills, laxatives or caffeine, without consulting your doctor.

POSSIBLE ADVERSE REACTIONS OR SIDE EFFECTS

SYMPTOMS	WHAT TO DO
Life-threatening: None expected.	
Common: None expected.	
Infrequent:	
• Dizziness, fainting, headache.	Discontinue. Call doctor right away.
• Red flush, rash, nausea, vomiting, cramps, weakness.	Continue. Call doctor when convenient.
Rare: None expected.	

WARNINGS & PRECAUTIONS

Don't take if:
- You are allergic to dipyridamole.
- You are recovering from a heart attack.

Before you start, consult your doctor:
- If you have low blood pressure.
- If you have liver disease.

Pregnancy:
No proven harm to unborn child. Avoid if possible.

Infants & children
Don't give to infants or young children unless prescribed and monitored by your physician.

Prolonged use:
No age-related problems expected.

Skin & sunlight:
No age-related problems expected.

Driving or hazardous activities:
Avoid if you feel dizzy. Otherwise, no problems expected.

Discontinuing:
Don't discontinue without doctor's advice until you complete prescribed dose, even though symptoms diminish or disappear.

Others:
Drug increases your ability to be active without angina pain. Avoid excessive physical exertion that might injure heart.

POSSIBLE INTERACTION WITH OTHER DRUGS

GENERIC NAME OR DRUG CLASS	COMBINED EFFECT
Anticoagulants (oral, see Drugs Glossary)	Increased anticoagulant effect. Bleeding tendency.
Aspirin	Increased dipyridamole effect. Dose may need adjustment.

POSSIBLE INTERACTION WITH OTHER SUBSTANCES

INTERACTS WITH	COMBINED EFFECT
Alcohol:	May lower blood pressure excessively.
Beverages:	None expected.
Cocaine (or crack):	No additional problems due to dipyridamole.
Foods:	Decreased dipyridamole absorption unless taken 1 hour before eating.
Marijuana:	Daily use—Decreased dipyridamole effect.
Tobacco: Nicotine.	May decrease dipyridamole effect.

DISOPYRAMIDE

BRAND NAMES

Norpace	Rythmodan
Norpace CR	Rythmodan-LA

BASIC INFORMATION

Habit forming? No
Prescription needed? Yes
Available as generic? Yes
Drug class: Antiarrhythmic

USES

Corrects heart rhythm disorders.

DOSAGE & USAGE INFORMATION

How to take:
Extended-release tablet or capsule—Swallow with liquid. If you can't swallow whole, open capsule and take with liquid or food.

When to take:
At the same times each day.

If you forget a dose:
Take as soon as you remember up to 2 hours late. If more than 2 hours, wait for next scheduled dose (don't double this dose).

What drug does:
Delays nerve impulses to heart to regulate heartbeat.

Time lapse before drug works:
Begins in 30 to 60 minutes. Must use for 5 to 7 days to determine effectiveness.

Continued next column

Don't take with:
Any other medicines, even over-the-counter drugs such as cough and cold medicines, nose drops, diet pills, laxatives or caffeine, without consulting your doctor.

OVERDOSE

SYMPTOMS:
Blood-pressure drop, irregular heartbeat, apnea, loss of consciousness.
WHAT TO DO:
- **Dial 0 (operator) or 911 (emergency) for an ambulance or medical help. Then give first aid immediately.**
- **If the child is unconscious and not breathing, give mouth-to-mouth breathing. If there is no heartbeat, use cardiac massage and mouth-to-mouth breathing (CPR). Don't try to make the child vomit. If you can't get help quickly, take the child to nearest emergency facility.**
- **See emergency information at the back of this book.**

POSSIBLE ADVERSE REACTIONS OR SIDE EFFECTS

SYMPTOMS	WHAT TO DO
Life-threatening:	
Hives, rash, intense itching, faintness soon after a dose (anaphylaxis).	Seek emergency treatment immediately.
Common:	
• Hypoglycemia.	Discontinue. Call doctor right away.
• Dry mouth, constipation, painful or difficult urination, rapid weight gain, blurred vision.	Continue. Call doctor when convenient.
Infrequent:	
• Dizziness, fainting, confusion, nervousness, depression, chest pain, slow or fast heartbeat.	Discontinue. Call doctor right away.
• Swollen feet.	Continue. Call doctor when convenient.
Rare:	
• Shortness of breath, psychosis.	Discontinue. Seek emergency treatment.
• Rash, sore throat, fever, headache, jaundice, muscle weakness.	Discontinue. Call doctor right away.
• Eye pain, diminished sex drive, swollen breasts in men, numbness or tingling of hands and feet, bleeding tendency.	Continue. Call doctor when convenient.

WARNINGS & PRECAUTIONS

Don't take if:
- You are allergic to disopyramide or any antiarrhythmic.
- You have second-or third-degree heart block.
- You have heart failure.

Before you start, consult your doctor:
- If you react unfavorably to other antiarrhythmic drugs.
- If you have had heart disease.
- If you have low blood pressure.
- If you have liver disease.
- If you have glaucoma.
- If you have enlarged prostate.
- If you have myasthenia gravis.
- If you take digitalis preparations or diuretics.

Pregnancy:
No proven harm to unborn child. Avoid if possible.

Infants & children:
Don't give to infants or young children unless prescribed and monitored by your physician.

Prolonged use:
No age-related problems expected.

Skin & sunlight:
No age-related problems expected.

Driving or hazardous activities:
Don't drive or pilot aircraft until you learn how medicine affects you. Don't work around dangerous machinery. Don't climb ladders or work in high places. Danger increases if you drink alcohol or take medicine affecting alertness and reflexes, such as antihistamines, tranquilizers, sedatives, pain medicine, narcotics, or mind-altering drugs.

Discontinuing:
Don't discontinue without doctor's advice until you complete prescribed dose, even though symptoms diminish or disappear.

Others:
If new illness, injury or surgery occurs, tell doctors of disopyramide use.

POSSIBLE INTERACTION WITH OTHER DRUGS

GENERIC NAME OR DRUG CLASS	COMBINED EFFECT
Antiarrhythmics (see Drugs Glossary)	May increase effect and toxicity of each drug.
Anticholinergics (see Drugs Glossary)	Increased anticholinergic effect.
Anticoagulants (oral, see Drugs Glossary)	Possible increased anticoagulant effect.
Antihypertensives (see Drugs Glossary)	Increased antihypertensive effect.
Encainide	Increased effect of toxicity on the heart muscle.
Flecainide	Possible irregular heartbeat.
Phenobarbital	Increased metabolism, decreased disopyramide effect.
Phenytoin	Increased metabolism, decreased disopyramide effect.
Rifampin	Increased metabolism, decreased disopyramide effect.
Tocainide	Increased likelihood of adverse reactions with either drug.

POSSIBLE INTERACTION WITH OTHER SUBSTANCES

INTERACTS WITH	COMBINED EFFECT
Alcohol:	Decreased blood pressure and blood sugar. Use caution.
Beverages:	None expected.
Cocaine (or crack):	Irregular heartbeat.
Foods:	None expected.
Marijuana:	Unpredictable. May decrease disopyramide effect.
Tobacco:	May decrease disopyramide effect.

DIURETICS, LOOP

BRAND & GENERIC NAMES

Apo-Furosemide	Lasix
BUMETANIDE	Lasix Special
Bumex	Neo-Renal
Edecrin	Novosemide
ETHACRYNIC ACID	SK-Furosemide
FUROSEMIDE	Uritol
Furoside	

BASIC INFORMATION

Habit forming? No
Prescription needed? Yes
Available as generic? Yes
Drug class: Diuretic, antihypertensive

USES

- Lowers high blood pressure.
- Decreases fluid retention.

DOSAGE & USAGE INFORMATION

How to take:
Tablet or liquid—Swallow with liquid. If you can't swallow whole, crumble tablet and take with liquid or food.

When to take:
- 1 dose a day—Take after breakfast.
- More than 1 dose a day—Take last dose no later than 6 p.m. unless otherwise directed.

If you forget a dose:
- 1 dose a day—Take as soon as you remember up to 12 hours late. If more than 12 hours, wait for next scheduled dose (don't double this dose).
- More than 1 dose a day—Take as soon as you remember up to 2 hours late. If more than 2 hours, wait for next scheduled dose (don't double this dose).

Continued next column

OVERDOSE

SYMPTOMS:
Weakness, lethargy, dizziness, confusion, nausea, vomiting, leg-muscle cramps, thirst, stupor, deep sleep, weak and rapid pulse, cardiac arrest.
WHAT TO DO:
- **Dial 0 (operator) or 911 (emergency) for an ambulance or medical help. Then give first aid immediately.**
- **See emergency information at the back of this book.**

What drug does:
Increases elimination of sodium and water from body. Decreased body fluid reduces blood pressure.

Time lapse before drug works:
1 hour to increase water loss. Requires 2 to 3 weeks to lower blood pressure.

Don't take with:
Any other medicines, even over-the-counter drugs such as cough and cold medicines, nose drops, diet pills, laxatives or caffeine, without consulting your doctor.

POSSIBLE ADVERSE REACTIONS OR SIDE EFFECTS

SYMPTOMS	WHAT TO DO
Life-threatening: None expected.	
Common: Dizziness.	Continue. Call doctor when convenient.
Infrequent: Mood change, fatigue, appetite loss, diarrhea, irregular heartbeat, muscle cramps, weakness, abdominal pain, low blood pressure.	Discontinue. Call doctor right away.
Rare: Rash or hives, yellow vision, ringing in ears, hearing loss, sore throat, fever, dry mouth, thirst, side or stomach pain, nausea, vomiting, unusual bleeding or bruising, joint pain, jaundice, numbness or tingling in hands or feet.	Discontinue. Call doctor right away.

WARNINGS & PRECAUTIONS

Don't take if:
You are allergic to loop diuretics.

Before you start, consult your doctor:
- If you are allergic to any sulfa drug.
- If you have liver or kidney disease.
- If you have gout, diabetes or impaired hearing.
- If you will have surgery within 2 months, including dental surgery, requiring general or spinal anesthesia.

Pregnancy:
Risk to unborn child outweighs drug benefits. Don't use.

Infants & children:
Use only under medical supervision.

Prolonged use:
- Impaired balance of water, salt and potassium in blood and body tissues.
- Possible diabetes.

Skin & sunlight:
May cause rash or intensify sunburn in areas exposed to sun or sunlamp.

Driving or hazardous activities:
No age-related problems expected.

Discontinuing:
Don't discontinue without doctor's advice until you complete prescribed dose, even though symptoms diminish or disappear.

Others:
Frequent laboratory studies to monitor potassium level in blood recommended. Eat foods rich in potassium or take potassium supplements. Consult doctor.

POSSIBLE INTERACTION WITH OTHER DRUGS

GENERIC NAME OR DRUG CLASS	COMBINED EFFECT
ACE inhibitors: captopril, enalapril, lisinopril (see Drugs Glossary)	Possible excessive potassium in blood.
Allopurinol	Decreased allopurinol effect.
Amiodarone	Increased risk of heartbeat irregularity due to low potassium.
Anticoagulants (see Drugs Glossary)	Abnormal clotting.
Antidepressants, tricyclic (TCA, see Drugs Glossary)	Excessive blood-pressure drop.
Antidiabetics (oral, see Drugs Glossary)	Decreased antidiabetic effect.
Antihypertensives (see Drugs Glossary)	Increased antihypertensive effect. Dosages may require adjustment.
Barbiturates (see Drugs Glossary)	Low blood pressure.
Beta-adrenergic blockers (see Drugs Glossary)	Increased antihypertensive effect. Dosages may require adjustment.
Calcium supplements (see Drugs Glossary)	Decreased calcium in blood.
Corticosteroids	Decreased potassium.
Cortisone drugs	Excessive potassium loss.
Digitalis preparations (see Drugs Glossary)	Excessive potassium loss could lead to serious heart rhythm disorders.
Digoxin	Increased possibility of digitalis toxicity.

See Additional Drug Interactions Section.

POSSIBLE INTERACTION WITH OTHER SUBSTANCES

INTERACTS WITH	COMBINED EFFECT
Alcohol:	Blood-pressure drop. Avoid.
Beverages:	None expected.
Cocaine (or crack):	Dangerous blood-pressure drop. Avoid.
Foods:	None expected.
Marijuana:	Increased thirst and urinary frequency, fainting.
Tobacco:	Decreased loop diuretic effect.

DIURETICS, THIAZIDE

BRAND & GENERIC NAMES

See complete list of brand and generic names in the Brand & Generic Name Directory.

BASIC INFORMATION

Habit forming? No
Prescription needed? Yes
Available as generic? Yes
Drug class: Antihypertensive, diuretic (thiazide)

USES

- Controls, but doesn't cure, high blood pressure.
- Reduces fluid retention (edema).

DOSAGE & USAGE INFORMATION

How to take:
Tablet or liquid—Swallow with liquid. If you can't swallow whole, crumble tablet and take with liquid or food.

When to take:
At the same time each day.

If you forget a dose:
Take as soon as you remember up to 2 hours late. If more than 2 hours, wait for next scheduled dose (don't double this dose).

What drug does:
- Forces sodium and water excretion, reducing body fluid.
- Relaxes muscle cells of small arteries.
- Reduced body fluid and relaxed arteries lower blood pressure.

Time lapse before drug works:
4 to 6 hours. May require several weeks to lower blood pressure.

Don't take with:
Any other medicines, even over-the-counter drugs such as cough and cold medicines, nose drops, diet pills, laxatives or caffeine, without consulting your doctor.

OVERDOSE

SYMPTOMS:
Cramps, weakness, drowsiness, weak pulse, coma.
WHAT TO DO:
- **Dial 0 (operator) or 911 (emergency) for an ambulance or medical help. Then give first aid immediately.**
- **See emergency information at the back of this book.**

POSSIBLE ADVERSE REACTIONS OR SIDE EFFECTS

SYMPTOMS	WHAT TO DO
Life-threatening: None expected.	
Common: None expected.	
Infrequent:	
• Blurred vision, severe abdominal pain, nausea, vomiting, irregular heartbeat, weak pulse.	Discontinue. Call doctor right away.
• Dizziness, mood change, headache, weakness, tiredness, weight changes.	Continue. Call doctor when convenient.
• Dry mouth, thirst.	Continue. Tell doctor at next visit.
Rare:	
• Rash or hives.	Discontinue. Seek emergency treatment.
• Sore throat, fever, jaundice.	Discontinue. Call doctor right away.

WARNINGS & PRECAUTIONS

Don't take if:
You are allergic to any thiazide diuretic drug.

Before you start, consult your doctor:
- If you are allergic to any sulfa drug.
- If you have gout.
- If you have liver, pancreas or kidney disorder.

Pregnancy:
Risk to unborn child outweighs drug benefits. Don't use.

Infants & children:
No age-related problems expected.

Prolonged use:
You may need medicine to treat high blood pressure for the rest of your life.

Skin & sunlight:
May cause rash or intensify sunburn in areas exposed to sun or sunlamp.

Driving or hazardous activities:
Don't drive or pilot aircraft until you learn how medicine affects you. Don't work around dangerous machinery. Don't climb ladders or work in high places. Danger increases if you drink alcohol or take medicine affecting alertness and reflexes, such as antihistamines, tranquilizers, sedatives, pain medicine, narcotics and mind-altering drugs.

Discontinuing:
Don't discontinue without medical advice.

Others:
• Hot weather and fever may cause dehydration and drop in blood pressure. Dose may require temporary adjustment. Weigh daily and report any unexpected weight decreases to your doctor.
• May cause rise in uric acid, leading to gout.
• May cause blood-sugar rise in diabetics.

POSSIBLE INTERACTION WITH OTHER DRUGS

GENERIC NAME OR DRUG CLASS	COMBINED EFFECT
ACE inhibitors: captopril, enalapril, lisinopril (see Drugs Glossary)	Decreased blood pressure.
Allopurinol	Decreased allopurinol effect.
Amiodarone	Increased risk of heartbeat irregularity due to low potassium.
Amphotericin B	Increased potassium.
Antidepressants, tricyclic (TCA, see Drugs Glossary)	Dangerous drop in blood pressure. Avoid combination unless under medical supervision.
Antidiabetic agents (oral, see Drugs Glossary)	Increased blood sugar.
Antihypertensives (see Drugs Glossary)	Increased hypertensive effect.
Barbiturates (see Drugs Glossary)	Increased diuretic effect.
Beta-adrenergic blockers (see Drugs Glossary)	Increased antihypertensive effect. Dosages of both drugs may require adjustments.
Calcium supplements (see Drugs Glossary)	Increased calcium in blood.
Cholestyramine	Decreased diuretic effect.
Colestipol	Decreased diuretic effect.
Cortisone drugs	Excessive potassium loss that causes dangerous heart rhythms.
Digitalis preparations (see Drugs Glossary)	Excessive potassium loss that causes dangerous heart rhythms.
Diuretics (thiazide, see Drugs Glossary)	Increased effect of other thiazide diuretics.
Indapamide	Increased diuretic effect.
Indomethacin	Decreased diuretic effect.
Labetolol	Increased anti-hypertensive effects.
Lithium	Increased effect of lithium.
MAO inhibitors (see Drugs Glossary)	Increased diuretic effect.

See Additional Drug Interactions Section

POSSIBLE INTERACTION WITH OTHER SUBSTANCES

INTERACTS WITH	COMBINED EFFECT
Alcohol:	Dangerous blood-pressure drop.
Beverages:	None expected.
Cocaine (or crack):	None expected.
Foods: Licorice.	Excessive potassium loss that causes dangerous heart rhythms.
Marijuana:	May increase blood pressure.
Tobacco:	None expected.

ENALAPRIL & HYDROCHLOROTHIAZIDE

BRAND NAMES

Vaseretic

BASIC INFORMATION

Habit forming? No
Prescription needed? Yes
Available as generic? No
Drug class: Antihypertensive, diuretic, ACE inhibitor (see Drugs Glossary)

USES

• Treatment for high blood pressure and congestive heart failure.
• Reduces fluid retention.

DOSAGE & USAGE INFORMATION

How to take:
Tablet—Swallow with liquid. These tablets are long-acting. Food does not alter normal absorption from the gastrointestinal tract.

When to take:
Usually once a day.

If you forget a dose:
Take as soon as you remember up to 18 hours late. If more than 18 hours, wait for next scheduled dose (don't double this dose).

What drug does:
• Forces sodium and water excretion, reducing body fluid.
• Relaxes muscle cells of small arteries.
• Reduced body fluid and relaxed arteries lower blood pressure.
• Reduces resistance in arteries.
• Strengthens heartbeat.

Continued next column

OVERDOSE

SYMPTOMS:
Cramps, weakness, drowsiness, weak pulse, fever, chills, sore throat, fainting, convulsions, coma.
WHAT TO DO:
• Dial 0 (operator) or 911 (emergency) for an ambulance or medical help. Then give first aid immediately.
• See emergency information at the back of this book.

Time lapse before drug works:
4 to 6 hours. May require several weeks to lower blood pressure.

Don't take with:
Any other medicines, even over-the-counter drugs such as cough and cold medicines, nose drops, diet pills, laxatives or caffeine, without consulting your doctor.

POSSIBLE ADVERSE REACTIONS OR SIDE EFFECTS

SYMPTOMS	WHAT TO DO
Life-threatening:	
Irregular heartbeat (fast or uneven); difficulty breathing; hives, rash, intense itching, faintness soon after a dose (anaphylaxis).	Discontinue. Seek emergency treatment.
Common:	
• Dry mouth, thirst, tiredness, weakness, muscle cramps, vomiting, chest pain, skin rash, coughing.	Discontinue. Call doctor right away.
• Taste loss, dizziness.	Continue. Call doctor when convenient.
Infrequent:	
• Face, mouth, hands swelling.	Discontinue. Call doctor right away.
• Nausea, diarrhea.	Continue. Call doctor when convenient.
Rare:	
None expected.	

WARNINGS & PRECAUTIONS

Don't take if:
• You are allergic to enalapril, captopril, or any thiazide diuretic drug.
• You have any autoimmune disease, including AIDS or lupus.
• You are receiving blood from a blood bank.
• You take drugs for cancer.
• You will have surgery within 2 months, including dental surgery, requiring general or spinal anesthesia.

Before you start, consult your doctor:
• If you have had a stroke.
• If you have angina, heart or blood-vessel disease, a high level of potassium in blood, lupus, gout, liver, pancreas or kidney disorder.
• If you are on a severe salt-restricted diet.
• If you are allergic to any sulfa drug.

Pregnancy:
Risk to unborn child outweighs drug benefits. Don't use.

Infants & children
Don't give to infants or young children unless prescribed and monitored by your physician.

Prolonged use:
May decrease white cells in blood or cause protein loss in urine. Request periodic laboratory blood counts and urine tests.

Skin & sunlight:
May cause rash or intensify sunburn in areas exposed to sun or sunlamp.

Driving or hazardous activities:
Don't drive or pilot aircraft until you learn how medicine affects you. Don't work around dangerous machinery. Don't climb ladders or work in high places. Danger increases if you drink alcohol or take medicine affecting alertness and reflexes, such as antihistamines, tranquilizers, sedatives, pain medicine, narcotics and mind-altering drugs.

Discontinuing:
Don't discontinue without consulting doctor. Dose may require gradual reduction if you have taken drug for a long time. Doses of other drugs may also require adjustment.

Others:
- Hot weather and fever may cause dehydration and drop in blood pressure. Dose may require temporary adjustment. Weigh daily and report any unexpected weight decreases to your doctor.
- May cause rise in uric acid, leading to gout.
- May cause blood-sugar rise in diabetics.

POSSIBLE INTERACTION WITH OTHER DRUGS

GENERIC NAME OR DRUG CLASS	COMBINED EFFECT
Allopurinol	Decreased allopurinol effect.
Amiloride	Possible excessive potassium in blood.
Antidepressants, tricyclic (TCA, see Drugs Glossary)	Dangerous drop in blood pressure. Avoid combination unless under medical supervision.
Antihypertensives (other, see Drugs Glossary)	Increased antihypertensive effect. Dosage of each may require adjustment.
Barbiturates (see Drugs Glossary)	Increased hydrochlorothiazide effect.
Beta-adrenergic blockers (see Drugs Glossary)	Increased antihypertensive effect Dosages of both drugs may require adjustments.
Chloramphenicol	Possible blood disorders.
Cholestyramine	Decreased hydrochlorothiazide effect.
Cortisone drugs	Excessive potassium loss that causes dangerous heart rhythms.
Digitalis preparations (see Drugs Glossary)	Excessive potassium loss that causes dangerous heart rhythms.
Diuretics (thiazide, see Drugs Glossary)	Increased effect of other thiazide diuretics.
Indapamide	Increased diuretic effect.
Lithium	Increased effect of lithium.
MAO inhibitors (see Drugs Glossary)	Increased hydrochlorothiazide effect.
Nitrates	Excessive blood-pressure drop.
Non-steroidal anti-inflammatory drugs (NSAIDs, see Drugs Glossary)	Decreased enalapril effect.

See Additional Drug Interactions Section

POSSIBLE INTERACTION WITH OTHER SUBSTANCES

INTERACTS WITH	COMBINED EFFECT
Alcohol:	Dangerous blood-pressure drop. Avoid.
Beverages: Low-salt milk.	Possible excessive potassium in blood.
Cocaine (or crack):	Increased dizziness, chest pain.
Foods: Salt substitutes.	Possible excessive potassium.
Marijuana:	Increased dizziness, may increase blood pressure.
Tobacco:	May decrease enalapril effect.

ERYTHROMYCINS

BRAND & GENERIC NAMES

See complete list of brand and generic names in the Brand & Generic Name Directory.

BASIC INFORMATION

Habit forming? No
Prescription needed? Yes
Available as generic? Yes
Drug class: Antibiotic (erythromycin)

USES

Treatment of infections responsive to erythromycin.

DOSAGE & USAGE INFORMATION

How to take:
- Tablet or capsule—Swallow with liquid.
- Extended-release tablets or capsules—Swallow each dose whole. If you take regular tablets, you may chew or crush them.
- Liquid, drops, granules, skin ointment, eye ointment, skin solution— Follow prescription label directions.

When to take:
At the same times each day, 1 hour before or 2 hours after eating.

If you forget a dose:
- If you take 3 or more doses daily—Take as soon as you remember. Return to regular schedule.
- If you take 2 doses daily—Take as soon as you remember. Wait 5 to 6 hours for next dose. Return to regular schedule.

What drug does:
Prevents growth and reproduction of susceptible bacteria.

Continued next column

OVERDOSE

SYMPTOMS:
Nausea, vomiting, abdominal discomfort, diarrhea.
WHAT TO DO:
Overdose unlikely to threaten life. If child takes much larger amount than prescribed, call doctor, poison-control center or hospital emergency room for instructions.

Time lapse before drug works:
2 to 5 days.

Don't take with:
Any other medicines, even over-the-counter drugs such as cough and cold medicines, nose drops, diet pills, laxatives or caffeine, without consulting your doctor.

POSSIBLE ADVERSE REACTIONS OR SIDE EFFECTS

SYMPTOMS	WHAT TO DO
Life-threatening:	
None expected.	
Common:	
Gastrointestinal upset.	Discontinue. Call doctor right away.
Infrequent:	
• Diarrhea, nausea, stomach cramps, discomfort, vomiting.	Discontinue. Call doctor right away.
• Skin dryness, irritation, itch, stinging with use of skin solution, sore mouth or tongue.	Continue. Call doctor when convenient.
Rare:	
• Jaundice in adults, hearing loss.	Discontinue. Call doctor right away.
• Unusual tiredness or weakness.	Continue. Call doctor when convenient.

WARNINGS & PRECAUTIONS

Don't take if:
- You are allergic to any erythromycin.
- You have had liver disease or impaired liver function.

Before you start, consult your doctor:
If you have taken erythromycin estolate in the past.

Pregnancy:
No proven harm to unborn child. Avoid if possible.

Infants & children:
Use only under medical supervision.

Prolonged use:
You may become more susceptible to infections caused by germs not responsive to erythromycin.

Skin & sunlight:
No age-related problems expected.

Driving or hazardous activities:
No age-related problems expected.

Discontinuing:
You must take full dose at least 10 consecutive days for streptococcal or staphylococcal infections.

Others:
No age-related problems expected.

POSSIBLE INTERACTION WITH OTHER DRUGS

GENERIC NAME OR DRUG CLASS	COMBINED EFFECT
Aminophylline	Increased effect of aminophylline in blood.
Lincomycins	Decreased lincomycin effect.
Oxtriphylline	Increased level of oxtriphylline in blood.
Penicillins (see Drugs Glossary)	Decreased penicillin effect.
Theophylline	Increased level of theophylline in blood.

POSSIBLE INTERACTION WITH OTHER SUBSTANCES

INTERACTS WITH	COMBINED EFFECT
Alcohol:	Possible liver damage.
Beverages:	None expected.
Cocaine (or crack):	None expected.
Foods:	None expected.
Marijuana:	None expected.
Tobacco:	None expected.

ESTROGEN

BRAND & GENERIC NAMES

See complete list of brand and generic names in the Brand & Generic Name Directory.

BASIC INFORMATION

Habit forming? No
Prescription needed? Yes
Available as generic? Yes
Drug class: Female sex hormone (estrogen)

USES

- Treatment for symptoms of menopause and menstrual-cycle irregularity.
- Treatment for estrogen-deficiency osteoporosis (bone softening from calcium loss).
- Treatment for DES-induced cancer.
- Treatment for atrophic vaginitis.

DOSAGE & USAGE INFORMATION

How to take:
- Tablet or capsule—Swallow with liquid. If you can't swallow whole, crumble tablet or open capsule and take with liquid or food.
- Vaginal cream or suppositories—Use as directed on label.

When to take:
At the same time each day.

If you forget a dose:
Take as soon as you remember up to 12 hours late. If more than 12 hours, wait for next scheduled dose (don't double this dose).

What drug does:
Restores normal estrogen level in tissues.

Time lapse before drug works:
10 to 20 days.

Continued next column

OVERDOSE

SYMPTOMS:
Nausea, vomiting, fluid retention, breast enlargement and discomfort, abnormal vaginal bleeding.
WHAT TO DO:
Overdose unlikely to threaten life. If child takes much larger amount than prescribed, call doctor, poison-control center or hospital emergency room for instructions.

Don't take with:
Any other medicines, even over-the-counter drugs such as cough and cold medicines, nose drops, diet pills, laxatives or caffeine, without consulting your doctor.

POSSIBLE ADVERSE REACTIONS OR SIDE EFFECTS

SYMPTOMS	WHAT TO DO
Life-threatening: None expected.	
Common:	
• Stomach cramps.	Discontinue. Call doctor right away.
• Appetite loss.	Continue. Call doctor when convenient.
• Nausea; diarrhea; swollen feet and ankles; tender, swollen breasts.	Continue. Tell doctor at next visit.
Infrequent:	
• Rash, stomach or side pain.	Discontinue. Call doctor right away.
• Depression, dizziness, headache, irritability, vomiting, breast lumps.	Continue. Call doctor when convenient.
• Brown blotches, hair loss, vaginal discharge or bleeding, changes in sex drive.	Continue. Tell doctor at next visit.
Rare:	
Jaundice, hypercalcemia in breast cancer, intolerance of contact lenses.	Discontinue. Call doctor right away.

WARNINGS & PRECAUTIONS

Don't take if:
- You are allergic to any estrogen-containing drugs.
- You have impaired liver function.
- You have had blood clots, stroke or heart attack.
- You have unexplained vaginal bleeding.

Before you start, consult your doctor:
• If you have had cancer of breast or reproductive organs, fibrocystic breast disease, fibroid tumors of the uterus or endometriosis.
• If you have had migraine headaches, epilepsy or porphyria.
• If you have diabetes, high blood pressure, asthma, congestive heart failure, kidney disease or gallstones.
• If you plan to become pregnant within 3 months.

Pregnancy:
Risk to unborn child outweighs drug benefits. Don't use.

Infants & children
Don't give to infants or young children unless prescribed and monitored by your physician.

Prolonged use:
Increased growth of fibroid tumors of uterus. Possible association with cancer of uterus.

Skin & sunlight:
May cause rash or intensify sunburn in areas exposed to sun or sunlamp.

Driving or hazardous activities:
No age-related problems expected.

Discontinuing:
You may need to discontinue estrogens periodically. Consult your doctor.

Others:
• In rare instances, may cause blood clot in lung, brain or leg. Symptoms are *sudden* severe headache, coordination loss, vision change, chest pain, breathing difficulty, slurred speech, pain in legs or groin. Seek emergency treatment immediately.
• Carefully read the paper called "Information for the Patient" that was given to you with your prescription. If you lose it, ask your pharmacist for a copy.

POSSIBLE INTERACTION WITH OTHER DRUGS

GENERIC NAME OR DRUG CLASS	COMBINED EFFECT
Anticoagulants (oral, see Drugs Glossary)	Decreased anticoagulant effect.
Anticonvulsants (see Drugs Glossary)	Decreased estrogen effect.
Antidepressants, tricyclic (TCA, see Drugs Glossary)	Increased toxicity of antidepressants.
Antidiabetics (oral, see Drugs Glossary)	Unpredictable increase or decrease in blood sugar.
Carbamazepine	Decreased estrogen effect.
Clofibrate	Decreased clofibrate effect.
Guanfacine	May decrease antihypertensive effects of guanfacine.
Insulin	Possible decreased insulin effect. May require dosage adjustment.
Meprobamate	Increased estrogen effect.
Phenobarbital	Decreased estrogen effect.
Primidone	Decreased estrogen effect.
Rifampin	Decreased estrogen effect.
Thyroid hormones	Decreased thyroid effect.
Vitamin C	Possible increased estrogen effect.

POSSIBLE INTERACTION WITH OTHER SUBSTANCES

INTERACTS WITH	COMBINED EFFECT
Alcohol:	None expected.
Beverages:	None expected.
Cocaine (or crack):	No proven problems.
Foods:	None expected.
Marijuana:	Possible menstrual irregularities and bleeding between periods.
Tobacco:	Increased risk of blood clots leading to stroke or heart attack.

FOLIC ACID (VITAMIN B-9)

BRAND NAMES

Apo-Folic
Folvite
Novofolacid
Numerous other multiple vitamin-mineral supplements.

BASIC INFORMATION

Habit forming? No
Prescription needed?
High strength: Yes
Vitamin mixtures: No
Available as generic? Yes
Drug class: Vitamin supplement

USES

• Dietary supplement to promote normal growth, development and good health.
• Treatment for anemias due to folic-acid deficiency occurring from alcoholism, liver disease, hemolytic anemia, sprue, infants on artificial formula, pregnancy, breast-feeding and oral-contraceptive use.

DOSAGE & USAGE INFORMATION

How to take:
Tablet—Swallow with liquid or food to lessen stomach irritation. If you can't swallow whole, crumble tablet and take with liquid or food.

When to take:
At the same time each day.

If you forget a dose:
Take when you remember. Don't double next dose. Resume regular schedule.

What drug does:
Essential to normal red-blood-cell formation.

Time lapse before drug works:
Not determined.

Don't take with:
Any other medicines, even over-the-counter drugs such as cough and cold medicines, nose drops, diet pills, laxatives or caffeine, without consulting your doctor.

OVERDOSE

SYMPTOMS:
None expected.
WHAT TO DO:
Overdose unlikely to threaten life.

POSSIBLE ADVERSE REACTIONS OR SIDE EFFECTS

SYMPTOMS	WHAT TO DO
Life-threatening:	
None expected.	
Common:	
Large dose may produce yellow urine.	Continue. Tell doctor at next visit.
Infrequent:	
None expected.	
Rare:	
Rash, itching, bronchospasm.	Discontinue. Call doctor right away.

WARNINGS & PRECAUTIONS

Don't take if:
You are allergic to any B vitamin.

Before you start, consult your doctor:
• If you have liver disease.
• If you have pernicious anemia. (Folic acid corrects anemia, but nerve damage of pernicious anemia continues.)

Pregnancy:
No problems expected.

Infants & children:
No age-related problems expected.

Prolonged use:
No problems expected.

Skin & sunlight:
No problems expected.

Driving or hazardous activities:
No problems expected.

Discontinuing:
Don't discontinue without doctor's advice until you complete prescribed dose, even though symptoms diminish or disappear.

Others:
• Folic acid removed by kidney dialysis. Dialysis the childs should increase intake to 300% of RDA.
• A balanced diet should provide all the folic acid a healthy child needs and make supplements unnecessary. Best sources are green, leafy vegetables, fruits, liver and kidney.

POSSIBLE INTERACTION WITH OTHER DRUGS

GENERIC NAME OR DRUG CLASS	COMBINED EFFECT
Analgesics	Decreased effect of folic acid.
Anticonvulsants (see Drugs Glossary)	Decreased effect of folic acid. Possible increased seizure frequency.
Chloramphenicol	Possible decreased folic acid effect.
Contraceptives (oral, see Drugs Glossary)	Decreased effect of folic acid.
Cortisone drugs	Decreased effect of folic acid.
Methotrexate	Decreased effect of folic acid.
Para-aminosalicylic acid (PAS)	Decreased effect of folic acid.
Pyrimethamine	Decreased effect of folic acid.
Sulfasalazine	Decreased dietary absorption of folic acid.
Triamterene	Decreased effect of folic acid.
Trimethoprim	Decreased effect of folic acid.
Zinc	Decreased zinc effect.

POSSIBLE INTERACTION WITH OTHER SUBSTANCES

INTERACTS WITH	COMBINED EFFECT
Alcohol:	None expected.
Beverages:	None expected.
Cocaine (or crack):	None expected.
Foods:	None expected.
Marijuana:	None expected.
Tobacco:	None expected.

HALOPERIDOL

BRAND NAMES

Apo-Haloperidol
Haldol
Haldol Decanoate
Haldol LA
Novoperidol
Peridol

BASIC INFORMATION

Habit forming? No
Prescription needed? Yes
Available as generic? Yes
Drug class: Tranquilizer (antipsychotic)

USES

Reduces severe anxiety, agitation and psychotic behavior.

DOSAGE & USAGE INFORMATION

How to take:
• Tablet or extended-release capsule—Swallow with liquid. If you can't swallow whole, crumble tablet and take with liquid or food.
• Drops—Dilute dose in beverage before swallowing.

When to take:
At the same times each day.

If you forget a dose:
Take as soon as you remember up to 2 hours late. If more than 2 hours, wait for next scheduled dose (don't double this dose).

What drug does:
Corrects an imbalance in nerve impulses from brain.

Continued next column

OVERDOSE

SYMPTOMS:
Weak, rapid pulse; shallow, slow breathing; very low blood pressure; convulsions; deep sleep ending in coma.
WHAT TO DO:
• Dial 0 (operator) or 911 (emergency) for an ambulance or medical help. Then give first aid immediately.
• If the child is unconscious and not breathing, give mouth-to-mouth breathing. If there is no heartbeat, use cardiac massage and mouth-to-mouth breathing (CPR). Don't try to make the child vomit. If you can't get help quickly, take the child to nearest emergency facility.
• See emergency information at the back of this book.

Time lapse before drug works:
3 weeks to 2 months for maximum benefit.

Don't take with:
Any other medicines, even over-the-counter drugs such as cough and cold medicines, nose drops, diet pills, laxatives or caffeine, without consulting your doctor.

POSSIBLE ADVERSE REACTIONS OR SIDE EFFECTS

SYMPTOMS	WHAT TO DO
Life-threatening:	
Uncontrolled muscle movements of tongue, face and other muscles (neuroleptic malignant syndrome, rare).	Discontinue. Seek emergency treatment.
Common:	
• Blurred vision.	Discontinue. Call doctor right away.
• Shuffling, stiffness, jerkiness, shakiness, constipation.	Continue. Call doctor when convenient.
• Dry mouth.	No action necessary.
Infrequent:	
• Rash, circling motions of tongue.	Discontinue. Call doctor right away.
• Dizziness, faintness, drowsiness, difficult urination, decreased sexual ability, nausea or vomiting.	Continue. Call doctor when convenient.
Rare:	
Sore throat, fever, jaundice, abdominal pain, constipation.	Discontinue. Call doctor right away.

WARNINGS & PRECAUTIONS

Don't take if:
• You have ever been allergic to haloperidol.
• You are depressed.
• You have Parkinson's disease.
• Patient is younger than 3 years old.

Before you start, consult your doctor:
• If you take sedatives, sleeping pills, tranquilizers, antidepressants, antihistamines, narcotics or mind-altering drugs.
• If you have a history of mental depression.
• If you have had kidney or liver problems.
• If you have diabetes, epilepsy, glaucoma, high blood pressure or heart disease, prostate trouble.
• If you drink alcoholic beverages frequently.

Pregnancy:
Risk to unborn child outweighs drug benefits. Don't use.

Infants & children
Don't give to infants or young children unless prescribed and monitored by your physician.

Prolonged use:
May develop tardive dyskinesia (involuntary movements of jaws, lips and tongue).

Skin & sunlight:
May cause rash or intensify sunburn in areas exposed to sun or sunlamp.

Driving or hazardous activities:
Don't drive or pilot aircraft until you learn how medicine affects you. Don't work around dangerous machinery. Don't climb ladders or work in high places. Danger increases if you drink alcohol or take medicine affecting alertness and reflexes.

Discontinuing:
Don't discontinue without consulting doctor. Dose may require gradual reduction if you have taken drug for a long time. Doses of other drugs may also require adjustment.

Others:
No age-related problems expected.

POSSIBLE INTERACTION WITH OTHER DRUGS

GENERIC NAME OR DRUG CLASS	COMBINED EFFECT
Anticholinergics (see Drugs Glossary)	Increased anticholinergic effect. May cause pressure within the eye.
Anticonvulsants (see Drugs Glossary)	Changed seizure pattern.
Antidepressants (see Drugs Glossary)	Excessive sedation.
Antihistamines (see Drugs Glossary)	Excessive sedation.
Antihypertensives (see Drugs Glossary)	May cause severe lood-pressure drop.
Barbiturates (see Drugs Glossary)	Excessive sedation.
Dronabinol	Increased effects of both drugs. Avoid.
Ethinamate	Dangerous increased effects of ethinamate. Avoid combining.
Fluoxetine	Increased depressant effects of both drugs.
Guanethidine	Decreased guanethidine effect.
Guanfacine	May increase depressant effects of either drug.
Loxapine	May increase toxic effects of both drugs.
Leucovorin	High alcohol content of leucovorin may cause adverse effects.
Levodopa	Decreased levodopa effect.
Lithium	Increased toxicity.
Methyldopa	Possible psychosis.
Methyprylon	Increased sedative effect, perhaps to dangerous level. Avoid.
Narcotics (see Drugs Glossary)	Excessive sedation.
Phenindione	Decreased anticoagulant effect.
Procarbazine	Increased sedation.
Sedatives (see Drugs Glossary)	Excessive sedation.
Tranquilizers (see Drugs Glossary)	Excessive sedation.

POSSIBLE INTERACTION WITH OTHER SUBSTANCES

INTERACTS WITH	COMBINED EFFECT
Alcohol:	Excessive sedation and depressed brain function. Avoid.
Beverages:	None expected.
Cocaine (or crack):	Decreased effect of haloperidol. Avoid.
Foods:	None expected.
Marijuana:	Occasional use—Increased sedation. Frequent use—Possible toxic psychosis.
Tobacco:	None expected.

HYDROXYZINE

BRAND & GENERIC NAMES

See complete list of brand and generic names in the Brand & Generic Name Directory.

BASIC INFORMATION

Habit forming? No
Prescription needed? Yes
Available as generic? Yes
Drug class: Tranquilizer, antihistamine

USES

- Treatment for anxiety, tension and agitation.
- Relieves itching from allergic reactions.

DOSAGE & USAGE INFORMATION

How to take:
• Tablet, syrup or capsule—Swallow with liquid. If you can't swallow whole, crumble tablet or open capsule and take with liquid or food.
• Liquid—If desired, dilute dose in beverage before swallowing.

When to take:
At the same times each day.

If you forget a dose:
Take as soon as you remember up to 2 hours late. If more than 2 hours, wait for next scheduled dose (don't double this dose).

What drug does:
May reduce activity in areas of the brain that influence emotional stability.

Time lapse before drug works:
15 to 30 minutes.

Don't take with:
Any other medicines, even over-the-counter drugs such as cough and cold medicines, nose drops, diet pills, laxatives or caffeine, without consulting your doctor.

OVERDOSE

SYMPTOMS:
Drowsiness, unsteadiness, agitation, purposeless movements, tremor, convulsions.
WHAT TO DO:
• Dial 0 (operator) or 911 (emergency) for an ambulance or medical help. Then give first aid immediately.
• See emergency information at the back of this book.

POSSIBLE ADVERSE REACTIONS OR SIDE EFFECTS

SYMPTOMS	WHAT TO DO
Life-threatening: None expected.	
Common: Drowsiness, difficult urination, dry mouth.	Continue. Tell doctor at next visit.
Infrequent: Headache.	Continue. Tell doctor at next visit.
Rare: Tremor, rash.	Discontinue. Call doctor right away.

WARNINGS & PRECAUTIONS

Don't take if:
You are allergic to any antihistamine.

Before you start, consult your doctor:
• If you have epilepsy.
• If you will have surgery within 2 months, including dental surgery, requiring general or spinal anesthesia.

Pregnancy:
Studies inconclusive on harm to unborn child. Animal studies show fetal abnormalities. Decide with your doctor whether drug benefits justify risk to unborn child.

Infants & children:
Use only under medical supervision.

Prolonged use:
Tolerance develops and reduces effectiveness.

Skin & sunlight:
No age-related problems expected.

Driving or hazardous activities:
Don't drive or pilot aircraft until you learn how medicine affects you. Don't work around dangerous machinery. Don't climb ladders or work in high places. Danger increases if you drink alcohol or take medicine affecting alertness and reflexes, such as antihistamines, tranquilizers, sedatives, pain medicine, narcotics and mind-altering drugs.

Discontinuing:
Don't discontinue without consulting doctor. Dose may require gradual reduction if you have taken drug for a long time. Doses of other drugs may also require adjustment.

Others:
No age-related problems expected.

POSSIBLE INTERACTION WITH OTHER DRUGS

GENERIC NAME OR DRUG CLASS	COMBINED EFFECT
Antidepressants, tricyclic (TCA, see Drugs Glossary)	Increased effect of both drugs.
Antihistamines (see Drugs Glossary)	Increased hydroxyzine effect.
Dronabinol	Increased effects of both drugs. Avoid.
Ethinamate	Dangerous increased effects of ethinamate. Avoid combining.
Fluoxetine	Increased depressant effects of both drugs.
Guanfacine	May increase depressant effects of either drug.
Leucovorin	High alcohol content of leucovorin may cause adverse effects.
Methyprylon	Increased sedative effect, perhaps to dangerous level. Avoid.
Narcotics (see Drugs Glossary)	Increased effect of both drugs.
Pain relievers	Increased effect of both drugs.
Sedatives (see Drugs Glossary)	Increased effect of both drugs.
Sleep inducers (see Drugs Glossary)	Increased effect of both drugs.
Tranquilizers (see Drugs Glossary)	Increased effect of both drugs.

POSSIBLE INTERACTION WITH OTHER SUBSTANCES

INTERACTS WITH	COMBINED EFFECT
Alcohol:	Increased sedation and intoxication. Use with caution.
Beverages: Caffeine drinks.	Decreased tranquilizer effect of hydroxyzine.
Cocaine (or crack):	Decreased hydroxyzine effect. Avoid.
Foods:	None expected.
Marijuana:	None expected.
Tobacco:	None expected.

ISOETHARINE

BRAND NAMES

Arm-a-Med Isoetharine
Beta-2
Bisorine
Bronkometer
Bronkosol
Dey-Dose Isoetharine
Dey-Dose Isoetharine S/F
Dey-Lute Isoetharine
Dilabron
Disorine
Dispos-a Med Isoetharine

BASIC INFORMATION

Habit forming? No
Prescription needed? Yes
Available as generic? Yes
Drug class: Sympathomimetic (bronchodilator)

USES

Eases breathing difficulty from bronchial asthma attacks, bronchitis and emphysema.

DOSAGE & USAGE INFORMATION

How to take:
Aerosol—Use only as directed on label. Don't inhale medicine more than twice per dose unless otherwise directed by doctor.

When to take:
As needed, no more often than every 3 hours.

If you forget a dose:
Take as soon as you remember if you need it. Never double dose.

Continued next column

OVERDOSE

SYMPTOMS:
Nervousness, anxiety, dizziness, palpitations, tremor, rapid heartbeat, spasm of bronchial tubes, cardiac arrest.
WHAT TO DO:
- **Dial 0 (operator) or 911 (emergency) for an ambulance or medical help. Then give first aid immediately.**
- **If the child is unconscious and not breathing, give mouth-to-mouth breathing. If there is no heartbeat, use cardiac massage and mouth-to-mouth breathing (CPR). Don't try to make the child vomit. If you can't get help quickly, take the child to nearest emergency facility.**
- **See emergency information at the back of this book.**

What drug does:
Dilates constricted bronchial tubes so air can pass.

Time lapse before drug works:
1 to 2 minutes.

Don't take with:
Any other medicines, even over-the-counter drugs such as cough and cold medicines, nose drops, diet pills, laxatives or caffeine, without consulting your doctor.

POSSIBLE ADVERSE REACTIONS OR SIDE EFFECTS

SYMPTOMS	WHAT TO DO
Life-threatening: None expected.	
Common: Dizziness, agitation, headache, insomnia, nausea, fast or pounding heartbeat.	Continue. Call doctor when convenient.
Infrequent: • Constriction of bronchial tubes, particularly after overuse.	Discontinue. Call doctor right away.
• Weakness.	Continue. Call doctor when convenient.
Rare: None expected.	

WARNINGS & PRECAUTIONS

Don't take if:
- You are allergic to any sympathomimetic drug.
- You have a heart-rhythm disorder.
- You have taken MAO inhibitors in past 2 weeks.

Before you start, consult your doctor:
- If you use epinephrine for asthma.
- If you have diabetes.
- If you have an overactive thyroid gland.
- If you take a digitalis preparation, have high blood pressure or heart disease.

Pregnancy:
No proven harm to unborn child. Avoid if possible.

Infants & children:
Don't give to infants younger than 2. For older children, use only under medical supervision.

Prolonged use:
No age-related problems expected.

Skin & sunlight:
No age-related problems expected.

Driving or hazardous activities:
No age-related problems expected. Use caution if you feel nervous or dizzy.

Discontinuing:
Discontinue if drug fails to provide relief. Don't increase dose or frequency.

Others:
May increase blood-and urine-sugar levels, particularly in diabetics.

POSSIBLE INTERACTION WITH OTHER DRUGS

GENERIC NAME OR DRUG CLASS	COMBINED EFFECT
Antidepressants, tricyclic (TCA, see Drugs Glossary)	Increased isoetharine effect.
Beta-adrenergic blockers (see Drugs Glossary)	Decreased effects of both drugs.
Ephedrine	Increased ephedrine effect. Excessive heart stimulation.
Epinephrine	Excessive heart stimulation.
Isoproterenol	Excessive heart stimulation.
MAO inhibitors (see Drugs Glossary)	Dangerous mixture. Avoid.
Nitrates	Possible decreased effects of both drugs.
Theophylline	Possible increased effect and toxicity of both drugs.

POSSIBLE INTERACTION WITH OTHER SUBSTANCES

INTERACTS WITH	COMBINED EFFECT
Alcohol:	None expected.
Beverages: Caffeine drinks.	May cause irregular or fast heartbeat.
Cocaine (or crack):	Excessive stimulation. Avoid.
Foods: Chocolates.	May cause irregular or fast heartbeat.
Marijuana:	Improves drug's antiasthmatic effect.
Tobacco:	None expected.

MEDICATIONS

LOPERAMIDE

BRAND NAMES

Imodium

BASIC INFORMATION

Habit forming? No, unless taken in high doses for long periods.
Prescription needed? Yes
Available as generic? No
Drug class: Antidiarrheal

USES

Relieves diarrhea and reduces volume of discharge from ileostomies and colostomies.

DOSAGE & USAGE INFORMATION

How to take:
- Capsule—Swallow with food to lessen stomach irritation.
- Liquid—Follow label instructions and use marked dropper.

When to take:
No more often than directed on label.

If you forget a dose:
Take as soon as you remember up to 2 hours late. If more than 2 hours, wait for next scheduled dose (don't double this dose).

What drug does:
Blocks digestive tract's nerve supply, which reduces irritability and contractions in intestinal tract.

Time lapse before drug works:
1 to 2 hours.

Don't take with:
Any other medicines, even over-the-counter drugs such as cough and cold medicines, nose drops, diet pills, laxatives or caffeine, without consulting your doctor.

OVERDOSE

SYMPTOMS:
Constipation, lethargy, drowsiness or unconsciousness.
WHAT TO DO:
Overdose unlikely to threaten life. If child takes much larger amount than prescribed, call doctor, poison-control center or hospital emergency room for instructions.

POSSIBLE ADVERSE REACTIONS OR SIDE EFFECTS

SYMPTOMS	WHAT TO DO
Life-threatening: None expected.	
Common: None expected.	
Infrequent:	
• Rash.	Discontinue. Call doctor right away.
• Drowsiness, dry mouth, bloating, constipation, appetite loss, stomach pain.	Continue. Call doctor when convenient.
Rare:	
Unexplained fever.	Discontinue. Call doctor right away.

WARNINGS & PRECAUTIONS

Don't take if:
• You have severe colitis.
• You have colitis resulting from antibiotic treatment or infection.

Before you start, consult your doctor:
• If you are dehydrated from fluid loss caused by diarrhea.
• If you have liver disease.

Pregnancy:
No proven harm. Avoid if possible.

Infants & children:
Don't give to infants or toddlers. Use only under doctor's supervision for children older than 2.

Prolonged use:
Habit forming at high dose.

Skin & sunlight:
No age-related problems expected.

Driving or hazardous activities:
Don't drive or pilot aircraft until you learn how medicine affects you. Don't work around dangerous machinery. Don't climb ladders or work in high places. Danger increases if you drink alcohol or take medicine affecting alertness and reflexes.

Discontinuing:
May be unnecessary to finish medicine. Follow doctor's instructions.
After discontinuing, consult doctor if you experience muscle cramps, nausea, vomiting, trembling, stomach cramps or unusual sweating.

Others:
• Follow warnings on package.
• If acute diarrhea lasts longer than 48 hours, discontinue and call doctor. In chronic diarrhea, loperamide is unlikely to be effective if diarrhea doesn't improve in 10 days.

POSSIBLE INTERACTION WITH OTHER DRUGS

GENERIC NAME OR DRUG CLASS	COMBINED EFFECT
Antibiotics (cephalosporins, clindamycins, lincomycins, penicillins, see Drugs Glossary)	May delay removal of toxins from colon in cases of diarrhea caused by side effects of these antibiotics.

POSSIBLE INTERACTION WITH OTHER SUBSTANCES

INTERACTS WITH	COMBINED EFFECT
Alcohol:	Depressed brain function. Avoid.
Beverages:	None expected.
Cocaine (or crack):	Decreased loperamide effect.
Foods:	None expected.
Marijuana:	None expected.
Tobacco:	None expected.

MEDICATIONS

METHYLDOPA & THIAZIDE DIURETICS

BRAND NAMES

Aldoclor
Aldomet
Aldoril
Dopamet
Medimet-250
Novodoparil
Novomedopa
PMS Dopazide

BASIC INFORMATION

Habit forming? No
Prescription needed? Yes
Available as generic? Yes
Drug class: Antihypertensive, diuretic (thiazide)

USES

- Controls, but doesn't cure, high blood pressure.
- Reduces fluid retention (edema).

DOSAGE & USAGE INFORMATION

How to take:
Tablet—Swallow with liquid. If you can't swallow whole, crumble tablet and take with liquid or food.

When to take:
At the same times each day.

If you forget a dose:
Take as soon as you remember up to 2 hours late. If more than 2 hours, wait for next scheduled dose (don't double this dose).

Continued next column

OVERDOSE

SYMPTOMS:
Drowsiness; exhaustion; cramps; weakness; stupor; confusion; slow, weak pulse; coma.
WHAT TO DO:
- **Dial 0 (operator) or 911 (emergency) for an ambulance or medical help. Then give first aid immediately.**
- **If the child is unconscious and not breathing, give mouth-to-mouth breathing. If there is no heartbeat, use cardiac massage and mouth-to-mouth breathing (CPR). Don't try to make the child vomit. If you can't get help quickly, take the child to nearest emergency facility.**
- **See emergency information at the back of this book.**

What drug does:
- Relaxes walls of small arteries to decrease blood pressure.
- Forces sodium and water excretion, reducing body fluid.
- Reduced body fluid and relaxed arteries lower blood pressure.

Time lapse before drug works:
Continual use for 2 to 4 weeks may be necessary to determine effectiveness.

Don't take with:
Any other medicines, even over-the-counter drugs such as cough and cold medicines, nose drops, diet pills, laxatives or caffeine, without consulting your doctor.

POSSIBLE ADVERSE REACTIONS OR SIDE EFFECTS

SYMPTOMS	WHAT TO DO
Life-threatening:	
Irregular heartbeat, weak pulse.	Discontinue. Seek emergency treatment.
Common:	
Depression, nightmares, drowsiness, weakness, stuffy nose, dry mouth, swollen feet and ankles, dizziness, sedation.	Continue. Call doctor when convenient.
Infrequent:	
• Fast heartbeat, change in vision, abdominal pain, nervousness.	Discontinue. Call doctor right away.
• Insomnia, nausea, vomiting, diarrhea, headache, constipation.	Continue. Call doctor when convenient.
Rare:	
• Rash; jaundice; hives; sore throat, fever, mouth sores; sore or "black" tongue; severe abdominal pain; decreased mental activity; memory impairment; facial paralysis; slow heartbeat; chest pain; drug-induced systemic lupus erythematosus.	Discontinue. Call doctor right away.
• Weight gain or loss.	Continue. Call doctor when convenient.

WARNINGS & PRECAUTIONS

Don't take if:
- You are allergic to any thiazide diuretic drug.
- If you will have surgery within 2 months, including dental surgery, requiring general or spinal anesthesia.

Before you start, consult your doctor:
- If you are allergic to any sulfa drug.
- If you have gout, liver, pancreas or kidney disorder.

Pregnancy:
Risk to unborn child outweighs drug benefits. Don't use.

Infants & children
Don't give to infants or young children unless prescribed and monitored by your physician.

Prolonged use:
- May cause anemia.
- Severe edema (fluid retention).

Skin & sunlight:
May cause rash or intensify sunburn in areas exposed to sun or sunlamp.

Driving or hazardous activities:
Don't drive or pilot aircraft until you learn how medicine affects you. Don't work around dangerous machinery. Don't climb ladders or work in high places. Danger increases if you drink alcohol or take medicine affecting alertness and reflexes, such as antihistamines, tranquilizers, sedatives, pain medicine, narcotics and mind-altering drugs.

Discontinuing:
Don't discontinue without consulting doctor. Dose may require gradual reduction if you have taken drug for a long time. Doses of other drugs may also require adjustment.

Others:
- Hot weather and fever may cause dehydration and drop in blood pressure. Dose may require temporary adjustment. Weigh daily and report any unexpected weight decreases to your doctor.
- May cause rise in uric acid, leading to gout.
- May cause blood-sugar rise in diabetics.
- Avoid heavy exercise, exertion, sweating.

POSSIBLE INTERACTION WITH OTHER DRUGS

GENERIC NAME OR DRUG CLASS	COMBINED EFFECT
Acebutolol	Increased antihyper tensive effect. Dosages of both drugs may require adjustments.
ACE inhibitors: captopril, enalapril, lisinopril (see Drugs Glossary)	Possible excessive potassium in blood.
Allopurinol	Decreased allopurinol effect.
Amphetamines (see Drugs Glossary)	Decreased methyldopa effect.
Anticoagulants (oral, see Drugs Glossary)	Increased anticoagulant effect.
Antidepressants, tricyclic (TCA, see Drugs Glossary)	Dangerous changes in blood pressure. Avoid combination unless under medical supervision.
Antihypertensives (see Drugs Glossary)	Increased antihypertensive effect.
Barbiturates (see Drugs Glossary)	Increased hydrochlorothiazide effect.

See Additional Drug Interactions Section

POSSIBLE INTERACTION WITH OTHER SUBSTANCES

INTERACTS WITH	COMBINED EFFECT
Alcohol:	Increased sedation. Excessive blood-pressure drop. Avoid.
Beverages:	None expected.
Cocaine (or crack):	Decreased methyldopa effect.
Foods:	
Licorice.	Excessive potassium loss that causes dangerous heart rhythms.
Marijuana:	May increase blood pressure.
Tobacco:	Possible increased blood pressure.

METHYLPHENIDATE

BRAND NAMES

Methidate
Ritalin
Ritalin SR

BASIC INFORMATION

Habit forming? Yes
Available as generic? Yes
Prescription needed? Yes
Drug class: Sympathomimetic (see Drugs Glossary)

USES

• Treatment for hyperactive children.
• Treatment for narcolepsy (uncontrollable attacks of sleepiness).

DOSAGE & USAGE INFORMATION

How to take:
Tablet or extended-release tablet—Swallow with liquid or food to lessen stomach irritation. If you can't swallow whole, crumble tablet and take with liquid or food.

When to take:
At the same times each day.

Don't take with:
Any other medicines, even over-the-counter drugs such as cough and cold medicines, nose drops, diet pills, laxatives or caffeine, without consulting your doctor.

Continued next column

OVERDOSE

SYMPTOMS:
Rapid heartbeat, fever, confusion, vomiting, agitation, hallucinations, convulsions, coma.
WHAT TO DO:
• Dial 0 (operator) or 911 (emergency) for an ambulance or medical help. Then give first aid immediately.
• If the child is unconscious and not breathing, give mouth-to-mouth breathing. If there is no heartbeat, use cardiac massage and mouth-to-mouth breathing (CPR). Don't try to make the child vomit. If you can't get help quickly, take the child to nearest emergency facility.
• See emergency information at the back of this book.

If you forget a dose:
Take as soon as you remember up to 2 hours late. If more than 2 hours, wait for next scheduled dose (don't double this dose).

What drug does:
Stimulates brain to improve alertness, concentration and attention span. Calms the hyperactive child.

Time lapse before drug works:
• 1 month or more for maximum effect on child.
• 30 minutes to stimulate adults.

POSSIBLE ADVERSE REACTIONS OR SIDE EFFECTS

SYMPTOMS	WHAT TO DO
Life-threatening:	
None expected.	
Common:	
• Mood change.	Continue. Call doctor when convenient.
• Nervousness, insomnia, dizziness, headache, appetite loss.	Continue. Tell doctor at next visit.
Infrequent:	
• Rash or hives; chest pain; fast, irregular heartbeat; unusual bruising; joint pain; psychosis; uncontrollable movements; unexplained fever.	Discontinue. Call doctor right away.
• Nausea, abdominal pain.	Continue. Call doctor when convenient.
Rare:	
• Blurred vision, sore throat, fever, red spots under skin.	Discontinue. Call doctor right away.
• Unusual tiredness.	Continue. Call doctor when convenient.

WARNINGS & PRECAUTIONS

Don't take if:
- You are allergic to methylphenidate.
- You have glaucoma.
- Patient is younger than 6.

Before you start, consult your doctor:
- If you have epilepsy.
- If you have high blood pressure.
- If you take MAO inhibitors.

Pregnancy:
No proven harm to unborn child. Avoid if possible.

Infants & children:
Use only under medical supervision for children 6 or older.

Prolonged use:
Rare: possibility of physical growth retardation.

Skin & sunlight:
No age-related problems expected.

Driving or hazardous activities:
No age-related problems expected.

Discontinuing:
Don't discontinue abruptly. Don't discontinue without doctor's advice until you complete prescribed dose, even though symptoms diminish or disappear.

Others:
Dose must be carefully adjusted by doctor.

POSSIBLE INTERACTION WITH OTHER DRUGS

GENERIC NAME OR DRUG CLASS	COMBINED EFFECT
Acebutolol	Decreased effects of both drugs.
Anticholinergics (see Drugs Glossary)	Increased anticholinergic effect.
Anticoagulants (oral, see Drugs Glossary)	Increased anticoagulant effect.
Anticonvulsants (see Drugs Glossary)	Increased anticonvulsant effect.
Antidepressants, tricyclic (TCA, see Drugs Glossary)	Increased antidepressant effect. Decreased methylphenidate effect.
Antihypertensives (see Drugs Glossary)	Decreased antihypertensive effect.
Guanadrel	Decreased guanadrel effect.
Guanethidine	Decreased guanethidine effect.
MAO inhibitors (see Drugs Glossary)	Dangerous rise in blood pressure.
Minoxidil	Decreased minoxidil effect.
Nitrates	Possible decreased effects of both drugs.
Oxprenolol	Decreased effects of both drugs.
Oxyphenbutazone	Increased oxyphenbutazone effect.
Phenylbutazone	Increased phenylbutazone effect.

POSSIBLE INTERACTION WITH OTHER SUBSTANCES

INTERACTS WITH	COMBINED EFFECT
Alcohol:	None expected.
Beverages: Caffeine drinks.	May raise blood pressure.
Cocaine (or crack):	Overstimulation. Avoid.
Foods: Foods containing tyramine (see Glossary).	May raise blood pressure.
Marijuana:	None expected.
Tobacco:	None expected.

METOCLOPRAMIDE

BRAND NAMES

Clopra
Emex
Maxeran
Maxolon
Reclomide
Reglan

BASIC INFORMATION

Habit forming? No
Prescription needed? Yes
Available as generic? Yes
Drug class: Antiemetic; dopaminergic blocker (see Drugs Glossary)

USES

- Relieves nausea and vomiting caused by chemotherapy and drug related postoperative factors.
- Relieves symptoms of esophagitis and stomach swelling in people with diabetes.

DOSAGE & USAGE INFORMATION

How to take:
Tablet or syrup—Swallow with liquid or food to lessen stomach irritation.

When to take:
30 minutes before symptoms expected, up to 4 times a day.

If you forget a dose:
Take as soon as you remember up to 2 hours late. If more than 2 hours, wait for next scheduled dose (don't double this dose).

Continued next column

OVERDOSE

SYMPTOMS:
Severe drowsiness, mental confusion, trembling, seizure, coma.
WHAT TO DO:
- **Dial 0 (operator) or 911 (emergency) for an ambulance or medical help. Then give first aid immediately.**
- **If the child is unconscious and not breathing, give mouth-to-mouth breathing. If there is no heartbeat, use cardiac massage and mouth-to-mouth breathing (CPR). Don't try to make the child vomit. If you can't get help quickly, take the child to nearest emergency facility.**
- **See emergency information at the back of this book.**

What drug does:
- Prevents smooth muscle in stomach from relaxing.
- Affects vomiting center in brain.

Time lapse before drug works:
30 to 60 minutes.

Don't take with:
Any other medicines, even over-the-counter drugs such as cough and cold medicines, nose drops, diet pills, laxatives or caffeine, without consulting your doctor.

POSSIBLE ADVERSE REACTIONS OR SIDE EFFECTS

SYMPTOMS	WHAT TO DO
Life-threatening:	
None expected.	
Common:	
• Drowsiness, restlessness.	Continue. Call doctor when convenient.
• Rash.	Continue. Call doctor when convenient.
Infrequent:	
• Wheezing, shortness of breath.	Discontinue. Call doctor right away.
• Dizziness; headache; insomnia; tender, swollen breasts; increased milk flow.	Continue. Call doctor when convenient.
Rare:	
• Abnormal, involuntary movements of jaw, lips and tongue; depression; Parkinson syndrome.	Discontinue. Call doctor right away.
• Constipation, diarrhea, nausea.	Continue. Call doctor when convenient.

WARNINGS & PRECAUTIONS

Don't take if:
You are allergic to procaine, procainamide or metoclopramide.

Before you start, consult your doctor:
- If you have Parkinson's disease.
- If you have liver or kidney disease.
- If you have epilepsy.
- If you have bleeding from gastrointestinal tract or intestinal obstruction.
- If you will have surgery within 2 months, including dental surgery, requiring general or spinal anesthesia.

Pregnancy:
No proven harm to unborn child. Avoid if possible.

Infants & children:
Adverse reactions more likely to occur than in adults.

Prolonged use:
Adverse reactions including muscle spasms and trembling hands more likely to occur.

Skin & sunlight:
No age-related problems expected.

Driving or hazardous activities:
Don't drive or pilot aircraft until you learn how medicine affects you. Don't work around dangerous machinery. Don't climb ladders or work in high places. Danger increases if you drink alcohol or take medicine affecting alertness and reflexes, such as antihistamines, tranquilizers, sedatives, pain medicine, narcotics and mind-altering drugs.

Discontinuing:
May be unnecessary to finish medicine. Follow doctor's instructions.

Others:
No age-related problems expected.

POSSIBLE INTERACTION WITH OTHER DRUGS

GENERIC NAME OR DRUG CLASS	COMBINED EFFECT
Acetaminophen	Increased absorption of acetaminophen.
Anticholinergics (see Drugs Glossary)	Decreased metoclopramide effect.
Aspirin	Increased absorption of aspirin.
Bromocriptine	Decreased bromocriptine effect.
Butyophenone	Increased chance of muscle spasm and trembling.
Central nervous system depressants (see Drugs Glossary)	Excess sedation.
Digitalis preparations (see Drugs Glossary)	Decreased absorption of digitalis.
Ethinamate	Dangerous increased effects of ethinamate. Avoid combining.
Fluoxetine	Increased depressant effects of both drugs.
Guanfacine	May increase depressant effects of either drug.
Insulin	Unpredictable changes in blood glucose. Dosages may require adjustment.
Leucovorin	High alcohol content of leucovorin may cause adverse effects.
Levodopa	Increased absorption of levodopa.
Lithium	Increased absorption of lithium.
Loxapine	May increase toxic effects of both drugs.
Methyprylon	Increased sedative effect, perhaps to dangerous level. Avoid.
Narcotics (see Drugs Glossary)	Decreased metoclopramide effect.
Phenothiazines	Increased chance of muscle spasm and trembling.
Tetracycline	Slow stomach emptying.
Thiothixines (see Drugs Glossary)	Increased chance of muscle spasm and trembling.

POSSIBLE INTERACTION WITH OTHER SUBSTANCES

INTERACTS WITH	COMBINED EFFECT
Alcohol:	Excess sedation. Avoid.
Beverages:	
Coffee.	Decreased metoclopramide effect.
Cocaine (or crack):	Decreased metoclopramide effect.
Foods:	None expected.
Marijuana:	Decreased metoclopramide effect.
Tobacco:	Decreased metoclopramide effect.

NARCOTIC & ACETAMINOPHEN

BRAND & GENERIC NAMES

See complete list of brand and generic names in the Brand & Generic Name Directory.

BASIC INFORMATION

Habit forming? Yes
Prescription needed? Yes
Available as generic? Yes
Drug class: Narcotic, analgesic

USES

Relieves pain.

DOSAGE & USAGE INFORMATION

How to take:
- Tablet or capsule—Swallow with liquid. If you can't swallow whole, crumble tablet or open capsule and take with liquid or food.
- Drops or liquid—Dilute dose in beverage before swallowing.

When to take:
When needed. No more often than every 4 hours.

If you forget a dose:
Take as soon as you remember. Wait 4 hours for next dose.

Continued next column

OVERDOSE

SYMPTOMS:
Stomach upset; irritability; sweating, anorexia, convulsions; deep sleep; slow breathing; slow pulse; flushed, warm skin; constricted pupils; coma.
WHAT TO DO:
- **Dial 0 (operator) or 911 (emergency) for an ambulance or medical help. Then give first aid immediately.**
- **If the child is unconscious and not breathing, give mouth-to-mouth breathing. If there is no heartbeat, use cardiac massage and mouth-to-mouth breathing (CPR). Don't try to make the child vomit. If you can't get help quickly, take the child to nearest emergency facility.**
- **See emergency information at the back of this book.**

What drug does:
- May affect hypothalamus—the part of the brain that helps regulate body heat and receives body's pain messages.
- Blocks pain messages to brain and spinal cord.
- Reduces sensitivity of brain's cough-control center.

Time lapse before drug works:
15 to 30 minutes. May last 4 hours.

Don't take with:
Any other medicines, even over-the-counter drugs such as cough and cold medicines, nose drops, diet pills, laxatives or caffeine, without consulting your doctor.

POSSIBLE ADVERSE REACTIONS OR SIDE EFFECTS

SYMPTOMS	WHAT TO DO
Life-threatening:	
Irregular or slow heartbeat, difficult breathing.	Discontinue. Seek emergency treatment.
Common:	
Dizziness, agitation, tiredness.	Continue. Call doctor when convenient.
Infrequent:	
Abdominal pain, constipation, vomiting.	Discontinue. Call doctor right away.
Rare:	
• Fatigue; itchy skin; rash; sore throat, fever, mouth sores; bruising and bleeding increased; painful or difficult urination; blood in urine; anemia; blurred vision.	Discontinue. Call doctor right away.
• Depression.	Continue. Call doctor when convenient.

WARNINGS & PRECAUTIONS

Don't take if:
- You are allergic to any narcotic or acetaminophen.
- Your symptoms don't improve after 2 days use. Call your doctor.

Before you start, consult your doctor:
- If you have bronchial asthma, kidney disease or liver damage.
- If you will have surgery within 2 months, including dental surgery, requiring general or spinal anesthesia.

Pregnancy:
Decide with your doctor whether drug benefits justify risk to unborn child. Abuse by pregnant woman will result in addicted newborn. Withdrawal of newborn can be life-threatening.

Infants & children
Don't give to infants or young children unless prescribed and monitored by your physician.

Prolonged use:
• Causes psychological and physical dependence (addiction).
• May affect blood stream and cause anemia. Limit use to 5 days for children 12 and under, and 10 days for adults.

Skin & sunlight:
May cause rash or intensify sunburn in areas exposed to sun or sunlamp.

Driving or hazardous activities:
Don't drive or pilot aircraft until you learn how medicine affects you. Don't work around dangerous machinery. Don't climb ladders or work in high places. Danger increases if you drink alcohol or take medicine affecting alertness and reflexes, such as antihistamines, tranquilizers, sedatives, pain medicine, narcotics and mind-altering drugs.

Discontinuing:
Discontinue in 2 days if symptoms don't improve.

Others:
No age-related problems expected.

POSSIBLE INTERACTION WITH OTHER DRUGS

GENERIC NAME OR DRUG CLASS	COMBINED EFFECT
Analgesics (other, see Drugs Glossary)	Increased analgesic effect.
Anticoagulants (other, see Drugs Glossary)	May increase anticoagulant effect. Prothrombin times should be monitored.
Anticholinergics (see Drugs Glossary)	Increased anticholinergic effect.
Antidepressants (see Drugs Glossary)	Increased sedative effect.
Antihistamines (see Drugs Glossary)	Increased sedative effect.
Mind-altering drugs (see Drugs Glossary)	Increased sedative effect.
Narcotics (other) (see Drugs Glossary)	Increased narcotic effect.
Nitrates (see Drugs Glossary)	Excessive blood-pressure drop.
Phenobarbital and other barbiturates	Quicker elimination and decreased effect of acetaminophen.
Phenothiazines (see Drugs Glossary)	Increased phenothiazine effect.
Sedatives (see Drugs Glossary)	Increased sedative effect.
Sleep inducers (see Drugs Glossary)	Increased sedative effect.
Terfenadine	Possible oversedation.
Tetracyclines (see Drugs Glossary)	May slow tetracycline absorption. Space doses 2 hours apart.
Tranquilizers (see Drugs Glossary)	Increased sedative effect.
Zidovudine	Increased toxicity of zidovudine.

POSSIBLE INTERACTION WITH OTHER SUBSTANCES

INTERACTS WITH	COMBINED EFFECT
Alcohol:	Increases alcohol's intoxicating effect. Long-term use may cause toxic effect in liver. Avoid.
Beverages:	None expected.
Cocaine (or crack):	Increased cocaine toxic effects. Avoid.
Foods:	None expected.
Marijuana:	Impairs physical and mental performance. Avoid.
Tobacco:	None expected.

NARCOTIC ANALGESICS

BRAND & GENERIC NAMES

See complete list of brand and generic names in the Brand & Generic Name Directory.

BASIC INFORMATION

Habit forming? Yes
Prescription needed? Yes
Available as generic? Yes
Drug class: Narcotic

USES

- Relieves pain.
- Suppresses cough.
- Relieves diarrhea.

DOSAGE & USAGE INFORMATION

How to take:
- Tablet, capsule or extended-release tablet—Swallow with liquid. If you can't swallow whole, crumble tablet or open capsule and take with liquid or food.
- Drops or liquid—Dilute dose in beverage before swallowing.

When to take:
When needed. No more often than every 4 hours.

If you forget a dose:
Take as soon as you remember. Wait 4 hours for next dose.

Continued next column

OVERDOSE

SYMPTOMS:
Deep sleep, slow breathing; slow pulse; respiratory arrest; flushed, warm skin; constricted pupils.
WHAT TO DO:
- **Dial 0 (operator) or 911 (emergency) for an ambulance or medical help. Then give first aid immediately.**
- **If the child is unconscious and not breathing, give mouth-to-mouth breathing. If there is no heartbeat, use cardiac massage and mouth-to-mouth breathing (CPR). Don't try to make the child vomit. If you can't get help quickly, take the child to nearest emergency facility.**
- **See emergency information at the back of this book.**

What drug does:
- Blocks pain messages to brain and spinal cord.
- Reduces sensitivity of brain's cough-control center.

Time lapse before drug works:
30 minutes.

Don't take with:
Any other medicines, even over-the-counter drugs such as cough and cold medicines, nose drops, diet pills, laxatives or caffeine, without consulting your doctor.

POSSIBLE ADVERSE REACTIONS OR SIDE EFFECTS

SYMPTOMS	WHAT TO DO
Life-threatening:	
Hives, rash, intense itching, faintness soon after a dose (anaphylaxis); morphine by injection.	Seek emergency treatment immediately.
Common:	
Dizziness, flushed face, difficult urination, unusual tiredness.	Continue. Call doctor when convenient.
Infrequent:	
Severe constipation, abdominal pain, vomiting, nausea.	Discontinue. Call doctor right away.
Rare:	
• Hives, rash, itchy skin, face swelling, slow heartbeat, irregular breathing, hallucinations, disorientation, fainting.	Discontinue. Call doctor right away.
• Depression, blurred vision, decreased mental performance, anxiety, insomnia, weakness and faintness when arising from bed or chair, euphoria.	Continue. Call doctor when convenient.

WARNINGS & PRECAUTIONS

Don't take if:
- You are allergic to any narcotic.
- Diarrhea is due to toxic effect of drugs or poisons.

Before you start, consult your doctor:
- If you have impaired liver or kidney function.
- If you will have surgery within 2 months, including dental surgery, requiring general or spinal anesthesia.
- If you have asthma.

Pregnancy:
Decide with your doctor whether drug benefits justify risk to unborn child. Abuse by pregnant woman will result in addicted newborn. Withdrawal of newborn can be life-threatening.

Infants & children
Don't give to infants or young children unless prescribed and monitored by your physician.

Prolonged use:
Causes psychological and physical dependence (addiction).

Skin & sunlight:
May cause rash or intensify sunburn in areas exposed to sun or sunlamp.

Driving or hazardous activities:
Don't drive or pilot aircraft until you learn how medicine affects you. Don't work around dangerous machinery. Don't climb ladders or work in high places. Danger increases if you drink alcohol or take medicine affecting alertness and reflexes, such as antihistamines, tranquilizers, sedatives, pain medicine, narcotics and mind-altering drugs.

Discontinuing:
May be unnecessary to finish medicine. Follow doctor's instructions.

Others:
Some products contain tartrazine dye. Avoid, especially if you are allergic to aspirin.

POSSIBLE INTERACTION WITH OTHER DRUGS

GENERIC NAME OR DRUG CLASS	COMBINED EFFECT
Analgesics (other, see Drugs Glossary)	Increased analgesic effect.
Anticoagulants (oral, see Drugs Glossary)	Possible increased anticoagulant effect.
Anticholinergics (see Drugs Glossary)	Increased anticholinergic effect.
Antidepressants (see Drugs Glossary)	Increased sedative effect.
Antihistamines (see Drugs Glossary)	Increased sedative effect.
Butorphanol	Possibly precipitates withdrawal with chronic narcotic use.
Carbamazepine	Increased carbamazepine effect with propoxyphene possible.
Cimetidine	Possible increased narcotic effect and toxicity.
Ethinamate	Dangerous increased effects of ethinamate. Avoid combining.
Fluoxetine	Increased depressant effects of both drugs.

See Additional Drug Interactions Section

POSSIBLE INTERACTION WITH OTHER SUBSTANCES

INTERACTS WITH	COMBINED EFFECT
Alcohol:	Increases alcohol's intoxicating effect. Avoid.
Beverages:	None expected.
Cocaine (or crack):	Increased cocaine toxic effects. Avoid.
Foods:	None expected.
Marijuana:	Impairs physical and mental performance. Avoid.
Tobacco:	None expected.

NARCOTIC ANALGESICS & ASPIRIN

BRAND & GENERIC NAMES

See complete list of brand and generic names in the Brand & Generic Name Directory.

BASIC INFORMATION

Habit forming? Yes
Prescription needed? Yes
Available as generic? No
Drug class: Analgesic

USES

- Reduces pain.
- Relieves swelling, stiffness, joint pain of arthritis or rheumatism.
- Suppresses cough.

DOSAGE & USAGE INFORMATION

How to take:
- Tablet or capsule—Swallow with liquid.
- Extended-release tablets or capsules—Swallow each dose whole.
- Suppositories—Remove wrapper and moisten suppository with water. Gently insert into rectum, large end first.

When to take:
As needed, no more often than every 4 hours.

If you forget a dose:
Pain, fever—Take as soon as you remember up to 2 hours. Wait 4 hours for next dose.

What drug does:
- Affects hypothalamus, the part of the brain which regulates temperature by dilating small blood vessels in skin.
- Suppresses body's pain messages.
- Reduces sensitivity of brain's cough control center.

Continued next column

OVERDOSE

SYMPTOMS:
Ringing in ears; nausea; vomiting; dizziness; fever; deep, unusually rapid or unusually slow breathing; constricted pupils, hallucinations; convulsions; coma.
WHAT TO DO:
- **Dial 0 (operator) or 911 (emergency) for an ambulance or medical help. Then give first aid immediately.**
- **See emergency information at the back of this book.**

Time lapse before drug works:
30 minutes for pain or fever.

Don't take with:
Any other medicines, even over-the-counter drugs such as cough and cold medicines, nose drops, diet pills, laxatives or caffeine, without consulting your doctor.

POSSIBLE ADVERSE REACTIONS OR SIDE EFFECTS

SYMPTOMS	WHAT TO DO
Life-threatening:	
Black or bloody vomit; blood in urine; difficulty breathing; hives, rash, intense itching, faintness soon after a dose (anaphylaxis).	Seek emergency treatment immediately.
Common:	
• Nausea, vomiting.	Discontinue. Seek emergency treatment.
• Heartburn, indigestion.	Continue. Call doctor when convenient.
• Ringing in ears.	Continue. Tell doctor at next visit.
Infrequent:	
None expected.	
Rare:	
• Black stools, unexplained fever, blood in urine, difficult urination.	Discontinue. Seek emergency treatment.
• Rash, hives, itch, diminished or blurred vision, shortness of breath, difficult breathing, wheezing, jaundice, mental confusion, unusual tiredness, euphoria.	Discontinue. Call doctor right away.
• Drowsiness.	Continue. Call doctor when convenient.

WARNINGS & PRECAUTIONS

Don't take if:
- You are allergic to any narcotic.
- You need to restrict sodium in your diet. Buffered effervescent tablets and sodium salicylate are high in sodium.
- You are sensitive to aspirin.
- You have a bleeding disorder.

Before you start, consult your doctor:
- If you have had stomach or duodenal ulcers.
- If you have had gout.
- If you have asthma or nasal polyps.

Pregnancy:
Risk to unborn child outweighs drug benefits. Don't use.

Infants & children:
- Overdose frequent and severe. Keep bottles out of children's reach.
- Consult doctor before giving to persons under age 18 who have fever and discomfort of viral illness, especially chickenpox and influenza. Probably increases risk of Reye's syndrome.

Prolonged use:
- Psychological and physical dependence.
- Kidney damage. Periodic kidney-function test recommended.

Skin & sunlight:
Aspirin combined with sunscreen may decrease sunburn.

Driving or hazardous activities:
No restrictions unless you feel drowsy.

Discontinuing:
For chronic illness—Don't discontinue without doctor's advice until you complete prescribed dose, even though symptoms diminish or disappear.

Others:
- Aspirin can complicate surgery, pregnancy, labor and delivery, and illness.
- Urine tests for blood sugar may be inaccurate.

POSSIBLE INTERACTION WITH OTHER DRUGS

GENERIC NAME OR DRUG CLASS	COMBINED EFFECT
Acebutolol	Decreased antihypertensive effect of acebutolol.
ACE inhibitors: captopril, enalapril, lisinopril (see Drugs Glossary)	Decreased ACE inhibitor effect.
Allopurinol	Decreased allopurinol effect.
Antacids (see Drugs Glossary)	Decreased aspirin effect.
Anticoagulants (see Drugs Glossary)	Increased anticoagulant effect. Abnormal bleeding.
Antidiabetics (oral, see Drugs Glossary)	Low blood sugar.
Aspirin (other)	Likely aspirin toxicity.
Bumetanide	Possible aspirin toxicity.
Cortisone drugs (see Drugs Glossary)	Increased cortisone effect. Risk of ulcers and stomach bleeding.
Ethacrynic acid	Possible aspirin toxicity.

See Additional Drug Interactions Section

POSSIBLE INTERACTION WITH OTHER SUBSTANCES

INTERACTS WITH	COMBINED EFFECT
Alcohol:	Increases alcohol's intoxicating effect. Avoid.
Beverages:	None expected.
Cocaine (or crack):	Increased cocaine toxic effects. Avoid.
Foods:	None expected.
Marijuana:	Impairs physical and mental performance. Avoid.
Tobacco:	None expected.

NITRATES

BRAND & GENERIC NAMES

See complete list of brand and generic names in the Brand & Generic Name Directory.

BASIC INFORMATION

Habit forming? No
Prescription needed? Yes
Available as generic? Yes
Drug class: Antianginal (nitrate)

USES

• Reduces frequency and severity of angina attacks.
• Treats congestive heart failure.

DOSAGE & USAGE INFORMATION

How to take:
• Extended-release tablets or capsules—Swallow each dose whole with liquid.
• Chewable tablet—Chew tablet at earliest sign of angina, and hold in mouth for 2 minutes.
• Regular tablet or capsule—Swallow whole with liquid. Don't crush, chew or open.
• Buccal tablets (Nitrogard)—Allow to dissolve in side of mouth.
• Translingual spray (nitrolingual)—Spray under tongue according to instructions enclosed with prescription.
• Ointment—Apply as directed.
• Patches—Apply to skin according to package instructions.
• Sublingual tablets—Place under tongue every 3 to 5 minutes at earliest sign of angina. If you don't have complete relief with 3 or 4 tablets, call doctor.

Continued next column

When to take:
• Swallowed tablets—Take at the same times each day, 1 or 2 hours after meals.
• Sublingual tablets or spray—At onset of angina.
• Ointment—Follow prescription directions.
• Patches—According to physician's instructions.

If you forget a dose:
Take as soon as you remember up to 2 hours late. If more than 2 hours, wait for next scheduled dose (don't double this dose).

What drug does:
Relaxes blood vessels, increasing blood flow to heart muscle.

Time lapse before drug works:
• Sublingual tablets and spray—1 to 3 minutes.
• Other forms—15 to 30 minutes. Will not stop an attack, but may prevent attacks.

Don't take with:
Any other medicines, even over-the-counter drugs such as cough and cold medicines, nose drops, diet pills, laxatives or caffeine, without consulting your doctor.

OVERDOSE

SYMPTOMS:
Dizziness; blue fingernails and lips; fainting; shortness of breath; weak, fast heartbeat; convulsions.
WHAT TO DO:
• **Dial 0 (operator) or 911 (emergency) for an ambulance or medical help. Then give first aid immediately.**
• **See emergency information at the back of this book.**

POSSIBLE ADVERSE REACTIONS OR SIDE EFFECTS

SYMPTOMS	WHAT TO DO
Life-threatening: None expected.	
Common: Headache, flushed face and neck, dry mouth, nausea, vomiting, rapid heartbeat.	Continue. Tell doctor at next visit.
Infrequent:	
• Fainting.	Discontinue. Call doctor right away.
• Restlessness, blurred vision.	Continue. Call doctor when convenient.
Rare:	
• Rash.	Discontinue. Call doctor right away.
• Severe irritation, peeling.	Continue. Call doctor when convenient.

WARNINGS & PRECAUTIONS

Don't take if:
You are allergic to nitrates, including nitroglycerin.

Before you start, consult your doctor:
• If you are taking non-prescription drugs.
• If you plan to become pregnant within medication period.
• If you have glaucoma.
• If you have reacted badly to any vasodilator drug.
• If you drink alcoholic beverages or smoke marijuana.

Pregnancy:
No proven harm to unborn child. Avoid if possible.

Infants & children
Don't give to infants or young children unless prescribed and monitored by your physician.

Prolonged use:
Drug may become less effective and require higher doses.

Skin & sunlight:
No age-related problems expected.

Driving or hazardous activities:
Don't drive or pilot aircraft until you learn how medicine affects you. Don't work around dangerous machinery. Don't climb ladders or work in high places. Danger increases if you drink alcohol or take medicine affecting alertness and reflexes.

Discontinuing:
Except for sublingual tablets, don't discontinue without doctor's advice until you complete prescribed dose, even though symptoms diminish or disappear.

Others:
• If discomfort is not caused by angina, nitrate medication will not bring relief. Call doctor if discomfort persists.
• Periodic urine and laboratory blood studies of white cell counts recommended if you take nitrates.
• Keep sublingual tablets in original container. Always carry them with you, but keep from body heat if possible.
• Sublingual tablets produce a burning, stinging sensation when placed under the tongue. Replace supply if no burning or stinging is noted.

POSSIBLE INTERACTION WITH OTHER DRUGS

GENERIC NAME OR DRUG CLASS	COMBINED EFFECT
Anticholinergics (see Drugs Glossary)	Increased internal-eye pressure.
Antidepressants, tricyclic (TCA, see Drugs Glossary)	Excessive blood-pressure drop.
Antihypertensives (see Drugs Glossary)	Excessive blood-pressure drop.
Beta-adrenergic blockers (see Drugs Glossary)	Excessive blood-pressure drop.
Calcium channel blockers (see Drugs Glossary)	Decreased blood pressure.
Cholinergics (see Drugs Glossary)	Decreased cholinergic effect.
Ephedrine	Decreased nitrate effect.
Guanfacine	Increased effect of both drugs.
Narcotics (see Drugs Glossary)	Excessive blood-pressure drop.
Phenothiazines (see Drugs Glossary)	May decrease blood pressure.
Sympathomimetics (see Drugs Glossary)	Possible reduced effects of both medicines.

POSSIBLE INTERACTION WITH OTHER SUBSTANCES

INTERACTS WITH	COMBINED EFFECT
Alcohol:	Excessive blood-pressure drop.
Beverages:	None expected.
Cocaine (or crack):	Flushed face and headache. Avoid.
Foods:	None expected.
Marijuana:	Decreased nitrate effect.
Tobacco:	Decreased nitrate effect.

NITROFURANTOIN

BRAND NAMES

Apo-Nitrofurantoin	Nephronex
Cyantin	Nifuran
Furadantin	Nitrex
Furalan	Nitrodan
Furaloid	Novofuran
Furantoin	Sarodant
Furatine	Trantoin
Macrodantin	Urotoin

BASIC INFORMATION

Habit forming? No
Prescription needed? Yes
Available as generic? Yes
Drug class: Antimicrobial (see Drugs Glossary)

USES

Treatment for urinary-tract infections.

DOSAGE & USAGE INFORMATION

How to take:
• Tablet or capsule—Swallow with food or milk to lessen stomach irritation. If you can't swallow whole, crumble tablet or open capsule and take with liquid or food.
• Liquid—Shake well and take with food. Use a measuring spoon to ensure accuracy.

When to take:
At the same times each day.

If you forget a dose:
Take as soon as you remember up to 2 hours late. If more than 2 hours, wait for next scheduled dose (don't double this dose).

What drug does:
Prevents susceptible bacteria in the urinary tract from growing and multiplying.

Continued next column

OVERDOSE

SYMPTOMS:
Nausea, vomiting, abdominal pain, diarrhea.
WHAT TO DO:
Overdose unlikely to threaten life. If child takes much larger amount than prescribed, call doctor, poison-control center or hospital emergency room for instructions.

Time lapse before drug works:
1 to 2 weeks.

Don't take with:
Any other medicines, even over-the-counter drugs such as cough and cold medicines, nose drops, diet pills, laxatives or caffeine, without consulting your doctor.

POSSIBLE ADVERSE REACTIONS OR SIDE EFFECTS

SYMPTOMS	WHAT TO DO
Life-threatening:	
Hives, rash, intense itching, faintness soon after a dose (anaphylaxis).	Seek emergency treatment immediately.
Common:	
• Diarrhea, appetite loss, nausea, vomiting, chest pain, cough, difficult breathing, chills or unexplained fever.	Discontinue. Call doctor right away.
• Rusty colored or brown urine.	No action necessary.
Infrequent:	
• Rash, itchy skin, numbness, tingling or burning of face or mouth, fatigue, weakness.	Discontinue. Call doctor right away.
• Dizziness, headache, drowsiness, paleness (in children), discolored teeth (from liquid form).	Continue. Call doctor when convenient.
Rare:	
Jaundice.	Discontinue. Call doctor right away.

WARNINGS & PRECAUTIONS

Don't take if:
- You are allergic to nitrofurantoin.
- You have impaired kidney function.
- You drink alcohol.

Before you start, consult your doctor:
- If you are prone to allergic reactions.
- If you are pregnant and within 2 weeks of delivery.
- If you have had kidney disease, lung disease, anemia, nerve damage, or G6PD deficiency (a metabolic deficiency).
- If you have diabetes. Drug may affect urine sugar tests.

Pregnancy:
Risk to unborn child outweighs drug benefits, especially in last month of pregnancy. Don't use.

Infants & children:
Don't give to infants younger than 1 month. Use only under medical supervision for older children.

Prolonged use:
Chest pain, cough, shortness of breath.

Skin & sunlight:
No age-related problems expected.

Driving or hazardous activities:
Avoid if you feel dizzy or drowsy. Otherwise, no problems expected.

Discontinuing:
Don't discontinue without consulting doctor. Dose may require gradual reduction if you have taken drug for a long time. Doses of other drugs may also require adjustment.

Others:
Periodic blood counts, liver-function tests, and chest X-rays recommended.

POSSIBLE INTERACTION WITH OTHER DRUGS

GENERIC NAME OR DRUG CLASS	COMBINED EFFECT
Nalidixic acid	Decreased nitrofurantoin effect.
Phenobarbital	Decreased nitrofurantoin effect.
Probenecid	Increased nitrofurantoin effect.
Sulfinpyrazone	Possible nitrofurantoin toxicity.

POSSIBLE INTERACTION WITH OTHER SUBSTANCES

INTERACTS WITH	COMBINED EFFECT
Alcohol:	Possible disulfiram reaction (see Drugs Glossary). Avoid.
Beverages:	None expected.
Cocaine (or crack):	No proven problems.
Foods:	None expected.
Marijuana:	None expected.
Tobacco:	None expected.

PANTOTHENIC ACID (VITAMIN B-5)

BRAND & GENERIC NAMES

CALCIUM PATOTHENATE	Durasil
Dexol T.D.	Pantholin
	PANTOTHENIC ACID

Ingredients in numerous multiple vitamin-mineral supplements.

BASIC INFORMATION

Habit forming? No
Prescription needed? No
Available as generic? Yes
Drug class: Vitamin supplement

USES

Prevents and treats vitamin B-5 deficiency.

DOSAGE & USAGE INFORMATION

How to take:
Tablet—Swallow with liquid.

When to take:
At the same times each day.

If you forget a dose:
Take as soon as you remember, then resume regular schedule.

What drug does:
Acts as co-enzyme in carbohydrate, protein and fat metabolism.

Time lapse before drug works:
15 to 20 minutes.

Don't take with:

- Levodopa—Small amounts of pantothenic acid will nullify levodopa effect. Carbidopa-levodopa combination not affected by this interaction.
- *Any* other medicines, even over-the-counter drugs such as cough and cold medicines, nose drops, diet pills, laxatives or caffeine, without consulting your doctor.

OVERDOSE

SYMPTOMS:
None expected.
WHAT TO DO:
Overdose unlikely to threaten life.

POSSIBLE ADVERSE REACTIONS OR SIDE EFFECTS

SYMPTOMS	WHAT TO DO
Life-threatening: None expected.	
Common: Heartburn.	Discontinue. Seek emergency treatment.
Infrequent: Cramps.	Discontinue Call doctor right away.
Rare: Rash, hives, difficult breathing.	Discontinue. Seek emergency treatment.

WARNINGS & PRECAUTIONS

Don't take if
You are allergic to pantothenic acid.

Before you start, consult your doctor
If you have hemophilia.

Pregnancy
Don't exceed recommended dose.

Infants & children
Don't exceed recommended dose.

Prolonged use
Large doses for more than 1 month may cause toxicity.

Skin & sunlight
No age-related problems expected.

Driving or hazardous activities
No age-related problems expected.

Discontinuing
No age-related problems expected.

Others
Regular pantothenic acid supplements are recommended if you take chloramphenicol, cycloserine, ethionamide, hydralazine, immunosuppressants, isoniazid or penicillamine. These, taken alone, decrease pantothenic acid absorption and can cause anemia or tingling and numbness in hands and feet.

POSSIBLE INTERACTION WITH OTHER DRUGS

GENERIC NAME OR DRUG CLASS	COMBINED EFFECT
None expected.	

POSSIBLE INTERACTION WITH OTHER SUBSTANCES

INTERACTS WITH	COMBINED EFFECT
Alcohol:	None expected.
Beverages:	None expected.
Cocaine (or crack):	None expected.
Foods:	None expected.
Marijuana:	None expected.
Tobacco:	May decrease pantothenic acid absorption. Decreased pantothenic acid effect.

PENICILLINS

BRAND & GENERIC NAMES

See complete list of brand and generic names in the Brand & Generic Name Directory.

BASIC INFORMATION

Habit forming? No
Prescription needed? Yes
Available as generic? Yes
Drug class: Antibiotic (penicillin)

USES

Treatment of bacterial infections that are susceptible to penicillins.

DOSAGE & USAGE INFORMATION

How to take:
- Tablet—Swallow with liquid on an empty stomach 1 hour before or 2 hours after eating.
- Liquid—Take with cold beverage. Liquid form is perishable and effective for only 7 days at room temperature. Effective for 14 days if stored in refrigerator. Don't freeze.

When to take:
Follow instructions on prescription label or side of package. Doses should be evenly spaced. For example, 4 times a day means every 6 hours.

If you forget a dose:
Take as soon as you remember. Continue regular schedule.

What drug does:
Destroys susceptible bacteria. Does not kill viruses.

Time lapse before drug works:
May be several days before medicine affects infection.

Continued next column

OVERDOSE

SYMPTOMS:
Severe diarrhea, nausea or vomiting.
WHAT TO DO:
Overdose unlikely to threaten life. If child takes much larger amount than prescribed, call doctor, poison-control center or hospital emergency room for instructions.

Don't take with:
Any other medicines, even over-the-counter drugs such as cough and cold medicines, nose drops, diet pills, laxatives or caffeine, without consulting your doctor.

POSSIBLE ADVERSE REACTIONS OR SIDE EFFECTS

SYMPTOMS	WHAT TO DO
Life-threatening:	
Hives, rash, intense itching, faintness soon after a dose (anaphylaxis).	Seek emergency treatment immediately.
Common:	
Dark or discolored tongue.	Continue. Tell doctor at next visit.
Infrequent:	
Mild nausea, vomiting, diarrhea.	Continue. Call doctor when convenient.
Rare:	
Unexplained bleeding.	Discontinue. Call doctor right away.

WARNINGS & PRECAUTIONS

Don't take if:
You are allergic to penicillins, cephalosporin antibiotics, other penicillins. Life-threatening reaction may occur.

Before you start, consult your doctor:
If you are allergic to any substance or drug.

Pregnancy:
Studies inconclusive on harm to unborn child. Animal studies show fetal abnormalities. Decide with your doctor whether drug benefits justify risk to unborn child.

Infants & children:
No age-related problems expected.

Prolonged use:
You may become more susceptible to infections caused by germs not responsive to penicillins.

Skin & sunlight:
No age-related problems expected.

Driving or hazardous activities:
Usually not dangerous. Most hazardous reactions likely to occur a few minutes after taking penicillins.

Discontinuing:
Don't discontinue without doctor's advice until you complete prescribed dose, even though symptoms diminish or disappear.

Others:
Urine sugar test for diabetes may show false positive result.

POSSIBLE INTERACTION WITH OTHER DRUGS

GENERIC NAME OR DRUG CLASS	COMBINED EFFECT
Beta-adrenergic blockers (see Drugs Glossary)	Increased chance of anaphylaxis (see emergency information at the back of this book).
Calcium supplements (see Drugs Glossary)	Decreased penicillin effect.
Chloramphenicol	Decreased effect of both drugs.
Cholestyramine	May decrease penicillin effect.
Colestipol	May decrease penicillin effect.
Contraceptives (oral, see Drugs Glossary)	Possible decreased contraceptive effect.
Erythromycins (see Drugs Glossary)	Decreased effect of both drugs.
Paromomycin	Decreased effect of both drugs.
Probenecid	Possible decreased penicillin effect.
Tetracyclines (see Drugs Glossary)	Decreased effect of both drugs.
Troleandomycin	Decreased effect of both drugs.

POSSIBLE INTERACTION WITH OTHER SUBSTANCES

INTERACTS WITH	COMBINED EFFECT
Alcohol:	Occasional stomach irritation.
Beverages:	None expected.
Cocaine (or crack):	No proven problems.
Foods:	Decreased effect of penicillins.
Marijuana:	No proven problems.
Tobacco:	None expected.

PENTOXIFYLLINE

BRAND NAMES

Trental

BASIC INFORMATION

Habit forming? No
Prescription needed? Yes
Available as generic? No
Drug class: Hemorrheologic agent (see Drugs Glossary)

USES

Reduces pain in legs caused by poor circulation.

DOSAGE & USAGE INFORMATION

How to take:
Extended-release tablets—Swallow whole with water and food.

When to take:
At mealtimes. Taking with food decreases the likelihood of irritating the stomach and cause nausea.

If you forget a dose:
Take as soon as you remember up to 3 hours late. If more than 3 hours, wait for next scheduled dose (don't double this dose).

What drug does:
- Reduces "stickiness" of red blood cells and improves flexibility of the red cells.
- Improves blood flow through blood vessels.

Time lapse before drug works:
1 hour. Several weeks for full effect on circulation.

Don't take with:
- Tobacco or medicines to treat hypertension.
- *Any* other medicines, even over-the-counter drugs such as cough and cold medicines, nose drops, diet pills, laxatives or caffeine, without consulting your doctor.

OVERDOSE

SYMPTOMS:
Drowsiness, flushed face, fainting, nervousness, convulsions, coma.
WHAT TO DO:
- **Dial 0 (operator) or 911 (emergency) for an ambulance or medical help. Then give first aid immediately.**
- **See emergency information at the back of this book.**

POSSIBLE ADVERSE REACTIONS OR SIDE EFFECTS

SYMPTOMS	WHAT TO DO
Life-threatening:	
Chest pain, irregular heartbeat.	Discontinue. Seek emergency treatment.
Common:	
None expected.	
Infrequent:	
• Dizziness, headache, nausea, vomiting. low blood pressure, nose bleed, swollen feet and ankles, viral-like syndrome, nasal congestion, laryngitis, rash, itchy skin, blurred vision.	Discontinue. Call doctor right away.
• Insomnia, nervousness, red eyes.	Continue. Call doctor when convenient.
Rare:	
None expected.	

WARNINGS & PRECAUTIONS

Don't take if:
You are allergic to pentoxifylline.

Before you start, consult your doctor:
- If you are allergic to caffeine, theophylline, theobromine, aminophyllin, dyphyllin, oxtriphylline, theobromine.
- If you have angina.

Pregnancy:
Safety to unborn child unestablished. Avoid if possible.

Infants & children
Don't give to infants or young children unless prescribed and monitored by your physician.

Prolonged use:
No age-related problems expected.

Skin & sunlight:
No age-related problems expected.

Driving or hazardous activities:
Wait to see if drug causes drowsiness or dizziness. If none, no problems expected.

Discontinuing:
No age-related problems expected.

Others:
Don't smoke.

POSSIBLE INTERACTION WITH OTHER DRUGS

GENERIC NAME OR DRUG CLASS	COMBINED EFFECT
Anticoagulants (oral, see Drugs Glossary)	Possible decreased effect of anticoagulant.
Anithypertensives (see Drugs Glossary)	Possible increased effect of hypertensive medication.

POSSIBLE INTERACTION WITH OTHER SUBSTANCES

INTERACTS WITH	COMBINED EFFECT
Alcohol:	Unknown. Best to avoid.
Beverages: Coffee, tea or other caffeine-containing beverages.	May decrease effectiveness of pentoxifylline.
Cocaine (or crack):	Reduces pentoxifylline effect.
Foods:	None expected.
Marijuana:	Decreased effect of pentoxifylline.
Tobacco:	Decreased effect of pentoxifylline.

PERPHENAZINE & AMITRIPTYLINE

BRAND NAMES

Etrafon
PMS Levazine
Triavil

BASIC INFORMATION

Habit forming? No
Prescription needed? Yes
Available as generic? Yes
Drug class: Tranquilizer (phenothiazine), antidepressant

USES

- Decreases nausea, vomiting, hiccups.
- Gradually relieves, but doesn't cure, symptoms of depression, anxiety, agitation.
- Pain relief (sometimes).

DOSAGE & USAGE INFORMATION

How to take:
Tablet or liquid—Swallow with liquid.

When to take:
At the same time each day.

If you forget a dose:
Bedtime dose—If you forget your once-a-day bedtime dose, don't take it more than 3 hours late. If more than 3 hours, wait for next scheduled dose (don't double this dose).

What drug does:
- Suppresses brain's vomiting center.
- Suppresses brain centers that control abnormal emotions and behavior.
- Probably affects part of brain that controls messages between nerve cells.

Continued next column

OVERDOSE

SYMPTOMS:
Stupor, convulsions, hallucinations, coma.
WHAT TO DO:
- **Dial 0 (operator) or 911 (emergency) for an ambulance or medical help. Then give first aid immediately.**
- **If the child is unconscious and not breathing, give mouth-to-mouth breathing. If there is no heartbeat, use cardiac massage and mouth-to-mouth breathing (CPR). Don't try to make the child vomit. If you can't get help quickly, take the child to nearest emergency facility.**
- **See emergency information at the back of this book.**

Time lapse before drug works:
- Nausea and vomiting—1 hour or less.
- Nervous and mental disorders—4-6 weeks.
- Begins in 1 to 2 weeks. May require 4 to 6 weeks for maximum benefit.

Don't take with:
Any other medicines, even over-the-counter drugs such as cough and cold medicines, nose drops, diet pills, laxatives or caffeine, without consulting your doctor.

POSSIBLE ADVERSE REACTIONS OR SIDE EFFECTS

SYMPTOMS	WHAT TO DO
Life-threatening:	
Seizures; irregular heartbeat; weak pulse; fainting; muscle spasms; uncontrolled muscle movements of tongue, face and other muscles (neuroleptic malignant syndrome, rare).	Discontinue. Seek emergency treatment.
Common:	
• Headache, constipation, nausea, vomiting, irregular heartbeat, drowsiness.	Discontinue. Call doctor right away.
• Insomnia, dry mouth, "sweet tooth," decreased sweating, runny nose, constipation.	Continue. Call doctor when convenient.
Infrequent:	
• Hallucinations, dizziness, tremor, blurred vision, eye pain, vomiting, inflamed tongue, joint pain, back pain, hiccups.	Discontinue. Call doctor right away.
• Frequent urination, diminished sex drive, breast swelling, menstrual irregularities, nasal congestion.	Continue. Call doctor when convenient.
Rare:	
• Rash; itchy skin; jaundice; change in vision; sore throat, fever, mouth sores; abdominal pain; constipation.	Discontinue. Call doctor right away.
• Fatigue, weakness.	Continue. Call doctor when convenient.

WARNINGS & PRECAUTIONS

Don't take if:
- You are allergic to any phenothiazine, tricyclic antidepressant.
- You have a blood or bone-marrow disease, glaucoma, prostate trouble.
- You drink alcohol.
- You have had a heart attack within 6 weeks.
- You have taken MAO inhibitors within 2 weeks.
- Patient is younger than 12.

Before you start, consult your doctor:
- If you have asthma, emphysema or other lung disorder.
- If you have an enlarged prostate, heart disease, high blood pressure, stomach or intestinal problems, overactive thyroid, liver disease.
- If you take non-prescription ulcer medicine, asthma medicine or amphetamines.
- If you will have surgery within 2 months, including dental surgery, requiring general or spinal anesthesia.

Pregnancy:
Risk to unborn child outweighs drug benefits. Don't use.

Infants & children:
Don't give to children younger than 12.

Prolonged use:
May lead to tardive dyskinesia (involuntary movement of jaws, lips, tongue, chewing).

Skin & sunlight:
May cause rash or intensify sunburn in areas exposed to sun or sunlamp. Skin may remain sensitive for 3 months after discontinuing.

Driving or hazardous activities:
Don't drive or pilot aircraft until you learn how medicine affects you. Don't work around dangerous machinery. Don't climb ladders or work in high places. Danger increases if you drink alcohol or take medicine affecting alertness and reflexes, such as antihistamines, tranquilizers, sedatives, pain medicine, narcotics and mind-altering drugs.

Discontinuing:
- Nervous and mental disorders—Don't discontinue without doctor's advice until you complete prescribed dose, even though symptoms diminish or disappear.
- Dose may require gradual reduction if you have taken drug for a long time. Doses of other drugs may also require adjustment.

Others:
No age-related problems expected.

POSSIBLE INTERACTION WITH OTHER DRUGS

GENERIC NAME OR DRUG CLASS	COMBINED EFFECT
Anticholinergics (see Drugs Glossary)	Increased anticholinergic effect, increased sedation.
Anticoagulants (oral, see Drugs Glossary)	Increased anticoagulant effect.
Antihistamines (see Drugs Glossary)	Increased antihistamine effect.
Appetite suppressants (see Drugs Glossary)	Decreased suppressant effect.
Barbiturates (see Drugs Glossary)	Decreased anti-depressant effect. Increased sedation.
Cimetidine	Possible increased effect and toxicity of perphenazine and amitriptyline.
Clonidine	Possible decreased clonidine effect.
Dronabinol	Increased effect of both drugs.
Ethchlorvynol	Delirium.

See Additional Drug Interactions Section

POSSIBLE INTERACTION WITH OTHER SUBSTANCES

INTERACTS WITH	COMBINED EFFECT
Alcohol: Beverages or medicines with alcohol.	Excessive intoxication. Avoid.
Beverages: Coffee.	Reduces effectiveness.
Cocaine (or crack):	Excessive intoxication. Avoid.
Foods:	None expected.
Marijuana:	Excessive drowsiness. Avoid.
Tobacco:	None expected.

POTASSIUM SUPPLEMENTS

BRAND & GENERIC NAMES

See complete list of brand and generic names in the Brand & Generic Name Directory.

BASIC INFORMATION

Habit forming? No
Prescription needed? Yes
Available as generic? Yes
Drug class: Mineral supplement (potassium)

USES

• Treatment for potassium deficiency from diuretics, cortisone or digitalis medicines.
• Treatment for low potassium associated with some illnesses.

DOSAGE & USAGE INFORMATION

How to take:
• Tablet or capsule—Swallow with liquid or food to lessen stomach irritation. You may chew or crush tablet.
• Extended-release tablets or capsules—Swallow each dose whole with liquid.
• Effervescent tablets, granules, powder or liquid—Dilute dose in water.

When to take:
At the same time each day, preferably with food or immediately after meals.

If you forget a dose:
Take as soon as you remember. Don't double next dose.

Continued next column

OVERDOSE

SYMPTOMS:
Paralysis of arms and legs, irregular heartbeat, blood-pressure drop, convulsions, coma, cardiac arrest.
WHAT TO DO:
• Dial 0 (operator) or 911 (emergency) for an ambulance or medical help. Then give first aid immediately.
• See emergency information at the back of this book.

What drug does:
Preserves or restores normal function of nerve cells, heart and skeletal-muscle cells, kidneys, and stomach-juice secretions.

Time lapse before drug works:
1 to 2 hours. Full benefit may require 12 to 24 hours.

Don't take with:
Any other medicines, even over-the-counter drugs such as cough and cold medicines, nose drops, diet pills, laxatives or caffeine, without consulting your doctor.

POSSIBLE ADVERSE REACTIONS OR SIDE EFFECTS

SYMPTOMS	WHAT TO DO
Life-threatening: None expected.	
Common: None expected.	
Infrequent: Diarrhea, nausea, vomiting, stomach discomfort, skin rash.	Continue. Call doctor when convenient.
Rare: • Confusion; irregular heartbeat; difficult breathing; unusual fatigue; weakness; heaviness of legs; small bowel ulcers, hemorrhage, perforation with enteric-coated tablets (rarely with wax matrix tablets); esophageal ulceration with tablets.	Discontinue. Call doctor right away.
• Numbness or tingling in hands or feet.	Continue. Call doctor when convenient.

WARNINGS & PRECAUTIONS

Don't take if:
- You are allergic to any potassium supplement.
- You have acute or chronic kidney disease.

Before you start, consult your doctor:
- If you have Addison's disease or familial periodic paralysis.
- If you have heart disease.
- If you have intestinal blockage.
- If you have a stomach ulcer.
- If you use diuretics.
- If you use heart medicine.
- If you use laxatives or have chronic diarrhea.
- If you use salt substitutes or low-salt milk.

Pregnancy:
No age-related problems expected if you adhere strictly to prescribed dose.

Infants & children:
Use only under doctor's supervision.

Prolonged use:
- Slows absorption of vitamin B-12. May cause anemia.
- Request frequent lab tests to monitor potassium levels in blood, especially if you take digitalis preparations.

Skin & sunlight:
No age-related problems expected.

Driving or hazardous activities:
No age-related problems expected.

Discontinuing:
Don't discontinue without consulting doctor. Dose may require gradual reduction if you have taken drug for a long time. Doses of other drugs may also require adjustment.

Others:
- Overdose or underdose serious. Frequent EKGs and laboratory blood studies to measure serum electrolytes and kidney function recommended.
- Prolonged diarrhea may call for increased dosage of potassium.
- Serious injury may necessitate temporary *decrease* in potassium.
- Some products contain tartrazine dye. Avoid, especially if you are allergic to aspirin.

POSSIBLE INTERACTION WITH OTHER DRUGS

GENERIC NAME OR DRUG CLASS	COMBINED EFFECT
ACE inhibitors: captopril, enalapril, lisinopril (see Drugs Glossary)	Possible increased potassium effect.
Amiloride	Dangerous rise in blood potassium.
Anticholinergics (other, see Drugs Glossary)	Increased possibility of intestinal ulcers, which sometimes occur with oral potassium tablets.
Atropine	Increased possibility of intestinal ulcers, which sometimes occur with oral potassium tablets.
Belladonna	Increased possibility of intestinal ulcers, which sometimes occur with oral potassium tablets.
Cortisone medicines (see Drugs Glossary)	Decreased effect of potassium.

See Additional Drug Interactions Section

POSSIBLE INTERACTION WITH OTHER SUBSTANCES

INTERACTS WITH	COMBINED EFFECT
Alcohol:	None expected.
Beverages: Salty drinks such as tomato juice, commercial thirst quenchers.	Increased fluid retention.
Cocaine (or crack):	May cause irregular heartbeat.
Foods: Salty foods.	Increased fluid retention.
Marijuana:	May cause irregular heartbeat.
Tobacco:	None expected.

PRAZOSIN

BRAND NAMES

Minipress

BASIC INFORMATION

Habit forming? No
Prescription needed? Yes
Available as generic? No
Drug class: Antihypertensive

USES

- Treatment for high blood pressure.
- May improve congestive heart failure.
- Treatment for Raynaud's disease.

DOSAGE & USAGE INFORMATION

How to take:
Tablet or capsule—Swallow with liquid. If you can't swallow whole, crumble tablet or open capsule and take with liquid or food.

When to take:
At the same times each day.

If you forget a dose:
Take as soon as you remember up to 2 hours late. If more than 2 hours, wait for next scheduled dose (don't double this dose).

What drug does:
Expands and relaxes blood-vessel walls to lower blood pressure.

Continued next column

OVERDOSE

SYMPTOMS:
Extreme weakness; loss of consciousness; cold, sweaty skin; weak, rapid pulse; coma.
WHAT TO DO:
- **Dial 0 (operator) or 911 (emergency) for an ambulance or medical help. Then give first aid immediately.**
- **If the child is unconscious and not breathing, give mouth-to-mouth breathing. If there is no heartbeat, use cardiac massage and mouth-to-mouth breathing (CPR). Don't try to make the child vomit. If you can't get help quickly, take the child to nearest emergency facility.**
- **See emergency information at the back of this book.**

Time lapse before drug works:
30 minutes.

Don't take with:
Any other medicines, even over-the-counter drugs such as cough and cold medicines, nose drops, diet pills, laxatives or caffeine, without consulting your doctor.

POSSIBLE ADVERSE REACTIONS OR SIDE EFFECTS

SYMPTOMS	WHAT TO DO
Life-threatening: None expected.	
Common:	
• Rapid heartbeat.	Discontinue. Call doctor right away.
• Vivid dreams, drowsiness, dizziness.	Continue. Call doctor when convenient.
Infrequent:	
• Rash or itchy skin, blurred vision, shortness of breath, difficult breathing, chest pain.	Discontinue. Call doctor right away.
• Appetite loss, constipation or diarrhea, stomach pain, nausea, vomiting, fluid retention, joint or muscle aches, weakness and faintness when arising from bed or chair.	Continue. Call doctor when convenient.
• Headache, irritability, depression, dry mouth, stuffy nose, increased urination.	Continue. Tell doctor at next visit.
Rare:	
Decreased sexual function.	Continue. Call doctor when convenient.

WARNINGS & PRECAUTIONS

Don't take if:
- You are allergic to prazosin.
- You are depressed.
- You will have surgery within 2 months, including dental surgery, requiring general or spinal anesthesia.

Before you start, consult your doctor:
- If you experience lightheadedness or fainting with other antihypertensive drugs.
- If you are easily depressed.
- If you have impaired brain circulation or have had a stroke.
- If you have coronary heart disease (with or without angina).
- If you have kidney disease or impaired liver function.

Pregnancy:
Studies inconclusive on harm to unborn child. Animal studies show fetal abnormalities. Decide with your doctor whether drug benefits justify risk to child.

Infants & children
Don't give to infants or young children unless prescribed and monitored by your physician.

Prolonged use:
No age-related problems expected.

Skin & sunlight:
No age-related problems expected.

Driving or hazardous activities:
Don't drive or pilot aircraft until you learn how medicine affects you. Don't work around dangerous machinery. Don't climb ladders or work in high places.

Discontinuing:
Don't discontinue without doctor's advice until you complete prescribed dose, even though symptoms diminish or disappear.

Others:
First dose likely to cause fainting. Take it at night and get out of bed slowly next morning.

POSSIBLE INTERACTION WITH OTHER DRUGS

GENERIC NAME OR DRUG CLASS	COMBINED EFFECT
Amphetamines (see Drugs Glossary)	Decreased prazosin effect.
Antihypertensives, (other, see Drugs Glossary)	Increased antihypertensive effect. Dosages may require adjustments.
Estrogen	Decreased effect of prazosin.
Guanfacine	Increased effect of both medicines.
MAO inhibitors (see Drugs Glossary)	Blood-pressure drop.
Nifedipine	Weakness and faintness when arising from bed or chair.
Nitrates (see Drugs Glossary)	Possible excessive blood-pressure drop.
Non-steroidal anti-inflammatory drugs (NSAIDs, see Drugs Glossary)	Decreased effect of prazosin.
Sympathomimetics (see Drugs Glossary)	Decreased effect of prazosin.
Verapamil	Weakness and faintness when arising from bed or chair.

POSSIBLE INTERACTION WITH OTHER SUBSTANCES

INTERACTS WITH	COMBINED EFFECT
Alcohol:	Excessive blood-pressure drop.
Beverages:	None expected.
Cocaine (or crack):	Decreased prazosin effect. Avoid.
Foods:	None expected.
Marijuana:	Possible fainting. Avoid.
Tobacco:	Possible spasm of coronary arteries. Avoid.

PROBENECID

BRAND NAMES

Benacen	Col-Probenecid
Benemid	Polycillin-PRB
Benuryl	Probalan
ColBENEMID	SK-Probenecid

BASIC INFORMATION

Habit forming? No
Prescription needed? Yes
Available as generic? Yes
Drug class: Antigout (uricosuric)

USES

- Treatment for chronic gout.
- Increases blood levels of penicillins and cephalosporins.

DOSAGE & USAGE INFORMATION

How to take:
Tablet—Swallow with liquid or food to lessen stomach irritation. If you can't swallow whole, crumble tablet and take with liquid or food.

When to take:
At the same time each day.

If you forget a dose:
Take as soon as you remember up to 12 hours late. If more than 12 hours, wait for next scheduled dose (don't double this dose).

What drug does:
- Forces kidneys to excrete uric acid.
- Reduces amount of penicillin excreted in urine, so increases blood level.

Time lapse before drug works:
May require several months of regular use to prevent acute gout.

Continued next column

OVERDOSE

SYMPTOMS:
Breathing difficulty, severe nervous agitation, vomiting, seizures, convulsions, delirium, coma.
WHAT TO DO:
- **Dial 0 (operator) or 911 (emergency) for an ambulance or medical help. Then give first aid immediately.**
- **See emergency information at the back of this book.**

Don't take with:
Any other medicines, even over-the-counter drugs such as cough and cold medicines, nose drops, diet pills, laxatives or caffeine, without consulting your doctor.

POSSIBLE ADVERSE REACTIONS OR SIDE EFFECTS

SYMPTOMS	WHAT TO DO
Life-threatening: None expected.	
Common: Headache, appetite loss, nausea, vomiting.	Continue. Call doctor when convenient.
Infrequent: • Blood in urine, low back pain. worsening gout.	Discontinue. Call doctor right away.
• Dizziness, flushed face, itchy skin.	Continue. Call doctor when convenient.
• Painful or frequent urination.	Continue. Tell doctor at next visit.
Rare: Sore throat; difficult breathing; unusual bleeding or bruising; red, painful joint; jaundice; fever.	Discontinue. Call doctor right away.

WARNINGS & PRECAUTIONS

Don't take if:
- You are allergic to any uricosuric.
- You have acute gout.
- Patient is younger than 2.

Before you start, consult your doctor:
- If you have had kidney stones or kidney disease.
- If you have a peptic ulcer.
- If you have bone-marrow or blood-cell disease.

Pregnancy:
Studies inconclusive on harm to unborn child. Animal studies show fetal abnormalities. Decide with your doctor whether drug benefits justify risk to unborn child.

Infants & children
Don't give to infants or young children unless prescribed and monitored by your physician.

Prolonged use:
Possible kidney damage.

Skin & sunlight:
No age-related problems expected.

Driving or hazardous activities:
Avoid if you feel dizzy. Otherwise, no problems expected.

Discontinuing:
Don't discontinue without consulting doctor. Dose may require gradual reduction if you have taken drug for a long time. Doses of other drugs may also require adjustment.

Others:
If signs of gout attack develop while taking medicine, consult doctor.

POSSIBLE INTERACTION WITH OTHER DRUGS

GENERIC NAME OR DRUG CLASS	COMBINED EFFECT
Allopurinol	Increased effect of each drug.
Anticoagulants (oral, see Drugs Glossary)	Increased anticoagulant effect.
Aspirin	Decreased probenecid effect.
Cephalosporins (see Drugs Glossary)	Increased cephalosporin effect.
Dapsone	Increased dapsone effect. Increased toxicity.
Diuretics (thiazide, see Drugs Glossary)	Decreased probenecid effect.
Hypoglycemics (oral, see Drugs Glossary)	Increased hypoglycemic effect.
Indomethacin	Increased adverse effects of indomethacin.
Methotrexate	Increased methotrexate toxicity.
Nitrofurantoin	Incresed effect of nitrofurantoin.
Para-aminosalicylic	Increased effect of acid (PAS)para-aminosalicylic acid.
Penicillins (see Drugs Glossary)	Enhanced penicillin effect.
Pyrazinamide	Decreased probenecid effect.
Salicylates (see Drugs Glossary)	Decreased probenecid effect.
Sulfa drugs	Slows elimination. May cause harmful accumulation of sulfa.

POSSIBLE INTERACTION WITH OTHER SUBSTANCES

INTERACTS WITH	COMBINED EFFECT
Alcohol:	Decreased probenecid effect.
Beverages: Caffeine drinks.	Loss of probenecid effectiveness.
Cocaine (or crack):	None expected.
Foods:	None expected.
Marijuana:	Daily use—Decreased probenecid effect.
Tobacco:	None expected.

PROCAINAMIDE

BRAND NAMES

Procan	Pronestyl
Procan SR	Pronestyl SR
Procamide	Rhythmin
Procapan	Sub-Quin
Promine	

BASIC INFORMATION

Habit forming? No
Prescription needed? Yes
Available as generic? Yes
Drug class: Antiarrhythmic

USES

Stabilizes irregular heartbeat.

DOSAGE & USAGE INFORMATION

How to take:
• Tablet or capsule—Swallow with liquid.
• Extended-release tablets—Swallow each dose whole. Do not crush them.

When to take:
Best taken on empty stomach, 1 hour before or 2 hours after meals. If necessary, may be taken with food or milk to lessen stomach upset.

If you forget a dose:
Take as soon as you remember up to 2 hours late. If more than 2 hours, wait for next scheduled dose (don't double this dose).

What drug does:
Slows activity of pacemaker (rhythm-control center of heart) and delays transmission of electrical impulses.

Time lapse before drug works:
30 to 60 minutes.

Continued next column

OVERDOSE

SYMPTOMS:
Fast and irregular heartbeat, confusion, stupor, decreased blood pressure, fainting, cardiac arrest.
WHAT TO DO:
• Dial 0 (operator) or 911 (emergency) for an ambulance or medical help. Then give first aid immediately.
• See emergency information at the back of this book.

Don't take with:
Any other medicines, even over-the-counter drugs such as cough and cold medicines, nose drops, diet pills, laxatives or caffeine, without consulting your doctor.

POSSIBLE ADVERSE REACTIONS OR SIDE EFFECTS

SYMPTOMS	WHAT TO DO
Life-threatening:	
Hives, rash, intense itching, faintness soon after a dose (anaphylaxis).	Seek emergency treatment immediately.
Common:	
Diarrhea, appetite loss, nausea, vomiting, bitter taste.	Continue. Call doctor when convenient.
Infrequent:	
• Joint pain, painful breathing.	Discontinue. Call doctor right away.
• Dizziness.	Continue. Call doctor when convenient.
Rare:	
• Hallucinations, depression, confusion, psychosis, itchy skin, rash, sore throat, fever, jaundice, convulsions.	Discontinue. Call doctor right away.
• Headache, fatigue.	Continue. Call doctor when convenient.

WARNINGS & PRECAUTIONS

Don't take if:
- You are allergic to procainamide.
- You have myasthenia gravis.

Before you start, consult your doctor:
- If you are allergic to local anesthetics that end in "caine."
- If you have had liver or kidney disease or impaired kidney function.
- If you have had lupus.
- If you take digitalis preparations.
- If you will have surgery within 2 months, including dental surgery, requiring general or spinal anesthesia.

Pregnancy:
No proven harm to unborn child. Avoid if possible.

Infants & children
Don't give to infants or young children unless prescribed and monitored by your physician.

Prolonged use:
May cause lupus-like illness.

Skin & sunlight:
No age-related problems expected.

Driving or hazardous activities:
Use caution if you feel dizzy or weak. Otherwise, no problems expected.

Discontinuing:
Don't discontinue without doctor's advice until you complete prescribed dose, even though symptoms diminish or disappear.

Others:
Some products contain tartrazine dye. Avoid, especially if you are allergic to aspirin.

POSSIBLE INTERACTION WITH OTHER DRUGS

GENERIC NAME OR DRUG CLASS	COMBINED EFFECT
Acetazolamide	Increased procainamide effect.
Ambenonium	Decreased ambenonium effect.
Aminoglycosides (see Drugs Glossary)	Possible severe muscle weakness, impaired breathing.
Antiarrhythmics (other, see Drugs Glossary)	Increased likelihood of adverse reactions with either drug. Possible increased effect of both drugs.
Anticholinergics (see Drugs Glossary)	Increased anticholinergic effect.
Antihypertensives (see Drugs Glossary)	Increased antihypertensive effect.
Antimyasthenics (see Drugs Glossary)	Decreased antimyasthenic effect.
Cimetidine	Increased procainamide effect.
Encainide	Increased effect of toxicity on heart muscle.
Guanfacine	Increased effect of both medicines.
Kanamycin	Possible severe muscle weakness, impaired breathing.
Neomycin	Possible severe muscle weakness, impaired breathing.

POSSIBLE INTERACTION WITH OTHER SUBSTANCES

INTERACTS WITH	COMBINED EFFECT
Alcohol:	None expected.
Beverages: Caffeine drinks, iced drinks.	Irregular heartbeat.
Cocaine (or crack):	Decreased procainamide effect.
Foods:	None expected.
Marijuana:	None expected.
Tobacco:	Decreased procainamide effect.

PROGESTINS

BRAND & GENERIC NAMES

See complete list of brand and generic names in the Brand & Generic Name Directory.

BASIC INFORMATION

Habit forming? No
Prescription needed? Yes
Available as generic? No
Drug class: Female sex hormone (progestin)

USES

• Treatment for menstrual or uterine disorders caused by progestin imbalance.
• Contraceptive.

DOSAGE & USAGE INFORMATION

How to take:
Tablet—Swallow with liquid or food to lessen stomach irritation. You may crumble tablet or open capsule.

When to take:
At the same time each day.

If you forget a dose:
• Menstrual disorders—Take up to 2 hours late. If more than 2 hours, wait for next dose (don't double this dose).
• Contraceptive—Consult your doctor. You may need to use another birth-control method until next period.

What drug does:
• Creates a uterine lining similar to pregnancy that prevents bleeding.
• Suppresses a pituitary gland hormone responsible for ovulation.
• Stimulates cervical mucus, which stops sperm penetration and prevents pregnancy.

Continued next column

OVERDOSE

SYMPTOMS:
Nausea, vomiting, fluid retention, breast discomfort or enlargement, vaginal bleeding.
WHAT TO DO:
Overdose unlikely to threaten life. If child takes much larger amount than prescribed, call doctor, poison-control center or hospital emergency room for instructions.

Time lapse before drug works:
• Menstrual disorders—24 to 48 hours.
• Contraception—3 weeks.

Don't take with:
Any other medicines, even over-the-counter drugs such as cough and cold medicines, nose drops, diet pills, laxatives or caffeine, without consulting your doctor.

POSSIBLE ADVERSE REACTIONS OR SIDE EFFECTS

SYMPTOMS	WHAT TO DO
Life-threatening:	
Blood clot in leg, brain or lung; hives, rash, intense itching, faintness soon after a dose (anaphylaxis).	Seek emergency treatment immediately.
Common:	
Appetite or weight changes, swollen ankles or feet, unusual tiredness or weakness.	Continue. Tell doctor at next visit.
Infrequent:	
• Prolonged vaginal bleeding.	Discontinue. Call doctor right away.
• Depression.	Continue. Call doctor when convenient.
• Acne, increased facial or body hair, nausea, breast tenderness.	Continue. Tell doctor at next visit.
Rare:	
• Rash, stomach or side pain, jaundice, fever.	Discontinue. Call doctor right away.
• Insomnia, hair loss, amenorrhea.	Continue. Call doctor when convenient.

WARNINGS & PRECAUTIONS

Don't take if:
- You are allergic to any progestin hormone.
- You may be pregnant.
- You have liver or gallbladder disease.
- You have had thrombophlebitis, embolism or stroke.
- You have unexplained vaginal bleeding.
- You have had breast or uterine cancer.

Before you start, consult your doctor:
- If you have heart or kidney disease.
- If you have diabetes.
- If you have a seizure disorder.
- If you suffer migraines.
- If you are easily depressed.

Pregnancy:
May harm child. Discontinue at first sign of pregnancy.

Infants & children:
Use only for female children under medical supervision.

Prolonged use:
No age-related problems expected.

Skin & sunlight:
No age-related problems expected.

Driving or hazardous activities:
No age-related problems expected.

Discontinuing:
Consult doctor. This medicine stays in the body and causes fetal abnormalities. Wait at least 3 months before becoming pregnant.

Others:
- Children with diabetes must be monitored closely.
- Symptoms of blood clot in leg, brain or lung are: chest, groin, leg pain; sudden, severe headache; loss of coordination; vision change; shortness of breath; slurred speech.

POSSIBLE INTERACTION WITH OTHER DRUGS

GENERIC NAME OR DRUG CLASS	COMBINED EFFECT
Hypoglycemics (oral, see Drugs Glossary)	Decreased effect of oral hypoglycemics.
Insulin	Decreased effect of insulin.
Oxyphenbutazone	Decreased progestin effect.
Phenobarbital	Decreased progestin effect.
Phenothiazines (see Drugs Glossary)	Increased phenothiazine effect.
Phenylbutazone	Decreased progestin effect.

POSSIBLE INTERACTION WITH OTHER SUBSTANCES

INTERACTS WITH	COMBINED EFFECT
Alcohol:	None expected.
Beverages:	None expected.
Cocaine (or crack):	Decreased norethindrone effect.
Foods: Salt.	Fluid retention.
Marijuana:	Possible menstrual irregularities or bleeding between periods.
Tobacco:	Possible blood clots in lung, brain, legs. Avoid.

PSORALENS

BRAND & GENERIC NAMES

METHOXSALEN	**Oxsoralen (Topical)**
Methoxsalen Lotion (Topical)	**TRIOXSALEN**
Oxsoralen	**Trisoralen**
Oxsoralen-Ultra	**UltraMOP**

BASIC INFORMATION

Habit forming? No
Prescription needed? Yes
Available as generic? No
Drug class: Repigmenting agent (psoralen)

USES

- Repigmenting skin affected with vitiligo (absence of skin pigment).
- Treatment for psoriasis, when other treatments haven't helped.
- Treatment for mycosis fungoides.

DOSAGE & USAGE INFORMATION

How to take: or apply:
- Tablet or capsule—Swallow with liquid or food to lessen stomach irritation.
- Topical—As directed by doctor.

When to take: or apply:
2 to 4 hours before exposure to sunlight or sunlamp.

If you forget a dose:
Take as soon as you remember. Delay sun exposure for at least 2 hours after taking.

What drug does:
Helps pigment cells when used in conjunction with ultraviolet light.

Time lapse before drug works:
- For vitiligo, 6 to 9 months.
- For psoriasis, 10 weeks or longer.
- For tanning, 3 to 4 days.

Continued next column

OVERDOSE

SYMPTOMS:
Blistering skin, swelling feet and legs.
WHAT TO DO:
Overdose unlikely to threaten life. If child takes much larger amount than prescribed, call doctor, poison-control center or hospital emergency room for instructions.

Don't take with:
- Any other medicine which causes skin sensitivity to sun. Ask pharmacist.
- *Any* other medicines, even over-the-counter drugs such as cough and cold medicines, nose drops, diet pills, laxatives or caffeine, without consulting your doctor.

POSSIBLE ADVERSE REACTIONS OR SIDE EFFECTS

SYMPTOMS	WHAT TO DO
Life-threatening: None expected.	
Always:	
• Increased skin sensitivity to sun.	Always protect from overexposure.
• Increased eye sensitivity to sunlight.	Always protect with wrap-around sunglasses.
Infrequent: None expected.	
Rare: Hepatitis with jaundice, blistering and peeling.	Discontinue. Call doctor right away.

WARNINGS & PRECAUTIONS

Don't take if:
- You are allergic to any other psoralen.
- You are unwilling or unable to remain under close medical supervision.

Before you start, consult your doctor:
- If you have heart or liver disease.
- If you have allergy to sunlight.
- If you have cataracts.
- If you have albinism.
- If you have lupus erythematosis, porphyria, chronic infection, skin cancer or peptic ulcer.
- If you will have surgery within 2 months, including dental surgery, requiring general or spinal anesthesia.

Pregnancy:
Risk to unborn child outweighs drug benefits. Don't use.

Infants & children
Don't give to infants or young children unless prescribed and monitored by your physician.

Prolonged use:
Increased chance of toxic effects.

Skin & sunlight:
Too much can burn skin. Cover skin for 24 hours before and 8 hours following treatments.

Driving or hazardous activities:
No age-related problems expected. Protect eyes and skin from bright light.

Discontinuing:
Skin may remain sensitive for some time after treatment stops. Use extra protection from sun.

Others:
- Use sunblock on lips.
- Don't use just to make skin tan.

POSSIBLE INTERACTION WITH OTHER DRUGS

GENERIC NAME OR DRUG CLASS	COMBINED EFFECT
Any medicine causing sensitization to sunlight, such as: acetohexamide, amitriptyline, anthralin, barbiturates, bendroflumethiazide, carbamazepine, chlordiazepoxide, chloroquine, chlorothiazide, chloropromazine, chloropropamide, chlortetracycline, chlorthalidone, clindamycin, coal tar derivatives, cyproheptadine, demeclocycline, desipramine, diethylstilbrestrol, diphenhydramine, doxepin, doxycycline, estrogen, fluphenazine, gold preparations, glyburide, griseofulvin, hydrochlorothiazide, hydroflumethiazide, imipramine, lincomycin, mesoridazine, methacycline, nalidixic acid, nortriptyline, oral contraceptives, oxyphenbutazone, oxytetracycline, perphenazine, phenobarbital, phenylbutazone, phenytoin, prochlorperazine, promazine, promethazine, protriptyline, pyrazinamide, sulfonamides, tetracycline, thioridazine, thiazide diuretics, tolazamide, tolbutamide, tranylcypromine, triamterene, trifluoperazine, trimeprazine, trimipramine, triprolidine.	Greatly increased likelihood of extreme sensitivity to sunlight.

POSSIBLE INTERACTION WITH OTHER SUBSTANCES

INTERACTS WITH	COMBINED EFFECT
Alcohol:	May increase chance of liver toxicity.
Beverages: Lime drinks.	Avoid—toxic.
Cocaine (or crack):	Increased chance of toxicity. Avoid.
Foods: Those containing furocoumarin (limes, parsley, figs, parsnips, carrots, celery, mustard).	May cause toxic effects to psoralens.
Marijuana:	Increased chance of toxicity. Avoid.
Tobacco:	May cause uneven absorption of medicine. Avoid.

PYRIDOXINE (VITAMIN B-6)

BRAND NAMES

Alba-Lybe	Hexa-Betalin
Al-Vite	Hexacrest
Beelith	Hexavibex
Beesix	Mega-B
Bendectin	Nu-Iron-V
Eldertonic	Pyroxine
Glutofac	Rodex
Hemo-vite	Tex Six T.R.
Herpecin-L	Vicon

BASIC INFORMATION

Habit forming? No
Prescription needed?
High strength: Yes
Low strength: No
Available as generic? Yes
Drug class: Vitamin supplement

USES

- Prevention and treatment of pyridoxine deficiency.
- Treatment of some forms of anemia.
- Treatment of INH (isonicotinic acid hydrozide), cycloserine poisoning.

DOSAGE & USAGE INFORMATION

How to take:
- Tablets—Swallow with liquid.
- Extended-release capsules—Swallow each dose whole with liquid.

When to take:
At the same times each day.

If you forget a dose:
Take as soon as you remember, then resume regular schedule.

What drug does:
Acts as co-enzyme in carbohydrate, protein and fat metabolism.

Time lapse before drug works:
15 to 20 minutes.

Continued next column

OVERDOSE

SYMPTOMS:
None expected.
WHAT TO DO:
Overdose unlikely to threaten life.

Don't take with:
- Levodopa—Small amounts of pyridoxine will nullify levodopa effect. Carbidopa-levodopa combination not affected by this interaction.
- *Any* other medicines, even over-the-counter drugs such as cough and cold medicines, nose drops, diet pills, laxatives or caffeine, without consulting your doctor.

POSSIBLE ADVERSE REACTIONS OR SIDE EFFECTS

SYMPTOMS	WHAT TO DO
Life-threatening:	
None expected.	
Common:	
None expected.	
Infrequent:	
Nausea, headache.	Discontinue. Call doctor right away.
Rare:	
Numbness or tingling in hands or feet (large doses).	Discontinue. Call doctor right away.

WARNINGS & PRECAUTIONS

Don't take if:
You are allergic to pyridoxine.

Before you start, consult your doctor:
If you are pregnant or breast-feeding.

Pregnancy:
Don't exceed recommended dose.

Infants & children:
Don't exceed recommended dose.

Prolonged use:
Large doses for more than 1 month may cause toxicity.

Skin & sunlight:
No age-related problems expected.

Driving or hazardous activities:
No age-related problems expected.

Discontinuing:
No age-related problems expected.

Others:
Regular pyridoxine supplements recommended if you take chloramphenicol, cycloserine, ethionamide, hydralazine, immunosuppressants, isoniazid or penicillamine. These decrease pyridoxine absorption and can cause anemia or tingling and numbness in hands and feet.

POSSIBLE INTERACTION WITH OTHER DRUGS

GENERIC NAME OR DRUG CLASS	COMBINED EFFECT
Contraceptives (oral, see Drugs Glossary)	Decreased pyridoxine effect.
Cycloserine	Decreased pyridoxine effect.
Hydralazine	Decreased pyridoxine effect.
Hypnotics (barbiturates) (see Drugs Glossary)	Decreased hypnotic effect.
Immunosuppressants (see Drugs Glossary)	Decreased pyridoxine effect.
Isoniazid	Decreased pyridoxine effect.
Levodopa	Decreased levodopa effect.
Penicillamine	Decreased pyridoxine effect.
Phenobarbital	Possible decreased phenobarbital effect.
Phenytoin	Decreased phenytoin effect.

POSSIBLE INTERACTION WITH OTHER SUBSTANCES

INTERACTS WITH	COMBINED EFFECT
Alcohol:	None expected.
Beverages:	None expected.
Cocaine (or crack):	None expected.
Foods:	None expected.
Marijuana:	None expected.
Tobacco:	May decrease pyridoxine absorption. Decreased pyridoxine effect.

QUINIDINE

BRAND NAMES

Apo-Quinidine
Biquin Durules
Cardioquin
Cin-Quin
Duraquin
Novoquinidin
Quinaglute Dura-Tabs
Quinalan
Quinate
Quinidex Extentabs
Quinobarb
Quinora
SK-Quinidine Sulfate

BASIC INFORMATION

Habit forming? No
Prescription needed?
U.S.: Yes
Canada: No
Available as generic? Yes
Drug class: Antiarrhythmic

USES

Corrects heart-rhythm disorders.

DOSAGE & USAGE INFORMATION

How to take:
• Tablet or capsule—Swallow with liquid or food to lessen stomach irritation.
• Extended-release tablets—Swallow each dose whole. Don't crush them.

Continued next column

OVERDOSE

SYMPTOMS:
Confusion, severe blood-pressure drop, lethargy, breathing difficulty, fainting, seizures, coma.
WHAT TO DO:
• Dial 0 (operator) or 911 (emergency) for an ambulance or medical help. Then give first aid immediately.
• If the child is unconscious and not breathing, give mouth-to-mouth breathing. If there is no heartbeat, use cardiac massage and mouth-to-mouth breathing (CPR). Don't try to make the child vomit. If you can't get help quickly, take the child to nearest emergency facility.
• See emergency information at the back of this book.

When to take:
At the same times each day.

If you forget a dose:
Take as soon as you remember up to 2 hours late. If more than 2 hours, wait for next scheduled dose (don't double this dose).

What drug does:
Delays nerve impulses to the heart to regulate heartbeat.

Time lapse before drug works:
2 to 4 hours.

Don't take with:
Any other medicines, even over-the-counter drugs such as cough and cold medicines, nose drops, diet pills, laxatives or caffeine, without consulting your doctor.

POSSIBLE ADVERSE REACTIONS OR SIDE EFFECTS

SYMPTOMS	WHAT TO DO
Life-threatening:	
Hives, rash, intense itching, faintness soon after a dose (anaphylaxis).	Seek emergency treatment immediately.
Common:	
Bitter taste, diarrhea, nausea, vomiting.	Discontinue. Call doctor right away.
Infrequent:	
• Dizziness, lightheadedness, fainting, headache, confusion, rash, change in vision, difficult breathing, rapid heartbeat.	Discontinue. Call doctor right away.
• Ringing in ears.	Continue. Call doctor when convenient.
Rare:	
• Unusual bleeding or bruising, difficulty or pain on swallowing, fever, joint pain, jaundice, hepatitis.	Discontinue. Call doctor right away.
• Weakness.	Continue. Call doctor when convenient.

WARNINGS & PRECAUTIONS

Don't take if:
- You are allergic to quinidine.
- You have an active infection.

Before you start, consult your doctor:
About any drug you take, including non-prescription drugs.

Pregnancy:
Risk to unborn child outweighs drug benefits. Don't use.

Infants & children:
No age-related problems expected.

Prolonged use:
No age-related problems expected.

Skin & sunlight:
No age-related problems expected.

Driving or hazardous activities:
Don't drive or pilot aircraft until you learn how medicine affects you. Don't work around dangerous machinery. Don't climb ladders or work in high places. Danger increases if you drink alcohol or take medicine affecting alertness and reflexes, such as antihistamines, tranquilizers, sedatives, pain medicine, narcotics and mind-altering drugs.

Discontinuing:
Don't discontinue without doctor's advice until you complete prescribed dose, even though symptoms diminish or disappear.

Others:
No age-related problems expected.

POSSIBLE INTERACTION WITH OTHER DRUGS

GENERIC NAME OR DRUG CLASS	COMBINED EFFECT
Alkaline urine	Slows quinidine elimination, increases effect and toxicity.
Antiarrhythmics (see Drugs Glossary)	May increase or decrease effect or toxicity of quinidine.
Anticholinergics (see Drugs Glossary)	Increased anticholinergic effect.
Anticoagulants (oral, see Drugs Glossary)	Possible increased anticoagulant effect.
Antihypertensives (see Drugs Glossary)	Increased antihypertensive effect.
Beta-adrenergic blockers (see Drugs Glossary)	May slow heartbeat excessively.
Cholinergics (see Drugs Glossary)	Decreased cholinergic effect.
Cimetidine	Increased quinidine effect.
Digitalis preparations (see Drugs Glossary)	May slow heartbeat excessively. Dose adjustments may be needed.
Encainide	Increased effect of toxicity on heart muscle.
Flecainide	Possible irregular heartbeat.
Guanfacine	Increased effect of both medicines.
Nifedipine	Possible decreased quinidine effect.
Phenobarbital	Decreased quinidine effect.
Phenothiazines (see Drugs Glossary)	Possible increased quinidine effect.
Phenytoin	Decreased quinidine effect.
Rauwolfia alkaloids (see Drugs Glossary)	Possibly disturbs heart rhythms.
Tocainide	Increased possibility of adverse reactions from either drug.
Rifampin	Decreased quinidine effect.
Verapamil	Hypotension.

POSSIBLE INTERACTION WITH OTHER SUBSTANCES

INTERACTS WITH	COMBINED EFFECT
Alcohol:	None expected.
Beverages: Caffeine drinks.	Causes rapid heartbeat. Use sparingly.
Cocaine (or crack):	Irregular heartbeat. Avoid.
Foods:	None expected.
Marijuana:	Can cause fainting.
Tobacco:	Irregular heartbeat. Avoid.

RANITIDINE

BRAND NAMES

Zantac

BASIC INFORMATION

Habit forming? No
Prescription needed? Yes
Available as generic? No
Drug class: Histamine H2 antagonist

USES

- Treatment for duodenal ulcer.
- Decreases acid in stomach.

DOSAGE & USAGE INFORMATION

How to take:
Tablets—Swallow with liquid.

When to take:
At same times each day.

If you forget a dose:
Take as soon as you remember up to 2 hours late. If more than 2 hours, wait for next scheduled dose (don't double this dose).

What drug does:
Decreases stomach-acid production.

Time lapse before drug works:
2 to 3 hours.

Don't take with:
- Alcohol.
- *Any* other medicines, even over-the-counter drugs such as cough and cold medicines, nose drops, diet pills, laxatives or caffeine, without consulting your doctor.

OVERDOSE

SYMPTOMS:
Muscular tremors, vomiting, rapid breathing, coma.
WHAT TO DO:
- **Dial 0 (operator) or 911 (emergency) for an ambulance or medical help. Then give first aid immediately.**
- **If the child is unconscious and not breathing, give mouth-to-mouth breathing. If there is no heartbeat, use cardiac massage and mouth-to-mouth breathing (CPR). Don't try to make the child vomit. If you can't get help quickly, take the child to nearest emergency facility.**
- **See emergency information at the back of this book.**

POSSIBLE ADVERSE REACTIONS OR SIDE EFFECTS

SYMPTOMS	WHAT TO DO
Life-threatening: None expected.	
Common: None expected.	
Infrequent:	
• Rash, confusion, diarrhea.	Discontinue. Call doctor right away.
• Headache, dizziness, constipation, nausea, abdominal pain.	Continue. Call doctor when convenient.
Rare:	
Jaundice.	Discontinue. Call doctor right away.

WARNINGS & PRECAUTIONS

Don't take if:
You are allergic to any histamine H2 antagonist.

Before you start, consult your doctor:
If you have kidney disease.

Pregnancy:
No proven harm to unborn child. Avoid if possible.

Infants & children
Don't give to infants or young children unless prescribed and monitored by your physician.

Prolonged use:
Not recommended. Use for short term only.

Skin & sunlight:
No age-related problems expected.

Driving or hazardous activities:
Avoid if you feel dizzy. Otherwise, no problems expected.

Discontinuing:
Don't discontinue without consulting doctor until you finish prescribed dose, even though symptoms diminish or disappear.

Others:
Drug interactions with ranitidine may occur in a small number of the patients, compared to cimetidine.

POSSIBLE INTERACTION WITH OTHER DRUGS

GENERIC NAME OR DRUG CLASS	COMBINED EFFECT
Antacids (see Drugs Glossary)	Decreased absorption of ranitidine if taken simultaneously.
Glipizide	Possible increased glipizide effect.
Ketoconazole	Decreased absorption of ranitidine.
Procainamide	Increased procainamide effect and toxicity.
Theophylline	Possible increased theophylline effect.
Warfarin	Increased warfarin effect.

POSSIBLE INTERACTION WITH OTHER SUBSTANCES

INTERACTS WITH	COMBINED EFFECT
Alcohol:	Decreased ranitidine effect.
Beverages:	None expected.
Cocaine (or crack):	No proven problems.
Foods:	None expected.
Marijuana:	No proven problems.
Tobacco:	Decreased ranitidine effect.

RIBOFLAVIN (VITAMIN B-2)

BRAND NAMES

Riobin-50

Many multivitamin preparations.

BASIC INFORMATION

Habit forming? No
Prescription needed? No
Available as generic? Yes
Drug class: Vitamin supplement

USES

- Dietary supplement to ensure normal growth and health.
- Dietary supplement to treat symptoms caused by deficiency of B-2: sores in mouth, eyes sensitive to light, itching and peeling skin.

DOSAGE & USAGE INFORMATION

How to take:
Tablet—Swallow with liquid or food to lessen stomach irritation. If you can't swallow whole, crumble tablet and take with liquid or food.

When to take:
At the same times each day.

If you forget a dose:
Take as soon as you remember. Resume regular schedule. Don't double dose.

What drug does:
Promotes normal growth and health.

Time lapse before drug works:
Requires continual intake.

Don't take with:
Any other medicines, even over-the-counter drugs such as cough and cold medicines, nose drops, diet pills, laxatives or caffeine, without consulting your doctor.

OVERDOSE

SYMPTOMS:
Dark urine, nausea, vomiting.
WHAT TO DO:
Overdose unlikely to threaten life. If child takes much larger amount than prescribed, call doctor, poison-control center or hospital emergency room for instructions.

POSSIBLE ADVERSE REACTIONS OR SIDE EFFECTS

SYMPTOMS	WHAT TO DO
Life-threatening: None expected.	
Common: Urine yellow in color.	No action necessary.
Infrequent: None expected.	
Rare: None expected.	

WARNINGS & PRECAUTIONS

Don't take if:
- You are allergic to any B vitamin.
- You have chronic kidney failure.

Before you start, consult your doctor:
If you are pregnant or plan pregnancy.

Pregnancy:
Recommended. Consult doctor.

Infants & children:
Consult doctor.

Prolonged use:
No age-related problems expected.

Skin & sunlight:
No age-related problems expected.

Driving or hazardous activities:
No age-related problems expected.

Discontinuing:
No age-related problems expected.

Others:
A balanced diet should provide all the vitamin B-2 a healthy person needs and make supplements unnecessary during periods of good health. Best sources are milk, meats and green leafy vegetables.

POSSIBLE INTERACTION WITH OTHER DRUGS

GENERIC NAME OR DRUG CLASS	COMBINED EFFECT
Anticholinergics (see Drugs Glossary)	Possible increased riboflavin absorption.
Antidepressants, tricyclic (TCA, see Drugs Glossary)	Decreased riboflavin effect.
Phenothiazines (see Drugs Glossary)	Decreased riboflavin effect.
Probenecid	Decreased riboflavin effect.

POSSIBLE INTERACTION WITH OTHER SUBSTANCES

INTERACTS WITH	COMBINED EFFECT
Alcohol:	Prevents uptake and absorption of vitamin B-2.
Beverages:	None expected.
Cocaine (or crack):	None expected.
Foods:	None expected.
Marijuana:	None expected.
Tobacco:	Prevents absorption of vitamin B-2 and other vitamins and nutrients.

MEDICATIONS

SUCRALFATE

BRAND NAMES

Carafate
Sulcrate

BASIC INFORMATION

Habit forming? No
Prescription needed? Yes
Available as generic? No
Drug class: Anti-ulcer

USES

Treatment of duodenal ulcer.

DOSAGE & USAGE INFORMATION

How to take:
Tablet—Swallow with liquid or food to lessen stomach irritation. If you can't swallow whole, crumble tablet or place tablet in water before taking with liquid or food.

When to take:
1 hour before meals and at bedtime. Allow 2 hours to elapse before taking other prescription medicines.

If you forget a dose:
Take as soon as you remember up to 2 hours late. If more than 2 hours, wait for next scheduled dose (don't double this dose).

What drug does:
Covers ulcer site and protects from acid, enzymes and bile salts.

Time lapse before drug works:
Begins in 30 minutes. May require several days to relieve pain.

Don't take with:
Any other medicines, even over-the-counter drugs such as cough and cold medicines, nose drops, diet pills, laxatives or caffeine, without consulting your doctor.

OVERDOSE

SYMPTOMS:
No data available yet for this drug.
WHAT TO DO:
Overdose unlikely to threaten life. If child takes much larger amount than prescribed, call doctor, poison-control center or hospital emergency room for instructions.

POSSIBLE ADVERSE REACTIONS OR SIDE EFFECTS

SYMPTOMS	WHAT TO DO
Life-threatening: None expected.	
Common: Constipation.	Continue. Call doctor when convenient.
Infrequent: • Diarrhea.	Discontinue. Call doctor right away.
• Dizziness, sleepiness, rash, itchy skin, abdominal pain, indigestion, vomiting, nausea, back pain.	Continue. Call doctor when convenient.
Rare: None expected.	

WARNINGS & PRECAUTIONS

Don't take if:
You are allergic to sucralfate.

Before you start, consult your doctor:
If you will have surgery within 2 months, including dental surgery, requiring general or spinal anesthesia.

Pregnancy:
No proven harm to unborn child. Avoid if possible.

Infants & children:
Don't give to infants or young children unless prescribed and monitored by your physician.

Prolonged use:
Request blood counts if medicine needed longer than 8 weeks.

Skin & sunlight:
No age-related problems expected.

Driving or hazardous activities:
Don't drive or pilot aircraft until you learn how medicine affects you. Don't work around dangerous machinery. Don't climb ladders or work in high places. Danger increases if you drink alcohol or take medicine affecting alertness and reflexes, such as antihistamines, tranquilizers, sedatives, pain medicine, narcotics and mind-altering drugs.

Discontinuing:
Don't discontinue without consulting doctor. Dose may require gradual reduction if you have taken drug for a long time. Doses of other drugs may also require adjustment.

Others:
No age-related problems expected.

POSSIBLE INTERACTION WITH OTHER DRUGS

GENERIC NAME OR DRUG CLASS	COMBINED EFFECT
Cimetidine	Possible decreased absorption of cimetidine if taken simultaneously.
Phenytoin	Possible decreased absorption of phenytoin if taken simultaneously.
Tetracyclines (see Drugs Glossary)	Possible decreased absorption of tetracycline if taken simultaneously.

POSSIBLE INTERACTION WITH OTHER SUBSTANCES

INTERACTS WITH	COMBINED EFFECT
Alcohol:	Irritates ulcer. Avoid.
Beverages: Caffeine.	Irritates ulcer. Avoid.
Cocaine (or crack):	May make ulcer worse. Avoid.
Foods:	None expected.
Marijuana:	May make ulcer worse. Avoid.
Tobacco:	May make ulcer worse. Avoid.

SULFONAMIDES

BRAND & GENERIC NAMES

See complete list of brand and generic names in the Brand & Generic Name Directory.

BASIC INFORMATION

Habit forming? No
Prescription needed? Yes
Available as generic? Yes
Drug class: Sulfa (sulfonamide)

USES

Treatment for urinary tract infections responsive to this drug.

DOSAGE & USAGE INFORMATION

How to take:
• Tablet—Swallow with liquid. Instructions to take on empty stomach mean 1 hour before or 2 hours after eating.
• Liquid—Shake carefully before measuring.

When to take:
At the same times each day, evenly spaced.

If you forget a dose:
Take as soon as you remember up to 2 hours late. If more than 2 hours, wait for next scheduled dose (don't double this dose).

What drug does:
Interferes with a nutrient (folic acid) necessary for growth and reproduction of bacteria. Will not attack viruses.

Time lapse before drug works:
2 to 5 days to affect infection.

Don't take with:
Any other medicines, even over-the-counter drugs such as cough and cold medicines, nose drops, diet pills, laxatives or caffeine, without consulting your doctor.

OVERDOSE

SYMPTOMS:
Less urine, bloody urine, coma.
WHAT TO DO:
• Dial 0 (operator) or 911 (emergency) for an ambulance or medical help. Then give first aid immediately.
• See emergency information at the back of this book.

POSSIBLE ADVERSE REACTIONS OR SIDE EFFECTS

SYMPTOMS	WHAT TO DO
Life-threatening: None expected.	
Common:	
• Itchy skin, rash.	Discontinue. Call doctor right away.
• Headache, nausea, vomiting, diarrhea, appetite loss.	Continue. Call doctor when convenient.
Infrequent:	
• Red, peeling or blistering skin; sore throat; fever; swallowing difficulty; unusual bruising; aching joints or muscles; jaundice.	Discontinue. Call doctor right away.
• Dizziness.	Continue. Call doctor when convenient.
Rare:	
Painful urination; low back pain; numbness, tingling, burning feeling in feet and hands.	Discontinue. Call doctor right away.

WARNINGS & PRECAUTIONS

Don't take if:
You are allergic to any sulfa drug.

Before you start, consult your doctor:
- If you are allergic to carbonic anhydrase inhibitors, oral antidiabetics or thiazide or loop diuretics.
- If you are allergic by nature.
- If you have liver or kidney disease.
- If you have porphyria.
- If you have developed anemia from use of any drug.

Pregnancy:
Risk to unborn child outweighs drug benefits. Don't use.

Infants & children:
Don't give to infants younger than 1 month.

Prolonged use:
- May enlarge thyroid gland.
- You may become more susceptible to infections caused by germs not responsive to this drug.
- Request frequent blood counts, liver-and kidney-function studies.

Skin & sunlight:
May cause rash or intensify sunburn in areas exposed to sun or sunlamp.

Driving or hazardous activities:
Avoid if you feel dizzy. Otherwise, no problems expected.

Discontinuing:
Don't discontinue without doctor's advice until you complete prescribed dose, even though symptoms diminish or disappear.

Others:
- Drink 2 quarts of liquid each day to prevent adverse reactions.
- If you require surgery, tell anesthetist you take sulfa. Pentothal anesthesia should not be used.

POSSIBLE INTERACTION WITH OTHER DRUGS

GENERIC NAME OR DRUG CLASS	COMBINED EFFECT
Aminobenzoate potassium	Possible decreased sulfa effect.
Anticoagulants (oral, see Drugs Glossary)	Increased anticoagulant effect.
Anticonvulsants (hydantoin, see Drugs Glossary)	Toxic effect on brain.
Aspirin	Increased sulfa effect.
Calcium supplements (see Drugs Glossary)	Decreased sulfa effect.
Isoniazid	Possible anemia.
Methenamine	Possible kidney blockage.
Methotrexate	Increased methotrexate effect.
Oxyphenbutazone	Increased sulfa effect.
Para-aminosalicylic acid (PAS)	Decreased sulfa effect.
Penicillins (see Drugs Glossary)	Decreased penicillin effect.
Phenylbutazone	Increased sulfa effect.
Probenecid	Increased sulfa effect.
Sulfinpyrazone	Increased sulfa effect.
Sulfonureas (see Drugs Glossary)	May increase hypoglycemic action.
Trimethoprim	Increased sulfa effect.

POSSIBLE INTERACTION WITH OTHER SUBSTANCES

INTERACTS WITH	COMBINED EFFECT
Alcohol:	Increased alcohol effect.
Beverages: Less than 2 quarts of fluid daily.	Kidney damage.
Cocaine (or crack):	None expected.
Foods:	None expected.
Marijuana:	None expected.
Tobacco:	None expected.

TERBUTALINE

BRAND NAMES

Brethaire
Brethine
Bricanyl

BASIC INFORMATION

Habit forming? No
Prescription needed? Yes
Available as generic? No
Drug class: Sympathomimetic (see Drugs Glossary)

USES

Treatment of bronchial asthma, bronchitis and emphysema.

DOSAGE & USAGE INFORMATION

How to take:
• Tablet—Swallow with liquid or food to lessen stomach irritation.
• Aerosol—Use according to package instructions.

When to take:
At the same times each day.

If you forget a dose:
Take as soon as you remember up to 2 hours late. If more than 2 hours, wait for next scheduled dose (don't double this dose).

What drug does:
Dilates constricted bronchial tubes.

Time lapse before drug works:
30 minutes.

Continued next column

OVERDOSE

SYMPTOMS:
Rapid heartbeat, chest pain, tremors.
WHAT TO DO:
• Dial 0 (operator) or 911 (emergency) for an ambulance or medical help. Then give first aid immediately.
• If the child is unconscious and not breathing, give mouth-to-mouth breathing. If there is no heartbeat, use cardiac massage and mouth-to-mouth breathing (CPR). Don't try to make the child vomit. If you can't get help quickly, take the child to nearest emergency facility.
• See emergency information at the back of this book.

Don't take with:
Any other medicines, even over-the-counter drugs such as cough and cold medicines, nose drops, diet pills, laxatives or caffeine, without consulting your doctor.

POSSIBLE ADVERSE REACTIONS OR SIDE EFFECTS

SYMPTOMS	WHAT TO DO
Life-threatening: None expected.	
Common: Headache, nervousness, restlessness, trembling.	Continue. Call doctor when convenient.
Infrequent: • Drowsiness, nausea, vomiting, fast or pounding heartbeat, cramps, weakness.	Discontinue. Call doctor right away.
• Unusual sweating.	Continue. Call doctor when convenient.
Rare: None expected.	

WARNINGS & PRECAUTIONS

Don't take if:
You are allergic to any sympathomimetic.

Before you start, consult your doctor:
- If you have diabetes.
- If you have heart disease or high blood pressure.
- If you have overactive thyroid.
- If you have had seizures.
- If you take non-prescription amphetamines or other asthma medicines.

Pregnancy:
No proven harm to unborn child. Avoid if possible. May prolong labor and delivery.

Infants & children:
Use only under medical supervision.

Prolonged use:
No age-related problems expected.

Skin & sunlight:
No age-related problems expected.

Driving or hazardous activities:
Avoid if you feel drowsy. Otherwise, no problems expected.

Discontinuing:
May be unnecessary to finish medicine. Follow doctor's instructions.

Others:
If troubled breathing does not improve or worsens after using medicine, don't increase dose. Consult doctor.

POSSIBLE INTERACTION WITH OTHER DRUGS

GENERIC NAME OR DRUG CLASS	COMBINED EFFECT
Albuterol	Increased effect of both drugs, especially harmful side effects.
Antidepressants, tricyclics (TCA, see Drugs Glossary)	Increased terbutaline effect.
Beta-adrenergic blockers (see Drugs Glossary)	Decreased effects of both drugs.
Ephedrine	Increased terbutaline effect. Excess heart stimulation.
Epinephrine	Increased terbutaline effect. Excess heart stimulation.
MAO inhibitors (see Drugs Glossary)	Increased terbutaline effect. Dangerous. Avoid.
Nitrates (see Drugs Glossary)	Possible decreased effects of both drugs.
Sympathomimetics (see Drugs Glossary)	Increased terbutaline effect.
Theophylline	Possible increased effect and toxicity of both drugs.

POSSIBLE INTERACTION WITH OTHER SUBSTANCES

INTERACTS WITH	COMBINED EFFECT
Alcohol:	None expected.
Beverages:	None expected.
Cocaine (or crack):	Overstimulation.
Foods:	None expected.
Marijuana:	Possible increased therapeutic effect of terbutaline. May cause lung disorders to worsen.
Tobacco:	No interactions expected, but smoking may slow body's recovery. Avoid.

TERFENADINE

BRAND NAMES

Seldane

BASIC INFORMATION

Habit forming? No
Prescription needed? Yes
Available as generic? No
Drug class: Antihistamine, hi-receptor antagonist

USES

Reduces allergic symptoms such as hay fever, hives, rash or itching. Less likely to cause drowsiness than most other antihistamines.

DOSAGE & USAGE INFORMATION

How to take:
Tablet—Swallow with water or food to lessen stomach irritation.

When to take:
Follow prescription instructions.

If you forget a dose:
Take as soon as you remember up to 2 hours late. If more than 2 hours, wait for next scheduled dose (don't double this dose).

What drug does:
Blocks effects of histamine, a chemical produced by the body as a result of contact with an allergen.

Time lapse before drug works:
1 to 2 hours; maximum effect at 3 to 4 hours.

Don't take with:
Any other medicines, even over-the-counter drugs such as cough and cold medicines, nose drops, diet pills, laxatives or caffeine, without consulting your doctor.

OVERDOSE

SYMPTOMS:
Headache, nausea, confusion, heartbeat rhythm disturbance.
WHAT TO DO:
- **Dial 0 (operator) or 911 (emergency) for an ambulance or medical help. Then give first aid immediately.**
- **See emergency information at the back of this book.**

POSSIBLE ADVERSE REACTIONS OR SIDE EFFECTS

SYMPTOMS	WHAT TO DO
Life-threatening: None expected.	
Common: None expected.	
Infrequent:	
• Nausea, vomiting, sore throat, itching.	Discontinue. Call doctor right away.
• Drowsiness, fatigue, headache, dizziness, weakness.	Continue. Call doctor when convenient.
Rare:	
• Swollen lips, difficult breathing.	Discontinue. Seek emergency treatment.
• Irregular heartbeat, nightmares, frequent urination.	Discontinue. Call doctor right away.
• Thinning hair.	Continue. Call doctor when convenient.

WARNINGS & PRECAUTIONS

Don't take if:
You are allergic to terfenadine.

Before you start, consult your doctor:
- If you are allergic to other antihistamines.
- If you have an enlarged prostate or glaucoma.
- If you are under age 12.
- If you are allergic to any substance or any medicine.
- If you are pregnant or expect to become pregnant.
- If you have asthma.
- If you will have surgery within 2 months, including dental surgery, requiring general or spinal anesthesia.
- If you plan to have skin tests for allergies.

Pregnancy:
No proven harm to unborn child. Avoid if possible.

Infants & children:
Safety and effectiveness in children under age 12 have not been established.

Prolonged use:
Take only on advice of your doctor.

Skin & sunlight:
No age-related problems expected.

Driving or hazardous activities:
Don't drive or pilot aircraft until you learn how medicine affects you. Sedation and dizziness are less likely to occur with terfenadine than with other antihistamines.

Discontinuing:
No age-related problems expected.

Others:
No age-related problems expected.

POSSIBLE INTERACTION WITH OTHER DRUGS

GENERIC NAME OR DRUG CLASS	COMBINED EFFECT
None.	

POSSIBLE INTERACTION WITH OTHER SUBSTANCES

INTERACTS WITH	COMBINED EFFECT
Alcohol:	Possible oversedation.
Beverages:	None expected.
Cocaine (or crack):	Decreased terfenadine effect.
Foods:	None expected.
Marijuana:	None expected.
Tobacco:	None expected.

MEDICATIONS

TETRACYCLINES

BRAND & GENERIC NAMES

See complete list of brand and generic names in the Brand & Generic Name Directory.

BASIC INFORMATION

Habit forming? No
Prescription needed? Yes
Available as generic? Yes
Drug class: Antibiotic (tetracycline)

USES

• Treatment for infections susceptible to any tetracycline. Will not cure virus infections such as colds or flu.
• Treatment for acne.

DOSAGE & USAGE INFORMATION

How to take:
• Tablet or capsule—Take on empty stomach 1 hour before or 2 hours after eating. If you can't swallow whole, crumble tablet or open capsule and take with liquid or food.
• Liquid—Shake well. Take with measuring spoon.

When to take:
At the same times each day, evenly spaced.

If you forget a dose:
Take as soon as you remember up to 2 hours late. If more than 2 hours, wait for next scheduled dose (don't double this dose).

What drug does:
Prevents germ growth and reproduction.

Time lapse before drug works:
• Infections—May require 5 days to affect infection.
• Acne—May require 4 weeks to affect acne.

Continued next column

OVERDOSE

SYMPTOMS:
Severe nausea, vomiting, diarrhea.
WHAT TO DO:
Overdose unlikely to threaten life. If child takes much larger amount than prescribed, call doctor, poison-control center or hospital emergency room for instructions.

Don't take with:
Any other medicines, even over-the-counter drugs such as cough and cold medicines, nose drops, diet pills, laxatives or caffeine, without consulting your doctor.

POSSIBLE ADVERSE REACTIONS OR SIDE EFFECTS

SYMPTOMS	WHAT TO DO
Life-threatening:	
Hives, rash, intense itching faintness soon after a dose (anaphylaxis).	Seek emergency treatment immediately.
Common:	
• Sore mouth or tongue, nausea, vomiting, diarrhea, abdominal burning.	Discontinue. Seek emergency treatment.
• Itching around rectum and genitals.	Discontinue. Call doctor right away.
• Vaginal discharge due to yeast.	Continue. Call doctor when convenient.
• Dark tongue.	Continue. Tell doctor at next visit.
Infrequent:	
• Headache, rash.	Discontinue. Call doctor right away.
• Excessive thirst, increased urination, dizziness (minocycline).	Continue. Call doctor when convenient.
Rare:	
Blurred vision, jaundice.	Discontinue. Call doctor right away.

WARNINGS & PRECAUTIONS

Don't take if:
You are allergic to any tetracycline antibiotic.

Before you start, consult your doctor:
- If you have kidney or liver disease.
- If you have lupus.
- If you have myasthenia gravis.

Pregnancy:
Risk to unborn child outweighs drug benefits. Don't use.

Infants & children:
May cause permanent teeth malformation or discoloration in children less than 8 years old. Don't use.

Prolonged use:
- You may become more susceptible to infections caused by germs not responsive to tetracycline.
- May cause rare problems in liver, kidney or bone marrow. Periodic laboratory blood studies, liver-and kidney-function tests recommended if you use drug a long time.

Skin & sunlight:
May cauce rash or intensify sunburn in areas exposed to sun or sunlamp.

Driving or hazardous activities:
No age-related problems expected.

Discontinuing:
Don't discontinue without doctor's advice until you complete prescribed dose, even though symptoms diminish or disappear.

Others:
Avoid using outdated drug.

POSSIBLE INTERACTION WITH OTHER DRUGS

GENERIC NAME OR DRUG CLASS	COMBINED EFFECT
Antacids (see Drugs Glossary)	Decreased tetracycline effect.
Anticoagulants (oral, see Glossary)	Increased anticoagulant effect.
Calcium supplements (see Drugs Glossary)	Decreased tetracycline effect.
Contraceptives (oral, see Glossary)	Decreased contraceptive effect.
Digitalis preparations (see Drugs Glossary)	Increased digitalis effect.
Etretinate	Increased chance of adverse reactions of etretinate.
Lithium	Increased lithium effect.
Mineral supplements (iron, calcium, magnesium, zinc)	Decreased tetracycline absorption. Separate doses by 1 to 2 hours.
Penicillins (see Drugs Glossary)	Decreased penicillin effect.
Sodium bicarbonate	Decreased tetracycline effect.

POSSIBLE INTERACTION WITH OTHER SUBSTANCES

INTERACTS WITH	COMBINED EFFECT
Alcohol:	Possible liver damage. Avoid.
Beverages: Milk.	Decreased tetracycline absorption. Take dose 2 hours after or 1 hour before drinking.
Cocaine (or crack):	No proven problems.
Foods: Dairy products.	Decreased tetracycline absorption. Take dose 2 hours after or 1 hour before eating.
Marijuana:	No interactions expected, but marijuana may slow body's recovery. Avoid.
Tobacco:	None expected.

THIAMINE (VITAMIN B-1)

BRAND NAMES

Betalin S
Betaxin
Bewon
Biamine
Pan-B-1
Numerous other multiple vitamin-mineral supplements.

BASIC INFORMATION

Habit forming? No
Prescription needed? No
Available as generic? Yes
Drug class: Vitamin supplement

USES

• Dietary supplement to promote normal growth, development and health.
• Treatment for beri-beri (a thiamine-deficiency disease).
• Dietary supplement for alcoholism, cirrhosis, overactive thyroid, infection, breast-feeding, absorption diseases, pregnancy, prolonged diarrhea, burns.

DOSAGE & USAGE INFORMATION

How to take:
Tablet or liquid—Swallow with beverage or food to lessen stomach irritation.

When to take:
At the same time each day.

If you forget a dose:
Take when remembered. Return to regular schedule.

What drug does:
• Promotes normal growth and development.
• Combines with an enzyme to metabolize carbohydrates.

Time lapse before drug works:
15 minutes.

Continued next column

OVERDOSE

SYMPTOMS:
Increased severity of adverse reactions and side effects.
WHAT TO DO:
Overdose unlikely to threaten life. If child takes much larger amount than prescribed, call doctor, poison-control center or hospital emergency room for instructions.

Don't take with:
Any other medicines, even over-the-counter drugs such as cough and cold medicines, nose drops, diet pills, laxatives or caffeine, without consulting your doctor.

POSSIBLE ADVERSE REACTIONS OR SIDE EFFECTS

SYMPTOMS	WHAT TO DO
Life-threatening:	
Hives, rash, intense itching, faintness soon after a dose (anaphylaxis).	Seek emergency treatment immediately.
Common:	
None expected.	
Infrequent:	
None expected.	
Rare:	
• Wheezing.	Discontinue. Seek emergency treatment.
• Rash or itchy skin.	Discontinue. Call doctor right away.

WARNINGS & PRECAUTIONS

Don't take if:
You are allergic to any B vitamin.

Before you start, consult your doctor:
If you have liver or kidney disease.

Pregnancy:
No age-related problems expected.

Infants & children:
No age-related problems expected.

Prolonged use:
No age-related problems expected.

Skin & sunlight:
No age-related problems expected.

Driving or hazardous activities:
No age-related problems expected.

Discontinuing:
No age-related problems expected.

Others:
A balanced diet should provide enough thiamine for healthy people to make supplement unnecessary. Best dietary sources of thiamine are whole-grain cereals and meats.

POSSIBLE INTERACTION WITH OTHER DRUGS

GENERIC NAME OR DRUG CLASS	COMBINED EFFECT
Barbiturates (see Drugs Glossary)	Decreased thiamine effect.

POSSIBLE INTERACTION WITH OTHER SUBSTANCES

INTERACTS WITH	COMBINED EFFECT
Alcohol:	None expected.
Beverages: Carbonates, citrates (additives listed on many beverage labels).	Decreased thiamine effect.
Cocaine (or crack):	None expected.
Foods: Carbonates, citrates (additives listed on many food labels).	Decreased thiamine effect.
Marijuana:	None expected.
Tobacco:	None expected.

TIMOLOL

BRAND NAMES

Blocadren
Timolide
Timoptic

BASIC INFORMATION

Habit forming? No
Prescription needed? Yes
Available as generic? No
Drug class: Beta-adrenergic blocker, antiglaucoma agent

USES

- Reduces angina attacks.
- Stabilizes irregular heartbeat.
- Lowers blood pressure.
- Reduces frequency of migraine headaches. (Does not relieve headache pain.)
- Decreases internal-eye pressure of glaucoma (ophthalmic drops).
- After myocardial infarction, prevents another heart attack.

DOSAGE & USAGE INFORMATION

How to take:
- Eye drops—Wash hands. Apply slight pressure with finger to inside corner of eye. Pull lower eyelid down. Put drop just above lowered eyelid. Close eye gently for 2 minutes. Don't blink.
- Tablet—Swallow with liquid or crumble and take with food.

When to take:
- Tablet—With meals or immediately after.
- Eye drops—Follow prescription directions.

If you forget a dose:
Take as soon as you remember. Return to regular schedule, but allow 3 hours between doses.

Continued next column

What drug does:
- Blocks certain actions of sympathetic nervous system.
- Lowers heart's oxygen requirements.
- Slows nerve impulses through heart.
- Reduces blood vessel contraction in heart, scalp and other body parts.
- Eye drops lower pressure inside eye.

Time lapse before drug works:
1 to 4 hours.

Don't take with:
Any other medicines, even over-the-counter drugs such as cough and cold medicines, nose drops, diet pills, laxatives or caffeine, without consulting your doctor.

OVERDOSE

SYMPTOMS:
Weakness; slow or weak pulse; blood-pressure drop; fainting; difficulty breathing, convulsions; cold, sweaty skin.
WHAT TO DO:
- **Dial 0 (operator) or 911 (emergency) for an ambulance or medical help. Then give first aid immediately.**
- **See emergency information at the back of this book.**

POSSIBLE ADVERSE REACTIONS OR SIDE EFFECTS

SYMPTOMS	WHAT TO DO
Life-threatening:	
Congestive heart failure.	Discontinue. Seek emergency treatment.
Common:	
• Pulse slower than 50 beats per minute.	Discontinue. Call doctor right away.
• Drowsiness, fatigue, numbness or tingling of fingers or toes, dizziness, diarrhea, nausea, weakness.	Continue. Call doctor when convenient.
• Cold hands or feet; dry mouth, eyes and skin.	Continue. Tell doctor at next visit.
Infrequent:	
• Hallucinations, nightmares, insomnia, headache, difficult breathing.	Discontinue. Call doctor right away.
• Confusion, reduced alertness, depression. impotence.	Continue. Call doctor when convenient.
• Constipation.	Continue. Tell doctor at next visit.
Rare:	
• Rash, sore throat, fever.	Discontinue. Call doctor right away.
• Unusual bleeding and bruising; dry, burning eyes.	Continue. Call doctor when convenient.

WARNINGS & PRECAUTIONS

Don't take if:
- You are allergic to any beta-adrenergic blocker.
- You have asthma or hay fever symptoms.
- You have taken MAO inhibitors in past 2 weeks.

Before you start, consult your doctor:
- If you have heart disease or poor circulation to the extremities.
- If you have hay fever, asthma, chronic bronchitis, emphysema.
- If you have overactive thyroid function.
- If you have impaired liver or kidney function.
- If you will have surgery within 2 months, including dental surgery, requiring general or spinal anesthesia.
- If you have diabetes or hypoglycemia.

Pregnancy:
Risk to unborn child outweighs drug benefits. Don't use.

Infants & children
Don't give to infants or young children unless prescribed and monitored by your physician.

Prolonged use:
Weakens heart muscle contractions.

Skin & sunlight:
No age-related problems expected.

Driving or hazardous activities:
Don't drive or pilot aircraft until you learn how medicine affects you. Don't work around dangerous machinery. Don't climb ladders or work in high places. Danger increases if you drink alcohol or take medicine affecting alertness and reflexes.

Discontinuing:
Don't discontinue without consulting doctor. Dose may require gradual reduction if you have taken drug for a long time. Doses of other drugs may also require adjustment.

Others:
- May mask hypoglycemia.
- Side effects, such as burning or stinging of the eye, may also occur with timolol used as eye drops.

POSSIBLE INTERACTION WITH OTHER DRUGS

GENERIC NAME OR DRUG CLASS	COMBINED EFFECT
ACE inhibitors: captopril, enalapril, lisinopril (see Drugs Glossary)	Increased antihypertensive effects of both drugs. Dosages may require adjustment.
Antidiabetics (see Drugs Glossary)	Increased antidiabetic effect.
Antihistamines (see Drugs Glossary)	Decreased antihistamine effect.
Antihypertensives (see Drugs Glossary)	Increased antihypertensive effect.
Barbiturates (see Drugs Glossary)	Increased barbiturate effect. Dangerous sedation.
Beta-agonists (see Drugs Glossary)	Decreased beta-agonist effect.
Betaxolol eyedrops	Possible increased timolol effect.
Digitalis preparations (see Drugs Glossary)	Increased or decreased heart rate. Improves irregular heartbeat.
Encainide	Increased effect of toxicity on heart muscle.
Indomethacin	Decreased timolol effect.
Insulin	Hypoglycemic effects may be prolonged.
Levobunolol eyedrops	Possible increased timolol effect.
Narcotics (see Drugs Glossary)	Increased narcotic effect. Dangerous sedation.
Nitrates (see Drugs Glossary)	Possible decreased blood pressure.

See Additional Drug Interactions Section

POSSIBLE INTERACTION WITH OTHER SUBSTANCES

INTERACTS WITH	COMBINED EFFECT
Alcohol:	Excessive blood-pressure drop. Avoid.
Beverages:	None expected.
Cocaine (or crack):	Irregular heartbeat. Avoid.
Foods:	None expected.
Marijuana:	Daily use—Impaired circulation to hands and feet.
Tobacco:	Possible irregular heartbeat.

TRAZODONE

BRAND NAMES

Desyrel
Desyrel Dividose
Trialodine

BASIC INFORMATION

Habit forming? No
Prescription needed? Yes
Available as generic? Yes
Drug class: Antidepressant (non-tricyclic)

USES

- Treats mental depression.
- Treats anxiety.

DOSAGE & USAGE INFORMATION

How to take:
Tablet—Swallow with liquid or food to lessen stomach irritation. If you can't swallow whole, crumble tablet and take with liquid or food.

When to take:
According to prescription directions. Bedtime dose usually higher than other doses.

If you forget a dose:
Take as soon as you remember up to 2 hours late. If more than 2 hours, wait for next scheduled dose (don't double this dose).

What drug does:
Inhibits serotonin uptake in brain cells.

Time lapse before drug works:
2 to 4 weeks for full effect.

Continued next column

OVERDOSE

SYMPTOMS:
Fainting, irregular heartbeat, respiratory arrest, chest pain, seizures, coma.
WHAT TO DO:
- **Dial 0 (operator) or 911 (emergency) for an ambulance or medical help. Then give first aid immediately.**
- **If the child is unconscious and not breathing, give mouth-to-mouth breathing. If there is no heartbeat, use cardiac massage and mouth-to-mouth breathing (CPR). Don't try to make the child vomit. If you can't get help quickly, take the child to nearest emergency facility.**
- **See emergency information at the back of this book.**

Don't take with:
Any other medicines, even over-the-counter drugs such as cough and cold medicines, nose drops, diet pills, laxatives or caffeine, without consulting your doctor.

POSSIBLE ADVERSE REACTIONS OR SIDE EFFECTS

SYMPTOMS	WHAT TO DO
Life-threatening: None expected.	
Common: Drowsiness.	Continue. Call doctor when convenient.
Infrequent: • Prolonged penile erections.	Seek emergency treatment immediately.
• Tremor, fainting, incoordination, blood pressue rise or drop, rapid heartbeat, shortness of breath.	Discontinue. Call doctor right away.
• Dizziness on standing, disorientation, confusion, fatigue, excitement, headache, nervousness, rash, itchy skin, blurred vision, ringing in ears, dry mouth, bad taste, diarrhea, nausea, vomiting, constipation, aching, menstrual changes, diminished sex drive, nightmares, vivid dreams, seizures.	Continue. Call doctor when convenient.
Rare: None expected.	

WARNINGS & PRECAUTIONS

Don't take if:
- You are allergic to trazodone.
- You are thinking about suicide.

Before you start, consult your doctor:
- If you have heart rhythm problem.
- If you have any heart disease.
- If you will have surgery within 2 months, including dental surgery, requiring general or spinal anesthesia.

Pregnancy:
Risk to unborn child outweighs drug benefits. Don't use.

Infants & children
Don't give to infants or young children unless prescribed and monitored by your physician.

Prolonged use:
Occasional blood counts, especially if you have fever and sore throat.

Skin & sunlight:
No age-related problems expected.

Driving or hazardous activities:
Don't drive or pilot aircraft until you learn how medicine affects you. Don't work around dangerous machinery. Don't climb ladders or work in high places. Danger increases if you drink alcohol or take medicine affecting alertness and reflexes, such as antihistamines, tranquilizers, sedatives, pain medicine, narcotics and mind-altering drugs.

Discontinuing:
Don't discontinue without consulting doctor. Dose may require gradual reduction if you have taken drug for a long time. Doses of other drugs may also require adjustment.

Others:
Electroshock therapy should be avoided.

POSSIBLE INTERACTION WITH OTHER DRUGS

GENERIC NAME OR DRUG CLASS	COMBINED EFFECT
Antidepressants, other (see Drugs Glossary)	Excess drowsiness.
Antihistamines (see Drugs Glossary)	Excess drowsiness.
Antihypertensives (see Drugs Glossary)	Possible too low blood pressure. Avoid.
Barbiturates (see Drugs Glossary)	Too low blood pressure. Avoid.
Digitalis preparations (see Drugs Glossary)	Possible increased digitalis level in blood.
Ethinamate	Dangerous increased effects of ethinamate. Avoid combining.
Fluoxetine	Increased depressant effects of both drugs.
Guanfacine	Increased effect of both medicines.
Leucovorin	High alcohol content of leucovorin may cause adverse effects.
MAO inhibitors (see Drugs Glossary)	May add to toxic effect of each.
Methyprylon	Increased sedative effect, perhaps to dangerous level. Avoid.
Narcotics (see Drugs Glossary)	Excess drowsiness.
Phenytoin	Possible increased phenytoin level in blood.
Sedatives (see Drugs Glossary)	Excess drowsiness.
Tranquilizers (see Drugs Glossary)	Excess drowsiness.

POSSIBLE INTERACTION WITH OTHER SUBSTANCES

INTERACTS WITH	COMBINED EFFECT
Alcohol:	Excess sedation. Avoid.
Beverages: Caffeine.	May add to heartbeat irregularity. Avoid.
Cocaine (or crack):	May add to heartbeat irregularity. Avoid.
Foods:	None expected.
Marijuana:	May add to heartbeat irregularity. Avoid.
Tobacco:	May add to heartbeat irregularity. Avoid.

MEDICATIONS

TRETINOIN

BRAND NAMES

Retin-A
Retinoic Acid
StieVAA
Vitamin A Acid

BASIC INFORMATION

Habit forming? No
Prescription needed? Yes
Available as generic? Yes
Drug class: Antiacne (topical)

USES

Treatment for acne, psoriasis, ichthyosis, keratosis, folliculitis, flat warts and skin wrinkles.

DOSAGE & USAGE INFORMATION

How to use:
Wash skin with non-medicated soap, pat dry, wait 20 minutes before applying.
- Cream or gel—Apply to affected areas with fingertips and rub in gently.
- Solution—Apply to affected areas with gauze pad or cotton swab. Avoid getting too wet so medicine doesn't drip into eyes, mouth, lips or inside nose.
- Follow manufacturer's directions on container.

When to use:
At the same time each day.

If you forget an application:
Use as soon as you remember.

What drug does:
Increases skin-cell turnover so skin layer peels off more easily.

Time lapse before drug works:
2 to 3 weeks. May require 6 weeks for maximum improvement.

Continued next column

OVERDOSE

SYMPTOMS:
None expected.
WHAT TO DO:
If person swallows drug, call doctor, poison-control center or hospital emergency room for instructions.

Don't use with:
- Benzoyl peroxide. Apply 12 hours apart.
- *Any* other medicines, even over-the-counter drugs such as cough and cold medicines, nose drops, diet pills, laxatives or caffeine, without consulting your doctor.

POSSIBLE ADVERSE REACTIONS OR SIDE EFFECTS

SYMPTOMS	WHAT TO DO
Life-threatening:	
None expected.	
Common:	
• Pigment change in treated area, warmth or stinging, peeling.	Continue. Tell doctor at next visit.
• Senstivity to wind or cold.	No action necessary.
Infrequent:	
Blistering, crusting, severe burning, swelling.	Discontinue. Call doctor right away.
Rare:	
None expected.	

WARNINGS & PRECAUTIONS

Don't take if:
- You are allergic to tretinoin.
- You are sunburned, windburned or have an open skin wound.

Before you start, consult your doctor:
If you have eczema.

Pregnancy:
No proven harm to unborn child. Avoid if possible.

Infants & children
Don't give to infants or young children unless prescribed and monitored by your physician.

Prolonged use:
No age-related problems expected.

Skin & sunlight:
- May cause rash or intensify sunburn in areas exposed to sun or sunlamp.
- In some animal studies, tretinoin caused skin tumors to develop faster when treated area was exposed to ultraviolet light (sunlight or sunlamp). No proven similar effects in humans.

Driving or hazardous activities:
No age-related problems expected.

Discontinuing:
Don't discontinue without doctor's advice until you complete prescribed dose, even though symptoms diminish or disappear.

Others:
Acne may get worse before improvement starts in 2 or 3 weeks. Don't wash face more than 2 or 3 times daily.

POSSIBLE INTERACTION WITH OTHER DRUGS

GENERIC NAME OR DRUG CLASS	COMBINED EFFECT
Antiacne topical preparations (other, see Drugs Glossary)	Severe skin irritation.
Cosmetics (medicated)	Severe skin irritation.
Etretinate	Increased chance of toxicity of each drug.
Skin preparations with alcohol	Severe skin irritation.
Soaps or cleansers (abrasive)	Severe skin irritation.

POSSIBLE INTERACTION WITH OTHER SUBSTANCES

INTERACTS WITH	COMBINED EFFECT
Alcohol:	None expected.
Beverages:	None expected.
Cocaine (or crack):	None expected.
Foods:	None expected.
Marijuana:	None expected.
Tobacco:	None expected.

TRIAMTERENE & HYDROCHLOROTHIAZIDE

BRAND NAMES

Apo-Triazide
Dyazide
Maxzide
Novotriamzide

BASIC INFORMATION

Habit forming? No
Prescription needed? Yes
Available as generic? Yes
Drug class: Diuretic (potassium-sparing)

USES

- Reduces fluid retention (edema).
- Reduces potassium loss.
- Controls, but doesn't cure, high blood pressure.

DOSAGE & USAGE INFORMATION

How to take:
Tablet or capsule—Swallow with liquid. If you can't swallow whole, crumble tablet or open capsule and take with liquid or food.

When to take:
- 1 dose per day—Take after breakfast.
- More than 1 dose per day—Take last dose no later than 6 p.m.

If you forget a dose:
Take as soon as you remember up to 6 hours late. If more than 6 hours, wait for next scheduled dose (don't double this dose).

Continued next column

OVERDOSE

SYMPTOMS:
Lethargy, irregular heartbeat, cramps, nausea, vomiting, hypotension, weakness, drowsiness, weak pulse, coma.
WHAT TO DO:
- **Dial 0 (operator) or 911 (emergency) for an ambulance or medical help. Then give first aid immediately.**
- **If the child is unconscious and not breathing, give mouth-to-mouth breathing. If there is no heartbeat, use cardiac massage and mouth-to-mouth breathing (CPR). Don't try to make the child vomit. If you can't get help quickly, take the child to nearest emergency facility.**
- **See emergency information at the back of this book.**

What drug does:
- Increases urine production to eliminate sodium and water from body while conserving potassium.
- Forces sodium and water excretion, reducing body fluid.
- Relaxes muscle cells of small arteries.
- Reduced body fluid and relaxed arteries lower blood pressure.

Time lapse before drug works:
4 to 6 hours. May require several weeks to lower blood pressure.

Don't take with:
Any other medicines, even over-the-counter drugs such as cough and cold medicines, nose drops, diet pills, laxatives or caffeine, without consulting your doctor.

POSSIBLE ADVERSE REACTIONS OR SIDE EFFECTS

SYMPTOMS	WHAT TO DO
Life-threatening:	
Irregular heartbeat, weak pulse, shortness of breath; hives, rash, intense itching, faintness soon after a dose (anaphylaxis).	Discontinue. Seek emergency treatment.
Common:	
• Mood change, muscle cramps.	Discontinue. Call doctor right away.
• Numbness or tingling in hands or feet.	Continue. Call doctor when convenient.
Infrequent:	
• Blurred vision, abdominal pain, nausea, vomiting, kidney stones.	Discontinue. Call doctor right away.
• Dizziness, mood change, headache, dry mouth, weakness, tiredness, weight gain or loss.	Continue. Call doctor when convenient.
Rare:	
• Sore throat, fever, mouth sores; jaundice; rash; joint or muscle pain; hives; unexplained bleeding or bruising.	Discontinue. Call doctor right away.
• Corners of mouth cracked, weakness.	Continue. Call doctor when convenient.

WARNINGS & PRECAUTIONS

Don't take if:
- If you are allergic to triamterene or any thiazide diuretic drug.
- If you have had severe liver or kidney disease.

Before you start, consult your doctor:
- If you have gout, diabetes, liver, pancreas or kidney disorder.
- If you are allergic to any sulfa drug.
- If you will have surgery within 2 months, including dental surgery, requiring general or spinal anesthesia.

Pregnancy:
Risk to unborn child outweighs drug benefits. Don't use.

Infants & children:
Don't give to infants or young children unless prescribed and monitored by your physician.

Prolonged use:
Potassium retention which may lead to heart-rhythm problems.

Skin & sunlight:
May cause rash or intensify sunburn in areas exposed to sun or sunlamp.

Driving or hazardous activities:
Don't drive or pilot aircraft until you learn how medicine affects you. Don't work around dangerous machinery. Don't climb ladders or work in high places. Danger increases if you drink alcohol or take medicine affecting alertness and reflexes, such as antihistamines, tranquilizers, sedatives, pain medicine, narcotics and mind-altering drugs.

Discontinuing:
Don't discontinue without consulting doctor. Dose may require gradual reduction if you have taken drug for a long time. Doses of other drugs may also require adjustment.

Others:
- Hot weather and fever may cause dehydration and drop in blood pressure. Dose may require temporary adjustment. Weigh daily and report any unexpected weight decreases to your doctor.
- May cause rise in uric acid, leading to gout.
- May cause blood-sugar rise in diabetics.

POSSIBLE INTERACTION WITH OTHER DRUGS

GENERIC NAME OR DRUG CLASS	COMBINED EFFECT
ACE inhibitors: captopril, enalapril, lisinopril (see Drugs Glossary)	Decreased blood pressure.
Allopurinol	Decreased allopurinol effect.
Amiloride	Dangerous retention of potassium.
Amphotericin B	Increased potassium.
Antidepressants (see Drugs Glossary)	Dangerous drop in blood pressure. Avoid combination unless under medical supervision.
Antihypertensives (see Drugs Glossary)	Increased hypertensive effect.
Barbiturates (see Drugs Glossary)	Increased hydro-chlorothiazide effect.
Beta-adrenergic blockers (see Drugs Glossary)	Increased antihyper-tensive effect. Dosages of both drugs may require adjustment.
Cholestyramine	Decreased hydro-chlorothiazide effect.

See Additional Drug Interactions Section

POSSIBLE INTERACTION WITH OTHER SUBSTANCES

INTERACTS WITH	COMBINED EFFECT
Alcohol:	Dangerous blood-pressure drop.
Beverages:	None expected.
Cocaine (or crack):	Decreased triamterene effect.
Foods: Salt.	Don't restrict unless directed by doctor.
Marijuana:	Daily use—Fainting likely.
Tobacco:	Decreases drug's effectiveness.

TRICYCLIC ANTIDEPRESSANTS

BRAND & GENERIC NAMES

See complete list of brand and generic names in the Brand & Generic Name Directory.

BASIC INFORMATION

Habit forming? No
Prescription needed? Yes
Available as generic? Yes
Drug class: Antidepressant (tricyclic, see Drugs Glossary)

USES

- Gradually relieves, but doesn't cure, symptoms of depression.
- Imipramine is also used to decrease bedwetting.
- Pain relief (sometimes).

DOSAGE & USAGE INFORMATION

How to take:
Tablet, capsule or syrup—Swallow with liquid.

When to take:
At the same time each day, usually at bedtime.

If you forget a dose:
Bedtime dose—If you forget your once-a-day bedtime dose, don't take it more than 3 hours late. If more than 3 hours, wait for next scheduled dose. Don't double this dose.

Continued next column

OVERDOSE

SYMPTOMS:
Hallucinations, respiratory failure, fever, cardiac arrhythmias, convulsions, coma.
WHAT TO DO:

- **Dial 0 (operator) or 911 (emergency) for an ambulance or medical help. Then give first aid immediately.**
- **If the child is unconscious and not breathing, give mouth-to-mouth breathing. If there is no heartbeat, use cardiac massage and mouth-to-mouth breathing (CPR). Don't try to make the child vomit. If you can't get help quickly, take the child to nearest emergency facility.**
- **See emergency information at the back of this book.**

What drug does:
Probably affects part of brain that controls messages between nerve cells.

Time lapse before drug works:
Begins in 1 to 2 weeks. May require 4 to 6 weeks for maximum benefit.

Don't take with:
Any other medicines, even over-the-counter drugs such as cough and cold medicines, nose drops, diet pills, laxatives or caffeine, without consulting your doctor.

POSSIBLE ADVERSE REACTIONS OR SIDE EFFECTS

SYMPTOMS	WHAT TO DO
Life-threatening:	
Seizures.	Seek emergency treatment immediately.
Common:	
• Tremor.	Discontinue. Call doctor right away.
• Headache, dry mouth or unpleasant taste, constipation or diarrhea, nausea, indigestion, fatigue, weakness, drowsiness, nervousness, anxiety, excessive sweating	Continue. Call doctor when convenient.
• Insomnia, "sweet tooth."	Continue. Tell doctor at next visit.
Infrequent:	
• Convulsions.	Discontinue. Seek emergency treatment.
• Hallucinations, shakiness, dizziness, fainting, blurred vision, eye pain, vomiting, irregular heartbeat or slow pulse, inflamed tongue, abdominal pain, jaundice, hair loss, rash, fever, chills, joint pain, palpitations, hiccups, visual changes.	Discontinue. Call doctor right away.
• Difficult or frequent urination; decreased libido; muscle aches; abnormal dreams; nasal congestion; weakness and faintness when arising from bed or chair; back pain; absent, painful or heavy menstruation.	Continue. Call doctor when convenient.

Rare:

Itchy skin; sore throat; involuntary movements of jaw, lips and tongue; nightmares; confusion; swollen breasts in males; decreased potassium by blood test.	Discontinue. Call doctor right away.

WARNINGS & PRECAUTIONS

Don't take if:
- You are allergic to any tricyclic antidepressant.
- You drink alcohol.
- You have had a heart attack within 6 weeks.
- You have glaucoma.
- You have taken MAO inhibitors within 2 weeks.
- Patient is younger than 12.

Before you start, consult your doctor:
- If you will have surgery within 2 months, including dental surgery, requiring general or spinal anesthesia.
- If you have an enlarged prostate.
- If you have heart disease or high blood pressure.
- If you have stomach or intestinal problems.
- If you have an overactive thyroid.
- If you have asthma.
- If you have liver disease.

Pregnancy:
- Studies inconclusive on harm to unborn child. Animal studies show fetal abnormalities. Decide with your doctor whether drug benefits justify risk to unborn child.

Infants & children:
Don't give to children younger than 12.

Prolonged use:
No age-related problems expected.

Skin & sunlight:
May cause rash or intensify sunburn in areas exposed to sun or sunlamp.

Driving or hazardous activities:
Don't drive or pilot aircraft until you learn how medicine affects you. Don't work around dangerous machinery. Don't climb ladders or work in high places. Danger increases if you drink alcohol or take medicine affecting alertness and reflexes.

Discontinuing:
Don't discontinue without consulting doctor. Dose may require gradual reduction if you have taken drug for a long time. Doses of other drugs may also require adjustment.

Others:
No age-related problems expected.

POSSIBLE INTERACTION WITH OTHER DRUGS

GENERIC NAME OR DRUG CLASS	COMBINED EFFECT
Anticoagulants (oral, see Drugs Glossary)	Possible increased anticoagulant effect.
Anticholinergics (see Drugs Glossary)	Increased anticholinergic effect.
Antihistamines (see Drugs Glossary)	Increased antihistamine effect.
Barbiturates (see Drugs Glossary)	Decreased antidepressant effect. Increased sedation.
Benzodiazepines (see Drugs Glossary)	Increased sedation.
Cimetidine	Possible increased tricyclic antidepressant effect and toxicity.
Clonidine	Possible decreased clonidine effect.
Disulfiram	Delirium.
Ethchlorvynol	Delirium.
Ethinamate	Dangerous increased effects of ethinamate. Avoid combining.
Fluoxetine	Increased depressant effects of both drugs.

See Additional Drug Interactions Section

POSSIBLE INTERACTION WITH OTHER SUBSTANCES

INTERACTS WITH	COMBINED EFFECT
Alcohol: Beverages or medicines with alcohol.	Excessive intoxication. Avoid.
Beverages:	None expected.
Cocaine (or crack):	Excessive intoxication. Avoid.
Foods:	None expected.
Marijuana:	Excessive drowsiness. Avoid.
Tobacco:	Possible decreased tricyclic antidepressant effect.

TRIMETHOPRIM

BRAND NAMES

Apo-Sulfatrim
Bactrim
Cotrim
Novotrimel
Proloprim
Protrin
Rovbac
Septra
SMZ-TMP
Syraprim
Trimpex

BASIC INFORMATION

Habit forming? No
Prescription needed? Yes
Available as generic? Yes
Drug class: Antimicrobial

USES

- Treatment for urinary-tract infections susceptible to trimethoprim.
- Helps prevent recurrent urinary-tract infections if taken once a day.

DOSAGE & USAGE INFORMATION

How to take:
Tablet—Swallow with liquid or food to lessen stomach irritation.

When to take:
Space doses evenly in 24 hours to keep constant amount in urine.

If you forget a dose:
Take as soon as possible. Wait 5 to 6 hours before next dose. Then return to regular schedule.

What drug does:
Stops harmful bacterial germs from multiplying. Will not kill viruses.

Time lapse before drug works:
2 to 5 days.

Don't take with:
Any other medicines, even over-the-counter drugs such as cough and cold medicines, nose drops, diet pills, laxatives or caffeine, without consulting your doctor.

OVERDOSE

SYMPTOMS:
Nausea, vomiting, diarrhea.
WHAT TO DO:
Overdose unlikely to threaten life. If child takes much larger amount than prescribed, call doctor, poison-control center or hospital emergency room for instructions.

POSSIBLE ADVERSE REACTIONS OR SIDE EFFECTS

SYMPTOMS	WHAT TO DO
Life-threatening: None expected.	
Common: Rash, itchy skin.	Discontinue. Seek emergency treatment.
Infrequent: • Diarrhea, nausea, vomiting, abdominal pain.	Discontinue. Call doctor right away.
• Headache.	Continue. Call doctor when convenient.
Rare: • Blue fingernails, lips and skin; difficult breathing.	Discontinue. Seek emergency treatment.
• Sore throat, fever, anemia, jaundice.	Discontinue. Call doctor right away.

WARNINGS & PRECAUTIONS

Don't take if:
- You are allergic to trimethoprim or any sulfa drug.
- You are anemic due to folic acid deficiency.

Before you start, consult your doctor:
If you have had liver or kidney disease.

Pregnancy:
Studies inconclusive on harm to unborn child. Animal studies show fetal abnormalities. Decide with your doctor whether drug benefits justify risk to unborn child.

Infants & children:
Use under medical supervision only.

Prolonged use:
Anemia.

Skin & sunlight:
May cause rash or intensify sunburn in areas exposed to sun or sunlamp.

Driving or hazardous activities:
No age-related problems expected.

Discontinuing:
Don't discontinue without doctor's advice until you complete prescribed dose, even though symptoms diminish or disappear.

Others:
No age-related problems expected.

POSSIBLE INTERACTION WITH OTHER DRUGS

GENERIC NAME OR DRUG CLASS	COMBINED EFFECT
Diuretics, thiazide (see Drugs Glossary)	Unusual bleeding or bruising.
Flecainide	Possible decreased blood-cell production in bone marrow.
Sulfamethoxazole	Beneficial increase of sulfamethoxazole effect.
Tocainide	Possible decreased blood-cell production in bone marrow.

POSSIBLE INTERACTION WITH OTHER SUBSTANCES

INTERACTS WITH	COMBINED EFFECT
Alcohol:	Increased alcohol effect with Bactrim or Septra.
Beverages:	None expected.
Cocaine (or crack):	No proven problems.
Foods:	None expected.
Marijuana:	None expected.
Tobacco:	None expected.

VITAMIN A

BRAND NAMES

Acon
Afaxin
Alphalin
Aquasol A
Dispatabs
Sust-A
Numerous multiple vitamin-mineral supplements.

BASIC INFORMATION

Habit forming? No
Prescription needed? No
Available as generic? Yes
Drug class: Vitamin supplement

USES

• Dietary supplement to ensure normal growth and health, especially eyes and skin.
• Beta carotene form (Solatene) decreases severity of sun exposure in the patients with porphyria.

DOSAGE & USAGE INFORMATION

How to take:
• Drops or capsule—Swallow with liquid. If you can't swallow whole, open capsule and take with liquid or food.
• Oral solution—Swallow with liquid.

When to take:
At the same time each day.

If you forget a dose:
Take as soon as you remember. Resume regular schedule.

What drug does:
• Prevents night blindness.
• Promotes normal growth and health.

Time lapse before drug works:
Requires continual intake.

Continued next column

OVERDOSE

SYMPTOMS:
Increased adverse reactions and side effects. Jaundice (rare, but may occur with large doses), malaise, anorexia, vomiting, irritability.
WHAT TO DO:
Overdose unlikely to threaten life. If child takes much larger amount than prescribed, call doctor, poison-control center or hospital emergency room for instructions.

Don't take with:
Any other medicines, even over-the-counter drugs such as cough and cold medicines, nose drops, diet pills, laxatives or caffeine, without consulting your doctor.

POSSIBLE ADVERSE REACTIONS OR SIDE EFFECTS

SYMPTOMS	WHAT TO DO
Life-threatening: None expected.	
Common: None expected.	
Infrequent:	
Confusion; dizziness; drowsiness; headache; irritability; dry, cracked lips; peeling skin; hair loss.	Continue. Call doctor when convenient.
Rare:	
• Bulging soft spot on baby's head, double vision.	Discontinue. Call doctor right away.
• Diarrhea, appetite loss, nausea, vomiting.	Continue. Call doctor when convenient.

WARNINGS & PRECAUTIONS

Don't take if:
You have chronic kidney failure.

Before you start, consult your doctor:
If you have any kidney disorder.

Pregnancy:
Don't take more than 6,000 units daily.

Infants & children:
- Avoid large doses.
- Keep vitamin-mineral supplements out of children's reach.

Prolonged use:
No age-related problems expected.

Skin & sunlight:
No age-related problems expected.

Driving or hazardous activities:
No age-related problems expected.

Discontinuing:
Don't discontinue without doctor's advice until you complete prescribed dose, even though symptoms diminish or disappear.

Others:
- Don't exceed dose. Too much over a long time may be harmful.
- A balanced diet should provide all the vitamin A a healthy person needs and prevent need for supplements. Best sources are liver, yellow-orange fruits and vegetables, dark-green, leafy vegetables, milk, butter and margarine.

POSSIBLE INTERACTION WITH OTHER DRUGS

GENERIC NAME OR DRUG CLASS	COMBINED EFFECT
Anticoagulants (see Drugs Glossary)	Increased anticoagulant effect with large doses (over 10,000 I.U.) of vitamin A.
Calcium supplements (see Drugs Glossary)	Decreased vitamin effect.
Cholestyramine	Decreased vitamin A absorption.
Colestipol	Decreased vitamin absorption.
Contraceptives (oral, see Drugs Glossary)	Increased vitamin A levels.
Mineral oil (long term)	Decreased vitamin A absorption.
Neomycin	Decreased vitamin absorption.
Vitamin A derivatives (other)	Increased toxicity risk.
Vitamin E (excess dose)	Vitamin A depletion.

POSSIBLE INTERACTION WITH OTHER SUBSTANCES

INTERACTS WITH	COMBINED EFFECT
Alcohol:	None expected.
Beverages:	None expected.
Cocaine (or crack):	None expected.
Foods:	None expected.
Marijuana:	None expected.
Tobacco:	None expected.

VITAMIN B-12 (CYANOCOBALAMIN)

BRAND & GENERIC NAMES

See complete list of brand and generic names in the Brand & Generic Name Directory.

BASIC INFORMATION

Habit forming? No
Prescription needed? No
Available as generic? Yes
Drug class: Vitamin supplement

USES

- Dietary supplement for normal growth, development and health.
- Treatment for nerve damage.
- Treatment for pernicious anemia.
- Treatment and prevention of vitamin B-12 deficiencies in people who have had stomach or intestines surgically removed.
- Prevention of vitamin B-12 deficiency in strict vegetarians and persons with absorption diseases.

DOSAGE & USAGE INFORMATION

How to take:
- Tablets—Swallow with liquid.
- Injection—Follow doctor's directions.

When to take:
- Oral—At the same time each day.
- Injection—Follow doctor's directions.

If you forget a dose:
Take when remembered. Don't double next dose. Resume regular schedule.

What drug does:
Acts as enzyme to promote normal fat and carbohydrate metabolism and protein synthesis.

Time lapse before drug works:
15 minutes.

Continued next column

OVERDOSE

SYMPTOMS:
Increased adverse reactions and side effects.
WHAT TO DO:
Overdose unlikely to threaten life. If child takes much larger amount than prescribed, call doctor, poison-control center or hospital emergency room for instructions.

Don't take with:
Any other medicines, even over-the-counter drugs such as cough and cold medicines, nose drops, diet pills, laxatives or caffeine, without consulting your doctor.

POSSIBLE ADVERSE REACTIONS OR SIDE EFFECTS

SYMPTOMS	WHAT TO DO
Life-threatening:	
Hives, rash, intense itching, faintness soon after a dose (anaphylaxis).	Seek emergency treatment immediately.
Common:	
None expected.	
Infrequent:	
None expected.	
Rare:	
• Itchy skin, wheezing.	Discontinue. Call doctor right away.
• Diarrhea.	Continue. Call doctor when convenient.

VITAMIN B-12 (CYANOCOBALAMIN)

WARNINGS & PRECAUTIONS

Don't take if:
You have Leber's disease (optic nerve atrophy).

Before you start, consult your doctor:
- If you have gout.
- If you have heart disease.

Pregnancy:
No age-related problems expected.

Infants & children:
No age-related problems expected.

Prolonged use:
No age-related problems expected.

Skin & sunlight:
No age-related problems expected.

Driving or hazardous activities:
No age-related problems expected.

Discontinuing:
Don't discontinue without doctor's advice until you complete prescribed dose, even though symptoms diminish or disappear.

Others:
- A balanced diet should provide all the vitamin B-12 a healthy person needs and make supplements unnecessary. Best sources are meat, fish, egg yolk and cheese.
- Tablets should be used only for diet supplements. All other uses of vitamin B-12 require injections.
- Don't take large doses of vitamin C (1,000mg or more per day) unless prescribed by your doctor.

POSSIBLE INTERACTION WITH OTHER DRUGS

GENERIC NAME OR DRUG CLASS	COMBINED EFFECT
Anticonvulsants (see Drugs Glossary)	Decreased absorption of vitamin B-12.
Chloramphenicol	Decreased vitamin B-12 effect.
Cimetidine	Decreased absorption of vitamin B-12
Colchicine	Decreased absorption of vitamin B-12.
Famotidine	Decreased absorption of vitamin B-12.
H2 antagonists (see Drugs Glossary)	Decreased absorption of vitamin B-12.
Neomycin	Decreased absorption of vitamin B-12.
Para-aminosalicylic acid (PAS)	Decreased effects of PAS.
Potassium (extended-release forms)	Decreased absorption of vitamin B-12.
Ranitidine	Decreased absorption of vitamin B-12.
Vitamin C (ascorbic acid)	Destroys vitamin B-12 if taken at same time. Take 2 hours apart.

POSSIBLE INTERACTION WITH OTHER SUBSTANCES

INTERACTS WITH	COMBINED EFFECT
Alcohol:	Decreased absorption of vitamin B-12.
Beverages:	None expected.
Cocaine (or crack):	None expected.
Foods:	None expected.
Marijuana:	None expected.
Tobacco:	None expected.

VITAMIN C (ASCORBIC ACID)

BRAND & GENERIC NAMES

See complete list of brand and generic names in the Brand & Generic Name Directory.

BASIC INFORMATION

Habit forming? No
Prescription needed? No
Available as generic? Yes
Drug class: Vitamin supplement

USES

- Prevention and treatment of scurvy and other vitamin-C deficiencies.
- Treatment of anemia.
- Maintenance of acid urine.

DOSAGE & USAGE INFORMATION

How to take:
- Tablets, capsules, liquid—Swallow with 8 oz. water.
- Extended-release tablets—Swallow whole.
- Drops—Squirt directly into mouth or mix with liquid or food.
- Chewable tablets—Chew well before swallowing.

When to take:
1, 2 or 3 times per day, as prescribed on label.

If you forget a dose:
Take as soon as you remember. Return to regular schedule.

What drug does:
- May help form collagen.
- Increases iron absorption from intestine.
- Contributes to hemoglobin and red-blood-cell production in bone marrow.

Time lapse before drug works:
1 week.

Continued next column

OVERDOSE

SYMPTOMS:
Diarrhea, vomiting, dizziness.
WHAT TO DO:
Overdose unlikely to threaten life. If child takes much larger amount than prescribed, call doctor, poison-control center or hospital emergency room for instructions.

Don't take with:
Any other medicines, even over-the-counter drugs such as cough and cold medicines, nose drops, diet pills, laxatives or caffeine, without consulting your doctor.

POSSIBLE ADVERSE REACTIONS OR SIDE EFFECTS

SYMPTOMS	WHAT TO DO
Life-threatening: None expected.	
Common: None expected.	
Infrequent:	
• Mild diarrhea, nausea, vomiting.	Discontinue. Call doctor right away.
• Flushed face.	Continue. Call doctor when convenient.
Rare:	
• Kidney stones with high doses, anemia.	Discontinue. Call doctor right away.
• Headache.	Continue. Tell doctor at next visit.

WARNINGS & PRECAUTIONS

Don't take if:
You are allergic to vitamin C.

Before you start, consult your doctor:
- If you have sickle-cell or other anemia.
- If you have had kidney stones.
- If you have gout.

Pregnancy:
No proven harm to unborn child. Avoid large doses.

Infants & children:
- Avoid large doses.
- Keep vitamin-mineral supplements out of children's reach.

Prolonged use:
Large doses for longer than 2 months may cause kidney stones.

Skin & sunlight:
No age-related problems expected.

Driving or hazardous activities:
No age-related problems expected.

Discontinuing:
No age-related problems expected.

Others:
- Store in cool, dry place.
- May cause inaccurate tests for sugar in urine or blood in stool.
- May cause crisis in patients with sickle-cell anemia.
- A balanced diet should provide all the vitamin C a healthy person needs and make supplements unnecessary. Best sources are citrus, strawberries, cantaloupe and raw peppers.
- Don't take large doses of vitamin C (1,000mg or more per day) unless prescribed by your doctor.
- Some products contain tartrazine dye. Avoid, especially if you are allergic to aspirin.

POSSIBLE INTERACTION WITH OTHER DRUGS

GENERIC NAME OR DRUG CLASS	COMBINED EFFECT
Amphetamines (see Drugs Glossary)	Possible decreased amphetamine effect.
Anticholinergics (see Drugs Glossary)	Possible decreased anticholinergic effect.
Anticoagulants (oral, see Drugs Glossary)	Possible decreased anticoagulant effect.
Antidepressants, tricyclic (TCA, see Drugs Glossary)	Possible decreased antidepressant effect.
Aspirin	Decreased vitamin C effect and salicylate excretion.
Barbiturates (see Drugs Glossary)	Decreased vitamin C effect. Increased barbiturate effect.
Contraceptives (oral, see Drugs Glossary)	Decreased vitamin C effect.
Estrogens (see Drugs Glossary)	Increased likelihood of adverse effects from estrogen with 1gm or more of vitamin C per day.
Iron supplements (see Drugs Glossary)	Increased iron absorption.
Mexiletine	Possible decreased effectiveness of mexiletine.
Quinidine	Possible decreased quinidine effect.
Salicylates (see Drugs Glossary)	Decreased vitamin C effect and salicylate excretion. May lead to salicylate toxicity.
Tranquilizers (phenothiazine, see Drugs Glossary)	May decrease phenothiazine effect if no vitamin C deficiency exists.

POSSIBLE INTERACTION WITH OTHER SUBSTANCES

INTERACTS WITH	COMBINED EFFECT
Alcohol:	None expected.
Beverages:	None expected.
Cocaine (or crack):	None expected.
Foods:	None expected.
Marijuana:	None expected.
Tobacco:	Increased requirement for vitamin C.

VITAMIN D

BRAND NAMES

Calciferol	Dihydrotachysterol
Calcifidiol	Drisdol
Calcijex	Ergocalciferol
Calcitriol	Hytakerol
Calderol	Ostoforte
Deltalin	Radiostol
DHT	Radiostol Forte
DHT Intensol	Rocaltrol

Numerous other multiple vitamin-mineral supplements.

BASIC INFORMATION

Habit forming? No
Prescription needed?
Low strength: No
High strength: Yes
Available as generic? Yes
Drug class: Vitamin supplement

USES

- Dietary supplement.
- Prevention of rickets (bone disease).
- Treatment for hypocalcemia (low blood calcium) in kidney disease.
- Treatment for postoperative muscle contractions.

DOSAGE & USAGE INFORMATION

How to take:
- Tablet, capsule or liquid—Swallow with liquid.
- Drops—Dilute dose in beverage.
- Injection—Take under doctor's supervision.

When to take:
As directed, usually once a day at the same time each day.

Continued next column

OVERDOSE

SYMPTOMS:
Severe stomach pain, nausea, vomiting, weight loss; bone and muscle pain; increased urination, cloudy urine; mood or mental changes (possible psychosis); high blood pressure, irregular heartbeat; eye irritation or light sensitivity; itchy skin.
WHAT TO DO:
Overdose unlikely to threaten life. If child takes much larger amount than prescribed, call doctor, poison-control center or hospital emergency room for instructions.

If you forget a dose:
Take up to 12 hours late. If more than 12 hours, wait for next dose (don't double this dose).

What drug does:
Maintains growth and health. Prevents rickets. Essential so body can use calcium and phosphate.

Time lapse before drug works:
2 hours. May require 2 to 3 weeks of continual use for maximum effect.

Don't take with:
Any other medicines, even over-the-counter drugs such as cough and cold medicines, nose drops, diet pills, laxatives or caffeine, without consulting your doctor.

POSSIBLE ADVERSE REACTIONS OR SIDE EFFECTS

SYMPTOMS	WHAT TO DO
Life-threatening: None expected.	
Common: None expected.	
Infrequent: Headache, metallic taste in mouth, thirst, dry mouth, constipation, appetite loss, nausea, vomiting, weakness.	Continue. Call doctor when convenient.
Rare: • Increased urination, increased thirst, pink eye, psychosis, severe abdominal pain, fever.	Discontinue. Call doctor right away.
• Muscle pain, bone pain.	Continue. Tell doctor when convenient.

WARNINGS & PRECAUTIONS

Don't take if:
You are allergic to medicine containing vitamin D.

Before you start, consult your doctor:
- If you plan to become pregnant while taking vitamin D.
- If you have epilepsy.
- If you have heart or blood-vessel disease.
- If you have kidney disease.

Pregnancy:
Risk to unborn child outweighs drug benefits. Don't use.

Infants & children:
- Avoid large doses.
- Keep vitamins out of children's reach.

Prolonged use:
No age-related problems expected.

Skin & sunlight:
No age-related problems expected.

Driving or hazardous activities:
No age-related problems expected.

Discontinuing:
Don't discontinue without doctor's advice until you complete prescribed dose, even though symptoms diminish or disappear.

Others:
- Don't exceed dose. Too much over a long time may be harmful.
- A balanced diet should provide all the vitamin D a healthy person needs and make supplements unnecessary. Best sources are fish and vitamin-D fortified milk and bread.
- Some products contain tartrazine dye. Avoid, especially if you are allergic to aspirin.

POSSIBLE INTERACTION WITH OTHER DRUGS

GENERIC NAME OR DRUG CLASS	COMBINED EFFECT
Antacids (magnesium-containing, see Drugs Glossary)	Possible excess magnesium.
Anticonvulsants (hydantoin, see Drugs Glossary)	Decreased vitamin D effect.
Calcium (high doses)	Excess calcium in blood.
Calcium-channel blockers (see Drugs Glossary)	Possible decreased effect of calcium-channel blockers.
Calcium supplements (see Drugs Glossary)	Excessive absorption of vitamin D.
Cholestyramine	Decreased vitamin D effect.
Colestipol	Decreased vitamin D absorption.
Cortisone	Decreased vitamin D effect.
Digitalis preparations (see Drugs Glossary)	Heartbeat irregularities.
Diuretics, thiazide (see Drugs Glossary)	Possible increased calcium.
Mineral oil	Decreased vitamin D effect.
Neomycin	Decreased vitamin D absorption.
Phenobarbital	Decreased vitamin D effect.
Phosphorous preparations (see Drugs Glossary)	Accumulation of excess phosphorous.
Rifampin	Possible decreased vitamin D effect.
Vitamin D (other)	Possible toxicity.

POSSIBLE INTERACTION WITH OTHER SUBSTANCES

INTERACTS WITH	COMBINED EFFECT
Alcohol:	None expected.
Beverages:	None expected.
Cocaine (or crack):	None expected.
Foods:	None expected.
Marijuana:	None expected.
Tobacco:	None expected.

VITAMIN E

BRAND NAMES

Aquasol E	Eprolin
Chew-E	Epsilan-M
Daltose	Pheryl-E
E-Ferol	Viterra E

Numerous other multiple vitamin-mineral supplements.

BASIC INFORMATION

Habit forming? No
Prescription needed? No
Available as generic? Yes
Drug class: Vitamin supplement

USES

- Dietary supplement to promote normal growth, development and health.
- Treatment and prevention of vitamin-E deficiency, especially in premature or low birth weight infants.
- Treatment for fibrocystic disease of the breast.
- Treatment for circulatory problems to the lower extremities.
- Treatment for sickle-cell anemia.
- Treatment for lung toxicity from air pollution.

DOSAGE & USAGE INFORMATION

How to take:
- Tablet or capsule—Swallow with liquid or food to lessen stomach irritation.
- Drops—Dilute dose in beverage before swallowing or squirt directly into mouth.
- Injection—Take under doctor's supervision.

When to take:
At the same times each day.

If you forget a dose:
Take when you remember. Don't double next dose.

What drug does:
- Promotes normal growth and development.
- Prevents oxidation in body.

Continued next column

OVERDOSE

SYMPTOMS:
Nausea, vomiting, fatigue.
WHAT TO DO:
Overdose unlikely to threaten life. If child takes much larger amount than prescribed, call doctor, poison-control center or hospital emergency room for instructions.

Time lapse before drug works:
Not determined.

Don't take with:
Any other medicines, even over-the-counter drugs such as cough and cold medicines, nose drops, diet pills, laxatives or caffeine, without consulting your doctor.

POSSIBLE ADVERSE REACTIONS OR SIDE EFFECTS

SYMPTOMS	WHAT TO DO
Life-threatening: None expected.	
Common: None expected.	
Infrequent:	
Nausea, stomach pain, muscle aches, pain in lower legs, fever, tiredness, weakness.	Continue. Call doctor when convenient.
Rare:	
Blurred vision, diarrhea.	Discontinue. Call doctor right away.

WARNINGS & PRECAUTIONS

Don't take if:
You are allergic to vitamin E.

Before you start, consult your doctor:
- If you have had blood clots in leg veins (thrombophlebitis).
- If you have liver disease.

Pregnancy:
No age-related problems expected with normal daily requirements. Don't exceed prescribed dose.

Infants & children:
Use only under medical supervision.

Prolonged use:
Toxic accumulation of vitamin E. Don't exceed recommended dose.

Skin & sunlight:
No age-related problems expected.

Driving or hazardous activities:
No age-related problems expected.

Discontinuing:
No age-related problems expected.

Others:
A balanced diet should provide all the vitamin E a healthy person needs and make supplements unnecessary. Best sources are vegetable oils, whole-grain cereals, liver.

POSSIBLE INTERACTION WITH OTHER DRUGS

GENERIC NAME OR DRUG CLASS	COMBINED EFFECT
Anticoagulants (oral, see Drugs Glossary)	Increased anticoagulant effect.
Cholestyramine	Decreased vitamin E absorption.
Colestipol	Decreased vitamin E absorption.
Iron supplements (see Drugs Glossary)	Possible decreased effect of iron supplement in patients with iron-deficiency anemia. Decreased vitamin E effect in healthy persons.
Mineral oil	Decreased vitamin E effect.
Neomycin	Decreased vitamin E absorption.
Vitamin A	Recommended dose of vitamin E. Increased benefit and decreased toxicity of vitamin A. Excess dose of vitamin E. Vitamin A depletion.

POSSIBLE INTERACTION WITH OTHER SUBSTANCES

INTERACTS WITH	COMBINED EFFECT
Alcohol:	None expected.
Beverages:	None expected.
Cocaine (or crack):	None expected.
Foods:	None expected.
Marijuana:	None expected.
Tobacco:	None expected.

VITAMIN K

BRAND NAMES

AquaMEPHYTON
Konakion
Menadione
Menadiol
Mephyton
Phytonadione
Synkayvite

BASIC INFORMATION

Habit forming? No
Prescription needed? No
Available as generic? No
Drug class: Vitamin supplement

USES

- Dietary supplement.
- Treatment for bleeding disorders and malabsorption diseases due to vitamin K deficiency.
- Treatment for hemorrhagic disease of the newborn.
- Treatment for bleeding due to overdose of oral anticoagulants (usually by injection).

DOSAGE & USAGE INFORMATION

How to take:
- Usually given by injection in hospital or doctor's office.
- Tablet—Swallow with liquid. If you can't swallow whole, crumble tablet and take with liquid or food.

When to take:
At the same time each day.

If you forget a dose:
Take as soon as you remember up to 12 hours late. If more than 12 hours, wait for next scheduled dose (don't double this dose).

What drug does:
- Promotes growth, development and good health in nutritionally-deprived children.
- Supplies a necessary ingredient for blood clotting.

Continued next column

OVERDOSE

SYMPTOMS:
Nausea, vomiting.
WHAT TO DO:
Overdose unlikely to threaten life. If child takes much larger amount than prescribed, call doctor, poison-control center or hospital emergency room for instructions.

Time lapse before drug works:
15 to 30 minutes to support blood clotting.

Don't take with:
Any other medicines, even over-the-counter drugs such as cough and cold medicines, nose drops, diet pills, laxatives or caffeine, without consulting your doctor.

POSSIBLE ADVERSE REACTIONS OR SIDE EFFECTS

SYMPTOMS	WHAT TO DO
Life-threatening:	
None expected.	
Common:	
None expected.	
Infrequent:	
Unusual taste.	Continue. Call doctor when convenient.
Rare:	
Rash, hives.	Discontinue. Call doctor right away.

WARNINGS & PRECAUTIONS

Don't take if:
- You are allergic to vitamin K.
- You have G6PD deficiency.
- You have liver disease.

Before you start, consult your doctor:
If you are pregnant.

Pregnancy:
Don't exceed dose.

Infants & children:
Phytonadione is the preferred form for hemorrhagic disease of the newborn.

Prolonged use:
No age-related problems expected.

Skin & sunlight:
No age-related problems expected.

Driving or hazardous activities:
No age-related problems expected.

Discontinuing:
No age-related problems expected.

Others:
- Tell all doctors and dentists you consult that you take this medicine.
- Don't exceed dose. Too much over a long time may be harmful.
- A balanced diet should provide all the vitamin K a healthy person needs and make supplements unnecessary. Best sources are green, leafy vegetables, meat or dairy products.

POSSIBLE INTERACTION WITH OTHER DRUGS

GENERIC NAME OR DRUG CLASS	COMBINED EFFECT
Anticoagulants (oral, see Drugs Glossary)	Decreased anticoagulant effect.
Cholestyramine	Decreased vitamin K effect.
Colestipol	Decreased vitamin K absorption.
Mineral oil (long term)	Vitamin K deficiency.
Neomycin	Decreased vitamin K absorption.
Sulfa drugs (see Drugs Glossary)	Vitamin K deficiency.

POSSIBLE INTERACTION WITH OTHER SUBSTANCES

INTERACTS WITH	COMBINED EFFECT
Alcohol:	None expected.
Beverages:	None expected.
Cocaine (or crack):	None expected.
Foods:	None expected.
Marijuana:	None expected.
Tobacco:	None expected.

XANTHINE BRONCHODILATORS

BRAND & GENERIC NAMES

See complete list of brand and generic names in the Brand & Generic Name Directory.

BASIC INFORMATION

Habit forming? No
Prescription needed?
Canada—No
U.S.: High strength—Yes
Low strength—No
Available as generic? Yes
Drug class: Bronchodilator (xanthine)

USES

Treatment for bronchial asthma symptoms.

DOSAGE & USAGE INFORMATION

How to take:

- Tablet or capsule—Swallow with liquid.
- Extended-release tablets or capsules—Swallow each dose whole. If you take regular tablets, you may chew or crush them.
- Suppositories—Remove wrapper and moisten suppository with water. Gently insert larger end into rectum. Push well into rectum with finger.
- Syrup—Take as directed on bottle.
- Enema—Use as directed on label.

When to take:
Most effective taken on empty stomach 1 hour before or 2 hours after eating. However, may take with food to lessen stomach upset.

If you forget a dose:
Take as soon as you remember up to 2 hours late. If more than 2 hours, wait for next scheduled dose (don't double this dose).

Continued next column

What drug does:
Relaxes and expands bronchial tubes.

Time lapse before drug works:
15 to 30 minutes.

Don't take with:
Any other medicines, even over-the-counter drugs such as cough and cold medicines, nose drops, diet pills, laxatives or caffeine, without consulting your doctor.

OVERDOSE

SYMPTOMS:
Restlessness, irritability, confusion, delirium, convulsions, rapid pulse, coma.
WHAT TO DO:

- **Dial 0 (operator) or 911 (emergency) for an ambulance or medical help. Then give first aid immediately.**
- **See emergency information at the back of this book.**

POSSIBLE ADVERSE REACTIONS OR SIDE EFFECTS

SYMPTOMS	WHAT TO DO
Life-threatening:	
None expected.	
Common:	
Headache, irritability, nervousness, nausea, restlessness, insomnia, vomiting, stomach pain.	Continue. Call doctor when convenient.
Infrequent:	
• Rash or hives, flushed face, diarrhea, appetite loss, rapid breathing, irregular heartbeat.	Discontinue. Call doctor right away.
• Dizziness or lightheadedness.	Continue. Call doctor when convenient.
Rare:	
Frequent urination.	Continue. Call doctor when convenient.

WARNINGS & PRECAUTIONS

Don't take if:
- You are allergic to any bronchodilator.
- You have an active peptic ulcer.

Before you start, consult your doctor:
- If you have had impaired kidney or liver function.
- If you have gastritis.
- If you have a peptic ulcer.
- If you have high blood pressure or heart disease.
- If you take medication for gout.

Pregnancy:
Risk to unborn child outweighs drug benefits. Don't use.

Infants & children:
Use only under medical supervision.

Prolonged use:
Stomach irritation.

Skin & sunlight:
No age-related problems expected.

Driving or hazardous activities:
Avoid if lightheaded or dizzy. Otherwise, no problems expected.

Discontinuing:
May be unnecessary to finish medicine. Follow doctor's instructions.

Others:
No age-related problems expected.

POSSIBLE INTERACTION WITH OTHER DRUGS

GENERIC NAME OR DRUG CLASS	COMBINED EFFECT
Allopurinol	Increased allopurinol effect.
Aminoglutethimide	Possible decreased bronchodilator effect.
Beta-agonists (see Drugs Glossary)	Increased effect of both drugs.
Beta-adrenergic blockers (see Drugs Glossary)	Decreased bronchodilator effect.
Cimetidine	Increased bronchodilator effect.
Clindamycin	May increase bronchodilator effect.
Corticosteroids	Possible increased bronchodilator effect.
Erythromycin	Increased bronchodilator effect.
Furosemide	Increased furosemide effect.
Lincomycin	May increase bronchodilator effect.
Lithiuim	Decreased lithiuim effect.
Phenobarbital	Decreased bronchodilator effect.
Phenytoin	Decreased bronchodilator effect.
Probenecid	Increased effect of dyphylline.
Ranitidine	Possible increased bronchodilator effect and toxicity.
Rauwolfia alkaloids (see Drugs Glossary)	Rapid heartbeat.
Rifampin	Decreased bronchodilator effect.
Sulfinpyrazone	Increased effect of dyphylline.
Sympathomimetics (see Drugs Glossary)	Possible increased bronchodilator effect.
Troleandomycin	Increased bronchodilator effect.

POSSIBLE INTERACTION WITH OTHER SUBSTANCES

INTERACTS WITH	COMBINED EFFECT
Alcohol:	None expected.
Beverages: Caffeine drinks.	Nervousness and insomnia.
Cocaine (or crack):	Excess stimulation. Avoid.
Foods:	None expected.
Marijuana:	Slightly increased anti-asthmatic effect of bronchodilator. Decreased effect with chronic use.
Tobacco:	Decreased bronchodilator effect.

BRAND & GENERIC NAME DIRECTORY

The following drugs are alphabetized by generic name or drug class, shown in large capital letters. The brand and generic names that follow each title in this list are the complete list referred to on the drug charts. Generic names are in all capital letters on the lists.

ACETAMINOPHEN

A'Cenol
Acephen
Aceta
Ace-Tabs
Aceta w/Codeine
Acetaco
Acetaminophen w/Codeine
Acetaminophen Uniserts
Actamin
Algisin
Amacodone
Amaphen
Amphenol
Anacin-3
Anapap
Anaphen
Anoquan
Anuphen
Apacet
Apamide Tablets
APAP
Apo-Acetaminophen
Arthralgen
Aspirin-Free Excedrin
Atasol
Axotal
Bancap w/Codeine
Banesin
Banesin Forte
Bayapap
Bromo-Seltzer
C2A
Cafadol
Campain
Capital
Capital w/Codeine
Chlorzone Forte
Co-Gesic
Co-Tylenol
Coastaldyne
Coastalgesic
Codalan
Codap
Colrex
Compal
Comtrex
Conacetol
Congespirin
Covangesic
D-Sinus
Dapa
Dapase
Darvocet-N
Datril
Dia-Gesic
Dialog
Dolacet
Dolanex
Dolene AP-65
Dolor
Dolprin
Dorcol
Dorcol Children's Fever and Pain Reducer
Dristan
Duadacin
Dularin
Duradyne DHC
Dynosal
Empracet w/Codeine
Endecon
Esgic
Excedrin
Exdol
Febrigesic
Febrinol
Febrogesic
Fendol
G-1
G-2
G-3
Gaysal
Genapap
Genebs
Genetabs
Guaiamine
Halenol
Hasacode
Hi-Temp
Hyco-Pap
Hycomine Compound
Korigesic
Liquiprin
Liquix-C
Lorcet
Lyteca
Meda Cap
Meda Tab
Mejoral without aspirin
Mejoralito
Metrogesic
Midol PMS
Midrin
Migralam
Minotal
Myapap
Naldegesic
NAPAP
Nebs
Neopap
Oraphen-PD
Ornex
Ossonate-Plus
Pacaps
Pain Relief without aspirin
Panadol
Panasorb
Panex
Paracetamol
Parafon Forte
Paraphen
Pavadon
Pedric
Peedee Dose Aspirin
Percocet-5
Percogesic
Phenaphen
Phenaphen w/Codeine
Phendex
Phrenilin
Presalin
Prodolor
Protid
Proval
Repan
Rhinocaps
Robigesic
Ronuvex
Rounox
S-A-C
SK-65 APAP
SK-APAP
SK-Oxycodone w/Acetaminophen
Salatin
Saleto

Salimeph Forte
Salphenyl
Sedapap
Sinarest
Sine-Aid
Sine-Off
Singlet
Sinubid
Sinulin
Sinutab
St. Joseph Aspirin Free
Stopayne
Strascogesic
Sudoprin
Summit
Supac
Suppap
Sylapar
T.P.I.
Talacen
Tapanol
Tapar
Temlo
Tempra
Tenlap
Tenol
Triaminicin
Trigesic
Trind Sryup
Two-Dyne
Ty Caplets
Ty Pap
Ty-tabs
Tylenol
Tylenol w/Codeine
Tylox
Valadol
Valorin
Vanquish
Vicodin
Wygesic

ADRENOCORTICOIDS (TOPICAL)

Acticort
Adcortyl
Adcortyl in Orabase
Aeroseb-Dex
Aeroseb-HC
Alphatrex
Aristocort
Aristocort A
Aristocort C
Aristocort D
Aristocort R
Bactine Hydrocortisone
Barriere-HC
Beben
Benisone
Beta-Val
Betacort
Betacort Scalp Lotion
Betaderm
Betaderm Scalp Lotion
Betatrex
Betnesol
Betnovate
CaldeCORT
Caldecort Anti-Itch
Carmol-HC
Celestoderm-V
Celestone
Cetacort
Clinicort
Cloderm
Cordran
Cordran SP
Cort-Dome
Cortaid
Cortate
Cortef
Corticaine
Corticosporin
Corticreme
Cortifoam
Cortiment
Cortisol
Cortizone
Cortoderm
Cortril
Cremocort
Cyclocort
Decaderm
Decadron
Decaspray
Delacort
Dermacort
DermiCort
Dermolate
Dermophyl
Dermovate
Dermovate Scalp Application
Dermtex HC
DesOwen
Dioderm
Diprolene
Diprosone
Drenison
EF cortelan
Ectosone
Ectosone Scalp Lotion
Eldecort
Emo-Cort
Epifoam
Florone
Fluocet
Fluoderm
Fluolar
Fluolean
Fluonid
Fluonide
Flurosyn
Flutex
Flutone
Gynecort
H2 Cort
HC-Jel
Halciderm
Halog
Halog E
Hexadrol
Hi-Cor
Hi-Cort
Hyderm
Hydro-Corilean
Hydro-Tex
Hydrocortone
Hytone
Kenalog
Kenalog-E
Kenalog-H
Kenalog in Orabase
Lacticare-HC
Lanacort
Lidemol
Lidex
Lidex-E
Locoid
Locacorten
Lyderm
Maxiflor
Medrol
Metaderm
Meti-Derm
Metosyn
Metosyn FAPG
Neo-Cortef
Neo-Decadron
Novobetamet
Novohydrocort
Nutracort
Orabase HCA
Oxylone
Penecort

Pharma-Cort
Proctocort
Psorcon
Psorcon-E
Racet-SE
Rectocort
Rhulicort
Spencort
Stie-Cort
Synacort
Synalar
Synamol
Synandone
Synemol
Temovate
Texacort
Topicort
Topsyn
Triacet
Triaderm
Trianide
Triderm
Tridesilon
Trymex
Unicort
Uticort
Valisone
Valisone Scalp Lotion
Vioform
Westcort
Some of these brands are available as oral medicine. Look under specific generic name for each brand.

ANTICONVULSANTS, HYDANTOIN

Dantoin
Dilantin
Dilantin Infatabs
Dilantin Kapseals
Dilantin-125
Dilantin-30-Pediatric
Di-Phen
Diphenylan
Diphenylhydantoin
ETHOTOIN
MEPHENYTOIN
Mesantoin
Novophenytoin
Peganone
PHENYTOIN

ANTIDIABETICS, ORAL

ACETOHEXAMIDE
Apo-Chlorpropamide
Apo-Tolbutamide
CHLORPROPAMIDE
DiaBeta
Diabinese
Dimelor
Dymelor
Euglucon
Glibenclamide
GLIPIZIDE
Glucamide
Glucotrol
GLYBURIDE
Micronase
Mobenol
Novobutamide
Novopropamide
Oramide
Orinase
Ronase
SK-Tolbutamide
TOLAZAMIDE
TOLBUTAMIDE
Tolinase

ANTIHISTAMINES

Actidil
Aller-Chlor
Allerid-O.D.
Apo-Dimenhydrinate
AZATADINE
Bayidyl
Beldin
Bena-D
Benadryl
Benadryl Children's Allergy
Benadryl Complete Allergy
Benahist
Benoject-10
Benylin
Bromamine
Brombay
BROMODIPHENHYDRAMINE
Bromphen
BROMPHENIRAMINE
Calm X
CARBINOXAMINE
Chlo-Amine
Chlor-100
Chlor-Mal
Chlor-Niramine
Chlor-Pro
Chlor-Trimeton
Chlor-Trimeton Repetabs
Chlor-Tripolon
Chlorphed
Chlorphen
CHLORPHENIRAMINE
Chlorspan
Chlortab
CLEMASTINE
Clistin
Compoz
CYPROHEPTADINE
Dehist
DEXCHLORPHENIRAMINE
Diahist
Dihydrex
DIMENHYDRINATE
Dimentabs
Dimetane
Dimetane Extentabs
Dimetane-Ten
Dinate
Diphen
Diphenacen
Diphenadril
DIPHENHYDRAMINE
DIPHENYLPYRALINE
Dommanate
Dormarex
DOXYLAMINE
Dramamine
Dramilin
Dramocen
Dramoject
Dymenate
Fenylhist
Fynex
Gravol
Hal-Chlor
Hispril
Histaject Modified
Histrey
Hydramine
Hydrate
Hydril
Hyrexin-50
HYDROXYZINE
Insomnal
Marmine
Motion-Aid
Nasahist B
Nauseatol
ND-Stat Revised
Nervine Nighttime Sleep-Aid

Nolahist
Noradryl
Nordryl
Novodimenate
Novopheniram
Nytol with DPH
Optimine
Oraminic II
PBZ
PBZ-SR
Periactin
Phenetron
Phenetron Lanacaps
PHENINDAMINE
PMS-Dimenhydrinate
Polaramine
Polaramine Repetabs
PROMETHAZINE
PYRILAMINE
Reidamine
Robalyn
Seldane
Sleep-Eze 3
Sominex
Sominex Formula 2
Somnicaps
Tavist
T.D. Alermine
Teldrin
Travamine
TRIMEPRAZINE
TRIPELENNAMINE
TRIPROLIDINE
Trymegen
Tusstat
Twilite
Unisom Nighttime
Sleep-Aid
Valdrene
Veltane
Wehamine
Wehdryl

ANTI-INFLAMMATORY ANALGESICS, NON-STEROIDAL

Advil
Amersol
Anaprox
Apo-Ibuprofen
Apo-Naproxen
Apo-Piroxicam
Apsifen
Apsifen-F
ASPIRIN
ASPIRIN, BUFFERED
Brufen
CHOLINE SALICYLATE
CHOLINE & MAGNESIUM SALICYLATES
Clinoril
DIFLUNISAL
Dolobid
Feldene
FENOPROFEN
Fenopron
Haltran
IBUPROFEN
Ifen
INDOMETHACIN
KETOPROFEN
MAGNESIUM SALICYLATE
MECLOFENAMATE
Meclomen
Medipren
MEFENAMIC ACID
Midol 200
Motrin
Nalfon
Naprosyn
NAPROXEN
Naxen
Neuvil
Novonaprox
Novopirocam
Novoprofen
Nuprin
Pamprin IB
PHENYLBUTAZONE
PIROXICAM
Ponstan
Ponstel
Progesic
Rufen
SALICYLAMIDE
SALSALATE
SODIUM SALICYLATE
SULINDAC
Synflex
Tolectin
Tolectin DS
TOLMETIN
Trendar

APPETITE SUPPRESSANTS

Adipex-D
Adipex-P
Adipost
Adphen
Anorex
Bacarate
BENZPHETAMINE
B.O.F.
Bontril PDM
Bontril Slow Release
Chlor-Tripolon
Chlorophen
CHLORPHENTERMINE
CLORTERMINE
Dapex
Dapex-37.5
Delcozine
D.E.P.—75
Depletite
Dexatrim
Di-Ap-Trol
Didrex
Dietec
DIETHYLPROPION
Dyrexan-OD
Elephemet
Ex-Obese
Fastin
FENFLURAMINE
Hyrex
Hyrex-105
Inifast Unicelles
Ionamin
Limit
Limitite
MASINDOL
Mazanor
Melfiat
Menrium
Metra
Minus
Nobesine
Nobesine-75
Nu-Dispoz
Obalan
Obe-Nil TR
Obe-Nix
Obephen
Obermine
Obestin
Obestin-30
Obestrol
Obeval
Obezine
Oby-Trim
Parmine
Penderal Pacaps
Phenazine-35
Phendiet

BRAND & GENERIC NAME DIRECTORY

PHENDIMETRAZINE
PHENMETRAZINE
Phentamine
PHENTERMINE
Phentrol
Phenzine
Plegine
Ponderal
Ponderal Pacaps
Pondimin
Pondimin Extentabs
Pre-Sate
Prelu-2
Preludin
Propion
P.S.P.R.X. 1, 2 & 3
Reducto
Regibon
Ro-Diet
Sanorex
Slim-Tabs
Slynn-LL
Span-RD
Sprx-1
Sprx-105
Sprx-3
Statobex
Statobex-G
Symetra
Tenuate
Tenuate Dospan
Tepanil
Tepanil Ten-Tab
Teramine
Tora
Trimcaps
Trimstat
Trimtabs
Unicelles
Unifast
Voranil
Wehless
Weightrol
Wilpowr
X-Trozine
X-Trozine LA

ASPIRIN

4-Way Cold Tablets
8-Hour Bayer Timed Release
Acetophen
Acetylsalicylic Acid
Alka Seltzer
Alka-Seltzer
Alka-Seltzer Effervescent Pain Reliever & Antacid
Aluminum ASA
Amytal and Aspirin
Anacin
Anaphen
Ancasal
Anexsia w/Codeine
A.P.C.
A.P.C. w/Codeine
Apo-Asen
Arthinol
Arthritis Bayer Timed-Release
Arthritis Pain Formula
A.S.A.
A.S.A. & Codeine Compound
A.S.A. Compound
A.S.A. Enseals
Ascodeen-30
Ascriptin
Ascriptin A/D
Ascriptin w/Codeine
Asperbuf
Aspergum
Aspir-10
Aspirin Compound w/Codeine
Aspirjen Jr.
Astrin
Axotal
Bancap w/Codeine
Bayer
Bayer Timed-Release Arthritic Pain Formula
Bexophene
Buff-A
Buff-A-Comp
Buffaprin
Buffered ASA
Bufferin
Buffex
Buffinol
Buf-Tabs
Calciphen
Cama Arthritis Reliever
Cama Inlay
Causalin
Cefinal
Cirin
Codalan
Codasa
Congespirin
Coralsone
Coricidin D
Coryphen
Cosprin
Darvon Compound
Dasicon
Decagesic
Dia-Gesic
Dihydrocodein Compound
Dolene Compound-65
Dolor
Dolprn
Dynosal
Easprin
Ecotrin
Elder 65 Compound
Emagrin
Empirin
Empirin Compound
Empirin Compound w/Codeine
Emprazil
Encaprin
Entrophen
Equagesic
Excedrin
Fiorinal
Fiorinal w/Codeine
Hiprin
Histadyl and ASA Compound
Hyco-Pap
ICN 65 Compound
Kengesin
Lanorinal
Lemidyne w/Codeine
Magnaprin
Maprin
Maprin I-B
Measurin
Mepro Compound
Metrogesic
Mobidin
Norgesic
Norwich Aspirin
Nova-Phase
Novasen
Pabirin Buffered
P-A-C Compound
P-A-C Compound w/Codeine
Pargesic Compound 65
Percodan
Persistin
Phenodyne w/Codeine
Poxy Compound-65

Presalin
Progesic Compound-65
Propoxychel Compound
Propoxyphene HCl Compound
Repro Compound 65
Rhinocaps
Riphen-10
Safety Coated APF Arthritis Pain Formula
St. Joseph
St. Joseph Aspirin for Children
Sal-Adult
Salatin
Salatin w/Codeine
Saleto
Salimeph Forte
Sal-Infant
Salocol
Salsprin
SK-65 Compound
Soma Compound
Soma Compound w/Codeine
Stero-Darvon
Supac
Supasa
Synalgos
Talwin Compound
Triaminic
Triaphen-10
Trigesic
Vanquish
Verin
Wesprin Buffered
Zorprin

BARBITURATES

Alurate
AMOBARBITAL
Amytal
APROBARBITAL
Barbased
Barbita
BUTABARBITAL
Butalan
Buticaps
Butisol
Day-Barb
Gardenal
Gemonil
Lotusate
Luminal
Mebaral
MEPHOBARBITAL
METHARBITAL
Nembutal
Neo-Barb
Novopentobarb
Novosecobarb
PENTOBARBITAL
PHENOBARBITAL
Sarisol No. 2
SECOBARBITAL
SECOBARBITAL & AMOBARBITAL
Seconal
Solfoton
TALBUTAL
Tuinal

BELLADONNA ALKALOIDS & BARBITURATES

Anaspaz PB
Antrocol
ATROPINE, HYOSCYAMINE, SCOPOLAMINE & BUTABARBITAL
ATROPINE, HYOSCYAMINE, SCOPOLAMINE & PHENOBARBITAL
ATROPINE & PHENOBARBITAL
Barbidonna
Barophen
Bay-Ase
Belap
Belladenal
Belladenal-S
Belladenal Spacetabs
BELLADONNA & BUTABARBITAL
BELLADONNA & PHENOBARBITAL
Bellalphen
Bellastal
Bellkatal
Butibel
Chardonna-2
Donnapine
Donna-Sed
Donnatal
Donnatal Extentabs
Donphen
Hybephen
HYOSCYAMINE & PHENOBARBITAL
HYOSCYAMINE, SCOPOLAMINE & PHENOBARBITAL
Hyosophen
Kinesed
Levsinex with Phenobarbital Timecaps
Levsin-PB
Levsin with Phenobarbital
Malatal
Palbar No. 2
Pheno-Bella
Relaxadon
Seds
Spaslin
Spasmolin
Spasmophen
Spasquid
Susano
Vanodonnal

BENZODIAZEPINES

ALPRAZOLAM
Alzapam
Apo-Chlordiazepoxide
Apo-Diazepam
Apo-Flurazepam
Apo-Lorazepam
Apo-Oxazepam
Ativan
Centrax
CHLORDIAZEPOXIDE
CLONAZEPAM
CLORAZEPATE
Dalmane
DIAZEPAM
D-Tran
Durapam
E-Pam
FLURAZEPAM
HALAZEPAM
Halcion
Klonopin
Libritabs
Librium
Lipoxide
Loraz
LORAZEPAM
Medilium
Meval
MIDAZOLAM
Neo-Calme
Novoclopate
Novodipam
Novoflupam

Novolorazem
Novopoxide
Novoxapam
OXAZEPAM
Ox-Pam
Paxipam
PRAZEPAM
Q-Pam
Razepam
Reposans
Restoril
Rival
Rivotril
Serax
Sereen
Serenack
SK-Lygen
Solium
Som-Pam
Somnol
Stress-Pam
Temaz
TEMAZEPAM
Tranxene
Tranxene T-Tab
Tranxene-SD
TRIAZOLAM
Valium
Valrelease
Vivol
Xanax
Zapex

BETA-ADRENERGIC BLOCKING AGENTS

ACEBUTOLOL
Apo-Metoprolol
Apo-Propranolol
ATENOLOL
Betaloc
Betaloc Durules
Blocadren
Corgard
Detensol
ESMOLOL
Inderal
Inderal LA
Inderide
LABETALOL
Lopresor
Lopresor SR
Lopressor
METOPROLOL
Monitan
NADOLOL
Normodyne
Novometoprol
Novopranol
OXPRENOLOL
Panolol
PINDOLOL
pms-Propranolol
PROPRANOLOL
Sectral
Slow-Trasicor
Sotacor
SOTALOL
Tenormin
TIMOLOL
Trandate
Trasicor
Visken

CEPHALOSPORINS

Ancef
Anspor
Ceclor
CEFACLOR
CEFADROXIL
Cefadyl
CEFAMANDOLE
CEFAZOLIN
Cefizox
Cefobid
Cefobine
CEFONICID
CEFOPERAZONE
CEFORANIDE
Cefotan
CEFOTAXIME
CEFOTETAN
CEFOXITIN
CEFTAZIDIME
CEFTIZOXIME
CEFTRIAXONE
CEFUROXIME
CEPHALEXIN
CEPHALOTHIN
CEPHAPIRIN
CEPHRADINE
Ceporacin
Ceporex
Claforan
Duricef
Fortaz
Keflet
Keflex
Keflin
Keflin Neutral
Kefurox
Kefzol
Lamoxactam
Latamoxef
Magnacef
Mandol
Mefoxin
Monocid
MOXALACTAM
Moxam
Novolexin
Oxalactam
Precef
Rocephin
Seffin Neutral
Tazicef
Tazidime
Ultracef
Velosef
Zinacef

DICYCLOMINE

Antispas
A-Spas
Baycyclomine
Bentyl
Bentylol
Byclomine
Cyclobec
Cyclocen
Dibent
Dicen
Di-Cyclonex
Dilomine
Di-Spaz
Dyspas
Formulex
Lomine
Menospasm
Neoquess
Nospaz
Or-Tyl
Protylol
Spasmoban
Spasmoject
Triactin
Viscerol

DIURETICS, THIAZIDE

Anhydron
Apo-Chlorthalidone
Apo-Hydro
Aquamox
Aquatag
Aquatensen
BENDROFLUMETHIAZIDE

BENZTHIAZIDE
CHLOROTHIAZIDE
CHLORTHALIDONE
CYCLOTHIAZIDE
Diucardin
Diuchlor H
Diulo
Diuril
Duretic
Enduron
Esidrix
Exna
Fluidil
Hydrex
HYDROCHLOROTHIAZIDE
Hydrochlorothiazide Intensol
HYDROFLUMETHIAZIDE
HydroDIURIL
Hydromox
Hygroton
Metahydrin
METHYCLOTHIAZIDE
METOLAZONE
Mictrin
Naqua
Natrimax
Naturetin
Neo-Codema
Novohydrazide
Novothalidone
Oretic
POLYTHIAZIDE
QUINETHAZONE
Renese
Saluron
Thalitone
Thiuretic
TRICHLORMETHIAZIDE
Uridon
Urozide
Zaroxolyn

ERYTHROMYCINS

Apo-Erythro-S
A/T/S
Bristamycin
Dowmycin
E-Biotic
E.E.S.
E-Mycin
E-Mycin E
Eryc
Eryc Sprinkle
Ery-derm
EryPed
Erymax
Erypar
Ery-Tab
Erythrocin
Erythrocin Ethyl Succinate
Erythromid
ERYTHROMYCIN
ERYTHROMYCIN ESTOLATE
ERYTHROMYCIN ETHYLSUCCINATE
ERYTHROMYCIN GLUCEPTATE
ERYTHROMYCIN LACTOBIONATE
ERYTHROMYCIN STEARATE
Ethril
Ilosone
Ilosone Estolate
Ilotycin
Ilotycin Gluceptate
Kesso-mycin
Novorythro
PCE Dispersatabs
Pediazole
Pediamycin
Pendiamycin
Pfizer-E
Robimycin
RP-Mycin
SK-Erythromycin
Staticin
T-Star
Wyamycin
Wyamycin E
Wyamycin S

ESTROGEN

Amnestrogen
C.E.S.
Clinestrone
Conjugated Estrogens
C.S.D.
Delestrogen
DES
DIENESTROL (vaginal)
DV (vaginal)
Estinyl
Estomed
Estrace
Estrace (vaginal)
ESTRADIOL (vaginal)
Estraguard (vaginal)
Estratab
Estrocon
ESTROGENS, CONJUGATED (vaginal)
ESTRONE (vaginal)
ESTROPIPATE (vaginal)
Estrovis
Evex
Feminone
Femogen
Formatrix
Hormonin
Menest
Menotrol
Menrium
Milprem
Oagen
Oestrilin
Oestrilin (vaginal)
Ogen
Ogen (vaginal)
Ortho Dienestrol (vaginal)
Piperazine Estrone Sulfate (vaginal)
PMB-200
PMB-400
Premarin
Premarin (vaginal)
Progens
Stilphostrol
Theogen

HYDROXYZINE

Anxanil
Atarax
Ataraxoid
Atozine
Cartrax
Durrax
Enarax
E-Vista
Hydroxacen
Hy-Pam
Hyzine
Marax
Multipax
Neucalm 50
Orgatrax
Quiess
T.E.H. Tablets
Theozine
Vamate
Vistacon
Vistaject
Vistaquel
Vistaril

Vistazine
Vistrax

NARCOTIC & ACETAMINOPHEN

Acetaco
ACETAMINOPHEN & CODEINE
Aceta with Codeine
Amacodone
Anexsia
APAP with Codeine
Atasol with Codeine
Bancap-HC
Bayapap with Codeine
Capital with Codeine
Codap
Co-gesic
Compal
Cotabs
Damacet-P
Darvocet-N
Demerol-APAP
Dolacet
Dolene-AP
Dolo-Pap
Duradyne DHC
Empracet with Codeine
Emtec
Exdol with Codeine
Hycodaphen
Hydrocet
HYDROCODONE & ACETAMINOPHEN
Hydrocone with APAP
Hydrogesic
HY-PHEN
Lenoltec
Lorcet
Lorcet-HD
Lortab
Lortab 5
Lortab 7
MEPERIDINE & ACETAMINOPHEN
Norcet
Oxycocet
OXYCODONE & ACETAMINOPHEN
PENTAZOCINE & ACETAMINOPHEN
Percocet
Percocet-Demi
Phenaphen with Codeine
Propacet
Propain-HC
PROPOXYPHENE & ACETAMINOPHEN
Proval
Rounox with Codeine
Roxicet
SK-APAP with Codeine
SK-Oxycodone and Acetaminophen
SK-65 APAP
Stopayne
Talacen
T-Gesic Forte
Tylenol with Codeine
Tylox
Ty-Tabs
Vicodin
Wygesic

NARCOTIC ANALGESICS

642
Aceta w/Codeine
Acetaco
Acetaminophen w/Codeine
Actifed-C
Actifed-C Expectorant
Adatuss
Algodex
Ambenyl
Anaphen
A.P.C. w/Codeine Phosphate Tablets
A.P.C. w/Codeine Phosphate
Arthralgen
Ascriptin w/Codeine
Aspirin Compound w/Codeine
Astramorph
Astramorph-PF
Axotal
Bancap w/Codeine
Banesin Forte
BUTORPHANOL
Calcidrine
Calcidrine Syrup
Capital w/Codeine
Cetro Cirose
Cheracol
Coastaldyne
Coastalgesic
Codalan
Codalex
Codap
CODEINE
Codeine Sulfate
Codimal PH
Coditrate
Codone
Colrex Compound
Copavin
Corutol DH
Cotussis
Co-Xan
Dapase
Darvocet-N 100
Darvon
Darvon-N
Demer-Idine
Demerol
Depronal-SA
Dialog
Dicodid
Dihydromorphinone
Dilaudid
Dilaudid-HP
Dimetane-DC
Dimetane Expectorant-DC
Dolene
Dolophine
Dolor
Doloxene
Doxaphene
Dromoran
Dularin
Duramorph PF
Dynosal
Empirin w/Codeine
Empracet w/Codeine
Emprazil-C
Ephedrol w/Codeine
Epimorph
Esgic
FL-Tussex
Fiorinal w/Codeine
Fortral
Gaysal
G-2
G-3
Hasacode
Hycodan
Hycotuss
HYDROCODONE
HYDROMORPHONE
Isoclor
Laudanum
Levo-Dromoran
Levorphan
LEVORPHANOL

Liquix-C
Lo-Tussin
Maxigesic
Mepergan Fortis
MEPERIDINE
METHADONE
Methadose
Metrogesic
Minotal
MORPHINE
Morphitec
M.O.S.
M.O.S. Syrup
MS Contin
MSIR
MST Continus
NALBUPHINE
Novahistine DH
Novahistine Expectorant
Novopropoxyn
Nubain
Numorphan
OPIUM
Ossonate-Plus
OXYCODONE
OXYMORPHONE
Pantapon
PAREGORIC
Pargesic
Pavadon
Paveral
Pediacof
PENTAZOCINE
Percodan
Pethadol
Pethidine
Phenaphen w/Codeine
Phenergan
Phrenilin
Physeptone
Poly-Histine w/Codeine
Presalin
Prodolor
Profene
Promethazine HCl w/Codeine
PROPOXYPHENE
Pro-65
Proxagesic
Proxene
Prunicodeine
RMS Uniserts
Robidone
Robitussin A-C
Roxanol
Roxanol SR
Roxicodone
S-A-C
Salatin
Saleto
Salimeph Forte
Sedapap
SK-65
SK-APAP w/Codeine
Soma Compound w/Codeine
Sorbase II
Stadol
Statex
Strascogesic
Supac
Supeudol
Sylapar
Synalgos-DC
Talwin
Talwin-NX
Terpin Hydrate w/Codeine
Triaminic w/Codeine
Trigesic
Tussar
Tussend
Tussi-Organidin
Tylenol w/Codeine
Tylox
Vicodin
Wygesic

NARCOTIC ANALGESICS & ASPIRIN

222
282
292
293
692
A&C with Codeine
A.C.&C.
Anacin with Codeine
Ancasal
Anexsia with Codeine
Anexsia-D
A.S.A. and Codeine Compound
Ascriptin with Codeine
ASPIRIN & CODEINE
ASPIRIN, CODEINE & CAFFEINE
Bexophene
BUFFERED ASPIRIN & CODEINE
Codoxy
Coryphen with Codeine
C2 with Codeine
C2 Buffered with Codeine
Damason-P
Darvon Compound
Darvon-N Compound
Darvon with A.S.A.
Darvon-N with A.S.A.
Dolene Compound
Doxaphene Compound
Drocade and Aspirin
DROCODE, ASPIRIN & CAFFEINE
Emcodeine
Empirin with Codeine
HYDROCODONE, ASPIRIN & CAFFEINE
Instantine Plus
Novo AC&C
Oxycodan
OXYCODONE & ASPIRIN
PENTAZOCINE & ASPIRIN
Percodan
Percodan-Demi
PROPOXYPHENE & ASPIRIN
PROPOXYPHENE ASPIRIN & CAFFEINE
SK-65 Compound
SK-Oxycodone with Aspirin
Synalgos-DC
Talwin Compound
Talwin Compound-50

NITRATES

AMYL NITRITE
Ang-O-Span
Apo-ISDN
Cardilate
Coronex
Deponit
Dilatrate SR
Duotrate
ERYTHRITYL TETRANITRATE
Iso-Bid
Isochron
Isonate
Isonate TR
Isordil
ISOSORBIDE DINITRATE
Isotrate
Klavikordal
Naptrate

N-G-C
Niong
Nitro-Bid
Nitrobon
Nitrocap
Nitrocap T.D.
Nitrocardin
Nitrodisc
Nitro-Dir
Nitro-Dur II
Nitrogard
Nitrogard SR
NITROGLYCERIN
Nitroglyn
Nitrol
Nitrolin
Nitrolingual
Nitro-Long
Nitronet
Nitrong
Nitrong SR
Nitrospan
Nitrostabilin
Nitrostat
Nitro-Time
Novosorbide
NTS
Onset
PENTAERYTHRITOL TETRANITRATE
Pentol
Pentol S.A.
Pentraspan SR
Pentritol
Pentylan
Peritrate
Peritrate Forte
Peritrate SA
Sorate
Sorbide T.D.
Sorbitrate
Sorbitrate SA
Transderm-Nitro
Tridil

PENICILLINS

Amcill
AMDINOCILLIN
AMOXICILLIN
AMOXICILLIN & CLAVULANATE
Amoxil
AMPICILLIN
Ampicin
Ampilean
Apo-Amoxi
Apo-Ampi
Apo-Cloxi
Apo-Pen-VK
Augmentin
Ayercillin
Azlin
AZLOCILLIN
BACAMPICILLIN
Bactocill
Baypen
Beepen-VK
Betapen-VK
Bicillin
Bicillin L-A
CARBENICILLIN
Clavulin
CLOXACILLIN
Cloxapen
Coactin
Crystapen
Crysticillin
CYCLACILLIN
Cyclapen-W
DICLOXACILLIN
Duracillin A.S.
Dycill
Dynapen
Geocillin
Geopen
Geopen Oral
Ledercillin VK
Mecillinam
Megacillin
METHICILLIN
Mezlin
MEZLOCILLIN
NAFCILLIN
NaMPICIL
Nadopen-V
Nafcil
Nallpen
Novamoxin
Novoampicillin
Novocloxin
Novopen-G
Novopen-VK
Omnipen
Omnipen-N
Orbenin
OXACILLIN
P-50
Pathocil
Pen Vee K
Penapar VK
Penbritin
Penglobe
PENICILLIN G
PENICILLIN V
Penioral
Pentids
Permapen
Pfizerpen
Pfizerpen G
Pfizerpen-AS
PIPERACILLIN
Pipracil
Polycillin
Polycillin-N
Polymox
Principen
Prostaphlin
PVF K
Pyopen
Robicillin VK
SK-Penicillin G
Spectrobid
Staphcillin
Sumox
Supen
Tegopen
Ticar
TICARCILLIN
TICARCILLIN & CLAVULANATE
Timentin
Totacillin
Totacillin-N
Trimox
Unipen
Utimox
V-Cillin K
VC-K
Veetids
Wycillin
Wymox

POTASSIUM SUPPLEMENTS

Apo-K
Bayon
Bi-K
Cena-K
K-10
Kalium Durules
Kaochlor
Kaochlor-Eff
Kaochlor S-F
Kaon
Kaon-Cl

Kao-Nor
Kato
Kay Ciel
Kaylixir
KCL
K-Dur
K-G Elixir
K-Long
K-Lor
Klor-10%
Klor-Con
Klor-Con/25
Klor-Con/EF
Klorvess
Klotrix
K-Lyte
K-Lyte/Cl
K-Lyte DS
K-Lyte/Cl Powder
Kolyum
K-Tab
Micro-K
Neo-K
Novolente-K
Potachlor
Potage
Potasalan
Potassine
POTASSIUM ACETATE
POTASSIUM BICARBONATE
POTASSIUM BICARBONATE & POTASSIUM CHLORIDE
POTASSIUM BICARBONATE & POTASSIUM CITRATE
POTASSIUM CHLORIDE
POTASSIUM CHLORIDE, POTASSIUM BICARBONATE & POTASSIUM CITRATE
POTASSIUM GLUCONATE
POTASSIUM GLUCONATE & POTASSIUM CHLORIDE
POTASSIUM GLUCONATE & POTASSIUM CITRATE
POTASSIUM GLUCONATE, POTASSIUM CITRATE & AMMONIUM CHLORIDE
Potassium-Rougier
Potassium-Sandoz
Roychlor
Royonate
Rum-K
Slo-Pot
Slow-K
Ten-K
Tri-K
TRIKATES
Twin-K
Twin-K-Cl

PROGESTINS

Aygestin
Lo-Ovral
Micronor
Modicon 21
Nor-O.D.
Nor-Q.D.
Norinyl 1+35 21-Day Tablets
Norlestrin
Norlutate
Norlutate Acetate
Norlutin
Ortho-Novum 1/35
Ovcon
Ovral
Ovrette
Tri-Norinyl

SULFONAMIDES

Apo-Sulfamethoxazole
Apo-Sulfatrim
Azo Gantanol
Bactrim
Cetamide
Co-trimoxazole
Cotrim
Cotrim D.S.
Gantanol
Gantrisin
Lipo-Gantrisin
Methoxanol
Novosoxazole
Novotrimel
Protrin
Renoquid
Roubac
Septra
SK-Soxazole
SMZ-TMP
SULFACYTINE
Sulfafurazole
Sulfamethoprim
SULFAMETHOXAZOLE
SULFAMETHOXAZOLE & TRIMETHOPRIM
SULFISOXAZOLE
Sulmeprim

TETRACYCLINES

Achromycin
Achromycin V
Achrostatin V
Apo-Tetra
Bicycline
Bio-Tetra
Bristacycline
Cefracycline
Centet
Comycin
Cyclopar
Declomycin
DEMECLOCYCLINE
Desamycin
Doxy
Doxy-Caps
Doxychel
DOXYCYCLINE
Doxy-Lemmon
Doxy-Tabs
Fed-Mycin
G-Mycin
Kesso-Tetra
Lemtrex
Maytrex-BID
Medicycline
METHACYCLINE
Minocin
MINOCYCLINE
Muracine
Mysteclin F
Neo-Tetrine
Nor-tet
Novotetra
Oxlopar
Oxy-Kesso-Tetra
OXYTETRACYCLINE
Paltet
Panmycin
Piracaps
PMS Tetracycline
Q'Dtet
Retet
Retet-S
Robitet
Ro-Cycline
Rondomycine
Sarocyclin
Scotrex
SK-Tetracycline
Sumycin
T-Caps
TETRACYCLINE
Terramycin

Tet-Cy
Tetet
Tetrachel
Tetra-Co
Tetracrine
Tetracyn
Tetracyrine
Tetralean
Tetram
Tetramax
Tetramine
Tetrastatin M
Tetrex
Tetrex-S
Topicycline
Trexin
Ultramycin
Urobiotic
Vibramycin
Vibratabs

TRICYCLIC ANTIDEPRESSANTS

Adapin
Amitid
Amitril
AMITRIPTYLINE
AMOXAPINE
Anafranil
Anemtyl
Apo-Amitriptyline
Apo-Imipramine
Ascendin
Aventyl
CLOMIPRAMINE
DESIPRAMINE
DOXEPIN
Elavil
Emitrip
Endep
Enovil
Etrafon
IMIPRAMINE
Impril
Janimine
Levate
Meravil
Norpramin
NORTRIPTYLINE
Novopramine
Novotriptyn
Pamelor
Pertofrane
Presamine
PROTRIPTYLINE
Sinequan
SK-Amitriptyline
SK-Pramine
Surmontil
Tipramine
Tofranil
Tofranil-PM
Triadapin
Triavil
TRIMIPRAMINE
Triptil
Vivactil

VITAMIN B-12 (CYANOCOBALAMIN)

Acti-B-12
Alphamin
Alpha Redisol
Anocobin
Bedoz
Berubigen
Betalin 12
Betalin 12 Crystalline
Codroxomin
Cyanabin
Droxomin
Kaybovite
Kaybovite-1000
Neo-Betalin
Neo-Rubex
Redisol
Rubion
Rubramin
Rubramin-PC
Sytobex
Numerous other multiple vitamin-mineral supplements.

VITAMIN C (ASCORBIC ACID)

Adenex
Apo-C
Arco-Cee
Ascorbajen
Ascorbicap
Ascoril
Calscorbate
Cecon
Cemill
Cenolate
Ceri-Bid
Cetane
Cevalin
Cevi-Bid
Ce-Vi-Sol
Cevita
C-Ject
Flavorcee
Liqui-Cee
Megascorb
Redoxon
Numerous other multiple vitamin-mineral supplements.

XANTHINE BRONCHODILATORS

Accurbron
Aerolate
Aerophylline
Airet
Amesec
Aminodur
Aminodur Dura-tabs
Aminophyl
Aminophyllin
AMINOPHYLLINE
Aminophylline and Amytal
Aminophylline-Phenobarbital
Amodrine
Amoline
Amophylline
Apo-Oxtriphylline
Aquaphyllin
Asbron
Asma
Asmalix
Asminyl
Asthmophylline
Bronchobid Duracaps
Broncholate
Brondecon
Brondilate
Bronkodyl
Bronkodyl S-R
Bronkolixir
Bronkotabs
Brosema
Choledyl
Choledyl SA
Chophylline
Constant-T
Corophyllin
Corophylline
Co-Xan
Dilin
Dilor
Dilor-G
Droxine

Droxine L.A.
Droxine S.F.
Duovent
Duraphyl
Dyflex
Dyline
DYPHILLINE
Dy-Phyl-Lin
Elixicon
Elixomin
Elixophyllin
Elixophyllin SR
Emfaseem
G-Bron
Iso-Asminyl
Isuprel Compound
Klophyllin
LABID
Lanophyllin
Liquophylline
Lixaminol
Lixaminol AT
Lixolin
Lodrane
Luasmin
Luftodil
Lufyllin
Marax
Marax DF
Mersalyl-Theophylline
Mini-Lix
Mudrane
Neospect
Neothylline
Neothylline-G
Novotriphyl
Numa-Dura-Tabs
Orthoxine & Aminophylline
OXTRIPHYLLINE
Oxystat
Palaron
Phenylin
Phyldrox
Phyllocontin
Physpan
PMS Theophylline
Primatene, M Formula
Primatene, P Formula
Protophylline
Pulmophylline
Quadrinal
Quibron
Quibron Plus
Quibron-T
Quibron-T Dividose
Quibron-T/SR Dividose
Respbid
Slo-Phyllin GG
Slo-Phyllin Gyrocaps
Slo-bid Gyrocaps
Slophyllin
Somophyllin
Somophyllin-12
Somophyllin-CRT
Somophyllin-DF
Somophyllin-T
Sudolin
Sustaire
Synophylate
Synophylate-GG
Tedfern
Tedral
T.E.H.
Thalfed
Theobid
Theobid Duracaps
Theobid Jr. Duracaps
Theochron
Theoclear
Theoclear L.A. Cenules
Theo-Dur
Theo-Dur Sprinkle
Theofedral
Theo-Guaia
Theolair
Theolair-Plus
Theolair-SR
Theolixir
Theon
Theo-Nar 100
Theo-Organidin
Theophyl
Theophyl-SR
THEOPHYLLINE
Theophylline Choline
Theospan
Theospan SR
Theostat
Theostate 80
Theotabs
Theo-Time
Theo-24
Theovent Long-acting
Theozine
Truphylline
Uniphyl

ADDITIONAL DRUG INTERACTIONS

The following list of drugs and their interactions with other drugs are continuations of lists found in the alphabetized drug charts. These lists are alphabetized by generic name or drug class name, shown in large capital letters. Only those lists too long for the drug charts are included in this section. For complete information about any generic drug, see the alphabetical charts.

ANTICOAGULANTS, ORAL

GENERIC NAME OR DRUG CLASS	COMBINED EFFECT
Calcium supplements	Decreased anticoagulant effect.
Carbamazepine	Decreased effect of anticoagulant.
Fluoxetine	May cause confusion, agitation, convulsions and high blood pressure. Avoid combining.
Griseofulvin	Decreased effect of anticoagulant.
Non-steroidal anti-inflammatory drugs (NSAIDs, see Drugs Glossary)	Increased risk of bleeding.
Phenytoin	Decreased phenytoin levels.
Rifampin	Decreased effect of anticoagulant.
Suprofen	Increased risk of bleeding.
Vitamin K	Decreased effect of anticoagulant.

ANTICONVULSANTS, HYDANTOIN

GENERIC NAME OR DRUG CLASS	COMBINED EFFECT
Furosemide	Decreased furosemide effect.
Gold compounds (see Drugs Glossary)	Increased phenytoin blood levels. Phenytoin dose may require adjustment.
Griseofulvin	Increased griseofulvin effect.
Hypoglycemics (oral, see Drugs Glossary)	Possible decreased hypoglycemic effect.
Isoniazid	Increased phenytoin effect.
Leucovorin	May counteract the effect of phenytoin or any hydantoin anticonvulsant.
Loxapine	Decreased anticonvulsant effect of phenytoin or any hydantoin anticonvulsant.
MAO inhibitors (see Drugs Glossary)	Increased polythiazide effect.
Methadone	Decreased methadone effect.
Methylphenidate	Increased phenytoin effect.
Molindone	Increased phenytoin effect.
Nitrates (see Drugs Glossary)	Excessive blood-pressure drop.
Oxyphenbutazone	Increased phenytoin effect.
Para-aminosalicylic acid (PAS)	Increased phenytoin effect.
Phenothiazines (see Drugs Glossary)	Increased phenytoin effect.
Phenylbutazone	Increased phenytoin effect.
Potassium supplements (see Drugs Glossary)	Decreased potassium effect.
Probenecid	Decreased probenecid effect.
Propranolol	Increased propranolol effect.
Quinidine	Increased quinidine effect.

ADDITIONAL DRUG INTERACTIONS

GENERIC NAME OR DRUG CLASS	COMBINED EFFECT	GENERIC NAME OR DRUG CLASS	COMBINED EFFECT

ANTICONVULSANTS, HYDANTOIN Continued

GENERIC NAME OR DRUG CLASS	COMBINED EFFECT	GENERIC NAME OR DRUG CLASS	COMBINED EFFECT
Sedatives (see Drugs Glossary)	Increased sedative effect.	**Theophylline**	Reduced anticonvulsant effect.
Sulfa drugs (see Drugs Glossary)	Increased phenytoin effect.	**Trimethoprim**	Increased phenytoin effect.
		Valproic acid	Unpredictable change in seizure control.

ASPIRIN

GENERIC NAME OR DRUG CLASS	COMBINED EFFECT	GENERIC NAME OR DRUG CLASS	COMBINED EFFECT
Furosemide	Possible aspirin toxicity. May decrease furosemide effect.	**Phenobarbital**	Decreased aspirin effect.
Gold compounds (see Drugs Glossary)	Increased likelihood of kidney damage.	**Phenytoin**	Increased phenytoin effect.
Indomethacin	Risk of stomach bleeding and ulcers.	**Probenecid**	Decreased probenecid effect.
Ketoprofen	Increased risk of stomach ulcer.	**Propranolol**	Decreased aspirin effect.
Methotrexate	Increased methotrexate effect.	**Rauwolfia alkaloids (see Drugs Glossary)**	Decreased aspirin effect.
Minoxidil	Decreased minoxidil effect.	**Salicylates (other)**	Likely aspirin toxicity.
Non-steroidal anti-inflammatory drugs (NSAIDs, see Drugs Glossary)	Risk of stomach bleeding and ulcers.	**Spironolactone**	Decreased spironolactone effect.
Oxprenolol	Decreased antihypertensive effect of oxprenolol.	**Sulfinpyrazone**	Decreased sulfinpyrazone effect.
Para-aminosalicylic acid (PAS)	Possible aspirin toxicity.	**Terfenadine**	May conceal symptoms of aspirin overdose, such as ringing in ears.
Penicillins (see Drugs Glossary)	Increased effect of both drugs.	**Vitamin C (large doses)**	Possible aspirin toxicity.
		Valproic acid	May increase valproic acid effect.

BARBITURATES

GENERIC NAME OR DRUG CLASS	COMBINED EFFECT	GENERIC NAME OR DRUG CLASS	COMBINED EFFECT
Molindone	Increased sedative effect.	**Non-steroidal anti-inflammatory drugs (NSAIDs, see Drugs Glossary)**	Decreased anti-inflammatory effect.
Narcotics (see Drugs Glossary)	Dangerous sedation. Avoid.	**Pain relievers (see Drugs Glossary)**	Dangerous sedation. Avoid.

ADDITIONAL DRUG INTERACTIONS

BARBITURATES Continued

GENERIC NAME OR DRUG CLASS	COMBINED EFFECT
Quinidine	Decreased quinidine effect.
Rifampin	Possible decreased barbiturate effect.
Sedatives (see Drugs Glossary)	Dangerous sedation. Avoid.
Sleep inducers (see Drugs Glossary)	Dangerous sedation. Avoid.
Tranquilizers (see Drugs Glossary)	Dangerous sedation. Avoid.
Valproic acid	Increased barbiturate effect.

BELLADONNA ALKALOIDS & BARBITURATES

GENERIC NAME OR DRUG CLASS	COMBINED EFFECT
Cortisone drugs (see Drugs Glossary)	Increased internal-eye pressure. Decreased cortisone effect.
Digitoxin	Decreased digitoxin effect.
Doxycycline	Decreased doxycycline effect.
Dronabinol	Increased effects of both drugs. Avoid.
Furosemide	Possible orthostatic hypotension.
Griseofulvin	Decreased griseofulvin effect.
Haloperidol	Increased internal-eye pressure.
Indapamide	Increased indapamide effect.
MAO inhibitors (see Drugs Glossary)	Increased belladonna and barbiturate effect.
Meperidine	Increased belladonna effect.
Methylphenidate	Increased belladonna effect.
Metronidazole	Decreased metronidazole effect.
Mind-altering drugs (see Drugs Glossary)	Dangerous sedation. Avoid.
Narcotics (see Drugs Glossary)	Dangerous sedation. Avoid.
Nitrates (see Drugs Glossary)	Increased internal-eye pressure.
Non-steroidal anti-inflammatory drugs (NSAIDs, see Drugs Glossary)	Decreased anti-inflammatory effect.
Orphenadrine	Increased belladonna effect.
Pain relievers (see Drugs Glossary)	Dangerous sedation. Avoid.
Phenothiazines (see Drugs Glossary)	Increased belladonna effect. Danger of oversedation.
Pilocarpine	Loss of pilocarpine effect in glaucoma treatment.
Potassium supplements (see Drugs Glossary)	Possible intestinal ulcers with oral potassium tablets.
Quinidine	Increased belladonna effect.
Sedatives (see Drugs Glossary)	Dangerous sedation. Avoid.
Sleep inducers (see Drugs Glossary)	Dangerous sedation. Avoid.
Tranquilizers (see Drugs Glossary)	Dangerous sedation. Avoid.
Valproic acid	Increased barbiturate effect.
Vitamin C	Decreased belladonna effect. Avoid large doses of vitamin C.

BETA-ADRENERGIC BLOCKING AGENTS

GENERIC NAME OR DRUG CLASS	COMBINED EFFECT
Indomethacin	Decreased effect of beta-adrenergic blockers.
Insulin	Hypoglycemic effects may be prolonged.
Levobunolol eyedrops	Possible increased beta-adrenergic blocker effect.
Molindone	Increased tranquilizer effect.
Narcotics (see Drugs Glossary)	Increased narcotic effect. Dangerous sedation.
Nitrates (see Drugs Glossary)	Possible excessive blood-pressure drop.
Non-steroidal anti-inflammatory drugs (NSAIDs, see Drugs Glossary)	Decreased antihypertensive effect of beta-adrenergic blockers.
Phenytoin	Decreased beta-adrenergic blocker effect.
Quinidine	Slows heart excessively.
Reserpine	Increased reserpine effect. Excessive sedation and depression.
Rifampin	Decreased beta-adrenergic blocker effect.
Timolol eyedrops	Possible increased beta-adrenergic blocker effect.
Tocainide	May worsen congestive heart failure.
Verapamil	Increased effects of both drugs.

BETA-ADRENERGIC BLOCKING AGENTS & THIAZIDE DIURETICS

GENERIC NAME OR DRUG CLASS	COMBINED EFFECT
Antihypertensives (see Drugs Glossary)	Increased antihypertensive effect.
Barbiturates (see Drugs Glossary)	Increased barbiturate effect. Dangerous sedation.
Beta-adrenergic blockers (see Drugs Glossary)	Increased antihypertensive effect. Dosages of both drugs may require adjustments.
Bumetanide	Increased diuretic effect.
Cholestyramine	Decreased hydrochlorothiazide effect.
Cortisone drugs (see Drugs Glossary)	Excessive potassium loss that causes dangerous heart rhythms.
Digitalis preparations (see Drugs Glossary)	Excessive potassium loss that causes dangerous heart rhythms. Can either increase or decrease heart rate. Improves irregular heartbeat.
Diuretics (thiazide, see Drugs Glossary)	Increased effect of other thiazide diuretics.
Ethacrynic acid	Increased diuretic effect.
Furosemide	Increased diuretic effect.
Guanfacine	Increased effect of both drugs.
Hypoglycemics (oral, see Drugs Glossary)	Decreased ability to lower blood glucose.
Indapamide	Increased diuretic effect.
Insulin	Decreased ability to lower blood glucose.

ADDITIONAL DRUG INTERACTIONS

BETA-ADRENERGIC BLOCKING AGENTS & THIAZIDE DIURETICS continued

GENERIC NAME OR DRUG CLASS	COMBINED EFFECT
MAO inhibitors (see Drugs Glossary)	Increased hydrochlorothiazide effect.
Metolazone	Increased diuretic effect.
Narcotics (see Drugs Glossary)	Increased narcotic effect. Dangerous sedation.
Nitrates (see Drugs Glossary)	Excessive blood-pressure drop.
Non-steroidal anti-inflammatory drugs (NSAIDs, see Drugs Glossary)	Decreased anti-inflammatory effect.
Phenytoin	Increased beta-adrenergic effect.
Potassium supplements (see Drugs Glossary)	Decreased potassium effect.
Probenecid	Decreased probenecid effect.
Quinidine	Slows heart excessively.
Reserpine	Increased reserpine effect. Excessive sedation and depression.
Tocainide	May worsen congestive heart failure.

BUTALBITAL & ASPIRIN (Also contains caffeine)

GENERIC NAME OR DRUG CLASS	COMBINED EFFECT
Beta-adrenergic blockers (see Drugs Glossary)	Decreased effect of beta-adrenergic blocker.
Contraceptives (oral, see Drugs Glossary)	Decreased contraceptive effect.
Cortisone drugs (see Drugs Glossary)	Increased cortisone effect. Risk of ulcer and stomach bleeding.
Digitoxin	Decreased digitoxin effect.
Doxycycline	Decreased doxycycline effect.
Dronabinol	Increased effect of both drugs.
Furosemide	Possible aspirin toxicity.
Gold compounds (see Drugs Glossary)	Increased likelihood of kidney damage.
Griseofulvin	Decreased griseofulvin effect.
Indapamide	Increased indapamide effect.
Indomethacin	Risk of stomach bleeding and ulcers.
MAO inhibitors (see Drugs Glossary)	Increased butalbital effect.
Methotrexate	Increased methotrexate effect.
Mind-altering drugs (see Drugs Glossary)	Dangerous sedation. Avoid.
Minoxidil	Decreased minoxidil effect.
Narcotics (see Drugs Glossary)	Dangerous sedation. Avoid.
Non-steroidal anti-inflammatory drugs (NSAIDs, see Drugs Glossary)	Risk of stomach bleeding and ulcers.
Pain relievers (see Drugs Glossary)	Dangerous sedation. Avoid.
Rifampin	May decrease butalbital effect.
Salicylates (others) (see Drugs Glossary)	Likely aspirin toxicity.
Sedatives (see Drugs Glossary)	Dangerous sedation. Avoid.
Sleep inducers (see Drugs Glossary)	Dangerous sedation. Avoid.
Spironolactone	Decreased spironolactone effect.
Sulfinpyrazone	Decreased sulfinpyrazone effect.

BUTALBITAL & ASPIRIN (Also contains caffeine) Continued

GENERIC NAME OR DRUG CLASS	COMBINED EFFECT
Terfenadine	May conceal symptoms of aspirin overdose, such as ringing in ears.
Tranquilizers (see Drugs Glossary)	Dangerous sedation. Avoid.
Valproic acid	Increased butalbital effect.
Vitamin C (large doses)	Possible aspirin toxicity.

CALCIUM CHANNEL BLOCKING AGENTS

GENERIC NAME OR DRUG CLASS	COMBINED EFFECT
Disopyramide	May cause dangerously slow, fast or irregular heartbeat.
Diuretics (see Drugs Glossary)	Dangerous blood-pressure drop.
Lithium	Possible decreased lithium effect.
Nitrates	Reduced angina attacks.
Phenytoin	Possible decreased calcium channel blocker effect.
Quinidine	Increased quinidine effect.
Rifampin	Decreased calcium channel blocker effect.
Theophylline	May increase theophylline effect and toxicity.
Tocainide	Increased likelihood of adverse reactions from either drug.
Vitamin D (large doses)	Decreased calcium channel blocker effect.

CAPTOPRIL & HYDROCHLOROTHIAZIDE

GENERIC NAME OR DRUG CLASS	COMBINED EFFECT
Non-steroidal anti-inflammatory drugs (NSAIDs, see Drugs Glossary)	Decreased captopril effect.
Potassium supplements (see Drugs Glossary)	Excessive potassium in blood.
Probenecid	Decreased probenecid effect.
Spironolactone	Possible excessive potassium in blood.
Triamterene	Possible excessive potassium in blood.

CARBAMAZEPINE

GENERIC NAME OR DRUG CLASS	COMBINED EFFECT
Guanfacine	May increase depressant effects of either drug.
Isonicotinic hydrazide (INH)	May increase carbamazepine effect.
Leucovorin	High alcohol content of leucovorin may cause adverse effects.
MAO inhibitors (see Drugs Glossary)	Dangerous overstimulation. Avoid.
Mebendazole	Decreased effect of mebendazole.
Methyprylon	Increased sedative effect, perhaps to dangerous level. Avoid.
Phenytoin	Decreased carbamazepine effect.
Phenobarbital	Decreased carbamazepine effect.
Primidone	Decreased carbamazepine effect.
Tranquilizers (benzodiazepine, see Drugs Glossary)	Increased carbamazepine effect.
Verapamil	Possible increased carbamazepine effect.

ADDITIONAL DRUG INTERACTIONS

GENERIC NAME OR DRUG CLASS	COMBINED EFFECT
CIMETIDINE	
Morphine	Increased effect and toxicity of morphine.
Phenytoin	Increased effect and toxicity of phenytoin.
Procainamide	Increased effect and toxicity of procainamide.
Propranolol	May increase propranolol effect.
Quinidine	Increased quinidine effect.
Theophylline	Increased theophylline effect.
Triazolam	Increased effect and toxicity of triazolam.
Verapamil	Increased effect and toxicity of verapamil.
CLONIDINE	
Guanfacine	Blood-pressure control impaired.
Leucovorin	High alcohol content of leucovorin may cause adverse effects.
Methyprylon	Increased sedative effect, perhaps to dangerous level. Avoid.
Nitrates	Possible excessive blood-pressure drop.
DIGITALIS PREPARATIONS	
Quinidine	Increased digitalis effect.
Rauwolfia alkaloids (see Drugs Glossary)	Increased digitalis effect.
Rifampin	Possible decreased digitalis effect.
Sulfasalazine	Decreased digitalis absorption.
Tetracycline	May increase digitalis absorption.
Thyroid hormones	Digitalis toxicity.
Trazodone	Possible increased digitalis toxicity.
Triamterene	Possible decreased digitalis effect.
Verapamil	Increased digitalis effect.
DIURETICS, LOOP	
Diuretics (other, see Drugs Glossary)	Increased diuretic effect.
Insulin	Decreased insulin effect.
Lithium	Increased lithium toxicity.
Narcotics	Dangerous low blood pressure. Avoid.
Nitrates	Excessive blood-pressure drop.
Non-steroidal anti-inflammatory drugs (NSAIDs, see Drugs Glossary)	Decreased loop diuretic effect.
Phenytoin	Decreased loop diuretic effect.
Potassium supplements (see Drugs Glossary)	Decreased potassium effect.
Probenecid	Decreased probenecid effect.
Salicylates (including aspirin)	Dangerous salicylate retention.
Sedatives (see Drugs Glossary)	Increased loop diuretic effect.

ADDITIONAL DRUG INTERACTIONS

DIURETICS, THIAZIDE

GENERIC NAME OR DRUG CLASS	COMBINED EFFECT
Nitrates	Excessive blood-pressure drop.
Opiates	Dizziness or weakness when standing up after sitting or lying down.
Oxprenolol	Increased antihypertensive effect. Dosages of both drugs may require adjustments.
Potassium supplements (see Drugs Glossary)	Decreased potassium effect.
Probenecid	Decreased probenecid effect.

ENALAPRIL & HYDROCHLOROTHIAZIDE

GENERIC NAME OR DRUG CLASS	COMBINED EFFECT
Potassium supplements (see Drugs Glossary)	Possible increased potassium in blood.
Probenecid	Decreased probenecid effect.
Spironolactone	Possible excessive potassium in blood.
Triamterene	Possible excessive potassium in blood.

METHYLDOPA & THIAZIDE DIURETICS

GENERIC NAME OR DRUG CLASS	COMBINED EFFECT
Cholestyamine	Decreased hydrochlorothiazide effect.
Cortisone drugs	Excessive potassium loss that causes dangerous heart rhythms.
Digitalis preparations (see Drugs Glossary)	Excessive potassium loss that causes dangerous heart rhythms.
Diuretics (thiazide, see Drugs Glossary)	Increased effect of both drugs.
Haloperidol	Increased sedation, possibly dementia.
Indapamide	Increased diuretic effect.
Levodopa	Increased effect of both drugs.
Lithium	Increased lithium effect.
MAO inhibitors (see Drugs Glossary)	Dangerous blood-pressure changes.
Nitrates (see Drugs Glossary)	Excessive blood-pressure drop.
Phenobenzanine	Urinary retention.
Potassium supplements (see Drugs Glossary)	Decreased potassium effect.
Propranolol	Increased blood pressure (rarely).
Tolbutamide	Increased tolbutamide effect.

NARCOTIC ANALGESICS

GENERIC NAME OR DRUG CLASS	COMBINED EFFECT
Guanfacine	May increase depressant effects of either drug.
Leucovorin	High alcohol content of leucovorin may cause adverse effects.
MAO inhibitors (see Drugs Glossary)	Serious toxicity (including death).
Methyprylon	Increased sedative effect, perhaps to dangerous level. Avoid.
Mind-altering drugs (see Drugs Glossary)	Increased sedative effect.
Molindone	Increased narcotic effect.

ADDITIONAL DRUG INTERACTIONS

GENERIC NAME OR DRUG CLASS	COMBINED EFFECT
NARCOTIC ANALGESICS Continued	
Nalbuphine	Possibly precipitates withdrawal with chronic narcotic use.
Naltrexone	Precipitates withdrawal symptoms. May lead to respiratory arrest, coma and death.
Narcotics (other, see Drugs Glossary)	Increased narcotic effect.
Nitrates (see Drugs Glossary)	Excessive blood-pressure drop.
Non-steroidal anti-inflammatory drugs (NSAIDs, see Drugs Glossary)	Increased narcotic effect.
Pentazocine	Possibly precipitates withdrawal with chronic narcotic use.
Phenothiazines (see Drugs Glossary)	Increased sedative effect.
Phenytoin	Possible decreased narcotic effect.
Rifampin	Possible decreased narcotic effect.
Sedatives (see Drugs Glossary)	Increased sedative effect.
Sleep inducers (see Drugs Glossary)	Increased sedative effect.
Tranquilizers (see Drugs Glossary)	Increased sedative effect.

NARCOTIC ANALGESICS & ASPIRIN

GENERIC NAME OR DRUG CLASS	COMBINED EFFECT
Furosemide	Possible aspirin toxicity. May decrease furosemide effect.
Gold compounds (see Drugs Glossary)	Increased likelihood of kidney damage.
Indomethacin	Risk of stomach bleeding and ulcers.
Ketoprofen	Increased risk of stomach ulcer.
Methotrexate	Increased methotrexate effect.
Minoxidil	Decreased minoxidil effect.
Non-steroidal anti-inflammatory drugs (NSAIDs, see Drugs Glossary)	Risk of stomach bleeding and ulcers.
Oxprenolol	Decreased antihypertensive effect of oxprenolol.
Para-aminosalicylic acid (PAS)	Possible aspirin toxicity.
Penicillins (see Drugs Glossary)	Increased effect of both drugs.
Phenobarbital	Decreased aspirin effect.
Phenytoin	Increased phenytoin effect.
Probenecid	Decreased probenecid effect.
Propranolol	Decreased aspirin effect.
Rauwolfia alkaloids (see Drugs Glossary)	Decreased aspirin effect.
Salicylates (other)	Likely aspirin toxicity.
Phenobarbital	Decreased aspirin effect.
Phenytoin	Increased phenytoin effect.
Probenecid	Decreased probenecid effect.
Propranolol	Decreased aspirin effect.
Rauwolfia alkaloids (see Drugs Glossary)	Decreased aspirin effect.
Salicylates (other, see Drugs Glossary)	Likely aspirin toxicity.
Sedatives (see Drugs Glossary)	Increased sedative effect.
Sleep inducers (see Drugs Glossary)	Increased sedative effect. Sleep inducer.

NARCOTIC ANALGESICS & ASPIRIN Continued

GENERIC NAME OR DRUG CLASS	COMBINED EFFECT
Spironolactone	Decreased spironolactone effect.
Sulfinpyrazone	Decreased sulfinpyrazone effect.
Terfenadine	Possible excessive sedation. May conceal symptoms of aspirin overdose, such as ringing in ears.
Tranquilizers (see Drugs Glossary)	Increased sedative effect.
Valproic acid	May increase valproic acid effect.
Vitamin C (large doses)	Possible aspirin toxicity.

PERPHENAZINE & AMITRIPTYLINE

GENERIC NAME OR DRUG CLASS	COMBINED EFFECT
Guanabenz	Possible decreased guanabenz effect.
Guanethidine	Decreased guanethidine effect.
Guanfacine	Possible decreased guanfacine effect.
Levodopa	Decreased levodopa effect.
Lithium	Possible decreased seizure threshold.
MAO inhibitors (see Drugs Glossary)	Fever, delirium, convulsions.
Methyldopa	Possible decreased methyldopa effect.
Methylphenidate	Possible increased antidepressant effect.
Mind-altering drugs (see Drugs Glossary)	Increased effect of mind-altering drugs.
Narcotics (see Drugs Glossary)	Increased narcotic effect and dangerous sedation.
Phenothiazines (see Drugs Glossary)	Possible increased antidepressant effect.
Procainamide	Possible irregular heartbeat.
Procarbazine	Increased sedation.
Quinidine	Impaired heart function. Dangerous mixture.
Sedatives (see Drugs Glossary)	Dangerous oversedation.
Sympathomimetics (see Drugs Glossary)	Increased sympathomimetics effect.
Thyroid hormones	Irregular heartbeat.
Tranquilizers (other, see Drugs Glossary)	Increased tranquilizer effect.

POTASSIUM SUPPLEMENTS

GENERIC NAME OR DRUG CLASS	COMBINED EFFECT
Digitalis preparations (see Drugs Glossary)	Possible irregular heartbeat.
Diuretics (thiazide, loop, see Drugs Glossary)	Decreased potassium effect.
Laxatives (see Drugs Glossary)	Possible decreased potassium effect.
Spironolactone	Dangerous rise in blood potassium.
Triamterene	Dangerous rise in blood potassium.
Vitamin B-12	Extended-release tablets may decrease vitamin B-12 absorption and increase vitamin B-12 requirements.

ADDITIONAL DRUG INTERACTIONS

TIMOLOL

GENERIC NAME OR DRUG CLASS	COMBINED EFFECT
Non-steroidal anti-inflammatory drugs (NSAIDs, see Drugs Glossary)	Decreased antihypertensive effect of timolol.

TRIAMTERINE & HYDROCHOLOROTHIAZIDE

GENERIC NAME OR DRUG CLASS	COMBINED EFFECT
Cortisone drugs (see Drugs Glossary)	Excessive potassium loss that causes dangerous heart rhythms.
Digitalis preparations (see Drugs Glossary)	Excessive potassium loss that causes dangerous heart rhythms.
Diuretics, thiazide (see Drugs Glossary)	Increased effect of other thiazide diuretics.
Indapamide	Increased diuretic effect.
Indomethacin	Possible acute renal failure.
Lithium	Increased lithium effect.
MAO inhibitors (see Drugs Glossary)	Increased hydrochlorothiazide effect.
Nitrates (see Drugs Glossary)	Excessive blood-pressure drop.
Opiates	Weakness and faintness when arising from bed or chair.
Potassium supplements	Possible excessive potassium retention.
(see Drugs Glossary)	Decreased potassium effect.
Probenecid	Decreased probenecid effect.
Spironolactone	Dangerous retention of potassium.

TRICYCLIC ANTIDEPRESSANTS

GENERIC NAME OR DRUG CLASS	COMBINED EFFECT
Guanabenz	Decreased guanabenz effect.
Guanfacine	May increase depressant effects of either drug.
Guanethidine	Decreased guanethidine effect.
Leucovorin	High alcohol content of leucovorin may cause adverse effects.
Levodopa	May increase blood pressure.
Lithium	Possible decreased seizure threshold.
Loxapine	May increase toxic effects of both drugs.
MAO inhibitors (see Drugs Glossary)	Fever, delirium, convulsions.
Methyprylon	Increased sedative effect, perhaps to dangerous level. Avoid.
Methyldopa	Possible decreased methyldopa effect.
Methylphenidate	Possible increased tricyclic antidepressant effect and toxicity.
Molindone	Increased molindone effect.
Narcotics (see Drugs Glossary)	Oversedation.
Phenothiazines (see Drugs Glossary)	Possible increased tricyclic antidepressant effect and toxicity.
Phenytoin	Decreased phenytoin effect.

GENERIC NAME OR DRUG CLASS	COMBINED EFFECT
TRICYCLIC ANTIDEPRESSANTS Continued	
Procainamide	Possible irregular heartbeat.
Quinidine	Possible irregular heartbeat.
Sedatives (see Drugs Glossary)	Dangerous oversedation.
Sympathomimetics (see Drugs Glossary)	Increased sympathomimetic effect.
Thyroid hormones	Irregular heartbeat.

DRUGS GLOSSARY

The following medical terms are found in the drug charts. Where drug names are listed, the generic or drug class is first, with brand names following in parentheses.

A

ACE Inhibitors—Angiotensin-Converting Enzyme (ACE)—A family of drugs used to treat hypertension and congestive heart failure. Inhibitors decrease the rate of conversion of Angiotensin I into Angiotensin II, which is the normal process for the angiotensin-converting enzyme. These drugs include: captopril (Capoten), enalapril (Vasotec), and lisinopril.

Acute—Having a short and relatively severe course.

Addiction—Psychological or physiological dependence upon a drug.

Addison's Disease—Changes in the body caused by a deficiency of hormones manufactured by the adrenal gland. Usually fatal if untreated. See chart in Illnesses section.

Adrenal Cortex—Outer layer of adrenal gland.

Adrenal Gland—Gland next to the kidney that produces cortisone and epinephrine (adrenalin).

Alkalizers—These drugs neutralize acidic properties of the blood and urine by making them more alkaline (or basic). Systemic alkalizers include: potassium citrate and citric acid, sodium bicarbonate, sodium citrate and citric acid, and tricitrates. Urinary alkalizers include: potassium citrate, potassium citrate and citric acid, potassium citrate and sodium citrate, sodium citrate and citric acid.

Alkylating Agent—Chemical used to treat malignant diseases.

Allergy—Excessive sensitivity to a substance.

Amebiasis—Infection with amoebas, one-celled organisms. Causes diarrhea, fever and abdominal cramps. See chart in Illnesses section.

Aminoglycosides—A family of antibiotics used for serious infections. Their usefulness is limited because of relative toxicity compared to some other antibiotics. These drugs include: amikacin, gentamicin, kanamycin, neomycin, netilmicin, streptomycin, tobramycin.

Amphetamines—A family of drugs that stimulates the central nervous system, prescribed to treat attention-deficit disorders in children and also for narcolepsy. They are habit-forming, controlled under U.S. law, and are no longer prescribed as appetite suppressants. These drugs include: amphetamine, dextroamphetamine, methamphetamine. They may be ingredients of several combination drugs.

Analgesic—Agent that reduces pain without reducing consciousness.

Anaphylaxis—Severe allergic response to a substance. Symptoms are wheezing, itching, hives, nasal congestion, intense burning of hands and feet, collapse, loss of consciousness and cardiac arrest. Symptoms appear within a few seconds or minutes after exposure. Anaphylaxis is a severe medical emergency. Without appropriate treatment, it can cause death. Instructions for home treatment for anaphylaxis are in the emergency information section at the back of this book. Also see chart in Illnesses section.

Androgens—A family of drugs that possess masculinizing properties. In the U.S., they are most frequently and inappropriately used by male and female athletes in hopes of increasing performance, muscle strength, or muscle bulk. These reasons are unacceptable and hazardous. Side effects include fluid retention, reduction in normal growth before puberty, suppression of normal sperm production, shriveling of the testicles, menstrual disturbances in females, and increased chance of liver cancer. All these adverse factors outweigh any possible benefits and make the use of androgens extremely undesirable. These drugs include: fluoxymesterone (Android-F, Halotestin, Ora-Testryl, Testolin); methyltestosterone (Android, Metandren, Metandren Linguets, Oreton Methyl, Testred, Virilon); testosterone (Andro, Andro-Cyp, Android-T, Andro-LA, Andronaq, Andronaq-LA, Andronate, Andryl, Delatestryl, depAndro, Depotest, Depo-Testosterone, Duratest, Durathate, Everone, Histerone, Malogen, Malogex, T-Cypionate, Tesionate, Testa-C, Testaqua, Testex, Testoject, Testoject-LA, Testone L.A., Testrin PA).

Anemia—Not enough healthy red blood cells in the bloodstream or too little hemoglobin in the red blood cells. Anemia is caused by imbalance of blood loss and blood production. See Anemia charts in Illnesses section.

Anemia, Hemolytic—Anemia caused by a shortened lifespan of red blood cells. The body can't manufacture new cells fast enough to replace old cells. See chart in Illnesses section.

Anemia, Iron-Deficiency—Anemia caused when iron necessary to manufacture red blood cells is not available. See chart in Illnesses section.

Anemia, Pernicious—Anemia caused by a vitamin B-12 deficiency. Symptoms include weakness, fatigue, numbness and tingling of the hands or feet, and degeneration of the central nervous system.

Anemia, Sickle-Cell—Anemia caused by defective hemoglobin that deprives red blood cells of oxygen, making them sickle-shaped. See Sickle-Cell Anemia in Illnesses section.
Anesthesias, general—A drug or agent—gaseous, inhaled or intravenous— that is used to abolish the sensation of pain. Most general anesthetics bring about unconsciousness as well.
Anesthetic—Drug that eliminates the sensation of pain.
Angina (Angina Pectoris)—Chest pain with a sensation of suffocation and impending death. Caused by a temporary reduction in the amount of oxygen to the heart muscle through diseased coronary arteries.
Antacids—A large family of drugs prescribed to treat hyperacidity, peptic ulcer, esophageal reflux, and others. These drugs include: aluminum carbonate, basic (Basaljel); aluminum hydroxide (Alagel, ALternaGEL, Alu-Cap, Alu-Tab, Amphojel, Dialume, Nephrox); dihydroxyaluminum aminoacetate (Robalate); dihydroxyaluminum sodium carbonate (Rolaids); alumina, magnesia and calcium carbonate (Camalox); alumina, magnesium carbonate and calcium carbonate (Duracid); simethicone, alumina, calcium carbonate and magnesia (Tempo); alumina and magnesia (Algenic Alka Improved, Aludrox, Alumid, Amphojel 500, Creamalin, Delcid, Diovol Ex, Gelamal, Gelusil, Gelusil Extra Strength, Kolantyl, Kudrox, Maalox Maalox No. 1, Maalox No. 2, Maalox TC, Magmalin, Mintox, Mylanta 2 Plain, Neutralca-S, Rolox, Rulox, Rulox No. 1, Rulox No. 2, Univol, WinGel); alumina, magnesia and simethicone (Almacone, Almacone II, Alma-Mag Improved, Alma-Mag #4 Improved, Alumid Plus, Amphojel Plus, AntaGel, AntaGel-II, Di-Gel, Diovol, Gelusil, Gelusil-II, Gelusil-M, Maalox Plus, MiAcid, Mygel, Mygel II, Mylanta, Mylanta-II, Mylanta-2, Mylanta-2 Extra Strength, Newtrogel II, Silain-Gel, Simaal Gel, Simaal 2 Gel, Simeco); alumina and magnesium carbonate (Gaviscon, Liquimint, Magnagel, Remegel); alumina and magnesium trisilicate (Gaviscon, Gaviscon-2); dihydroxyaluminum aminoacetate, magnesia and alumina (Tralmag); magnesium trisilicate, alumina and magnesia (Magnatril); magnesium trisilicate, alumina and magnesium carbonate (Escot); simethicone, alumina, magnesium carbonate and magnesia (Amphojel Plus, Di-Gel); alumina, magnesium trisilicate and sodium bicarbonate (Gas-is-gon, Triconsil); calcium carbonate (Alka-Mints, Amitone, Chooz, Calcilac, Calglycine, Dicarbosil, Equilet, Gustalac, Pama No. 1, Titracin, Titralac, Tums, Tums E-X); calcium carbonate and magnesia (Bisodol, Calcitrel); calcium carbonate, magnesia and simethicone (Advanced Formula Di-Gel); calcium and magnesium carbonates (Marblen, Noralac, Spastosed); calcium and magnesium carbonates and magnesium oxide (Alkets); magaldrate (Lowsium, Riopan); magaldrate and simethicone (Riopan Plus, Lowsium); magnesium hydroxide (M.O.M., Phillips' Milk of Magnesia); magnesium oxide (Mag-Ox 400, Maox, Par-Mag, Uro-Mag); magnesium carbonate and sodium bicarbonate (Bisodol).
Anthelmintic—A family of drugs used to treat intestinal parasites. Names of these drugs include: niclosamide, piperazine, pyrantel, pyrvinium, quinacrine, mebendazole, metronidazole, oxamniquine, praziquantel, thiabendazole.
Antianginal—A group of drugs used to treat *angina pectoris* (chest pain that comes and goes, caused by coronary artery disease). These drugs include: acebutolol, amyl nitrite, atenolol, diltiazem, erythrityl tetranitrate, isosorbide dinitrate, labetalol, metoprolol, nadolol, nifedipine, nitroglycerin, oxprenolol, pentaerythritol tetranitrate, pindolol, propranolol, sotalol, timolol, verapamil.
Antianxiety Agents or Drugs—A group of drugs prescribed to treat anxiety. These drugs include: alprazolam, bromazepam, buspirone, chlordiazepoxide, chlorpromazine, clomipramine, clorazepate, diazepam, halazepam, hydroxyzine, imipramine, ketazolam, lorazepam, meprobamate, mesoridazine, oxazepam, prazepam, prochlorperazine, thioridazine, trifluoperazine.
Antiarrhythimc—A group of drugs used to treat heartbeat irregularities (arrhythmias). These drugs include: acebutolol, amiodarone, atenolol, atropine, bretylium, deslanoside, digitalis, digitoxin, disopyramide, edrophonium, encainide, esmolol, flecainide, glycopyrrolate, hyoscyamine, lidocaine, methoxamine, metoprolol, mexiletine, nadolol, oxprenolol, phenytoin, procainamide, propranolol, quinidine, scopolamine, sotalol, timolol, tocainide, verapamil.
Antiasthmatics (Antasthmatic)—Any drug that relieves the spasm in bronchial tubes caused by asthma. These drugs include: beclomethasone, dexamethasone, flunisolide, triamcinolone, xanthines, sympathomimetics.

DRUGS GLOSSARY

Antibacterial—A group of drugs prescribed to treat infections. These drus include: amdinocillin, amikacin, amoxicillin, amoxicillin and clavulanate, ampicillin, azlocillin, aztreonam, bacampicillin, carbenicillin, cefaclor, cefadroxil, cefamandole, cefazolin, cefonicid, cefoperazone, ceforanide, cefotaxime, cefotetan, cefoxitin, ceftazidime, ceftizoxime, ceftriaxone, cefuroxime, cephalexin, cephalothin, cephapirin, cephradine, chloramphenicol, cinoxacine, clindamycin, cloxacillin, cyclacillin, cycloserine, demeclocycline, dicloxacillin, doxycycline, erythromycin, erythromycin and sulfisoxazole, flucloxacillin, fusidic acid, gentamicin, imipenem and cilastatin, kanamycin, lincomycin, methacycline, methenamine, methicillin, metronidazole, mezlocillin, minocycline, moxalactam, nafcillin, nalidixic acid, netilmicin, nitrofurantoin, norfloxacin, oxacillin, oxytetracycline, penicillin G, penicillin V, piperacillin, pivampicillin, rifampin, spectinomycin, streptomycin, sulfacytine, sulfadiazine and trimethoprim, sulfamethoxazole, sulfamethoxazole and trimethoprim, sulfisoxazole, tetracycline, ticarcillin, ticarcillin and clavulanate, tobramycin, trimethoprim, vancomycin.

Antibiotic—Chemical that inhibits the growth of or kills germs.

Anticholinergics—Drugs that block the effects of acetylcholine in the body. The primary usefulness is in treatment of peptic ulcer disease in the stomach, duodenum, and esophagus. These drugs include: anisotropine; atropine; atropine, hyoscyamine, scopolamine and butabarbital; atropine, hyoscyamine, scopolamine and phenobarbital; atropine and phenobarbital; belladonna; belladonna and butabarbital; belladonna and phenobarbital; chlordiazepoxide and clidinium; clidinium; glycopyrrolate; hexocyclium; homatropine; hyoscyamine; hyoscyamine and phenobarbital; hyoscyamine and scopolamine; hyoscyamine, scopolamine and phenobarbital; isopropamide; mepenzolate; methantheline; methscopolamine; oxyphencyclimine; oxyphenonium; pirenzepine; propantheline; tridihexethyl.

Anticoagulants—A family of drugs prescribed to slow the rate of blood-clotting. These drugs include: acenocoumarol, anisindione, dicumarol, heparin, warfarin, dihydroergotamine and heparin.

Anticonvulsants—A group of drugs prescribed to treat or prevent seizures (convulsions). These drugs include: amobarbital, carbamazepine, clonazepam, clorazepate, diazepam, divalproex, ethosuximide, ethotoin, lorazepam, magnesium sulfate, mephenytoin, mephobarbital, metharbital, methsuximide, nitrazepam, paraldehyde, paramethadione, pentobarbital, phenobarbital, phensuximide, phenytoin, primidone, secobarbital, trimethadione, valproic acid.

Antidepressants—A group of medicines prescribed to treat mental depression. These drugs include: amitriptyline, amoxapine, clomipramine, desipramine, doxepin, imipramine, isocarboxazid, maprotiline, nortriptyline, phenelzine, protriptyline, tranylcypromine, trazodone, trimipramine.

Antidepressants, MAO (Monamine Oxidase Inhibitors)—A special group of drugs prescribed for mental depression. These are not as popular as in years past because of a relatively high incidence of adverse effects. These drugs include: isocarboxazid (Marplan), phenelzine (Nardil), tranylcypromine (Parnate).

Antidepressants, Tricyclic (TCA)—A group of medicines with similar chemical structure and pharmacologic activity used to treat mental depression. These drugs include: amitriptyline (Amitril, Apo-Amitriptyline, Elavil, Emitrip, Endep, Levate, Meravil, Novotriptyn); amoxapine (Asendin); clomipramine (Anafranil); desipramine (Pertofrane, Norpramin); doxepin (Adapin, Sinequan, triadapin); imipramine (Apo-Imipramine, Impril, Janimine, Novopramine, Tipramine, Tofranil, Tofranil-PM); nortriptyline (Aventyl, Pamelor); protriptyline (Triptil, Vivactil); trimipramine (Surmontil).

Antidiabetic—A group of drugs used in the treatment of *diabetes mellitus*. These medicines all reduce blood sugar. These drugs include: acetohexamide, chlorpropamide, glipizide, glyburide, insulin, metformin, tolazamide, tolbutamide.

Antidyskinetic—A group of drugs used for treatment of Parkinsonism (paralysis agitans) and drug-induced extrapyramidal reactions (see elsewhere in Drugs Glossary). These drugs include: amantadine, benztropine, biperiden, bromocriptine, carbidopa and levodopa, diphenhydramine, ethopropazine, levodopa, levodopa and benserazide.

Antiemetic—A group of drugs used to treat nausea and vomiting. These drugs include: buclizine, cyclizine, chlorpromazine, dimenhydrinate, diphenhydramine, diphenidol, domperidone, dronabinol, haloperidol, hydroxyzine, meclizine, metoclopramide, nabilone, perphenazine, prochlorperazine, promethazine, scopolamine, triflupromazine, trimethobenzamide.

Antifungal—A group of drugs used to treat fungus infection. Those listed as systemic are taken orally or given by injection. Those listed as topical are applied directly to the skin and include liquids, powders, creams, ointments and liniments. Those listed as vaginal are used topically inside the vagina and sometimes on the vaginal lips. These drugs include: Systemic—amphotericin B, miconazole, flucytosine, griseofulvin, ketoconazole, potassium iodide. Topical—carbol-fuchsin; ciclopirox; clioquinol; clotrimazole; econazole; haloprogin; ketoconzaole; miconazole; nystatin; salicylic acid, sulfur and coal; tolnaftate. Vaginal—butoconazole, clotrimazole, gentian violet, miconazole, nystatin.

Antiglaucoma—Medicines used to treat glaucoma. Those listed as systemic are taken orally or given by injection. Those listed as ophthalmic are used as eye drops. These drugs include: Systemic—acetazolamide, dichlorphenamide, glycerin, mannitol, methazolamide, timolol, urea. Ophthalmic—betaxolol, carbachol ophthalmic solution, demecarium, dipivefrin, echothiophate, epinephrine, epinephrine bitartrate, epinephryl borate, isoflurophate, levobunolol, physostigmine, pilocarpine, timolol.

Antihistamines—A family of drugs used to treat allergic conditions, such as hay fever, allergic conjunctivitis, itching, sneezing, runny nose, motion sickness, dizziness, sedation, insomnia and others. These drugs include: azatadine (Optimine); brompheniramine (Bromamine, Brombay, Bromphen, Chlorphed, Dehist, Dimetane, Dimetane Extentabs, Dimetane-Ten, Histaject Modified, Nasahist B, ND-Stat Revised, Oraminic II, Veltane); carbinoxamine (Clistin); chlorpheniramine (Aller-Chlor, Allerid-O.D., Chlo-Amine, Chlor-100, Chlor-Mal, Chlor-Niramine, Chlorphen, Chlor-Pro, Chlorspan, Chlortab, Chlor-Trimeton, Chlor-Trimeton Repetabs, Chlor-Tripolon, Hal-Chlor, Histrey, Novopheniram, Phenetron, Phenetron Lanacaps, T.D. Alermine, Teldrin, Trymegen); clemastine (Tavist); cyproheptadine (Periactin); dexchlorpheniramine (Polaramine, Polaramine Repetabs); dimenhydrinate (Apo-Dimenhydrinate, Calm X, Dimentabs, Dinate, Dommanate, Dramamine, Dramilin, Dramocen, Dramoject, Dymenate, Gravol, Hydrate, Marmine, Motion-Aid, Nauseatol, Novodimenate, PMS-Dimenhydrinate, Reidamine, Travamine, Wehamine); diphenhydramine (Beldin, Benadryl, Benadryl Children's Allergy, Benadryl Complete Allergy, Bendylate, Benylin, Compoz, Diahist, Diphen, Diphenadril, Fenylhist, Fynex, Hydramine, Hydril, Insomnal, Nervine Nighttime Sleep-Aid, Noradryl, Nordryl, Nytol with DPH, Robalyn, Sleep-Eze 3, Sominex Formula 2, Tusstate, Twilite, Valdrene); diphenylpyraline (Hispril); doxylamine (Unisom Nighttime Sleep-Aid); phenindamine (Nolahist); pyrilamine (Dormarex, Somnicaps, Sominex); terfenadine (Seldane); tripelennamine (PBZ, PBZ- SR); triprolidine (Actidil, Bayidyl).

Antihypertensives—Drugs used to treat high blood pressure. These medicines can be used singly or in combination with other drugs. They work best if accompanied by a low-salt, low-fat diet plus an active exercise program. These drugs include: acebutolol, alseroxylon, amiloride, amiloride and hydrochlorothiazide, atenolol, atenolol and chlorthalidone, bendroflumethiazide, benzthiazide, bumetanide, captopril, captopril and hydrochlorothiazide, chlorothiazide, chlorthalidone, clonidine, clonidine and chlorthalidone, cyclothiazide, debrisoquine, deserpidine, deserpidine and hydrochlorothiazide, deserpidine and methyclothiazide, diazoxide, diltiazem, enalapril, enalapril and hydrochlorothiazide, ethacrynic acid, furosemide, guanabenz, guanadrel, guanethidine, guanethidine and hydrochlorothiazide, guanfacine, hydralazine, hydralazine and hydrochlorothiazide, hydrochlorothiazide, hydroflumethiazide, indapamide, labetalol, labetalol and hydrochlorothiazide, mecamylamine, methyclothiazide, methyldopa, methyldopa and chlorothiazide, methyldopa and hydrochlorothiazide, metolazone, metoprolol, metoprolol and hydrochlorothiazide, minoxidil, nadolol, nadolol and bendroflumethiazide, nifedipine, nitroglycerin, nitroprusside, oxprenolol, pargyline, pargyline and methyclothiazide, pindolol, pindolol and hydrochlorothiazide, polythiazide, prazosin, prazosin and polythiazide, propranolol, propranolol and hydrochlorothiazide, quinethazone, rauwolfia serpentina, rauwolfia serpentina and bendroflumethazide, reserpine, reserpine and chlorothiazide, reserpine and chlorthalidone, reserpine and hydralazine, reserpine, hydralazine and hydrochlorothiazide, reserpine and hydrochlorothiazide, reserpine and hydroflumethiazide, reserpine and methyclothiazide, reserpine and polythiazide, reserpine and quinethazone, reserpine and trichlormethiazide, sotalol, spironolactone, spironolactone and hydrochlorothiazide, terazosin, timolol, timolol and hydrochlorothiazide, triamterene, triamterene and hydrochlorothiazide, trichlormethiazide, trimethaphan, verapamil.

Anti-Inflammatory, Non-Steroidal (NSAIDs)—Drugs that decrease inflammation wherever it occurs in the body. Used for treatment of pain, fever, arthritis, gout, menstrual cramps and vascular headaches. These drugs include: aspirin; aspirin, alumina and magnesia tablets; buffered aspirin; bufexamac; choline salicylate; choline and magnesium salicylates; diflunisal; fenoprofen; ibuprofen; indomethacin; ketoprofen; magnesium salicylate; meclofenamate; naproxen; piroxicam; salsalate; sodium salicylate; sulindac; tolmetin.

Anti-Inflammatory, Steroidal—A family of drugs with similar pharmacologic characteristics of cortisone and cortisone-like drugs. They are used for many purposes to help the body deal with inflammation no matter what the cause. Steroidal drugs may be used orally or by injection (systemic), as local applications for the skin, eyes, ears, bronchial tubes (topical), and for others. These drugs include: Nasal—beclomethasone, dexamethasone, flunisolide. Ophthalmic (eyes)—betamethasone, dexamethasone, fluorometholone, hydrocortisone, medrysone, prednisolone. Otic (ears)—betamethasone, desonide and acetic acid, dexamethasone, hydrocortisone, hydrocortisone and acetic acid, prednisolone. Systemic—betamethasone, cortisone, dexamethasone, hydrocortisone, methylprednisolone, paramethasone, prednisolone, prednisone, triamcinolone. Topical—alclometasone; amcinonide; beclomethasone; betamethasone; clobetasol; clobetasone; clocortolone; desonide; desoximetasone; dexamethasone; diflorasone; diflucortolone; flumethasone; fluocinolone; fluocinonide; fluocinonide, procinonide and ciprocinonide; flurandrenolid; halcinonide; hydrocortisone; methylprednisolone; mometasone; triamcinolone.

Antimalarials (also called Antiprotozoals)—A group of drugs used to treat malaria. The choice depends on the precise type of malaria organism and its developmental state. These drugs include: amphotericin B, chloroquine, dapsone, demeclocycline, doxycycline, hydroxychloroquine, iodoquinol, methacycline, metronidazole, minocycline, oxytetracycline, pentamidine, primaquine, pyrimethamine, quinacrine, quinine, sulfadoxine and pyrimethamine, sulfamethoxazole, sulfamethoxazole and trimethoprim, sulfisoxazole, tetracycline.

Antimuscarines—Drugs that block the muscarinic action of acetylcholine and therefore decrease spasm of smooth muscles. They are prescribed for peptic ulcers, dysmenorrhea, dizziness, seasickness, bedwetting, slow heart rate, treatment of toxicity from pesticides made from organophosphates, and other medical problems. These drugs include: anisotropine, atropine, belladonna, clidinium dicyclomine, glycopyrrolate, hexocyclium, homatropine, hyoscyamine, hyoscyamine and scopolamine, isopropamide, mepenzolate, methantheline, methscopolamine, oxyphencyclimine, oxyphenonium, pirenzepine, propantheline, scopolamine, tridihexethyl.

Antimyasthenics—A family of drugs effective in treating the symptoms caused by myasthenia gravis. These drugs include: ambenonium, neostigmine, pyridostigmine.

Antineoplastic—Potent drugs used for malignant disease, they are listed here for completeness. Some of these are *not* described in this book. These drugs include: Systemic—aminoglutethimide, amsacrine, asparaginase, bleomycin, busulfan, carboplatin, carmustine, chlorambucil, chlorotrianisene, chromic phosphate, cisplatin, cyclophosphamide, cyproterone, cytarabine, dacarbazine, dactinomycin, daunorubicin, diethylstilbestrol, doxorubicin, dromostanolone, epirubicin, estradiol, estradiol valerate, estramustine, estrogens (conjugated and esterified), estrone, ethinyl estradiol, etoposide, floxuridine, fluorouracil, flutamide, fluoxymesterone, hexamethylmelamine, hydroxyprogesterone, hydroxyurea, interferon alfa-2a and alfa-2b (recombinant), ketoconazole, leuprolide, levothyroxine, liothyronine, liotrix, lomustine, mechlorethamine, medroxyprogesterone, megestrol, melphalan, methyltestosterone, mercaptopurine, methotrexate, mitomycin, mitotane, mitoxantrone, nandrolone phenpropionate, plicamycin, procarbazine, sodium iodide I 131, sodium phosphate P 32, streptozocin, tamoxifen, teniposide, testolactone, testosterone, thioguanine, thiotepa, thyroglobulin, thyroid, thyrotropin, uracil mustard, vinblastine, vincristine, vindesine. Topical—fluorouracil, mechlorethamine.

Antipsychotic—A group of drugs used to treat the mental disease of psychosis, such as schizophrenia, manic-depressive illness, anxiety states, severe behavior problems and others. These drugs include: acetophenazine, carbamazepine, chlorpromazine, chlorprothixene, fluphenazine, flupenthixol, fluspirilene, haloperidol, loxapine, mesoridazine, methotrimeprazine, molindone, pericyazine, perphenazine, pipotiazine, prochlorperazine, promazine, thioridazine, thiothixene, trifluoperazine, triflupromazine.
Antitussive—A group of drugs used to suppress cough. These drugs include: chlophedianol, codeine (oral), dextromethorphan, diphenhydramine syrup, hydrocodone, hydromorphone, methadone, morphine.
Antiulcer—A group of medicines used to treat peptic ulcer in the stomach, duodenum or the lower end of the esophagus. These drugs include: cimetidine, doxepin, famotidine, ranitidine, sucralfate, trimipramine.
Antiviral—A group of drugs to treat viral infection. These drugs include: Ophthalmic (eye)—idoxuridine, trifluridine, vidarabine. Systemic—acyclovir, amantadine, ribavirin, zidovudine. Topical— acyclovir.
Appendicitis—Inflammation or infection of the appendix. Symptoms include loss of appetite, nausea, low-grade fever and tenderness in the lower right of the abdomen. See chart in Illnesses section.
Appetite Suppressants—A group of drugs used to decrease the appetite as part of an overall treatment for obesity. These drugs include: benzphetamine, cyproheptadine, diethylpropion, fenfluramine, mazindol, phendimetrazine, phenmetrazine, phentermine, phenylpropanolamine.
Artery—Blood vessel carrying blood away from the heart.
Asthma—Recurrent attacks of breathing difficulty due to spasms and contractions of the bronchial tubes. See Asthma charts in Illnesses section.

B

Bacteria—Microscopic organism. Some bacteria contribute to health; others (germs) cause disease.
Barbiturates—A family of drugs used as sedatives to induce rest or sleep, anticonvulsants, and as adjuncts for anesthesia. Their use to relieve anxiety, tension, or apprehension has been abandoned because barbiturates are habit-forming. Another drug family, benzodiazepines, has replaced barbiturates for daytime sedation. Barbiturates include: amobarbital (Amytal); aprobarbital (Alurate); butabarbital (Barbased, Butalan, Buticaps, Butisol, Day-Barb, Neo-Barb, Sarisol No. 2); mephobarbital (Mebaral); metharbital (Gemonil); pentobarbital (Nembutal, Novopentobarb); phenobarbital (Barbita, Gardenal, Luminal, Solfoton); secobarbital (Novosecobarb, Seconal); secobarbital and amobarbital (Tuinal); talbutal (Lotusate).
Basal Area of Brain—Part of the brain that regulates muscle control and tone.
Beta-Agonists—A group of drugs that act directly on cells in the body (beta-adrenergic receptors) to relieve spasm of the bronchial tubes and other organs consisting of smooth muscles. These drugs include: albuterol, bitolerol, isoetharine, isoproterenol, methproterenol, terbutaline.
Beta-blockers (beta-adrenergic blocking agents)—A family of drugs with similar pharmacological actions with some variations. These drugs are prescribed for angina, heartbeat irregularities (arrhythmias), high blood pressure, hypertrophic subaortic stenosis, vascular headaches (as a preventative, not to treat once the pain begins), and others. Timolol is prescribed for treatment of open-angle glaucoma. These drugs include: acebutolol (Monitan, Sectral); atenolol (Esmolol); labetalol (Normodyne, Trandate); metoprolol (Apo-Metoprolol, Betaloc, Betaloc Durules, Lopresor, Lopresor SR, Lopressor, Novometoprol); nadolol (Corgard); oxprenolol (Trasicor, Slow-Trasicor); pindolol (Visken); propranolol (Apo-Propranolol, Detensol, Inderal, Inderal LA, Novopranol, pms-Propranolol); sotalol (Sotacor); timolol (Blocadren).
Benzodiazepines—A family of drugs prescribed to treat anxiety, alcohol withdrawal, and sometimes for sedation. These drugs include: alprazolam, chlordiazepoxide, clonazepam, clorazepate, diazepam, flurazepam, halazepam, lorazepam, midazolam, oxazepam, prazepam, temazepam, triazolam.
Birth Control Pills—See Contraceptives, Oral.
Blood Count—Laboratory studies to count white blood cells, red blood cells, platelets and other elements of the blood. See Blood Count appendix.
Blood Pressure, Diastolic—Pressure (usually recorded in millimeters of mercury) in the large arteries of the body when the heart muscle is relaxed and filling for the next contraction.

Blood Pressure, Systolic—Pressure (usually recorded in millimeters of mercury) in the large arteries of the body at the instant the heart muscle contracts.

Blood Sugar (Blood Glucose)—Necessary element in the blood to sustain life.

Bronchodilators—A group of drugs used to dilate the bronchial tubes to treat such problems as asthma, emphysema, bronchitis, bronchiectasis, allergies and others. These drugs include: albuterol, aminophylline, bitolterol, dyphylline, ephedrine, epinephrine, ethylnorepinephrine, fenoterol, ipratropium, isoetharine, isoproterenol, metaproterenol, oxtriphylline, oxtriphylline and guaifenesin, terbutaline, theophylline, theophylline and guaifenesin.

Bronchodilators, Xanthine Derivative—Drugs of similar chemical structure and pharmacological activity. They are prescribed to dilate bronchial tubes in disorders such as asthma, bronchitis, emphysema and other chronic lung diseases. These drugs include: aminophylline, dyphylline, oxtriphylline, theophylline.

C

Carbonic Anyhdrase Inhibitors—A family of drugs used to treat epilepsy, altitude sickness, and glaucoma. These drugs include: acetazolamide (Acetazolam, Ak-Zol, Apo-Acetazolamide, Dazamide, Diamox, Diamox Sequels); dichlorphenamide (Daranide); methazolamide (Neptazane).

Cataract—Loss of transparency in the lens of the eye.

Cell—Unit of protoplasm, the essential living matter of all plants and animals.

Central Nervous System (CNS) Depression-Producing Medications—These drugs cause sedation or otherwise diminish brain activity and other parts of the nervous system. These drugs include: alcohol, aminoglutethimide, anesthetics (general and injection-local), anticonvulsants, antidepressants (MAO inhibitors, TCA), antidyskinetics (except amantadine), antihistamines, apomorphine, baclofen, barbiturates, benzodiazepines, buclizine, carbamazepine, chloral hydrate, chlorzoxazone, clonidine, cyclizine, difenoxin and atropine, diphenoxylate and atropine, disulfiram, dronabinol, ethchlorvynol, ethinamate, etomidate, fenfluramine, flavoxate, glutethimide, guanabenz, guanfacine, haloperidol, hydroxyzine, interferon, loxapine, magnesium sulfate (injection), maprotiline, meclizine, meprobamate, methyldopa, methyprylon, metoclopramide, metyrosine, mitotane, molindone, opioid (narcotic) analgesics, oxybutynin, paraldehyde, paregoric, pargyline, phenothiazines, pimozide, procarbazine, promethazine, propiomazine, rauwolfia alkaloids, scopolamine, skeletal muscle relaxants (centrally acting), thioxanthenes, trazodone, trimeprazine, trimethobenzamide.

Central Nervous System (CNS) Stimulants—Drugs that cause excitation, anxiety, nervousness or otherwise stimulate the brain and other parts of the central nervous system. These drugs include: amantadine, amphetamines, anesthetics (local), appetite suppressants (except fenfluramine), bronchodilators (xanthine-derivative), caffeine, chlophedianol, cocaine, doxapram, methylphenidate, pemoline, sympathomimetics.

Cephalosporins—Potent drugs (antibiotics) that fight various infections. These drugs include: cefaclor (Ceclor); cefadroxil (Duricef, Ultracef); cefamandole (Mandol); cefazolin (Ancef, Kefzol); cefonicid (Monocid); cefoperazone (Cefobid, Cefobine); ceforanide (Precef); cefotaxime (Claforan); cefotetan (Cefotan); cefoxitin (Mefoxin); ceftazidime (Fortaz, Magnacef, Tazicef, Tazidime); ceftizoxime (Cefizox); ceftriaxone (Rocephin); cefuroxime (Kefurox, Zinacef); cephalexin (Ceporex, Keflet, Keflex, Novolexin); cephalothin (Ceporacin, Keflin, Keflin Neutral, Seffin Neutral); cephapirin (Cefadyl); cephradine (Anspor, Velosef); moxalactam (Moxam, Oxalactam).

Cholinergic (also Parasympathomimetic)—Drugs that mimic the activity of acetylcholine in the body. These drugs include: bethanechol, atropine, glycopyrrolate, hyoscyamine, ambenonium, edrophonium, neostigmine, physostigmine, pyridostigmine.

Chronic—Long-term, continuing. Chronic illnesses may not be curable, but they can often be prevented from becoming worse. Symptoms usually can be alleviated or controlled.

Cirrhosis—Disease that scars and destroys liver tissue.

Cold Urticaria—Hives that appear in areas of the body exposed to the cold. See Hives chart in Illnesses section.

Colitis, Ulcerative—Chronic, recurring ulcers of the colon for unknown reasons. See chart in Illnesses section.

Collagen—Support tissue of skin, tendon, bone, cartilage and connective tissue.

Colostomy—Surgical opening from the colon, the large intestine, to the outside of the body.

Congestive—Excess accumulation of blood. In congestive heart failure, congestion occurs in the lungs, liver, kidney and other parts of the body to cause shortness of breath, swelling of the ankles and feet, rapid heartbeat and other symptoms.
Constriction—Tightness or pressure.
Contraceptives (Birth-Control Pills)—A group of hormones used to prevent ovulation, therefore preventing pregnancy. These hormones include: ethynodiol diacetate and ethinyl estradiol, ethynodiol diacetate and mestranol, levonorgestrel and ethinyl estradiol, medroxyprogesterone, norethindrone tablets, norethindrone acetate and ethinyl estradiol, norethindrone and ethinyl estradiol, norethindrone and mestranol, norethynodrel and mestranol, norgestrel, norgestrel and ethinyl estradiol. *Note:* Law requires that written information be given to the patient at the same time that the pills are dispensed. Study this information carefully.
Convulsions—Violent, uncontrollable contractions of the voluntary muscles.
Corticosteroid (Adrenocorticosteroid)—Steroid hormones produced by the body's adrenal cortex or their synthetic equivalents.
Cortisone (Adrenocorticoids, Glucocorticoids) and other adrenal steroids—Medicines that mimic the action of the steroid hormone cortisone, manufactured in the cortex of the adrenal gland. These drugs decrease the effects of inflammation within the body. They are available for injection, oral use, topical use for the skin and nose and inhalation for the bronchial tubes. These drugs include: alclometasone; amcinonide; beclomethasone; benzyl benzoate; betamethasone; bismuth; clobetasol; clobetasone 17-butyrate; clocortolone; cortisone; desonide; desoximetasone; desoxycorticosterone; dexamethasone; diflorasone; diflucortolone; fludrocortisone; flumethasone; flunisolide; fluocinonide; fluocinonide, procinonide and ciprocinonide; fluorometholone; flurandrenolide; halcinonide; hydrocortisone; medrysone; methylprednisolone; mometasone; paramethasone; peruvian balsam; prednisolone; prednisone; triamcinolone; zinc oxide.
Cystitis—Inflammation of the urinary bladder.

D

Decongestants—Drugs used to open nasal passages by shrinking swollen lining membranes in the nose. These drugs include: Cough-suppressing—phenylephrine and dextromethorphan, phenylpropanolamine and caramiphen, phenylpropanolamine and dextromethorphan, phenylpropanolamine and hydrocodone, pseudoephedrine and codeine, pseudoephedrine and dextromethorphan, pseudoephedrine and hydrocodone. Cough-suppressing and pain-relieving—phenylpropanolamine, dextromethorphan and acetaminophen. Cough-suppressing and sputum-thinning—phenylephrine, dextromethorphan and guaifenesin; phenylephrine, hydrocodone and guaifenesin; phenylpropanolamine, codeine and guaifenesin; phenylpropanolamine, dextromethorphan and guaifenesin; pseudoephedrine, codeine and guaifenesin; pseudoephedrine, dextromethorphan and guaifenesin; pseudoephedrine, hydrocodone and guaifenesin; phenylephrine, dextromethorphan, guaifenesin and acetaminophen; pseudoephedrine, dextromethorphan, guaifenesin and acetaminophen. Sputum-thinning—ephedrine and guaifenesin; ephedrine and potassium iodide; phenylephrine, phenylpropanolamine and guaifenesin; phenylpropanolamine and guaifenesin; pseudoephedrine and guaifenesin. Nasal—ephedrine (oral), phenylpropanolamine, pseudoephedrine. Ophthalmic (eye)—naphazoline, oxymetazoline, phenylephrine. Topical—oxymetazoline, phenylephrine, xylometazoline.
Delirium—Temporary mental disturbance characterized by hallucinations, agitation and incoherence.
Diabetes—Metabolic disorder in which the body can't use carbohydrates efficiently. This leads to a dangerously high level of glucose (a carbohydrate) in the blood. See Diabetes charts in Illnesses section.
Dialysis—Procedure to filter waste products from the bloodstream of patients with kidney failure.
Digitalis Preparations (Digitalis Glycosides)—Important drugs to treat heart disease, such as congestive heart failure, heartbeat irregularities and cardiogenic shock. These drugs include: deslanoside (Cedilanid); powdered digitalis (Crystodigin); digoxin (Lanoxin, Lanoxicaps).
Dilation—Enlargement.

DRUGS GLOSSARY

Disulfiram Reaction—Disulfiram (Antabuse) is a drug to treat alcoholism. When alcohol in the bloodstream interacts with disulfiram, it causes a flushed face, severe headache, chest pains, shortness of breath, nausea, vomiting, sweating and weakness. Severe reactions may cause death. A disulfiram reaction is the interaction of any drug with alcohol or another drug to produce these symptoms.

Diuretics—Drugs that act on the kidneys to prevent reabsorption of electrolytes, especially chlorides. They are used to treat edema, high blood pressure, congestive heart failure, kidney and liver failure and others. These drugs include: amiloride, amiloride and hydrochlorothiazide, bendroflumethiazide, benzthiazide, bumetanide, chlorothiazide, chlorthalidone, cyclothiazide, ethacrynic acid, furosemide, glycerin, hydrochlorothiazide, hydroflumethiazide, indapamide, mannitol, methyclothiazide metolazone, polythiazide, quinethazone, spironolactone, sprionolactone and hydrochlorothiazide, triamterene, triamterene and hydrochlorothiazide, trichlormethiazide, urea.

Diuretics, Loop—Drugs that act on the kidneys to prevent reabsorption of electrolytes, especially chlorides. They are used to treat edema, high blood pressure, congestive heart failure, kidney and liver failure and others. These drugs include: bumetanide, ethacrynic acid, furosemide.

Diuretics, Thiazide—Drugs that act on the kidneys to prevent reabsorption of electrolytes, especially chlorides. They are used to treat edema, high blood pressure, congestive heart failure, kidney and liver failure and others. These drugs include: bendroflumethiazide (Naturetin); benzthiazide (Aquatag, Exna, Hydrex); chlorothiazide (Diuril); chlorthalidone (Apo-Chlorthalidone, Hygroton, Novothalidone, Thalitone, Uridon); cyclothiazide (Anhydron, Fluidil); hydrochlorothiazide (Apo-Hydro, Diuchlor H, Esidrix, Hydrochlorothiazide Intensol, HydroDIURIL, Mictrin, Natrimax, Neo-Codema, Novohydrazide, Oretic, Thiuretic, Urozide); hydroflumethiazide (Diucardin, Saluron); methyclothiazide (Aquatensen, Duretic, Enduron); metolazone (Diulo, Zaroxolyn); polythiazide (Renese); quinethazone (Aquamox, Hydromox); trichlormethiazide (Metahydrin, Naqua).

Diuretics, Potassium-Sparing—Drugs that act on the kidneys to prevent reabsorption of electrolytes, especially chlorides. They are used to treat edema, high blood pressure, congestive heart failure, kidney and liver failure and others. This particular group of diuretics does not allow the unwanted side effect of low potassium in the blood to occur. These drugs include: amiloride, spironolactone, triamterene.

Duodenum—The first 12 inches of the small intestine.

E

Eczema—Disorder of the skin with redness, itching, blisters, weeping and abnormal pigmentation. See chart in Illnesses section.

Electrolyte—Substance that can transmit electrical impulses when dissolved in body fluids.

Embolism—Sudden blockage of an artery by a clot or foreign material in the blood.

Emphysema—Disease in which the lung's air sacs lose elasticity, and air accumulates in the lungs.

Endometriosis—Condition in which uterus tissue is found outside the uterus. Can cause pain, abnormal menstruation and infertility.

Enzyme—Protein chemical that can accelerate a chemical reaction in the body.

Epilepsy—Episodes of brain disturbance that cause convulsions and loss of consciousness. See chart in Illnesses section.

Erythromycins—A group of drugs with similar structure used to treat infections. These drugs include: erythromycin (Eryc, Eryc Sprinkle, Erythromid, Novorythro, E-Mycin, Ery-Tab, Ilotycin, PCE Dispersatabs, Robimycin, RP-Mycin); erythromycin estolate (Ilosone, Novorythro); erythromycin ethylsuccinate (E.E.S., E-Mycin E, Pediamycin, Wyamycin E, EryPed); erythromycin gluceptate (Ilotycin); erythromycin lactobionate (Erythrocin); erythromycin stearate (ApoErythro-S).

Esophagitis—Inflammation of the lower part of the esophagus, the tube connecting the throat and the stomach. See Esophageal Stricture in Illnesses section.

Estrogens—Female hormones used to replenish the body's stores after the ovaries have been removed or become non-functional after menopause. Also used with progesterone in some birth-control pills and for other purposes. These drugs include: Systemic—chlorotrianisene, diethylstilbestrol, estradiol, estrogens (conjugated and esterified), estrone, estropipate, ethinyl estradiol, quinestrol. Vaginal—dienestrol, estradiol, estrogens (conjugated), estrone, estropipate.

Eustachian Tube—Small passage from the middle ear to the sinuses and nasal passages.

Extrapyramidal Reactions—Drugs that may cause abnormal reactions in the power and coordination of posture and muscular movements. Movements are not under voluntary control. Some drugs associated with producing extrapyramidal reactions include: antidepressants (tricyclic), droperidol, haloperidol, loxapine, methyldopa, metoclopramide, metyrosine, molindone, pemoline, phenothiazines, pimozide, rauwolfia alkaloids, thioxanthenes.

Extremity—Arm, leg, hand or foot.

F

Fecal Impaction—Condition in which feces become firmly wedged in the rectum. See chart in Illnesses section.

Fibrocystic Breast Disease—Overgrowth of fibrous tissue in the breast, producing non-malignant cysts.

Fibroid Tumors—Non-malignant tumors of the muscular layer of the uterus.

Flu (Influenza)—A virus infection of the respiratory tract that lasts three to ten days. Symptoms include headache, fever, runny nose, cough, tiredness and muscle aches. See Influenza chart in Illnesses section.

Folliculitis—Inflammation of a follicle. See chart in Illnesses section.

G

G6PD—Deficiency of glucose 6-phosphate, necessary for glucose metabolism.

Gastritis—Inflammation of the stomach. See chart in Illnesses section.

Gastrointestinal—Stomach and intestinal tract.

Gland—Cells that manufacture and excrete materials not required for their own metabolic needs.

Glaucoma—Eye disease in which increased pressure inside the eye damages the optic nerve, causes pain and changes vision. See chart in Illnesses section.

Gold Compounds—A family of drugs used to treat rheumatoid arthritis. Their base is the metal gold. These drugs include: auranofin (Ridaura); aurothioglucose (Solganal); gold sodium thiomalate (Myochrysine, Myocrisin). They are usually administered by injection, but auranofin may be taken orally.

Glucagon—Injectable drug that immediately elevates blood sugar by mobilizing glycogen from the liver.

H

H2 Antagonist (H2 Receptor Antagonist)—Medicines that block the production of stomach acid by inhibiting the normal action of histamine at H2 receptor sites in stomach cells. It also inhibits production of stomach acid that has been stimulated by eating food. These drugs include: cimetidine (Apo-Cimetidine, Novocimetidine, Peptol, Tagamet); famotidine (Pepsid); ranitidine (Zantac).

Hangover Effect—The same feelings as a "hang-over" after too much alcohol consumption. Symptoms include headache, irritablity and nausea.

Hemochromatosis—Disorder of iron metabolism in which excessive iron is deposited in and damages body tissues, particularly liver and pancreas.

Hemoglobin—Pigment that carries oxygen in red blood cells.

Hemorrhage—Heavy bleeding.

Hemosiderosis—Increase of iron deposits in body tissues without tissue damage.

Hepatitis—Inflammation of liver cells, usually accompanied by jaundice. See chart in Illnesses section.

Hepatotoxic—Medications that can possibly cause toxicity or decreased normal function of the liver. These drugs include: acetaminophen (with long-term, high-dose use or acute overdose), 4-aminoquinolines, amiodarone, anabolic steroids, androgens, antithyroid agents, asparaginase, azlocillin, carbamazepine, carmustine, contraceptives (estrogen-containing, oral), dantrolene, daunorubicin, disulfiram, divalprocx, erythromycins, estrogens, etretinate, gold compounds, halothane, isoniazid, ketoconazole (oral), mercaptopurine, methotrexate, methyldopa, mezlocillin, naltrexone (with long-term, high-dose use), nitrofurans, phenothiazines, phenytoin, piperacillin, plicamycin, rifampin, sulfonamides (systemic), tetracycline (intravenous), valproic acid.

Hiatal Hernia—Section of stomach that protrudes into the chest cavity. See chart in Illnesses section.

Histamine—Chemical in body tissues that dilates the smallest blood vessels, constricts the smooth muscle surrounding the bronchial tubes and stimulates stomach secretions.

History—Past medical events in a patient's life.

Hives—Elevated patches on the skin that are redder or paler than surrounding skin and often itch severely. See chart in Illnesses section.

Hormone—Chemical substance produced in the body to regulate other body functions.

Hypertension—High blood pressure. See chart in Illnesses section.
Hypocalcemia—Abnormally low level of calcium in the blood.
Hypoglycemia—Low blood sugar (blood glucose). A critically low blood-sugar level will interfere with normal brain function and can damage the brain permanently. See Hypoglycemia charts in Illnesses section.
Hypoglycemics—Medications that reduce elevated blood sugar. Hypoglycemics are used especially by those who have diabetes mellitus. These drugs include: acetohexamide, insulin, chlorpropamide, glipizide, glyburide, metformin, tolazamide, tolbutamide.
Hypotension—Blood pressure decreased below normal. Symptoms may include weakness, lightheadedness, dizziness. Some medications that might cause hypotension include: alcohol, alprostadil, amantadine, anesthetics (general), angiotensin-converting enzyme inhibitors (ACE inhibitors), antidepressants (MAO inhibitors, tricyclic), antihypertensives, benzodiazepines used as preanesthetics, beta-adrenergic blocking agents, bromocriptine, calcium channel-blocking agents, captopril, diuretics, edetate calcium disodium, edetate disodium, enalapril, encainide, haloperidol, hydralazine, levodopa, lidocaine (systemic), loxapine, maprotiline, molindone, nitrates, nitrites, opioid analgesics (including fentanil, fentanyl and sufentanil), pentamidine, phenothiazines, pimozide, prazosin, procainamide, quinidine, radiopaques (materials used in x-ray studies), thioxanthenes, tocainide, trazodone. If you take any of these medications, be sure to tell a dentist, anesthesiologist or anyone else who intends to give you an anesthetic to put you to sleep.

I

Ichthyosis—Skin disorder with dryness, scaling and roughness.
Ileitis—Inflammation of the ileum, the last section of the small intestine.
Ileostomy—Surgical opening from the ileum, the end of the small intestine, to the outside of the body.
Impotence—Male's inability to achieve or sustain erection of the penis for sexual intercourse.
Immunosuppressants—Potent drugs that suppress the body's immune system. They are usually used with adrenocorticoids (cortisone drugs) to prevent and treat rejection of organ transplants, such as lung, heart, kidney and liver. Other uses include treatment for malignancies such as leukemia, breast cancer, and many others. Immunosuppressants are also sometimes used to treat autoimmune diseases such as rheumatoid arthritis. These drugs include: azathioprine, betamethasone, chlorambucil, corticotropin, cortisone, cyclophosphamide, cyclosporine, dexamethasone, hydrocortisone, mercaptopurine, methylprednisolone, muromonab-CD3, paramethasone, prednisolone, prednisone, triamcinolone.
Insomnia—Sleeplessness.
Interaction—Change in the body's response to one drug when another is taken. Interaction may decrease the effect of one or both drugs, decrease the effect of one or both drugs, or cause toxicity.
Iron Supplements—Any medication that contains elemental iron used to treat iron deficiencies. Iron is a frequent component of numerous vitamin-mineral supplements. Iron supplements include: ferrous fumarate (Femiron, Feostat, Fumasorb, Fumerin, Hemocyte, Ircon, Neo-Fer, Novofumar, Palafer, Palmiron, Span-FF); ferrous gluconate (Apo-Ferrous Gluconate, Fergon, Ferralet, Fertinic, Novoferrogluc, Simron); ferrous sulfate (Apo-Ferrous Sulfate, Feosol, Fer-In-Sol, Fer-Iron, Fero-Grad, Fero-Gradumet, Ferralyn, Ferra-TD, Fesofor, Mol-Iron, Novoferrosulfa, PMS Ferrous Sulfate, Slow Fe); iron-polysaccharide (Hytinic, Niferex, Niferex-150, Nu-Iron, Nu-Iron 150); iron dextran (Dextraron, Feostat, Feronim, Hematran, Hydextran, Imferon, Imfergen, Irodex, K-Feron, Nor-Feron, Proferdex).

J

Jaundice—Symptoms of liver damage, bile obstruction or red blood cell destruction. Symptoms include yellowed whites of the eyes, yellow skin, dark urine and light stool.

K

Keratosis—Growth that is an accumulation of cells from the outer skin layers. See chart in Illnesses section.
Kidney Stones—Small, solid stones made from calcium, cholesterol, cysteine and other body chemicals. See Kidney charts in Illnesses section.

L

Laxatives—Medicines prescribed to treat constipation. These medicines include: bisacodyl; bisacodyl and docusate; casanthranol; casanthranol and docusate; cascara sagrada; cascara sagrada and aloe; cascara sagrada and phenolphthalein; castor oil; danthron; danthron and docusate; danthron and poloxamer 188; dehydrocholic acid; dehydrocholic acid and docusate; docusate; docusate and phenolphthalein; docusate and mineral oil; docusate and phenolphthalein; docusate, carboxymethylcellulose and casanthranol glycerin; lactulose; magnesium citrate; magnesium hydroxide; magnesium hydroxide and mineral oil; magnesium oxide; magnesium sulfate; malt soup extract; malt soup extract and psyllium; methylcellulose; mineral oil; mineral oil and cascara sagrada; mineral oil and phenolphthalein; mineral oil, glycerin and phenolphthalein; phenolphthalein; poloxamer; polycarbophil; potassium bitartrate and sodium bicarbonate; psyllium; psyllium and senna; psyllium hydrophilic mucilloid; psyllium hydrophilic mucilloid and carboxymethylcellulose; psyllium hydrophilic mucilloid and sennosides; psyllium hydrophilic musilloid and senna; senna; senna and docusate; sennosides; sodium phosphate.

Lupus—Serious disorder of connective tissue that primarily affects women. Varies in severity with skin eruptions, joint inflammation, low white blood cells count and damage to internal organs, especially the kidney. See Lupus charts in Illnesses section.

Lymph Glands—Glands in the lymph vessels throughout the body that trap foreign and infectious matter and protect the bloodstream from infection.

M

MAO Inhibitors—See Antidepressants, MAO.

Manic-Depressive Illness—Psychosis with alternating cycles of excessive enthusiasm and depression.

Mast Cell—Connective-tissue cell.

Menopause—The end of menstruation in the female, often accompanied by irritability, hot flushes, changes in the skin and bones and vaginal dryness.

Metabolism—Process of using nutrients and energy to build and break down wastes.

Migraine—Periodic headaches caused by constriction of arteries to the skull. Symptoms include severe pain, vision disturbances, nausea, vomiting and light sensitivity. See Headache, Migraine charts in Illnesses section.

Mind-Altering Drugs—Any drug that decreases alertness, perception, concentration, contact with reality or muscular coordination. These drugs include: alcohol; amphetamines (dextroamphetamine, methamphetamine); anti-anxiety drugs (Valium, Librium); barbiturates (Seconal, Tuinal); benzodiazepines (Valium, Librium); phenothiazines (Thorazine, Compazine); cocaine; marijuana; opiates (herion, morphine); LSD; peyote; mescaline; methadone; inhalants (cleaning fluids, amyl nitrite, airplane glue). Signs of drug abuse include: abrupt change in attitude or mood; temper flares; increased borrowing of money from family or friends; stealing from home, school or employer; associating with a new group of friends; heightened secrecy; irresponsibility.

Myasthenia Gravis—Disease of the muscles characterized by fatigue and progressive paralysis. It is usually confined to muscles of the face, lips, tongue and neck. See chart in Illnesses section.

N

Narcotics—A group of habit-forming, addicting drugs used for treatment of pain, diarrhea, cough, acute pulmonary edema and others. They are all dervied from opium, a milky exudate in capsules of *Papaver somniferum*. Law requires licensed physicians to dispense by prescription. These drugs include: alfentanil, buprenorphine, butorphanol, codeine, fentanyl, hydrocodone, hydromorphone, levorphanol, meperidine, methadone, morphine, nalbuphine, opium, oxycodone, oxymorphone, pentazocine, propoxyphene, sufetanil.

Nephrotoxic Medications (Kidney-Poisoning)—Under some circumstances, these medicines can be toxic to the kidneys. These medicines include: acyclovir; aminoglycosides; amphotericin B (given internally); analgesic combinations containing acetaminophen and aspirin or other salicylates (with chronic high-dose use); anti-inflammatory analgesics (non-steroidal); bacitracin (given internally); capreomycin; captopril; carmustine; cisplatin; cyclosporine; demeclocycline (nephrogenic diabetes insipidus); edetate calcium disodium (with high doses); edetate disodium (with high dose); enalapril; gold compounds; lithium; methotrexate (with high dose therapy); methoxyflurane; neomycin (oral); penicillamine; pentamidine; plicamycin; polymyxins (given internally); radiopaques (materials used for special x-ray examinations); rifampin; streptozocin; sulfonamides; tetracyclines (other, except doxycycline and minocycline); vancomycin (given internally).

Neuromuscular Blocking Agents—A group of drugs prescribed to relax skeletal muscles. They are all given by injection and descriptions are not included in this book. These drugs include: atracurium, gallamine, metocurine, pancuronium, succinylcholine, tubocurarine, vecuronium.
Nitrates—Drugs used to treat heart disease, including congestive heart failure, high blood pressure, and angina pectoris. These drugs include: amyl nitrite; erythrityl tetranitrate (Cardilate); isosorbide dinitrate (Apo-ISDN, Coronex, Dilatrate SR, Iso-Bid, Isochron, Isonate, Isonate TR, Isordil, Isotrate, Novosorbide, Onset, Sorate, Sorbide T.D., Sorbitrate, Sorbitrate SA); nitroglycerin (Ang-O-Span, Deponit, Klavikordal, N-G-C, Niong, Nitro-Bid, Nitrobon, Nitrocap, Nitrocap T.D., Nitrocardin, Nitrodisc, Nitro-Dur, Nitro-Dur II, Nitrogard, Nitrogard SR, Nitroglyn, Nitrol, Nitrolin, Nitrolingual, Nitro-Long, Nitronet, Nitrong, Nitrong SR, Nitrospan, Nitrostabilin, Nitrostat, Nitro-Time, NTS, Transderm-Nitro, Tridil); pentaerythritol tetranitrate (Duotrate, Naptrate, Pentol, Pentol S.A., Pentraspan SR, Pentritol, Pentylan, Peritrate, Peritrate Forte, Peritrate SA).
Nutritional Supplements—Substances used to treat and prevent deficiencies when the body is unable to absorb them by eating a well-balanced, nutritional diet. These supplements include: Vitamins— ascorbic acid, ascorbic acid and sodium ascorbate, calcifediol, calcitriol, calcium pantothenate, cyanocobalamin, dihydrotachysterol, ergocalciferol, folate sodium, folic acid, hydroxoco-balamin, niacin, niacinamide, pantothenic, pyridoxine, riboflavin, sodium ascorbate, thiamine, vitamin A, vitamin E. Minerals—calcium carbonate, calcium citrate, calcium glubionate, calcium gluconate, calcium lactate, calcium phosphate (dibasic and tribasic), sodium fluoride. Other— levocarnitine, omega-3 polyunsaturated fatty acids.

O

Osteoporosis—Softening of bones caused by a loss of chemicals usually found in bone.
Ototoxic Medications—These medicines may possibly cause hearing damage. They include: aminoglycosides, 4-aminoquinolines, anti-inflammatory analgesics (non-steroidal), bumetanide, capreomyucin, cisplatin, deferoxamine, erythromycins, ethacrynic acid, furosemide, minocycline, quinine, salicylates, vancomycin.
Ovary—Female sexual gland where eggs mature and ripen for fertilization.

P

Pain Relievers—Any medication that decreases the perception of pain. These drugs include: aspirin, acetaminophen, narcotics, non-steroidal anti-inflammatory agents.
Palpitations—Rapid heartbeat noticeable to the patient.
Pancreatitis—Serious inflammation or infection of the pancreas that causes upper abdominal pain.
Parkinson's Disease—Disease of the central nervous system. Characteristics are a fixed, emotionless expression of the face, tremor, slower muscle movements, weakness, changed gait and a peculiar posture.
Pellagra—Disease caused by a deficiency of the water-soluble vitamin, thiamine (vitamin B-1). Symptoms include brain disturbance, diarrhea and skin inflammation. See Vitamin B Deficiency chart in Illnesses section.
Penicillin—Chemical substance (antibiotic) originally discovered as a product of mold, which can kill some bacterial germs.
Phenothiazines—A family of drugs used to treat anxiety, nausea, vomiting, and some psychoses.
Phlegm—Thick mucus secreted by glands in the respiratory tract.
Phosphorus Preparations (Phosphates)—Drugs used to acidify the urine (sometimes useful in treating kidney stones) and to replenish phosphorous deficiencies. These drugs include: potassium phosphates (K- Phos Original, Neutra-Phos-K); potassium and sodium phosphates (K-Phos M.F., K-Phos Neutral, K-Phos No. 2, Neutra-Phos, Uro-KP-Neutral); sodium phosphates.
Photosensitizing Medications—Medicines that can cause abnormally-heightened skin reactions to the effects of sunlight. These medicines include: amiodarone, anthralin, antidiabetic agents (oral), antihistamines, benzocaine, coal tar, contraceptives (estrogen-containing, oral), diuretics, thiazide, estrogens, ethionamide, etretinate, fluorouracil, furosemide, griseofulvin, isotretinoin, ketoprofen, methotrexate, methoxsalen, nalidixic acid, naproxen, phenothiazines, phenylbutazone, piroxicam, pyrazinamide, sulfonamides, sulindac, tetracyclines, thioxanthenes, tretinoin, trioxsalen.
Pinworms—Common intestinal parasite that causes rectal itching and irritation. See chart in Illnesses section.
Pituitary Gland—Gland at the base of the brain that secretes hormones to stimulate growth and other glands to produce hormones. See Pituitary charts in Illnesses section.

Platelet—Disc-shaped element of the blood, smaller than red or white blood cells, necessary for blood clotting.
Polyp—Growth on a mucous membrane.
Porphyria—Inherited metabolic disorder characterized by changes in the nervous system and kidney. See chart in Illnesses section.
Post-Partum—Following delivery of a baby.
Potassium—Important chemical found in body cells.
Potassium Foods—Foods high in potassium content, including dried apricots and peaches, lentils, raisins, citrus and whole-grain cereals.
Potassium Supplements—Medications to prevent potassium deficiencies in the body or to treat potassium deficiencies due to disease or a result of taking medications, such as diuretics and others, that deplete potassium stores. These supplements include: potassium acetate; potassium bicarbonate (Klor-Con/EF); potassium bicarbonate and potassium chloride (Klorvess, K-Lyte/Cl, Neo-K, Potassium-Sandoz); potassium bicarbonate and potassium citrate (K-Lyte, K-Lyte DS); potassium chloride (Apo-K, Cena-K, K-10, Kalium Durules, Kaochlor, Kaochlor S-F, Kaon-Cl, Kato, Kay Ciel, KCL, K-Dur, K-Long, K-Lor, Klor-10%, Klor-Con, Klor-Con/25, Klotrix, K-Lyte/Cl Powder, K-Tab, Micro-K, Novolente-K, Potachlor, Potage, Potasalan, Potassine, Roychlor, Rum-K, Slo-Pot, Slow-K, Ten-K); potassium chloride, potassium bicarbonate and potassium citrate (Kaochlor-Eff); potassium gluconate (Bayon, Bi-K, Kaon, Kao-Nor, Kaylixir, K-G Elixir, Potassium-Rougier, Royonate); potassium gluconate and potassium chloride (Kolyum); potassium gluconate and potassium citrate (Twin-K); potassium gluconate, potassium citrate and ammonium chloride (Twin-K-Cl); trikates (Tri-K).
Prostate—Gland in the male that surrounds the neck of the bladder and the urethra. The prostate gland produces a fluid that is added to sperm to produce semen.
Prothrombin—Blood substance essential in clotting.
Prothrombin Time—Laboratory study used to follow prothrombin activity and keep coagulation safe.
Psoriasis—Chronic, inherited skin disease. Symptoms are lesions with silvery scales on the edges.
Psychosis—Mental disorder characterized by deranged personality, loss of contact with reality and possible delusions, hallucinations or illusions.
Purine Foods—Foods that are metabolized into uric acid. Foods high in purines include anchovies, liver, brains, sweetbreads, sardines, kidney, oysters, gravy and meat extracts.

R

Rauwolfia Alkaloids—A family of drugs derived from the herb *rauwolfia serpentina*. At one time, rauwolfia alkaloids were used quite often for treating high blood pressure. Now they are not used as often because of the unacceptable frequency of side effects or adverse reactions. These drugs include: alseroxylon (Rauwiloid); deserpidine (Harmonyl); rauwolfia serpentina (Raudixin, Rauverid, Wolfina); reserpine (Novoreserpine, Releserp-5, Reserfia, Serpasil).
RDA—Recommended daily allowance of a vitamin or mineral.
Rebound Effect—Return of a condition, often with increased severity, once the prescribed drug is withdrawn.
Renal—Pertaining to the kidney.
Retina—Innermost covering of the eyeball on which the image is formed.
Reye's Syndrome—Rare, sometimes fatal, disease of children that cause brain and liver damage. See chart in Illnesses section.
Rickets—Bone disease caused by vitamin-D deficiency. Bones become bent and distorted during infancy or childhood.

S

Salicylates—Any salt of salicylic acid. The most frequently used salicylate is acetylsalicylic acid (aspirin). Salicylates are used to reduce pain, fever, inflammation, and clumping of platelets in the coronary arteries. These drugs include: aspirin (Apo-Asen, Arthrinol, A.S.A., A.S.A. Enseals, Aspergum, Astrin, Bayer Aspirin, Bayer Timed-Release Arthritic Pain Formula, Coryphen, Easprin, Ecotrin, Empirin, Encaprin, Entrophen, 8-Hour Bayer Timed-Release, Measurin, Norwich Aspirin, Novasen, Riphen-10, Safety Coated APF Arthritis Pain Formula, Sal-Adult, Sal-Infant, St. Joseph Aspirin for Children, Supasa, Triaphen-10, ZORprin; aspirin, buffered (Alka-Seltzer Effervescent Pain Reliever and Antacid, Asperbuf, Buffaprin, Bufferin, Buffex, Buffinol, Buf-Tabs, Cama Arthritis Reliever); choline salicylate (Arthropan); aspirin and caffeine (Accurate, Acotin, Alsidol, Anacin, Asafen, C2, CP-2, 812, Instantine, Major-cin, Neo-Tigol, Nervine, P- A-C Revised Formula, Paradol, 217, T-R-C Regular); aspirin, alumina and magnesia (Arthritic Pain Formula, Arthritis Pain Formula, Ascriptin, Ascriptin A/D, Magnaprin, Maprin, Maprin I-B, Wesprin

Buffered); choline and magnesium salicylates (Trilisate); diflunisal; magnesium salicylate (Doan's Pills, Magan, Mobidin); salicylamide (Uromide); salsalate (Artha-G, Disalcid, Mono-Gesic); sodium salicylate (Uracel).

Sedatives—Drugs that reduce excitement or anxiety. Depending on their use, there are various types of sedatives. These include: conscious sedation (diazepam, midazolam); sedation and amnesia (midazolam); alcohol withdrawal (carbamazepine, chlordiazepoxide, cloracepate, diazepam, hydroxyzine, lorazepam, oxazepam); anxiety (alprazolam, amoxapine, bromazepam, buspirone, chlordiazepoxide, chlordiazepoxide and amitriptyline, chlorpromazine, clomipramine, clorazepate, diazepam, doxepin, halazepam, hydroxyzine, imipramine, ketazolam, lorazepam, maprotiline, meprobamate, mesoridazine, oxazepam, perphenazine and amitriptyline, prazepam, prochlorperazine, thioridazine, trifluoperazine); insomnia (amobarbital, aprobarbital, butabarbital, chloral hydrate, diphenhydramine, doxylamine, ethchlorvynol, ethinamate, flurazepam, lorazepam, methyprylon, nitrazepam, pentobarbital, phenobarbital, pyrilamine, secobarbital, secobarbital and amobarbital, talbutal, temazepam, triazolam); sedation (chloral hydrate, diphenhydramine, hydroxyzine, methotrimeprazine, promethazine, trimeprazine).

Seizure—Brain disorder causing changes of consciousness or convulsions.

Sinusitis—Inflammation or infection of the sinus cavities in the skull. See Sinus Infection in Illnesses section.

Skeletal Muscle Relaxants—A group of drugs prescribed to treat spasm of skeletal muscles. These drugs include: carisoprodol, chlorphenesin, chlorzoxazone, cyclobenzaprine, diazepam, lorazepam, metaxalone, methocarbamol, orphenadrine, phenytoin.

Sleep Inducers—Any medication that aids sleep when it won't occur naturally. Barbiturates were formerly used for this purpose, but have mostly been abandoned in favor of benzodiazepines (see Drugs Glossary entry). Benzodiazepines are much safer, produce fewer adverse reactions, and are not as likely to be habit-forming.

Stimulants, Central Nervous System (CNS)—Drugs that stimulate the brain and spinal cord nerves. These drugs include: amphetamine, caffeine, caffeine (citrated), caffeine and sodium benzoate, cocaine, dextroamphetamine, ephedrine (oral), methamphetamine, methylphenidate, pemoline.

Streptococcus—Bacteria that causes infections in the throat, respiratory system and skin. Improperly treated, can lead to disease in the heart, joints and kidneys.

Stroke—Sudden, severe attack. Usually sudden paralysis from injury to the brain or spinal cord caused by a blood clot or hemorrhage in the brain.

Stupor—Near unconsciousness.

Sublingual—Under the tongue. Some drugs are absorbed almost as quickly this way as by injection.

Sulfa Drugs (Sulfonamides)—Drugs that treat various infections. These drugs include: sulfacytine (Renoquid); sulfamethoxazole (Gantanol, Methoxanol); sulfamethoxazole and trimethoprim (Apo-Sulfatrim, Bactrim, Cotrim, Novotrimel, Protrin, Roubac, Septra, SMZ-TMP, Sulfamethoprim, Sulmeprim); sulfisoxazole (Gantrisin, Lipo Gantrisin, Novosoxazole, SK-Soxazole).

Sulfonureas—A family of drugs taken orally to treat diabetes mellitus. These drugs include: acetohexamide, chlorpropamide, glipizide, glyburide, tolazamide, tolbutamide.

Sulfonamides—See Sulfa Drugs.

Sympathomimetics—A large group of drugs that mimic the effects of stimulation of the *sympathetic* part of the autonomic nervous system. These drugs include: adrenalin (epinephrine); norepinephrine; appetite suppressants (such as benzphetamine, diethylpropion, fenfluramine, mazindol, phendimetrazine, phenmetrazine, phentermine, phenylpropanolamine); aramine; dobutamine; ephedrine; mephentermine; methoxamine; phenylephrine; metaraminol; isoproterenol.

T

Tardive Dyskinesia—Involuntary movements of the jaw, lips and tongue caused by an unpredictable drug reaction.

Tartrazine Dye—A dye used in foods and medicine preparations that may cause an allergic reaction in some people.

Tetracyclines—A group of medicines with similar chemical structure used to treat infections. These drugs include: demeclocycline, doxycycline, methacycline, minocycline, oxytetracycline, tetracycline.

Thrombophlebitis—Inflammation of a vein caused by a blood clot in the vein.

Thyroid—Gland in the neck that manufactures and secretes several hormones.

Tic-douloureux—Painful condition caused by inflammation of a nerve in the face.

Toxicity—Poisonous reaction to a drug that impairs body functions or damages cells.
Tranquilizers—Drugs that calm or quiet without clouding consciousness. The most commonly used medications for this purpose are in the drug family called benzodiazepines. See Benzodiazepines.
Tremor—Involuntary trembling.
Trichomoniasis—Infestation of the vagina by *trichomonas*, an infectious organism. The infection causes itching, vaginal discharge and irritation. See Vaginitis, Trichomonal, in Illnesses section.
Triglyceride—Fatty chemical manufactured from carbohydrates for storage in fat cells.
Tyramine—Normal chemical component of the body that helps sustain blood pressure. Can rise to fatal levels in combination with some drugs. Tyramine is found in many foods: Beverages—Alcohol beverages, especially Chianti or robust red wines, vermouth, ale, beer. Breads—Homemade bread with a lot of yeast and breads or crackers containing cheese. Fats—Sour cream. Fruits—Bananas, red plums, avocados, figs, raisins. Meats and meat substitutes—Aged game, liver, canned meats, salami, sausage, cheese, salted dried fish, pickled herring. Vegetables—Italian broad beans, green-bean pods, eggplant. Miscellaneous—Yeast concentrates or extracts, marmite, soup cubes, commercial gravy, soy sauce, any protein food that has been stored improperly or is spoiled.

U

Ulcer, Peptic—Open sore on the mucous membrane of the esophagus, stomach or duodenum caused by stomach acid. See Peptic Ulcer in Illnesses section.
Urethra—Hollow tube through which urine (and semen in men) is discharged.
Urethritis—Inflammation or infection of the urethra. See chart in Illnesses section.
Uterus—Also called womb. A hollow muscular organ in the female in which the embryo develops into a fetus.

V

Vascular—Pertaining to blood vessels.
Vascular Headache (Preventative)—Medicines prescribed to prevent the occurrence of or reduce the frequency and severity of vascular headache such as migraine. These drugs include: atenolol; clonidine; ergotamine, belladonna alkaloids and phenobarbital; fenoprofen; ibuprofen; indomethacin; lithium; mefenamic acid; methysergide; metoprolol; nadolol; naproxen; pizotyline; propranolol; timolol.
Vascular Headache (Treatment)—Medicine prescribed to treat vascular headaches such as migraine. These drugs include: dihydroergotamine; ergotamine; ergotamine and caffeine; ergotamine, caffeine, belladonna alkaloids and pentobarbital; fenoprofen; ibuprofen; indomethacin (capsules, oral suspension, rectal); isometheptene, dichloralphenazone and acetaminophen; naproxen. See Headache, Tension or Vascular, in Illnesses section.
Virus—Infectious organism that reproduces in the cells of the infected host.

Y

Yeast—A single-cell organism that can cause infections of the mouth, vagina, skin and parts of the gastrointestinal system.

Appendices

APPENDIX 1

Immunizations

Immunizations protect children and adults from serious diseases that can be fatal. The schedule below is the current recommendation of the Centers for Disease Control, an agency of the U.S. Public Health Service.

Don't consider the recommended ages as absolute. For example, "2 months" can mean a range of 6 to 10 weeks. Immunizations may not be a good idea at the recommended time if your child is ill or taking immunosuppressants or cortisone. Rely on the judgment of informed professionals.

SCHEDULE OF IMMUNIZATIONS

Age Recommended	Vaccines
2 months	DPT 1 [Diphtheria, Pertussis (whooping cough), Tetanus] OPV 1 (Oral Polio Vaccine)
4 months	DPT 2, OPV 2
6 months	DPT 3
15 months	MMR [Measles, Mumps, Rubella (German Measles)]
18 months	DPT 4, OPV 3, HIB (Hemophilus Influenza B)
Anytime under age 2	Influenza
4 to 6 years	DPT 5, OPV 4
14 to 16 years	Td (Adult Tetanus and Diphtheria toxoid combined)
Every 10 years thereafter	Td

Vaccines are also available to protect against pneumococcal pneumonia, influenza, hepatitis, rabies, typhoid fever and other diseases. These vaccines are given only under special circumstances.

Ask your doctor, health department, or travel agent about vaccinations required or recommended before your family travels in another country. Inquire several months before your expected departure.

APPENDIX 2

Medical History Form

Before the next visit to your child's physician, go over this checklist to remind yourself of events or symptoms that might be very important for accurate diagnosis and your child's future health care.

1. Has a doctor ever said your child has had the following: (Check all that apply.)
   - ☐ Allergies (asthma, hives, hay fever)
   - ☐ Anemia
   - ☐ Bleeding tendency
   - ☐ Diabetes
   - ☐ Convulsions
   - ☐ Rheumatic fever
   - ☐ Pneumonia
   - ☐ Heart murmur
   - ☐ Urinary infection

2. Is your child receiving medications for any of the above problems or any other reasons? Yes ☐ No ☐ If yes, the medication and dose if possible: ________
   Is your child allergic to any medications? Yes ☐ No ☐
   Is your child receiving vitamins? Yes ☐ No ☐ If yes, what type? ________

3. Has your child been hospitalized at any time since birth? Yes ☐ No ☐
   If yes, the hospital, date, and reason, if possible: ________

4. Has the child's school work been satisfactory this past year? Yes ☐ No ☐
   As good as the previous year? Yes ☐ No ☐
   If no, what do you think is the reason? ________
   How many days was your child absent from school? ________
   What was the major reason for the child missing school? ________

5. How many colds has your child had during the past year? ________
   Were they severe? Yes ☐ No ☐ How long did they last? ________

6. Does your child appear to see and hear adequately? Yes ☐ No ☐
   Has the child's vision and hearing been tested? Yes ☐ No ☐
   If yes, when? ________
   Has the child's hearing been tested? Yes ☐ No ☐ If yes, when? ________
   Has the child complained of earaches? Yes ☐ No ☐
   Draining ears? Yes ☐ No ☐
   Nosebleeds? Yes ☐ No ☐
   Sore throats? Yes ☐ No ☐
   Red eyes? Yes ☐ No ☐
   Do the child's eyes ever turn in or out? Yes ☐ No ☐

7. Does your child have a chronic cough? Yes ☐ No ☐
   Does it awaken the child? Yes ☐ No ☐
   Does it cause vomiting? Yes ☐ No ☐
   Does the child have it now? Yes ☐ No ☐
   Has the child ever been wheezing? Yes ☐ No ☐
   Has the child had croup? Yes ☐ No ☐
   Has the child experienced shortness of breath? Yes ☐ No ☐

8. Has your child ever had a heart murmur? Yes ☐ No ☐
   When was it first heard? ________
   Can the child run and play as well as friends of the same age? Yes ☐ No ☐
   Does the child tire easily? Yes ☐ No ☐
   Does the child ever get a blue color to his skin? Yes ☐ No ☐

9. How is your child's appetite? ☐ Good ☐ Fair ☐ Poor
   Has the child lost weight recently? Yes ☐ No ☐
   Has the child been troubled with:
   Chronic diarrhea Yes ☐ No ☐
   Vomiting Yes ☐ No ☐
   Constipation Yes ☐ No
   Abdominal pain Yes ☐ No ☐
   Hernia Yes ☐ No ☐

10. Does your son have a good urinary stream? Yes ☐ No ☐
    Does your son or daughter urinate more frequently than normal? Yes ☐ No ☐
    Does the child complain of pain on urination? Yes ☐ No ☐
    Has the child ever had blood or pus in an examined urine specimen? Yes☐ No ☐

11. Is your child's gait (manner of walking) normal? Yes ☐ No ☐
    Does the child ever complain of joint pains? Yes ☐ No ☐

12. Does your child complain of headaches? Yes ☐ No ☐
    Has there ever been a severe head trauma? Yes ☐ No ☐
    Was the child unconscious during the trauma or at any other time? Yes ☐ No ☐
    Is the child nervous? Yes ☐ No ☐
    Has the child ever had a convulsion with or without fever? Yes ☐ No ☐
    Does the child have any of these habits:
    ☐ Thumbsucking
    ☐ Temper tantrums
    ☐ Tics
    ☐ Inability to get along with other children
    ☐ Bedwetting
    ☐ Watching TV excessively
    ☐ Masturbating excessively
    Are there any habits not mentioned that your child has? Yes ☐ No ☐
    If yes, explain: ______________________________

13. Is your child pale? Yes ☐ No ☐
    Is the child susceptible to rashes? Yes ☐ No ☐

14. Has your child had any contagious diseases since last seen by a doctor? Yes ☐ No ☐
    If yes, which of these:
    ☐ Chickenpox
    ☐ Mumps
    ☐ Measles
    ☐ Scarlet fever
    ☐ Strep throat
    ☐ German measles
    ☐ Roseola

15. In the past week, has your child had any of these symptoms:
    ☐ Nasal congestion
    ☐ Cough
    ☐ Sneezing
    ☐ Diarrhea
    ☐ Vomiting
    ☐ Abdominal cramps
    ☐ Fever
    ☐ Rash
    ☐ Contact with contagious diseases

APPENDIX 3

Health Record

Date recorded: ____________________

Fill out a copy of this record for each child and share it with your physician.

Name ______________________________ Birthdate ____________

Weight __________ Height __________

Family history of importance ______________________________

____

IMMUNIZATIONS & TESTS

1. Diphtheria-Whooping Cough-Tetanus: 1. ______ 2. ______ 3. ______
   Boosters: ____________ Td Boosters: ____________
2. Oral Polio trivalent: 1. ______ 2. ______ 3. ______
   Boosters: ____________ 5. Mumps: ____________
3. Tuberculin tests: ____________ 6. Rubella: ____________
4. Measles vaccine: ____________ 7. Hemophilus influenza: ____________

CONTAGIOUS DISEASE DATES

Measles: ____________ Mumps: ____________

Scarlet Fever: ____________ Whooping Cough: ____________

German Measles (Rubella): ____________ Chickenpox: ____________

Roseola: ____________

PAST ILLNESS DATES (Significant Illnesses)

____

ALLERGIES

____

INJURIES

____

HOSPITALIZATIONS (Dates & diagnoses)

____

OPERATIONS

Tonsillectomy & Adenoidectomy: ____________

Others: ____

Heart Surgery: ____________________

LABORATORY TESTS

Last hemoglobin or CBC (date): ____________ Last urinalysis (date): ____________

Last weight & height (date): ______________________________

Birth defects or special needs of your child: ______________________________

Additional information: ______________________________

____

Parent Questionnaire

If you plan to take your child to a new or different pediatrician or family physician, fill out a copy of this form before your appointment to give the new physician a quick profile of your child's health, growth, and development.

ABILITIES OF THE CHILD

1. Evaluate. Much above average (4+), above average (3+), average (2+), below average (1+), much below average (0):

   Reading ____________ Special interests ____________
   Spelling ____________ Writing ____________
   Arithmetic ____________ Athletics ____________
   Art ____________ Activity preferred ____________
   Music ____________ Activity avoided ____________

2. What special placement or help has the child had? (Check all that apply.)

   ☐ Upgraded ☐ Remedial reading
   ☐ Sight saving ☐ Repeater Grade: ______
   ☐ Special class ☐ Speech correction
   ☐ Tutoring Subject: ______

3. From your observation, disregarding achievement, consider the child's abilities in the following areas:

   General information ____________
   Self-expression ____________
   Grasp of concepts ____________
   Curiosity and desire to gain information ____________

4. Do you feel the child is working up to mental capacity? ☐ Yes ☐ No

ATTENTION SPAN (Check all that apply.)

☐ Listens ☐ Is easily distracted
☐ Observes ☐ Has short attention span
☐ Sticks to tasks ☐ Has long attention span
☐ Sustains interest in self-initiated projects

HOME BEHAVIOR (Check all that apply and add anything you consider important.)

☐ Sits fiddling with objects (fidgety) ☐ Steals
☐ Hums and makes odd sounds ☐ Is destructive
☐ Falls apart under stress ☐ Is annoying
☐ Has poor coordination ☐ Is aggressive
☐ Is restless and overactive ☐ Is submissive
☐ Is excitable ☐ Talks excessively
☐ Is inattentive ☐ Talks very little
☐ Has difficulty in concentration ☐ Acts without thought (impulsive)
☐ Is immature ☐ Is fearful
☐ Has temper outbursts ☐ Is dependent
☐ Daydreams ☐ Is cooperative
☐ Is sullen or sulky ☐ Bites nails
☐ Disturbs other children ☐ Sucks thumb
☐ Is quarrelsome ☐ Seeks unusual amount of attention
☐ Has tics (odd movements) ☐ Other ____________
☐ Tells lies

APPENDIX 4 (continued)

GROUP BEHAVIOR (Check and answer all that apply.)

☐ Enjoys companionship
☐ Is not accepted by other children
☐ Teases other children
☐ Injures other children
☐ Prefers to be with adults
☐ Possesses no sense of fair play
☐ Prefers solitary play
☐ Prefers younger children
☐ Prefers mother, father

How do classmates feel about the child? ______
How do members of the household feel about the child? ______
How do neighborhood children feel about the child? ______

LANGUAGE AND SPEECH (Check all that apply.)

☐ Follows directions
☐ Repeats directions given
☐ Expresses self in sentences
☐ Uses expressive vocabulary
☐ Recalls new words
☐ Enunciates clearly
☐ Exhibits immature speech
☐ Stutters

COORDINATION (Check all that apply.)

Gross:

☐ Is well coordinated
☐ Runs well
☐ Walks well
☐ Skips
☐ Hops
☐ Rides a tricycle or bicycle

Fine:

☐ Draws well
☐ Colors well
☐ Does a puzzle well
☐ Writes own name well
☐ Holds pencil correctly
☐ Reverses letters or words
☐ Draws and writes neatly

Handed:

☐ Right ☐ Left ☐ Both

PERIODS OF STRESS IN THE CHILD'S LIFE

Hospitalizations: ______
Significant injuries: ______
Marital problems of parents: ______
Changes in the household (new baby, others living in the household): ______
Moving to a new home: ______
How do the parents react to the child's failures? ______
What are the child's successes? ______
How do the parents react to the child's successes? ______
Are there books, a dictionary, other learning materials in the home? ☐ Yes ☐ No
Does the child have a fear of going to school: ______

HIGHEST GRADE OF SCHOOL COMPLETED BY

Mother ______
Father ______
Brothers ______
Sisters ______

SCHOOL RECORD

Days tardy __________ Days absent __________

Visits to the school nurse's office during the past year __________

Visits to the doctor's office during the past year __________

Is the child robust or sickly? __________

Did brothers, sisters, parents, or close relatives have an educational problem?

☐ Yes ☐ No If yes, what was it? ____________________________________

How does this child differ from other children? ______________________________

APPENDIX 5

Blood Count

A blood count is a laboratory test that measures the number and characteristics of the red and white blood cells and the platelets in a drop of blood.

• Red blood cells carry oxygen from inhaled air in the lungs to all parts of the body and return carbon dioxide to the child's lungs for elimination through the exhaled air.

• White blood cells fight infection and perform many other functions. The white blood cell count may help to determine if a child's infection is viral or bacterial by the total number of cells. A high white blood cell count suggests a bacterial infection that may be helped by antibiotics. A low white blood cell count may indicate a virus disease, which usually does not respond to antibiotics.

• Platelets are small white blood cells that play an important role in blood clotting.

The blood count is done in several parts, including the *hematocrit*, the *hemoglobin*, and the *blood smear*.

• The hematocrit measures the proportion of red cells in a unit of blood. This test is done with blood in a centrifuge (a machine that spins its contents at a very rapid speed for the purpose of separating substances of differing densities). When the tube is spun, the blood is separated into the cells and the plasma. The proportion of the centrifuged column of blood occupied by the red blood cells is known as the hematocrit.

• The hemoglobin test measures the quantity of hemoglobin (the red chemical contained in the red blood cells that binds oxygen and carbon dioxide) in a unit volume of blood.

• The blood smear measures a number of components, including the number of white cells per cubic centimeter of blood and the differential white count (the proportion of the various kinds of white cells present). A drop of blood is placed on a glass slide and spread thin. The smear is stained with a special dye that colors the red blood cells, the white blood cells, and the platelets, making them more visible. One hundred white blood cells are counted and classified according to cell type. The shape, size, and intensity of coloration of the red blood cells and the number of platelets can also be determined.

Blood counts frequently help establish a precise diagnosis. However, the history of the illness and the physical examination are equally important.

APPENDIX 6 (continued on next page)

Urinalysis

Urinary tract infections are the second most frequent infections (upper respiratory infections are first) that occur in children. These infections may be present and cause no symptoms, or they may cause obvious symptoms such as fever, frequent urination, and burning during urination. Some infections of the urinary tract may start as unexplained fever with no other obvious cause.

A *urinalysis* is a routine examination of a urine specimen in an office or laboratory that includes the study of:

- The urine pH (acidity or alkalinity of the urine), which serves as a clue to urinary tract infection, urine stones, and disturbances in the body's acid-base balance.
- Protein in the urine, which may be a sign of kidney disease.
- Glucose (sugar) in the urine, which may be an indicator of diabetes.
- Ketones in the urine, which indicate the status of body fat metabolism.
- Blood in the urine, which is a sign of kidney or urinary tract disease.
- Pus cells and bacteria, which may indicate urinary infection.

A *colony count* is a special test that checks for bacteria (germs) in urine cultured for 24 to 48 hours. Counting the number of bacteria that grow in a calculated amount of urine for a specified length of time aids the doctor in determining the presence of infection.

The colony count is more reliable than a routine urinalysis in detecting urinary tract infection. Urine that contains germs is either *infected* (from germs in the bladder or kidney) or *contaminated* from germs normally on the skin being washed along with the urine stream. If 2 or more different types of germs are found, contamination is the usual cause. Infection is usually caused by a single type of germ.

It is important to determine whether the urine is infected or merely contaminated, because prescribing medicine and referring to a urologist may be decided from the test. If the child does not have specific urinary symptoms, but the "count" is positive, your physician may wish to re-examine the urine and even catheterize the patient before labeling the problem a urinary tract infection.

Most authorities recommend X-ray studies of the urinary tract for boys after the first urinary infection is diagnosed, and for girls after the second. However, this is determined by each child's particular circumstances. Hospitalization may be necessary for some of the tests.

In addition to the urinalysis, colony counts, and X-rays, parents should observe their babies and young children for the following signs that may indicate a problem with the urinary tract.

- Straining with urination. This is normal with the passage of gas and bowel movements in babies, but not with urination.
- A thin, weak urinary stream or one that is interrupted (stops and starts with no reason), dribbles out, is divided, or is misdirected.
- Any pain or burning during urination.
- Frequent urination so the diaper or underclothes are continually wet.

Routine urinalysis screening is done annually at the regular checkup, whenever a child has fever without an apparent cause, or if there are any symptoms of a urinary tract infection.

Protein in the urine (proteinuria) may be a sign of renal (kidney) disease. The kidney acts as a sieve that allows only very small amounts of protein to pass into the urine, normally too little to show up as more than a trace on the chemical tests used for urine. Thus when protein shows up in the urine, your physician must be certain not to overlook a renal problem.

Some adolescents and older children who are growing rapidly may show protein in their urine only when they are standing, but not when they are lying down. This condition, called "orthostatic albuminuria," is not usually a renal problem, although it must be followed carefully by your physician.

To test whether orthostatic albuminuria or a renal problem is present, your child should follow these instructions:

- Urinate and empty the bladder just before going to sleep at night.
- Urinate upon awakening in the morning, into a jar while still lying flat in bed, if possible.
- Urinate again into another jar after moving around for a few hours.
- Do this for 2 days and take each urine specimen to the lab, labeled as to the time and position taken (lying flat or standing), to be tested for protein in the urine.

Children with orthostatic albuminuria should have a complete urinalysis every 6 months to make sure no renal problem is developing. Baseline kidney tests may be ordered.

TO COLLECT A STERILE URINE SPECIMEN

- Use a proper sterile container. Obtain an open-neck jar (peanut butter, jam, etc.) and wash and thoroughly rinse the jar and lid. Place the jar with the lid lying beside it in boiling water and let them boil for 15-20 minutes. Let the jar air dry. Shake the water out of the jar, but do not wipe it out, because this may introduce germs. The purity of the urine is the important part, not the exact amount. If some water droplets remain in the jar, it is not important.

- Cleanse the child.
  —Boys: Using a non-irritating antiseptic solution such as pHisoHex, saturate a cotton ball and thoroughly but gently cleanse the end of the penis if the child is toilet trained. If the boy is not circumcised, draw the foreskin back as much as possible, cleanse the area, and collect urine in the clean jar, with the foreskin drawn back. For an infant, cleanse the entire penis and surrounding area that fits into the urine collection bag your doctor will prescribe.
  —Girls: Proper collection of a clean-catch midstream urine specimen requires that a sample be obtained after the urethra (opening to the bladder) and surrounding area have been thoroughly cleansed with a non-irritating antiseptic solution, then rinsed with sterile water and gently wiped dry with a sterile towel prior to voiding. For an infant, use the sterile urine collection bag your doctor will prescribe. Being careful not to touch the inside of the bag, peel off the adhesive, spread the child's labia (the outer lips of the genitals) after cleansing as described above, and stick the bag on the open area.

- Important points:
—Midstream urine: Ideally the collection of urine from a girl should be done after voiding is started and before urination stops, from the "middle of the stream." This is done by having the girl squat over the sterile container after she has begun to urinate.
—Storage: If not immediately taken to the doctor's office or laboratory, the urine should be placed in the refrigerator (not in the freezer). Urine should not stand unrefrigerated more than 2 hours before analysis.
—The first morning specimen is preferred, but urine collected at other times is also acceptable. When the specimen is brought to the office or laboratory, be sure to tell the nurse or technician that it is for a *colony count*, if that is what your physician has ordered. Otherwise, only a simple, routine urinalysis will be done.

APPENDIX 7

Evaluation of Your Child's Pain

To aid in understanding your child's pain, make and record observations of the following factors. Report them to your doctor:

• **Location of pain:** Be as precise as possible. Ask the child to point with one finger where it hurts the most. If it isn't in one spot, note this also.

• **Severity:** (How bad is the pain?) Compare it with other hurts or pains the child has experienced. Is it disabling? Does it interfere with sleep? Can the child be distracted from the pain? Is it present when the child is at rest or only when moving?

• **Nature:** (Description of the type of pain.) An older child may be able to describe the pain as burning, sharp, throbbing, cramp-like. Does the pain come and go or is it there all the time?

• **Response of pain to treatment:** (What relieves the pain or makes the pain worse?) Is it better or worse at rest or with moving about? Do certain positions relieve or make the child's pain worse? Is it worse with deep breathing, running, or resting? Do any drugs relieve the pain? Does a bowel movement relieve the pain?

• **Associated symptoms:** Are there any other sensations or symptoms associated with the pain, such as hunger, dizziness, cramps, diarrhea, pallor (paleness), fever, eating, eating certain foods, running, coughing, or nasal congestion?

• **Timing of the pain:** What time of the day does the child's pain occur? What days of the week? Is it related to school? Do other symptoms occur before, during or after the episode of pain? Did vomiting occur before or after or during the abdominal pain or headache? Does vomiting relieve the pain?

• **Precipitating factor:** Is there anything that appears to bring on the child's pain? Fever, emotional upset or tension, hunger?

• **Duration:** How long does the pain last? How often do episodes of pain occur?

• **Onset:** Does the pain start suddenly or gradually? Ask the child to try to recall the exact day and time the pain began.

• **Radiation:** Does the child's pain begin at one point and spread to other areas? If so, when?

• **Family history:** Is there anyone at home who has recently had or is presently suffering from a similar pain? Is there a family history of similar pain?

• **When the child is busy or distracted,** such as watching a favorite TV show or playing a game, does the pain seem to go away or get better?

APPENDIX 8

Testicular Pain Without A Specific Diagnosis

Testicular pain is unusual in a young boy, but when it occurs it can be serious.

CAUSES AND TREATMENT

• **Injury or direct blow to the groin**—The pain is often severe, leading to crying and doubling up. An ice pack will relieve the discomfort, which should be gone in an hour. If the boy's pain persists or worsens, particularly if there is swelling and discoloration, contact your son's physician.

• **Twisting of the spermatic cord (torsion) THIS IS AN EMERGENCY!**—The spermatic cord is a tube attached to the upper pole of the testes. It contains the vas deferens (which transports sperm), blood vessels, nerves, and muscle. If it twists, the blood supply to the testis is cut off and there is a danger of infarction (death) of the testicular tissue from poor circulation. As this develops, the testis swells and becomes painful. Later a fever, abdominal pain, and vomiting develop. The only treatment is emergency surgery to untwist the spermatic cord and fix the testis to the scrotum so that retwisting cannot occur.

• **Twisting of the small testicular appendage**—More common is a twist of a testicular appendage (torsion of the appendix testis). This is a small, normal structure that protrudes from the testis. It may twist and die, causing symptoms that are indistinguishable from a twisting of the entire testis. The testis in this condition remains alive. Surgery may be necessary to rule out the possibility of torsion of the entire testis and to alleviate the pain this condition causes.

• **Bacterial infection**—Bacterial infection of the epididymis (an elongated, cordlike structure along the back of the testis) occurs in adolescence and occasionally in younger children. Often it is associated with a urinary tract infection.

• **Testicular tumors**—Testicular tumors are rare causes of pain in the testes.

• **Mumps**—Testicular pain can occur with mumps but is almost never seen in children who have not reached puberty.

HOME CARE

When the exact diagnosis is not clear, call your doctor if:

• Your son's temperature continues to rise.
• The testicle becomes harder.
• The testicle becomes larger.
• The pain continues to get worse.
• Nausea or vomiting begin.

APPENDIX 9

Childhood Headache—Investigating the Cause

An investigation to determine the cause of your child's headaches may be extensive and include several laboratory studies as well as a complete physical examination. Even so, perhaps the most important part of the investigation will be collecting detailed information regarding several factors. You can help this part a great deal if you will complete a copy of the following questionnaire and share the information with your physician.

DESCRIPTION OF PAIN

1. At what age did the headaches begin? ____________
2. Where is the headache located? (front, side, top, back of neck, all over?) ________
3. Does the pain begin in one area and spread to a different area? ☐ Yes ☐ No
   If so, where? ____________
4. How severe is the pain? Does it awaken the child from sleep, interfere with school work, sports, TV? ____________
5. What is the nature of the pain? Pressure, band around the head, throbbing, ache?
   ____
6. Are there any symptoms occurring before the headache? ☐ Yes ☐ No
   If yes, specify:
   - ☐ Light sensitivity
   - ☐ Mood changes
   - ☐ Weakness
   - ☐ Spots before eyes
   - ☐ Irritability
   - ☐ "Tightening up" and "relaxing" movements
   - ☐ Unusual odors
   - ☐ Others ____________
7. How often does the headache occur? ____________
8. How long does it last?
   Minutes ________ Hours ________ Days ________ Weeks ________
9. When does it occur?
   - ☐ Mornings
   - ☐ On weekdays
   - ☐ On weekends
   - ☐ On holidays
   - ☐ At night
   - ☐ On vacation
   - ☐ During school
   - ☐ Afternoon
   - ☐ Before meals
   - ☐ Evening
   - ☐ While reading

FAMILY HISTORY

1. Does anyone else in the family have headaches? ☐ Yes ☐ No
2. Type of headaches: Migraine ________ Tension ________ Other ____________
3. Relationship to patient: ____________
4. History of allergy in family? ☐ Yes ☐ No
5. Does any member of the family have diseases involving the head?
   ☐ Yes ☐ No If yes, specify: ☐Tumor ☐Stroke ☐Other ____________

MENTAL STATUS

(Check those that apply.)

☐ Acts normal during attack
☐ Acts differently during attack
☐ After headache, drowsiness or sleep
☐ Other ____________

APPENDIX 9 (continued)

FACTORS INFLUENCING HEADACHE

(Check those that apply.)

1. Caused by:
   - ☐ Movies, TV, sunlight, strobe lights
   - ☐ Anxiety and stress (exams, arguments, illness, exercise, allergy)
   - ☐ Reading
   - ☐ Changes in position
   - ☐ Coughing or sneezing
   - ☐ Temperature change
   - ☐ Recent head injury
   - ☐ Other ______
2. Relieved by:
   - ☐ Non-prescription pain medicine (name/dosage) ______
   - ☐ Distraction
   - ☐ Quiet/darkened room
   - ☐ Sleep/bed rest
   - ☐ Other (cold compresses) ______
   - ☐ Other (drugs—name them) ______

______

ASSOCIATED SYMPTOMS

(Check those that apply.)

- ☐ Abdominal pain
- ☐ Pallor, blueness, flushing
- ☐ Sweating
- ☐ Dizziness (vertigo)
- ☐ Nausea/vomiting
- ☐ Neck or shoulder soreness
- ☐ Double or blurred vision
- ☐ Numbness
- ☐ Stuffy or runny nose
- ☐ Chills
- ☐ Fatigue
- ☐ Sinus pain
- ☐ Fever
- ☐ Change in sense of smell
- ☐ Hearing loss/ringing in ears
- ☐ Weakness

Other ______

PHYSICAL HISTORY

(Check those that apply.)

- ☐ Loss of appetite
- ☐ Fatigue or tiredness
- ☐ Abdominal pain when younger
- ☐ Burning or tearing of eyes
- ☐ Teeth clenching or grinding
- ☐ Recent dental work
- ☐ Unexplained fevers
- ☐ Staggering
- ☐ Nervous tremor
- ☐ Seizures
- ☐ Weakness
- ☐ Drugs
- ☐ Allergies
- ☐ Behavior change
- ☐ Seeing double
- ☐ Birth injury
- ☐ Nightmares/phobias
- ☐ Runny nose
- ☐ Head trauma

APPENDIX 10

Back Care Instructions for Your Child

EXERCISES WHILE BACK PAIN IS PRESENT

While lying on your back:

• Bring one knee up to your chest. Lower it slowly, but do not straighten your leg. Relax. Repeat with each leg 10 times.
• Bring both knees slowly up to your chest. Tighten the abdominal muscles and press your back flat against the bed. Hold your knees to your chest 20 seconds, then lower slowly. Relax. Repeat 5 times. This exercise gently stretches shortened muscles of the lower back, while strengthening abdominal muscles. Clasp your knees, bring them up to your chest, at the same time coming to a sitting position. Rock back and forth.

EXERCISES AFTER BACK PAIN SUBSIDES

Use these inconspicuous exercises whenever you have a spare moment during the day, both to reduce tension and improve the tone of important muscle groups.

• Rotate your shoulders, forward and backward.
• Turn your head slowly side to side.
• Turn your head down and to the right as if stretching to see your right armpit. Stretch your neck slowly up, around and down, switching to a gaze at your left armpit. Repeat, starting on the left side.
• Slowly, touch left ear to left shoulder, then right ear to right shoulder. Raise both shoulders to touch ears, then drop them as far down as possible.
• At any pause in the day (such as waiting for class to begin), pull in the abdominal muscles, tighten and hold for the count of 8 without breathing. Relax slowly. Increase the count gradually after the first week, and practice breathing normally with the abdomen flat and contracted. Do this while sitting, standing, and walking.

RULES TO PREVENT RECURRENT BACK PAIN

• Never bend from the waist only. Bend both hips and knees.
• Never lift a heavy object higher than your waist.
• Always turn and face the object you wish to lift.
• Avoid carrying unbalanced loads. Hold heavy objects close to your body.
• Never carry anything heavier than you can easily manage.
• Never lift or move heavy furniture alone. Get help from someone who knows the principles of leverage.
• Avoid sudden movements that "overload" muscles. Learn to move deliberately, swinging the legs from the hips.
• Train yourself to use your abdominal muscles to flatten your lower abdomen. In time, this muscle contraction will become a habit.
• For good posture, concentrate on strengthening "nature's corset," the abdominal and buttock muscles.
• For proper bed posture, a firm mattress is essential. If you have a soft mattress, you need a ¾-inch piece of plywood under it. Lie and sleep on your side with the knees flexed.
• Learn to keep your head in line with your spine when standing, sitting, and lying in bed.
• Don't sit in soft chairs and deep couches. During prolonged sitting, cross your legs to rest your back.
• Use a rocking chair. Rocking rests the back.
• Avoid exercise that arches or overstrains the lower back, such as backward bends, forward bends, or touching your toes with your knees straight.

APPENDIX 11

How to Treat Diarrhea with Clear Liquids

One of the best treatments for diarrhea is letting the bowel rest. An already inflamed bowel can quickly heal itself if it is left alone for a day or two.

However, a child can't be starved for 2 days, and a child must have fluids, so how can the bowel be given a rest? The answer is with frequent small feedings of clear liquids (such as those listed below).

- For infants under 1 year, give ½ ounce (no more), every 20 minutes.
- For children over 1 year, give 1 ounce (no more), every 30 minutes.

For the first few hours, this diet will not satisfy your child. The child will almost certainly want more, but don't give in. Soon the diarrhea will stop and the child will begin to catch up on lost fluids. You may have to continue giving your child fluids in this manner for most of the waking hours of 1 or 2 days. The child will let you know when the thirst is quenched.

A few words of caution:
- Offer only the amount of fluid you intend for the child to have at one time. A thirsty baby can down 4 ounces of fluid in almost no time at all.
- Do not supplement the clear fluids with milk (which makes curds) or with solid foods.
- Call your doctor if the diarrhea continues in spite of several hours of frequent small clear-liquid feedings.
- Do not use Kaopectate or other stool-firming agents. They usually don't work well in children and often make things worse.

When your child has been diarrhea-free for 1 whole day, offer a single "solid" feeding from the list of low-residue foods (such as those listed below). If no diarrhea occurs in the next 2 hours, feed the child from this list for the rest of the day. If all goes well, give your child a regular diet after that.

Danger signals are a black tarry-looking stool or bright red blood in the stool. Call your doctor right away if either should happen.

Clear Liquid Foods:

Sweetened tea
Apple, grape, or cranberry juice
Coke, Pepsi, Dr. Pepper, etc.
Jello or Jello-water

16 oz. (1 pint) water plus—
— ¼ level teaspoon salt
— 1 level tablespoon sugar
1 bouillon cube/per quart of water

Low-Residue Foods:

Melon
Banana
Applesauce (cooked)
Cherries (cooked)
Peaches (cooked)
Pears (cooked)
Eggs
Ground Meat
Peanut Butter

Bread
Rice, Noodles
Carrots (cooked)
Peas (cooked)
Canned Tomatoes (cooked)
Potatoes
Sugar Cookies
Lollipops

APPENDIX 12

Care of the Sick Child at Home

• The person taking care of a sick child should wear clothing that can be laundered (for example, a coverall apron that can be worn and left in the sickroom). Wash the hands with soap and running water immediately after each handling of the sick child. Ignore suggestions of neighbors and relatives. Visitors should not be allowed because they could be carrying infections that the now run-down patient cannot resist.

• A separate room, well-ventilated, well-lit, and near the bathroom is best. The temperature the patient prefers is important. For a child too young to express a preference, it is best to keep the temperature between 68 and 72 degrees while the patient is sleeping. It is helpful to put the child in warm clothing and to ventilate the room 3 times a day—on arising, after lunch, and before retiring. Lighting can be adjusted depending on the patient's preference.

• The room should contain a minimum of equipment:
—Comb, brush, washcloths, towels, toothbrush and toothpaste, and a basin, if needed, for vomitus.
—A clinical thermometer, 70% alcohol, tissues for nose and throat discharges, a paper or plastic bag to discard the used tissues. (The top of this bag should be tied before careful disposal.)
—Take medications with you when you leave a child's room, and lock them in the medicine cabinet for safety.
—Bed clothing should be made of light, washable materials. Change a baby's diapers frequently. For children not in diapers who cannot control body discharges while they are ill, protection such as a vinyl mattress cover, rubber sheet, oil cloth, or even newspapers under the sheet can be used. A plastic case under a cloth pillowcase helps to prevent contamination of the pillow. Sheets can be washed and then sterilized by hot ironing.
—Eating utensils should be the disposable type, or else should be kept separate and boiled for 5 minutes before putting them back with the family dishes.

• Give the child a light, warm sponge bath and a clean set of sleeping garments on arising and retiring. Clean the child's teeth and comb the hair—important points for general morale.

• Use toys and books that are washable. Otherwise, air them for 24 hours after the illness, or discard them.

• After an illness of the virus type, airing the room for 6 to 12 hours will be sufficient to kill the virus. After bacterial infection such as streptococcus, wash down the walls and furniture with disinfectant washes.

• The child who feels well enough can spend time out of bed and can even be taken out in the car.

• Unless there is an emergency, report on the following during your doctor's "call hours" the next day:
- —The child's temperature.
- —Quality and duration of sleep.
- —Bowel movements.
- —Amount of urine passed (in babies, the diapers were dry for how long?).
- —Amount of liquids taken.
- —Attitude or mood of the child (irritable, cheerful, etc.).
- —Any new symptoms, such as rash, pain and its locations, diarrhea, vomiting, cough, nasal congestion.

• Outdoor activities such as an airing, a ride in a car, or ventilating the room may be beneficial even for a child with fever. Keep a sick child away from people, because they can transmit new diseases when the child is run-down.

• Playing outdoors with other children or going back to school or daycare depends upon the disease, how fast the patient responds to treatment, and the results of appropriate laboratory tests. In most instances the child should not associate with others for a minimum of 2 days after any fever and 5 days after a streptococcal infection. Also, the child should be as active as during the previously healthy state before being allowed in contact with others. Call your physician during call hours to discuss this aspect of the child's care.

APPENDIX 13

When Your Child Is Ill (Observation Checklist)

Be a good communicator. When you think or know your child is ill, be prepared to answer questions about the child. The knowledge gained from the answers will help your physician decide what to do.

• When you call, give the full name of the child, the age, and any known allergies or reactions to medication used in the past.
• Write down what seems to be wrong. This will help clarify the problem in your mind.
• Have your druggist's phone number available.

To assist in preparing answers to most of the questions your physician may ask, use the following list of observations. Note them before placing the call.

CHECKLIST OF OBSERVATIONS OF YOUR CHILD WHEN ILL

Important: For any positive answer, tell how long the observation has been present.

1. Temperature:
   Is there fever? Yes ☐ No ☐
   What is it now? ____________________
   What was the highest degree? ____________________
   Have you given the child medicine to reduce it? Yes ☐ No ☐
   When did you last give this medicine? ____________________
   What did you give? ____________________
2. Eyes:
   Is there a discharge of pus? Yes ☐ No ☐
   Are they red? Yes ☐ No ☐
3. Nose:
   Is it running or stuffy? Yes ☐ No ☐
4. Ears:
   Is there an indication of pain? Yes ☐ No ☐
   Is there a discharge? Yes ☐ No ☐
5. Mouth:
   Is there a complaint of sore throat? Yes ☐ No ☐
   Difficulty in swallowing? Yes ☐ No ☐
   Can the child swallow water? Yes ☐ No ☐
6. Neck:
   Is it stiff or painful? Yes ☐ No ☐
   Can the chin be bent to touch the chest? Yes ☐ No ☐
   Are the glands swollen? Yes ☐ No ☐
7. Chest:
   Is it heaving? Yes ☐No ☐
   Pulling in? Yes ☐ No ☐
   Is there a wheeze? Yes ☐ No ☐
   Is there a cough? Yes ☐ No ☐
   Is the cough dry, moist, barking? Circle the most appropriate.
   When does the cough occur? ____________________
   Does the cough produce vomiting or awaken the child from sleep? Yes ☐ No ☐
   Is there rapid breathing? Yes ☐ No ☐
   (Count the child's breathing rate for 1 full minute and report.)
   Is there hoarseness? Yes ☐ No ☐

APPENDIX 13 (continued)

8. Abdomen:
   Is vomiting present? Yes ☐ No ☐
   How many times the past day? ______
   Is diarrhea present? Yes ☐ No ☐
   How many times the past day? ______
   When did the child urinate last? ______
   Did the bowel movement contain mucus or blood? Yes ☐ No ☐
   Where is it tender when you press on it? ______
   Is the abdomen bulging? Yes ☐ No ☐
   Is there a bulging in the groin? Yes ☐ No ☐
   If yes, where? ☐ navel
   ☐ upper right
   ☐ upper left
   ☐ lower right
   ☐ lower left
   Is there a bulging in the scrotum? Yes ☐ No ☐
9. Limbs:
   Can the child's limbs be moved freely without pain? Yes ☐ No ☐
   Is there a limp? Yes ☐ No ☐
   Is there swelling? Yes ☐ No ☐
10. Skin:
    Is there a rash? Yes ☐ No ☐
    Is it red, pink, purple, blistered, raw? Circle the most appropriate.
    Is it painful, tender, itchy? Yes ☐ No ☐
    Does it remain in one spot or change areas? Yes ☐ No ☐
11. Contact:
    Are any family members ill? Yes ☐ No ☐
    Is there any illness in the neighborhood or school? Yes ☐ No ☐
    Has there been any contact with a contagious disease? Yes ☐ No ☐
12. In what way is the child acting differently? ______
    ______
13. Have you given any medication for this illness? Yes ☐ No ☐
    If yes, what?
    For how long?
    Do you think it helped? Yes ☐ No ☐

APPENDICES

APPENDIX 14

Vaporizers for Cool Mist

Coughing is often caused by thick, sticky mucus getting on the vocal cords. This irritates the vocal cords and triggers a coughing reflex—a natural way to keep foreign material out of the lungs.

Handling a Cough

- Suppressing the cough reflex with a cough syrup that contains codeine or dextromethorphan may result in pneumonia.
- Helping the cough become more effective by making mucus thin and less sticky is a better practice. There are cough syrups that are supposed to do this, but they don't work very well. The best remedy for coughing (and certainly the safest and cheapest) is a cool mist vaporizer. By putting water into the air, the vaporizer allows the child's mucus to become less sticky, the coughing to be more effective, and the lungs to be protected.

Do's and Don'ts about Vaporizers

- Do get a cool mist vaporizer.
- Don't get a hot mist vaporizer or "steamer." They are dangerous and can cause serious burns.
- Don't put anything but cool water in your cool mist vaporizer. Commercial compounds and oils do no good at all and may ruin your vaporizer.
- Do get a large vaporizer, preferably one with a 1½- to 2-gallon capacity.
- Don't confuse a vaporizer with a humidifier. A good vaporizer puts out an easily visible column of mist, makes the whole room feel moist, and is designed for intermittent use (as when your child has a cold). A humidifier puts out much less vapor, is designed for constant use in a dry climate and adds very little water to the air.
- Don't use the vaporizer all the time. Mold will grow on your wallpaper and window sills, and your furniture will be damaged. (This is particularly important for children with allergies to molds.)
- When you do use the vaporizer, close the windows and doors and turn the equipment on as high as it will go.
- Clean the vaporizer thoroughly after each use and dry it inside and out before putting it away. Never store the vaporizer with water in it.

APPENDIX 15

Baby with a Cold: How to Clean the Nose

Small infants (especially those under 5 or 6 months of age) become particularly miserable when they catch a cold. The principal reason is that *until* they are about 5 or 6 months old, babies may be unable to breathe through their mouths when their noses get plugged up with mucus. Thus, they can't sleep and they can't relax.

To help remedy this situation, you may need to clean out your baby's nose from time to time, especially when the baby is ready for sleep. Follow this technique:

• Obtain a bottle of "isotonic saline nose drops," or prepare your own by adding ½ teaspoon of salt to 8 ounces of water), boil for 15 minutes, and allow to cool. Have close by a dropper, a soft rubber bulb ear syringe, and a person to help.

• Request the helper to hold the baby's face upward with the child's head between the helper's knees. Hold the head and arms still.

• Squirt a dropperful of the saline nose drops gently into one nostril.

• Insert the soft rubber tip of the nose syringe into the baby's nostril and gently but thoroughly suck out the mucus. The child will probably object.

• Repeat the previous 2 steps, several times if necessary, until both of the baby's nostrils are clear and clean. You can use as many dropperfuls of the saline nose drops as you need to clean the baby's nose.

• Put your child to bed with a cool mist vaporizer.

CAUTION:
• Don't use regular adult nose drops, which are too strong for a baby.
• A baby with a fever should be seen by your doctor.
• A baby that "looks sick" should be seen by your doctor.
• A baby with a significant cough should be seen by your doctor.

APPENDIX 16

How to Give Nose Drops

- Lay your child down on his back on a bed or sofa.

- Bend his head over the edge of the bed so that his nostrils are pointing toward the ceiling.

- Quickly squirt about ¾ of a dropperful of the prescribed children's nose drops well into each nostril.

- The child will probably object strenuously because it stings a little.

- Continue holding your child down while you count slowly to 20. This will give the nose drops time to drain well down into the nasal passages.

- Repeat no oftener than every 4 hours.

- Do not give nose drops for more than 3 consecutive days. Children quickly lose their responsiveness to them and, after 3 days, drops just irritate the nose!

- Never use any strong adult nose drops in your child.

- Do not use nose drops with an oil base in infants. Check the label carefully.

APPENDIX 17

How to Reduce Your Child's Fever

DON'T GIVE ASPIRIN TO A CHILD TO REDUCE FEVER!
Fever is the body's reaction to infection or inflammation. It is not a disease in itself, but rather a sign of a problem.

The normal temperature in children varies with activity, eating, and the time of day, ranging from 99F (37.2C) to 100F (37.8C) *rectally* in healthy children. Rectal thermometers are the most accurate and are the preferred method of taking temperature in children under 10 years old. The thermometer has its line at 98.6F (37C), which is *not* the normal rectal temperature.

FLUIDS
Fluids are the only important requirement in the diet of a child with fever. Provide your child with water, weak tea, ginger ale, broth, nectar, or liquid Jello. Some of the best-tolerated foods are saltines, cereal, applesauce, bananas, carrots, and lean meat. Offer food, but don't force it. Fluids in small, frequent doses are all that is important for the first few days.

HOW TO REDUCE FEVER
If your child's temperature rises to 103F (39.4C) or above, your doctor may recommend sponging the child's body with warm water to reduce the fever temporarily. This is one common technique:

- Remove all clothing and lay the child down on a towel.
- Fill a basin with warm water.
- Dip a washcloth (preferably a new one that is still a little bit rough) into the warm water. Wring it out until it is damp but not soggy.
- Using the washcloth, begin massaging all over the body, covering as much surface as you can. The child should not be dripping wet, but should feel moist all over.
- Continue constant gentle massaging. This increases the flow of warm blood to the skin.
- When the washcloth begins to cool off, dip it into the warm water and wring it out again.
- Repeat massages. In 5 to 15 minutes, the child's temperature will probably be on its way down.
- Don't use a fan, alcohol, ice, or cold water, and don't use cold baths or leave your child covered with wet towels!
- Don't give the child aspirin because of the danger of developing Reye's syndrome. (See Reye's syndrome in Illnesses section.)
- When giving acetaminophen, follow dosage instructions on the package carefully.

APPENDIX 18

Safe Use of Medicine for Your Child

Some suggestions for wise, safe use of medicine apply to all medicines. Your doctor and dentist must have complete information to prescribe drugs wisely for your child or any member of your family. Always give the following information to your physician, dentist, or other health-care professional:

YOUR CHILD'S COMPLETE MEDICAL HISTORY

Tell the important facts of your child's medical history dealing with medicines. Include allergic reactions, side effects, or adverse reactions your child has experienced in the past. Describe the allergic problems your child has, such as hay fever, asthma, eye watering and itching, throat irritation and reactions to food. Children who have allergies to common substances are more likely to develop side effects or adverse reactions to drugs.

MEDICINES YOUR CHILD IS TAKING NOW

List all prescription and non-prescription drugs. Don't forget common ones such as laxatives; vitamin or mineral supplements; skin, rectal or vaginal medicines; antacids; antihistamines; cold and cough remedies; aspirin and aspirin-containing pain pills; motion sickness remedies; weight-loss aids; salt and sugar substitutes; caffeine (in coffee, tea, cola drinks, and cocoa); oral contraceptives; sleeping pills; or "tonics."

KNOW THIS INFORMATION BEFORE GIVING YOUR CHILD ANY MEDICINE

- Generic names and brand names of all the medicines your child takes. Write them down to help you remember. If a drug is a mixture of two or more generic ingredients, learn the names of each.
- Uses for each medicine your child takes.
- How to take each medicine—for example, with or without water, or with food.
- When to take the medicine.
- What to do if your child forgets a dose.
- How each drug works in your child's body.
- Time lapse before the drug works.
- Symptoms and treatment of overdose.
- Possible adverse reactions and side effects and what to do if they occur.
- Interactions with other drugs and other substances such as alcohol, food, beverages, cocaine, marijuana, and tobacco. When mixed with some medicines, these substances can sometimes cause life-threatening interactions in your child.
- Know all warnings and precautions that apply to special circumstances, such as:
  1. Reasons not to take the drug in the presence of some medical conditions. These reasons are called *contraindications*.
  2. Special considerations for infants, children, and pregnant or breast-feeding women.
  3. Implications for prolonged use; exposure to sun and sunlight; driving; flying in airplanes; hazardous activities.
  4. Instructions before discontinuing the drug.

OTHER SAFETY TIPS FOR YOUR CHILD

- Before giving any prescribed medicine to a child, discuss with your doctor any plans for elective surgery or other problems.
- Don't hesitate to ask questions about a drug. Your doctor, nurse, and pharmacist will be able to provide more information if they are familiar with you and your family's past medical history, especially regarding medicines.
- Never give or take medicine in the dark! It is always possible to take the wrong one. Recheck the label each time you or your child use a drug.
- Tell your doctor about any new or unexpected symptoms your child develops while taking medicine. You may need to change medicines or have a dose adjustment.
- Store all medicines out of children's reach. Keep drugs in a cool, dry place, such as a kitchen cabinet or bedroom. Avoid medicine cabinets in bathrooms—they get too moist and warm at times. Keep medicine in its original container, tightly closed. Don't remove the label! If the directions call for refrigeration, keep the medicine cool but don't freeze it.
- Don't save leftover oral or injectable medicine to use later. Discard it before or on the expiration date shown on the container. Dispose of it safely to protect children and pets.
- Study any information you can find about the specific drugs your child takes. An excellent reference is *Complete Guide to Prescription and Non-Prescription Drugs,* published by The Body Press, a division of Price Stern & Sloan, Inc.
- Don't give your child any drug prescribed for someone else.
- Prior to any surgery (including oral surgery or simple dental procedures), tell your doctor or dentist about all medicines your child takes or has taken in the past few weeks.

APPENDIX 19

How to Help Your Child Cope with Stress and Psychosomatic Illness

Changes in lifestyle and disruptions in the normal routine of people in all age groups can bring about stress. Some of the common causes of a child's stress are:

- Recent death of a loved one—parent, grandparent, sibling, friend.
- Loss of anything valuable to the child.
- Injuries or severe illness.
- Parents' divorce or separation.
- Changing schools.
- Recent move to a new home.
- Regular conflict between your child and another family member, close friend, or school teacher.
- Constant fatigue brought about by inadequate rest, sleep, or recreation.

STRESS-RELATED DISORDERS

A certain amount of stress is not always bad. It varies from child to child how much stress one can handle easily. Sometimes, stress can push a child on to greater achievement. But excessive stress can be self-defeating. Too much stress in your child's life can also lead to any of the following disorders:

- Mental and emotional upheavals.
- Skin eruptions, such as eczema and neurodermatitis.
- Digestive system problems, including peptic ulcers, colitis, and irritable colon.
- Eating disorders, such as anorexia nervosa and bulimia.
- Endocrine disorders, including overactive thyroid, adrenal- or pituitary-gland overactivity or underactivity, changes in menstrual patterns, impotence and premature ejaculation in males, or orgasmic dysfunction in females.
- Lung disorders associated with spasm of the bronchial tubes, such as in asthma.
- Pain syndromes, such as chronic or recurrent disabling headaches or back pain.

Many doctors believe that stress has a role in almost any disorder. Practically no one doubts that stress can complicate any illness in your child by preventing normal recovery, prolonging pain, and sustaining disability.

SELF-HELP TIPS FOR COPING

Here are some tips that may help your child reduce stress:

- Learn a meditation technique and practice it regularly—daily if possible. There are many methods available. Most of them include "tuning in to" and giving complete attention to a word, sound, sentence, or concept that you silently repeat to yourself. Don't try to banish other thoughts that enter your mind during your period of concentration, but don't focus on them enough to stop you from meditating. The purpose of meditation is to empty your mind of all disturbing thoughts for a given period of time to encourage mental relaxation. Mental relaxation, in turn, will help reduce stress.

- Take a short period of time away from any stressful situation you encounter during a day. Practice a muscle-tensing and muscle-relaxing technique. Close your eyes. Take a series of deep breaths. Then start with the muscle groups in your face. Consciously tense them and hold the contraction for a few seconds. Then consciously relax them.

Continue through all major muscle groups in the body: neck, shoulders, hands, abdomen, back, and legs. When you become skillful, you can use this technique to produce relaxation quickly any time you need to and in almost any environment.

• Adopt an exercise program. If you stay in good physical condition you are less likely to suffer the negative effects of stress, anxiety, or depression.

• Avoid taking your problems to bed with you. At the end of the day, spend a few minutes reviewing your entire day's experiences, event by event, as if you're replaying a tape. Release all negative emotions you have harbored (anger, feelings of insecurity, or anxiety). Relish all good energy or emotion (loving thoughts, praise, feeling good about your accomplishments or yourself). Reach a decision about unfinished events, and release mental or muscular tension. Now you're ready for a relaxing and emotionally healing sleep.

PSYCHOSOMATIC ILLNESS

We can't separate our children's bodies from their minds or their spirits. Most departures from good health have some connection with these elements.

• *Psychosomatic illness* is a term used to describe an illness in which factors other than physical ones are dominant. They may also play an important part in complications. Such illnesses are real—not imagined, as many people think. The links between mind, spirit, and body may be poorly defined at times, but they are provable by accepted scientific methods.

• Although medical researchers are beginning to understand the basic mechanisms, we still have much to learn about pschosomatic illness. One group of researchers believes that mental, emotional or spiritual stress can trigger almost any illness in a child or any person genetically predisposed to that illness. Such illnesses include asthma, cancer, digestive disturbances, heart disease—all these and others are more common in certain families. However, not all members of the same genetic makeup succumb to the same illnesses.

SUGGESTIONS

Here are some simple suggestions to help your child improve, prevent, or cope with psychosomatic illness:

• Define and resolve all personal conflicts. Define and confront areas of personal conflict in spiritual, emotional, school, occupational, or recreational involvements. If you can't resolve these conflicts alone, seek help from family, friends, or competent counselors.
• Be moderate in all your activities.
• Seek a balanced life of study, work, intellectual and physical challenges, recreation, friendship and intimacy, reflection, and rest.
• Be of good humor whenever possible.
• Be a friend to others both inside and outside your family.
• Give and receive love.
• Keep a positive outlook on life. Considerate, respectful and loving attitudes toward yourself and others are powerful allies.

APPENDIX 20

Infants of Mothers with Diabetes Mellitus

The Mother

Meticulous diabetes control in a mother with diabetes mellitus is the most critical factor in producing a healthy infant. This means early, frequent contact with her physician, with her obstetrician and, as delivery approaches, with a pediatrician. Neither the duration of the diabetes nor the amount of insulin the mother takes affects the baby.

For a successful pregnancy, there should be no insulin reactions. No ketosis. No acidosis. As normal as possible blood sugar. No infections. Careful prenatal care. All are important. It may not be possible to attain these objectives completely, but every effort should be made.

The Baby

Most information suggests that the newborn baby does best if delivered between the 36th and 37th weeks of pregnancy. Regardless of the time of birth, about 40% to 60% of the infants of diabetic mothers have no more problems than do other infants. Most doctors consider *all* infants of diabetic mothers to be very fragile, even when the newborn weighs 9 or 10 pounds. These infants are usually kept in incubators, unclothed for careful observation, in a special nursery.

The most common complication is respiratory distress or difficulty in breathing. This sometimes requires that the baby be given oxygen, fluids administered intravenously, and (less frequently) assisted ventilation of the lungs or artificial respiration. Diagnostic procedures such as X-rays and repeated blood and urine samples for ordinary and special analyses are often necessary. Some infants may have very low blood sugars. Others may develop jaundice, kidney complications, or muscle spasms from low calcium levels. Many have too much blood and occasionally may require the removal of blood.

Some of the babies may become jaundiced (too yellow) and may require an exchange transfusion to reduce the jaundice, as is done in the Rh-incompatible baby. Others may develop heart failure and may require oxygen, digitalis, and diuretics (medicines which promote the loss of water and salt by the kidneys). For these reasons, the baby should be under the care of a pediatrician familiar with the special problems that may develop during the first hours and days after birth. The causes of many of the complications occurring in a small percentage of these infants are not yet known.

The baby is *not* diabetic at birth and usually does not develop diabetes mellitus. Once beyond the first days and weeks of life, most will do as well as any infant.

If the baby's father is diabetic and the mother is not, the new-born will have no more problems than any other infant. Diabetes in the father alone requires no special care for the mother or the newborn baby.

APPENDIX 21

Diabetes: Hypoglycemia Differentiated from Oncoming Diabetic Coma (Ketoacidosis)

The following table can serve as a reminder for your child or other members of your family of the various factors associated with hypoglycemia and diabetic coma. Below are separate columns for each of these conditions to explain symptoms. Keep this table to refer to in case unexpected symptoms begin, which may mean that either of these conditions is developing.

Recognition of Hypoglycemia and Its Differentiation from Oncoming Diabetic Coma (Ketosis)

	Hypoglycemia	Diabetic Ketoacidosis
Cause	Too much insulin or not enough food	Not enough insulin
General appearance of patient	A well person who has fainted	Very ill
Breathing	Normal	Rapid and deep
Onset	Rapid (minutes)	Slow (at least 8 hrs.)
Hunger	Great	Loss of appetite
Thirst	None	Great
Vomiting	Rare	Common
Eyes	Staring, double vision common	Sunken
Headache	Common	Infrequent
Skin	Wet	Dry
Muscle twitching	Common	Absent
Complicating infections	Absent	Common
Pain in abdomen	None	Common
Sugar in urine	None after residual urine is discarded	Present
Blood sugar	Below 60 mg.%	Above 200 mg.%
Ketones in urine	Absent	Present—usually 4+
Ketones in blood plasma	None detectible	Present

* From Duncan, Garfield G. *A Modern Pilgrim's Progress for Diabetics*. Philadelphia, W.B. Saunders Company, reviewed 1980.

APPENDICES

APPENDIX 22

Delayed and Faulty Speech

A child usually has a vocabulary of 1 word by 10 months and 2 or 3 words by a year. Boys are generally slower than girls. At 18 months the average vocabulary is about 18 words, which the child is beginning to put into phrases. A 2-year-old can speak in simple sentences, but sometimes they are difficult to understand. A child's speech should be intelligible to strangers by 3 years of age. If the child is a year behind normal speech development, then it may be time to evaluate the child's intellectual development and hearing and finally to start training in verbal sound production.

CAUSES OF DELAYED SPEECH

- Personality. The cautious, sensitive child who decides it is safer not to walk early in life may also decide to delay speaking.
- Environment. The child who is surrounded by adults or older children who monopolize the conversation or who anticipate needs before the child has to speak may be helped by going to nursery school.
- The parent who uses complicated words, talks too fast, and does not repeat simple words may be causing the delay.
- Medical handicaps can cause speech disorders: congenital malformations, abnormal hearing and vision, injuries, infection, cerebral palsy and other central nervous system disorders, brain damage, and mental retardation. In these situations, other signs are present. The speech deficiency is only one of the signs.

CAUSES OF FAULTY SPEECH

- Use of baby talk, lisping, and immature speech to win points in child-parent controversies. It may be prolonged by parents who think it is "cute." Baby talk characterizes 80% of the speech defects in school-age children and clears up without extensive speech training.
- Playmate jargon.
- A bilingual home or foreign-born parents. Do not discourage the child from learning both languages; minor speech faults are not significant.

CHECKLIST OF SPEECH DEFECTS NEEDING INVESTIGATION

- No intelligible speech after 3 years old.
- Missing consonants after 3 years old.
- No sentences after 3 years old.
- Verbalization decreasing after having been normal.
- Word endings still dropped after 5 years old.
- Faulty sentence structure after 5 years old.
- Stuttering after 5 years old.
- A loud, monotone voice.
- Pitch that is inappropriate for age and sex.
- Hypernasality or lack of nasal resonance (abnormal nasal sound).
- Abnormal rhythm, rate, or inflection after 5 years old.

SPEECH PROBLEMS

Just as stumbling and falling are part of learning to walk, speaking imperfectly, repeating words, or stammering in the first few years of talking is perfectly normal.

STUTTERING

Parents with close relatives who stutter are often particularly concerned about early signs in their child. However, many children go through a stuttering stage. In most it lasts only a few days, but in the more sensitive it may last longer. The age for these episodes is 3 to 4 years. Following are some suggestions to relieve the strain and anxiety that may be the cause of a child's stuttering:

- Ignore the stuttering and request others to do the same. Make no remarks like "speak slowly" or "take a deep breath and start again."
- Do not deal with the child's hesitation by "shushing" everyone else, scolding other children who tease your child, or fearing to interrupt your child's talking.
- Do not seek advice about stuttering from friends, relatives, teachers, magazines, or nonprofessional books.
- Avoid parental arguments about how to deal with the problem, particularly in the presence of the child.
- Make your child feel adequate and acceptable by giving the child as much love, affection and security as you can.
- Build the child's ego by concentrating on abilities.
- Do not be afraid to say to the child: "It upsets me when you have difficulty in speaking, but when you are older and more relaxed it will get better."
- If the problem persists and becomes progressively worse, consultation with a speech therapist may be necessary.

APPENDIX 23

Hypospadias

DESCRIPTION

This relatively common birth defect affects the external genitalia of both sexes, in varying degrees of severity. It occurs in males more often than females. The exact cause is not known.

• **In males**—The urethral opening appears on the underside of the boy's penis and not at the tip; the shaft of the penis may be bent downward; the prepuce (or foreskin) may be defective or altogether absent on the underside, giving the penis a hooded appearance. In the most common form, which requires no treatment, the urethral opening will be just below the normal site. In severe cases, it may occur anywhere along the shaft, to as far back as the juncture of the penis and scrotum. In rare instances, the scrotum is divided in two with the urethral opening between the sections. About one-third of patients with hypospadias may also have other disorders of the urinary tract. If your son has hypospadias, X-ray examination of the kidneys, ureter, and bladder is in order.

• **In females**—Displacement of the urethra is not so noticeable and may be discovered only in a gynecological examination. In the most severe cases, the opening may occur in the girl's vagina and manifest itself by causing difficulty in urination.

CAUSES

Possibly an abnormality of the hormonal environment prior to birth. The external genitalia (penis, vagina, clitoris, scrotum) should be carefully examined to determine the exact sex of the baby. Other studies may be needed as well. A boy should not have a circumcision if this condition is present, because the foreskin may be needed in the surgical correction of the deformity.

TREATMENT

The more severe forms of hypospadias may interfere with sexual activity in your child's adult life and have definite psychological implications for a male. The treatment is surgical, the results of which are uniformly good, though more than one operation may be required. Beginning with the first procedure at age 2, total correction can and should be completed before the child starts school.

APPENDIX 24

Well-Balanced Diet

The well-balanced diet is for all people whose condition does not require dietary treatment. There are no restrictions in types of foods that may be consumed as part of this diet. Quantities consumed depend upon your child's size and age.

This diet provides the Recommended Dietary Allowances (RDA) established by the Food and Nutrition Board of the National Research Council.

BASIC FOUR FOOD GROUPS
Amounts vary according to your child's age and development. Consult your pediatrician for recommended quantities.

- **Milk and Milk Products Group**—Milk, cheese, yogurt, ice cream.

- **Meat Group**—Lean meats, poultry, fish, eggs, beans.

- **Vegetable and Fruit Group.**

- **Bread and Cereals Group**—Unrefined, unsweetened, whole-grain cereals and breads.

Most dietetic experts recommend a regular diet with increased fiber (roughage) to promote normal bowel function. Increased roughage also protects against diverticulosis, some forms of intestinal cancer and perhaps even atherosclerosis—thus protecting your child against heart attack and stroke later in life.

Daily fat intake should not exceed 30% of total calories in the child's regular diet. A low-fat diet (see Appendix 28) will help control obesity and decrease the likelihood of your child developing atherosclerosis later in life.

For optimal health, reduce intake of refined sugars, such as those in candy, in the child's regular diet. Your child should eat unrefined sugars such as those found in fresh fruits, vegetables, potatoes, and whole-grain breads and cereals.

A healthy, well-balanced diet for your child should include minimum salt; reduced fat; lots of complex carbohydrates and fiber; more fish, seafood, and poultry; less red meat; and less fatty, salty, prepared meats and snacks.

APPENDIX 25

Nutrition for Athletes

Good nutrition at all times is essential for excellent athletic performance, even if competition is only seasonal. The basic nutritional requirements for athletes and fitness enthusiasts are the same as those for the general population. However, a few minor modifications prior to competition may enhance your child's athletic performance.

Two decades ago, athletes were advised to eat a high protein diet, eat little on days of competition, stay away from refreshments and cold drinks during competition, take salt tablets during periods of heavy sweating, consume large doses of vitamins, and eat less than usual for a day following competition. These recommendations have proven more harmful than helpful, and have been discredited in recent years.

PRESENT DIETARY GUIDELINES

Following are the general guidelines advocated currently by nutritionists for a well-balanced diet for athletes and fitness enthusiasts. These guidelines may also be modified eventually as research provides additional information about nutrition and athletic performance, but they represent sound nutritional sense.

- **Protein**—Contrary to what many coaches and athletes believe, the protein requirement for athletes is not significantly greater than it is for others. Most persons need about 1 gram of protein for each kilogram of weight. This amount is easily obtained in a diet in which protein comprises 10 to 15 percent of total calories.
- **Carbohydrates**—The recommended percentage of total daily caloric intake for carbohydrates is 65%. Complex carbohydrates—as opposed to simple carbohydrates (sugar)—should make up the majority of the carbohydrate requirement. Complex carbohydrates are found in potatoes, brown rice, dried beans, fresh fruits and vegetables, and whole-grain breads and cereals. These foods also provide dietary fiber, an important element in regulating bowel function. In addition, complex carbohydrates provide the liver and muscle cells with glucose. This is stored as glycogen and converted back to glucose for use when needed during exercise.
- **Fat**—No more than 20% of the dietary calories should come from fat.
- **Special Diets**—Many good books provide detailed dietary and diet supplement-regimens for athletes. However, beware of advice given by anyone making extraordinary claims for fad foods or for protein, vitamin and mineral supplements. Most of these are not based on sound nutritional research, and are not recommended by nutritionists.
- **Weight-Loss Diets**—Athletes engaged in vigorous physical activity should not skimp on their diets to "lose weight." Vigorous exercise will replace some body fat with muscle at the same time the body weight remains constant. A strenuous exercise program is accompanied by an increased metabolic rate, requiring an increased caloric intake. If your child stops exercising for any reason, be sure to reduce caloric intake. Otherwise, the child may gain weight rapidly.

ADDITIONAL RECOMMENDATIONS FOR WOMEN ATHLETES

Some supplements may be necessary for females.

- Calcium supplements are recommended for women who exercise so strenuously (as in marathon running) that menstrual periods cease. These women are at a higher risk of developing osteoporosis (softening of the bones) at an early age.

• Iron supplements are also recommended for some females. Normally, iron stores are not diminished directly by exercise. However, if iron-deficiency anemia develops from other causes (such as excessive menstruation), an iron supplement is essential to assure normal physical performance in women.

EATING SCHEDULES FOR ATHLETES

• **Before Competition**—Your child should eat a meal 3 to 5 hours before competition. This meal should contain lots of carbohydrates (pasta, fruits, cooked vegetables, gelatin desserts), decreased fats, decreased protein (small amounts of lean meat, fish, or poultry are acceptable), and decreased foods that cause extra "gas." The food can be digested in the 3 to 5 hours before competition, allowing nutrients to be stored before excitement begins.
• **After Competition**—Glucose stores in the liver and muscles diminish during strenuous exercise. To replenish these, your child should increase carbohydrate intake for 3 days following competition. Otherwise, training should be reduced during that time.

FLUID INTAKE & EXERCISE—INSTRUCTIONS FOR YOUR CHILD

• **Water**—Drink cold water during competition. It is absorbed faster and is less likely to cause cramps than warm water. In addition to drinking extra water during competition, drink at least eight 8-ounce glasses of water a day. An occasional soft drink or cup of tea or coffee is not harmful, but these should not make up the major portion of your daily fluid intake. Clear, pure water is best to meet your daily fluid requirement.
• **Fluid and Glucose Replacement**—During extended athletic activity, such as jogging or running a marathon, fluid and glucose must be replaced as they are used by the body. The recommended concentration of glucose is 2 to 2.5 grams of glucose (sugar) to each deciliter of water. Don't drink more than 800ml of fluid during any hour of endurance activity. To exceed this will overload your stomach and may impair performance.

APPENDIX 26

Allergy Diet

Many children suffer allergic reactions after eating certain foods. This diet is used to prevent or reduce those reactions by eliminating the offending foods from your child's diet.

FOODS	ALLOWED	OMITTED
Highly Seasoned Foods		Highly seasoned foods.
Beverages	Tea; carbonated beverages; cereal beverages, such as Ovaltine.	Coffee; cola beverages; chocolate-flavored beverages.
Meats	Any except those in omitted column; cottage cheese.	Highly seasoned meats (such as cold cuts); fresh pork; fish; shellfish; eggs*; other cheeses; peanut butter; corned beef; cheese spreads.
Fats	Any except those in omitted column.	Cream cheese; nuts; salad dressings made with eggs or cheese.
Milk	Milk; milk drinks.	Chocolate milk; eggnog; hot cocoa.
Bread	Any except those in omitted column.	Commercially prepared mixes; any bread made with eggs or nuts; cornbread.
Vegetables	Any except those in omitted column.	Tomatoes; tomato products (puree, sauce, catsup, etc.).
Fruits	Any except those in omitted column.	Fresh or frozen: apples; cherries; berries**. Fresh, frozen, dried or cooked: bananas; grapes; mangoes; papayas; pineapple; rhubarb; raisins.
Soups	Any except those in omitted column.	Any made with corn, tomatoes, or shellfish.
Desserts	Any except those in omitted column.	Any made with chocolate, cocoa, eggs, nuts, or omitted fruits; commercially prepared mixes.
Sweets	Any except those in omitted column.	Jelly, jam, or marmalade made with omitted fruits; candy with chocolate, eggs, nuts, or omitted fruits.

FOODS	ALLOWED	OMITTED
Miscellaneous	Salt, spices, herbs except those omitted; vinegar; pickles; gravy; white sauce.	Garlic; strong spices; chocolate; cocoa.

*Avoid serving your allergic child eggs in any form. Later, as an adult, your child may be able to tolerate small amounts of cooked eggs, such as those found in most desserts. The allergic protein in eggs is denatured by cooking.

**Cooking denatures some allergens. Therefore, your child may be able to tolerate *cooked* apples, cherries, and berries. Other fruits may be extremely allergenic in some children, and cooking does not denature the allergens.

(Adapted from the Mayo Clinic Diet Manual, Fourth and Fifth Editions. Philadelphia, W. B. Saunders Company)

APPENDIX 27

Cholesterol and Triglyceride Problems

DESCRIPTION

Both substances are important parts of the liquid part of blood and all body cells. They are produced by the liver but also enter a child's body in foods containing fats. Problems may develop later in your child's life when levels of either, or both, are too high. High levels can cause plaques to develop in the arteries of the heart, brain, kidney, and other areas. These plaques can eventually cause clogging, removing nutrition and depriving important tissues of the body of oxygen.

CAUSES

Heredity, stress, medicines, and diet can all cause elevated levels. A child's diet that contains high levels of saturated fats (found in eggs, fatty meats, butter, some margarines, some oils, nuts, and whole milk products) can lead to high levels of cholesterol and triglycerides in the body's circulatory system.

TREATMENT

Keep fat intake to 28% or less of your older child's total diet. Do not modify the diet of a child under 2 years. After that give the child 3 eggs per week or less, use skim milk and low-fat dairy products, and use corn or olive oil instead of coconut or palm oil. If dietary restrictions aren't helpful, medication is available. Consult your pediatrician regarding the best diet for your child.

APPENDIX 28 (continued on next page)

Low-Fat Diet

Most diet experts agree that Americans eat too much fat. A low-fat diet in children beyond infancy can help prevent obesity and the dangers it causes to health. Use the diet suggestions below for general good health or for dietary treatment of your child's condition as recommended by your doctor. Portions recommended are for children age 10 or older. Younger children should eat proportionately less.

FOODS	ALLOWED	OMITTED
Beverages	Coffee; tea; carbonated beverages.	No restrictions.
Breads and Cereals	4 servings or more a day of whole-grain or enriched cereals; white, whole wheat, rye, or French bread; plain rolls; saltines; graham crackers; wheat crackers; corn or flour tortillas.	Biscuits, cornbread, pancakes and waffles, unless made with allowed vegetable oils, egg white, and skim milk or buttermilk; doughnuts; commercial coffee cakes; cheese crackers; pretzels; rusks.
Desserts	Angel food cake; cakes and cookies made with skim milk, oil, and egg whites; fruit (preferred); fruit pie and cobblers (or pastry made with allowed oils); fruit whips; fruit meringues; gelatin desserts; puddings and custards made with skim milk; sherbet; fruit ices.	Desserts containing butter or margarine, chocolate, cream, egg yolk (unless from day's allowance), shortening or whole milk (such as ice cream and regular puddings); commercial cakes, cookies, and pastries.
Eggs	Egg whites as desired, but limit egg yolks to not more than 3 per week, including those used in cooking; low-cholesterol egg substitute.	
Fats (Use sparingly)	Corn oil; cottonseed oil; safflower oil; soybean oil; non-hydrogenated vegetable-oil margarine; sunflower seed oil; commercial mayonnaise and salad dressings; peanut oil, olive oil.	All visible fat on meats; butter; chocolate; coconut oil; cream; lard; hydrogenated (hardened) fats; margarine (except non-hydrogenated vegetable oil); bacon drippings.
Fruits	2 servings or more a day.	Avocado.

APPENDIX 28 (continued)

FOODS	ALLOWED	OMITTED
Meats and Meat Substitutes	5 ounces daily total of lean meat, fish, or poultry (trim all visible fat from meat before cooking); low-fat cottage cheese; sapsago cheese; mozzarella cheese; specially prepared low-cholesterol cheeses; mature shelled beans and peas; peanut butter (for second entree when possible); barbecue (using only sauce without fat), broil, boil, or roast on a rack so that fat will drip out; nuts (particularly peanuts and walnuts if caloric allowance permits); tripe; beef or veal liver once a month.	Liver; duck; goose; bacon; salt pork; sausage; lunch meat; frankfurters; brisket; shortribs; club, porterhouse and T-bone steaks; prime rib roasts; cheese (except those allowed); any fish prepared with fats other than allowed oils; cashew nuts.
Milk	1½ pints a day of skim milk or buttermilk; cocoa prepared with skim milk.	Whole milk; evaporated milk; Bulgarian buttermilk; beverages containing chocolate (note: cocoa is allowed); ice cream; ice milk; eggs; cream.
Miscellaneous	Herbs; catsup; mustard; pickles; spices; gravies made from pan drippings skimmed free of fat (let stand in refrigerator until fat forms); popcorn cooked in oil or non-hydrogenated vegetable-oil margarine; olives (use sparingly).	Coconut; buttered popcorn.
Potato or Substitute	White or sweet potato; brown or restored rice; corn; hominy; enriched grits; macaroni or noodles; dried beans and peas.	Fried potatoes and potato chips (unless not cooked in oil).
Soups	Meat and chicken soups (soups should be cooled and fat removed from the top before reheating and serving); fat-free broth and bouillon; soups made with skim milk and allowed vegetable-oil margarine.	Any soup made with butter, ordinary margarine or whole milk; most canned soups.

FOODS	ALLOWED	OMITTED
Sweets	Gumdrops; hard candy; homemade candies made without cream, whole milk, chocolate, or butter; honey; jam; jelly; jelly beans; marshmallows; mints made with allowed ingredients; molasses; syrup; sugar.	Candies containing fats such as butter, chocolate, cocoa butter, coconut, or cream.
Vegetables	2 servings or more of any vegetable. Do not cook vegetables with meat; season with non-hydrogenated vegetable-oil margarine.	Any vegetables prepared with butter, ordinary margarine, cream, salt pork, or bacon grease.

(Adapted from The Arizona Diet Manual, by the Diet Therapy Section of The Arizona Dietetic Association, Inc.)

APPENDIX 29

Low-Salt Diet

This is a normal diet, restricted only in certain foods that have excessive salt or sodium. Avoid serving your child canned and prepared frozen foods. Read all labels carefully. Attempt to keep the child's total sodium intake below 3.5 grams (about 1/7 ounce) per day.

FOODS	ALLOWED	OMITTED
Beverages	All tea, coffee, milk (sodium-free).	No restrictions.
Bread and Cereals	Regular bread and cereals.	Crackers with salted tops; pretzels; salted popcorn.
Desserts	All, in moderation.	No restrictions.
Fats	All except those in omitted column.	Bacon and bacon fat; salt pork; olives; prepared meats.
Fruits	All.	No restrictions.
Meat and Meat Substitutes	Meat; fish; poultry; eggs; cottage cheese; dried beans and peas; all cheeses except those omitted; cured meats and fish may be consumed once a week.	Any meat, fish or poultry that is smoked, brine-cured or salted, including: bacon; bologna; chipped beef; corned beef; frankfurters; luncheon meats; ham; kosher meats; salt pork; sausages; salted or smoked fish such as herring, sardines, anchovies or salted codfish; processed cheese; cheese spreads; or cheese such as Roquefort or Camembert.
Potatoes and Substitutes	All except potato chips.	Potato chips.
Seasonings and Flavorings	A small amount of salt or other seasoning may be used in cooking.	Salt at the table; catsup; pickles; relishes; soy sauce.
Soups	Cream soups; canned soups.	Bouillon cubes, prepared soup bases, and canned soups containing smoked or salty meats.
Vegetables	All except those in omitted column.	Sauerkraut and other vegetables prepared in brine.

(Adapted from The Arizona Diet Manual, by the Diet Therapy Section of The Arizona Dietetic Association, Inc.)

APPENDIX 30

Milk-Restricted Diet

This diet is used to treat a child's lactose intolerance and milk allergy.

Lactose Intolerance—Lactose intolerance is caused by a deficiency of the enzyme lactase, which breaks down lactose, the form of sugar found in milk. This intolerance is commonly found in several ethnic groups, including blacks, American Indians, Mexican-Americans, and Orientals.

For infants, the substitution of formulas that do not contain lactose, such as soybean formula, will relieve symptoms of lactose intolerance.

Children and pregnant women should take a calcium supplement if they consume only small amounts of milk products.

Milk Allergy—A milk allergy is a reaction caused by hypersensitivity to the protein found in milk. This allergy may occur more frequently in infants than in older children and adults, and can frequently cause an allergic reaction.

Milk allergy is treated with a diet using soybean or meat-based formulas that contain no milk. Commercially available soybean formulas vary considerably in mineral content, and deficiencies of both vitamin A and thiamine have been reported in infants consuming these formulas. Ask your doctor about vitamin supplements for your child.

Some children who are allergic to milk in one form may be able to use milk that has been boiled, evaporated or dried, because these processes change the protein. Milk is an important source of calcium, protein, vitamins A and D, and riboflavin. Foods rich in these nutrients should be selected when milk has been excluded from the child's diet. When milk products are excluded from the child's diet, high-calcium foods from the list below should be substituted.

More than 1,000 mg. per serving size
¾ cup dry barley, oatmeal, or rice cereal

More than 100 mg. per serving size
½ cup collard greens
¾ cup kale
½ cup mustard greens
12 oysters
3½ oz. salmon (if bones are eaten)
12 shrimp
1 cup cooked instant creamed wheat (no milk added)
½ cup cooked barley cereal (no milk added)

More than 50 mg. per serving size
½ cup broccoli
1 cup Brussels sprouts

(Adapted from The Arizona Diet Manual, by the Diet Therapy Section of The Arizona Dietetic Association, Inc.)

APPENDIX 31

Obesity: Guidelines for Losing Weight

Consult your doctor before starting your child on a diet or strenuous exercise program.

EXERCISE

Daily exercise to the point of breathing hard can increase your child's rate of weight loss and sense of physical well-being.

Instructions for your child:

Take advantage of your gym program in school. Spend 10 minutes per day exercising in your room. If possible, walk places instead of riding in a car. Use the stairs instead of elevators. Limit your TV time to 2 hours or less per day. As you lose weight, exercise will be less tiring. Attempt to learn new sports that especially appeal to you. Swimming, bicycling, skiing, and jogging are sports that burn the most calories.

DIET

A reasonable diet allows a child to have 3 meals a day and eat average-size portions. There are no forbidden foods; the dieter can have a serving of anything family or friends are eating. However, there are forbidden amounts. While reducing, your child must learn to leave the table a little bit hungry. Shortcuts such as fasting, crash diets, or diet pills rarely work and may be dangerous. Calorie counting is helpful for some children, but usually it just doesn't work for most dieters.

Instructions for your child:

- Fluids: Take all milk as skim milk. Limit it to 16 oz. per day, as milk has lots of calories. All other fluid intake should be either water, unsweetened tea, or diet drinks. Drink at least 6 glasses of water per day.
- Meals: Eat average portions. No seconds.
- Desserts: Eat smaller than average portions. No seconds. Try to eat Jello or fresh fruit more often.
- Snacks: Eliminate them. If this is impossible, use only the special filler foods listed below and no more than twice a day.
- Types of food: If you have a choice, eat protein in preference to carbohydrates or fats. Proteins are the best food for depressing the appetite (for example, cheese, meat, eggs).
- Vitamins: Take 1 multivitamin tablet per day while reducing.
- Reminders: Put a note up on the refrigerator, bathroom mirror, etc., which says, "EAT LESS."

Filler foods:

These special low-calorie foods can be eaten fairly freely. They are especially useful if your child gets an urge to eat a larger quantity of food than usual, as everyone does at times.

- Diet soft drinks, Kool-Aid, coffee, or tea.
- Diet Kool-Aid popsicles.
- Bouillon soup in cold weather.
- Raw vegetables—some that are particularly good with flavored salts are raw carrot sticks, celery sticks, raw potato sticks, cucumbers, pickles, cauliflower.

• Raw fruits—these contain more calories than raw vegetables, but some acceptable ones are apples, oranges, cantaloupe, and strawberries.
• Popcorn—minimal calories if popped in little or no oil. No butter.
• Desserts—Jello or diet desserts.
• Sugar-free gum can be useful for lessening the appetite.

Helpful hints about family eating patterns:

• The overweight child should be allowed to eat the same foods as the rest of the family. Snacks must be discontinued for the entire family, not just for that child. Rich desserts should be decreased for the whole family. If other people in the family are overweight, they should try to set a good example for the child by restricting their servings of the main course.
• High-calorie foods that might be eaten as snacks should not be purchased so that the temptation to eat them need not arise (e.g., corn chips, potato chips, regular pop, cookies, cakes, candy).
• Food should not be kept in any room of the house other than the kitchen.
• Eating while watching TV should be discontinued for everyone.
• Diet pop and other filler foods should be kept available in the home.
• If any diet is being used with a younger child, it must be one that can be tolerated by the child. The parents can encourage the child to stick to it, but they must never use force. Imposed diets can cause lots of problems.

APPENDIX 32

Pregnancy and Breast-Feeding Diet

General guidelines for you or your daughter during pregnancy:

- Increase your normal caloric intake about 10% above what you should normally consume if you were not pregnant.
- Except under unusual circumstances, don't try to lose weight during pregnancy. The average weight gain in an uncomplicated pregnancy is 22 to 27 pounds.
- Make sure your diet contains adequate protein during pregnancy and during breast-feeding. Protein is the "building block" of body tissue.
- Iron, vitamins, minerals, and calcium supplements are helpful to maintain proper nutrition. Follow your doctor's recommendations. Remember that calcium tablets are not a substitute for milk.
- Use iodized salt.
- Avoid caffeine during pregnancy. Either eliminate coffee, cola, cocoa, tea, and other caffeine-containing substances from your diet, or reduce the amount you consume drastically.

DAILY DIET FOR PREGNANCY AND BREAST-FEEDING

Foods	During First Half of Pregnancy	During Second Half of Pregnancy	During Breast-Feeding
Milk Group			
Pasteurized milk includes: whole, skim, evaporated, reliquified dry or buttermilk	2 cups (to drink or use in cooking)	4 to 6 cups (to drink or use in cooking)	4 to 6 cups (to drink or use in cooking)
(1½ ounces cheddar cheese may be substituted for each cup of milk)			

The diet as directed during pregnancy and breast-feeding supplies adequate nutrients as recommended by the National Research Council, with the possible exception of vitamin D. The daily need for vitamin D may be met by consuming 1 quart of vitamin D milk or a prescribed supplement.

Foods	During First Half of Pregnancy	During Second Half of Pregnancy	During Breast-Feeding
Meat Group			
Lean cooked meat, fish, poultry (include liver frequently)	1 serving (2 to 3 ounces)	1 to 2 servings (5 ounces)	1 to 2 servings (5 ounces)
Meat alternate: 1 serving of any variety cheese; mature shelled beans or peas (dried or fresh); nuts; or peanut butter			
Egg	1	1	1

Vegetable and Fruit Group			
Vitamin A—Dark green vegetables and fruits	1 serving	1 serving	1 to 2 servings
Other vegetables or fruits	1 serving	2 servings	2 servings
Vitamin C-rich foods: **Good Sources**—citrus fruit or juice (fresh, frozen, or canned); cantaloupe; strawberries; broccoli; green pepper; sweet red pepper **Fair Sources**—honeydew melon; tangerines; watermelon; asparagus; Brussels sprouts; raw cabbage; greens; potatoes and sweet potatoes cooked in their skins; spinach; strawberries; tomatoes or tomato juice; watercress	1 good source or 2 fair sources	1 good source and 2 fair sources or 2 good sources	1 good source and 2 fair sources or 2 good sources
Bread and Cereals Group			
Whole-grain or enriched cereal	1 serving	1 serving	1 serving
Whole-grain or enriched bread	2 to 3 slices	2 to 3 slices	3 slices
Butter or Fortified Margarine	As caloric intake permits	As caloric intake permits	As caloric intake permits

(Adapted from The Arizona Diet Manual, by the Diet Therapy Section of The Arizona Dietetic Association, Inc.)

APPENDIX 33

Disqualifying Medical Conditions for Sports Participation

NON-COLLISION, NON-CONTACT SPORTS

Competitive running or marathons; track and field events; racket sports; competitive swimming; bowling; golf; archery.

Temporary Disqualifications

- Active infection including:
  - — Respiratory infection.
  - — Kidney infection.
  - — Infectious mononucleosis.
  - — Hepatitis.
  - — Acute rheumatic fever.
  - — Active tuberculosis.
- Joint inflammation resulting from infection or recent injury.

Permanent Disqualifications

- Chronic diseases, including:
  - — Those that involve serious bleeding tendencies, such as hemophilia.
  - — Inadequately controlled diabetes.
  - — Severe chronic obstructive pulmonary disease.
  - — Valvular heart disease (mitral stenosis, aortic stenosis).
  - — Previous heart surgery (sometimes).
  - — High blood pressure with a known cause, such as chronic kidney disease, coarctation (constriction of a small segment) of the aorta, adrenal tumors, or congenital arteriosclerosis. This disqualification does not include essential hypertension or high blood pressure from an unknown cause that is under control with medication. Vigorous exercise after adequate training is recommended for children with this condition.

Exceptions

Children with mild forms of the preceding conditions may benefit from non-contact, non-collision exercise programs if they have medical supervision and frequent monitoring of their conditions. Consult your doctor for guidance if your child has any of the following:

- High blood pressure.
- Asthma.
- Early obstructive pulmonary disease.
- Well-controlled diabetes.
- Convulsive disorders controlled by medication.
- Absence of one kidney.
- Absence of one testicle or undescended testicles.
- Previous heart surgery.

COLLISION AND CONTACT SPORTS

Football; hockey; rugby; lacrosse; baseball; basketball; soccer; wrestling; boxing.

Temporary Disqualifications

- Active infection including:
  - — Respiratory infection.
  - — Kidney infection.
  - — Infectious mononucleosis.
  - — Hepatitis.
  - — Acute rheumatic fever.
  - — Active tuberculosis.
- Joint inflammation resulting from infection or recent injury.
- Skin disease in an active phase (boils, impetigo, herpes).

Permanent Disqualifications

- Physical immaturity in comparison with others competing in the same group.
- Chronic diseases, including:
  - — Those that involve serious bleeding tendencies, such as hemophilia.
  - — Inadequately controlled diabetes.
  - — Severe chronic obstructive pulmonary disease.
  - — Valvular heart disease (mitral stenosis, aortic stenosis).
  - — Previous heart surgery (sometimes).
  - — High blood pressure with a known cause, such as chronic kidney disease, coarctation (constriction of a small segment) of the aorta, adrenal tumors, or congenital arteriosclerosis. This disqualification does not include essential hypertension or high blood pressure from an unknown cause that is under control with medication. Vigorous exercise after adequate training is recommended for children with this condition.
- Hernia (no disqualification after successful surgical repair).
- Congenital musculo-skeletal abnormalities that prevent competitive function, such as clubfoot or osteogenesis imperfecta.
- Loss of one eye or blindness in one eye.
- Repeated head injuries or repeated concussions accompanied by unconsciousness.
- Epilepsy or other convulsive disorder not controlled with medication.
- Previous head or brain surgery.
- Absence of one kidney.
- Absence of one testicle.

APPENDIX 34

Drugs in Sports

The use of drugs by amateur and professional athletes has received much publicity in recent years. Many athletes believe that drugs are essential for optimum performance. The issue of whether drugs can enhance physical performance remains controversial and unresolved. However, the physiological effects that drugs have on the body can be documented. This section is devoted to examining the most-common drugs used by athletes. Questions of legality or ethics are best answered by the prevailing view in sports medicine: The use of drugs is generally considered unethical—in some cases illegal—and such use is usually forbidden by organizations that govern competitive athletics.

ANABOLIC STEROID HORMONES

Some athletes take synthetic male hormones (anabolic steroids) in the hope of increasing strength or muscle mass. The most common synthetic male hormones taken by athletes include testosterone, methandrostenolone, and nandrolone.

Effects in Females—Muscle mass increases when the hormone is taken for a sufficiently long period of time. However, side effects and adverse reactions include the following:

- Growth of hair on the face and other body parts.
- Enlargement of the clitoris.
- Deepening of the voice.
- Acne.
- Baldness.
- Change in sex drive (usually increased).
- Irregular menstrual periods.
- Depression.

Effects in Males—Strength and body weight sometimes increase. However, many side effects and adverse reactions are possible. These include:

- Decreased levels of FSH (follicle-stimulating hormone) and leutenizing hormone. These in turn cause decreased male-hormone production, decreased sperm production, and testicular atrophy.
- A decrease in high-density lipoprotein, which may increase the likelihood of hardening of the arteries, stroke, and kidney disease.
- Increased incidence of liver tumors.
- Increased aggressiveness.
- Acne.
- Depression.
- Change in sex drive (sometimes lessened, sometimes increased).

The consensus among medical experts is that the use of anabolic steroids by both males and females poses greater risk and danger from adverse effects than is justified by any possible benefit. Physicians uniformly advise against using them. Their use is condemned by the Medical Commission of the International Olympic Committee.

APPENDIX 34 (continued on next page)

AMPHETAMINES

These drugs are central-nervous-system stimulants. Athletes take them believing they will help performance in competition. Studies show that performance is actually diminished, despite the feeling on the part of the athlete that performance is outstanding. The toxic effects of amphetamines are:

- Tremor.
- Confusion.
- Restlessness.
- Loss of appetite.
- Delusions and hallucinations.
- High blood pressure.
- Heartbeat irregularities.

Amphetamines are particularly dangerous if taken with other stimulants such as cocaine, appetite suppressants, and caffeine.

CAFFEINE

Caffeine is also a central-nervous-system stimulant. When taken in small, infrequent doses, caffeine seems to have few if any long-lasting ill effects. However, new evidence suggests a correlation between consumption of any coffee—including decaffeinated coffee—and an increase in low-density lipoproteins. High levels of these fatty elements in the blood are known to increase the likelihood that arteriosclerosis (hardening of the arteries), heart disease, kidney disease and stroke will develop later in your child's life. This effect is noted with the consumption of as little as 2 cups of coffee per day.

The immediate effects of caffeine consumption vary from person to person, depending on individual factors. Most adults can tolerate 2 cups of caffeine-containing liquid a day, but children should avoid caffeine, which is present in many carbonated soft drinks. Too much caffeine will produce the following:

- Nervousness, irritability, and rapid heartbeat.
- Insomnia.
- Increased urine output.
- Symptoms of low blood sugar (hypoglycemia), including tremor, weakness, and increased irritability.

Some people believe caffeine consumption relieves fatigue, but this is an artificial effect. Use of caffeine does not result in increased athletic performance.

COCAINE

This central-nervous-system stimulant has similar effects to those of amphetamines and caffeine—except stronger. Cocaine is illegal and addicting. Its use can lead to delusions, psychosocial problems, tremor, restlessness, and damage to nasal tissues (if "snorted"). An overdose of cocaine can be fatal. Its damaging effects on the central nervous system increase greatly when it is taken with other stimulants such as amphetamines, appetite suppressants, or caffeine. Medical experts have documented no benefits from the use of cocaine among athletes.

NICOTINE

This is the addicting factor in tobacco smoke that makes smoking cessation so difficult for many persons. Nicotine causes constriction of peripheral blood vessels. It also causes an increase in heart rate that does not result in increased cardiac output. The result of these two effects is increased fatigue and diminished athletic performance.

PRESCRIPTION AND NONPRESCRIPTION DRUGS

All effective medications have potential side effects for at least some individuals. Your child should not expect to be able to perform at his accustomed level if he is taking any medication.

Safety precautions for athletes are similar to those for the general population. The most important additional precaution for athletes relates to fluid loss that accompanies heavy sweating. Drugs most likely to become dangerous under these conditions are:

- Digitalis (a heart medicine).
- Diuretics (medicine to treat high blood pressure and heart problems).
- Steroid hormones.

All the above can cause excessive loss of sodium and potassium from the body. The effect of these drugs may be accelerated by fluid loss, as in heavy sweating, diarrhea, and vomiting, particularly in hot weather. Excessive sweating from any cause may require a dose modification of digitalis, diuretics, or hormones. Let your doctor know if your child exercises vigorously.

APPENDIX 35

Mental Retardation, Sports and Exercise

Athletic activity and recreation are important for everyone, regardless of mental capacity. Sports and athletic activities can make a positive difference in problems experienced by mentally retarded children. These problems include poor physical fitness, obesity, restlessness, boredom, hyperactivity, and social immaturity. Most health professionals and social workers believe that mild to moderately retarded children and adults can and should participate safely in many athletic activities, as long as they are supervised adequately. This section presents guidelines to parents or guardians of mentally retarded children and adults who are considering an exercise program or athletic competition for them.

RECOMMENDATIONS

• Encourage and stress activities that require gross motor (large-muscle) coordination rather than fine motor coordination.

• Stress the right kinds of activities. Mentally retarded children find more satisfaction and success in participating in dual and individual sports rather than team sports. Retarded children may benefit from non-competitive sports with normal children.

• Teach and encourage games, which are more interesting than exercises. The following sports and activities are recommended: tennis, folk-dancing, shooting baskets, running races, playing catch, boating, bicycling, and hiking. Less suitable activities that are not recommended include basketball, football, or baseball.

• Match competitors evenly so each child has a chance to win sometimes. Have children participate with each other according to developmental age rather than chronological age. Otherwise, some individuals may fail repeatedly, damaging their self-esteem—and turning a positive situation into a negative one.

• Keep records of improvement, and share them with the retarded child.

• Support development of athletic opportunities at the community level. For more information about programs for the mentally retarded, contact either of the following:

The Special Olympics, Inc.
1350 New York Ave., N.W., Suite 500
Washington, D.C. 20005
202-347-7233

Division of Innovation and Development
Department of Education
Donahue Bldg., Rm. 3159
400 Maryland Ave., S.W.
Washington, D.C. 20202
202-732-3366

APPENDIX 36

Benefits of Exercise and Physical Fitness

Regular exercise can play a key role in helping your child stay healthy or get healthier. Exercise can be an important part of treating many medical problems, such as hypertension, sleep disorders, depression, anxiety, diabetes, and high blood-fat levels (especially high levels of low-density cholesterol).

Regular exercise also can help improve your child's body image and increase the child's energy level. It can help control weight, reduce stress, and protect the child from heart and blood-vessel disease.

EXERCISE PRESCRIPTION

After obtaining a medical history and performing a physical examination, your doctor may address four components of your child's exercise "prescription."

Type of Exercise—Popular ones include brisk walking, swimming, bike riding, jogging.
Frequency of Exercise—It's best for the child to start at about three exercise sessions per week, then increase gradually to four, five, or more.
Duration of Exercise—The ideal duration is 30 minutes of continuous activity. It's best to begin with 10 or 15 minutes and increase as your child's tolerance for exercise improves.
Intensity of Exercise—This component varies greatly depending on your child's age, sex, and medical condition. If your doctor prescribes an exercise program, there will be specific instructions that uniquely apply to your child after a physical checkup.

KEYS TO SUCCESS OF AN EXERCISE PROGRAM

Instructions for your child:

- Fit exercise into your normal daily schedule.
- Exercise regularly—increase your pace gradually.
- Recruit a friend to make exercise fun.
- Consider trying out for sports teams at your school.
- Vary your activity. Alternate forms of exercise to avoid boredom.
- Increase exercise in easy, day-by-day activities. Walking up a flight of stairs to your classes in school is good exercise, as is riding a bicycle with friends after school.

AEROBIC EXERCISE

An exercise is aerobic if it provides your child with the following:

- Sustained physical activity that uses major muscle groups of the body.
- Regulated intensity, long-duration exercise for 20 minutes or more.

Medical experts recommend aerobic exercise as a good program for achieving and maintaining cardio-pulmonary-vascular fitness—strong and healthy heart, lungs, and blood vessels. Proper aerobic benefit is based on sufficient exercise to accelerate the child's heart rate to a prescribed level and keep it there a certain length of time. Most exercise routines call for aerobic sessions three to five times per week for maximum benefit.

The best forms of aerobic exercise for your child include brisk walking, swimming, bike riding, jogging, rope jumping, and rowing. Sports such as tennis and golf have good recreational effects, but they do not require enough effort to reach sustained aerobic levels.

Good sources for additional reading about aerobics include *The New Aerobics* by Dr. Kenneth Cooper, a recognized international authority on the subject. *MuscleAerobics: The Ultimate Workout For Body Shaping,* by Patricia Patano and Linette Savage, published by The Body Press, is a new approach that combines aerobics with the use of body-shaping hand weights.

APPENDIX 37 (continued on next page)

Safe Use of Crutches

Crutches are often a necessary aid to walking when a person has injured a foot, ankle, leg, or hip. Proper use of crutches can allow safe, satisfactory mobility for your child. Improper use can cause further accidents.

INSTRUCTIONS FOR YOUR CHILD:

BEFORE YOU USE CRUTCHES

• Practice using crutches under supervision before trying them out on your own.
• Reread these instructions frequently while getting used to crutches until using the crutches becomes automatic.
• Use a backpack to carry necessary belongings while using crutches. Never try to carry anything in your hands or arms.

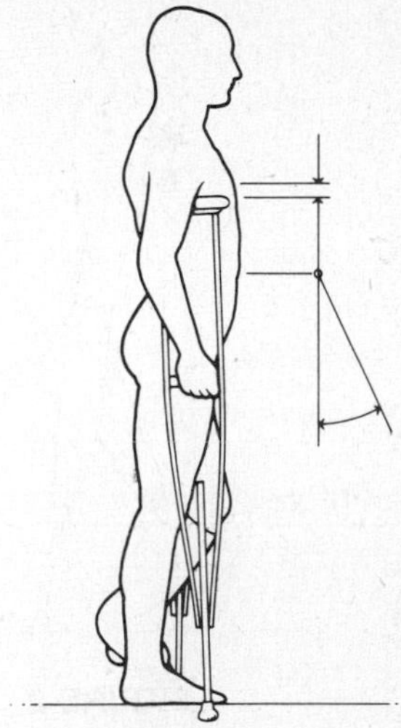

FIGURE 1

FITTING CRUTCHES

You will be fitted for your crutches at the place where you rent or buy them—usually a medical-supply store. The following points are important in ensuring a proper fit:

1. Stand straight.
2. Adjust the length of the crutches so 2 or 3 fingers can fit between the top of the crutch and the armpit (about 2 inches).
3. Adjust the hand grip so your elbow bends about 25 degrees, as shown in Figure 1. **Warning:** Don't bear any weight in the armpits. This can cause permanent damage to the nerves of the arm and hand.

MOVING ON CRUTCHES

• There are 4 major gaits used by people who need crutches:

— *Swing-through Gait*—Fastest and most difficult.
— *Swing-to Gait*—Slower and easier, and good to use until you become skillful with crutches and can advance to a faster gait.
— *Shuffle Gait*—Slowest of all, and most appropriate for older people.
— *3-Point Gait*—Can be used only when a slight amount of weight can be borne on the weak side.

• The last three gaits are described here. When you are ready to progress to a faster gait, such as the swing-through gait, you will need instructions and supervision from your trainer, nurse, or doctor. Also described are instructions on ascending and descending stair and curbs. These are general suggestions that apply to everyone on crutches.

SWING-TO GAIT

This is a good gait for beginners.

1. Place both crutches forward simultaneously, 12 inches in front of your feet, 6 to 8 inches wider than your toes on both sides (see Figure 2).
2. Push your hands down against the handles and shift your weight forward.
3. Swing your body to a point directly between the crutches. Let the heel on the healthy side land first.
   Note: The Swing-through Gait is the same as the Swing-to Gait except that the body swings through and lands in front of the crutches (see Figure 3).

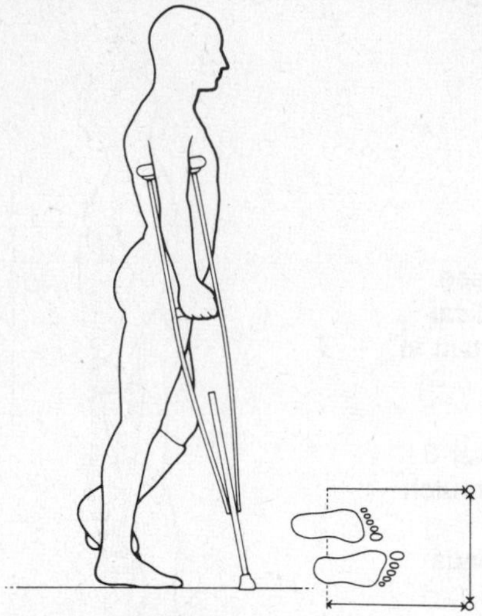

FIGURE 2

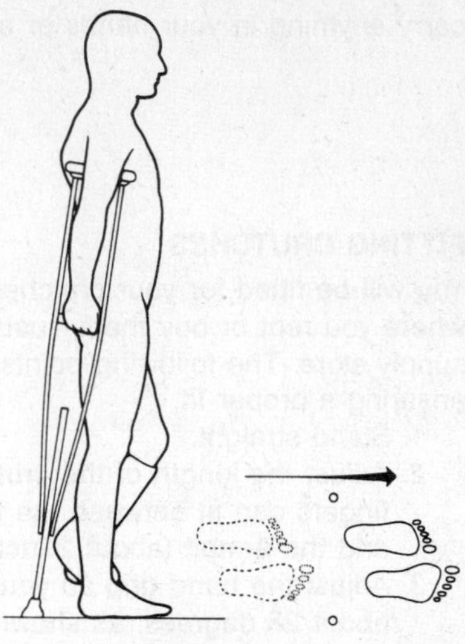

FIGURE 3

SHUFFLE GAIT

This gait should be used when the Swing-to Gait is too difficult:

1. Place both crutches forward simultaneously, 12 inches in front of your feet, 6 to 8 inches wider than your toes on both sides (see Figure 4).
2. Push hands down against the handles as you shift your body weight forward.
3. Slide the strong leg forward a few inches to a point between the crutches.
4. Follow with the weak leg, ending with the legs together.

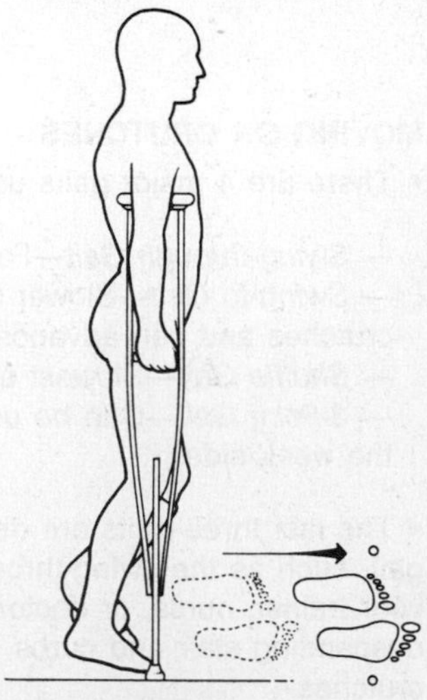

FIGURE 4

3-POINT GAIT

Use this gait only when you are able to bear slight, increasing weight on the weak leg (see Figure 5).

1. Place both crutches and the weak foot forward simultaneously, with the weak foot between the crutches. The weight is borne on the strong foot.
2. Push against the handles and shift your weight forward.
3. Swing your body forward with weight on your hands, and bear a slight amount of weight on the weak foot.
4. End with the strong foot ahead of the crutches.

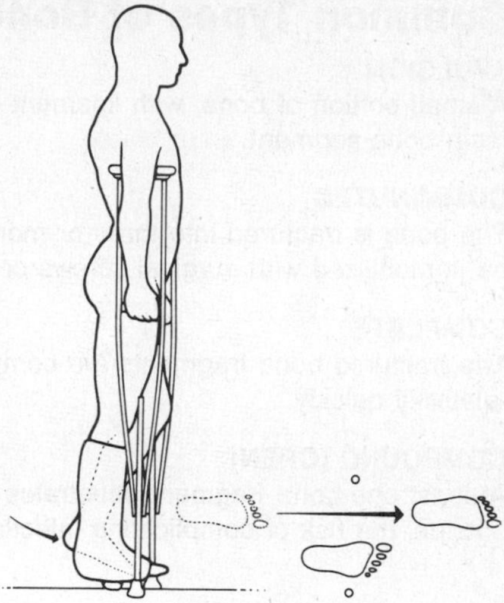

FIGURE 5

ASCENDING STEPS AND CURBS

1. Keep crutches on the lower step. Body weight is on the hands.
2. Raise the strong foot to the step above, trailing the weak leg (see Figure 6).
3. Straighten the strong leg and advance the crutches to the next step above.

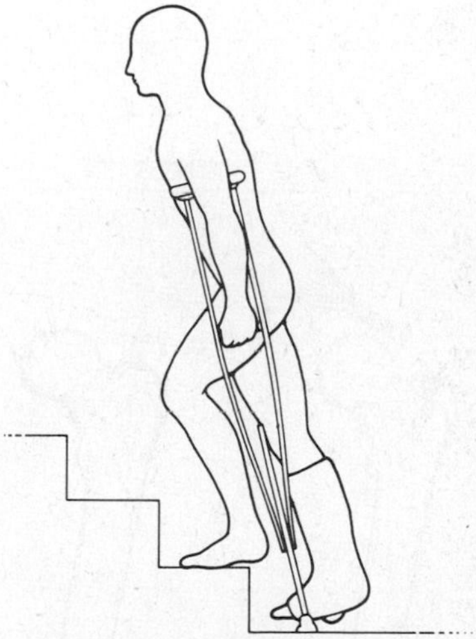

FIGURE 6

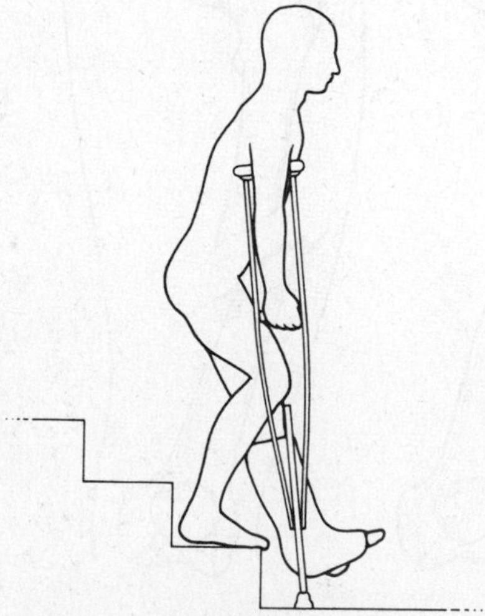

FIGURE 7

DESCENDING STEPS AND CURBS

1. Place crutches on the lower step, and extend the weak leg forward. Body weight is on the hands (see Figure 7).
2. Bend the strong leg and slowly lower the body.
3. Quickly move the strong leg to the lower step.

Reminder for ascending and descending steps with crutches:
"The good goes up, the bad goes down."

APPENDIX 38

Common Types of Bone Fractures

AVULSION
A small portion of bone, with ligament or tendon attached, is pulled away from the main bone segment.

COMMINUTED
The bone is fractured into three or more segments. This type of fracture usually must be immobilized with surgical screws or pins for healing.

COMPLETE
The fractured bone fragments are completely separated. A clean break usually heals relatively quickly.

COMPOUND (OPEN)
At least one bone fragment penetrates the skin. By opening the injury area to the outside, the risk of complicating infections increases.

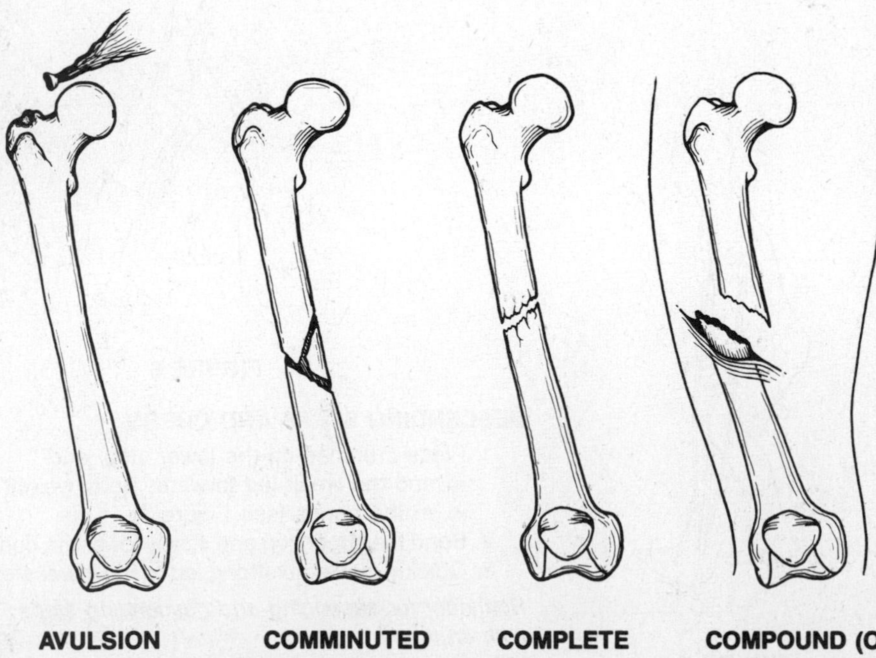

AVULSION COMMINUTED COMPLETE COMPOUND (OPEN)

COMPRESSION
Fracture occurs when the mass of bones is compressed, usually by forces in opposite directions. Compression fractures are most common in the spinal vertebrae.

FATIGUE
A complete or incomplete hairline fracture that develops after repeated stress to the bone.

GREENSTICK
This is an incomplete fracture, with bone fragments joined by at least some bone. Greenstick fractures heal more quickly than other fractures.

SPIRAL
Shearing forces cause the fractured segments to separate in a spiral fashion.

STRESS (SEE FATIGUE)

TRANSVERSE (WITH DISPLACEMENT)
The complete fractured bone segments are displaced in relation to each other. These fractures require strength and skill to return bone fragments to a functional position for healing.

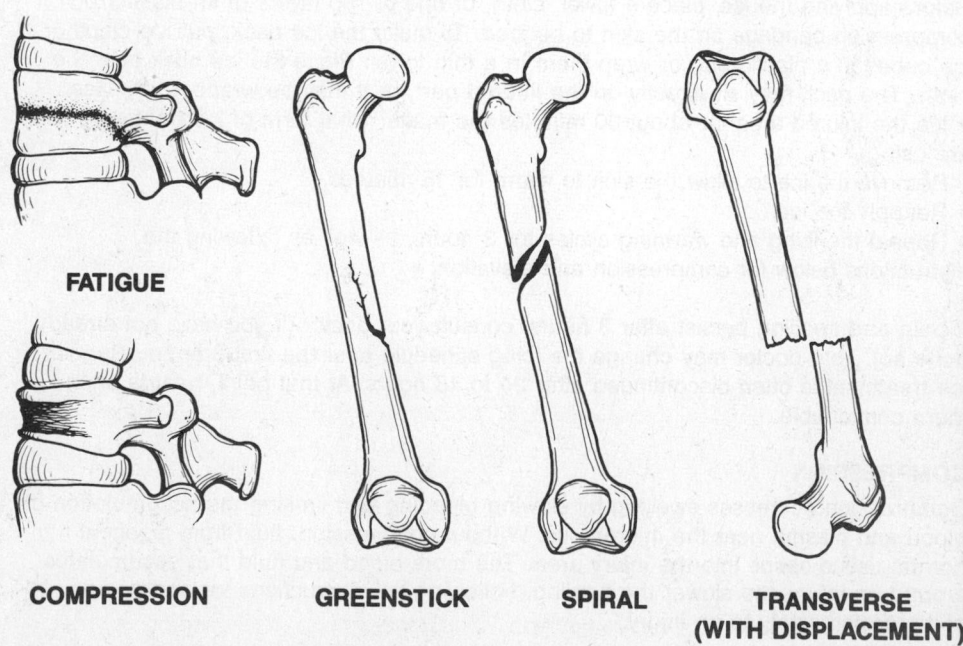

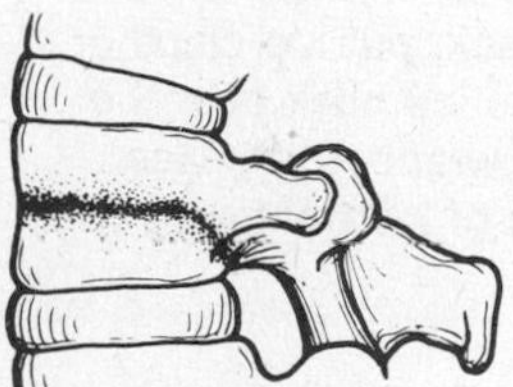

FATIGUE

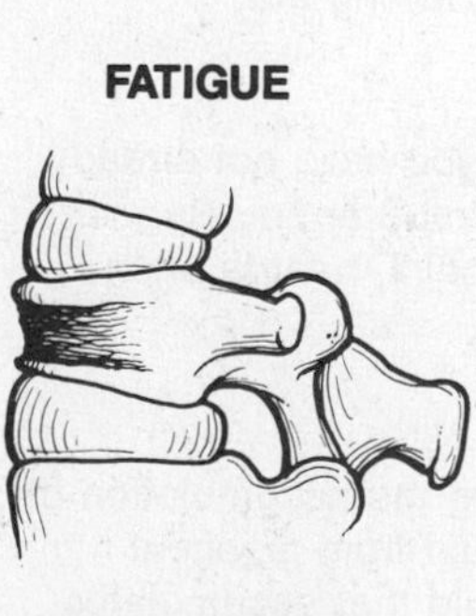

COMPRESSION

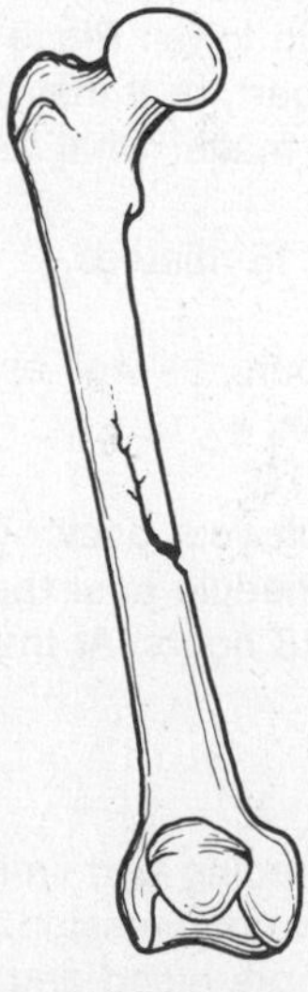

GREENSTICK

SPIRAL

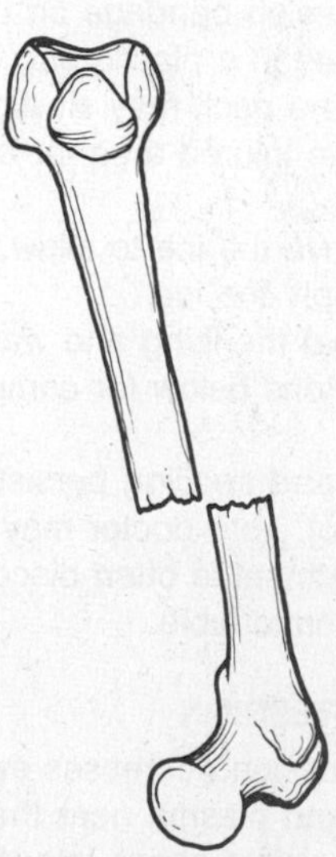

TRANSVERSE (WITH DISPLACEMENT)

APPENDIX 39

R.I.C.E. (Rest, Ice, Compression, Elevation)

R.I.C.E. is an acronym (a word coined from first letters) for the most important elements—*rest, ice, compression* and *elevation*—in first aid of many injuries. This acronym appears repeatedly throughout this book—and in medical literature in general—in reference to athletic injuries. Use the word R.I.C.E. to jog your memory when your child is faced with such injuries as contusions, sprains, strains, dislocations, or uncomplicated fractures.

REST

Your child should stop using the injured part and rest it as soon as an injury has taken place. Continued exercise or other activity could cause further injury, delay healing, increase pain, and stimulate bleeding. The child can use crutches to avoid bearing weight on injuries of the foot, ankle, knee, or leg and splints for injuries of the hand, wrist, elbow, or arm. After medical treatment, the injured part may require immobilization with splints or a cast to keep the area at rest until it heals.

ICE

Ice helps stop internal bleeding from injured blood vessels and capillaries. Sudden cold causes small blood vessels to contract. This contraction of blood vessels decreases the amount of blood that can collect around the child's wound. The more blood that collects, the longer the healing time. Ice can be safely applied in several ways using the following instructions:

- For injuries to small areas, such as a finger, toe, foot, or wrist, immerse the injured area in a bucket of ice water. Use ice cubes to keep the water cold as ice dissolves.
- For injuries to larger areas, use ice packs. Avoid placing ice directly on the skin. Before applying the ice, place a towel, cloth, or one or two layers of an elasticized compression bandage on the skin to be iced. To make the ice pack, put ice chips or ice cubes in a plastic bag or wrap them in a thin towel. Place the ice pack over the cloth. The pack may sit directly on the injured part, or it may be wrapped in place.
- Ice the injured area for about 30 minutes (no matter what form of ice treatment you are using).
- Remove the ice to allow the skin to warm for 15 minutes.
- Reapply the ice.
- Repeat the icing and warming cycles for 3 hours, as well as following the instructions below for compression and elevation.

If pain and swelling persist after 3 hours, consult your doctor (if you have not already done so). Your doctor may change the icing schedule after the first 3 hours. Regular ice treatment is often discontinued after 24 to 48 hours. At that point, heat is often more comfortable.

COMPRESSION

Compression decreases swelling by slowing bleeding and limiting the accumulation of blood and plasma near the injured site. Without compression, fluid from adjacent normal tissue seeps into the injury area. The more blood and fluid that accumulates around an injury, the slower the healing. Following are instructions for applying compression safely to an injury.

Use an elasticized bandage (Ace bandage) on the child for compression, if possible. If you do not have one available, any kind of cloth will suffice for a short time. Wrap the injured part firmly, wrapping over the ice also. Begin wrapping below the injury site and extend above the injury site. Be careful not to compress the area so tightly that the blood supply is impaired. Signs of blood-supply deprivation include pain, numbness, cramping, and blue or dusky-colored nails. Remove the compression bandage immediately if any of these symptoms appear. Leave the bandage off the child until all signs of impaired circulation disappear. Then rewrap the area—less tightly this time.

ELEVATION

Elevating the injured part above the level of the child's heart is another way to decrease swelling and pain at the injury site. Elevate the iced, compressed area in whatever way is most convenient. Prop an injured leg on solid objects or pillows. Elevate an injured arm by having the child lie down and placing pillows under the arm, or placing them on the chest with the arm folded across. The whole upper part of the child's body may be elevated gently with pillows by having the child sit in a reclining chair or by raising the top of the child's bed on blocks.

APPENDIX 40

Physical Therapy Methods and Techniques

• Rehabilitation, when applied to athletic injuries, means to restore to health. Traditionally this has meant exercising muscles to restore strength, endurance, and normal range of motion. A broader interpretation includes other methods and techniques that facilitate the healing process in your child.

• Physical agents such as heat, cold, massage, and electric current can be used in conjunction with exercise programs—and sometimes, medications—to hasten rehabilitation. The first three can often be used at home under the supervision of a doctor, physical therapist, or trainer. These trained professionals can oversee your child's progress, shifting from one type of exercise to another when advisable. The different methods are explained in greater detail below. Electrical current can only be performed with specialized equipment in a clinical setting, but it is very effective in muscle retraining and restoration of strength.

HEAT

• When heat is applied to an injury, it dilates (enlarges) small blood vessels in the area, increasing blood flow. The increased blood supply nourishes the tissues and hastens healing. Heat also reduces pain in an injured area and reduces muscle spasm. But heat increases the chance that small capillaries will leak blood and plasma into soft tissues around the injury. While dilation of the blood vessels and increased blood flow are desirable in healing, capillary leakage is undesirable. It leads to greater fluid accumulation and swelling, which retards the healing process. To be beneficial, heat should not be applied until the capillaries have had a chance to seal and stop leaking. This usually requires 24 to 48 hours following your child's injury—if ice, compression, and elevation were used immediately.

• Depending on the type of injury, heat can be applied in several ways: hot compresses, hydrocollator packs (see Glossary), heat lamps, heating pads, whirlpool baths or hot tubs, ultrasound, or diathermy (seldom used now—see Glossary).

• Your doctor or therapist must prescribe the best program for your child and provide supervision and guidance throughout the child's rehabilitation program. You and your child will need instructions about when to start, how long to apply heat during each treatment, and how long to continue with heat treatments. These factors are determined by many variables, such as type and extent of injury, previous medical history, and healing rate.

COLD (CRYOTHERAPY)

• During the past several years, cold treatment has been used increasingly in first aid and in rehabilitation of athletic injuries. Localized cold treatments provide these important benefits:

— Reduction and control of swelling (edema).

— Facilitation of active or passive joint motion, allowing the child to return to exercising sooner than is possible without cryotherapy. Ice is applied before exercise during the healing phase.

— Reduction of pain and muscle spasm.

• Because ice can be applied prior to exercise, reducing your child's pain and muscle spasm, muscle and joint movements can start sooner without interfering with the healing process. A thin margin of safety regarding when exercise should start and continue makes clinical supervision necessary during rehabilitation.

• Ice can be applied as ice packs, ice compresses, or ice massage. Ice massage is particularly helpful for sore muscles or muscles in spasm.
• Techniques of ice massage:
— Fill a large Styrofoam cup with water and freeze.
— Tear a small amount of foam from the top so ice protrudes.
— Massage firmly over the injured area in a circle about the size of a softball.
— Do this for 15 minutes at a time, 3 or 4 times a day, and before workouts or competition.

MASSAGE

Gentle massage is useful for treating your child's sore muscles. It consists of gentle or firm stroking of the injured area. Strokes should be directed toward the heart. The appropriate amount of pressure and length of the massage should be determined by the person receiving the massage. Massage that increases pain is too hard. When properly administered, massage can reduce fluid accumulation and swelling around an injury. It will stimulate circulation through the veins and lymphatic vessels. However, *overzealous* massage can aggravate a child's injury and increase bleeding.

APPENDIX 41

Care of Casts

• A cast immobilizes a part of the body that has been injured. Casts are used most commonly after bone fractures.
• Casts are usually applied by placing a splint along the injured part and wrapping it with gauze saturated with plaster of Paris. Before the injury heals, it may be necessary to change the child's cast one or more times. The time needed for healing determines how long a cast remains in place. Some casts are needed for only 2 weeks. Others are necessary for several months.
• X-rays through your child's cast reveal whether bone alignment is satisfactory. They are also used in later stages to check for signs of healing.

AFTER YOU LEAVE THE DOCTOR'S OFFICE

• Don't allow pressure on any part of the child's cast—no matter what type of casting material was used—until it is completely dry. Any depression that develops will create pressure on the skin underneath, making ulcer formation likely. Drying time varies depending on the type of material used, thickness of the cast, temperature, and humidity. Drying can require 24 hours or longer.
• Keep the child's cast dry, especially at first. If the cast accidentally gets wet and a soft area appears, return to the doctor's office, emergency room, or outpatient surgical facility for repairs.
• Whenever possible, raise the body part enclosed in the cast. This decreases the chance of tissue swelling inside the cast. Prop a leg in a cast on a pillow when the child is in bed, and on a footstool or chair when the child is sitting. Prop an arm in a cast on a pillow placed on the chest. Elevate the foot of the bed at night for any injury requiring a cast below the child's abdomen.

SWELLING INSIDE A CAST

No matter how carefully the injured tissues are handled, and no matter how expertly the cast is applied, swelling sometimes occurs inside a cast. Swelling should be reported immediately to the doctor. The following are common symptoms and signs of swelling:

• Severe, persistent pain.
• Change in color of tissues beyond the cast, such as a change to blue or gray under the fingernails or toenails.
• Coldness of the tissues beyond the cast, even though the rest of the child's body is warm.
• Numbness or complete loss of feeling in the skin beyond the cast.
• Feeling of tightness under the cast after it dries.
• For a leg cast, inability to raise the big toe.

INFECTION INSIDE A CAST

Sometimes the injured area becomes infected during healing. Detecting the infection in early stages may be difficult if the infected area is covered by a cast. Infection should be reported immediately to the child's doctor. Following are common signs and symptoms of infection:

• Leakage of fluid through the cast.
• Pain or soreness of the skin under the cast.
• Fever accompanied by a general ill feeling.

ITCHING INSIDE A CAST

Itching can be a maddening problem for a child with a cast—especially during hot weather. Even if it is possible to reach the itch, urge your child not to scratch the skin inside the cast. Because the skin is in a hot, moist environment, it is very vulnerable to damage. Scratching is more likely to injure the skin than under normal circumstances. If no incision was made, you may sprinkle cornstarch into the cast to relieve itching. If an incision was made, consult your doctor for pain medication. Itching is a form of mild pain.

BATHING WITH A CAST

Your child may find bathing difficult when wearing a cast. The cast must be kept dry at all times, so the child should not take showers. If the cast is on a limb, such as the arm or leg, the child may take tub baths. Position a chair or other support by the tub so you can prop the injured part out of the water while the child is bathing. If the cast is on the trunk of the body, your child should take sponge baths until the cast is removed.

APPENDIX 42

Drugs of Abuse

• Each of the drug charts in the Medications section lists the interactions of alcohol, marijuana, and cocaine with the therapeutic drug in a child's bloodstream. These three drugs are singled out because of their widespread use and abuse. The information is factual, not judgmental.
• The many long-term effects of alcohol and tobacco abuse have been well-publicized. Information is provided here as a reminder to your child of the inherent dangers of these drugs.
• Drugs of potential abuse include those that are addictive and harmful. They usually produce a temporary, false sense of well-being. The long-term effects, however, are harmful and can be devastating to the body and psyche of the addict.
These are the most common drugs of abuse:

TOBACCO (NICOTINE)

• **What it does to your child:** Tobacco smoke contains noxious and cancer-producing ingredients. They include nicotine, carbon monoxide, ammonia, and a variety of harmful tars. Carcinogens in smoke probably come from the tars. Most are present in chewing tobacco and snuff as well as smoke from cigarettes, cigars, and pipes. Tobacco smoke interferes with the immune mechanisms of the body.
• **Short-term effects of average amount:** Relaxation of mood in a steady smoker. Constriction of blood vessels.
• **Short-term effects of large amount inhaled:** Headache, loss of appetite, nausea.
• **Long-term effects:** Greatly enhanced chances of developing lung cancer later in your child's life. Impaired breathing and chronic lung disease (asthma, emphysema, bronchiectasis, lung abscess and others) much more likely. Heart and blood vessel disease more frequent and more severe when they happen later in a child's life. These include myocardial infarction (heart attack), coronary artery disease, heartbeat irregularities, generalized arteriosclerosis (hardening of the arteries making the brain, heart, and kidney more vulnerable to disease), peripheral vascular disease such as intermittent claudication, Buerger's disease, and others. Tobacco and nicotine lead to an increased incidence of abortion and significantly reduce the birth weight of babies brought to term and delivered of women who smoke during pregnancy. Tobacco smoking causes higher frequency not only of lung cancer, but also increases the likelihood of developing cancer of the throat, larynx, mouth, esophagus, bladder, and pancreas later in a child's life.

ALCOHOL

• **What it does to your child's**
— **Central nervous system:** It *depresses*, it does *not* stimulate, the action of all parts of the central nervous system, including the depression of normal mental activity and normal muscle function. Short-term effects of an average amount: relaxation, breakdown of inhibitions, euphoria, decreased alertness. Short-term effects of large amounts: nausea, stupor, hangover, unconsciousness, even death.
— **Gastrointestinal system:** It increases stomach acid and poisons liver function. Chronic alcoholism frequently leads to permanent damage to the liver.
— **Heart and blood vessels:** It decreases normal function, leading to heart diseases such as cardiomyopathy and disorders of the blood vessels and kidney such as high blood pressure later in a child's life. Bleeding from the esophagus and stomach frequently accompany chronic alcoholism.

— **Unborn fetus (teratogenicity):** Alcoholism in the mother carrying a fetus causes *fetal alcohol syndrome (FAS)*, which includes the production of mental deficiency, facial abnormalities, slow growth, and other major and minor malformations in the newborn.

- **Signs of Use**

— **Early signs:** Prominent smell of alcohol on the child's breath, behavior changes (aggressiveness; passivity; acting out sexually; using poor judgment; outbursts of uncontrolled emotion, such as rage or tearfulness).

— **Intoxication signs:** Unsteady gait, slurred speech, poor performance of any brain or muscle function, stupor or coma in *severe* alcoholic intoxication with slow, noisy breathing, cold and clammy skin, heartbeat faster than usual.

- **Long-term effects**

— **Addiction:** Compulsive use of alcohol. Persons addicted to alcohol have severe withdrawal symptoms when alcohol is unavailable. Even with successful treatment, addiction to alcohol (and other drugs that cause addiction) has a high tendency to relapse. (Memory of euphoric feelings plus family, social, emotional, psychological, and genetic factors probably are all important factors in producing the addiction.)

— **Liver disease:** Usually cirrhosis later in a child's life; also, deleterious effects on the unborn child of an alcoholic mother.

— **Loss of sexual function:** Impotence, erectile dysfunction, loss of libido.

— **Increased incidence of cancer:** Mouth, pharynx, larynx, esophagus, liver, and lung later in a child's life.

— **Changes in blood:** Makes it less likely for blood to clot efficiently.

— **Heart disease:** Decreased normal function leading to possible damage and disease later in a child's life.

— **Stomach and intestinal problems:** Increased production of stomach acid.

— **Interference with expected or normal actions of many medications:** Detailed on every chart in this book, drugs such as sedatives, pain killers, narcotics, antihistamines, anticonvulsants, anticoagulants, and others.

MARIJUANA (CANNABIS, HASHISH)

- **What they do to your child:** Heighten perception, cause mood swings, relax mind and body.
- **Signs of use:** Red eyes, lethargy, uncoordinated body movements.
- **Long-term effects:** Decreased motivation. Possible brain, heart, lung, and reproductive system damage.

AMPHETAMINES

- **What they do to your child:** Speed up physical and mental processes to cause a false sense of energy and excitement. The moods are temporary and unreal.
- **Signs of use:** Dilated pupils, insomnia, trembling.
- **Long-term effects:** Violent behavior, paranoia, possible death from overdose.

BARBITURATES

- **What they do to your child:** Produce drowsiness and lethargy.
- **Signs of use:** Confused speech, lack of coordination and balance.
- **Long-term effects:** Disrupts normal sleep pattern. Possible death from overdose, especially in combination with alcohol.

COCAINE

• **What it does to your child:** Stimulates the nervous system, heightens sensations and may produce hallucinations.
• **Signs of use:** Trembling, intoxication, dilated pupils, constant sniffling.
• **Long-term effects:** Ulceration of nasal passages where sniffed. Itching all over the body, sometimes with open sores. Possible brain damage. Possible death from overdose.

OPIATES (CODEINE, HEROIN, METHADONE, MORPHINE, OPIUM)

• **What they do to your child:** Relieve pain, create temporary and false sense of well-being.
• **Signs of use:** Constricted pupils, mood swings, slurred speech, sore eyes, lethargy, weight loss, sweating.
• **Long-term effects:** Malnutrition, extreme susceptibility to infection, the need to increase drug amount to produce the same effects. Possible death from overdose.

PSYCHEDELIC DRUGS (LSD, MESCALINE)

• **What they do to your child:** Produce hallucinations, either pleasant or frightening.
• **Signs of use:** Dilated pupils, sweating, trembling, fever, chills.
• **Long-term effects:** Lack of motivation, unpredictable behavior, narcissism, recurrent hallucinations without drug use ("flashbacks"). Possible death from overdose.

VOLATILE SUBSTANCES (GLUE, SOLVENTS)

• **What they do to your child:** Produce hallucinations, temporary, false sense of well-being, and possible unconsciousness.
• **Signs of use:** Dilated pupils, flushed face, confusion.
• **Long-term effects:** Permanent brain, liver, kidney damage. Possible death from overdose.

APPENDIX 43

Child Abuse

What—Any kind of deprivation or mistreatment that adversely affects the welfare of an infant, child, or adolescent. Mistreatment can be physical or emotional. Annually, an estimated 2% to 6% of all children in the U.S. suffer injury from neglect or assault.

Who—It is estimated that 90% of child abuse is inflicted by a close relative, parent or brother or sister—usually the parent. Abusers come from all strata of society, all geographical areas, and all ethnic groups.

Why—Parents who abuse children usually do so as a response to *stress*. Abusers often were abused themselves as children.

Signs of Child Abuse—Bruises, welts, burns, bumps, cuts, bite marks, broken bones, black eyes. Emotional changes in the abused child may be manifested by failure to thrive, weight loss, weight gain, nightmares, inability to sleep, phobias, frequent illnesses, withdrawal, listlessness, passiveness, low self-esteem, anxiety and/or depression. Some abused children may become aggressive, disruptive, impulsive, hyperactive, or negative. They may participate in sexual aberrations, drug abuse, or prostitution.

Reporting to Authorities—Report to your local authorities or child protective agency any child in whom you observe signs of abuse. Many states have laws that charge you with being an accomplice to abuse or neglect if you see it and do not report it. If you suspect abuse or neglect, report it and let the authorities make the final decision. Your name will be kept confidential.

If You Were Abused—If you yourself were abused as a child, ask for guidance and counseling so you will not be likely to abuse your own child. You will find great satisfaction in breaking the abuse pattern. Help is available (see Support Services).

Treatment—Both parents and children: Psychotherapy, preferably long-term.

Support Services—Shelters are available in almost any area of the country. Call Parents Anonymous (1-800-882-1250) or Prevent Child Abuse (Box 2866, Chicago, IL 60690).

APPENDIX 44

Diseases Caused by Pets

Larva Migrans (Roundworm)—Caused by a child eating soil contaminated with feces from puppies or kittens. Treated with medication taken orally. See entry in Illnesses section.

Toxoplasmosis—Caused by a parasite transmitted when a child cleans a kitten's litter box or otherwise handles cat feces. Symptoms include muscle pain, swollen lymph glands, and skin rash. Toxoplasmosis in a more severe form can be transmitted by an infected mother passing on the disease in her bloodstream to the unborn child, through the placenta. Antibiotics can prevent on-going infection in the mother but will not prevent damage to the unborn child.

Pasteurella—Caused by bacteria entering the child's body through cat or dog bites. Usually treated with antibiotics.

Salmonellosis—Caused by bacteria often carried by pet turtles and other pets. Symptoms include fever, abdominal pain, and diarrhea. Treatment includes antibiotics for children under 1 year. In older children the disease is usually self-limited and requires no antibiotics.

Psittacosis—Caused by a germ carried in the droppings of infected birds, usually tropical birds such as parrots, macaws, or parakeets. Treated with antibiotics. See entry in Illnesses section.

Cat-Scratch Fever—See entry in Illnesses section.

Rabies—See entry in Illnesses section.

Leptospirosis—Caused by a germ in urine of infected dogs. Symptoms include fever, headache, muscle aches, nausea and vomiting, cramps, chills, and red eyes. Treatment requires antibiotics.

Rocky Mountain Spotted Fever—See entry in Illnesses section.

Lyme Disease—See entry in Illnesses section.

Toxocara—See entry in Illnesses section.

Histoplasmosis—See entry in Illnesses section.

APPENDIX 45

Dizziness Questionnaire

Work with your child to answer these questions so you can give accurate information to your physician.

1. What does dizziness mean to you: whirling, movement up and down or side to side, faintness, light headedness? Do *you* spin or does the *world* spin.

2. How does it start? Is it sudden or gradual?

3. How often does it occur?

4. How long does it last? Seconds, minutes, hours, days, weeks?

5. Is it influenced by your head or body movements?

6. Which of the following, if any, are associated with the dizziness? Nausea, vomiting, fainting, ringing in the ears, deafness, vision changes, convulsions, numbness?

7. Is your child taking any of these drugs: aspirin or pain killers, sedatives, tranquilizers, alcohol, hallucinogens?

8. Is your child exposed to any fumes at home or school?

9. Has your child had any recent illness, accident, or emotional upset?

10. Does your child have any ear complaints: ringing, drainage, sense of fullness, hearing loss?

11. Does your child have any palpitation of the heart?

APPENDIX 46

Visits to the Doctor

Most infants start to cry in the doctor's office at 5 to 6 months of age. This is a normal reaction. The fear of strangers will continue until the child is 2½ to 3 years old. Keep in mind that the child is undressed and being handled by giant-sized strangers in a strange place! Reassure your child, but remember that it is natural for a young child to be anxious and fearful and to put up some sort of protest.

Suggestions to Minimize the Protests

- Never tell your child there won't be an injection (shot). It is better to say nothing.
- Do not say, "Shut up or you'll get a shot." It is ill-advised to threaten your child in this way.
- If you tell your child "it will not hurt," the child probably will hear only the word "hurt" and may wonder why it was mentioned. The child may think that the *visit* will hurt.
- Try not to be overly sympathetic. It will prolong the pain and the child may use this as an attention-getting mechanism later.
- Do not refer to the doctor or nurse as "mean" or "bad."
- Empty your child's mouth of all gum, candy, fruit, and cookies.
- Do not tell your child that you are going for a treat and then end up unexpectedly at the doctor's office.
- Do not laugh at the child.

Constructive Dialogue and Actions

- Tell your child you know he's good, even when he's crying. Reassure the child that when he's older, it will be better.
- Let the older child know it's all right to cry or scream or say ouch if the shot hurts. You can explain that injections help keep children healthy and well even when they hurt.
- Respect the child's dignity and establish trust by telling the truth and explaining what to expect from a visit to the doctor's office.
- If your physician requests that you hold your child during an office procedure, do it securely.
- Watch an infant on an examining table at all times.
- Be on time for your child's appointment.

It is important to develop a relationship with physicians in whom you have confidence. Feel free to discuss any concerns you have, but do not take time with trivia. Regular checkups are no guarantee against ill health but they help to detect disease earlier.

Traveling

If you are going to travel without your child, a *written consent* to allow a doctor to perform any necessary medical or surgical treatment should be left with the person caring for the child. Avoid extensive traveling with an infant under the age of 3 months. If you must travel with your infant, approximately 10 days to 2 weeks before the trip:

- Take your infant for a medical checkup, including any injections that your pediatrician recommends. (But no measles vaccine or smallpox vaccination, which cause a reaction 6-12 days after injection.)
- Introduce any new foods.
- Have the infant sleep in a special traveling bed to get accustomed to it.
- Have the infant or any child traveling with you get used to a washable plastic toy. Leave the large furry animals home.

Clothing—The child's clothing should be light, soft, loose, easily washable and preferably the drip-dry type. Use disposable diapers.

Schedule—Write out your child's daily schedule and list the items used. Do this 10 days to 2 weeks before the trip is planned. Each day, as you perform the schedule, add other necessary things to the list. Examples:

- A waterproof bag for soiled clothes.
- Plenty of cleansing tissues, foil-packaged face and hand cleaners, and disposable wipes for your baby in diapers.
- For small children, a small portable toilet seat.
- A plastic table cloth to protect the bed from being soiled and to cover the carpet if the infant is fed in a hotel room.
- Several large bibs.
- Straws and plastic spoons.
- Most important—the necessary openers for the cans of food or formula.

Formulas and feedings—Buy distilled sterile water in ½-gallon bottles from the druggist. Buy "ready-to-use" formula in cans or disposable bottles, which contain the milk, sugar, and water already mixed. If you are preparing the formula yourself, pour the water and the approximate amount of sugar into the bottles and sterilize them by the terminal method before leaving, then add the evaporated milk from the can when the baby needs a bottle. If you are planning to go by train or airline, find out about the conveniences they offer for the baby. Disposable bottles are very useful. Choose foods your infant or child likes best, and throw away any used food. Expect your child to eat less on a trip.

Avoid weekend auto travel and traffic jams, particularly in the summertime. Start early and plan mid-morning, noon, and mid-afternoon stops, with a final stop before 4 p.m.

If there are any toddlers on the trip, pad all the door handles and use proper automobile restraining devices and padded car seats.

MOTION SICKNESS

- DO NOT USE ANY MEDICATION ON INFANTS UNDER ONE YEAR. Ask your physician about simple medicine for your child's motion sickness.
- Driving and flying at night will reduce visual stimulation to an infant.
- Have the child sit in a reclining position and occupy a seat toward the center of gravity.
- Don't let the child read during the journey.
- Closed eyes or colored glasses may help.
- Be sure there is adequate ventilation.
- Stop and let the child walk at frequent intervals if possible.
- Give the child a light meal before the journey and sips of water during the trip.
- Do not mention before or during the trip past episodes of motion sickness.

APPENDIX 48 (continued on next page)

Suggestions to Help Your Child Live Longer

The following list represents the conclusions of a group of researchers headed by Drs. Belloc and Breslow of the University of California at Los Angeles. They studied the physical health status and health practices of thousands of people.

The conclusions scientifically validate what we have known all along. Simple as they seem, they require accepting and reviewing and following—if you desire to maintain your child's optimum health and highest level of physical fitness, mental alertness, and creativity.

Here are some suggestions for your child for healthy living based on result of the study:

GET ENOUGH SLEEP

Get the right amount of sleep (average 8 hours for adolescents, more for younger children) each night. The right amount must also be coupled with the right *quality* of sleep. Consider some of these suggestions for good sleep:

- Use the bedroom for sleep only. Avoid taking private worries to bed with you. Avoid getting caught up in suspenseful reading or television while relaxing in bed. If you toss and turn on occasion and can't get to sleep, go to another room and do something productive.
- Learn relaxation techniques. Try meditation or breathing exercises, or alternate tensing and relaxing muscles. Use one or more of these techniques, followed by a warm bath, before going to bed at night.

EAT A GOOD BREAKFAST

Don't skip breakfast! Failing to eat because "you don't have time" or ill-advised reduction of calories per day can lead to poor health. The scientific evidence for this recommendation is convincing.

EAT THREE MEALS A DAY AT REGULAR TIMES

Regular meals keep the metabolic and digestive systems functioning at their most efficient levels. If you get hungry between meals, don't resort to fatty, salty, or refined-sugar snacks. Instead, eat fruit, raw vegetables, or whole-grain snacks.

EXERCISE REGULARLY

Exercise that you enjoy is most likely to be successful and continued.

CONTROL YOUR WEIGHT

Even small amounts of excessive weight can shorten your life! Extreme obesity is associated with many physical and mental disorders. If you are overweight but still growing taller, maintain your weight until you have grown up to it. If you need to reduce, do so. If your weight is ideal, work to keep it that way.

DON'T DRINK ALCOHOL!

Alcohol abuse can cause serious diseases, reduce your lifespan, and make your life miserable.

DON'T SMOKE!

There is overwhelming evidence that smoking damages the human body and shortens life. Cigarette smoking is a risk factor for many illnesses, particularly lung cancer, chronic lung disease, hardening of the arteries, heart attack, and damage to unborn children of pregnant women who smoke. Anyone who smokes is at greater risk of problems with anesthesia during surgery.

DON'T ABUSE DRUGS!

Evidence is mounting about the cumulative ill effects of drug abuse. Common sense dictates avoiding them if you want to stay mentally and physically healthy.

A

Abdominal Aorta — Section of the aorta that passes through the abdomen to supply blood to the lower part of the body.

Abscess — Swollen inflamed, tender area of infection containing pus.

Accident-Proneness — Tendency of some children to have more accidents than normal. It may be due to a risk factor such as poor vision, but unconscious factors are often the cause.

Acetaminophen — Non-prescription medication used to relieve minor pain and to reduce fever. Its analgesic effects are similar to aspirin, but it does not reduce inflammation or swelling. It is less irritating to the stomach than aspirin.

Achylasia — Condition of the esophagus that disrupts normal swallowing.

Acupuncture — Method of anesthesia and treatment of pain developed by the Chinese. Needles are inserted through the skin to stimulate prescise areas.

Acute — Beginning suddenly; also severe, but of short duration.

Addiction — Intense craving for substances such as alcohol, tobacco or narcotics, or a compulsive behavior such as gambling.

Adenoids — Infection-fighting tissue (part of the lymphatic system) in the upper throat, near the tonsils.

Adenoids, Enlarged — Adenoids that have swollen and impaired speech.

Adenovirus — Group of viruses that cause certain respiratory and eye infections.

Adhesions — Small strands of fibrous tissue that cause organs in the abdomen and pelvis to cling together abnormally, creating a risk of intestinal obstruction.

Adolescence — Time of life from the beginning of puberty until maturity.

Adrenal Glands — Two glands attached to the kidneys. Each has an outer layer (cortex) that produces steroid hormones and an inner layer (medulla) that produces adrenalin.

Adrenalin — Hormone produced by the adrenal glands that increases heart rate and prepares the body for crisis. Also called epinephrine.

Aging — The normal process of gradual physical and mental decline.

Airways — Tubular passages that air passes through to the lungs; the trachea (windpipe), bronchi, and bronchioles.

Albinism — A rare, inherited disorder characterized by a lack of normal coloration of eyes, hair, skin, and sometimes shortness. The eyes are intolerant of light, move back and forth, and are affected by astigmatism. There is no treatment, except total protection from exposure to sunlight.

Allergy Skin Tests — A series of tests in which various substances are injected into the skin in minute amounts for the purpose of ruling in or out a person's allergy to that substance.

Alveoli — Lung cells at ends of the airways where oxygen enters the blood and waste gases leave the blood.

Ambulatory Medical Center — A health-care facility for patients who do not require prolonged bed rest or hospitalization.

Amniocentesis — A surgical procedure using a laparoscope (a hollow instrument with a system of lenses) that is pushed through a small incision in the abdominal wall and thence into the uterus to obtain amniotic fluid for study.

Amniotic Sac — The thin, transparent membrane filled with fluid in which the fetus lives until born.

Amphetamine Drugs — Habit-forming drugs that stimulate the brain and central nervous system, increase blood pressure, reduce nasal stuffiness, or suppress appetite.

Amyloid Deposits — Abnormal protein material deposited in tissues, usually caused by diseases. These deposits cause impairment of certain organs.

Analgesics — Medications that relieve pain.

Anemia — Condition in which red blood cells or hemoglobin (oxygen-carrying substance in blood) is inadequate.

Anesthesia, General — Causing temporary loss of consciousness and inability to feel pain by use of inhaled gases or injected anesthetics.

GLOSSARY

Anesthesia, Local — Temporary prevention of pain by injecting medication (local anesthetic).
Anesthesia, Local (Nerve Block) — Injection of the local anesthetic near the nerves of the surgical area.
Aneurysm — Abnormal swelling or ballooning of a blood vessel.
Angiogram, Angiography — Study of arteries and veins by injecting material into them that X-rays can outline.
Anoscopy — Visual examination of the anus by means of a short tube called an anoscope, an optical instrument with lenses and a lighted tip.
Antacid — Medicine taken orally that reduces or neutralizes stomach acid.
Antiarrhythmics — Medications used to treat heartbeat irregularities (arrhythmias).
Antibiotics — Medications that attack germs and fight infection.
Antibiotics, Cephalosporin — Class of antibiotics related to penicillin, capable of destroying more kinds of germs than penicillin.
Antibiotics, Erythromycin — Class of antibiotics that destroys germs similar to those destroyed by penicillin. Often used to treat infections in patients who are allergic to penicillin.
Antibodies — Proteins created in blood and body tissue by the immune system to neutralize or destroy sources of disease.
Anticancer Drugs — Medications that weaken or destroy cancerous tissues without harming healthy tissues.
Anticholingergic Drugs — Medications that reduce nerve impulses in the parasympathetic nervous system. They control some activities of the gastrointestinal system, heart, bladder, and other organs.
Anticoagulants — Medications that slow or delay blood clotting.
Anticonvulsants — Medications that control seizures (convulsions), pain, or conditions in which the brain or nerves are overly sensitive.
Antidepressants — Medications that help control depression.
Antiemetic Drugs — Medications that prevent or stop nausea and vomiting.
Antifungal Drugs — Medications used to treat fungus diseases.
Antigens — Germs or other sources of disease that antibodies (produced by the immune system) neutralize or destroy.
Antihelminthic Drugs — Medications used to treat worms in the intestines.
Antihistamines — Medications used to treat allergies.
Antihyperlipidemic Drugs — Medications that reduce fat (cholesterol) in the blood. They help prevent blood-vessel disease.
Antihypertensives — Medications used to reduce blood pressure.
Anti-Inflammatory Drugs — Medications used to control inflammation not caused by infection.
Antimalarial Drugs — Medications used to prevent or treat malaria.
Antimetabolite Drugs — Medications that are used to treat some cancers and autoimmune diseases.
Antimicrobial Drugs — Same as *Antibiotics*.
Antinuclear Antibody — Substance that appears in the blood, indicating presence of an autoimmune disease.
Antiparkinsonism Drugs — Medications used to treat Parkinson's disease.
Antiprotozoal Drugs — Medications used in treatment of single-celled parasites (protozoa).
Antipruritic Drugs — Medications that reduce itching.
Antispasmodic Drugs — Medications that improve digestion and relieve intestinal cramps.
Anti-Streptococcal Titer — Blood test that measures body's response to infection by streptococcal bacteria.
Antithyroid Drugs — Medications used to counter the effects of an overactive thyroid gland.
Antiviral Drugs — Medications used to treat infections caused by viruses.
Anus — A muscular band at the end of the rectum that opens and expands to allow passage of feces.

Anus, Imperforate — Congenital abnormality of newborn infants in which the anus cannot pass feces.
Anxiety — Uncomfortable feeling that something unpleasant or dangerous will happen.
Aorta — Body's largest blood vessel, arising from the top of the heart. It carries blood from the heart to all parts of the body.
Appendage — Body part that has a minor role (or no role at all) in normal body function. For example, the appendix is an appendage to the colon that seems to have no function.
Arrhythmia — Any variation from a normal heartbeat. Many that occur in children require no treatment. Abnormal rhythms can be caused by diseases of the heart (congenital heart disease, rheumatic heart disease) or by other diseases that may affect the heart rate (examples: thyroid problems, blood clotting, some drugs such as digitalis). There may be no symptoms in a child or there may be a heart rate far too fast to count—300 or over. Other symptoms include faintness, dizziness, light-headedness. Treatment depends on the cause and must be supervised by a physician.
Arteriogram, Arteriography — Studying arteries by injecting material into them that X-rays can outline.
Artery — Blood vessels that carry blood from the heart to the body.
Arthrograms — X-rays of the joints taken with an arthroscope.
Arthroscope — Slender optical instrument with a lighted tip that allows direct visual examination of some joints. It can also be used to correct some defects in joints.
Artificial Limbs — Mechanical substitutions for amputated arms or legs.
Ascending Colon — First part of the large colon (intestine) extending from the lower end of the small intestine.
Asphyxia — Literally from the Greek: "a stopping of the pulse." Modern interpretation is the condition caused by lack of oxygen in breathed air, resulting in impending or actual cessation of life.
Aspiration — 1) Removal of accumulated pus or fluid with a needle. 2) Accidental inhalation of objects or fluids into the lungs.
Astigmatism — Visual impairment caused by abnormal eye shape.
Assymmetrical — Uneven in size, shape, or position.
Atria — Small chambers in the heart that pump blood into the ventricles. Also called auricles.
Atropine — Medication used to treat diseases of the eye, heart, gastrointestinal system and nervous system.
Audiogram, Audiometry — Test of hearing ability.
Autism — A developmental disorder characterized by a lack of responsiveness to other people and by deficits in development and use of language. Cause is unknown, but may appear in conjunction with birth defects such as congenital German measles, mental retardation, or encephalitis. Treatment requires special education, training, and constant care. For further information and help, contact: National Society for Autistic Children, 1234 Massachusetts Ave., NW, Washington, DC 20005, phone (202)783-0125.
Autoimmune Assays (ANA Tests) — Blood tests to identify autoimmune disease.
Autoimmune Disease, Autoimmunity — Disease in which a person's immune system attacks its own tissues.
Autoimmune Disorder — Disease in which the immune system produces antibodies that attack the body's own tissues.
Autonomic Nervous System — Part of the nervous system that controls organs that function involuntarily, such as the heart, lungs, digestive system, and blood vessels.

B

Back pain — A common human complaint, less likely to occur in children than in adolescents or adults. Causes include injuries such as muscle strains or sprains, muscle spasms caused by sports or auto injuries, bad mattresses, stress, urinary tract infections, influenza, fractures, dislocations, arthritis, ruptured disc, leg length discrepancies, and tumors. Treatment must be directed at the cause, under the supervision of your physician.

Bacteria — One-celled micro-organisms that can sometimes cause disease.

Bad Breath — An unpleasant mouth odor, rare in children. The cause is usually poor oral hygiene, but it may also occur as a result of thrush, sinusitis, congested nasal passages, and ilnesses with fever, such as colds and mononucleosis. Treatment consists of improving oral hygiene with careful brushing, using mouthwash and flossing teeth, gums, and tongue, or treating any underlying diseases.

Baldness or Hair Loss — Can occur at any stage of childhood. Hair present at birth usually falls out, but new hair grows during childhood. Causes of hair loss other than normal include pulling or twisting hair, burns, emotional upsets, hormone problems, iron deficiency, infections (such as ringworm of the scalp, impetigo), drastic weight loss, calcium deficiency, inherited factors. Treatment varies according to the underlying cause and should be under the direction of your physician.

Balloon Angioplasty — Treatment for obstructed arteries, especially those supplying blood to the heart and brain. A small uninflated balloon is passed up the artery to the obstruction, and then expanded to release the obstruction.

Barium Enema X-rays — Examining the colon by filling it with a barium solution that is detected by X-rays.

Bartholin's Glands — Small glands in the lips of the vagina that secrete a lubricating fluid, especially during sexual arousal.

Belladonna — Medication derived from a plant used to treat some diseases of the gastrointestinal system. It is similar to atropine.

Benign — 1) Tumor or growth that is neither cancerous nor located where it might impair normal function. 2) Harmless.

Beta-Adrenergic Blockers (Beta-Blockers) — Medications that reduce heart or blood-vessel overactivity to improve blood circulation. Also used to prevent migraine headaches, high blood pressure, and angina.

Bile — A digestive juice produced in the liver and stored in the gallbladder. Bile empties into the small intestine for digestive processes.

Bile Duct — A small tube that allows bile to pass from the gallbladder into the intestines.

Bilirubin — A yellowish, red blood cell waste product in bile that the blood caries to the liver. It contributes to urine's yellowish color and can cause jaundice if it builds up in the blood.

Biofeedback Training — The process of providing visual or auditory evidence to a person of the status of the autonomic nervous system. For example: the sounding of a tone when blood pressure is at a desirable level, so that the patient may exert control at future times to lower elevated blood pressure to satisfactory levels.

Biopsy — Removal of a small amount of tissue or fluid for laboratory examination that aids in diagnosis.

Biopsy Needle — Instrument often used to perform a biopsy.

Birth Canal — Passageway through the cervix and the vagina through which the baby passes during childbirth.

Birth Control — Two-thirds of adolescent males and one-half of adolescent females in America are sexually active. Make sure your youngster has adequate instruction in sex education and particularly birth control. Example of devices and methods include condoms, contraceptive foam, diaphragm, cervical cap, vaginal contraceptive sponge, birth control pills, intrauterine device (IUD). For further information write: American Academy of Pediatrics, Department of Publications, P.O. Box 927,

Elk Grove Village, IL 60007, or Imprints Magazine, Birth and Life Bookstore, 7001 Alonzo Avenue NW, P.O. Box 70625, Seattle, WA 98107.

Birthmarks — These are blemishes of the skin present at birth. They fit into two categories: pigmentary and vascular. Pigmentary types include nevocellular nevi, mongolian spots, cafe-au-lait spots, epithelial nevi, Becker's nevi, dysplastic melanocytic nevi, and white birthmarks. Vascular types include hemangiomas (also called strawberry birthmarks), port-wine stains, stork bites or salmon patches. Diagnosis requires identification by your physician. Treatment depends on the type. Most fade and disappear, others need surgical or medical treatment under a physician's guidance.

Bladder — An organ that holds fluids such as urine (urinary bladder) or bile (gallbladder).

Blastomycosis — Infection caused by organisms of the genus *Blastomyces*.

Blindness and Other Vision Problems — The absence of vision. It may occur singly or in conjunction with other disabling handicaps. 20/200 or worse in the better eye is the legal limit of blindness. Ophthalmologists are required by law to report newly diagnosed blind individuals to an appropriate state agency. Causes include retrolental fibroplasia, congenital cataracts, congenital glaucoma, disorders of the retina or the optic nerve, acquired eye disease, accidents, or diseases affecting the whole body, including cancer. A precise diagnosis must be established by a competent eye specialist (ophthalmologist), who also will monitor treatment for treatable causes. Most of the treatment for a blind child is educational and takes place at home and at school and involves parents and teachers. The goal in treatment is to make it possible for the sight-impaired child to learn to become as independent as possible. Many aids (tapes, computers, books in braille, etc.) exist other than personal ones to help bring about self-sufficiency and self-confidence.

Blood Cells, Red — Microscopic cells in the blood that carry oxygen to tissues of the body. One drop of blood contains about 200 million red cells.

Blood Cells, White — Microscopic cells in the blood that help fight infection by destroying germs. One drop of blood contains about 400,000 white cells.

Blood Chemistries — Tests that measure chemicals in the blood.

Blood Count — Counting red and white blood cells to aid in diagnosis of many diseases.

Blood Platelets — See *Platelet Count*.

Blood Studies — Examination of a blood sample to measure white blood cells, red blood cells, hemoglobin, hematocrit, and chemical substances. See *Blood Chemistries*.

Blood Vessels — Arteries, veins, and capillaries; the tubes in which blood circulates through the body.

Bone Bank — Facility where human bone is stored and made available for transplantation.

Bone Cancer — Over 100 diseases marked by uncontrolled growth of cells. Some names of cancer applied to bones include Ewing's sarcoma, osteogenic sarcoma, chondrosarcoma, non-Hodgkin's lymphoma of the bone. The cause is unknown. Injury in the vicinity of affected bone often *precedes the detection* of bone cancer, but there is no evidence that injury causes the cancer. Treatment must be individualized according to the cell type of the cancer, and the age and sex of the patient. Treatment methods include surgery, chemotherapy, and radiation therapy, either singly or in combination.

Bone Spurs — Abnormal and sometimes painful protrusions of bone with sharp points near joints or tendons.

Breasts — Fat and fibrous tissue, milk-producing glands, and milk-transporting ducts. *Development:* Most girls begin to develop breasts between 9 and 14 years of age. Average age is 10 or 11. Each girl develops at her own rate. The onset and rate of development and ultimate size are determined by heridity, level of female

hormones, and nutrition. *Disorders:* If breasts fail to develop, if one is excessively larger than the other, if there is a lump in the breast or discharge from the nipple, consult your physician.
Bronchial Tubes (Bronchi) — Hollow air passageways that branch from the windpipe (trachea) into the lungs. They carry oxygen into the lungs and pass waste gases (mostly carbon dioxide) out of the body.
Bronchioles — Small air passageways that serve the same purpose as bronchial tubes. Bronchioles are the smallest parts of the respiratory system.
Bronchodilator Drugs — Medications used to treat diseases of the bronchi that cause shortness of breath, such as asthma. The medicines help constricted tubes to relax.
Bronchogram — Diagnosing lung diseases by placing a material in the lung that X-rays can outline.
Bronchopulmonary Dysplasia Disease (BPD) — A chronic lung disease occurring in premature infants who have required oxygen and mechanical ventilation for a long period of time during treatment to sustain life after birth. Treatment consists of assisted breathing support, supplements of calcium and vitamin E, plus medicines to assist the heart and kidneys.
Bronchoscope — An optical instrument with a lighted tip that is passed into the windpipe, then into the bronchi.
Bruising — Discoloration under the skin caused by injury or bleeding.
Buerger's Disease — A disease characterized by an inflammatory reaction in the arteries, veins, and nerves, which leads to a thickening of the vessel walls. It occurs mostly in young men who smoke tobacco.

C

Calcification — A process in which calcium from the blood is deposited abnormally into tissues due to injury, infection, or aging. Often it is part of healing and not a sign of active disease.
Calcium-Channel Blocker Drugs — Medication used to treat angina, hypertension, and heartbeat irregularities.
Cancerous Growths — Extensions of cancerous tissues that invade nearby healthy tissues.
Cancers — Destructive tumors that can arise in almost all parts of the body. Cancer can destroy nearby healthy tissue and may spread to distant organs.
Capillaries — Microscopic vessels that supply all body cells and tissues with blood.
Carbohydrates, Complex — Starches, sugars, cellulose, and gums. Complex carbohydrates are those contained in whole grains, fresh fruits, and fresh vegetables. These are considered more nutritious than simple carbohydrates.
Carbohydrates, Simple — Refined carbohydrates (sugars) that have lower molecular weights than complex carbohydrates. They produce a quick rise in blood-sugar levels. Most nutrition counselors recommend that daily diets contain minimal amounts of refined sugars. So-called "junk foods" are frequently very high in simple carbohydrates.
Cardiac Catheter — A slender tube that is inserted into an artery or vein and then passed into the heart. It is used to artery or vein and then passed into the heart. It is used to examine the heart and nearby blood vessels by injecting material into the heart that X-rays can detect.
Cardiac Catheterization — Studying heart function with a cardiac catheter.
Cardiopulmonary Resuscitation (CPR) — Emergency treatment for a patient whose heart has stopped (cardiac arrest).
Cardiovascular — Relating to the heart and blood vessels.
Cardiovascular Surgeon — Doctor specially trained to operate on the heart and blood vessels.
Cardiovascular System — System that supplies the body with blood. It consists of the heart and blood vessels (arteries, capillaries, veins).

Carotid Arteries — Large arteries that supply much of the blood to the brain.
Cartilage — Rubbery, dense connective tissue that permits smooth movement of joints. It also helps shape flexible parts of the nose and external ear.
Caruncle — Small, red protrusion of tissue near a body opening. The most common caruncles arise from the urethra or cervix.
CAT (or CT) Scan (Computerized Axial Tomography) — A computerized X-ray procedure that provides exceptionally clear images of parts of the body. It aids in diagnosis of diseases that cannot be diagnosed by ordinary X-ray methods.
Catheter — A hollow tube used to introduce fluids into the body or to drain fluids away.
Caudal Anesthesia — Form of local (low-spinal) anesthesia used to reduce pain during childbirth and surgery on pelvic areas.
Cauterant — Chemical used to destroy abnormal or diseased cells on the skin.
Cauterization — The destruction of tissue with an electric current, a hot iron, or a caustic chemical substance.
Cautery — Destroying small areas of diseased tissue by burning with an electric needle or laser beam, freezing with low-temperature instruments or using a chemical that destroys tissuc.
Cecum — The part of the intestinal tract at the beginning of the large colon (intestine).
Central Nervous System — System that controls the body's voluntary acts. It consists of the brain and spinal cord.
Cervical Spine — Bones in the neck at the top of the spinal column.
Cervix — Lower third of the uterus, which protrudes into the vagina.
Cesarean Section — Delivery of a baby through incisions in the mother's abdomen and uterus. It is performed when normal vaginal delivery would be dangerous for the mother or baby.
Chancre — Hard, slightly ulcerated, painless lesion that forms where syphilis enters the body, usually on the genital lips.
Chemocautery — Destruction of abnormal tissue by means of acids, caustics, or poisons.
Chemotherapy — Treatment of cancer by injecting medications that kill cancer cells without harming healthy tissue. It is used to treat cancers that cannot be completely cured or treated with surgery or radiation.
Chiggers — Small red biting insects. Also called "red bugs."
Child — Person in the first 10 years of life.
Chiropractor — Practitioner of chiropractic treatment of disease, which involves massage and manipulations that chiropractors claim restore normal body functions.
Chokes — Severe breathing difficulty experienced by scuba divers and others who go from high to normal air pressure too rapidly. Bubbles of nitrogen develop in the blood stream and obstruct the blood supply to vital organs, sometimes resulting in severe injury or death.
Cholangiogram, Cholangiography — X-ray procedures to diagnose diseases of the bile system (liver, gallbladder, bile ducts). Special medications are used to make the bile system visible on X-rays.
Cholera — Acute, severe, infectious disease causing extreme diarrhea and dehydration.
Choroiditis — Inflammation of the part of the eye that supports the retina and supplies blood to it.
Chromosome — Structures inside the nucleus of living cells that contain hereditary information. Defects in chromosomes cause many birth defects and inherited diseases.
Chronic — Long-term, continuing. Chronic illnesses are usually not curable, but they can often be prevented from worsening. Symptoms usually can be controlled.
Cinematography — Form of motion-picture photography used to record a fast-moving series of X-ray images.
Circulatory System — The system that provides blood to the body, consisting of the heart, arteries, veins, and lymphatic system.

Clinician — Health-care professional who has direct contact with patients. The word literally means "someone who is at the patient's bedside."
Clips — See *Skin Clips.*
Clot Retraction Test — Measurement of the time necessary for a tube of blood to form a clot. Abnormal results often indicate a defect in blood platelets, cells important in blood coagulation.
Clotting — Activity of the blood and blood vessels that cause blood to form a jellylike clot, usually near an injury. Clotting helps stop bleeding. The body's clotting mechanism is slowed or reduced ("thinning the blood") with anticoagulants to treat certain diseases.
Clubfoot — Malformation at birth of foot and ankle bones. The heel turns in under the ankle, the inner edge of the foot turns upward, and the front of the foot turns in toward the other. Treatment consisting of straightening and holding the position in casts must start within a few days of birth. New casts are applied every week until age 3 months, then at longer intervals. If casting is not successful, surgery can correct the problem.
Coagulation — Same as *Clotting.*
Cocaine — Medication applied directly to mucous membranes to control pain in the nose and throat. Used illegally as a mind-altering drug, it is addicting and dangerous.
Colic, Colicky — A pain that recurs in a regular pattern every few second or minutes.
Collagen — A gelatinous protein from which body tissues are formed.
Colon — The last major portion of the gastrointestinal tract, where waste material is formed into feces and held for elimination. It is also known as the large intestine.
Colonoscopy — Method of diagnosing diseases of the colon by visual examination of the inside of the colon through a *flexible colonoscope,* a fiber-optic instrument with a lighted tip.
Color-Blindness — Inability to recognize red and green, which appear to be gray. It is usually hereditary.
Colposcopy — Visual examination of the cervix by means of a colposcope, a slender optical instrument with a lighted tip.
Coma (Latin: "Deep Sleep") — A state of unconsciousness from which a person cannot be aroused. Coma can be caused by any substance, disease, or injury that disrupts the brain system controlling alertness and awareness. Some specific causes are head injuries, meningitis, alcohol, sedatives, drugs of abuse, encephalitis, diabetic coma or hypoglycemia, seizures, congenital heart disease, anemias, hydrocephalus, stroke, brain tumors, hypothyroidism. Most of the time drowsiness, stupor, and deep stupor will precede coma. The pulse is slower than normal and blood pressure is frequently high. Treatment includes stabilization of circulation and breathing, lowering the pressure of fluid inside the skull, and monitoring all body functions. These may require medicines, surgery, or both.
Combined Immunodeficiency Disease — Serious inherited disease in which the immune system of infants is unable to defend against disease.
Complication — Undesirable event during disease or treatment that causes further symptoms and delay in recovery.
Compress — Cloth, sometimes soaked in warm water or coated with medication. It is applied to the skin to relieve discomfort.
Compression — Applying pressure to the surface of the body, usually to stop bleeding.
Compulsion, Compulsive — Intense, irrational urge to perform some action.
Condom — A thin sheath, usually of rubber, applied to the penis before sexual intercourse. It is used to prevent disease of the genitals and as a contraceptive.
Congenital — Abnormality of the body, present at birth, usually meaning a defect. Congenital defects may be inherited or caused by conditions occurring while the fetus grows in the uterus.

Congenital Hypoplastic Anemia — See *Hypoplastic Anemia.*
Conization of the Cervix — Removal of a cone of tissue from the cervix. Laboratory examination of the removed tissue identifies possible cancer.
Conjunctiva — The mucous membrane lining the outermost surface of the eye ("white of the eye").
Connective Tissue — Body's supporting framework of tissue consisting of strands of collagen, elastic fibers, and simple cells.
Contact Lenses — Small plastic lenses worn on the eyes to correct nearsightedness, farsightedness, or astigmatism.
Contagious — Disease or condition that spreads from one person to another.
Convalescence — Recovery from an illness or surgery.
COPD (Chronic Obstructive Pulmonary Disease) — Several usually incurable lung diseases associated with gradually increasing breathing difficulty.
Copious — Large in amount.
Cornea — Clear thickened surface of the eye through which light passes. It has no blood supply and can be transplanted without danger of rejection.
Coronary — Referring to the blood vessels supplying the heart. Sometimes, it refers to a heart attack resulting from coronary-artery obstruction.
Coronary Care Unit (CCU) — Area of a hospital equipped to care for patients who have suffered a heart attack or other life-threatening heart conditions.
Cortisone Drugs — Medications similar to natural hormones produced by the central core of the adrenal glands.
Cosmetic Surgery — Surgery to improve appearance.
Coxsackie Viruses — Group of viruses causing infections such as poliomyelitis, aseptic meningitis, herpangina, and myocarditis.
CPR — See *Cardiopulmonary Resuscitation.*
Craniotomy — An operation to open the cranium, the eight bones that form the vault to cradle the brain.
Cranium — Bones that make up the skull.
Cryosurgery — Destruction of abnormal tissue by applying freezing temperatures, usually with liquid nitrogen.
Cryotherapy — The use of cold (below -200F) temperatures in treatment.
CT Scan — See *CAT Scan.*
Culdocentesis — Piercing of the space deep in the vagina under the cervix, to obtain fluid. Laboratory examination of the removed fluid aids in diagnosis of ectopic pregnancy and other disorders.
Culdoscopy — Visual examination of the female pelvic organs by means of a slender instrument brought into the pelvic cavity by penetrating through the space deep in the vagina under the cervix.
Culture — Identification of bacteria, fungi and viruses. Material (pus, blood, or urine) from an area infected is collected, placed on nutrient material, and kept warm (usually in an incubator) until the infecting agent has grown. The resulting growth is examined with a microscope.
Curettage — Scraping process frequently used to obtain tissue from the lining of the uterus for laboratory examination. Laboratory examination of the removed tissue aids in diagnosis.
Curette — Instrument with a sharp end used to scrape tissue from the inner lining of the uterus and to scrape away skin lesions.
Cyst — Sac or cavity filled with fluid or diseased matter.
Cyst Aspiration — Removal of cyst contents for examination, or drainage for relief of symptoms.
Cystoscopy — Visual examination of the inside of the urinary bladder by means of a cystoscope, a slender optical instrument with a lighted tip.
Cytotoxic Drugs — Medications used to destroy cancerous cells with minimal harm to healthy cells.

GLOSSARY

D

D.C. Conversion — A procedure using paddles through which direct current passes. The current is carefully measured. The organ targeted is usually a diseased or injured heart with an abnormal rhythm or a heart that has stopped beating.

Debilitating — Causing a general weakening or deterioration in health.

Defibrillation, Cardiac — Applying an electric current to the chest over the heart to interrupt fibrillation, a disturbance of heartbeat.

Dehydration — Loss of essential fluids from the tissues and blood of the body.

Dependence — Condition in which a person requires substances such as narcotics or alcohol to remain comfortable. If the substances are not used, withdrawal symptoms develop.

Dermatome — Area of the skin to which feeling (sensation) is provided by a nerve to the spinal cord.

Descending Colon — The part of the colon in the left side of the abdomen that stores feces until they are passed from the body.

Diabetic Retinopathy — Degeneration of the retina that develops in patients with diabetes mellitus. It may cause vision impairment or blindness.

Diagnosis — Identifying disease. A complete diagnosis names the part of the body affected, the disease process (such as inflammation, cancer, or allergy) and the cause of disease.

Dialysis — Removal of natural wastes from the bloodstream. It is used to treat patients with kidney failure.

Diaphragm — Thin, broad sheet of muscle separating the chest cavity from the abdominal cavity.

Diathermy — Treatment in which mild heat is generated within the body by high-frequency radio waves.

Digestive System — Organs in which food is processed for absorption into the bloodstream. The major digestive organs are the mouth, esophagus, stomach, duodenum, small bowel (small intestine), colon (large intestine), and rectum. The liver, gallbladder, and pancreas are also considered parts of the digestive system.

Digitalis — A drug used to treat congestive heart failure and some other heart diseases.

Dilate, Dilation — To widen, expand, or open up.

Dilator — Instrument used to widen organs that have narrowed because of disease.

Discolored Teeth — A yellowish-brown discoloration of the teeth frequently occurring in infants whose mothers took tetracycline while pregnant. Children may also be affected if they take tetracycline before they have their permanent teeth.

Discomfort — Unpleasant physical or mental sensation.

Disease — Adverse change in health; sickness or ailment. A disease can be defined by the body part involved (for example, the heart or liver), by the abnormality present (cancer, infection, allergy, degeneration, etc.) or by its cause (bacteria, poisons, injury, etc.).

Disk — Same as *Intervertebral Disk.*

Disorder — Same as *Disease.*

Diuretics — Medications that force the kidneys to excrete more urine, sodium, and potassium than normal, which helps eliminate excessive body fluid.

Diverticulum — Small pouch or sac that develops in the wall of tubular organs such as the esophagus or colon.

Dizziness — Sensation of faintness, lightneadedness, or spinning (vertigo).

Donor — Person who gives to someone else. In transplantation surgery, the donor gives up an organ (such as a kidney) to be transplanted into the recipient.

Doppler Sonography — See *Sonogram*: this is one of several methods of sonography.

Dormant — Sleeping or inactive state of living things. Also, an inactive state of a disease.

Drainage — Passage of fluids out of the body through an opening or incision.

Ductus Arteriosus — Small blood vessel connecting the aorta and the pulmonary artery, which is the main artery to the lung.

The vessel is open during the time the fetus is in the uterus, but normally closes at birth.
Duodenum — First 12 inches of the small intestine.
Dupuytren's Contracture — Chronic condition in which scar tissue forms in the palms. In severe cases, it can impair use of the fingers.
Dwarfism — Condition of being undersized for one's age. It may be due to endocrine disorders, malnutrition, or an inherited defect.
Dysproteinemia — An abnormality of the protein content of the blood.

E

Ear Canal — Passageway extending from the outer ear inward to the eardrum.
Ear, Nose, and Throat (ENT) Specialist — A physician specially trained to treat diseases of the ears, nose, and throat.
Echocardiogram, Echocardiography — Studying the heart by examining sound waves created by an instrument placed on the chest. The waves reflected from the heart form an image (echocardiogram) on a minitor, aiding in diagnosis of heart diseases.
Edema — Accumulation of fluid under the skin, in the lungs, or elsewhere.
EEG (Electroencephalography) — Studying the brain by measuring electric activity ("brain waves") with an electroencephalograph. The record produced is the electroencephalogram.
EKG (Electrocardiography) — Method of diagnosing heart diseases by measuring electrical activity of the heart with an electrocardiograph. The record produced is called an electrocardiogram.
Electrocardiography — See *EKG*.
Electrocautery — Destruction of tissue by heat applied with a controlled electric current.
Electroencephalography — See *EEG*.
Electrolyte — A chemical that is dissolved in the blood and all other body fluids. Electrolytes play an essential tole in all body functions. The major electrolytes are: sodium, potassium, chloride, calcium, phosphorus, magnesium, and carbon dioxide. Electrolytes come from food. They are regulated mostly by the kidneys and lungs.
Electrolyte Measurement — Laboratory test on blood or urine to identify and measure the electrolytes present.
Electrolyte Supplements — Electrolytes taken to correct or to prevent body-fluid or electrolyte imbalance.
Electromyography — Studying nerve and muscle disorders by recording electrical activity of muscles with an electromyograph. The record produced is the electromyogram.
Electrosurgery — Minor surgery performed with an electric current sent through an electric cauterizing instrument. It not only destroys tissue, but also controls bleeding.
Endemic — Disease that is constantly present in a community or group of people. Endemic disease may affect only a few people at any one time.
Endocrine System — System of organs that secrete hormones into the blood to regulate basic functions of cells and tissues. The endocrine organs are the anterior and posterior pituitary glands, thyroid and parathyroid glands, pancreas, adrenal glands, ovaries (in women), and testicles (in men).
Endocrinologist — Doctor specially trained in diagnosis and treatment of endocrine disorders.
Endoscopy — Method of diagnosing diseases in hollow organs. An endoscope (an optical instrument with a lighted tip) is inserted into the organ, which allows visual examination of the cavity. Used in the abdomen, pelvis, lumen of the bronchial tubes, or intestines.
Endotracheal Tube — Tube temporarily placed in the grachea (windpipe) of patients who are unable to breathe normally because of disease or surgery.
Enteric — Relating to the small intestine. Enteric-coated medicine is coated with a hard shell that dissolves when it reaches the small intestine.

GLOSSARY

Enterostomy — Surgically created artificial opening for elimination of feces. An enterostomy nurse or enterostomy specialist is a professional who teaches patients how to care for the artificial opening.
Enzymes — Proteins manufactured by the body that regulate the rate of essential life processes (metabolism).
Epinephrine — Same as *Adrenalin.*
Episcleritis — Inflammation of tissues on the sclera (the "white of the eye").
Epithelial Horn — Thick, rough lesion protruding from the skin. It may become cancerous if not removed.
Equine Virus — Virus that causes a serious form of encephalitis in horses and man.
Ergot — Medication derived from a fungus that grows on rye plants. It is used to treat migraine headache and to increase the strength of uterine contractions during and immediately after childbirth.
Esophageal Varices — Enlarged veins on the lining of the esophagus. They are subject to severe bleeding and often appear in patients with severe liver disease.
Esophagoscopy — Method of diagnosing diseases of the esophagus by means of an esophagoscope, an optical instrument with lenses and a lighted tip.
Esophagus — Muscular tube connecting the throat and stomach.
Estrogen — Female sex hormone, primarily secreted by the ovaries. It can also be produced synthetically for use in estrogen replacement therapy.
Estrogen Receptor Value — Used in the study of breast-cancer cells to determine the best treatment.
Etiology — Cause or causes of a disease.
Eustachian Tubes — Slender passages between the throat and the middle ear that maintain normal air pressure in the middle ear.
Excise — To remove by cutting out.
Exploratory Laparotomy — Diagnosing abdominal disease by surgically opening the abdomen and examining its contents.
Extremities — Arms and legs.
Eye Bank — Facility where living corneas are stored and made available for transplantation.
Eyes, Crossed — Condition in which muscles controlling the eyes are unbalanced. The eyes point in different directions. Also called squint or strabismus.

F

Fallopian Tubes — Organs of the female reproductive tract through which an egg (ovum) passes from the ovary to the uterus. Tying these tubes (tubal ligation) accomplishes sterility.
Familial Polyposis — Inherited condition in which the lining of the intestines contains many polyps, some of which may become cancerous.
Family History — Information about illnesses that tend to occur within a family. This information is used to determine the likelihood of diseases occurring in other members of the family.
Farsightedness — Same as *Hypermetropia.*
Fascia — Sheet or band of tough, fibrous tissue that covers muscles and other body organs.
Fecal — Relating to feces, waste products eliminated through the lower intestinal tract.
Fecal-Oral — Pathway by which some fecal germs gain entry into the bloodstream. Sewage in drinking water, hand-to-mouth transmission after bowel movements or sexual contact can cause infection.
Feces — Body waste formed of undigested food that has passed through the gastrointestinal system to the colon. Feces are produced and stored in the colon until eliminated.
Fetal Monitoring — Measuring the heart rate of the fetus during labor.
Fetal-Scalp Electrodes — Fine wires attached to the scalp of a fetus to measure heart rate and rhythm during labor.
Fetal-Scalp Monitoring — Measuring the well-being of the fetus during labor by obtaining blood from the scalp or by measuring the heart rate of the fetus or contraction strength of the uterus.

Fever — A body temperature that is an elevation above normal of at least 1 degree. Critical points of fever that require treatment are as follows (all rectal temperatures): 6 months or younger—100F (37.8C) or higher; 6 months to 3 years—102F (38.8C); any age—fever accompanied by unusual drowsiness and loss of alertness, labored breathing, or otherwise appears ill. Fever is a *sign* of disease, not a disease itself. It may be caused by bacterial infections, viral infections, reactions to drugs, heatstroke, dehydration, or fevers of undetermined origin. Low-grade fever can be helpful by stimulating the production of white blood cells and speeding up the body's immune system—both providing useful defense mechanisms for fighting disease. Treatment of fever should be under the direction of your physician.
Fiber — A non-nutritious ingredient of many complex carbohydrates. Fiber increases bulk in the diet. Many nutritionists recommend including ample fiber in the diet. Experimental studies and clinical studies show that people who eat high-fiber diets are less likely to develop colon cancer, diverticulitis, atherosclerosis, and gallbladder disease.
Fiber Optics — System of transmitting light and images through thread-like strands of glass. Fiber-optic instruments make some examinations and surgical procedures simple, safe, and effective.
Fibrin — Protein formed by the action of blood clotting on fibrogen.
Fibrinogen — Protein in the blood needed for blood clotting.
Fibrositis — Inflammatory conditions affecting connective tissue of muscles, joints, ligaments, and tendons.
First Molars — First permanent flat teeth, used for grinding food, which appear at about age 6 to 7.
Fissure — Break in the skin or inner lining of organs.
Fistula — Abnormal passage between two organs or between the body and the outside.
Flank — Area on the side of the body below the ribs and above the hip.
Fleas — Tiny biting insects. Most cause minor skin irritation; some carry and transmit serious diseases such as plague and typhus.
Fluorescein-Dye Test — Method of diagnosis using fluorescein, a dye, to study tissues and germs. When these dyed tissues are exposed to ultraviolet light, they glow. Substances to which the dye does not cling do not glow.
Fluorescent Antibody Studies — Tests used to study some allergic and infectious conditions. When antibodies created by these conditions are present in the blood, they can be made to glow by using a dye and a microscope with ultraviolet light.
Fluoroscopy — Method of X-ray diagnosis in which moving organs (such as the heart or intestinal tract) can be studied in action.
Foley Catheter — Slender, flexible tube used to drain urine from the bladder of patients who are unable to urinate normally.
Forceps — Instrument with two blades and handles. It is used to grasp tissue, body parts, or sterile materials. Also used to deliver babies when progress of labor is slow.
Fracture — Break; usually used to refer to a bone or tooth.
Frei Test — Test used to make a precise diagnosis of lymphogranuloma, a sexually transmitted disease.
Friedreich's Ataxia — Rare, inherited nervous-system disease that causes loss of balance and coordination, awkward walking, speech difficulty, and tremors.
Frozen Section — A study in a pathology laboratory of fresh tissue that was removed during surgery. The purpose is to determine if a suspicious area is or is not cancerous.
Fungus — Mold or yeast that may infect skin, internal surfaces (mouth, vagina), or tissues.
Fungus Infection — Infection caused by fungus.
Fusiform Bacteria — Bacteria shaped like slender rods.

GLOSSARY

G

Galactorrhea — 1) Continued breast-milk flow after weaning. 2) Excess breast-milk flow during nursing.

Galactosemia — Inherited disease of infants in which milk cannot be digested. Milk should be eliminated from the infant's diet to prevent malnutrition, liver and kidney disease, and mental retardation.

Gallbladder — Small organ under the liver that stores bile. For digestion, the gallbladder contracts to empty bile into the intestines.

Gamma Globulin — Protein in the blood manufactured by the immune system to help destroy or neutralize infection-causing germs. Gamma globulin derived and concentrated from blood of other humans is used to help create temporary immunity to some diseases.

Gammaglobulinemia — Extremely low levels in the blood of gamma globulin brought about by a disease of the immune system. The deficiency causes increased susceptibility to many infections by bacteria, viruses, and fungi. Also called hypogammaglobulinemia.

Gangrene — Death of tissue, usually due to partial or total loss of blood supply.

Gastrectomy — Removal of part or all of the stomach.

Gastroenterologist — Doctor who specializes in the diagnosis and treatment of diseases of the gastrointestinal system.

Gastrointestinal Series (Upper GI Series) — X-rays of the upper digestive system (esophagus, stomach, and duodenum).

Gastrointestinal Tract — See *Digestive System.*

Gastroscopy — Visual examination of the inside of the stomach by means of a gastroscope, an optical instrument with a lighted tip.

Gene — Basic unit of protein molecules in chromosomes of cells. Genes transmit inherited characteristics such as eye color, blood type, gender, or body shape. Defective genes cause many kinds of birth defects and inborn diseases.

Gene, Dominant or Recessive — Dominant gene, if present in either the mother's egg or father's sperm, will transmit its characteristics to the newborn child. Recessive genes must be present in both parents before its characteristics will be transmitted.

General Surgeon — A doctor specially trained to perform operations.

Genetic Counseling — Counseling to help couples decide whether to have children or not when there is a risk of genetic disease being transmitted to the child.

Genetics — Science of determining inherited factors that result in the unique make-up of every human being; also, science that traces the appearance patterms to genetic (inherited) disease.

Genitourinary Tract — Body system that forms, stores, and eliminates urine. Also has a role in male and female reproductive functions. Organs include the kidneys, ureters, bladder, urethra, uterus, Fallopian tubes, ovaries, vagina, cervix, penis, scrotum, and testicles.

German Measles, Congenital — A virus infection in a fetus or newborn caused by a virus spreading in the bloodstream of the mother during pregnancy and passing through the placenta to the unborn child. Symptoms include prematurity, heart disease, visual problems, brain damage, hearing loss, pneumonia, thyroid problems, diabetes, hemolytic anemia, and others.

Germs — Organisms that cause infection such as bacteria, viruses, or fungi.

Gestation — Time spent in the mother's uterus by the fetus. Average gestation time for the human infant, from conception to delivery, is approximately 39 weeks.

Gigantism — Condition in which the body or a body part grows excessively, sometimes due to an overactive pituitary gland.

Glomerulonephritis — An inflammatory disorder of the kidney secondary to an allergic reaction to the streptococcus germ. This is one of the possible complications of a strep infection. It can usually be prevented by adequate treatment of the original strep infection with penicillin or other suitable antibiotic.

Glucagon — Hormone secreted by the pancreas that increases blood sugar. A synthetic form is sometimes used as emergency treatment for patients with diabetes who have temporarily low blood sugar.

Glucose — Major form of sugar in the blood, stored primarily in the liver. It provides energy to most tissues, organs, and systems.

Glucose-Tolerance Test — Method of diagnosing diabetes mellitus or functional hypoglycemia. The patient drinks a measured amount of glucose (sugar). The blood and urine are tested at measured intervals for glucose content.

Gluten — Protein found in wheat and other foods that cannot be digested by some persons because of genetic disease. A gluten-free diet allows persons with the disorder to digest food and grow normally.

Gonads — Parts of the reproductive system that produce and release female eggs (ovaries) or male sperm (testes).

Growing Pains — Harmless, normal, temporary aches and pains in a child's growing limbs. Vigorous use of incompletely developed muscles and bones causes the discomfort. Very common during ages 6 to 12 years. The discomfort most likely involves the thighs, calves, and feet, but also may affect the arms or back muscles. The pains occur only when the child is at rest. Most physicians recommend no treatment except gentle massage, heating pads, or warm-water soaks. There is no known way to prevent growing pains.

Growth Disorders — Conditions in children that result in underdevelopment or overdevelopment of the body. Diseases of the endocrine glands, nutritional problems, or genetic abnormalities are frequently the causes.

Gynecologist — Doctor specially trained to treat diseases of the female reproductive system.

H

H-2 Blocker Drugs — Class of antihistamines that reduce the production of stomach acid for treatment of peptic ulcers.

Hallucinogens — Substances that produce hallucinations, apparent sights, sounds, or other experiences that do not actually exist.

Hand Surgeon — Surgeon specially trained to treat hand diseases, injuries, infections, and arthritic conditions.

Hangover — Unpleasant aftereffects of excessive consumption of alcoholic beverages. Symptoms include irritability, headache, and nausea. Sometimes, the same feelings result from using certain medications.

Hashimoto's Thyroiditis — One of several kinds of inflammation of the thyroid gland.

Head Banging and Rocking — A common, usually harmless, habit. The child hits his head against a solid object in a rhythmical way. Head banging first appears between 6 and 12 months of age and disappears before 3 years. This habit is 3 times more common in boys than girls and occurs in 5-10% of all children. This habit is closely associated with *rocking*, also a harmless habit. The cause of either banging or rocking is unknown. Head banging may also be a part of the symptoms of children with other disorders, including autism, mental retardation, blindness, and hearing loss. If rhythmical behavior begins after 18 months, consult your physician.

Hearing Loss — An inability to hear the range of sounds that the human ear normally detects. Hearing loss comes in many degrees and may affect either or both ears—slight to total, temporary or permanent, congenital or acquired. Over half the time, no cause is found. Known causes of conductive loss include middle ear inflammation or infection, wax in the ear canal (easily curable), or a foreign body in the ear (curable). Causes of sensorineural loss (nerve deafness, due to malfunction of the internal ear, brain, or nervous system) include drug and alcohol abuse in the mother, lack of oxygen during birth, maternal German measles, herpes, chickenpox, syphilis, mumps, parasite infections such as toxoplasmosis, or severe jaundice during the newborn period. Treatment depends upon the underlying cause. See your physician for guidance. Treatments include hearing aids, learning sign language, finger spelling, body language, lip-reading, TTY machines. For more information, write: National Association of the Deaf, 814 Thayer Avenue, Silver Springs, MD 20910, (301) 587-1788. Preventing hearing loss: females of childbearing age should be immunized against German measles and other severe viruses *before* becoming pregnant. Don't allow children to put anything in their ears; prevent noise pollution by too loud rock music or headphones; prevent head injuries by having everyone in your family use auto restraints and insisting upon appropriate protective headgear for sports; treat your child's middle ear infections vigorously.

Heart Catheterization — Same as *Cardiac Catheterization.*

Heart Disease, Congenital — A heart defect present at birth, caused by abnormal development before birth. Many children with congenital heart disease have multiple congenital defects. Types of congenital heart disease include the following: *Septal defects*—abnormal openings in the wall that divides the right and left chambers of the heart. Sometimes treated with surgery. *Patent ductus arteriosus*—failure to close soon after birth of a special channel between the arteries that carry blood between the aorta and the pulmonary artery. Treated successfully with surgery. *Tetralogy of Fallot*—a combination of four different anatomical structures of the heart. Treated successfully with surgery. *Transposition of the great arteries*—the pulmonary artery arises from the left ventricle and the aorta arises from the right ventricle. Must be treated surgically promptly after delivery in order to preserve life. *Coarctation of the aorta*—a narrowing of the aorta (the main artery that carries blood from the heart to all parts of the body). Among other problems, this congenital defect causes high blood pressure. Coarctation of the aorta is curable with surgery. *Aortic and pulmonary stenosis*—narrow valves between the lower chambers (ventricles) and the two large arteries leading away from the heart. Surgery will cure.

Heart Murmur — Same as *Murmur.*

Heart Tumors — Rare tumors that grow in the heart wall or in the heart chambers, interfering with normal heart function.

Heart-Lung Machine — Complex mechanical device that provides artificial function of a patient's heart and lungs for a short time during open-heart surgery and heart or lung transplantation.

Hematocrit — Blood test used to detect anemia and other blood disorders. It is expressed as the percentage of blood made up of red blood cells (the remainder of the blood is made up of serum or plasma). The normal hematocrit range is approximately 35% to 45%, but it varies with age and sex.

Hematologist — Doctor specially trained to diagnose and treat diseases of the blood and blood-forming organs.

Hemochromatosis — Disease in which excessive iron accumulates in the liver, pancreas, and skin, resulting in liver disease, diabetes mellitus, and a bronzed skin color.

Hemoglobin, Hemoglobin Range — 1) Component that carries oxygen to body tissues. 2) Blood test used to detect anemia and other blood disorders, expressed in grams per 100 cubic centimeters. The normal hemoglobin range is approximately 12 to 18 grams per 100 cubic centimeters and varies according to age and sex.

Hirschsprung's Disease — Congenital defect of infants in which the colon cannot eliminate feces, resulting in severe constipation.

Histamine — Chemical in body tissues that dilates the smallest blood vessels, constricts the muscle around the bronchial tubes, stimulates stomach secretions, and produces an allergic response.

Holter Monitor — Instrument that detects heartbeat-rhythm abnormalities 24 hours or longer. The device is portable for patients to carry wherever they go.
Hormones — Powerful substances manufactured by the endocrine glands and carried by the blood to body tissues and organs. Hormones determine growth and structure of many organs (such as during growth and maturation) and also control many vital body functions.
Host — Person or animal with an infection that has been received from another person, animal or plant, or the environment.
Hyaline-Membrane Disease — Serious condition of premature infants in which the lungs can't expand normally. Cause is unknown.
Hydatidiform Mole — Disease occurring during early pregnancy resulting in death of the fetus and an overgrowth of tissue within the uterus.
Hydraminos and Polyhydraminos — Condition in which amniotic fluid (fluid in the uterus that surrounds the fetus until birth) becomes excessive.
Hygiene — Personal self-care and cleanliness that reduces the risk of infections and diseases.
Hyoid Bone — V-shaped bone located just above the larynx.
Hyperalimentation — Method of supplying total nutritional needs of patients unable to eat normally. The method (usually intravenous or by tube through the nose into the stomach) provides nutrients containing essential proteins, fats, carbohydrates, and vitamins.
Hyperbaric Chamber — Large, sealed room in which air pressure can be raised above normal levels. It is used primarily to treat patients with either decompression sickness or severe burns (sometimes).
Hypercalcemia — Presence of excessive calcium in the blood; occasionally a sign of malignancy.
Hyperlipoproteinemia — Condition in which excessive lipoproteins (cholesterol and other fatty materials) accumulate in the blood.
Hypermetropia — Seeing distant objects clearly while nearby objects appear blurred; also called farsightedness.
Hypersensitivity — Extreme sensitivity to any agent (drugs, pollens, chemicals, etc.) that causes allergic reactions. Some reactions can be life-threatening, but most are less serious.
Hypnotics — Medications that produce sleep.
Hypogammaglobulinemia — An abnormally low level of all classes of gamma globulin in the blood.
Hypoplastic Anemia (Aplastic Anemia) — Group of anemias that decrease blood-producing bone marrow. This can be life-threatening.
Hypothalamus — Part of the brain that regulates body functions such as temperature, blood pressure, appetite and thirst.
Hysteria — 1) Condition in which a person becomes anxious and excitable and experiences impaired sensory and motor abilities. Sometimes, hysterical persons simulate conditions of diseases such as deafness or blindness. 2) Outbreak of uncontrolled emotions, such as fits of laughing or crying.
Hysterosalpingography — Studying the uterus and Fallopian tubes by injecting material into the uterus that X-rays can detect. It is used primarily to determine if the passageway for the ovum (egg) is open all the way to the uterus. The X-ray image is the hysterosalpingogram.
Hysteroscope — An instrument with lens system and lighted tip used in direct visual examination of the cervix and the cavity of the uterus.
Hysterostomy — Incision of the uterus to prepare for Cesarean-section delivery of a baby.

I

I-131 Uptake — Measuring thyroid activity with radioactive iodine and radiation emission counters.

GLOSSARY

Idiopathic — Condition caused by unknown factors.
Ileostomy — A surgical operation that creates an opening between the ilium (the last part of the small intestine) and the outside of the abdomen. Fecal contents will pass directly to the outside of the body after an iliostomy instead of progressing through the large intestine and rectum.
Ileum — Part of the small intestine just above the large intestine (colon).
Ileus — Condition of the small intestine in which either an obstruction or paralysis prevents material from passing through the intestine.
Iliac Arteries — Large arteries in the inner pelvis that supply blood to the legs.
Immune, Immunity — Resistance or protection against infection by the body's natural defenses. A person may be immune to one kind of infection but not immune to another. Some infections, such as measles, chickenpox, or mumps, cause the body to become immune permanently to that infection.
Immune System — Body's system of defense against infection.
Immunization — Producing immunity by giving a vaccine (orally or by injection) of germs that have been altered so they cannot produce significant disease. The vaccine causes the body's immune system to produce antibodies that create immunity.
Immunosuppressants — Drugs used in immunosuppression treatment to weaken the immune system and to inhibit immune response.
Immunosuppression — Prevention of the body from forming a normal immune response. It is used to treat diseases (especially when organs must be transplanted) where certain antibodies must be inactivated.
Impotence — Male's inability to achieve or to sustain an erection or to ejaculate sperm during sexual intercourse.
Incise, Incision — To cut open or cut into.
Incomplete Spontaneous Miscarriage — Naturally occurring miscarriage in which the fetus is expelled, but part of the placenta remains in the uterus. Excessive bleeding and infection can result unless the uterus is emptied, usually by dilatation and curettage of the uterus (D & C) or suction curettage.
Incubation Period — The time between exposure to an infecting germ and the appearance of symptoms indicating an infection. Also describes the period of bacterial growth in laboratory cultures.
Infant — Child between the ages of 2 weeks and 1 year.
Infection, Infectious — Disease caused by germs (bacteria, viruses, fungi) that enter the body and cause inflammation or other processes that have an adverse effect on health.
Inflammation, Inflammatory Process — Process by which the body attempts to overcome illness-producing causes such as germs, injuries such as burns, or diseases such as arthritis. The process causes increased body heat (fever or local warmth), swelling, pain, and tenderness. If the inflammation is near the skin, redness results.
Inhalation — Breathing air into the lungs.
Inherited — Body characteristic that is transmitted from one generation to the next by chromosomes in the mother's egg and father's sperm. Some inherited characteristics such as brown eyes are normal; others such as Down syndrome are disorders.
Inoculation — Injection of infected material such as pus into a nutrient medium where the germs will grow, or incubate. They are then stained and analyzed through a microscope. Also describes any kind of immunization.
Insufflation Test — See *Rubin's Insufflation Test.*
Intensive Care Unit (ICU) — Area of a hospital where patients who are seriously ill or recovering from serious surgery are given more care than is available in other hospital

units. As soon as the condition improves, the patient is transferred from the ICU to a regular hospital unit.

Intermittent — Happening only occasionally or under certain conditions.

Internist — Doctor specially trained in non-surgical diagnosis and treatment of diseases in adults.

Intervertebral Disk — Cartilage that connects adjacent vertebrae in the spinal column.

Intestinal Tract — All parts of the gastrointestinal tract except the mouth, esophagus, and stomach. The intestinal tract organs are: duodenum, small bowel, ileum, cecum, appendix, ascending colon, transverse colon, descending colon, sigmoid colon, rectum, and anus.

Intestine, Large — Last major portion of the gastrointestinal tract located just under the small intestine. It is also called the colon or large bowel. It processes waste material into feces, which are stored until eliminated from the body.

Intestine, Small — Longest section of the gastrointestinal tract, located just under the stomach and duodenum. It absorbs digested food into the bloodstream and passes waste material into the large intestine.

Intrauterine Death — Death of a fetus while inside the mother's uterus.

Intrauterine Device (IUD) — Birth-control method in which a small device placed permanently in the uterus prevents growth of fertilized eggs.

Intravenous — Within the vein. Fluids, medications, and nutrients that cannot be taken orally are given intravenously by a needle placed in a large vein near the surface of the skin.

Intravenous Pyelogram (IVP) — See *Pyelogram, Intravenous.*

IQ (Intelligence Quotient) — Supposedly a measure of a person's intelligence, rather than what one has learned. Recent research on intelligence raises questions about the accuracy and meaning of the I.Q. test.

Iridectomy — Surgery performed to treat some kinds of glaucoma.

Irrigation — Flooding with water or other liquid. It is used frequently to clean wounds or areas of the body that will undergo surgery.

Isolation, Reverse Isolation — Procedures to prevent spread of infection in a hospital. Isolation protects hospital staff and visitors from contracting a contagious disease from a patient. Reverse isolation protects a patient susceptible to infection because of immunosuppression from contracting infection from hospital staff or visitors.

IUD — See *Intrauterine Device.*

J

Jaundice — Yellow skin and whites of the eyes, dark urine and light stools, symptoms of diseases of the liver and blood.

Joint — Structure that enables two or more bones to move easily in relation to each other. A joint consists of ligaments and cartilage that hold bones together.

Joint Capsule — Tough, fibrous tissue that surrounds a joint.

Joint Replacement — Replacement of diseased joints with mechanical joints. The wrist, hip and knee joints are among the most common joints replaced.

K

Ketoacidosis — Serious complication of diabetes mellitus in which the body produces acids that cause fluid and electrolyte disorders, dehydration, and sometimes coma.

Klinefelter's Syndrome — Inherited disease of young males in which secondary sex characteristics are underdeveloped. The condition does not become evident until puberty. Mental deficiency and some female characteristics are present.

L

Laceration — Wound with jagged edges.

Lactiferous Ducts — Network of tubes in the female breast that collects milk and delivers it to the nipple.

GLOSSARY

Laparoscopy — Exploratory examination of the organs inside the abdominal cavity with a laparoscope, an optical instrument with a lighted tip. The laparoscope is inserted into the abdomen through a small incision. Visual examination can then be made of many abdominal organs.
Laparotomy — Exploratory surgery in the abdomen performed to diagnose and sometimes treat abdominal disease.
Laryngeal Nerve — Nerve located in the neck that controls the vocal cords and enables a person to speak.
Larynx — Structure of muscle and cartilage in the upper neck. It contains the vocal cords. Air passes through the larynx into the windpipe and then into the lungs. The "Adam's apple" is part of the larynx.
Laser Therapy — Using a laser beam to treat many diseases. Sharply focused laser light creates intense heat and is valuable in cutting tissue, destroying unwanted tissue, and joining tissue together. It is most often used to treat retinal detachment, endometriosis, or atherosclerosis.
Latent — Present but inactive; something that exists in an undeveloped form.
Laxatives — Medications used to treat constipation.
Lesion — General term for injury or damage to an organ or tissue.
Lethargy — Fatigue or lack of usual physical or mental energy.
Libido — Sexual desire.
Life Cycle — Growth and development from birth to death.
Ligaments — Strong, flexible cords of tissue near joints that hold bones together and permit bone motion.
Lipoproteins (High Density and Low Density) — Components of the fluid in blood that are measured to help predict the likelihood of atherosclerosis (hardening of the arteries).
Liquid Nitrogen — Nitrogen that has been cooled until it becomes a liquid. It is used most often in cryosurgery.
Local Anesthesia — See *Anesthesia, Local.*
Low-Residue Diet — Diet consisting of foods that are digested almost entirely, leaving minimal material to form feces.
Low-Spinal Anesthesia — Also called "saddle-block" anesthesia. An injection into the lower spinal canal provides anesthesia to the lower body.
Lower GI Series — Same as *Barium-Enema X-rays.*
Lumbar Puncture (Spinal Tap) — A diagnostic procedure in which a needle is inserted between 2 bones (vertebrae) of the lower spine to collect spinal fluid for laboratory examination.
Lumbar Spine — Lower part of the spine, from the lowest ribs to the bottom of the spine.
Lymph (or Lymphatic) System — Lymph channels and lymph glands considered as a single body system.
Lymph Channels — Tubes of tissue that carry lymph fluid away from tissues and back to the bloodstream. Lymph fluid is composed of proteins and water, varying in composition in different parts of the body.
Lymph Glands — Small collections of tissue (nodes) located along lymph channels in areas such as the elbow, armpit, or groin. When infection is present, nearby lymph glands enlarge, become tender, and destroy germs that enter lymph channels. Lymph glands also manufacture antibodies to help fight infection.
Lymphangiogram, Lymphangiography — Diagnostic method of studying the lymphatic system by infecting a material into the lymph channels that X-rays can detect. The image on X-ray film is the lymphangiogram.
Lymphatic Leukemia — Class of leukemias, involving primarily lymphatic cells, affecting children and adults.
Lymphocytes — One of several types of white blood cells that help fight infection.
Lymphosarcoma — Class of cancers of the lymphatic system.

M

Macular Degeneration of the Eye — Condition of the macula (area on the retina that provides detailed vision) in which impaired blood supply causes gradual vision loss.
Macule — General term for any discolored spot or patch on the skin, such as a freckle.
Magnetic Resonance Imaging (MRI) — This test relies on the magnetic properties of the body's atoms. It uses radiofrequency energy and a powerful magnetic field to produce computerized images in multiple planes with startling detail and resolution.
Malignant — Capable of causing great harm, including death. It usually refers to cancerous growth.
Mammogram, Mammography — Diagnostic method of studying the female breast by an X-ray technique that detects cancerous growths while they are still treatable. The image on X-ray film is the mammogram.
Manic-Depressive Illness — Mental illness in which behavior alternates between unrealistic enthusiasm and deep depression.
MAO Inhibitors — See *Monamine Oxidase Inhibitors.*
Marijuana — Mood-altering substance that is usually taken into the body by smoking. It is derived from Indian hemp or Cannabis leaves, stems, and seed pods.
Marrow — Core of many bones, where most of the body's blood cells are produced.
Mastoiditis — Infection of the mastoid (bony area just behind the ear).
Masturbation — Stimulation of the genitals for pleasure. Normal behavior in infants, children, adolescents, and adults. Generally satisfying, particularly during times of separation, such as at bedtime. Stimulation of genitals will help release sexual tensions and gratify fantasies and may help control sex drives.
Mediators — Substances that: 1) help nerve impulses travel from one cell to the next; 2) participate in the allergic process.
Medic-Alert — Non-profit agency that maintains a medical-record system. Subscribers receive a bracelet or pendant that states their medical condition and provides a toll-free number for more information. The service can save the life of a person with a major medical condition who may not be able to provide a medical history. For information write: Medic-Alert Foundation, P.O. Box 1009, Tulock, CA 95381.
Medical History — Essential facts about past and present medical conditions. Knowing your medical history enables your doctor to plan the best possible health care. Have your family carry a card stating essential health details in their purses or wallets, and consider joining the Medic-Alert program (see above).
Meibomian Glands — Small glands on the inner eyelid. They secrete a fluid that helps the eyelids move easily over the surface of the eye.
Membrane — Thin tissue lining a body cavity, covering an internal organ or dividing a space.
Meninges — Three-layered membrane covering the brain.
Mental Retardation — A disability in the area of thought, perception, and memory. These problems lead to slow development in language skills, learning, muscle control, poor social adaptation. Brain abnormalities from hundreds of diseases, genetic disorders, injuries, or physical deprivation. It may occur before birth or anytime after birth. Mental retardation cannot be cured, but disability can sometimes be reduced. Two good sources for support and detailed information: Association for Retarded Citizens/U.S., 2501 Avenue J, Arlington, TX 76011, (817)640-0204; Joseph P. Kennedy, Jr. Foundation, 1350 New York Avenue NW, Washington, DC 20005, (202)393-1250.
Mental System (Mind) — Functions of the brain that provide the abilities to perceive surroundings, to have emotions, imagination, memory and will, and to process information.
Metastases — Cancerous cells or infectious germs that spread from their original location to other parts of the body.

Metatarsal Bones — Bones in the middle of the foot.
Midwife — Nurse with special training and experience in childbirth.
Mole — Skin lesion, often dark-brown or black.
Monamine Oxidase (MAO) Inhibitors — Medications used to treat some forms of depression.
Motor Nerve — Nerve that transmits the stimulus that causes muscles to contract.
Mucous Membrane — Thin tissue lining internal cavities (nose, mouth, vagina) and tubular systems (respiratory and gastrointestinal) that produce mucus.
Mucus — Slippery liquid produced by the lining of internal cavities and tubular systems to protect tissue.
Murmur — Sound of blood rushing through the heart and blood vessels, detected by a stethoscope. Some murmurs are innocent, meaning they are not caused by disease. Other murmurs arise from heart disease or partial obstruction in the arteries.
Muscle — Tissue that contracts, often with considerable force, when stimulated by the motor-nerve impulses.
Muscle Biopsy — The surgical removal of a small amount of muscle tissue for laboratory microscopic examination.
Muscle Relaxants — Medications that relieve muscle spasms. They also can have significant side effects.
Muscle Tumors — Benign or cancerous tumors arising from muscle tissue.
Musculo-Skeletal System — The system of bones, muscles, ligaments, and tendons that enable the body to move.
Myelogram — Special X-ray of the spinal canal and spinal cord, requiring a spinal tap and injection of dye that is visible on X-ray film. Myelograms frequently are used to identify the location of ruptured disks.
Myoma — Tumor of the muscle.
Myopia — Disease of the eye in which close objects are clearly visible while distant objects are blurred. Also called nearsightedness.

N

Nail Biting — A frequent habit among children and adults. The majority of experts believe that nail biting results as a mechanism for discharging everyday tension, similar to thumb-sucking. Nail biting frequently accompanies fear, sadness, nervousness, or distress. *Treatment:* Try to provide an incentive to avoid nail biting, such as symbolic awards (stars on a calendar, etc.). Instill pride in good grooming. *Don't* scold or lavish attention for negative behavior.
Narcotics — Medications used to control severe pain. Narcotics should be used only when necessary because of their serious side effects: addiction; reduced breathing; nausea and vomiting; low blood pressure; reduced cough reflex; and constipation.
Naso-Gastric Tube — Slender tube passed through the nose into the stomach. It is used to drain away stomach secretions or to feed patients unable to eat normally.
Naturopathy — Health-care system relying on diet, sunshine, exercises, herbs, and other non-medicinal treatment.
Nausea — Unpleasant sensation of being about to vomit.
Nearsightedness — Same as *Myopia.*
Nebulizer — Device for administering medications used to treat asthma and similar conditions. It converts medication into a fine mist that is inhaled deeply into the lungs.
Needle Biopsy — A simplified form of removing tissue for microscopic examination using a needle inserted into the tissue to be studied. Tissue is removed by suction.
Nerve-Block Local Anesthesia — See *Anesthesia, Nerve Block or Local.*
Nerve-Conduction Test — Diagnostic test that measures the rate at which an electrical impulse moves along a nerve. It is used to diagnose disorders of the peripheral nerves and muscle.
Nervous Breakdown — Non-technical term for mental illness serious enough to interfere with daily activities.
Neuritis — Inflammation of a nerve.

Neuroblastoma — A solid cancerous tumor of a nerve tissue that may spread to chest, abdomen, or pelvis. Treatment combines surgery, radiation, and chemotherapy. Before age 1, 90% can be cured if treated vigorously.
Neurological — Relating to the body's nervous system.
Neurologist — Doctor specially trained to diagnose and treat diseases of the nervous system.
Neuroma — Tumor arising from nerve tissue.
Neuro-Muscular System — Nerves and muscles acting together as a system to control body movements.
Neurosis — Mental illness in which anxiety is controlled by avoidance, blaming others, developing bodily complaints, or other mechanisms.
Neurosurgeon — Doctor specially trained to diagnose and treat surgically diseases of the brain, spinal cord, and nerves.
Nodes — See *Lymph Glands.*
Nodule — Small, rounded lump or firm swelling underneath the skin.
Non-Steroidal Anti-Inflammatory Drugs — Medications that control inflammation other than that caused by infection. Usually used to treat conditions of the joints and muscles and pain such as menstrual cramps or headache. "Non-steroidal" means they are not steroid hormones such as cortisone, prednisone, dextramethasone, and others.
Nurse Practitioner (NP) — Registered nurse with additional medical training who can diagnose and treat common illness. Nurse practitioners usually work closely with a doctor, although in some states the practitioner can prescribe medicine and work independently of a physician.
Nutrient — Food or material containing elements needed to promote growth and development or to support life.

O

Obsessions — Unpleasant, frightening, senseless thoughts that won't go away despite reasoning.
Obstetrician-Gynecologist — Doctor specially trained to treat diseases of the female reproductive system and provide health care for pregnant mothers.
Obstructive Pulmonary Disease — See *COPD (Chronic Obstructive Pulmonary Disease).*
Occlusion — Closing or obstruction. Usually used to describe blockage in blood vessels. In dentistry, it means the way the teeth come together when the mouth is closed.
Oncologist — Doctor specially trained to diagnose and treat cancer.
Operative Death Rate — Percentage of patients who die as a result of a certain surgery. It provides a general measure of the risk of a particular surgery.
Ophthalmologist — Doctor specially trained to diagnose and treat diseases of the eyes.
Optic Neuritis — Inflammation of the nerve that conducts vision impulses from the eye to the brain.
Oral — Relating to the mouth.
Oral-Fecal — See *Fecal-Oral.*
Organic — Conditions or diseases resulting from change in body organs that can be measured or seen. Organic diseases are distinct from functional diseases in which no change can be observed in an organ that is not functioning normally.
Organic Psychosis — Mental illness that results from disease in the brain.
Orthodontia — Straightening teeth by applying temporary braces.
Orthopedic Surgeon (Orthopedist) — Doctor specially trained to diagnose and treat diseases of the muscles, bones, and joints, using surgical or mechanical means. A *rheumatologist* is an internist who diagnoses and treats similar conditions primarily with medications and other non-surgical means.
Osteogenesis Imperfecta — Inherited condition in which the bones are brittle and easily broken.
Otorhinolaryngologist or Otolaryngologist — See *Ear, Nose and Throat Specialist.*

Ovary — Female sexual gland where eggs mature and ripen for fertilization.
Ovulation — Monthly process in which an egg leaves the ovary for possible fertilization by a sperm cell.
Ovum — Egg produced by the ovary.

P

Pain — Unpleasant sensation arising from stimulation of sensory nerves located in almost every part of the body. Disease, injury, and strenuous activity can all cause pain.
Palate — Roof of the mouth, consisting of a bony front portion (hard palate) and a soft back portion (soft palate).
Palpitations — Irregular rapid heartbeat, noticeable to the patient.
Pancreas — Organ located on the back abdominal wall that produces and secretes digestive juices into the small intestine. It also produces and secretes insulin into the bloodstream to regulate the level of sugar and other nutrients.
Pap Smear — Test done to detect cancer of the cervix in an early and treatable stage.
Papule — Small, raised skin lesion. Papules may be red, brown, yellow, white, or skin-colored. They may be flat-topped, pointed, or dome-shaped.
Paranoia — Mental illness in which a person believes that he or she is being talked about or plotted against.
Parasite — Organism that lives within, upon, or at the expense of another living organism. Human parasites include disease-causing agents such as amoebas or worms that infect the digestive system, or fungi that live on the skin.
Parasympathetic Nervous System — System of nerves that controls digestion, heartbeat, and relaxation or contraction of small muscles.
Parathyroid Glands — Small glands that control calcium levels in the blood and bones. They are located within or next to the thyroid glands at the base of the neck.
Passive Exercises — Exercises in which a therapist moves the arms and legs of a patient while the patient relaxes. These exercises keep the joints limber until the patient is able to move without assistance.
Patency — Blood vessels or any hollow organs that clog or become blocked are said to lose their patency.
Pathological — Relating to an abnormal condition.
Pathological Examination — Laboratory study of abnormal tissue to establish or confirm a diagnosis.
Pediatrician — Doctor specially trained to care for children and adolescents, especially to foster normal growth and development.
Pediculicide — Medication that cures body lice (pediculosis). Usually applied to the skin.
Pelvic Examination — Examination of a woman's reproductive organs to diagnose pregnancy or detect diseases.
Pelvic Ultrasonography — Examination of a woman's reproductive organs that uses high-frequency sound waves to create an image. It is used to determine the age, size, and position of a fetus in the uterus or to diagnose disease of the pelvic organs.
Pelvis — Lower part of the trunk of the body.
Penis — Male organ used for urination and sexual intercourse.
Perforation — Abnormal hole or opening.
Perforation, Intestinal — Complication of conditions such as ulcers, cancers, or injury to the digestive system. When this occurs, intestinal contents enter the abdominal cavity, causing severe inflammation.
Perfusionist — Medical technician who controls the heart-lung machine to sustain a patient's life during open-heart and lung-transplant surgery.
Perineum — Area between the vulva and anus in females, and between the scrotum and anus in males.
Peripheral Neuropathy (also called Peripheral Neuritis) — A group of symptoms caused by abnormalities in motor or sensory nerves. Characteristics include:

tingling, numbness, pain, usually beginning in the feet and spreading to hands and other parts of the body.

Peripheral Nervous System — Nerves that connect to all parts of the body and carry information via electrical impulses to and from the brain and spinal cord.

Peripheral Vascular System — Network of arteries, veins, and lymphatic channels supplying the head, arms, and legs.

Perirectal — Skin and underlying tissue around the rectum.

Peristalsis — Rhythmic movements of hollow muscular organs (such as the intestines) that move contents (such as digestive material) in one direction.

Peritoneal Cavity — Space enclosed by the peritoneum.

Peritoneum — Very thin, two-layered tissue. One layer lines the outer surface of all the abdominal organs. The other layer lines the abdominal wall.

Peritonsillar Abscess — Abscess forming in the back of the throat near the tonsils.

Pessary — Small ring-shaped device that is inserted into the vagina to help maintain the uterus in a normal position.

pH Balance — Measure of blood's acidity or alkalinity. The pH is controlled by body fluids and electrolytes. Body tissues cannot function normally if the pH varies from a limited range.

Phenothiazine Drugs — Medications used to slow and regulate mental-system activity. Usually used to treat anxiety and other mental conditions; also useful in producing sleep.

Phlebotomy — Removing blood from the blood vessels. This was once believed to cure many diseases; today, it is done to remove blood for diagnostic testing.

Phobia — A powerful, unfounded, irrational fear. Young children, especially fragile ones, are especially likely to develop them. *Common examples:* fear of dogs, monsters, dreams, darkness, robbers, fear of school, fear of separation. *Causes:* The mingling of the real and the imaginary in a toddler's or child's mind usually triggered by anxiety due to illness, an accident, an unpleasant incident, quarreling within the family, and others. *Treatment:* Reassurance by parents, insistance on returning to school. Seek professional help when simpler measures fail.

Physical Therapy — Treatment of diseases of the bone, muscular and nervous systems to help restore normal function after disease or injury.

Physician's Assistant (PA) — Someone trained to do some of the simpler tasks ordinarily performed by a doctor. The PA works under the direction of the doctor.

Pigeon Toes (Toeing-in) — Description: Turning in of part or all of the foot. Occurs in all age groups. Usually disappears when a child grows and begins to walk. *Causes:* Normal part of a child's development. Sometimes a part of cerebral palsy. *Treatment:* For cases that do not disappear at the expected time, surgery may done at about age 6 or 7.

Pilocarpine — Medication used principally in eye drops to treat glaucoma.

Pituitary Gland — Small endocrine gland at the base of the brain that controls growth and regulates other endocrine glands.

Placenta — Disk-shaped organ that attaches and grows inside the uterus during pregnancy. It enables the fetus to receive nutrients from and transfer natural wastes to the mother's bloodstream. The umbilical cord connects the placenta to the fetus.

Plaque — 1) Small raised area of abnormal material on a surface such as the skin or lining of a blood vessel. 2) Mixtures of bacteria and calcium deposited on the teeth that can cause cavities and gum diseases.

Plasma — Liquid part of blood that remains when blood cells are removed.

Plastic and Reconstructive Surgeon (Plastic Surgeon) — Doctor specially trained to perform plastic and reconstructive surgery.

Plastic and Reconstructive Surgery — Special surgery to repair and change body parts to improve function or appearance. The face, hands, breasts, and skin are areas most frequently treated.

GLOSSARY

Platelet Count — Platelets are blood cells (much smaller than red or white blood cells) that assist in the blood-clotting process. A drop of blood contains about 12.5 million platelets. A platelet count determines if the number of platelets is normal.
Pleura — Thin tissue lining the lungs and chest cavity. Inflammation of the pleura (pleurisy) is a painful condition caused by lung diseases.
Pleural Effusion (Pleural Fluid Effusion) — Fluid that collects around the lungs, usually caused by inflammation of the lungs and pleura or congestive heart failure.
Podiatrist — Health-care professional trained in the medical and surgical treatment of foot diseases.
Polyp — A growth, often on a stalk arising from dry mucous membranes, such as in the nose, cervix, or colon.
Portal-Vein System — Veins that drain blood from the gastrointestinal system. The smaller veins empty into the portal vein, which transports blood into the liver.
Postmature Infant — Infant that spends 3 weeks or more beyond the normal 39 weeks of pregnancy in the womb.
Postoperative — Period of recuperation and return to normal health after surgery.
Postural Drainage — Exercises and body positions that promote drainage of fluid and secretions that collect in the lungs and airways.
Potassium — Electrolyte present in all body cells, blood, and body fluids. Potassium is important in maintaining normal heart contractions and the strength and contractions of all muscles. Foods high in potassium include dried apricots and peaches, whole-grain cereals, plain cocoa, dried lentils and peas, bananas, and molasses.
Precancerous — Characteristic of a growth that has the potential to become cancerous.
Predisposition — Tendency. For example, a person who gets many infections has a predisposition to infection.
Premature Labor — Labor beginning before the usual 39 weeks of pregnancy.
Prematurity — Premature babies are those born too soon—earlier than 37 weeks of gestation. Premature infants born after less than 25 weeks gestation usually don't survive. Most premature babies weigh less than 5-1/2 pounds at birth. *Causes:* Unknown, but socioecomonic and biological factors play a part. 7% of white newborns are premature; 18% of non-white newborns are premature. Medical factors that may play a part include maternal alcoholism, drug addiction, cigarette smoking, exposure to synthetic estrogen hormones (DES), stress, long-term illness, endocrine problems, toxemia, high blood pressure, infection, problems with the maternal uterus, or fetal malformations. *Treatment:* Incubators in neonatal intensive care units for medical and nursing special care. Before discharge home the baby should be able to eat by mouth, keep a normal temperature, and have steady heart and breathing rates.
Presbyopia — Form of nearsightedness that normally accompanies aging.
Primary Disorder — Basic disease that may result in complications. Diabetes mellitus, for example, is a primary disorder that often causes secondary complications involving the kidneys, blood vessels, and eyes.
Proctoscope, Proctoscopy — Method of examining the rectum and lower part of the colon with a proctoscope, an optical instrument with a lighted tip.
Prolapse — Pushing or falling out of a part or an organ from its normal position.
Prolapsed (Dropped) Uterus — Uterus that has moved from its normal position because of loose pelvic muscles and ligaments. In severe cases, it can protrude completely outside the vagina.
Prophylaxis — Measures taken to prevent an illness.
Prophylaxis, Dental — Regular care (including cleaning) of the teeth and gums that helps prevent tooth decay and gum inflammation.

Prostaglandins — Natural substances found in semen, menstrual fluid, and many body tissues. They are involved in basic body functions such as inflammation, immune response, and activities of the lungs, heart, kidneys, uterus, and digestive system.
Prostate (Prostate Gland) — Male sex gland located at the base of the urinary bladder. It produces a fluid that is added to sperm to produce semen.
Prosthesis — Artificial device used as a substitute for a missing or badly functioning part of the body.
Prothrombin Time — Test to measure one of the components of the body's blood-clotting mechanism. It is used to diagnose clotting diseases and to control blood-thinning (anticoagulation) in treatment of some diseases of the heart and blood vessels.
Psychiatrist — Doctor specially trained to diagnose and treat mental illness.
Psychoanalysis — Treatment of some mental illness that involves a detailed understanding of how past events in a person's life may have resulted in mental disturbances.
Psychologist — Health-care professional specially trained to diagnose and treat somc kinds of mental illness.
Psychopathy — Psychological or mental illness.
Psychosis — Mental illness characterized by deranged personality, loss of contact with reality, and possible delusions, hallucinations, or illusions.
Psychosocial — Influences of society on growth and development.
Psychosomatic Disorders — Diseases and symptoms not caused by physical factors. "Psycho"—the mind. "Somatic"—the relationship to the body. These disorders are not faked or imaginary, but are usually caused by family disharmony, poor parent-child relationships, and inability to express feelings. Almost any illness can be affected by situational and psychological factors. Examples: Recurrent abdominal pain and headaches; diarrhea. *Treatment:* Seek out and confront areas of stress; deal with it effectively within the family or seek outside support. Create an atmosphere of trust so the child can speak freely about concerns and fears.
Psychosomatic Illness — Illness in which thoughts and emotions play an important role.
Psychotherapist — Professional specially trained to diagnose and treat some mental illnesses.
Puberty — Period in early adolescence when hormonal changes bring about full sexual maturity and capacity to reproduce.
Pubic Bone — One of the bones of the pelvis located above the genitals in both sexes.
Pulmonary — Relating to the lungs and breathing.
Pulmonary Embolism — Blood clots that form elsewhere in the body and travel through the veins into the right heart and thence through the pulmonary artery into a vessel so small that it no longer can pass. Lung tissue beyond the embolus will not receive adequate blood supply to survive.
Pulmonary Hypertension — Increased pressure in the blood vessels of the lungs.
Pulse — Heartbeat (contraction of the heart) as felt in an artery. Heart rate is often measured by counting the pulse felt in the artery in the wrist.
Pus — Thick fluid, usually green or yellow, that forms to fight local infection. Pus often collects in an enclosed sac, an abscess, at the site of an infection.
Pyelogram, Intravenous — Method of studying the kidneys and urinary tract by injecting into the bloodstream a medication that X-rays can detect.
Pyelogram, Retrograde — Method of studying the kidneys, similar to an intravenous pyelogram, but in which the medication detected by X-rays is placed in the urinary system by a catheter inserted through the bladder into the ureters.

R

Radiation Therapy or Treatment — Use of high-energy waves (generated by special X-rays machines, cobalt machines, and other devices) to treat some forms of cancer.

Radiation destroys cancerous tissue but does little harm to healthy tissue.
Radioactive Chromium Studies — Diagnostic method used to measure total blood in the body.
Radioactive Fibrinogen — Fibrinogen treated with a radioactive substance for laboratory analysis.
Radioactive Iodine Uptake and Scan — Same as *Thyroid Scan.*
Radioactive Studies — Same as *Radioisotope Studies.*
Radioactive Technetium 99 Scan — Radioisotope scan method used to diagnose some disorders of the heart, liver, spleen, and other organs.
Radioisotope — Radioactive form of chemicals normally present in the body.
Radioisotope Scan — Scan of radioisotopes given orally or intravenously to a patient that become concentrated in organs such as the heart, lungs, or brain. Instruments measure the radiation given off by the radioisotopes and create a photographic image of the organ being studied.
Radioisotope Studies — Radioisotopes are chemical elements that give off radiation. A radioisotope of a chemical element normally present in the body (such as carbon), if injected into the body, will mix with the non-isotopes. The body doesn't know the difference, but radiation from the isotopes can be detected with special instruments. Determining where radioisotopes go in the body allows diagnosis of diseases that cannot be detected otherwise.
Radioisotope Therapy — Treatment of some cancers with radioisotopes.
Radiologist — Doctor specially trained to use X-rays and other kinds of radiation in diagnosis and treatment.
Radionuclide Scans (a Nuclear Medicine Procedure) — These tests use selected radioactive isotopes injected into patients. The isotope is selected to be picked up in increased amounts by the target organ, such as brain, lung, bone, thyroid glands, kidney, etc. The absorbed radioisotope produces a localized increase in concentration of the radioisotope tracer. Images are recorded on a scintillating camera.
Raynaud's Phenomenon — A circulatory system disorder affecting fingers and toes that is a complication of an underlying disease or emotional disturbance. Characteristics include fingers that turn pale when exposed to cold or stress. Paleness is followed by a bluish tinge and then redness.
Rebound Phenomenon — A reversed response on withdrawal of a stimulus. For example: Many times when using a nasal spray or nose drops to shrink the nasal tissues in order to facilitate breathing through the nose, a rebound phenomenon will occur. Upon withdrawal of the spray or drops, the congestion is worse than it was before using the drops or spray.
Recovery Room — Specially equipped and staffed area of a hospital for observing and caring for patients who have just undergone surgery. Postoperative patients usually remain in the recovery room until they are awake and their vital signs (blood pressure, pulse, and respiration) are satisfactory.
Rectum — End of the large intestine, located in the pelvis below the sigmoid colon and above the anus.
Regenerate — Ability of some parts of the body to grow back to normal after being damaged.
Regional Enteritis — Inflammation of a region of the small intestine, usually the last part of the small intestine where it empties into the large intestine.
Regurgitate — To vomit.
Relapse — Stage of illness in which the patient gets worse after having improved.
Remission — Stage of a chronic illness when the patient's condition improves.
Renal Dialysis — Mechanical and chemical method of removing normal wastes from the body of a patient whose kidneys cannot function adequately. It is also used to remove harmful poison or a drug overdose from the bloodstream.
Reproductive Organs, Female — Organs of a woman's body that enable her to become pregnant and deliver a baby. The major

organs are the vagina, uterus, Fallopian tubes, and ovaries.

Reproductive Organs, Male — Organs of a man's body that enables him to produce sperm and impregnate a woman. The major organs are the penis, testicles, seminal vesicles, and prostate gland.

Reproductive System — Body system enabling impregnation and delivery of a baby. It also provides characteristic male or female appearance.

Resect — Surgical removal of a part of the body.

Respiratory-Distress Syndrome (RDS, Hyaline Membrane Disease) — Breathing difficulty in a newborn infant. *Causes:* Prematurity, underdeveloped lungs, deficiency of moistening and lubricating fluid in lungs and bronchial tubes. *Symptoms:* Trouble with breathing (rapid, shallow breathing, chest retractions, grunting, flared nostrils, bluish tint to skin). Low blood pressure. Low body temperature. Increasing fatigue. RDS can lead to pneumonia, heartbeat irregularities, and apnea. *Treatment:* Treatment of the mother in premature labor to slow or halt labor or treatment of the mother with medication that stimulates the production of surfactant in the fetus. After birth treatment requires intensive care, an incubator, oxygen, intravenous fluids. Professional workers take care not to give an excess of oxygen to prevent problems of the eyes called retrolental fibroplasia.

Retained Placenta — Condition occurring immediately after childbirth in which part of the placenta remains attached to the uterus, creating a risk of serious bleeding or infection.

Retina — Light-senstitive part of the eye at the back of the eyeball on which the lens focuses images. The retina converts the image to impulses that go to the brain.

Retina-Vein Occlusion — Condition in which a clot forms in the vein supplying the retina with blood.

Retinoblastoma — Cancerous tumor that forms in the eye of an infant.

Retrolental Fibroplasia — A problem of the retina of the eyes of premature infants who required excessive amounts of oxygen to sustain life during intensive care following premature birth. If severe, retrolental fibroplasia can lead to severe visual problems or blindness.

Retrovirus — Group of viruses that cause AIDS (Acquired Immunodeficiency Syndrome) and some types of lymphoma and leukemia.

Rh and ABO Incompatibility — When a pregnant woman during her second pregnancy has Rh negative blood and her unborn infant has Rh positive blood, incompatibility can result, causing *erythroblastosis* in the child at birth. Since the 1960s, preventive treatment has existed, early detection is possible, and severe erythroblastosis can be prevented. A related but much less common problem exists when a mother has type O blood and the fetus has type A or B blood. When this problem occurs, treatment requires exchange transfusion of the newborn. Rh incompatibility can be prevented by giving RhoGAM to an Rh negative mother within 72 hours of delivery of her first Rh positive baby.

Rh Negative Blood — A subtype of red blood cells. Blood subtypes are inherited. The major subtypes are types A, B, O and Rh negative.

Rheumatologist — A specialist in internal medicine who subspecializes in medical diagnosis and treatment of rheumatic and arthritis disorders.

Rickets — A childhood disease characterized by soft, deformed bones due to a vitamin D deficiency. There is also a similar disorder caused by genetic factors called vitamin D-resistant rickets. *Causes of the deficiency:* Malabsorption, inadequate diet, absence of exposure to enough ultraviolet light from the sun, gastrointestinal infections, celiac disease, cystic fibrosis of the pancreas, liver diseases, or hypophosphatemia. *Treatment:* Large daily doses of vitamin D, monitored

by your physician. Treatment for vitamin D-resistant rickets requires combined treatment with phosphates and vitamin D.
Rinne Test — Test using a tuning fork to diagnose hearing disorders.
Rotator Cuff — The structure around the shoulder joint capsule composed of intermingled muscle and tendon fibers. The rotator cuff provides stability and strength to the shoulder joint.
Rubin's Insufflation Test — Test used in diagnosing fertility problems in women. A harmless gas is introduced into the uterus to determine if there is a blockage in the Fallopian tubes.
Rumination — A rare disorder among infants aged 3 to 12 months characterized by self-induced regurgitation of partially digested food. The infant makes sucking or chewing movements before or during regurgitation. After regurgitation, some food is dribbled or spit out and some is chewed and swallowed again. These children do not retch and are not nauseated or physically ill. Most children resolve these problems spontaneously; some require treatment. Treatment may require hospitalization to correct malnutrition and/or dehydration. Other treatment methods include physical and occupational therapy, holding an infant after eating, stimulation with parent-child eye contact and verbal communication, child care, family counseling, and other social service support services.

S

Sacroiliac Region — Area of the lower back where the spine meets the pelvic bone.
Saline — Salt-containing solution similar to normal body fluid that is given intravenously to help correct fluid and electrolyte imbalances.
Salivary Glands — Glands located inside the mouth around the jaw that secrete saliva into the mouth.
Saphenous-Femoral Vein System — Network of large veins in the legs that helps return blood from the leg to the inferior vena cava, then to the heart.
Sarcoidosis — A chronic, progressive disease involving the lungs, lymph nodes, and other tissues. There is no known treatment.
Scale, Scaling — Flakes of dried skin which form as whitish skin lesions.
Schizophrenia — Mental illness characterized by a distorted sense of reality, bizarre behavior, and fragmentation of the personality.
Sciatic Nerve — Large nerve that begins at the base of the spine and passes through the buttocks down the back side of the thigh and down the leg.
Sciatica — Painful condition resulting from irritation of the sciatic nerve.
Scleritis — Inflammation of the sclera (the white of the eye).
Scoliosis — Curvature of the spine.
Scopolamine — Medication used to treat hyperactive or spastic conditions of the digestive system and to prevent motion sickness.
Scrotum — Organ of the male reproductive system that contains the testicles, blood vessels, and the vas deferens.
Scurvy — Disease of bones, gums, and blood vessels caused by a deficiency of vitamin C.
Second Molars — Permanent grinding teeth that appear at about age 11 to 13.
Secondary Infection — Infection that results from some other problem. It may occur after surgery or develop during antibiotic treatment of another infection.
Sedative — Medication used to produce relaxation or sleep.
Sedative-Hypnotics — Class of medications that help relieve anxiety and promote sleep.
Sedimentation Rate — Blood test measuring the rate that blood settles in a test tube. It identifies infection, inflammation or tissue damage.
Self-Care — Treatment that patients can administer for themselves.
Seminal Vesicles — Small sacs next to the prostate that help make and store seminal fluid, and contract to eject semen.

Senile Dementia — Permanent loss of mental functions of older persons, resulting from conditions such as Alzheimer's disease and atherosclerosis (hardening of the arteries).
Senile Keratosis — Same as *Seborrheic Keratoses.* (See Illnesses section.)
Sensitivity Studies (Antibiotics) — Laboratory method of determining which antibiotic will most likely be successful in treating infections caused by bacteria.
Sensory — Ability to feel or experience sensations such as sound, light, or pain.
Septic — Infected.
Serological Tests — Tests of serum (blood without cells) used to diagnose a variety of diseases, especially infections and autoimmune conditions.
Serum — Liquid portion of blood that remains after blood cells and blood clots have been removed.
Serum Alkaline Phosphatase — Material present in excessive amounts in the blood of patients with some bone and liver diseases.
Serum Electrolytes — Same as *Electrolytes.*
Sesamoid Bones — Small oval-shaped bones in the tendons of the hands and feet.
Sever's Disease — Painful condition of the heel bone of growing children.
Sexual Dysfunction — Inability to participate in sexual relations that are satisfactory for both partners.
Shave Biopsy — Procedure to diagnose skin disorders in which a thin layer of tissue from under a skin lesion is shaved away for laboratory examination.
Shock — Condition in which the blood pressure falls below the level needed to supply blood to the body. Signs and symptoms include weakness, paleness, rapid heartbeat, dry mouth, cold sweat, and feelings of doom.
Sick-Sinus Syndrome — Form of heart-rhythm disorder (arrhythmia).
Sigmoid Colon — Lower part of the large colon (intestine) located in the pelvis just above the rectum.
Sigmoidoscope, Sigmoidoscopy — Same as *Proctoscope, Proctoscopy.*
Signs — Evidence of disease that can be observed and measured, in contrast to *symptoms,* which only patients can experience. For example, blood-pressure measurement or red tonsils are *signs;* headache or nausea are *symptoms.*
Silicone — Artificial compound used by plastic and reconstructive surgeons to reshape parts of the body, such as the breast.
Silver Nitrate — Chemical used for cautery.
Sims-Huhner Test — Test used in diagnosis of reasons for infertility in women in which the mucus from the cervix is examined, especially for the presence of sperm after sexual intercourse.
Skin Clips — Small U-shaped metal strips used instead of stitches to close skin that has been incised during surgery.
Skin Tests for Allergy — Diagnostic method used to determine whether a particular substance is causing allergic reactions. The test is carried out by introducing a small amount of the suspected material, such as pollen or dust, under the skin or on the skin. If inflammation results, the patient is allergic to the material.
Sleep Inducers — Medications used to produce sleep.
Sleep-Study Laboratory — Laboratory where persons are studied with sensitive instruments while asleep. Information from sleep study aids in diagnosis of sleep disorders.
Sleepwalking, Sleeptalking, Night Terrors — Not dreams, but crying, kicking, moaning, mumbling or running about. They occur during partial arousal from deep, non-dreaming sleep. Most common in children 2 to 5 years old. Each may last from a few seconds to 40 minutes or so, then the child awakens, goes back to sleep and doesn't remember the episode. Do not allow your child to become habitually accustomed to sleeping with a parent, but occasionally after sleepwalking or night terrors, it's okay to allow the child to crawl in for the remainder of that night. More information: Association of Sleep Disorder Centers, 604 Second Street SW, Rochester, MN 55905, (507)287-6006.

Slow Viruses — Group of viruses that infect the brain but do not cause disease until many years afterward.
Soaks — Applying moisture—either plain water or water with dissolved medicines—to an inflamed area of the skin.
Soft Palate — Fleshy part of the roof of the mouth close to the throat.
Sonogram, Sonography — Diagnostic method in which high-frequency (ultrasound) sound waves are transmitted into the body. Their reflections create images of body organs. This non-invasive test requires a technician to guide a transducer over the area of the body being studied. The transducer sends sound waves at frequencies the ear does not hear. These waves reflect back, convert into images, and allow the images to be amplified, displayed on a screen, and photographed.
Spasmodic — Sudden intermittent symptom, or intermittent muscle spasm.
Spastic, Spasticity — A description of muscles that are continuously contracting and in a state of excessive tension.
Speculum — Instrument used to examine the interior of openings such as the vagina, nose, ear, or rectum.
Sperm — Male reproductive cells manufactured in testicles and ejaculated in semen.
Spherocytosis — Abnormally shaped red blood cells caused by some anemias. These cells are sphere-shaped, in contrast to the doughnut shape of normal red blood cells.
Spikes, Temperature — High but brief episodes of fever.
Spina Bifida — Congenital (inherited) disorder in which the base of the spine remains open, sometimes exposing the spinal cord and nerves.
Spinal Anesthesia — Method to provide anesthesia to the lower body by injecting an anesthetic into the fluid in the space that surrounds the lower spinal cord.
Spirometry — Test of lung (pulmonary) function.
Spleen — A large organ in the upper abdomen on the left side, located close to the left side of the stomach. It is the largest structure of the lymph system. The spleen causes disintegration of old red blood cells in adults, manufactures red blood cells in the fetus and newborn, and serves as an important reservoir of blood.
Splenic-Vein Thrombosis — Clot in the major vein that carries blood away from the spleen.
Splints — Rigid supports, made of metal, plastic or plaster, used to immobilize an injured or inflamed part of the body. Splints are used temporarily in the case of injury, following some surgical procedures on joints or ligaments, or occasionally in the case of arthritis.
Spore — Microscopic seed form of fungi. Spores are extremely hardy, and survive extremes of temperature. If they enter the body of a susceptible person, they can cause fungal disease.
Sputum — Secretion of the lungs, coughed up in large amounts in some lung diseases.
Staphylococcus — Bacteria that frequently cause boils, abscesses, pneumonias, bone infections, and infections in other tissues or organs.
Staples — Small U-shaped metal wires used in place of stitches to close incised skin after some surgeries, especially in the digestive system. Also used to close off some portions of the stomach during operations for extreme obesity.
Sterilized — 1) Made completely free of all germs, usually by steam heat, toxic gas, or chemicals. All instruments used in surgeries are sterilized, as is most other medical equipment. 2) Made unable to conceive children.
Steroids — Medications that resemble hormones produced by the cortex of the adrenal glands, ovaries, and testicles.
Stethoscope — Instrument used to listen to the sounds produced by the heart, lungs, blood vessels, and pregnant uterus.
Still's Disease — Form of arthritis in children similar to rheumatoid arthritis in adults.
Stimulant Drugs — Medications that increase the activity of the brain and nervous system.

Stomatitis — Inflammation of the mouth.
Stool — Feces.
Streptococcus — Bacteria that cause illnesses such as laryngitis, cellulitis of the skin, pneumonia, meningitis, and others. If not treated, streptococcal infections may also cause serious heart and kidney diseases as complications that appear after the original infection has cleared.
Stress — A disruption of a person's physical or mental well-being or balance. Stress occurs in every life, but people respond in different ways.
Stuttering — A disruption in the natural rhythm and flow of speech with repeated sounds or syllables, prolongation of sounds, or blocked speech. Treatment includes parents controlling their own reaction to the child's stuttering. With severe problems a speech therapist may, with great patience, help a child over this language barrier.
Sublingual Salivary Glands — Small glands near the base of the tongue that secrete saliva into the mouth.
Submaxillary Salivary Glands — Small glands near the jaw that secrete saliva into the mouth.
Suicide — The third leading cause of death among adolescents, following accidents and homicides. Suicide occurs in all socioeconomic groups. All suicide threats or attempts must be taken seriously and dealt with immediately. Suicidal threats should be first addressed by the family with patient listening. As soon as a child feels that help is available, things get better with practical advice, emotional support, or professional help.
Sulfonamides (Sulfa Drugs) — Class of drugs used to fight infections.
Sulfonurea Drugs — Medications taken orally to treat some forms of diabetes mellitus.
Surgery — Treatment in which the body is restored to a healthy condition by physical methods (or operations) such as cutting, removing, replacing, straightening, repairing, or joining.
Surgical Suite — Group of rooms used to perform surgery. In addition to operating rooms, where surgery takes place, there are supply areas, a recovery room, administrative rooms, and a lounge for the staff to rest between surgeries.
Suture — Thread-like material used to hold tissues or skin edges together.
Symmetry, Symmetrical — Refers to the arrangement of the body in pairs, such as two arms, legs, kidneys, lungs, etc.
Sympathomimetics — Medications similar to adrenalin in their actions.
Symptoms — Effects of disease that only the patient can experience, such as pain, nausea, dizziness, anxiety, depression and others.
Synovial Membranes — Delicate tissue that lines the inside of joints.
Systemic — Conditions that affect most or all of the body, in contrast to conditions that affect only a limited area. For example, diabetes mellitus is a systemic condition; an abscess is a local condition.

T

Tampons — Absorbent material to insert into the vagina during menstruation. They may be used alone, or with pads. They are safe to use as soon as menstruation begins. They should be changed about every 4 hours or more frequently. Use the smallest size possible and wear pads instead at night. Continue to take daily baths and showers. Don't use feminine sprays or douches. If the odor is really bad or a heavy discharge develops, consult your physician.
Tartar — Hard deposit that forms on the teeth and causes inflammation of the gums.
Temperature Spike — See *Spikes, Temperature.*
Temporo-Mandibular Joint — Joint that joins the jaw to the other head bones.
Tenderness — Condition that causes pain when pressure is applied.
Tendon — Tough cord of tissue at the end of muscles that attach to bone. Tendons transmit the force of muscle contraction to cause movement.
Testes or Testicles — Male sex glands that produce sex hormones and sperm.

Therapeutic Trial — Form of diagnosis and treatment where medication is used even though the diagnosis is not firmly established. If the patient improves after treatment with a medication known to be useful in treating a specific condition, the improvement suggests that the specific disease was present. Therapeutic trials are somewhat risky and are used only when other forms of diagnosis and treatment have failed.
Therapist — Health-care professional specially trained to provide therapy.
Thermogram, Thermography — Method of diagnosis that measures body heat. The area being studied is scanned by a heat-sensitive instrument capable of producing an image (thermogram) of areas of increased heat. They are useful in studying female breast tumors and some blood-vessel conditions.
Thiazide Diuretics — Class of medications that promote excretion of excess fluids by the kidneys.
Third Molars — Permanent grinding teeth that appear at about age 17 to 25.
Thoracic Duct — The largest channel of the lymphatic system through which lymph fluid enters the vena cava.
Thoracic Spine — That part of the spinal column below the neck and above the back. Ribs attach to the thoracic spine.
Thoracic Surgeon — A surgeon who specializes in surgical treatment of disorders of the organs in the thorax (chest), including lungs, pericardium, heart, pleura (covering of lungs), bronchial tubes, and large blood vessels.
Thyroglossal Duct — Small passageway, normally closed, located in the upper neck. It extends from the back of the tongue to just above the larynx. If an abnormally open duct becomes filled with fluid, a *thyroglossal cyst* results.
Thyroid Cartilage — Larynx (also called the voice box, or Adam's apple), made of semihard cartilage.
Thyroid Gland — Endocrine gland located in the lower neck next to the trachea that produces hormones that regulate the rate at which all body cells function. Thyroid hormones are also essential for normal growth and development.
Thyroid Scan — Method of examination of the thyroid gland in which a small amount of radioactive iodine introduced into the body collects in the thyroid gland. An instrument passed over the thyroid produces an image of the gland based on the concentration of the radioactive iodine.
Ticks — Small biting insects that may cause inflammation of the skin or serious infections such as Rocky Mountain Spotted Fever.
Tics — Brief, uncontrollable muscle spasms.
Tissue — Building blocks of body organs; living cells all of one type.
Titer — The quantity of a substance required to produce a reaction with a given volume of another substance.
Tonsils — Lymphatic tissues that help fight infection located at the entrance of the throat. They frequently become infected, especially in children.
Topical — Medications applied to the skin, conjunctiva, or mucous membrane of the mouth, nose, vagina, or rectum.
Tourniquet — Cord or band wrapped around an arm or leg tightly enough to stop blood circulation temporarily.
Toxic, Toxicity — Harmful; capable of causing body damage.
Toxin — Poison. Usually refers to the chemicals produced by some living organisms that harm the human body.
Traction — Method of treating some conditions of bones, muscles, and ligaments by exerting a steady pull on the affected parts. Some bone fractures and back pain due to a ruptured disk are treated this way.
Tranquilizer — Medication used to help diminish anxiety and to produce calmness.
Tranquilizers, Benzodiazepine — Class of tranquilizers commonly used to treat anxiety, nervousness, or tension.
Transfuse — To give a patient blood, necessary in the treatment of some conditions.

Transfusion — Process of introducing blood through a needle placed in the patient's vein.
Transfusion Reaction — Undesirable symptom or condition resulting from a blood transfusion.
Transmission, Transmit — Passing a disease to another person.
Transplant — Living organ (such as kidney, cornea, heart, bone marrow, or skin), removed from one person (donor), and placed in the body of another (recipient).
Transverse Colon — Middle part of the colon (intestine), lying horizontally in the middle or upper abdomen.
Trauma — Force that injures or damages any part of the body.
Tricyclic Antidepressant Drugs (Tricyclics) — Class of medications used to treat depression.
Trophoblastic Tumors — See *Hydatidiform Mole*.
Tube Feeding — Providing nutrients through a small tube placed in the stomach of a patient who is unable to eat. The tube may pass through the nose to the stomach or be inserted through an incision in the stomach.
Tuberous Sclerosis — Rare inherited condition of the skin, nervous system, and other organs of the body.
Tumor — Literally, a swelling; usually used to refer to a benign or cancerous growth.
Turner's Syndrome — A disorder in girls characterized by an abnormal chromosome pattern—they lack one of the two sex hormones. *Signs and symptoms:* Low birth weight, skin and bone abnormalities, "webbed" neck, swollen hands and feet, broad chest, a low hairline at the nape of the neck, congenital heart disease (frequently), absence of breast development and menstruation, or short stature. *Treatment:* Female hormones beginning at age 13 to 15 years. Treatment is usually quite successful.

U

Ulceration — Wearing away of the surface or lining of an organ, exposing underlying tissue. Ulceration of the lining of the stomach exposes blood vessels, which may bleed. Ulceration may erode through the wall of an organ (perforation). Ulceration frequently affects the skin, if rubbed excessively or if diseased.
Ultrasonography — See *Sonography.*
Ultrasound Treatment — Method of treatment in which high-energy sound waves are focused on the affected area, producing mild heat that helps relieve inflammation. It is especially useful in treatment of muscular symptoms.
Underlying — Beneath, below, or more basic. Thus, losing weight may result from an underlying condition such as diabetes mellitus or cancer.
Upper Gastrointestinal Series — X-ray examination of the esophagus, stomach, and duodenum accomplished by having the patient swallow a barium solution that X-rays can detect.
Upper Respiratory System — Upper part of the breathing system, consisting of the nose, throat, larynx, trachea, and bronchial tubes.
Uremia — A serious condition associated with kidney failure in which body wastes build up in the blood and body tissues.
Ureters — Slender muscular tubes that carry urine from the kidneys to the urinary bladder, where it is stored until eliminated from the body.
Urethra — Tubular passageway extending from the urinary bladder to the outside of the body.
Uric Acid — Chemical normally produced in the body from metabolism or breakdown of protein and eliminated in the urine. If the level of uric acid rises in the body as a result of disease, gout or kidney stones may result.
Urinalysis — Laboratory test performed on a urine sample that helps diagnose diseases of the kidney and other parts of the body.
Urinary Bladder — Muscular sac in the lower abdomen that stores urine brought to it from the kidneys by the ureters. The bladder stores urine until it can be eliminated through the urethra by contractions of the bladder muscles.

Urinary studies — Laboratory or X-ray tests of the urinary tract.
Urinary Tract — Organs that produce, store, and eliminate urine. The organs are the kidneys, ureters, urinary bladder, and urethra.
Uterus — Organ of the female reproductive system on the wall of which the fertilized egg (ovum) attaches and develops to form a fetus.
Uveitis — Inflammation of the parts of the eyes that make up the iris (colored tissue encircling the clear center—the pupil).
Uvula — Soft tissue hanging down from the soft palate at the back of the throat.

V
Vaccination — Method of providing protection against disease (immunity) by giving a patient a small amount of the disease-causing germ that is weakened, killed, or otherwise modified so that it cannot itself cause disease. Same as *Immunization.*
Vaccine — Medication used to provide immunity by vaccination. Vaccines are given mostly by injection or by mouth.
Vagus Nerve — Long cranial nerve, arising in the base of the brain and passing to the chest and abdomen. It helps regulate heart rate, breathing, swallowing, digestion, and many other body functions.
Varicose — Swollen and twisting, usually used to describe varicose veins.
Vas Deferens — Tube that carries sperm manufactured by the testicles toward the prostate gland and seminal vesicles.
Vasculitis — Inflammation of blood vessels, the basis of any illnesses.
Vasoconstrictor Drugs — Medications that cause blood vessels to contract, tighten, or become smaller.
Vasodilator Drugs — Medications that cause small arteries to widen, providing more blood to an area of the body where the blood vessels are constricted by spasm, narrowed or obstructed.
Vector — 1) An imaginary line that represents both direction and quantity used to study electrocardiograms (EKGs). 2) An agent that transmits infectious germs from one organism to another.
Veins — Blood vessels that return blood from body organs to the heart and lungs. Veins are much thinner than arteries. Veins carry blood at a much lower pressure than do arteries.
Vena Cava — Largest vein in the body. It collects blood from the venous system and carries it to the heart.
Venereal — Related to sexual intercourse or sexual contact. Veneral diseases such as genital herpes, gonorrhea, or syphilis are now usually referred to as "sexually transmitted diseases."
Venous System — Network of veins that extend from all body organs and transport blood back to the heart.
Ventricles — Chambers containing fluid. The ventricles of the heart pump blood; ventricles of the brain contain cerebrospinal fluid.
Ventricular Aneurysm — Ballooning of the wall of the heart resulting from a weakening of the heart muscle, a complication of scarring from a previous heart attack.
Vertebrae — Bones of the spine that form the vertebral column (backbone).
Vertebral Column — The spine; the bones of the back.
Virulent — Extremely dangerous or harmful. Virulent bacteria are ones capable of causing diseases.
Viruses — Small germs responsible for a variety of infectious illnesses. Viruses are not alive until they enter cells of the body, where they grow and reproduce, causing viral illnesses.
Visual Acuity — Clarity with which objects are seen.
Vitamins — Chemical substances found in food that are necessary for healthy body growth, function, and tissue repair.
Vitreous — Clear fluid that fills much of the eye.

Vocal Cords — Two narrow bands of fibrous and muscular tissue in the larynx that vibrate to create the sounds of the voice.
Voiding Cystourethrography — An X-ray study made of the bladder and urethra after injection of a dye through a catheter inserted through the urethra into the bladder.
Volvulus — Twisting of loops of intestines, which beome closed off (obstructed) and may lose their blood supply.

W

Warts — Small, often hard and rough skin growths caused by viruses that infect the skin.
Wasting of Body or Muscles — Severe loss of body tissues (other than surplus fat), especially muscles and vital organs, resulting in weakness, susceptibility to infection, bone fractures, and sometimes death.
Weber Test — Hearing test performed with a tuning fork.
Wheezes — High-pitched sounds and whistles produced in the lungs where secretions have partially blocked air passages.
Whirlpool Treatment — Method of treating minor blood-vessel and musculo-skeletal diseases by immersion in a pool where jets of warm water enter and swirl under high pressure.
Wisdom Teeth — Same as *Third Molars.*
Wryneck (Torticollis) — A painful condition that causes a child to tip or tilt to one side. It may be present at birth (perhaps caused by injury at birth), or later in life may be caused by muscle inflammation caused by an accident, tumor, or disease. *Treatment:* Congenital form: A series of muscle-stretching exercises. The worst cases require surgery. Other forms: Treatment of the underlying condition.

X

Xeroradiogram — Method of X-ray diagnosis, usually of the female breast, which uses a process similar to that used to produce photocopies.
X-Rays — High energy, invisible waves capable of penetrating the body and creating shadows on photographic film. The shadows provide images of the body tissues through which the X-rays pass.

Z

Zoster— "Girdle," used to describe a form of virus infection (herpes zoster, shingles) that often produces bands of inflammation across the chest or abdomen.

RESOURCES FOR ADDITIONAL INFORMATION

AIDS

National AIDS Hot Line
800-342-AIDS
(general information recording)

Centers for Disease Control Office of Public Inquiries
1600 Clifton Rd., N.E.
Atlanta, GA 30333
404-329-3534

ALCOHOLISM

Alateen World Service Headquarters
1 Park Ave.
New York, NY 10016
212-481-6565

ARTHRITIS

American Juvenile Arthritis Organization
1314 Spring St. N.W.
Atlanta, GA 30309
404-872-7100

National Institute of Arthritis & Metabolic Diseases
Bldg. 31
9000 Rockville Pike
Bethesda, MD 20205

ASTHMA AND ALLERGY

Asthma & Allergy Foundation of America
1835 K St. N.W., Suite P-900
Washington, DC 20006
202-293-2950

AUTISM

National Society for Children and Adults with Autism
1234 Massachusetts Ave. N.W.
Suite 1017
Washington, DC 20005
202-783-0125

BIRTH DEFECTS

March of Dimes Birth Defects Foundation
1275 Mamaroneck Ave.
White Plains, NY 10605
914-428-7100

National Maternal and Child Health Clearinghouse
3520 Prospect St. N.W.
Washington, DC 20057
202-625-8410

BLINDNESS

American Foundation for the Blind (AFB)
15 W. 16th St.
New York, NY 10011
212-620-2000

Eye Bank Association of America
6560 Fannin, Level 9
Houston, TX 77030
713-790-5949

Helen Keller National Center for Deaf-Blind Youths and Adults
111 Middle Neck Rd.
Sands Point, NY 11050
516-944-8900

BREAST-FEEDING

La Leche League International, Inc.
9619 Minneapolis Ave.
Franklin Park, IL 60131
312-455-7730

BURNS

National Burn Victim Foundation
308 Main St.
Orange, NJ 07050
201-731-3112

National Institute of Burn Medicine
909 E. Ann St.
Ann Arbor, MI 48104
313-769-9000

RESOURCES FOR ADDITIONAL INFORMATION

CANCER

American Cancer Society (ACS)
90 Park Ave.
New York, NY 10016
212-599-8200

Association for Research of Childhood Cancer
P.O. Box 251
Buffalo, NY 14225
716-681-4433

Candlelighters Childhood Cancer Foundation
1901 Pennsylvania Ave. N.W. Suite 1001
Washington, DC 20006
202-659-5136

The National Cancer Institute
9000 Rockville Pike, Bldg. 31 Room 10A18
Bethesda, MD 20892
800-4-CANCER

CEREBRAL PALSY

National Easter Seal Society
2023 W. Ogden Ave.
Chicago, IL 60612
312-243-8400

United Cerebral Palsy Association (UCPA)
60 E. 34th St.
New York, NY 10016
212-481-2811

CESAREAN BIRTH (see also Childbirth)

Cesarean Birth Council International, Inc.
P.O. Box 6081
San Jose, CA 95150
415-343-4044

The Cesarean Prevention Movement
P.O. Box 152, University Station
Syracuse, NY 13210
312-424-1942

Council for Cesarean Awareness
5520 S.W. 92nd Ave.
Miami, FL 33165
305-596-2699

C/SEC, Inc. (Cesareans/Support, Education and Concern)
22 Forest Road
Framingham, MA 01701
617-877-8266

CHILD ABUSE

Parents Anonymous
2810 Artesia Blvd.
Redondo Beach, CA 90278
800-352-0386 or 800-421-0353

CHILDBIRTH

American Foundation for Maternal and Child Health
30 Beekman Place
New York, NY 10022
212-759-5510

International Association of Parents & Professionals for Safe Alternatives in Childbirth
Box 429
Marble Hill, MO 63764
314-238-2010

International Childbirth Education Assoc.
P.O. Box 20048
Minneapolis, MN 55420
612-854-8660

CLEFT PALATE

American Cleft Palate Association
331 Salk Hall
University of Pittsburgh
Pittsburgh, PA 15261
412-681-9620

CYSTIC FIBROSIS

Cystic Fibrosis Foundation
6000 Executive Blvd.
Suite 309
Rockville, MD 20852
301-881-9130

DEAFNESS (see Hearing and Speech Impairment)

RESOURCES FOR ADDITIONAL INFORMATION

DENTAL CARE

American Dental Association
211 E. Chicago Ave.
Chicago, IL 60611
312-440-2500

DIABETES

American Diabetes Association
1660 Duke St.
Alexandria, VA 22314
703-549-1500
800-232-3472

Juvenile Diabetes Foundation International
60 Madison Ave.
New York, NY 10010
212-889-7575

The National Diabetes Information Clearinghouse
Box NDIC
Bethesda, MD 20892
301-468-2162

DRUG ABUSE

National Clearinghouse for Drug Abuse Information
5600 Fisher's Lane
Room 10 A-43
Rockville, MD 20857
301-443-6500

DRUGS

Food & Drug Administration
5600 Fisher's Lane
Rockville, MD 20857

ENDOCRINE DISORDERS (Thyroid, Parathyroid, Pituitary, Sex Glands, Adrenals)

National Institute of Metabolic Disease
9650 Rockville Pike
Bethesda, MD 20205

EATING DISORDERS

American Anorexia Nervosa Association
133 Cedar La.
Teaneck, NJ 07666
201-836-1800

National Anorexic Aid Society
5796 Karl Rd.
Columbus, OH 43229
614-436-1112

The National Association of Anorexia Nervosa & Associated Disorders
Box 271
Highland Park, IL 60035
312-831-3438

EPILEPSY

Epilepsy Foundation of America (EFA)
4351 Garden City, Suite 406
Landover, MD 20785
301-459-3700

FOOT DISORDERS

American Podiatry Association
20 Chevy Chase Circle N.W.
Washington, DC 20015

GASTROINTESTINAL DISORDERS

American Digestive Disease Society
7720 Wisconsin Ave.
Bethesda, MD 20014
301-652-9293

HANDICAPPED

Goodwill Industries of America
9200 Wisconsin Ave.
Bethesda, MD 20814-3896
301-530-6500

National Easter Seal Society
2023 W. Ogden Ave.
Chicago, IL 60612
312-243-8400

National Society for Crippled Children & Adults
2023 W. Ogden Ave.
Chicago, IL 60612

HEARING AND SPEECH IMPAIRMENT

Alexander Graham Bell Association for the Deaf
3417 Volta Place N.W.
Washington, DC 20007
202-337-5220

American Society for Deaf Children
814 Thayer Ave.
Silver Spring, MD 20910
301-585-5400

American Speech-Language-Hearing Association
10801 Rockville Pike
Rockville, MD 20852
301-897-5700

Helen Keller National Center for Deaf-Blind Youths and Adults
111 Middle Neck Rd.
Sands Point, NY 11050
516-944-8900

HEART DISEASE

American Heart Association
7320 Greenville Ave.
Dallas, TX 75231
214-750-5300

HEMOPHILIA

National Hemophilia Foundation (NHF)
19 W. 34th St., Room 1204
New York, NY 10001
212-563-0211

World Federation of Hemophilia
Suite 2902
1155 Dorchester Blvd., W.
Montreal, Quebec H3B 2L3 Canada

HYPERTENSION (High Blood Pressure)

National High Blood Pressure Information Center
NIH 120/80
Bethesda, MD 20014

HYPOGLYCEMIA

Adrenal Metabolic Research Society of the Hypoglycemia Foundation, Inc.
153 Pawling Ave.
Troy, NY 12180
518-272-7154

INFECTIOUS DISEASES

Centers for Disease Control (CDC)
1600 Clifton Rd. N.E.
Atlanta, GA 30333
404-329-3311

KIDNEY DISEASE

National Association of Patients on Hemodialysis and Transplantation, Inc.
150 Nassau St.
New York, NY 10038
212-619-2727

National Kidney Foundation
2 Park Ave.
New York, NY 10016
212-889-2210

LEUKEMIA

Leukemia Society of America, Inc.
800 Second Ave.
New York, NY 10017
212-573-8484

LIVER DISEASE

Children's Liver Foundation
76 S. Orange Ave., Suite 202
South Orange, NJ 07079
201-761-1111

RESOURCES FOR ADDITIONAL INFORMATION

LUNG DISEASE

American Lung Association, National Headquarters
1740 Broadway
New York, NY 10019
212-315-8700

National Heart, Lung & Blood Institute Information Center
Bethesda, MD 20014
301-496-4236

LUPUS ERYTHEMATOSUS

American Lupus Society
23751 Madison St.
Torrance, CA 90505
213-373-1335

National Lupus Erythematotus Foundation (NLEF)
5430 Van Nuys Blvd., Suite 206
Van Nuys, CA 91401
213-885-8787

MENTAL HEALTH

Association for the Care of Children's Health
3615 Wisconsin Ave.
Washington, DC 20016
202-244-1801

National Mental Health Association
1800 N. Kent St.
Arlington, VA 22209
703-528-6405

MENTAL RETARDATION

Association for Children with Retarded Mental Development, Inc. (A/CRMD)
817 Broadway
New York, NY 10003
212-470-7200

President's Committee on Mental Retardation
Regional Office, Bldg. 3
7th & D Sts. S.W.
Washington, DC 20201
202-245-7634

MISCELLANEOUS

American Red Cross (ARC)
17th & D Sts. N.W.
Washington, DC 20006
202-737-8300

Medic Alert Foundation
Box K-7
Turlock, CA 95380

MULTIPLE SCLEROSIS

National Multiple Sclerosis Society (NMSS)
205 E. 42nd St.
New York, NY 10017
212-986-3240

MUSCULAR DYSTROPHY

Muscular Dystrophy Association, Inc.
810 7th Ave.
New York, NY 10019
212-586-0808

ORGAN TRANSPLANTS

Children's Transplant Association
P.O. Box 2106
Laurinburg, NC 28352
919-276-7171

PARENTING

Parent's Resources
P.O. Box 107, Planetarium Station
New York, NY 10024
212-866-4776

COPE (Coping with the Overall Pregnancy/Parenting Experience)
37 Clarendon St.
Boston, MA 02116
617-357-5588

PLASTIC SURGERY

Society for the Rehabilitation of the Facially Disfigured, Inc.
550 First Ave.
New York, NY 10016

PREGNANCY (see Childbirth)

PSORIASIS

National Psoriasis Foundation
6415 S.W. Canyon Court, Suite 200
Portland, OR 97221
503-297-1545

REYE'S SYNDROME

National Reye's Syndrome Foundation, Inc.
426 N. Lewis
P.O. Box 829
Bryan, OH 43506
419-636-2679

SCOLIOSIS

Scoliosis Association, Inc.
One Penn Plaza
New York, NY 10119
212-845-1760

SEX EDUCATION

Planned Parenthood Federation of America
810 Seventh Ave.
New York, NY 10019
212-541-7800

Sex Information and Education Council of the U.S. (SIECUS)
80 Fifth Ave., Suite 801
New York, NY 10011
212-929-2300

SICKLE-CELL ANEMIA

National Association for Sickle-Cell Disease
3460 Wilshire Blvd, Suite 1012
Los Angeles, CA 90010
213-731-1166

SLEEP DISORDERS

The American Narcolepsy Association
1139 Bush St., Suite D
San Carlos, CA 94070-2477

The Association of Sleep Disorders Centers National Office
P.O. Box 2604
Del Mar, CA 92014
619-755-7556

SPINA BIFIDA

Spina Bifida Association of America
343 S. Dearborn St.
Chicago, IL 60604
312-663-1562
800-621-3141

SPINAL INJURY

American Paralysis Association
P.O. Box 187
Short Hills, NJ 07078
201-379-2690
800-225-0292

American Spinal Injury Association
250 E. Superior, Room 619
Chicago, IL 60611
312-649-3425

National Spinal Cord Injury Assoc.
149 California St.
Newton, MA 02158
617-964-0521

SUDDEN INFANT DEATH SYNDROME

The Guild for Infant Survival
P.O. Box 3841
Davenport, IA 52808
319-326-4653

National Center for the Prevention of Sudden Infant Death Syndrome
330 N. Charles St.
Baltimore, MD 21201
301-547-0300

RESOURCES FOR ADDITIONAL INFORMATION

National Sudden Infant Death Syndrome Clearinghouse
8201 Greensboro Drive, Suite 600
McLean, VA 22102
703-821-8955
703-625-8410

National Sudden Infant Death Syndrome Foundation
8240 Professional Place, Suite 205
Landover, MD 20785
301-459-3388
800-221-SIDS

SUICIDE

National Committee on Youth Suicide Prevention
666 Fifth Ave., 13th Floor
New York, NY, 10103
212-957-9292

Youth Suicide National Center
1825 I St. N.W., Suite 400
Washington, DC 20006
202-429-0190

TAY-SACHS DISEASE

National Tay-Sachs & Allied Diseases Association, Inc. (NTSAD)
92 Washington Ave.
Cedarhurst, NY 11516
516-569-4300

MISCELLANEOUS RESOURCES

MAGAZINES

American Baby Magazine
P.O. Box 51194
Boulder, CO 80322-1194

Growing Child
22 N. Second St.
P.O. Box 1100
Lafayette, IN 47902

Mothering
P.O. Box 8410
Santa Fe, NM 87504

BOOKSTORES

Birth and Life Bookstore, Inc.
P.O. Box 70625
Seattle, WA 98107
206-789-4444
Puts out a quarterly catalog, called *Imprints,* which reviews current books on parenting topics. Mailed free to customers.

Cascade Birthing
P.O. Box 12203
Salem, OR 97309
503-378-7545

NAPSAC Bookstore
P.O. Box 429
Marble Hill, MO 63764
314-238-2010
NAPSAC publishes a newsletter about alternative childbirth. Write to be put on their mailing list.

SUGGESTED READING FOR ADDITIONAL INFORMATION

AIDS

Gone, Victor, ed. *Understanding AIDS: A Comprehensive Guide.* New Brunswick, NJ: Rutgers University Press, 1986.

ALCOHOLISM

Elkin, Michael. *Families Under the Influence: Changing Alcoholic Patterns.* New York: Norton, 1984.

ALLERGIES

Feldman, B. Robert. *The Complete Book of Children's Allergies: A Guide For Parents.* New York: Times Books, 1986.

ARTHRITIS

Fries, James F. *Arthritis: A Comprehensive Guide.* rev. ed. Reading, MA: Addison-Wesley, 1986.

BIRTH DEFECTS

Hales, Dianne, and Creasy, Robert K. *New Hope for Problem Pregnancies: Helping Babies Before They're Born.* New York: Berkley Pub., 1984.

BREAST-FEEDING

La Leche League. *The Womanly Art of Breastfeeding.* 4th rev. ed. Franklin Park, IL: La Leche League International, 1987.

Pryor, Karen. *Nursing Your Baby.* New York: Pocket Books, 1984.

BURNS

Nicosia, Jean, ed. *Manual of Burn Care.* New York: Raven Press, 1982.

CANCER

The American Cancer Society Cancer Book. New York: Doubleday, 1986.

Levitt, Paul. *The Cancer Reference Book: Direct and Clear Answers to Everyone's Questions.* rev. ed. New York: Facts on File, 1983.

Morra, Marion, and Potts, Eve. *Choices: Realistic Alternatives in Cancer Treatment.* rev. ed. New York: Avon Books, 1987.

Williams, Chris and Sue. *Cancer: A Patient's Guide.* New York: Wiley, 1986.

CEREBRAL PALSY

Schleichkorn, Jay. *Coping with Cerebral Palsy: Answers to Questions Parents Often Ask.* Baltimore: University Park Press, 1983.

CHILDBIRTH

Donovan, Bonnie. *The Cesarean Birth Experience.* rev. ed. Bostom: Beacon Press, 1986.

Gilgoff, Alice. *Home Birth: An Invitation & a Guide.* South Hadley, MA: Bergin & Garvey, 1988.

* Denotes that the book contains technical medical language.

SUGGESTED READING FOR ADDITIONAL INFORMATION

Greenfield, Ellen J. *You Can Have an Easier Delivery.* Chicago: Contemporary Books, 1988.

Savage, Beverly and Simkin, Diana. *Preparation for Birth: The Complete Guide to the Lamaze Method.* New York: Ballantine Books, 1987.

CHILDREN'S HEALTH

Berberich, Ralph. *The Available Pediatrician: Every Parent's Guide to Common Childhood Illnesses.* New York: Pantheon Books, 1988.

Boston Children's Hospital. *The New Child Health Encyclopedia: The Complete Guide for Parents.* New York: Delacorte, 1987.

Diagram Group. *Child's Body: A Parent's Manual.* New York: Paddington, 1987.

Pantell, Robert H., et al. *Taking Care of Your Child: A Parent's Guide to Medical Care.* rev. ed. Reading, MA: Addison-Wesley, 1984.

* Silver, Henry K. *Handbook of Pediatrics.* 15th ed., Los Altos, CA: Appleton & Lange, 1986.

Simon, Gilbert and Cohen, Marcia. *The Parent's Pediatric Companion.* New York: William Morrow, 1985.

Zuckerman, Barry S. *Child Health: A Pediatrician's Guide for Parents.* New York: Hearst Books, 1986.

DENTAL CARE

Hatfield, Denise. *Teeth and Gum Care.* Springhouse, PA: Springhouse Corporation, 1986.

DIABETES

Ducat, Leslie. *Diabetes: A New and Complete Guide to Healthier Living for Parents, Children and Young Adults with Insulin-Dependent Diabetes.* New York: Harper & Row, 1983.

Duncan, Theodore G. *The Diabetes Fact Book.* New York: Scribner, 1982.

DOWN SYNDROME

Pueschel, Siegfriend M. *The Young Child With Down Syndrome.* New York: Human Sciences Press, 1984.

DRUG ABUSE

Baron, Jason D. *Kids and Drugs: A Parent's Handbook of Drug Treatment and Prevention.* New York: Putnam Pub. Group, 1983.

DRUGS

Bindler, Ruth McGillis. *A Parent's Guide to Pediatric Drugs.* New York: Harper & Row, 1986.

Griffith, H. Winter. *Complete Guide to Prescription & Non-Prescription Drugs*, rev. ed. Los Angeles: The Body Press, 1988.

Physician's Desk Reference. 42nd ed. Oradell, N.J.: Medical Economics, 1988.

* Denotes that the book contains technical medical language.

SUGGESTED READING FOR ADDITIONAL INFORMATION

EATING DISORDERS

Arenson, Gloria. *Binge Eating: How to Stop It Forever.* New York: Rawson Associates, 1984.

Slade, Roger. *The Anorexia Nervosa Reference Book.* New York: Harper & Row, 1984.

EMERGENCY CARE

American Medical Association. *The American Medical Association's Handbook of First Aid and Emergency Care.* New York: Random, 1980.

Green, Martin I. *Lifesavers: The Complete Home Medical & Emergency Handbook.* New York: Ballantine, 1982.

EPILEPSY

Gumnit, Robert J. *The Epilepsy Handbook.* New York: Raven Press, 1983.

EXERCISE, POSTNATAL

Noble, Elizabeth. *Essential Exercises for the Childbearing Year.* Boston: Houghton, Mifflin, 1982.

Whiteford, Barbara and Polden, Margie. *The Postnatal Exercise Book.* New York: Pantheon, 1984.

EYE

Kavner, Richard S. *Your Child's Vision: A Parent's Guide to Seeing, Growing, and Developing.* New York: Fireside, 1985.

Zinn, Walter J. *The Complete Guide to Eyecare, Eyeglasses, and Contact Lenses.* rev. ed. Hollywood, FL: Frederick Fell Publishing, 1986.

FATHERHOOD

Bradley, Robert A. *Husband-Coached Childbirth.* 3rd ed. New York: Harper & Row, 1981.

Jones, Carl. *Sharing Birth: A Father's Guide to Giving Support During Labor.* New York: William Morrow, 1985.

GENERAL HEALTH ENCYCLOPEDIAS AND DICTIONARIES

The American Medical Association. *Family Medical Guide.* New York: Random, 1987.

**Dorland's Illustrated Medical Dictionary.* 27th ed. Philadelphia: Saunders, 1988.

Griffith, H. Winter. *Complete Guide to Symptoms, Illness & Surgery.* Los Angeles: Price Stern Sloan, 1989.

Horton, Edward, and Smart, Felicity, eds. *The Illustrated Encyclopedia of Family Health.* London: Marshall Cavendish Ltd., 1986. 24 vols.

* *Merck Manual of Diagnosis and Therapy.* 15th ed. Rahway, NJ: Merck, 1987.

* *Mosby's Medical and Nursing Dictionary.* 2nd ed. St. Louis MO: Mosby, 1985.

* Rakel, Robert E., ed. *Conn's Current Therapy.* Philadelphia: Saunders, 1988.

GROWTH & DEVELOPMENT

Brazelton, T. Berry. *Infants and Mothers: Differences in Development.* rev. ed. New York: Dell, 1986.

* Denotes that the book contains technical medical language.

SUGGESTED READING FOR ADDITIONAL INFORMATION

Brazelton, T. Berry. *What Every Baby Knows.* New York: Ballantine, 1988.

Cole, Joanna. *The New Baby at Your House.* New York: William Morrow, 1987.

Heins, Marilyn. *Child Care/Parent Care.* New York: Doubleday, 1987.

Leach, Penelope. *Your Growing Child: From Babyhood Through Adolescence.* New York: Knopf, 1986.

Spock, Benjamin. *Dr. Spock's Baby and Child Care.* New York: Simon & Schuster, 1985.

HEART DISEASE

Amsterdam, Ezra A. *Take Care of Your Heart.* New York: Facts on File, 1984.

Gasner, Douglas. *The American Medical Association's Book of Heart Care.* New York: Random. 1982.

INFECTIOUS DISEASES

* Top, F. H., and P. F. Wehrle, eds. *Communicable and Infectious Diseases,* 9th ed. St. Louis, MO: Mosby, 1981.

KIDNEY DISEASE

Cameron, Stewart. *Kidney Disease: The Facts.* 2nd ed. New York: Oxford University Press, 1986.

LUNG DISEASES

Lung Diseases of Children: An Introduction. New York: American Lung Association, 1986.

LUPUS ERYTHEMATOSUS, SYSTEMIC

Blau, Sheldon Paul. *Lupus: The Body Against Itself,* rev. ed. New York: Doubleday, 1984.

MEDICAL TESTS

Griffith, H. Winter. *Complete Guide to Medical Tests—Over-the-Counter and Doctor-Ordered.* Tucson, AZ: Fisher Books, 1988.

Haessler, Herbert. *How to Make Sure Your Baby is Well and Stays That Way: The First Guide to Over 400 Medical Tests and Treatment You Can Do At Home to Check Your Baby's Health and Growth.* New York: Rawson Assoc., 1984.

MENTAL HEALTH

Rubin, Theodore Isaac. *Not to Worry: The American Family Book of Mental Health.* New York: Viking, 1984.

MOTHERHOOD

DelliQuadri, Lyn, and Breckenridge, Kati. *The New Mother Care: Helping Yourself Through the Emotional & Physical Transitions of Motherhood.* Los Angeles: Tarcher, 1984.

* Denotes that the book contains technical medical language.

SUGGESTED READING FOR ADDITIONAL INFORMATION

MULTIPLE SCLEROSIS

Rosner, Louis J. *Multiple Sclerosis: New Hope and Practical Advice For People With MS and Their Families.* New York: Prentice Hall, 1987.

Scheinberg, Labe C., ed. *Multiple Sclerosis: A Guide For Patients and Their Families.* 2nd ed. New York: Raven, 1987.

NUTRITION

Griffith, H. Winter. *Complete Guide to Vitamins, Minerals & Supplements.* Tucson, AZ: Fisher Books, 1988.

Kirschmann, John D. *Nutrition Almanac.* 2nd ed. New York: McGraw Hill, 1984.

POISONING

* Dreisbach, Robert M. *Handbook of Poisoning: Prevention, Diagnosis and Treatment,* 12th ed. Los Altos, CA: Appleton & Lange, 1987.

PREGNANCY

Brewer, Gail. *The Very Important Pregnancy Program.* Emmaus, PA: Rodale Press, 1988.

Brewer, Gail. *What Every Pregnant Woman Should Know.* New York: Penguin Books, 1985.

Curtis, Lindsay. *Pregnant & Lovin' It.* rev. ed. Los Angeles: Price Stern Sloan, 1988.

Hotchner, Tracy. *Pregnancy & Childbirth: The Complete Guide for a New Life.* New York: Avon, 1988.

Kitzinger, Sheila. *Complete Book of Pregnancy and Childbirth.* New York: Knopf, 1980.

Samuels, Mike and Nancy. *The Well Pregnancy Book.* New York: Summit Books, 1986.

Tapley, Donald F., ed. *The Columbia University College of Physicians and Surgeons Complete Home Medical Guide to Pregnancy.* New York: Crown, 1988.

PREMATURE BABIES

Harrison, Helen, and Kositsky, Ann. *The Premature Baby Book: A Parent's Guide to Coping and Caring in the First Years.* New York: St. Martin's, 1984.

Sammons, William A.H., and Lewis, Jennifer M. *Premature Babies: A Different Beginning.* St. Louis, MO: Mosby, 1985.

PREMENSTRUAL SYNDROME (PMS)

Dalton, Katharina. *Dr. Katharina Dalton's Once a Month: The Original Premenstrual Syndrome Handbook.* 3rd ed. Claremont, CA: Hunter House, 1987.

SEX EDUCATION

Bell, Ruth. *Changing Bodies, Changing Lives: A Book For Teens on Sex and Relationships.* rev. ed. New York: Random House, 1987.

Kitzinger, Sheila. *Being Born* (for grades 2-5). New York: Putnam, 1986.

* Denotes that the book contains technical medical language.

Madaras, Lynda and Saavedra, Dane. *The What's Happening to My Body? Book for Boys.* new ed. New York: Newmarket Press, 1987.

Madaras, Lynda, and Area. *The What's Happening to My Body? Book for Girls.* new ed. New York: Newmarket Press, 1987.

Sheffield, Margaret. *Where Do Babies Come From?* (for 4-8 years old). New York: Knopf, 1978.

SKIN DISORDERS

Marks, Ronald A. *Psoriasis: A Guide to One of the Commonest Skin Diseases.* New York: Arco Publishing, 1981.

SPINAL CORD INJURIES

Phillips, Lyn, et al. *Spinal Cord Injury: A Guide for Patients and Their Families.* New York: Raven Press, 1986.

SUDDEN INFANT DEATH SYNDROME (SIDS)

Tyler, James W. *Sudden Infant Death (S.I.D.S.): Probable Causes and Simple Prevention.* New York: Sterling Impact Books, 1986.

TWINS

Gromada, Karen. *Mothering Multiples.* 2nd ed. Franklin Park, IL: La Leche League International, 1985.

Leigh, Gillian. *All About Twins: A Handbook for Parents.* New York: Methuen, Inc., 1984.

WOMEN'S HEALTH

Boston Women's Health Book Collective. *The New Our Bodies, Ourselves.* New York: Simon & Schuster, 1985.

Cherry, Sheldon H. *For Women of All Ages: A Gynecological Guide to Modern Female Health Care.* New York: Macmillan, 1979.

* Danforth, David N., ed. *Obstetrics and Gynecology,* 4th ed. New York: Harper, 1982.

Diagram Group. *Woman's Body: An Owner's Manual.* New York: Paddington, 1977.

Gifford-Jones, W. *What Every Woman Should Know About Hysterectomy.* New York: Funk & Wagnalls, 1977.

Holt, Linda Hughey. *The American Medical Association Guide to Womancare,* rev. ed. New York: Random, 1984.

Scott, Joseph W. *Woman, Know Thyself.* Thorofare, NJ: Charles B. Slack, 1976.

Stewart, Felicia Hance. *My Body, My Health: The Concerned Women's Guide to Gynecology.* New York: Bantam, 1981.

* Denotes that the book contains technical medical language.

TOLL FREE HEALTH HOT LINES

Acne Help Line — 800-222-SKIN.
In California: 800-221-SKIN.

AIDS (see listing under National AIDS Hot Line)

Alzheimer's Disease and Related Disorders Association — 800-621-0379.

American Academy of Facial Plastic and Reconstructive Surgery — 800-332-FACE.

American Academy of Pediatrics (AAP) — 800-421-0589.

American Association for Counseling and Development (AACD) — 800-345-2008.

American College of Physicians — 800-523-1546.

American Council of the Blind — 800-424-8666.

American Diabetes Association — 800-232-3472.

American Kidney Fund — 800-638-8299. In Maryland: 800-492-8361.

American Liver Foundation — 800-223-0179.

American Paralysis Association — 800-225-0292.

American Parkinson's Disease Association — 800-233-2732.

American Social Health Association (VD National Hot Line) — 800-982-5803.

American Society for Dermatologic Surgery — 800-441-ASDS.

American Society of Plastic and Reconstructive Surgeons — 800-635-0635.

American Trauma Society (ATS) — 800-556-7890.

American Tuberous Sclerosis Association — 800-446-1211.

Arthritis Medical Center — 800-327-3027. In Ft. Lauderdale, FL area: 305-739-3202.

Better Hearing Institute — 800-424-8576.

Bulimia and Anorexia Self Help — 800-762-3334. In St. Louis area: 314-768-3838.

Cancer Information Service — 800-4-CANCER. In Alaska: 800-638-6070.

Commission on Professional and Hospital Activities — 800-521-6210.

Consumer Product Safety Commission — 800-638-2772. In Maryland: 800-492-8363. In Alaska and Hawaii: 800-638-8333.

Contact Lens Manufacturers Association — 800-343-5367.

Cystic Fibrosis Foundation — 800-344-4823.

Deafness Research Foundation — 800-535-3323.

Department of Health and Human Services, Inspector General's Hot Line — 800-368-5779.

Dial-a-Hearing Screen Test — 800-222-EARS. In Pennsylvania: 800-345-3277.

Epilepsy Foundation of America — 800-EFA-1000. In Maryland: 301-459-3700.

Federal Emergency Management Agency (FEMA) — (Flood insurance inquiries) — 800-638-6620.

Gallaudet College (National Information Center on Deafness) — 800-672-6720.

Heartlife — 800-241-6993.

Huxley Institute for BioSocial Research/American Schizophrenia Association — 800-847-3802.

Institute of Logopedics (multiply handicapped children) — 800-835-1043.

Juvenile Diabetes Foundation (JDF) — 800-223-1138.

Living Bank (organ and body donations) — 800-528-2971.

Medic Alert Foundation International (emergency medical identification system) — 800-344-3226.

Metro-Help. National Runaway Switchboard — 800-621-4000. In Illinois: 800-972-6004.

National Abortion Federation — 800-772-9100.

National AIDS Hot Line — 800-342-AIDS.

National Alliance of Blind Students — 800-424-8666.

National Association for Hearing and Speech Action (NAHSA) — 800-638-8255.

National Association for Sickle Cell Disease — 800-421-8453.

National Association for the Education of Young Children — 800-424-2460.

National Center for Missing and Exploited Children — 800-843-5678.

National Center for Stuttering — 800-221-2483. In New York City: 212-532-1460.

National Cocaine Hot Line — 800-262-2463.

National Down Syndrome Congress — 800-446-3835. In Illinois: 232-NDSC.

National Down Syndrome Society — 800-221-4602.

National Federal of Parents for Drug-Free Youth — 800-554-5437.

National Gay Task Force — 800-221-7044.

National Health Information Clearinghouse — 800-336-4797.

National Hearing Aid Society — 800-521-5247.

National Highway Traffic Safety Administration — 800-424-9393.

National Information Center for Orphan Drugs and Rare Diseases — 800-336-4797.

National Institute on Drug Abuse — 800-662-4357.

National Jewish Hospital and Research Center/National Asthma Center — 800-222-5864.

National Library of Medicine — 800-638-8480.

National Migraine Foundation — 800-843-2256.

National Neurofibromatosis Foundation — 800-323-7938.

National Parkinson Foundation — 800-327-4545.

National Pesticide Telecommunications Network — 800-858-7378.

TOLL FREE HEALTH HOTLINES

National Rehabilitation Information Center — 800-34-NARIC.

National Retinitis Pigmentosa Foundation — 800-638-2300.

National Reye's Syndrome Foundation — 800-233-7393. In Ohio: 800-231-7393.

National Second Surgical Opinion Program — 800-638-6833. In Maryland: 800-492-6603.

National Sudden Infant Death Syndrome Foundation — 800-221-SIDS.

Office of Health Facilities — 800-638-0742.

Parents Anonymous (PA) — 800-421-0353. In California: 800-352-0386.

Recording for the Blind (RFB) — 800-221-4792.

Runaway Hot Line — 800-231-6946. In Texas: 800-392-3552.

Sexually Transmitted Disease Hot Line — 800-227-8922.

Simon Foundation (urinary incontinence) — 800-237-4666.

Spina Bifida Association of America — 800-621-3141.

Sudden Infant Death Syndrome Hot Line — 800-221-7437. In Maryland: 301-459-3388.

Women's Sport Foundation — 800-227-3988.

Y-Me Breast Cancer Support Program — 800-221-2141. In Chicago: 312-799-8228.

This information was compiled from a publication called "Health Hot Lines," put out by the National Library of Medicine. These telephone numbers are subject to change.

Guide to the Index

Alphabetized entries in the index include all the important topics of this book, such as illnesses, injuries and disorders; names of drug "families," drug brand names and drug generic names; other special pediatric topics found in the *Appendices* section; emergency first aid topics; and so on. The only exception is that *symptoms and signs* are not included in this index. All symptoms and signs are found in a special section called *Symptoms Guide*, pages 1-60, in the front of the book. Use that section the same way you would use an index to look up your child's symptoms and to find the illnesses or disorders that the symptoms may indicate.

INDEX

INDEX

INDEX

D

M

INDEX

O

P

INDEX

Q

R

INDEX

T

U

INDEX

Accidents cause 150,000 lives to be lost each year in the USA alone—the fourth leading cause of deaths. In infants, children, and adolescent males, accidents are the leading cause of death. In addition, 70 million or more Americans are injured seriously enough to require medical care. The number self-treated is even higher.

More than half of these can probably be prevented with simple, common-sense precautions such as:
1. Wear seat belts in the car.
2. Teach children proper safety habits.
3. Practice safety at home.
4. Follow fire prevention warnings.
5. Keep all medicines in a safe place away from the reach of children.
6. Keep children away from all power tools.
7. Teach bicycle safety, including wearing protective headgear.
8. Teach every child how to competently swim.
9. Wear life jackets in boats.
10. Heed weather reports when planning outdoor activity.

This section is not an all-inclusive checklist, but instead covers the most frequent, most serious, and most preventable accidents.

FIRST-AID SUPPLIES

Keep first-aid supplies readily available. Carry a set in the car and have another at home in your medical supply cabinet or shelf. Campers, hikers, bikers, and anyone who expects to spend time in a remote and unpopulated area should carry a portable first-aid kit. Carry a first-aid kit wrapped in a waterproof cover on all boats. These supplies should be checked periodically and replenished promptly. Specific items that should be on hand include:
- A pair of tweezers
- A roll of absorbent cotton
- A roll of adhesive bandage tape, 1 inch wide
- A tightly covered bottle of hydrogen peroxide
- Adhesive bandages in assorted sizes, including 4-inch-square compress pads
- Airtight packages of hand-cleansing disposable towels (optional)
- An antiseptic spray or cream
- Antidiarrheal medication
- Antihistamine tablets
- Containers of ipecac syrup and activated charcoal
- Cotton-tipped applicators
- Elastic bandages 2 and 3 inches wide
- Fever thermometer
- Paper tissues
- Precut triangular bandages of various sizes for slings, splints, and bandages
- Safety pins
- Several medium-sized boards to use as splints for an arm or leg
- Sharp scissors
- Sterile gauze pads
- Tongue depressors
- Two rolls of gauze, 1 inch and 2 inches wide

In addition, these items should be carried at all times in a car or boat:
- A clean, folded sheet
- A flashlight with fresh batteries
- A folded lightweight blanket (sometimes called a "space" blanket)
- A large waterproof cover (tarpaulin)
- A tightly capped plastic bottle of water
- Flares

If a person is hypersensitive to bee or insect stings, he or she also should have a kit containing a syringe of adrenaline, an antihistamine, and a hypodermic needle. These insect-sting kits must be prescribed by and used under the instruction and direction of a physician. Wear a *Medic-Alert* bracelet or necklace if you have diabetes, heart disease, serious allergies, or take special medicines. For information on how to obtain one, call collect in USA: 209-634-4917.

NOTE

Take a cardiopulmonary (CPR) course through the Red Cross or American Heart

Association. This will prepare you to administer CPR if it is ever needed.

ANAPHYLAXIS (Severe allergic reaction)

Description

Itching, rash, hives, runny nose, wheezing, paleness, cold sweats, low blood pressure, coma, and cardiac arrest.

Treatment

If Victim is Unconscious, Not Breathing:

1. Yell for help. Don't leave victim.
2. Begin mouth-to-mouth breathing immediately.
3. If there is no heartbeat, give external cardiac massage.
4. Have someone call O (operator) or 911 (emergency) for an ambulance or medical help.
5. Don't stop cardiopulmonary resuscitation (CPR) until help arrives.

If Victim is Unconscious and Breathing:

1. Dial O (operator) or 911 (emergency) for an ambulance or emergency medical help.
2. If you can't get help immediately, take patient to nearest emergency room or other facility with adequate equipment and personnel to care for medical emergencies.

BLEEDING

Description

Bleeding caused by any serious injury should be treated in an emergency facility. There is usually a lot of bright-red blood pumping from an injured artery, or darker blood if a large vein has been injured.

Treatment

1. Call for ambulance or take to emergency room. In the meantime render first aid yourself.
2. Cover entire injured area with cloth or bare hands if no cloth is available.
3. Apply strong pressure directly on injured area for 10 minutes while awaiting ambulance or transporting to emergency room.
4. If direct pressure doesn't control brisk bleeding and emergency assistance will not be available within 5 minutes, use a tourniquet *as a last resort* to prevent death from bleeding. Make a tourniquet from a length of cloth or similar material. Wrap and tie the tourniquet around extremity above the wound. Place a stick or other rigid object between the cloth and the extremity. Twist the rigid object several times until tight pressure has been applied and bleeding stops. Note how long the tourniquet is in place so emergency medical personnel will know.

BURNS

Description

First- and second-degree burns are not usually life-threatening.

First-degree burns cause only red skin and mild swelling.

Second-degree burns cause blisters, pain, and oozing.

Third-degree burns can be life-threatening if extensive. Skin turns white or appears charred.

Treatment

For First- and Second-Degree Burns:

1. Put the flames out as quickly as possible.
2. Apply lotion to cool first-degree burns. However, if marked swelling develops, seek emergency care.
3. Immerse small second- or third-degree burn areas (as from hot-grease splatters) in cold water for 10 minutes to reduce pain and swelling.
4. Keep the burn area clean. Soak in a tub or use warm compresses once a day. You may add 2 tablespoons of powdered detergent to the tub to help soak off crusting areas. Use plain water for compresses.
5. Prop the burn area higher than the rest of the body, if possible.
6. Use dressings on the burned area, if you wish.

For Third-Degree Burns:

1. Don't use ice to "relieve" pain!
2. Keep patient lying flat and lightly covered to prevent shock.
3. Remove clothes and jewelry unless they are sticking to burned skin.

4. Take to emergency room.

Special Instructions:
1. **Electrical Burns**—Turn off the source of electricity, if possible. If not, use a non-conductive material, such as a board or wooden chair, to pull the victim away from the electrical source. Don't use your bare hands. If the victim is not breathing, begin mouth-to-mouth breathing.
2. **Chemical Burns of the Eye or Skin**—Hold the victim's head or other burned area beneath a faucet. Turn on cool water at medium pressure. Rinse for at least 15 minutes, directing the water away from the unaffected area.
3. **For Burns of Large Areas**—Prepare a solution for the victim to drink on the way to the emergency room. Mix 1 quart of water with ⅓ teaspoon of salt and ⅓ teaspoon of baking soda. This may help prevent kidney failure.

CHOKING

Description

Clutching at throat. Gagging or gasping for air. Sudden collapse without previous illness. Unable to speak. Breathing labored and wheezing if breathing is possible at all.

Treatment
1. Stand behind child, bend child forward and give 3 or 4 sharp blows to back between shoulder blades.
2. If this doesn't dislodge obstruction, perform the Heimlich Maneuver as follows:

Heimlich Maneuver
1. Stand behind child, place both arms around his upper abdomen and grasp your wrists halfway between bottom of ribs and waistline, just above navel.
2. Give 3 or 4 quick forceful squeezes, pushing in and up.

FRACTURES AND DISLOCATIONS

Description

Extreme pain and tenderness in any injured area; change in appearance of injured part, such as swelling, protruding bone, or blood under skin. Extremity, such as finger, arm or leg, may be bent out of normal alignment.

Treatment
1. Immobilize any injured area and keep movement to minimum. For obvious fractures of fingers, wrists, arms, legs, ankles, or feet, improvise a splint from stiff rolled-up paper, scrap wood, or metal.
2. Attach splint firmly to injured extremity with strips of cloth, twine, or similar material to prevent movement.
3. If leg, back, or neck is severely injured and possibly fractured or dislocated, keep patient warm and still until ambulance arrives. **Don't move the victim.**

CARDIOPULMONARY RESUSCITATION

Description

To maintain life, everyone needs a constant supply of oxygen to survive—permanent brain damage can result after only 3 minutes without oxygen. If your child is unconscious and not breathing, you may be able to save his life by taking over his breathing and blood circulation. Cardiopulmonary resuscitation (CPR) is the term used to describe the techniques used to revive someone who is unconscious and not breathing.

It is always worth starting cardiopulmonary resuscitation; keep going until a doctor arrives or your child starts to breathe again on his own.

Treatment
1. Yell for help. Don't leave victim.
2. Begin mouth-to-mouth breathing immediately.
3. If there is no heartbeat, give external cardiac massage.
4. Have someone call O (operator) or 911 (emergency) for an ambulance or medical help.
5. Don't stop cardiopulmonary resuscitation (CPR) until help arrives.

Airway

The airway consists of the passages between your child's mouth and nose and his lungs. If your child is unconscious, particularly if he is lying face upward, breathing may be difficult. Air may not be able to get through to his lungs because: the tongue has fallen back and blocked the windpipe; the head has tilted forward, narrowing the top of the windpipe; fluid or vomit has collected at the back of the throat and is unable to drain.

Keep your fingers and hand away from the soft tissues under your child's chin and along his neck.

1. Lay your child on a firm surface. Place one hand on the child's forehead and one hand under the back of his neck. Tilt the head back. The neck and head are in the right position when you can see straight down the nostrils.
2. Place two fingers of one hand on your child's chin, and lift the jaw up so the chin juts forward. The tongue will come forward with the jaw, thus opening the airway.

Opening the Airway for Babies and Small Children

Babies have very short necks and soft windpipes, and if you tilt the head back too far, you can easily block the airway.

1. Lay your child on a firm surface. Place one hand on the child's forehead, and press very gently to tilt his head slightly.
2. Support the jaw by placing two fingers of the other hand on the bony part of the chin. Check breathing.

Clearing the Airway

If your child is not breathing after you have tilted his head back, take a look inside his mouth to see if there is something blocking the airway.

1. Turn your child's head to one side. Quickly, but carefully, run your index finger around the inside of his mouth. Remove anything you find.
2. Be very careful not to push anything farther down his throat.

IMPORTANT

With a young baby, don't put your finger in the baby's mouth unless you can see the foreign body clearly and you are sure there is no risk of pushing it down his throat. It's better to hold the baby upside down and slap the baby's back. If the child is still not breathing, immediately begin mouth-to-mouth resuscitation (see below).

Checking Breathing

If the child is unconscious, before you do anything else, **make sure he is breathing.** Open the airway.

1. With his head tilted back, place your ear as near to his mouth and nose as possible, and look along his chest at the same time.
2. If he is breathing, you will see his chest moving, and you will hear and feel his breath against your face.
3. If he is not breathing, try to clear the airway.

IMPORTANT

If your child is breathing, even slightly, leave him alone. Do not try to give him mouth-to-mouth resuscitation to try to increase the breathing rate. Just put him in a comfortable position, lying on his abdomen with head and face turned so air can enter mouth and nose.

MOUTH-TO-MOUTH RESUSCITATION

Start this whenever you find your child. If he is in the water, start mouth-to-mouth resuscitation there. If for any reason you can't put your mouth over your child's mouth, close off his mouth and breathe into his nose. If he is very small, it may be easier to place your mouth over his mouth and nose together. If the infant or child is not breathing, it is also likely that the heart is not beating. Begin cardiopulmonary resuscitation *immediately* and never stop until professional help arrives. At the same time that another person at the scene begins external chest compression (see below), begin mouth-to-mouth resuscitation as follows:

1. Tilt the child's head back to open the airway. If necessary clear the airway.
2. Support the child's jaw with one hand. Be careful not to rest your hand on his neck because you can close off the windpipe. Pinch your child's nostrils shut with two fingers of the other hand.
3. Take a deep breath. Open your mouth wide, and seal your lips around the child's mouth.
4. Breathe gently, but firmly, into his mouth. Blow from your lungs, not just your mouth, until you see the unconscious patient's chest rise. Look along the child's chest—you should see the chest fall again if you have been successful.

NOTE
If the chest has not risen, check to see if:
• The head is in the correct position. You should be able to see straight down his nostrils.
• You are pinching the nostrils shut and your mouth is forming an airtight seal around his mouth.
• Try again; if you're still unsuccessful, give him back slaps.
5. Repeat the breathing procedure 3 more times, as quickly as possible. Wait for the chest to fall between each breath. Then check your child's heartbeat.
6. If your child's heart is beating, continue rescue breathing at a rate of 15 to 20 breaths per minute until he can breathe by himself. Wait for the ambulance.
7. If your child's heart is not beating, continue external chest compression (also called external cardiac massage). See below for instructions.

Mouth-to-mouth for Infants and Small Children

The basic breathing techniques are the same. However, take the baby's smaller size into account when giving mouth-to-mouth resuscitation. The gap between the nose and mouth is small, so you may find it easier to place your mouth over the mouth and nose together. You'll only have to breathe a small amount of air into the lungs, at a slightly faster rate of 20 breaths per minute; don't breathe too hard.
1. Lay the child on his back. Tap the soles of his feet to make sure he really is unconscious. If there is no reaction, tilt his head back slightly by pressing on his forehead and supporting his chin with your fingers. Do not tilt the head too far.
2. Slide one hand under his back to support him and keep his head back. Put your mouth over his mouth and nose together. Breathe out gently until his chest rises. Repeat 3 more times, as quickly as possible, then check heartbeat.

NOTE
If you cannot inflate the lungs, check and see if the airway is open. If you still cannot force air in, hold him upside down and give him back slaps.

EXTERNAL CHEST COMPRESSION

Use this technique in conjunction with mouth-to-mouth resuscitation when a child is unconscious and not breathing and his heart is not beating. Chest compression is important because if the heart is not beating, the oxygen you breathe into your child will not get to the body tissues. Permanent brain damage can occur after only 3 minutes without oxygen.

How to Check for the Heartbeat

Check the pulse in the carotid arteries—the arteries that supply blood to the brain.
1. Find the front of the child's windpipe and slide the pads of three fingers across into the groove between it and the large muscle in the neck, just below the jaw and in line with the ear lobe.
2. Feel for about 5 seconds. If you can't feel anything, the heart has probably stopped beating.
3. If the child's heart has stopped beating, lay the child on a hard surface, and kneel beside him facing his chest. Find his breastbone (the bone that runs down the center of his chest). Feel for the top in the

groove between the two collarbones at the top of your child's chest; then find the center of the breastbone.

4. Place the heel of one hand over the lower half of the breastbone. Position yourself so your shoulders are directly over the child's breastbone. Depress it 1 to 1-½ inches (2.5 to 3.5 cm); then release the pressure.

5. Complete 5 compressions at a rate of about 80 to 100 compressions per minute (count "1-and-2-and-" as you go). Someone else should be administering mouth-to-mouth resuscitation simultaneously.

External Chest Compression for Babies and Small Children

The sequence of steps for giving chest compression to babies and small children under age 2 is the same as for large children, but you must use less pressure.

UNCONSCIOUSNESS

Description

Unconsciousness may occur from many causes such as high fever, head injury, epilepsy, an adverse reaction to too much insulin in diabetes, an adverse reaction to many other medications, syncopal or simple fainting episodes—and others.

Unconsciousness is always an emergency. Yell for help and call for an ambulance. **Don't ever leave an unconscious child.** Render CPR as described above if the child is not breathing or has no heartbeat.

Dealing with an Unconscious Infant

The procedure for treating an unconscious baby is the same as for an older child, except you should tap his feet to establish whether he is unconscious. He is unconscious if there is no response.

When opening the airway, don't tilt a baby's head back as far as for an older child. Blow gently into the mouth when giving mouth-to-mouth. Apply only gentle pressure when giving external chest compression.